# THE ONCOGENOMICS HANDBOOK

# CANCER DRUG DISCOVERY AND DEVELOPMENT

## BEVERLY A. TEICHER, SERIES EDITOR

# THE ONCOGENOMICS HANDBOOK

*Edited by*

## WILLIAM J. LaROCHELLE, PhD
## RICHARD A. SHIMKETS, PhD

*CuraGen Corporation*
*New Haven, CT*

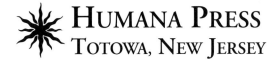
HUMANA PRESS
TOTOWA, NEW JERSEY

Cover design by Patricia F. Cleary
Cover illustrations: FOREGROUND: Regression of tumors after de-induction (*see* full caption and discussion on p. 250, Fig. 1, Chapter 16, and Color Plate 6, following p. 302). BACKGROUND: Reconstitution of a mammary gland (*see* full caption and discussion on p. 253, Fig. 2, Chapter 16, and Color Plate 6).

This publication is printed on acid-free paper. ∞
ANSI Z39.48-1984 (American National Standards Institute)
Permanence of Paper for Printed Library Materials

Printed in the United States of America.   10   9   8   7   6   5   4   3   2   1

eISBN 1-59259-893-5

**Library of Congress Cataloging-in-Publication Data**
Oncogenomics handbook / edited by William J. LaRochelle, Richard A. Shimkets.
    p. ; cm.
  Includes bibliographical references and index.
  ISBN 1-58829-425-0 (alk. paper)
   1. Cancer--Genetic aspects--Handbooks, manuals, etc. 2. Oncogenes--Handbooks, manuals, etc. 3. Genomics--Handbooks, manuals, etc. 4. Proteomics--Handbooks, manuals, etc. [DNLM: 1. Genomics. 2. Neoplasms--genetics. 3. Oncogenes--genetics. ] I. Larochelle, William J. II. Shimkets, Richard A.
  RC268.4.O54 2005
  616.99'4042--dc22                                                      2004027753

# PREFACE

Recent advances in genomic and proteomic research into the molecular biology and biochemistry of cancer have revealed critical differences between normal and malignant tissues. Exploiting these differences, investigators from academia as well as the biotechnology and pharmaceutical industries have underscored key processes that regulate the growth and progression of cancers. Bioinformatic integration of these findings within an evolving systems biology network has spearheaded the development of specific and selective therapeutics that target differentially expressed markers of pathways implicated in cellular proliferation, differentiation, metastasis, evasion of immune surveillance, angiogenesis, and apoptosis. These approaches have resulted in a modest clinical survival benefit for certain cancers, yet many challenges remain, including combinatorial approaches with standard cytotoxic chemotherapy as well as antiangiogenic therapy.

The main objective of *The Oncogenomics Handbook* is to provide a comprehensive update of a variety of perspectives and the consequential approaches toward advancing cancer therapy. Most importantly, we hope to paint with broad strokes and representative examples the drug development process as a network whose components are intimately linked with one another and progressing together from the discovered target to the ultimate therapeutic product. As an accurate reflection of the state of the art, we have brought together outstanding translational research from both academia and the biotechnology sectors.

This handbook is organized into seven parts. The first begins with a discussion of genomic databases and presents examples of elegant approaches to discover oncological targets. The second part expands the understanding of the tractable genome from the gene and transcript to the realm of proteomics that provides an understanding at the level of protein biochemistry. The third and fourth parts move from the chemical realm to that of the living cell and ultimately animal modeling, where preclinical cell biologists and animal pharmacologists translate proof of concept models toward clinical development. The fifth part of the book provides an overview of clinical diagnostics, bioanalytics, and biomarkers, as well as the importance of these molecules to therapeutic outcome. The sixth part of the book is divided into three sections that present antiangiogenic, supportive, immunomodulatory, and tumor-targeted approaches to cancer therapy. The final part of the book provides a systems biology bioinformatics overview of strategies and initiatives leading the post-genomic era. Although many of these approaches are in different stages of clinical development and present examples of future cancer therapies, several have resulted in some clinical benefit for certain cancers. Although many challenges are presented, optimism surrounds the potential use of combination therapies using approved cytotoxics, novel small molecule inhibitors, antiangiogenics, monoclonal antibodies, vaccines, immunomodulatory drugs, and radiation therapy. As always, much work needs to be done.

The *Handbook of Oncogenomics* should prove useful as a text for advanced undergraduate or graduate courses that focus on the drug development process from discovery to clinic. It may also be used as a complementary text for scientific professionals seeking to expand their knowledge of the rapidly progressing fields of cancer research. Finally, although many of the sections of the book focus on scientific professionals, the book covers concepts and issues appropriate to a wide range of professionals, including those involved in consulting services and marketing related to the specialized knowledge contained herein.

*William J. LaRochelle, PhD*
*Richard A. Shimkets, PhD*

# Contents

## PART VI. EMERGING APPROACHES TO CANCER THERAPY

### VI-A. TARGETING THE VASCULATURE

### VI-B. SUPPORTIVE AND ADJUVANT THERAPIES

### VI-C. TUMOR-TARGETED THERAPIES

# CONTRIBUTORS

JOAN ALBANELL, MD • *Medical Oncology Department, ICMHO & IDIBAPS, Hospital Clínic i Provincial de Barcelona, Barcelona, Spain*

GULSHAN ARA, PhD • *Oncology, Group Leader, Preclinical Development, CuraGen Corporation, Branford, CT*

BRUCE J. ARONOW, PhD • *Division of Pediatric Informatics, Children's Hospital Medical Center and, The University of Cincinnati College of Medicine, Cincinnati, OH*

NEIL H. BANDER, MD • *Department of Urology, Department of Medicine, Weill Medical College of Cornell University, New York, NY*

AMOS BARUCH, PhD • *Celera Genomics, South San Francisco, CA*

TAPAN K. BERA, PhD • *Laboratory of Molecular Biology, National Cancer Institute, National Institutes of Health, Bethesda, Maryland*

IVAR BLEUMER, MD • *Department of Urology, University Hospital St Radboud, Nijmegen, The Netherlands*

MATTHEW BOGYO, PhD • *Department of Pathology, Stanford University School of Medicine, Stanford, CA*

ROLF A. BREKKEN, PhD • *Hamon Center for Therapeutic Oncology Research, Department of Surgery, UT-Southwestern Medical Center, Dallas, TX*

LUCY A. CARVER, PhD • *Sidney Kimmel Cancer Center, San Diego, CA*

ANDREA CERUTTI, MD • *Department of Lymphoma and Myeloma, Unit 429, The University of Texas, M. D. Anderson Cancer Center, Houston, TX*

ARNAB CHAKRAVARTI, MD • *Massachusetts General Hospital, Department of Radiation Oncology, Boston, MA*

LIEPING CHEN, MD, PhD • *The Johns Hopkins University School of Medicine, Baltimore, MD*

SUZIE CHEN, PhD • *Susan Lehman Cullman Laboratory for Cancer Research, Ernest Mario School of Pharmacy, Rutgers, The State University of New Jersey, Piscataway, NJ*

PAMELA REILLY CONTAG, PhD • *President and Co-CEO, Xenogen Corporation, Alameda, CA*

JAMES C. CUSACK, JR., MD • *Division of Surgical Oncology, Massachusetts General Hospital, Boston, MA*

GENE CUTLER, PhD • *Tularik Inc., South San Francisco, CA*

PRADIP DATTA, PhD, DABCC • *Bayer Diagnostics, Tarrytown, NY*

C. GEOFFREY DAVIS, PhD • *Abgenix Inc., Fremont CA*

MUSTAPHA DIALLO, DiplBiol • *Kekule Institut für Organische Chemie und Biochemie, Universität Bonn, Bonn, Germany*

JOHN B. EASTON, PhD • *Department of Molecular Pharmacology, St. Jude Children's Research Hospital, Memphis, TN*

KRISTI A. EGLAND, PhD • *Laboratory of Molecular Biology, National Cancer Institute, National Institutes of Health, Bethesda, Maryland*

JEFF L. ELLSWORTH, PhD • *Department of Autoimmunity and Inflammation, ZymoGenetics Inc., Seattle, WA*

CATHERINE L. FARRELL, PhD • *Global Operations Planning, Amgen Inc., Thousand Oaks, CA*

ANDREW FELDHAUS, PhD • *Departments of Genetics, ZymoGenetics Inc., Seattle, WA*

CARLOS GARCÍA-ECHEVERRÍA, PhD • *Global Discovery Chemistry Oncology Research, Novartis Institutes for Biomedical Research, Basel, Switzerland*

PERE GASCON, MD • *Professor and Director, Division of Medical Oncology, ICMHO and IDIBAPS, Hospital Clínic i Provincial de Barcelona, Barcelona, Spain*

ARUNDHATI GHOSH, PhD • *George M. O'Brien Center for Urology Research, Department of Cancer Biology, Lerner Research Institute, Cleveland Clinic Foundation, Cleveland, OH*

STANLEY J. GOLDSMITH, MD • *Professor of Radiology and Medicine, Division of Nuclear Medicine, Department of Radiology, Weill Medical College of Cornell University, New York, NY*

JOHN R. GRIFFITHS, MB BS, DPhil • *CR UK Biomedical MR Research Group, Department of Basic Medical Sciences, St. George's Hospital Medical School, London, UK*

HEIKO HERMEKING, PhD • *Head of the Molecular Oncology Group, Max-Planck-Institute of Biochemistry, Martinsried/Munich, Germany*

WARREN D. W. HESTON, PhD • *George M. O'Brien Center for Urology Research, Department of Cancer Biology, Lerner Research Institute, and Glickman Urological Institute, Cleveland Clinic Foundation. Cleveland, OH*

JOERG HEYER, PhD • *Department of Model Development, GenPath Pharmaceuticals Inc., Cambridge, MA*

TIMOTHY HOEY, PhD • *Director, Biology Department, Tularik Inc., South San Francisco CA*

PETER J. HOUGHTON, PhD • *Department Molecular Pharmacology, St. Jude Children's Research Hospital, Memphis, TN*

XIANMING HUANG, PhD • *Hamon Center for Therapeutic Oncology Research, Department of Pharmacology, UT-Southwestern Medical Center, Dallas, TX*

STEVEN D. HUGHES, PhD • *PreClinical Development, ZymoGenetics Inc., Seattle, WA*

ROBIN C. HUMPHREYS, PhD • *Antibody Development and Discovery, Human Genome Sciences, Rockville, MD*

K. K. JAIN, MD, FRACS, FFPM • *Chief Executive Officer, Jain PharmaBiotech, Basel, Switzerland*

DOUGLAS A JEFFERY, PhD • *Celera Genomics, South San Francisco, CA*

GRZEGORZ KORPANTY, MD • *Hamon Center for Therapeutic Oncology Research, Department of Surgery, UT-Southwestern Medical Center, Dallas, TX*

LALE KOSTAKOGLU, MD • *Division of Nuclear Medicine, Department of Radiology, Weill Medical College of Cornell University, New York, NY*

WILLIAM J. LAROCHELLE, PhD • *Head of Oncology, Preclinical Development, CuraGen Corporation, Branford, CT*

MARTIN LEACH, PhD • *Vice President of Informatics, CuraGen Corporation, Branford, CT*

ALICE Y. LEE, MS • *H. Lee Moffitt Cancer Center, Tampa, FL*

B. K. LEE, PhD • *Laboratory of Molecular Biology, National Cancer Institute, National Institutes of Health, Bethesda, MD*

QIXIN LENG, PhD • *Department of Pathology, University of Maryland Baltimore, Baltimore, MD*

HEINZ-JOSEF LENZ, MD, FACP • *Division of Medical Oncology, University of Southern California, Norris Comprehensive Cancer Center, Los Angeles, CA*

ZHONGXING LIAO, MD • *Department of Radiation Oncology, The University of Texas M. D. Anderson Cancer Center, Houston, TX*

XUEFENG BRUCE LING, PhD • *Tularik Inc., South San Francisco, CA*

DAVID LJUNGMAN, MD • *Division of Surgical Oncology, Massachusetts General Hospital, Boston, MA*

JEFFREY J. MARTINO • *Susan Lehman Cullman Laboratory for Cancer Research, Ernest Mario School of Pharmacy, Rutgers, The State University of New Jersey, Piscataway, NJ*

KATHRYN A. MASON, MSc • *Experimental Radiation Oncology, The University of Texas M. D. Anderson Cancer Center, Houston, TX*

CINDY E. MCKINNEY, PhD • *Department of Animal Sciences, The Pennsylvania State University, University Park, PA*

LUKA MILAS, MD, PhD • *Experimental Radiation Oncology, The University of Texas M. D. Anderson Cancer Center, Houston, TX*

MATTHEW I. MILOWSKY, MD • *Division of Hematology and Medical Oncology, Department of Medicine, Weill Medical College of Cornell University, New York, NY*

A. JAMES MIXSON, MD • *Department of Pathology, University of Maryland Baltimore, Baltimore, MD*

ARTURO MOLINA, MD • *Medical Affairs Oncology/Hematology, Biogen Idec, San Diego, CA*

PETER F. A. MULDERS, MD, PhD • *Department of Urology, University Hospital St Radboud, The Netherlands*

ALEXANDER NAKEFF, PhD • *Drug Discovery and Development Program, Henry Ford Health System, Detroit, MI*

DAVID M. NANUS, MD • *Division of Hematology and Medical Oncology, Department of Medicine, Weill Medical College of Cornell University, New York, NY*

RÓNÁN C. O'HAGAN • *Department of Target Validation, GenPath Pharmaceuticals Inc., Cambridge, MA*

DAVID J. PARK, MD • *Division of Medical Oncology, University of Southern California, Norris Comprehensive Cancer Center, Los Angeles, CA*

IRA PASTAN, MD • *Laboratory of Molecular Biology, National Cancer Institute, National Institutes of Health, Bethesda, MD*

BHARVIN K. R. PATEL, PhD • *Principal Research Scientist, Cancer Research, Eli Lilly and Company, Indianapolis, IN*

LINDA PRONK, MD • *Division Pharma, F. Hoffmann-La Roche, Basel, Switzerland*

UMA RAJU, PhD • *Experimental Radiation Oncology, The University of Texas M. D. Anderson Cancer Center, Houston, TX*

WILLIAM M. RIDEOUT III, PhD • *Scientist, Department of Model Development, GenPath Pharmaceuticals Inc., Cambridge, MA*

BRIAN Z. RING, PhD • *Applied Genomics Inc., Sunnyvale, CA*

HUIJUN Z. RING, PhD • *ABMG, Molecular Genetics Program Manager, SRI International, Menlo Park, CA*

LORIN ROSKOS, PhD • *Abgenix Inc., Fremont CA*

JEFFREY S. ROSS, MD • *Department of Pathology and Laboratory Medicine, Albany Medical College, Albany, NY; Division of Molecular Medicine, Millennium Pharmaceuticals Inc., Cambridge, MA*

KRIS F. SACHSENMEIER, PhD • *Automated Cell Inc., Pittsburgh, PA*

FRANK A. SCAPPATICCI, MD, PhD • *Genentech Inc., South San Francisco, CA; University of California Davis Cancer Center, Davis, CA*

KATJA SCHMITZ, PhD • *Kekule Institut für Organische Chemie und Biochemie, Universität Bonn, Bonn, Germany*

UTE SCHEPERS, PhD • *Kekule Institut für Organische Chemie und Biochemie, Universität Bonn, Bonn, Germany*

JAN E. SCHNITZER, MD • *Vascular Biology and Angiogenesis Program, Sidney Kimmel Cancer Center, San Diego, CA*

GISELA SCHWAB, MD • *Abgenix Inc., Fremont CA*

COODUVALLI S. SHASHIKANT, PhD • *Department of Animal Sciences, The Pennsylvania State University, University Park, PA*

RICHARD SHIMKETS, PhD • *CuraGen Corporation, Branford, CT*

SUDHIR SRIVASTAVA, PhD • *Cancer Biomarkers Research Group, Division of Cancer Prevention, National Cancer Institute, National Institutes of Health, Rockville, MD*

GARY C. STARLING, PhD • *Inflammation, CuraGen Corporation, Branford, CT*

MARION STUBBS, DPhil • *CR UK Biomedical MR Research Group, Department of Basic Medical Sciences, St. George's Hospital Medical School, London, UK*

BALANEHRU SUBRAMANIAN, PhD • *Drug Discovery and Development Program, Henry Ford Health System, Detroit, MI*

JIMMY C. SUNG, MD, JD • *Department of Surgery, H. Lee Moffitt Cancer Center, Tampa, FL*

JONATHAN A. TERRETT, PhD • *CellTech, The Quadrant, Abingdon, United Kingdom*

FREDERICK VALERIOTE, PhD • *Drug Discovery and Development Program, Henry Ford Health System, Detroit, MI*

SHANKAR VALLABHAJOSULA, PhD • *Division of Nuclear Medicine, Department of Radiology, Weill Medical College of Cornell University, New York, NY*

MUKESH VERMA, PhD • *Cancer Biomarkers Research Group, Division of Cancer Prevention, National Cancer Institute, National Institutes of Health, Rockville, MD*

PING WEI, PhD • *Department of Hematology, Amgen Inc., Thousand Oaks, CA*

SUSANNE I. WELLS, PhD • *Division of Hematology/Oncology, Children's Hospital Medical Center, The University of Cincinnati College of Medicine, Cincinnati, OH*

SARAH S. WILLIAMS • *Division of Pediatric Informatics, Children's Hospital Medical Center, The University of Cincinnati College of Medicine, Cincinnati, OH*

MIN WU, PhD • *Department of Model Development, GenPath Pharmaceuticals Inc., Cambridge, MA*

CHEN XU, PhD • *Department of Cell Biology, The Scripps Research Institute, LaJolla, CA*

XIAODONG YANG, MD, PhD • *Abgenix Inc., Fremont CA*

SHENG YAO, PhD • *The Johns Hopkins University School of Medicine, Baltimore, MD*

JOHN R. YATES III, PhD • *Department of Cell Biology, The Scripps Research Institute, LaJolla, CA*

TIMOTHY J. YEATMAN, MD • *Clinical Investigations, H. Lee Moffitt Cancer Center, Tampa, FL*

ANAS YOUNES, MD • *Department of Lymphoma and Myeloma, The University of Texas, M. D. Anderson Cancer Center, Houston, TX*

GARY GUOTANG ZHAI, PhD • *Department of Radiation Oncology, Massachusetts General Hospital, Boston, MA*

HEPING ZHANG, PhD • *Department of Epidemiology and Public Health, Yale University School of Medicine, New Haven, CT*

YINGHUI ZHOU, PhD • *Department of Model Development, GenPath Pharmaceuticals Inc., Cambridge, MA*

# COLOR PLATES

Color Plates 1–4 follow p. 78 and 5–12 follow p. 302.

# I GENOMICS, CANCER TARGETS, TRANSCRIPTOMICS, AND GENE EXPRESSION ANALYSIS

# 1
# Genomic Resources for Cancer Biologists

*Xuefeng Bruce Ling, PhD,*
*Gene Cutler, PhD, and Timothy Hoey, PhD*

## CONTENTS

## SUMMARY

Cancer is fundamentally a genetic disease caused by a combination of several mutations that make a tumor cell distinct from a normal cell. The new generation of cancer therapies is aimed at targeting this difference, for example, by inhibiting the activity of the product of a hyperactive or overexpressed oncogene. The utilization of genomic approaches to identify cancer-causing mutations and understand the underlying biological mechanisms has made significant advances in recent years. Notably, profiling of gene expression in tumor samples by microarrays has provided new insights into the molecular characterization of many types of cancer. Other genomic approaches including genomewide profiling of amplifications and deletions and analysis of single-nucleotide polymorphisms (SNPs), hold the promise of enabling the systematic description of all mutations in a given tumor and, thus, the possibility of personalizing cancer diagnosis and treatment. Because of the explosion in the use of genomic approaches in the field, knowledge and expertise in the efficient utilization of bioinformatics resources and tools has become essential for cancer researchers. This chapter is intended to help cancer biologists navigate through the complexity of current genomic databases to find the information they need.

**Key Words:** Cancer; genomics; database; genome assembly; genetics; oncogene; tumor suppressor; microarray; CGH.

From: *Cancer Drug Discovery and Development: The Oncogenomics Handbook*
Edited by: W. J. LaRochelle and R. A. Shimkets © Humana Press Inc., Totowa, NJ

# 1. INTRODUCTION

"The completion of a high-quality, comprehensive sequence of the human genome, in this fiftieth anniversary year of the discovery of the double-helical structure of DNA, is a landmark event. The genome era is now a reality … and a revolution in biological research has begun" *(1)*. Undoubtedly, the unprecedented explosion of datasets (including genomes, transcriptomes, proteomes, allelic variability, mapping, synteny, mutational data, and various model organism genetic and phenotypic datasets) and tools (database interfaces and analysis software) has transformed biomedical research, drug discovery, and medical product development. Oncogenomics or cancer genomics, the application of genomics to understand, diagnose, and combat cancer, is no exception and has been making significant advances. For example, genome-scale profiling of gene expression in tumor samples has provided new insights into the molecular characterization of many types of cancer. Microarray technology and other genomic approaches including genotyping by analysis of single-nucleotide polymorphisms (SNPs) hold the promise of enabling us to systematically profile individuals' genomes, making it possible to personalize cancer diagnosis and treatment. Because cancer is fundamentally a genetic disease occurring as a result of mutations in the genome, it is anticipated that genomics will play a critical role in cancer research and medicine.

Despite all of the publicity about the new "genome era" and the great opportunities that have arisen, many biomedical researchers are still largely unaware of what these datasets and tools can do for them and of how to best use them *(2)*. The paradox arises because the new high-volume data now seem to be most useful only to specialists rather than to the larger research community. This problem will only become worse as the complexity of these databases continues to grow. The huge popular attention garnered by the Human Genome Project does have the beneficial effects of motivating and accelerating progress in the areas of genome sequencing, assembly, and annotation, aiming at turning the massive volumes of data into useful (and sometimes marketable) information. Nevertheless, the intense competition has also produced some undesirable results and hampered the use of these genomics resources *(3)*.

In order to assist bench scientists to navigate these rapidly growing genomic resources, human genome resource guides, including the hands-on guide from Nature Genetics *(4)*, the NCBI human genome resource fact sheets (http://www.nlm.nih.gov/pubs/factsheets/humangenome.html), the NCBI information project handbook (http://www.ncbi.nlm.nih.gov/books/bv.fcgi?call=bv.View..ShowSection&rid=handbook), and resources describing the various database collections *(5,6)* have been developed and are freely accessible through the Internet.

# 2. MAJOR PUBLIC SEQUENCE DATABASES AND GENOME BROWSERS

The International Nucleotide Sequence Database Collaboration, which consists of the following genome centers, is the primary organization responsible for collecting new protein and nucleotide sequences:

DDBJ: http://www.ddbj.nig.ac.jp
EMBL: http://www.ebi.ac.uk/embl/index.html
GenBank: http://www.ncbi.nlm.nih.gov

These centers exchange data on a daily basis so that all submitted data are mirrored across all sites. In addition to providing direct access to the datasets, these genome centers also provide various sequence search and analysis tools. Figure 1, modified after the EBI reference *(7)*, summarizes the services the centers provide through their Internet sites.

Major genome browsers, surviving through the initial genomic "gold rush" *(8)*, include the following:

Ensembl: http://www.ensembl.org
NCBI Map Viewer: http://www.ncbi.nlm.nih.gov/mapview/
UCSC Genome Browser: http://genome.ucsc.edu
RIKEN Genomic Sciences Center: http://hgrep.ims.u-tokyo.ac.jp
ORNL Genome Channel: http://compbio.ornl.gov/channel/
Celera Genomics: http://www.celeradiscoverysystem.com/index.cfm

Although each has its own unique annotation pipeline, manually reviewed datasets, and software application framework, all of these Internet portals have been competing to become "one-stop" genome gateways, integrating data from human, mouse, and other model organism genomes. In reality, almost all regular data mining queries *(4)* can be addressed using any of the above browsers as well as their associated tools and databases. Such queries include but are not limited to determining gene structure, identifying SNPs, mapping cDNA sequence to the genome and analyzing alternative splicing, locating gene family members, and discovering orthologs across multiple species.

Genome-scale data mining projects usually demand high-throughput computing power and complicated data handling processes, much more than what these portal genome browsers are designed to support. Unlike the commercial subscription-based genome access sites such as Celera Discovery System™ *(9)* and ERGO™ *(10)*, public-domain genome projects *(11,12)* remain entirely open-sourced with all data freely available and application code openly licensed for, at least, noncommercial research. Mailing lists, such as ensembl-dev@ensembl.org and genome@cse.ucsc.edu, provide forums for announcements of new releases and features, troubleshooting installation and code development, and general discussions. Thus, they serve as important networks connecting developers and users. The open-source nature of these projects allows for on-site, behind-firewall genome application installation *(11,12)*. In conjunction with an organization's in-house computing infrastructure, this greatly empowers bioinformaticians to succeed in their genome data mining efforts.

## 3. HUMAN GENOME ASSEMBLIES

In February 2001, the International Human Genome Sequencing Consortium (HGSC) and Celera Genomics simultaneously published descriptions of the sequencing, assembly, analysis, and gene annotation of the human genome *(13,14)*. The human genome assembly became a very controversial topic soon afterward. Both in scientific and public discussions, the sequencing and assembly by the public (HGSC) and private (Celera) groups have been portrayed as a race, and the use by Celera of public data to complete their assembly sparked controversy and discussion *(3,15–19)*. In the public domain, the UCSC, NCBI, and RIKEN groups each generated their own complete assemblies of the human genome using different approaches. Comparative studies showed significant discrepancies in the

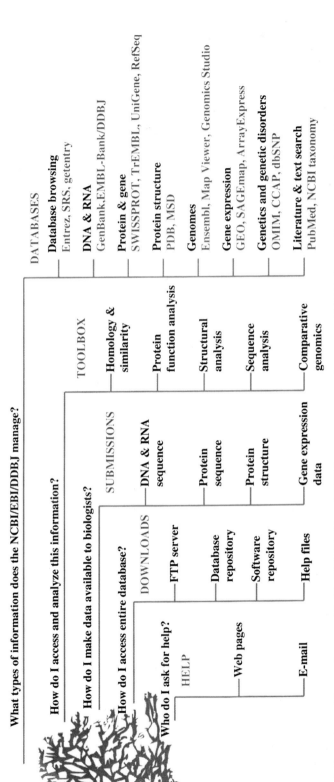

**Fig. 1.** Summary of the services provided by NCBI, EBI, and DDBJ genome centers. Acronyms: CCAP, Cancer Chromosome Aberration Project; DDBJ, DNA Data Bank of Japan; EBI, European Bioinformatics Institute; EMBL, European Molecular Biology Laboratory; GEO, Gene Expression Ommibus; MSD, Macromolecular Structures Database; NCBI, National Center for Biotechnology Information; OMIM, Online Mendelian Inheritance in Man; PDB, Protein Data Bank; SAGE, Serial Analysis of Gene Expression; SNP, single nucleotide polymorphism; SRS, sequence retrieval system.

sequence as well as in the order and orientation of GenBank entries used in constructing the initial NCBI and UCSC assemblies *(20)*. HGSC has decided to standardize on the NCBI assembly as the "official" public-domain human genome assembly *(4)*.

The genome assembly serves as an important source for the identification and characterization of novel therapeutic targets of medical and scientific interest and the quality of this assembly greatly affects the data mining efforts. Although both HGSC and Celera identified approx 30,000 genes *(13,14)*, a direct comparison of the Celera and HGSC (Ensembl) datasets revealed relatively little overlap between their novel predicted genes *(21)*. Parallel analysis of the two genome assemblies *(22)* showed that there are major differences between these two datasets, in the numbers, identities, and properties of predicted genes, and that assembly-level differences must be at least partly responsible for the gene set discrepancies.

In order to provide an up-to-date status report of the human genome assemblies, to understand how these assemblies have been evolving since their initial releases, and to compare the different assembly approaches and resulting gene datasets, Tularik Inc. (now Amgen) and the Genome Institute of Novartis Research Foundation (GNF) have collected all the available HGSC and Celera assembly releases and performed a systematic comparative analysis *(23)*.

Genome assemblies can vary because of differences in local sequence content as well as long-range differences resulting from differing sequence assembly. As a gage of the quality and completeness of the local sequence content in both genome assemblies, the BLAT algorithm *(24)* was used to map the NCBI RefSeq *(25,26)* and the Research Genetics cDNA database (http://mp.invitrogen.com/) against both the HGSC and Celera genome assemblies. Because a positive BLAT hit only requires a match of 40 nucleotides, this analysis should be largely insensitive to global assembly issues. A gradual increase in the number of mapped cDNA sequences for both HGSC and Celera assemblies was observed, leveling off for both at around 97%. These results suggest that the HGSC and Celera assemblies have had very similar local sequence content levels since their early releases.

Gene sets derived from the genome assemblies can vary because of differences in local sequence, global assembly, and the particular gene-prediction pipelines used. Because genes can span large sequence lengths, all gene-prediction algorithms, to some extent, will be sensitive to sequence coverage and assembly issues. To eliminate variability resulting from differing gene-prediction pipelines, the same gene-prediction algorithm, GENSCAN *(27,28)*, was used to generate gene sets from multiple releases of both genome assemblies. The "full-length" GENSCAN genes subsets were extracted from all of the predicted genes, including only those GENSCAN predictions containing both 5' promoter and 3' poly-adenylation signal sequence predictions. Because long-range sequence discontinuity in the assemblies can lead GENSCAN to predict partial genes that would lack 5' promoter and/or 3' poly-adenylation signal sequences, this full-length subset can be used to probe the quality of the genome assembly.

The total and full-length GENSCAN HGSC gene counts as well as the Celera full-length GENSCAN gene counts all showed modest and gradual increases over time (Fig. 2A). In contrast, the total GENSCAN gene counts for the Celera assemblies started out at levels more than twice as high as the HGSC gene sets, and only came down to comparable levels in the July 2001 release. Because gene prediction depends on not only local sequence content but also on long-range assembled sequence, the initially high total GENSCAN gene numbers for Celera were most likely the result of sequence fragmentation resulting

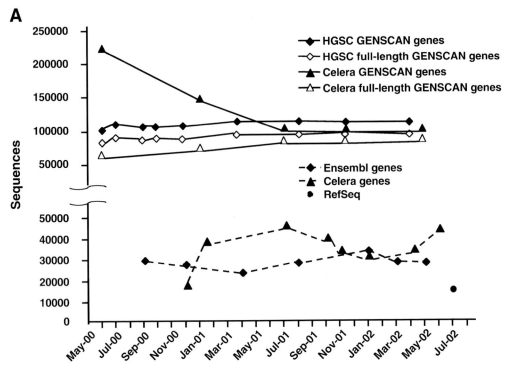

**Fig. 2.** Gene set distributions from multiple HGSC and Celera genome releases. (**A**) The numbers of pipeline-derived genes from various releases of Ensembl and Celera gene sets along with the numbers of total GENSCAN-predicted genes and full-length GENSCAN-predicted genes derived from various releases of the HGSC and Celera genomes are plotted based on release dates. For reference, the number of human genes in the July 2002 release of RefSeq is also shown.

in many individual genes being split into separate GENSCAN predictions. This apparent Celera genome fragmentation, perhaps because of gaps or assembly errors, might indicate a disadvantage of Celera's whole-genome shotgun (WGS) sequencing approach *(16,29)* in comparison to HGSC's hierarchical shotgun (HS) approach *(13)*.

## 4. HUMAN GENE BUILDING AND GENE DATABASES

The completion of the genome assembly in February 2001 did not give a definitive human transcriptome and gene count, which has been an issue of special interest to the biomedical research community. As shown in Fig. 2A, the early published agreement between HGSC and Celera *(13,14)* of the 30,000 genes in the human genome is purely coincidental, and significant disparities do exist in genome assembly *(15,16,22,23)* and associated gene set *(21,23)*. Both the Ensembl gene build system *(11)* and Celera's Otto pipeline *(14)* use several criteria for gene identification, including homology to known proteins, expressed sequence tags (ESTs) and *ab initio* gene prediction with algorithms including GENSCAN. Ensembl is more dependent on known human proteins from SPTREMBL, GENSCAN predictions, and gene-prediction hidden Markov models (HMMs), whereas Celera uses more data from outside of their genome such as cross-genome homology and

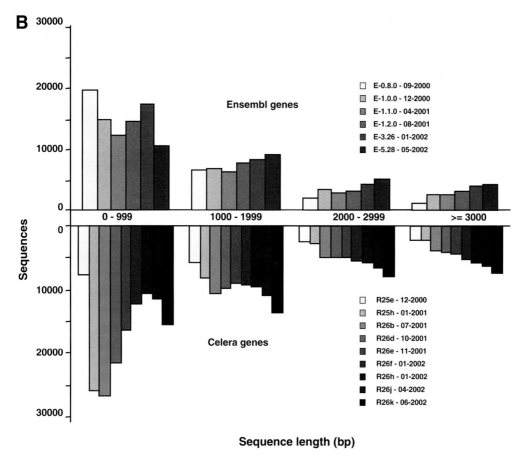

**Fig. 2. (B)** Multiple Ensembl and Celera gene sets were analyzed based on gene length. The numbers of sequences from each release that lie in the given gene-length bins are shown.

even the Ensembl gene set (ref. 62 in ref. *14*). Analyzing the length distributions of the Ensembl and Celera gene sets (Fig. 2B) shows a large decrease in short Celera genes accompanied by increases in the numbers of longer genes over time, similar but more pronounced than what is seen with the HGSC genes. A similar trend is seen with the GENSCAN-predicted gene sets, further reinforcing the notion that initial Celera assembly releases could have had comparatively high levels of fragmentation.

Ensembl, Celera, and RefSeq gene sets are overlapping *(21,23)* and have all provided different perspectives to our current knowledge of the human transcriptome. In order to estimate the total gene number, the Ensembl, Celera, and RefSeq gene sets were clustered via a permissive clustering algorithm and combined into a large superset (Fig. 3). The nonredundant gene number computed here should represent a lower limit for the true human gene count because nearly identical paralogs that are found in some gene families would not be distinguishable and genes that were missed by both Ensembl and Celera gene identification processes would not be included. This analysis of multiple gene sets together, coupled with the removal of redundancy, allows a more complete estimate of the total human gene content than has previously been described *(13,14)*.

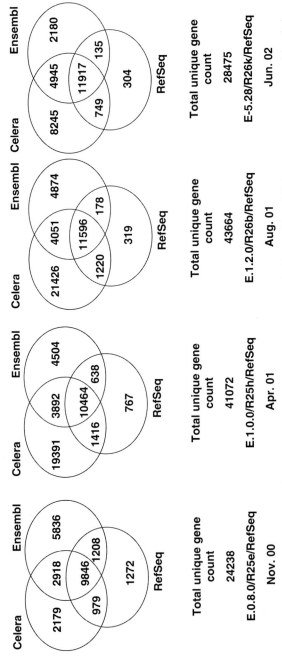

**Fig. 3.** Estimation of nonredundant gene count. For the releases shown, the Ensembl and Celera gene sets were combined along with the human subset of RefSeq. This combined gene set was clustered via a permissive clustering algorithm. The resulting gene cluster number represents the total number of unique genes in the Ensembl, Celera, and RefSeq gene sets that could be resolved by our BLAST analysis.

## 5. REFERENCE GENOMES PROVIDE
## ANCHORS FOR BIOLOGICAL INFORMATION

The availability of the human genome, along with numerous completed model organism genomes, presents challenges in the areas of efficient data storage, retrieval, and update when newer versions become available. On the other hand, genomes are natural data mining entry points, where genome assemblies can serve as common scaffolds upon which various biological datasets can be anchored and, thus, easily cross-referenced to each other. As a result, systematic chromosomal views of genomewide biology, including gene expression, chromosomal amplifications and deletions, SNPs, and evolutionary relationships to other species, become possible.

With the completion of the genome, all human genes can be accurately positioned on their chromosomes, enabling a high-resolution map in which the chromosomal positions of human expressed sequence tags (ESTs) (http://www.ncbi.nlm.nih.gov/dbEST) and mRNA belonging to UniGene clusters (http://www.ncbi.nlm.nih.gov/entrez/query.fcgi? db=unigene) are readily identified. Human transcriptome maps, integrating gene maps with genomewide messenger RNA expression profiles, can provide whole-genome views of gene expression to aid in identifying overexpressed or silenced chromosomal loci in cancer samples *(30,31)*. These expression maps include those based on EST abundance (dbEST, http://www.ncbi.nlm.nih.gov/dbEST/) and on serial analysis of gene expression tags (SAGE database, http://www.ncbi.nlm.nih.gov/SAGE/) measured in various normal or diseased tissues.

Because genomic changes are believed to be the primary causes of cancer, the characterization of gene amplification and deletion through the measurement of DNA copy-number changes in tumors is important for the basic understanding of cancer *(32,33)*, identification of therapeutic targets *(34–37)*, and cancer diagnosis *(38)*. Array-based comparative genomic hybridization *(38)* (CGH) has been developed for genomewide detection of chromosomal imbalances in tumor samples. The human genome sequence and genome-based high-resolution gene maps have greatly enhanced our ability to map DNA copy-number changes. In addition, the public CGH database (http://www.ncbi.nlm.nih.gov/sky/) has been set up to serve as a research platform for investigators to share and compare their datasets.

A key aspect of research in genetics is associating sequence variations with heritable phenotypes *(39)*. The most common variations are SNPs, which occur approximately once every 100–300 bases in the human genome. Comprehensive SNP maps (The Cold Spring Harbor SNP collection http://snp.cshl.org; dbSNP, http://www.ncbi.nlm.nih.gov/SNP/) can facilitate the cataloging and profiling of the unique sets of changes in different diseases. The availability of high-quality and high-density SNP maps has been enabled genome-scale correlations studies between SNPs and precancerous conditions *(40,41)*, drug resistance in chemotherapy *(42,43)*, cancer susceptibility *(44,45)*, and drug response *(46–49)*. This approach has the promise of significantly advancing our abilities to understand and treat cancer. A comprehensive review of the current SNP-related resources can be found at Human Genome Variation Database website (http://hgvbase.cgb.ki.se/databases.htm).

Thanks to technological advances, large-scale sequencing projects can efficiently generate high-quality and high-volume genome sequences, from yeast to chimpanzees, at reasonable costs. Comparative analysis between human and model organism genomes can reveal regions of similarity and difference helping scientists to better understand the structure and function of human genes. All of the genome browsers *(12,50,51)*, including Ensembl, UCSC genome browser, and NCBI map viewer, are organizing and integrating multispecies datasets of fine-grained DNA–DNA alignments, orthologous protein information, and large-scale synteny. Because the systematic comparison of genomic sequences from different organisms has become a central focus of current genome analysis, automatic comparative genome analysis and visualization will be a major focus of development for these genome browser projects.

## 6. INFORMATION-INTENSIVE "OMIC" RESOURCES

With a transcriptome of 30,000 protein-coding genes and an even larger proteome, "omic" (as in "gen-omic") methodologies *(52)*, aiming to systematically study biology in aggregate and powered by high-throughput data production, have become increasingly important. An example is the National Cancer Institute's anticancer drug-screening program analyzing over 70,000 chemical compounds and 60 cancer cell lines through genomic, proteomic, and tissue array profiling *(53–55)*. The resulting pharmacogenomic databases, plus tools for analysis and visualization of the data, are great resources for studying molecular pharmacology of cancer (http://discover.nci.nih.gov). Encouraged by the success of the Human Genome Project, there has been a growing desire and push *(56)* from the biomedical research community to establish public repositories with a consistent submission process, such as that seen in the Human Genome Project, to store and distribute interoperable high-throughput "omic" datasets. In reality, even though technological advances enable data production at unprecedented levels, none of the current datasets are sufficient and comprehensive enough to fully meet the goals of complex endeavors like multicellular disease research.

Comprehensive gene expression studies have been the useful of the genomic approaches in cancer research. The NCBI Gene Expression Omnibus (GEO) and EBI ArrayExpress (Fig. 1) have been established as centralized repositories for gene expression data *(56)*. Unfortunately, these microarray database portals are still primitive compared to the genome browsers because of such challenges as multiple incompatible array platforms producing different types and formats of data, a wide range of experimental designs, and uneven data quality. Thus, the "one-stop shop" implementation for microarray databases does not yet exist and the flourishing of primary and secondary microarray databases, including those listed in the Molecular Biology Database Collection *(5,6)*, continues. These expression databases, constructed by various academic institutions such as The National Cancer Institute Cancer Genome Anatomy Project (NCI CGAP http://cgap.nci.nih.gov/), the Stanford Microarray Database (http://genome-www5.stanford.edu/), the Whitehead Institute ChipDB (http://chipdb.wi.mit.edu/chipdb/public/), the Gene Expression Atlas from GNF (http://expression.gnf.org/cgi-bin/index.cgi), EpoDB from University of Pennsylvania (http://www.cbil.upenn.edu/EpoDB/), and commercial databases from the large microarray companies such as Affymetrix and GeneLogic remain the most useful sources of microarray data.

Gene expression profiling shows great promise for clinical cancer research, as the phenotypic diversity of different tumor types correlates well with corresponding diversities in gene expression patterns. The establishment of comprehensive tumor expression profiling databases and the databases of patient tumor expression "portraits" *(57)* can potentially lead to more accurate diagnosis and personalized treatment. Although a complete picture of the diversity of cancers is still a long way off, the current public-domain micro-array databases have already proven very useful. For example, high-quality open-source array databases like NCI60 *(55,58)* and GCM *(59)* have been used by many research groups to develop tumor classification methodologies for use in expression-based cancer diagnosis *(59–63)*.

## 7. OTHER INTERNET RESOURCES AND KNOWLEDGE INTEGRATION

There are now countless pages of information on nearly any topic available on the Internet: a recent Google search for the word "cancer" returned 83 million results. Thus, general search engines or broadly inclusive website guides like the cancer index http://www.cancerindex.org often prove inefficient. Furthermore, it is common for researchers to need to compile datasets from various sources for doing more advanced analysis. For example, Internet database resources pertinent to basic cancer genetics have been surveyed, summarized *(64)*, and updated (http://tumor.informatics.jax.org/cancer_links.html#biology) into the following categories: distributors and animal production services related to animal models; phenotypes for genetically defined and genetically engineered animals related to animal models; cancer genetics and genomics; pathology; reagents, services, laboratory protocols; cancer biology. These online resources can collectively be used to address the practical research needs for a particular cancer study.

In order to raise awareness and encourage the use of molecular biology databases that represent the best knowledge in particular research areas, the *Journal of Nucleic Acids Research* (http://nar.oupjournals.org/) has been compiling and updating the Molecular Biology Database Collection *(5,6)* in its January issue for the past 10 yr. This guide has been provided as a free resource to online users. Each of the listed databases focuses on a particular biological specialty such as metabolic pathways, protein motifs and structures, transgenics, RNA information, mutational databases, intermolecular interactions, and much more. The contents of these specialized databases are usually curated by domain experts and are often experimentally verified.

Despite the great utility of these individual data sources, the synthesis of these disparate databases would provide even more usefulness. The lack of interoperability between databases and knowledge-sharing solutions has emerged as a significant barrier to productivity in both drug development and basic research *(65,66)*. Many "bio-standards" groups, including OMG (http://www.omg.org/), I3C (http://www.i3c.org/), MGED (http://www.mged.org/), Biopathways (http://www.biopax.org/), Bio-ontologies http://www.cs.man.ac.uk/~stevensr/boc/), Open-Bio (http://open-bio.org/), and CDISC (http://www.cdisc.org/) have formulated data standards to address the representation and distilling of the complex biological data sets. To date, implementations of such standards and associated specifications have not been as effective as expected and promoted. Nevertheless, ontology-based database implementations *(67,68)* have proven to be useful in representing not only taxonomies, as is evidenced by the Gene Ontology database (http://www.geneontology.org) *(69)*, but also diverse concepts and complex relationships such as those seen in biochemical pathways *(70,71)*.

As with the genome sequences, the vast amount of knowledge found in the body of biomedical literature is another focus of intense data mining efforts. This work aims to computationally extract sequence–structure–function relationships in the literature. Emerging as a new field of research seeking to manage biomedical literature and generate specific predictions pertaining to gene function, natural language processing (NLP) *(72)* of biological data is expected to provide additional large-scale datasets and tools.

## 8. SUMMARY

The completion of the Human Genome Project, as well as the sequencing of the genomes of many model organisms, has led to the development of many sophisticated bioinformatics databases and applications. Although it has gained popularity with grand and, sometimes, unrealistic promises, the field of bioinformatics has gradually evolved into an indispensable tool for researchers. The utilization of online genomics resources, including nucleotide and protein sequences and structures, gene expression databases, and genetic linkage information, has become essential for almost any biological research project. Consequently, biomedical scientists have been challenged to acquire the computational and interdisciplinary skills necessary to utilize these resources for their particular research needs. As with any technologically driven advance, the novelty of these bioinformatics tools will wear off and the utility will increase as they become more integrated into the mainstream of biology research. The challenge that lies ahead is how to extract knowledge and insight from these vast amounts of data *(73)*.

## REFERENCES

1. Collins FS, Green ED, Guttmacher AE, Guyer MS. A vision for the future of genomics research. Nature 2003; 422:835–847.
2. Packer A. Spreading the word. Nature Genet 2003; 35(Suppl 1):1.
3. Green P. Whole-genome disassembly. Proc Natl Acad Sci USA 2002; 99:4143–4144.
4. Wolfsberg TG, Wetterstrand KA, Guyer MS, Collins FS, Baxevanis AD. A user's guide to the human genome. Nature Genet 2003; 35(Suppl 1):4.
5. Baxevanis AD. The Molecular Biology Database Collection: 2003 update. Nucleic Acids Res 2003; 31: 1–12.
6. Galperin MY. The Molecular Biology Database Collection: 2004 update. Nucleic Acids Res 2004;32: 1–12.
7. Brooksbank C, Camon E, Harris MA, Magrane M, Martin MJ, Mulder N, et al. The European Bioinformatics Institute's data resources. Nucleic Acids Res 2003; 31:43–50.
8. Knight J. Software firm falls victim to shifting bioinformatics needs. Nature 2002; 416:357.
9. Kerlavage A, Bonazzi V, di Tommaso M, Lawrence C, Li P, Mayberry F, et al. The Celera Discovery System. Nucleic Acids Res 2002; 30:129–136.
10. Overbeek R, Larsen N, Walunas T, D'Souza M, Pusch G, Selkov E Jr, et al. The ERGO genome analysis and discovery system. Nucleic Acids Res 2003; 31:164–171.
11. Hubbard T, Barker D, Birney E, Cameron G, Chen Y, Clark L, et al. The Ensembl genome database project. Nucleic Acids Res 2002; 30:38–41.
12. Karolchik D, Baertsch R, Diekhans M, Furey TS, Hinrichs A, Lu YT, et al. The UCSC Genome Browser Database. Nucleic Acids Res 2003; 31:51–54.
13. Lander ES, Linton LM, Birren B, et al. Initial sequencing and analysis of the human genome. Nature 2001; 409:860–921.
14. Venter JC, Adams MD, Myers EW, Li PW, Mural RJ, Sutton GG, et al. The sequence of the human genome. Science 2001; 291:1304–1351.
15. Waterston RH, Lander ES, Sulston JE. On the sequencing of the human genome. Proc Natl Acad Sci USA 2002; 99:3712–3716.
16. Myers EW, Sutton GG, Smith HO, Adams MD, Venter JC. On the sequencing and assembly of the human genome. Proc Natl Acad Sci USA 2002; 99:4145–4146.

17. Cozzarelli NR. Revisiting the independence of the publicly and privately funded drafts of the human genome. Proc Natl Acad Sci USA 2003; 100:3021.

18. Waterston RH, Lander ES, Sulston JE. More on the sequencing of the human genome. Proc Natl Acad Sci USA 2003; 100:3022–3024; author reply 3025–3026.

19. Adams MD, Sutton GG, Smith HO, Myers EW, Venter JC. The independence of our genome assemblies. Proc Natl Acad Sci USA 2003; 100:3025–3026.

20. Rouchka EC, Gish W, States DJ. Comparison of whole genome assemblies of the human genome. Nucleic Acids Res 2002; 30:5004–5014.

21. Hogenesch JB, Ching KA, Batalov S, Su AI, Walker JR, Zhou Y, et al. A comparison of the Celera and Ensembl predicted gene sets reveals little overlap in novel genes. Cell 2001; 106:413–415.

22. Li S, Liao J, Cutler G, Hoey T, Hogenesch JB, Cooke MP, et al. Comparative analysis of human genome assemblies reveals genome-level differences. Genomics 2002;80:138–139.

23. Li S, Cutler G, Liu JJ, Hoey T, Chen L, Schultz PG, et al. A comparative analysis of HGSC and Celera human genome assemblies and gene sets. Bioinformatics 2003; 19:1597–1605.

24. Kent WJ. BLAT—the BLAST-like alignment tool. Genome Res 2002; 12:656–664.

25. Maglott DR, Katz KS, Sicotte H, Pruitt KD. NCBI's LocusLink and RefSeq. Nucleic Acids Res 2000; 28:126–128.

26. Pruitt KD, Maglott DR. RefSeq and LocusLink: NCBI gene-centered resources. Nucleic Acids Res 2001; 29:137–140.

27. Burge C. Identification of genes in human genomic DNA. PhD thesis, Stanford University, 1997.

28. Burge C, Karlin S. Prediction of complete gene structures in human genomic DNA. J Mol Biol 1997; 268: 78–94.

29. Huson DH, Reinert K, Kravitz SA, Remington KA, Delcher AL, Dew IM, et al. Design of a compartmentalized shotgun assembler for the human genome. Bioinformatics 2001; 17:S132–S139.

30. Zhou Y, Luoh SM, Zhang Y, Watanabe C, Wu TD, Ostland M, et al. Genome-wide identification of chromosomal regions of increased tumor expression by transcriptome analysis. Cancer Res 2003; 63: 5781–5784.

31. Caron H, van Schaik B, van der Mee M, Baas F, Riggins G, van Sluis P, et al. The human transcriptome map: clustering of highly expressed genes in chromosomal domains. Science 2001; 291:1289–1292.

32. Lucito R, West J, Reiner A, Alexander J, Esposito D, Mishra B, et al. Detecting gene copy number fluctuations in tumor cells by microarray analysis of genomic representations. Genome Res 2000; 10:1726–1736.

33. Lucito R, Healy J, Alexander J, Reiner A, Esposito D, Chi M, et al. Representational oligonucleotide microarray analysis: a high-resolution method to detect genome copy number variation. Genome Res 2003; 13:2291–2305.

34. Pei L, Wiser O, Slavin A, Mu D, Powers S, Jan LY, et al. Oncogenic potential of TASK3 (Kcnk9) depends on K+ channel function. Proc Natl Acad Sci USA 2003; 100:7803–7807.

35. Pei L, Peng Y, Yang Y, Ling XB, Van Eyndhoven WG, Nguyen KC, et al. PRC17, a novel oncogene encoding a Rab GTPase-activating protein, is amplified in prostate cancer. Cancer Res 2002; 62: 5420–5424.

36. Li J, Yang Y, Peng Y, Austin RJ, van Eyndhoven WG, Nguyen KC, et al. Oncogenic properties of PPM1D located within a breast cancer amplification epicenter at 17q23. Nature Genet 2002; 31:133–134.

37. Mu D, Chen L, Zhang X, See LH, Koch CM, Yen C, et al. Genomic amplification and oncogenic properties of the KCNK9 potassium channel gene. Cancer Cell 2003; 3:297–302.

38. Pollack JR, Perou CM, Alizadeh AA, Eisen MB, Pergamenschikov A, Williams CF, et al. Genome-wide analysis of DNA copy-number changes using cDNA microarrays. Nature Genet 1999; 23:41–46.

39. Strausberg RL, Simpson AJ, Wooster R. Sequence-based cancer genomics: progress, lessons and opportunities. Nature Rev Genet 2003; 4:409–418.

40. Zhou W. Mapping genetic alterations in tumors with single nucleotide polymorphisms. Curr Opin Oncol 2003; 15:50–54.

41. Negm RS, Verma M, Srivastava S. The promise of biomarkers in cancer screening and detection. Trends Mol Med 2002; 8:288–293.

42. Haas DW, Wu H, Li H, Bosch RJ, Lederman MM, Kuritzkes D, et al. MDR1 gene polymorphisms and phase 1 viral decay during HIV-1 infection: an adult AIDS Clinical Trials Group study. J Acquir Immune Defic Syndr 2003; 34:295–298.

43. Kerb R, Hoffmeyer S, Brinkmann U. ABC drug transporters: hereditary polymorphisms and pharmacological impact in MDR1, MRP1 and MRP2. Pharmacogenomics 2001; 2:51–64.

44. Chang BL, Zheng SL, Isaacs SD, Turner AR, Bleecker ER, Walsh PC, et al. Evaluation of SRD5A2 sequence variants in susceptibility to hereditary and sporadic prostate cancer. Prostate 2003; 56:37–44.
45. Wang M, Lemon WJ, Liu G, Wang Y, Iraqi FA, Malkinson AM, et al. Fine mapping and identification of candidate pulmonary adenoma susceptibility 1 genes using advanced intercross lines. Cancer Res 2003; 63:3317–3324.
46. Liggett SB. Pharmacogenetic applications of the Human Genome Project. Nature Med 2001; 7:281–283.
47. Packer BR, Yeager M, Staats B, Welch R, Crenshaw A, Kiley M, et al. SNP500Cancer: a public resource for sequence validation and assay development for genetic variation in candidate genes. Nucleic Acids Res 2004; 32:D528–D532.
48. McLeod HL, Yu J. Cancer pharmacogenomics: SNPs, chips, and the individual patient. Cancer Invest 2003; 21:630–640.
49. Cyranoski D. Biologists take tentative steps towards bespoke cancer drugs. Nature 2003; 423:209.
50. Thomas JW, Touchman JW, Blakesley RW, Bouffard GG, Beckstrom-Sternberg SM, Margulies EH, et al. Comparative analyses of multi-species sequences from targeted genomic regions. Nature 2003; 424: 788–793.
51. Clamp M, Andrews D, Barker D, Bevan P, Cameron G, Chen Y, et al. Ensembl 2002: accommodating comparative genomics. Nucleic Acids Res 2003; 31:38–42.
52. Weinstein JN. "Omic" and hypothesis-driven research in the molecular pharmacology of cancer. Curr Opin Pharmacol 2003; 2002; 2:361–365.
53. Nishizuka S, Chen ST, Gwadry FG, Alexander J, Major SM, Scherf U, et al. Diagnostic markers that distinguish colon and ovarian adenocarcinomas: identification by genomic, proteomic, and tissue array profiling. Cancer Res 2003; 63:5243–5250.
54. Nishizuka S, Charboneau L, Young L, Major S, Reinhold WC, Waltham M, et al. Proteomic profiling of the NCI-60 cancer cell lines using new high-density reverse-phase lysate microarrays. Proc Natl Acad Sci USA 2003; 100:14,229–14,234.
55. Ross DT, Scherf U, Eisen MB, Perou CM, Rees C, Spellman P, et al. Systematic variation in gene expression patterns in human cancer cell lines. Nature Genet 2000; 24:227–235.
56. Brazma A, Robinson A, Cameron G, Ashburner M. One-stop shop for microarray data. Nature 2000; 403:699–700.
57. Perou CM, Sorlie T, Eisen MB, van de Rijn M, Jeffrey SS, Rees CA, et al. Molecular portraits of human breast tumours. Nature 2000; 406:747–752.
58. Staunton JE, Slonim DK, Coller HA, Tamayo P, Angelo MJ, Park J, et al. Chemosensitivity prediction by transcriptional profiling. Proc Natl Acad Sci USA 2001; 98:10,787–10,792.
59. Ramaswamy S, Tamayo P, Rifkin R, Mukherjee S, Yeang CH, Angelo M, et al. Multiclass cancer diagnosis using tumor gene expression signatures. Proc Natl Acad Sci USA 2001; 98:15,149–15,154.
60. Yeang CH, Ramaswamy S, Tamayo P, Mukherjee S, Rifkin RM, Angelo M, et al. Molecular classification of multiple tumor types. Bioinformatics 2001; 17(Suppl 1):S316–S322.
61. Su AI, Welsh JB, Sapinoso LM, Kern SG, Dimitrov P, Lapp H, et al. Molecular classification of human carcinomas by use of gene expression signatures. Cancer Biology 2001; 61:7388–7393.
62. Ooi CH, Tan P. Genetic algorithms applied to multi-class prediction for the analysis of gene expression data. Bioinformatics 2003; 19:37–44.
63. Peng S, Xu Q, Ling XB, Peng X, Du W, Chen L. Molecular classification of cancer types from microarray data using the combination of genetic algorithms and support vector machines. FEBS Lett 2003; 555: 358–362.
64. Bult CJ, Krupke DM, Tennent BJ, Eppig JT. A survey of web resources for basic cancer genetics research. Genome Res 1999; 9:397–408.
65. Neumann E, Thomas J. Knowledge assembly for the life sciences. Drug Discov Today 2002; 7:S160–S162.
66. Attwood TK. Genomics. The Babel of bioinformatics. Science 2000; 290:471–473.
67. Pouliot Y, Gao J, Su QJ, Liu GG, Ling XB. DIAN: a novel algorithm for genome ontological classification. Genome Res 2001; 11:1766–1779.
68. Diehn M, Sherlock G, Binkley G, Jin H, Matese JC, Hernandez-Boussard T, et al. SOURCE: a unified genomic resource of functional annotations, ontologies, and gene expression data. Nucleic Acids Res 2003; 31:219–223.
69. Ashburner M, Ball CA, Blake JA, Botstein D, Butler H, Cherry JM, et al. Gene ontology: tool for the unification of biology. The Gene Ontology Consortium. Nature Genet 2000; 25:25–29.
70. Karp PD. An ontology for biological function based on molecular interactions. Bioinformatics 2000; 16:269–285.

71. Karp PD. Pathway databases: a case study in computational symbolic theories. Science 2001; 293: 2040–2044.
72. Yandell MD, Majoros WH. Genomics and natural language processing. Nature Rev Genet 2002; 3: 601–610.
73. Brenner S. Ontology recapitulates philology. Scientist 2002; 16:12.

# 2

# Cancer Drug Target Identification by SAGE, LongSAGE, and Digital Karyotyping

*Heiko Hermeking, PhD*

## Contents

## Summary

Activated oncogenes are required for the initiation and maintenance of the cancer cell phenotype, and, therefore, represent attractive therapeutic targets. Specific inhibition of oncogene products was recently approved for cancer treatment. Oncogene activation often results from genomic amplification. The SAGE (serial analysis of gene expression) method has recently been adapted to the analysis of genomic alterations, including amplifications. As a first step in this direction, LongSAGE, which allows one to localize differentially expressed SAGE tags/mRNAs in the human genome, was devised. Subsequently, the LongSAGE protocol was adapted to the quantitative analysis of copy-number changes in genomic DNA. This new method, named Digital Karyotyping, identifies amplifications at an unprecedented resolution. In this chapter the SAGE-based quantification of gene expression and genomic copy-number changes is described as well as how it might be integrated into the identification of oncogenes and cancer drug targets.

**Key Words:** Oncogene; cancer therapy; Digital Karyotyping; SAGE; serial analysis of gene expression; drug target; tumor biology; tumor suppressor gene; amplification.

From: *Cancer Drug Discovery and Development: The Oncogenomics Handbook*
Edited by: W. J. LaRochelle and R. A. Shimkets © Humana Press Inc., Totowa, NJ

# 1. ALTERATIONS IN ONCOGENES
# AND TUMOR SUPPRESSOR GENES CAUSE CANCER

Cancer is a disease primarily caused by the genetic activation of oncogenes and inactivation of tumor suppressor genes *(1–4)*. In addition, epigenetic inactivation of tumor suppressors by CpG methylation of promoter sequences seems to occur at a substantial frequency *(5)*. In the last 20 yr, numerous oncogenes and tumor suppressor genes have been identified. Oncogenes were initially identified via analysis of retroviruses that cause cancer in mice and chicken *(1)*. These viruses were found to have incorporated cellular genes with mitogenic properties into their genomes. The cellular counterparts of these viral oncogenes turned out to be important components of mitogenic signaling pathways (e.g., *SRC, MYC, HER2/neu, FOS, MYB*). In human cancer, these genes, also called proto-oncogenes, are activated by genomic amplifications, translocations (with fusion to foreign promoters or protein-coding sequences), or point mutations.

# 2. ONCOGENES AS ANTICANCER DRUG TARGETS

Cancer therapy directed at specific, frequently occurring molecular alterations in signaling pathways of cancer cells has been validated through the clinical development and regulatory approval in the recent years *(6)*. An example of an approved therapeutic agent is Herceptin/trastazumab, a humanized antibody directed against the product of the *HER2/neu* oncogene, which is amplified in approx 20% of advanced breast cancer and encodes a receptor tyrosine kinase. Another example is the small-molecule drug Gleevec/imatinib, which inhibits the BCR-ABL tyrosine kinase and the c-kit tyrosine kinase receptor, and is currently used for treatment of chronic myelogenous leukemia and gastro-intestinal cancer.

It is anticipated that a wave of sophisticated "smart drugs" directed at activated or overexpressed oncogene products identified through genomic and proteomic techniques will fundamentally change the treatment of all cancers *(6)*. Tumor suppressor genes obviously represent more difficult targets because their products are lost or inactive in tumors. However, their loss could be exploited via the resulting increased sensitivity to DNA-damaging treatments or recombinant viruses, for example *(7–10)*. For several oncogenes, it was shown that they are not only involved in establishing the tumor, but that they are also necessary for maintaining the growth and proliferation of tumor cells; for example, conditional inactivation of c-MYC in an experimental c-MYC-induced tumor leads to differentiation of tumor cells *(11)*. Subsequent reactivation of the conditional c-MYC allele induced apoptosis, suggesting that even transient therapeutic inhibition of c-MYC could lead to a significant tumor reduction and even complete regression (reviewed in ref. *12)*. Although a number of oncogenes, which might serve as potential target proteins for further development of targeted therapeutics, are known, there is a shortage of targets for most of the common cancers. In the case of breast cancer, therapy with the anti ErbB2-antibody Herceptin is restricted to approx 20% of the breast cancer patients who have detectable *HER2* amplifications. Therefore, numerous efforts are ongoing to identify frequently occurring amplifications/mutations present in the remaining 80% of breast cancers.

# 3. TECHNIQUES USED FOR IDENTIFICATION
# OF ONCOGENIC AMPLIFICATIONS

A number of different techniques has been used in the past to identify oncogenes. As mentioned earlier, the pioneering work took advantage of the fact that murine and avian retroviruses had incorporated a number of cellular oncogenes. Several of these genes were shown to have undergone activating alterations in human cancer. Another approach was to directly identify and characterize genetic alterations in human cancer by using cytogenetic methods. This led to the discovery of oncogenic fusion proteins resulting from recurrent breakpoint fusions between different chromosomes. One famous example is the *BCR-ABL* fusion, which occurs in CML (chronic myeloid leukemia) as a result of the fusion of the chromosomal regions 9q34 to 22q11 *(13)*. Other oncogenes were identified as components of cytogenetically detectable amplifications of genetic material in the form of double minutes and homogenously staining regions (HSRs) *(14)*. The increase of gene dosage by DNA amplification is a common genetic mechanism for upregulating gene expression. DNA amplification has been detected in response to exposure to cytotoxic drugs *(15–17)* or during tumorigenesis *(18)*. Therefore, amplifications can also occur in response to chemotherapeutic cancer treatment and result in resistance (discussed later in this paragraph). The possible genetic mechanisms of gene amplification are discussed in ref. *19*. Interestingly, no instance of amplifications as a tissue culture artifact has been reported *(19)*. The region of amplification is often much larger than the oncogene targeted by the respective amplification event. The regions of amplification can range from several hundred Kbp to several Mbp. The size of the amplification unit often correlates with the tumor type. Small amplified regions, which can contain a single gene (N-*myc*), have been observed in 20% of neuroblastoma and correlate with more aggressive variants of neuroblastoma. N-*myc* amplification is currently used as a powerful marker to predict poor outcome in low-stage neuroblastoma *(19)*. Furthermore, amplification of N-*myc* is used to tailor therapeutic approaches. Larger amplification units usually contain several genes. In these cases, the coamplified genes might not convey any advantage for the affected cell. However, in some cases, syntenic coamplified genes might also play a role in tumor development; for example, the 12q13-14 amplification involves the *MDM2, CDK4,* and *GLI* genes, all of which have oncogenic activity when expressed alone. This amplification occurs in sarcomas *(20)* and in neuroblastoma *(21)*. Another famous example of an amplified oncogene is the *ErbB2/HER2/neu* gene, which encodes a receptor tyrosine kinase *(22)*. Approximately 20–25% of primary breast cancer showed amplified *HER2/neu* genes *(23)*. The level of observed amplifications was up to 20-fold. The *HER2/ neu* amplification was found to be a significant predictor of overall survival and time to relapse *(24)*. Generally, levels of amplifications in tumors can range from 5-fold to more than 500-fold. In most tumors, values around 50- to 100-fold are seen.

The development of the comparative genomic hybridization (CGH) method, which allows the genomewide analyses of copy-number changes at a resolution between 10 and 20 Mbp, supported the identification of amplified genomic regions harboring oncogenes. However, because of the low resolution of CGH, only a small number of oncogenes were identified via this route. One example is *PIK3CA (14)*. In the future, array-CGH (also referred to as matrix-CGH), which promises to have a resolution up to 50 kbp, will presumably aid in the identification of genomic amplifications and the critical proto-oncogenes involved. However, a number of technical problems have to be overcome before this technique becomes widely used *(25)*. Another approach used for the identification of oncogenes is RDA (representational difference analysis) *(26)*. Recently, *KCNK9* was identified by RDA as a gene amplified 3- to 10-fold in 10% of breast tumors *(27)*.

In rare cases, amplified oncogenes, such as *K-RAS*, were found by analysis of mRNA expression, which allowed the detection of overexpressed gene products *(28)*. Serial analysis of gene expression (SAGE) analysis of differential gene expression in distinct tumor stages has recently led to the identification of an amplified gene, which can be of therapeutic relevance: Saha et al. analyzed a number of different progression stages of colorectal cancers and found a subset of genes that were dramatically upregulated in metastatic lesions *(29)*. Among these was the gene encoding the tyrosine phosphatase PRL3. Because of the central role of signaling via tyrosine phosphorylation in cancer the *PRL3* gene was studied in more detail. Indeed, 3 out of 12 metastatic tumors analyzed showed a more than 100-fold amplification of *PRL3*. However, gene expression analysis is a rather indirect approach for identifying oncogenes, because cancer cells display a large number of deregulated genes when compared to their normal counterparts. Most of these tumor-specific changes in gene expression are secondary to the genetic and epigenetic changes in a few critical oncogenes or tumor suppressor genes.

## 4. FROM SAGE TO LONGSAGE: INCORPORATING THE GENOMIC LEVEL

Serial analysis of gene expression was devised to allow the analysis of mRNA expression without prior sequence information of the genes subjected to analysis *(30;* reviewed in ref. *31)*. A number of genes and pathways relevant for tumor biology were identified using SAGE *(7,31–35)*. The 14-bp tag, including four fixed positions (CATG), used during conventional SAGE is sufficient to distinguish 1,048,576 different mRNAs. Because human or murine mRNA populations contain 30,000–50,000 different mRNAs, the 14-bp SAGE tag allows one to identify and quantify the correct, corresponding cDNA as shown by numerous validations of differential SAGE-tag expression using independent methods as Northern blotting and quantitative real-time polymerase chain reaction (PCR) (e.g., ref. *36)*. Nonetheless, some ambiguities occurred when using SAGE because in some cases single SAGE tags match several different mRNAs. Furthermore, the 14-bp tag is not sufficient to map the SAGE tag to the genome and thereby determine position and exons of previously unknown cDNAs *(37)*. cDNAs representing genes expressed at low levels, which might have important regulatory functions, are often not represented in the expressed sequence tag (EST) databases and would be missed in a SAGE screen. Therefore, several techniques using the SAGE tag as a primer in an anchored PCR reaction to identify the cDNA in a gene-by-gene manner were proposed *(34,38)*. It was estimated that approx 15,000 exons have not been confirmed through EST sequencing projects to date *(37)*. Furthermore, calculations showed that a SAGE tag of 21-bp length would provide sufficient information to allow the direct mapping of the SAGE tag to the genome with a certainty of 99.83% *(37)*. Accordingly, the SAGE protocol was modified by changing the type IIS restriction enzyme, which is used to release the LongSAGE tag from the 3' ends of cDNAs, from *Bsf*mI to *Mme*I. This allowed one to retrieve SAGE tags of 21-bp size *(37)*. In a pilot experiment, a LongSAGE library of 27,737 tags was generated from a colorectal cancer cell line *(37)*. This library represented 3336 genes annotated in the Human Genome Project. However, an additional 1503 tags matched to exons, which had not been previously annotated, with 583 tags matching to internal exons and 920 to novel genes. In order to validate these results, the expression of 129 candidate genes was determined by reverse transcription (RT)–PCR. Thereby, the expression of 123 predicted genes was confirmed *(37)*. These results show that LongSAGE is a useful tool for the identification of novel genes overexpressed in cancer, which could include tumor markers or drug targets. An overview of the Long-SAGE approach is depicted in Fig. 1.

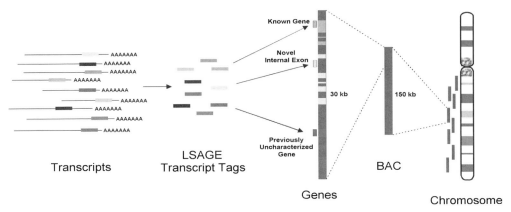

**Fig. 1.** Schematic of the LongSAGE method. Comparison of tag localizations to previously annotated genes can provide expression evidence for predicted genes and identify novel internal exons and previously uncharacterized genes. *See* text for details. (From ref. *37* with permission from Dr. Victor Velculescu, Nature publishing group: www.nature.com.)

## 5. DIGITAL KARYOTYPING: CHARTING CANCER CELL GENOMES

As mentioned earlier, the tumor-specific changes in the levels of protein and mRNA expression might be secondary to genetic alterations. Furthermore, gene expression is difficult to measure and might be very specific for each tumor or even the area of the tumor that is analyzed. In contrast, genetic alterations (genomic copy-numbers changes) are stable throughout the tumor cell population. Furthermore, it has been shown that they have a causal role in the development of cancer, because they contain oncogenes (amplifications) and tumor suppressor genes (deletions). Therefore, they provide valuable information about the pathogenetic mechanisms underlying the development of the respective tumor. However, the techniques for detection of these copy-number changes available today are still limited in their resolution. Therefore, Wang et al. recently developed Digital Karyotyping, which is based on the LongSAGE methodology *(39)* (*see* Fig. 2 for an overview of the Digital Karyotyping procedure [Color Plate 1, following p. 78]). As with SAGE, it is not necessary to clone probes for the sequences that are being analyzed. However, it is necessary that the genome of interest be completely sequenced and aligned. For Digital Karyotyping, the genomic DNA (approx 1 µg) is cleaved by the so-called mapping enzyme, a restriction enzyme with a 6-bp recognition sequence (e.g., *Sac*I), which results in fragments with an average size of 4096 bp. After ligation of biotinylated linkers to the DNA molecules, a digest with a 4-bp recognizing enzyme (*Nla*III, recognizes CATG) is performed. The DNA fragments containing the biotinylated linker are purified by magnetic streptavidin beads. An oligonucleotide harboring a type IIS restriction endonuclease (*Mme*I) recognition site is ligated to the free *Nla*III site. The LongSAGE tags are then released by cleavage with *Mme*I, which cleaves 21 bp from its recognition site. The released 21-bp tags are self-ligated, PCR-amplified, concatenated, cloned, and automatically sequenced. Sequencing of at least 160,000 tags is necessary to obtain interpretable karyotypes. Because approx 30 LongSAGE tags can be determined per reaction, sequencing of approx 5500 plasmids is required. The templates for these sequencing reactions can either be DNA plasmids

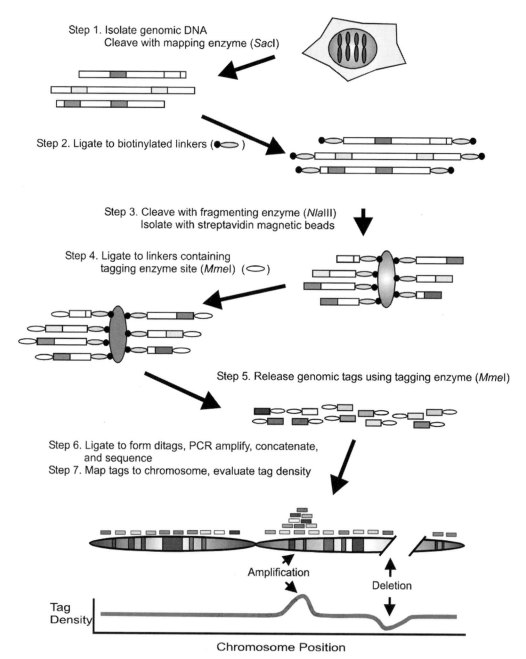

**Fig. 2.** Summary of the Digital Karyotyping procedure. Small, shaded squares represent genomic tags. Small ovals represent linkers. Large ovals represent streptavidin-coated magnetic beads. *See* text for details. (*See* Color Plate 1 following p. 78; from ref. *39* with permission from *PNAS*.)

or PCR products. By capillary sequencing, this task can be completed in 1–5 d, depending on the availability of a 96- or 384-format sequencer. The resulting sequence data are imported into a so-called SAGE library with the help of the SAGE2000 software and subse-

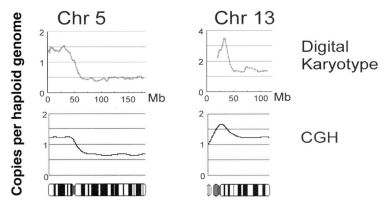

**Fig. 3.** Digital Karyotyping compared to CGH analysis. Genomic DNA derived from the colorectal cancer cell line DiFi was analyzed either by Digital Karyotyping (upper panel) or conventional CGH (lower panel). Ideograms of the normal human chromosomes 5 and 13 are depicted below the graphs. Values on the *y*-axis indicate genome copies per haploid genome. Values alone the *x*-axis represent positions along the chromosome (in megabasepairs). Digital Karyotype values represent exponentially smoothed ratios of DiFi tag densities, using a sliding window of 1000 virtual tags normalized to a diploid genome. An example of a smaller window size is shown in Fig. 4. For details, *see* the text. (From ref. *39* with permission from *PNAS*.)

quently matched with a virtual Digital Karyotyping library representing the tags occurring only once in the analyzed genome. In this way, any repetitive sequences are excluded from the analysis. This filtering results in a 40–50% decrease of sequenced tags that are used for the determination of copy-number changes (e.g., 171,795 collected genomic tags resulted in 107,515 filtered tags). The library of filtered tags is then analyzed with Digital Karyotyping software, which generates maps showing the tag densities across the genome. Examples of Digital Karyotyping results compared to conventional CGH analyses of chromosome 5 and 13 of a colorectal cancer cell line are shown at low resolution in Fig. 3. The Digital Karyotyping software allows to display the data at different resolutions and includes a bitmap viewer for maximal resolution and direct access to the raw data at any given chromosomal position. Figure 4 shows the resolution obtained using the bitmap viewer of the amplification on chromosome 7 shown in Fig. 3. The depicted amplification of the *EGFR* (*EGF-receptor*) protooncogene on chromosome 7 has been missed by the CGH analysis, which only indicates an slight increase in the DNA content (data not shown). The size of the amplicon was approx 500 kbp, which explains why it was not detected by CGH. The degree of amplification (approx 120-fold) was confirmed by quantitative PCR *(39)*. Furthermore, the software allows one to set cutoffs for the levels of amplifications and deletions, which should be regarded as relevant. Thereby, the most significant alterations can be rapidly identified. The software described here can be downloaded from the following websites: www.sagenet.org and http://www.digitalkaryotyping.org/. The copy-number values obtained by Digital Karyotyping were confirmed by quantitative real-time PCR (qPCR) for a number of amplifications and deletions, suggesting that the quantification achieved by Digital Karyotyping is very accurate *(39)*. Wang et al. estimated the positive predictive value of Digital Karyotyping data at a library size of 160,000 sequenced LongSAGE tags. Accordingly, a 10-fold amplification of only 100 kbp size is reliably

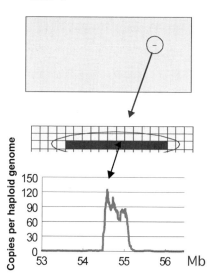

**Fig. 4.** High-resolution tag density maps of an *EGFR* gene amplification on chromosome 7. A bit-map viewer with the region containing the alteration encircled is depicted. The bitmap viewer is comprised of 39,000 pixels representing tag density values of each virtual tag on chromosome 7, determined from sliding windows of 50 virtual tags. Gray pixels correspond to copy numbers <110, and black pixels represent copy numbers >110. An enlarged view of the region of alteration is shown. (**Bottom**) A graphic representating the amplified region with values on the *y*-axis indicating genome copies per haploid genome and values on the *x*-axis representing positions along the chromosome (in Mbp). (From ref. *39* with permission from *PNAS.*)

detected by Digital Karyotyping *(39)*. In case of deletions, the resolution is significantly smaller. The minimal size of reliably detected homozygous deletions is in the range of 500 kbp. Therefore, Digital Karyotyping seems especially useful for the detection of small amplifications. As starting material, 1 µg genomic DNA is required for an analysis by Digital Karyotyping. Furthermore, several oligonucleotides, modifying and restriction enzymes, PCR and sequencing reagents, and the SAGE and Digital Karyotyping software have to be obtained. The first attempts to perform Digital Karyotyping should be accompanied by a confirmatory CGH analysis of the same tumor DNA, as the CGH results should be very similar to a low-resolution representation of Digital Karyotyping results. Similar to Wang et al. *(39)*, we were able to confirm Digital Karyotyping results by conventional CGH (Hermeking et al., unpublished results).

## 6. VALIDATION OF DIGITAL KARYOTYPING RESULTS

It is necessary to confirm the alterations detected by Digital Karyotyping using independent methods. In the case of amplifications qPCR or FISH (fluorescence *in situ* hybridization) should be employed to confirm the findings. For qPCR, several primer pairs should be used to confirm each alteration and determine the size of the alteration. Fine mapping the amplification is necessary to restrict the number of potential candidate genes. Generally, even small amplifications will harbor several candidate genes. The genes with functions similar to known oncogenes (e.g., kinases, transcriptions factors) represent the most promising candidates for playing a causal role in the detected amplification event. Primer pairs neighboring these genes should be used to screen genomic DNAs isolated from tumors of a larger number of patients (>50) in order to determine the frequency of the gene-amplification event in a particular type of cancer. This analysis will also define the smallest, amplified consensus region. Other types of tumor can be included in the analysis. Several of the classic oncogenes show moderate frequencies of amplification in a given tumor type; for example, c-*myc* and *HER2/neu* are amplified in approx 20% of all breast cancer cases analyzed *(19)*. For certain genes, an alternative to amplification can be activation by point mutation. Therefore, genes found to be amplified by Digital Karyotyping should be analyzed for point mutations in tumors showing no amplification. Interphase FISH using a gene-specific probe can be used to determine the frequency of amplifications in paraffin-embedded tumor sections *(40)*, which allows one to extend the observations made on a few tumors to larger cohorts of archival patient material.

In order to determine which gene is critically involved in the amplification, the encoded gene product should be inactivated by experimental means. For rapid, although partial, inactivation RNA interference (RNAi)-based techniques can be used *(41)*. Recently, a facile approach for the inactivation of specific genes by homologous recombination in human cell lines has been introduced, which can be used in cases were the complete inactivation of the candidate gene is necessary *(42)*. Alternatively, validation by (conditional) knockout approaches in mice can be useful. In Fig. 5, the possible steps and outcomes of a SAGE-based analysis of gene expression and genomic changes in tumors are summarized.

## 7. FURTHER APPLICATIONS OF DIGITAL KARYOTYPING IN CANCER RESEARCH

Digital Karyotyping has been recently used to show that the gene encoding thymidylate kinase (*TYMS*) is specifically amplified in tumors which underwent treatment with 5-fluorouracil (5-FU) *(40)*. This example shows that Digital Karyotyping can also be useful in identifying genes that modulate the outcome of current cancer therapeutic approaches: Patients with a *TYMS* amplification are largely resistant to treatment with 5-FU and have a considerably worse survival compared to similar patients without *TYMS* amplification *(40)*. Importantly, patients with *TYMS* amplifications, which is relatively easy to routinely detect in paraffin-embedded tumor samples, could be spared from treatment with 5-FU and the associated toxicity in the future. Instead, new drugs specifically targeting the elevated levels/activity of the TYMS protein should be developed.

Another application of Digital Karyotyping might be the detection of DNA, which is not normally present in the genome analyzed (e.g., viral DNA) *(39)*. Wang et al. showed that Epstein–Barr virus sequences could be readily detected Digital Karytyping of lymphoblastoid cell lines. As more viral genome sequences become available, it might be interesting to determine whether neoplastic cells contain any potentially pathogenic viral DNAs.

## 8. ALTERNATIVES TO DIGITAL KARYOTYPING

A recent improvement in the resolution of CGH was achieved by incorporating microarrays in the CGH analysis. Instead of hybridizing the tumor DNA to metaphase spreads of normal cells, the DNA is hybridized to BAC (bacterial artificial chromosome)

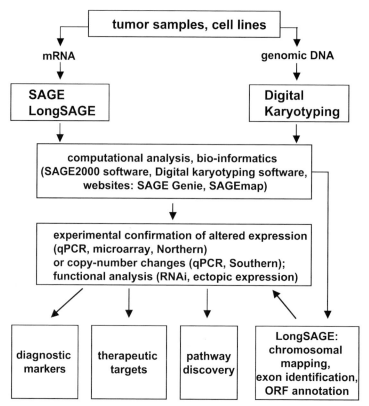

**Fig. 5.** SAGE analysis of cancer-specific alterations in gene expression and copy-number changes. Flowchart showing the possible steps and outcomes of a SAGE-based analysis of cancer cell genomes and transcriptomes. Website addresses are as follows: SAGEmap: http://www.ncbi.nlm.nih.gov/SAGE; SAGE Genie: http://cgap.nci.nih.gov/SAGE.

clones representing the human genome spotted on arrays. Dependent on the size and coverage of the BACs used, this technique allows a resolution of 50 kbp. However, currently the use of array-CGH is restricted to a small number of specialized laboratories. Furthermore, there might be significant difficulties because of the problems encountered with hybridizations of complex DNA mixtures.

In the future, a parallel analysis of tumor DNAs by Digital Karyotyping and array-CGH might generate a comprehensive picture of the analyzed cancer cell genome by complementation of the specific advantages of both approaches.

## REFERENCES

1. Bishop JM. Molecular themes in oncogenesis. Cell 1991; 64:235–248.
2. Hahn WC, Weinberg RA. Modelling the molecular circuitry of cancer. Nature Rev Cancer 2002; 2:331–341.
3. Hanahan D, Weinberg RA. The hallmarks of cancer. Cell 2000; 100:57–70.
4. Kinzler KW, Vogelstein B. Lessons from hereditary colorectal cancer. Cell 1996; 87:159–170.
5. Jones PA, Baylin SB. The fundamental role of epigenetic events in cancer. Nature Rev Genet 2002; 3: 415–428.

6. Shawver LK, Slamon D, Ullrich A. Smart drugs: tyrosine kinase inhibitors in cancer therapy. Cancer Cell 2002; 1:117–123.

7. Hermeking H. The 14-3-3 cancer connection. Nature Rev Cancer 2003; 3:931–943.

8. Chan TA, Hermeking H, Lengauer C, Kinzler KW, Vogelstein B. 14-3-3 Sigma is required to prevent mitotic catastrophe after DNA damage. Nature 1999; 401:616–620.

9. Chan TA, Hwang PM, Hermeking H, Kinzler KW, Vogelstein B. Cooperative effects of genes controlling the G(2)/M checkpoint. Genes Dev 2000; 14:1584–1588.

10. Lodygin D, Menssen A, Hermeking H. Induction of the Cdk inhibitor p21 by LY83583 inhibits tumor cell proliferation in a p53-independent manner. J Clin Invest 2002; 110:1717–1727.

11. Jain M, Arvanitis C, Chu K, et al. Sustained loss of a neoplastic phenotype by brief inactivation of MYC. Science 2002; 297:102–104.

12. Hermeking H. The MYC oncogene as a cancer drug target. Curr Cancer Drug Targets 2003; 3:163–175.

13. de Klein A, van Kessel AG, Grosveld G, et al. A cellular oncogene is translocated to the Philadelphia chromosome in chronic myelocytic leukaemia. Nature 1982; 300:765–767.

14. Shayesteh L, Lu Y, Kuo WL, et al. PIK3CA is implicated as an oncogene in ovarian cancer. Nature Genet 1999; 21:99–102.

15. Schimke RT. Gene amplification in cultured animal cells. Cell 1984; 37:705–713.

16. Stark GR, Wahl GM. Gene amplification. Annu Rev Biochem 1984; 53:447–491.

17. Stark GR, Debatisse M, Giulotto E, Wahl GM. Recent progress in understanding mechanisms of mammalian DNA amplification. Cell 1989; 57:901–908.

18. Alitalo K, Schwab M. Oncogene amplification in tumor cells. Adv Cancer Res 1986; 47:235–281.

19. Savelyeva L, Schwab M. Amplification of oncogenes revisited: from expression profiling to clinical application. Cancer Lett 2001; 167:115–123.

20. Khatib ZA, Matsushime H, Valentine M, Shapiro DN, Sherr CJ, Look AT. Coamplification of the CDK4 gene with MDM2 and GLI in human sarcomas. Cancer Res 1993; 53:5535–5541.

21. Corvi R, Savelyeva L, Breit S, et al. Non-syntenic amplification of MDM2 and MYCN in human neuroblastoma. Oncogene 1995; 10:1081–1086.

22. King CR, Kraus MH, Aaronson SA. Amplification of a novel v-erbB-related gene in a human mammary carcinoma. Science 1985; 229:974–976.

23. Slamon DJ, Clark GM, Wong SG, Levin WJ, Ullrich A, McGuire WL. Human breast cancer: correlation of relapse and survival with amplification of the HER-2/neu oncogene. Science 1987; 235:177–182.

24. Slamon DJ, Godolphin W, Jones LA, et al. Studies of the HER-2/neu proto-oncogene in human breast and ovarian cancer. Science 1989; 244:707–712.

25. Albertson DG, Pinkel D. Genomic microarrays in human genetic disease and cancer. Hum Mol Genet 2003; 12 (Spec No 2):R145–R152.

26. Lisitsyn N, Wigler M. Cloning the differences between two complex genomes. Science 1993; 259:946–951.

27. Mu D, Chen L, Zhang X, et al. Genomic amplification and oncogenic properties of the KCNK9 potassium channel gene. Cancer Cell 2003; 3:297–302.

28. Schwab M, Alitalo K, Varmus HE, Bishop JM, George D. A cellular oncogene (c-Ki-ras) is amplified, overexpressed, and located within karyotypic abnormalities in mouse adrenocortical tumour cells. Nature 1983; 303:497–501.

29. Saha S, Bardelli A, Buckhaults P, et al. A phosphatase associated with metastasis of colorectal cancer. Science 2001; 294:1343–1346.

30. Velculescu VE, Zhang L, Vogelstein B, Kinzler KW. Serial analysis of gene expression. Science 1995; 270:484–487.

31. Hermeking H. Serial analysis of gene expression and cancer. Curr Opin Oncol 2003; 15:44–49.

32. Hermeking H, Lengauer C, Polyak K, et al. 14-3-3 Sigma is a p53-regulated inhibitor of G2/M progression. Mol Cell 1997; 1:3–11.

33. He TC, Sparks AB, Rago C, et al. Identification of c-MYC as a target of the APC pathway. Science 1998; 281:1509–1512.

34. Polyak K, Xia Y, Zweier JL, Kinzler KW, Vogelstein B. A model for p53-induced apoptosis. Nature 1997; 389:300–305.

35. Yu J, Zhang L, Hwang PM, Rago C, Kinzler KW, Vogelstein B. Identification and classification of p53-regulated genes. Proc Natl Acad Sci USA 1999; 96:11,517–11,522.

36. Menssen A, Hermeking H. Characterization of the c-MYC-regulated transcriptome by SAGE: identification and analysis of c-MYC target genes. Proc Natl Acad Sci USA 2002; 99:6274–6279.

37. Saha S, Sparks AB, Rago C, et al. Using the transcriptome to annotate the genome. Nature Biotechnol 2002; 20:508–512.

38. Kannbley U, Kapinya K, Dirnagl U, Trendelenburg G. Improved protocol for SAGE tag-to-gene allocation. Biotechniques 2003; 34:1212–1214.

39. Wang TL, Maierhofer C, Speicher MR, et al. Digital karyotyping. Proc Natl Acad Sci USA 2002; 99: 16,156–16,161.

40. Wang TL, Diaz LA Jr, Romans K, et al. Digital karyotyping identifies thymidylate synthase amplification as a mechanism of resistance to 5-fluorouracil in metastatic colorectal cancer patients. Proc Natl Acad Sci USA 2004; 101:3089–3094.

41. Dykxhoorn DM, Novina CD, Sharp PA. Killing the messenger: short RNAs that silence gene expression. Nature Rev Mol Cell Biol 2003; 4:457–467.

42. Kohli M, Rago C, Lengauer C, Kinzler KW, Vogelstein B. Facile methods for generating human somatic cell gene knockouts using recombinant adeno-associated viruses. Nucleic Acids Res 2004; 32:e3.

# 3

# Identification of Novel Cancer Target Antigens Utilizing EST and Genome Sequence Databases

*Tapan K. Bera, PhD, Kristi A. Egland, PhD, B. K. Lee, PhD, and Ira Pastan, MD*

### CONTENTS

INTRODUCTION
STRATEGIES
DISCUSSION
ACKNOWLEDGMENTS
REFERENCES

### SUMMARY

Completion of the human genome sequence has opened up an enormous opportunity to researchers all over the world. The Human Genome Project, which includes the expressed sequence tags (ESTs) database and the genome sequence database, provides a huge source of data that can be used to study and identify molecular targets for a wide range of diseases, including cancer. Major efforts must now be devoted to develop strategies by which these databases will be mined efficiently to identify the hidden therapeutic treasures. We have utilized the EST and genome databases, different bioinformatics tools, and several experimental methods to identify tissue-specific genes for prostate and breast cancer. The genes identified can be used as novel targets for the diagnosis and treatment of prostate and breast cancer.

**Key Words:** TARP; NGEP; PAGE4; GDEP; PRAC; POTE; XAGE1; BASE; MAPcL.

## 1. INTRODUCTION

The identification of novel markers and therapeutic target antigens for specific cancers is critical for the diagnosis and the targeted therapy of cancer. Ideal targets for the immuno-based therapy of cancers are proteins that are expressed on the cancer at high levels but are not expressed in any essential normal tissues like the heart, brain, liver,

From: *Cancer Drug Discovery and Development: The Oncogenomics Handbook*
Edited by: W. J. LaRochelle and R. A. Shimkets © Humana Press Inc., Totowa, NJ

kidney, and so forth. Also, the target proteins must be located on the cell surface, where they are accessible to antibodies or antibody-based therapeutics. Our laboratory is interested in developing new immuno-based therapies for the treatment of cancer and, particularly, prostate and breast cancer.

Prostate cancer is a major public health problem and the second leading cause of death for men in the United States. It has been estimated that about one in five men in the United States will develop prostate cancer during their lifetime (1). Despite its distinction as the most frequently diagnosed noncutaneous cancer, little is known about the causes of this disease largely because of the cellular heterogeneity of the prostate and the lack of systematic analysis of the genes expressed in this tissue. To date, there are no curative therapies available for this disease after it has metastasized from its site of origin. Therefore, it is of great importance to identify specific molecular targets for prostate cancer, which can be used as early detection markers or for the targeted therapy of prostate cancer.

Breast cancer is the most common type of epithelial cancer among women in the United States. More than 180,000 women are diagnosed with breast cancer each year. About one in eight women in the United States (approx 12.8%) will develop breast cancer during her lifetime (http://cis.nci.nih.gov/fact/5-6.htm). At present, there are no curative therapies available for breast cancer that has metastasized from its site of origin, and there is urgent need for developing new targets for breast cancer therapy.

## 2. STRATEGIES

Several experimental methods have been used to identify genes that are selectively expressed in a particular cancer. These include differential display (2), subtractive hybridization (3), serial analysis of gene expression (4), and microarray analysis (5). The publication of the human genome sequence has provided a new era for cancer research (6). Using bioinformatics as a tool to mine the expressed sequence tags (ESTs) and human genome sequence databases, one can identify new genes that can serve either as targets for cancer therapy or improve our understanding of the essential biological pathways that control cell growth, differentiation, or transformation of normal cells into cancer cells. Our laboratory is particularly interested in discovering genes that can be used as targets for the therapy or diagnosis of prostate and breast cancer. We have employed three strategies to identify genes that are specifically expressed in prostate and breast cancers but not in any essential normal tissues like the brain, heart, liver, kidney, and so forth. The approaches are described and a short description of the genes identified by these strategies is summarized in Table 1.

### 2.1. Gene Identification by EST Database Mining

The Cancer Genome Anatomy Project (CGAP) of the NCI along with other consortiums support sequencing of ESTs from many cancers and their corresponding normal tissues (www.cgap.nci.nih.gov). We use this information to search for new genes and the proteins they encode (7). We search the human EST database (which now contains the sequences of over 5 million ESTs) for DNA sequences that have the following properties: (1) expressed in prostate cancers or breast cancers, (2) not associated with known genes, and (3) not expressed in any essential organ or tissue. These sequences are arranged into clusters based on sequence identity (Fig. 1A; see Color Plate 1 following p. 78) and a consensus sequence is produced. A typical EST cluster is shown in Fig. 1B.

Table 1

New Genes Discovered in Prostate and Breast Cancer

| Gene Location | mRNA (kb) | Protein (kDa) | Normal Tissue Expression | | | | Cancer Expression | | | Cell Lines | Localization |
|---|---|---|---|---|---|---|---|---|---|---|---|
| | | | PR | TE | PL | Other | PR | BR | Other | | |
| NGEP/S 2q37.3 | 0.9 | 18 | + | – | – | - | + | N.D. | N.D. | LNCaP | Cytosol |
| NGEP/L | 3.5 | 95 | + | – | – | Retina | + | N.D. | N.D. | LNCaP | Membrane |
| POTE 21q11.2 | 2.0 | 66 | + | + | + | Ovary | + | N.D. | N.D. | LNCaP | Plasma membrane |
| TARP 7p14.1 | 1.1 | 7 | + | – | – | Breast | + | + | N.D. | LNCaP, ZR-75-1, MCF7 | Mitochondria |
| GDEP/S 4q21.1 | 0.52 | 4.0 | + | – | – | - | + | – | – | No | N.D. |
| GDEP/L | 0.6 | 7.1 | + | – | – | - | + | – | – | No | Nuclear |
| PATE 11q24 | 1.5 | 14 | + | + | – | Adrenal | + | – | N.D. | No | Secreted |
| PRAC 17q21 | 0.38 | 6.0 | + | – | – | Rectum | + | – | Rectum, colon | LNCaP, PC3 | Nuclear |
| PRAC2 17q21 | 0.56 | 10.5 | + | – | – | Rectum, colon | + | – | Rectum, colon | LNCaP, PC3 | Nuclear |
| TEPP 16q13 | 1.0 | 30.7 | + | + | + | Rectum, colon | – | – | – | – | N.D. |
| PAGE 4 Xp11 | 0.5 | 16 | + | + | + | Uterus | + | – | Uterine | No | Cytosol |
| XAGE-1 Xp11.23 | 0.45–0.80 | 9 | – | + | – | Lung, breast | + | + | Lung Ewing's | LNCaP, Ewing's lung | N.D. |
| MRP8 16q12.1 | 4.5 | 150 | + | + | – | Breast, liver | + | + | N.D. | N.D. | Plasma membrane |
| MRP9V1 16q12.1 | 4.5 | 100 | – | + | – | Breast | N.D. | + | N.D. | CRL 1500 | Plasma membrane |
| MRP9V2 16q12.1 | 1.3 | 20 | + | + | – | Brain, ovary, SK muscle | N.D. | N.D. | N.D. | N.D. | N.D. |
| BASE 20q11.21 | 2.3 | 19.5 | – | – | – | Salivary gland | – | + | N.D. | SK-BR-3, ZR-75-1 | N.D. |

Abbreviations: PR, prostate; TE, testis; PL, placenta; BR, breast; N.D., not determined.

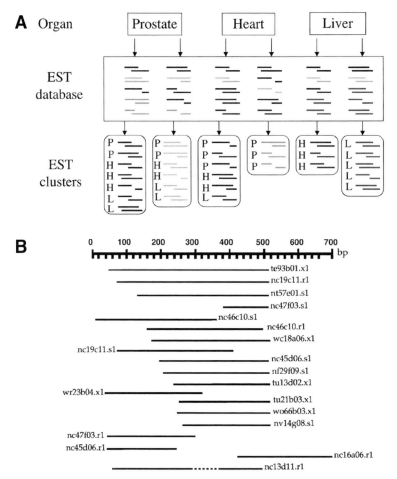

**Fig. 1.** Schematics showing ESTs and EST clusters. (**A**) Schematic description of ESTs from different tissue libraries and their corresponding clusters. Similar color lines represent ESTs from the same transcript, letters (P, prostate; H, heart; L, liver) represent the tissue from which the EST was generated. (**B**) Schematics of the EST cluster for *GDEP*. Each line represents one EST. The cluster consists of 19 ESTs, and the composite cluster is about 510 nucleotides in length. (*See* Color Plate 1 following p. 78.)

We use this consensus sequence to carry out the following experiments: (1) Design primers to determine if the RNA is expressed in essential normal tissues by reverse transcriptase–polymerase chain reaction (RT-PCR) using a panel of normal tissue samples (Fig. 2A) and by hybridization using a $^{32}$P-labeled cDNA probe on multitissue mRNA dot blots (Fig. 2B). (2) If no expression in essential tissues is found, we examine mRNAs from a set of prostate cancers by RT-PCR to determine if the gene is expressed in these cancers. If expression is frequently observed, we perform *in situ* hybridization of prostate cancer samples to be certain that expression is in the cancer cells and not in the extracellular matrix or other cell types in the specimen (Fig. 3; *see* Color Plate 2 following p. 78). For many of the genes, we also perform *in situ* analyses on multitissue arrays and, thus, verify that expression is present in many cancer samples. We also examine mRNA expression

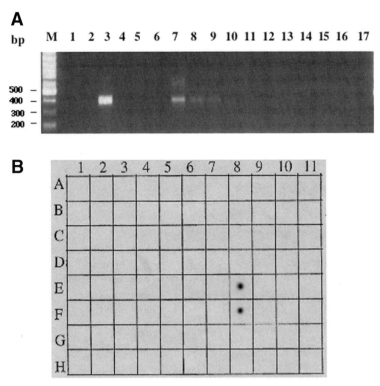

**Fig. 2.** Specificity of *POTE* expression in different tissues. (**A**) PCR analysis on cDNAs from 16 different human tissues. The expected size of the PCR product is 400-bp. A specific 400 bp PCR product is detected in the testis (lane 3), prostate (lane 7), and a very weak band is detected in the placenta (lane 8) and ovary (lane 9). A PCR product is not detected in the following: negative control (lane 1), thymus (lane 2), spleen (lane 4), skeletal muscle (lane 5), peripheral blood leukocyte (lane 6), pancreas (lane 10), lung (lane 11), liver (lane 12), kidney (lane 13), small intestine (lane 14), heart (lane 15), colon (lane 16), and brain (lane 17). (**B**) RNA hybridization of a multiple tissue dot blot containing mRNA from 76 normal human cell types or tissues using a cDNA probe. Strong expression is observed in the prostate (E8) and testis (F8). There is no detectable expression in the brain (A1), heart (A4), kidney (A7), liver (A9), lung (A8), and colon (A6).

in three prostate cancer cell lines, LNCaP (well differentiated, androgen dependent) and DU145 and PC3 (poorly differentiated). (3) If the gene is deemed interesting and worthy of further study, we then isolate a full-length cDNA after determining the transcript size by performing a Northern analysis. Finally, we determine the nucleotide sequence of the transcript and that of the predicted protein it encodes. The following genes have been isolated using this approach, a few of which encode membrane proteins and are potential candidates for antibody-based therapies. However, all of the prostate and breast specific candidates can be used for vaccine therapy.

### 2.1.1. *NGEP* (New Gene Expressed in Prostate)

*NGEP* was discovered as a cluster of five ESTs (three from a normal prostate and two from a prostate cancer library). The Northern blot analysis showed a small RNA (0.9 kb)

**1**                          **2**

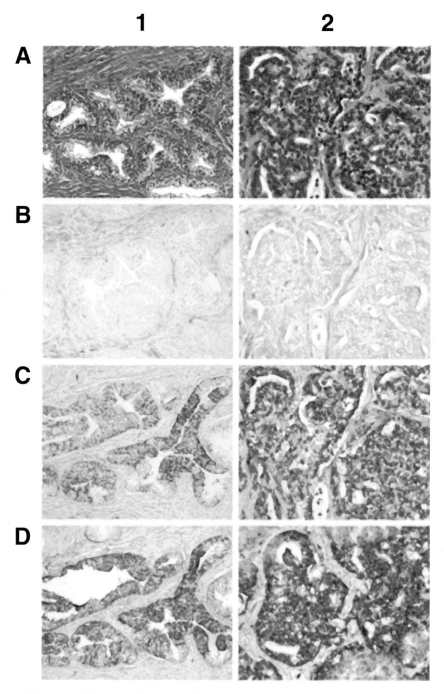

**Fig. 3.** Localization of *NGEP* mRNA in epithelial cells of prostate tissues. (**A**) Normal prostate (panel 1) and prostate cancer (panels 2) sections stained with hematoxylin and eosin (H&E) to show the morphology of the examined tissues. (**B**) Lymphocyte (B-lymphocyte)-specific gene, CD22, was used as a probe for a negative control for *in situ* hybridization. Note the absence of signal in the epithelial cells. (**C**) U6, a small nuclear RNA, was used as a probe for a positive control for *in situ* hybridization. The epithelial cells show a strong signal. (**D**) *NGEP* is used as a probe for determining which cell types express *NGEP* in the prostate tissue section. NGEP shows signals in the epithelial cells of normal prostate tissue (panel 1) as well as one representative adenocarcinoma (panel 2). (*See* Color Plate 2 following p. 78.)

and two larger RNAs around 3.5 kb in size, suggesting spliced forms. The short variant (NGEP-S) is derived from four exons and encodes a 20-kDa intracellular protein with possible phosphorylation sites. The long form (NGEP-L) is derived from 18 exons and encodes a 95-kDa protein that is predicted to contain 7 membrane-spanning regions. *In situ* hybridization analysis shows that *NGEP* mRNA is localized in epithelial cells of normal prostate and prostate cancers. Immunocytochemical analysis of cells transfected with a construct encoding a short NGEP with a Myc epitope tag at the C-terminus showed that the protein encoded by the short transcript is localized in the cytoplasm. A similar experiment using a cDNA corresponding to the long transcript showed the protein was localized on the plasma membrane. Because of its selective expression in prostate cancer and its presence on the cell surface, NGEP-L is a promising target for the immunotherapy of prostate cancer *(8)*.

### 2.1.2. *POTE* (Prostate, Ovary, Testis, and Placenta)

*POTE* was identified by EST database mining. It is only expressed in the prostate, testis, ovary, and placenta. One extremely unusual feature of *POTE* is that 10 paralogs have been identified in humans and are located on 8 different chromosomes with preservation of open reading frames and splice junctions *(9)*. The paralogs are 88–98% identical at the DNA level. Another unusual feature is that *POTE* paralogs are found in primates but have not yet been found in mice, suggesting that *POTE* might be a primate-specific gene family. At least five different paralogs are expressed in prostate and in testis. *In situ* hybridization analysis shows that the *POTE* is expressed in the prostate cancers and in the LNCaP prostate cancer cell line. The POTE protein contains seven ankyrin repeats between amino acids 140 and 380. The presence of ankyrin repeats indicates POTE interacts with other proteins probably to convey signals from the cell surface to the interior. Its selective expression in reproductive cells and gametes and maintenance of multiple functional genes suggest an important role in reproduction and, perhaps, speciation. Expression of *POTE* in prostate cancer and its undetectable expression in normal essential tissues make *POTE* a candidate for the immunotherapy of prostate cancer.

### 2.1.3. *TARP* (T-Cell Receptor-γ Alternate Reading Frame Protein)

*TARP* is expressed in normal prostate, prostate cancer, and breast cancers. It was also identified by EST database mining. It is a very unusual gene because it is located within the T-cell receptor-γ (TCRγ) gene. The *TARP* promoter, which contains androgen response elements, is located in an intron just upstream of the Jγ1.2 exon of the TCRγ gene (Fig. 4). The transcript found in prostate is spliced just like TCRγ transcripts and contains the Jγ1.2 exon and the three Cγ1 exons *(10)*. However, the reading frame used to make the TARP protein is different from that used for the TCRγ protein and encodes a small 7-kDa protein with a leucine zipper motif and a basic domain. The TARP protein also has homology to a yeast transcription factor, TUP1 *(11)*. *TARP* RNA is detected in almost all primary prostate cancers and at the same frequency as PSA (prostate-specific antigen) (unpublished data). Because of its wide expression in prostate and breast cancers, TARP is now being developed as a vaccine target for prostate and breast cancers *(12)*.

### 2.1.4. *GDEP* (Gene Differentially Expressed in Prostate)

*GDEP* was originally identified as a prostate-specific cluster containing 19 EST (Fig. 1B). There are currently 35 EST entries from normal prostate and prostate cancer libraries

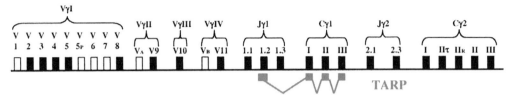

**Fig. 4.** Schematics showing the TARP transcript expressed from TCRγ locus. The transcript consists of four exons—one from Jγ1.2 and three exons from Cγ1.

for *GDEP*. *GDEP* mRNA is highly expressed in almost all human normal prostate samples examined, but not by any prostate cancer cell lines including LNCaP. The first GDEP transcript we characterized was 520 bp long *(13)*; recently, a longer alternatively spliced form was found, and we named it GDEP/L. The short form encodes a 4-kDa protein and the long form encodes a 7-kDa protein (unpublished data).

### 2.1.5. *PATE* (Prostate and Testis)

*PATE* was found as an EST cluster derived from prostate and testis libraries, and experimental analysis also showed expression in prostate cancers *(14)*. The protein is 14 kDa in size and has a signal sequence at the amino terminus. Examination of the human and mouse genome databases indicates that the human and mouse PATE-deduced amino acid sequences are very similar. Studies in which a construct encoding myc-tagged PATE was transfected into PC3 cells showed that PATE is found in the endoplasmic reticulum and in the cell culture medium, suggesting that PATE is a secreted protein. PATE has two interesting structural features. It has a phospholipase A2 motif and it has a series of conserved cysteine residues placing it in the three-finger toxin family. This family includes extracellular domains of some receptors as well as snake venom *(15,16)*.

### 2.1.6. *PRAC* and *PRAC-2* (Prostate, Rectum, and Colon)

Using a computer-based analysis, a cluster of homologous ESTs was identified that contained ESTs derived only from human prostate cDNA libraries. The tissue-specificity analysis by multiple tissue mRNA dot blots and RT-PCR indicates that *PRAC* is expressed in prostate but also in rectum and colon. The *PRAC* transcript is 382 bp and encodes a 6-kDa nuclear protein. The *PRAC* gene is located on chromosome 17 at position 17q21, about 4 kb downstream from the homeodomain *Hoxb-13* gene *(17)*. Homeodomain protein Hoxb-13 is a sequence-specific transcription factor and is involved in the developmental regulatory system that provides cells with specific positional identities on the anterior–posterior axis *(18)*. Recently, it has been reported that Hoxb-13 is required for normal differentiation and secretory function of the ventral prostate *(19)*.

Using the *PRAC* gene and the EST database as a guide, we identified the *PRAC2* gene, which is located between the *Hoxb-13* and *PRAC* genes on chromosome 17 at position 17q21 *(20)*. *PRAC2* is expressed in the prostate, rectum, distal colon, and testis. Weak expression was also found in the placenta, peripheral blood leukocytes, skin, and in two prostate cancer cell lines (LNCaP and PC-3). This transcript encodes a 10.5-kDa nuclear protein. Because the *PRAC* genes are located close to *Hoxb-13*, we believe they might have important roles in the embryonic development of prostate and surrounding tissues.

### 2.1.7. *TEPP* (Testis, Prostate, and Placenta)

The *TEPP* gene is specifically expressed in the testis, prostate, and placenta. The gene has one major transcript of 1.0 kb in size and encodes a 271-amino-acid protein with a molecular weight of 30.7 kDa. The amino-acid-sequence analysis of TEPP indicates that it has a signal peptide with a predicted cleavage site between amino acids 19 and 20, suggesting it might be a secreted protein. Analysis of the predicted TEPP orthologs from different species shows that these proteins are highly conserved in chordates. In addition, we have identified a splice variant of TEPP, which encodes a 37-kDa protein *(21)*. Selective expression of TEPP in the testis, prostate, and placenta with its high conservation among different species indicates that TEPP might have a role in reproductive biology.

### 2.1.8. *PAGE4*

PAGE4 is an X chromosome-linked cancer–testis antigen and was identified by EST database mining. It is expressed in the normal prostate, testis, uterus, placenta, and prostate cancer *(22)*. *PAGE4* is homologous to a family of genes encoding GAGE-like proteins. *PAGE4* encodes a 16-kDa protein that is localized in the cytoplasm of the cells *(23)*. The expression of *PAGE4* in prostate cancer and no expression in normal essential organs makes it a possible vaccine-based therapeutic target for prostate cancer.

### 2.1.9. *XAGE1*

*XAGE1* and several related genes were discovered by a technique termed homology walking in which EST sequences related to *PAGE4* were examined *(24)*. The initial EST database analysis showed that *XAGE1* was expressed in Ewing's sarcoma and this was confirmed by examining cell lines and cancer samples from patients with this disease and with osteosarcoma *(25)*. Subsequent experimental analysis showed *XAGE1* was expressed in many prostate, lung, breast, and other cancers *(26)*. Despite the high levels of *XAGE1* RNA detected in cell lines, the XAGE1 protein has not yet been detected in these cells using polyclonal antibodies prepared in rabbits against XAGE1.

## 2.2. Identification of Genes Encoding Membrane Proteins by Utilizing Both the EST Database and the Human Genome Sequence

In this approach, we identify EST clusters that are breast-specific or prostate cancer-specific, as described in the previous approach, and then align the assembled cluster sequence into the human genome using the "Golden Path" human genome browser (http://genome.ucsc.edu). We then analyze a region about 180 kb in size around the locus of the identified genomic sequences for genes predicted to encode membrane proteins using different gene-prediction programs. After the identification of the candidate genes, we experimentally validate the finding as described earlier and then isolate a full-length cDNA and obtain its sequence and that of the predicted protein. Two new members of the ABC transporter superfamily have been identified using this approach, one of which is a potential target for immuno-based therapy of breast cancer.

### 2.2.1. *MRP8* and *MRP9*

Expressed sequence tag database analysis followed by genome analysis using a gene-prediction program as described earlier identified a specific breast cancer gene designated *MRP8* (ABCC11). However, experimental data showed that *MRP8* was weakly expressed in the liver and brain *(27)*. Because some genes of the multidrug transporter family are adjacent to each other, probably as a result of evolution by gene duplication, we examined the human genome database for genes near *MRP8* and found a related gene, which we termed *MRP9* (ABCC12). *MRP9* has two transcripts associated with it. The long transcript (4.5 kb) encodes a 100-kDa protein with six transmembrane domains. The mRNA is detected only in breast cancer and normal testis *(28)*. The short transcript from *MRP9* (1.3 kb) is present in the brain and encodes a 25-kDa protein. The long *MRP9* transcript was detected in 9 of 12 breast cancer samples examined and is expressed in the ZR-75-1 breast cancer cell line, in which a 100-kDa protein is detected.

## *2.3. Identification of Genes Encoding Membrane Proteins by Generating a Membrane-Associated Polyribosomal cDNA Library*

Unlike for prostate cancer, the EST mining approach did not identify many breast cancer candidate genes. Taking advantage of the fact that there are many breast cancer cell lines that accurately reflect the properties of the parental cancer (which is not the case with prostate cancer), we decided to use breast cancer cell lines to search for new membrane-associated proteins. Our strategy was to isolate membrane-associated polysomal RNA from several phenotypically diverse breast cancer cell lines with different properties such as ER positive, ER negative, erbB2 positive, and erbB2 negative. This RNA, which is enriched in transcripts encoding membrane and secreted proteins, was then used to generate a large high-quality cDNA library with an average insert size of 2 kb. We call this library MAPcL (Membrane Associated Polyribosomal cDNA Library). Sequencing of 900 clones confirmed that the library was greatly enriched for the desired mRNAs. The cDNA library was then subtracted with RNA from five essential normal tissues (brain, liver, kidney, lung, and skeletal muscle) to remove RNAs that are widely expressed. We obtained a large "subtracted" cDNA library with $1.3 \times 10^7$ colony-forming units and an average insert size of 1.8 kb. To determine the nature of the genes represented in this library, a single 5' sequencing reaction was performed on over 25,000 clones, and these sequences were compared with the human genome sequence and the EST database.

Analysis of the sequencing results confirmed that we had successfully made a library enriched in genes encoding membrane and secreted proteins that are highly expressed in breast cancer *(29)*. Some of the encoded membrane proteins might be targets for immunotherapies and the secreted proteins could be used as diagnostic markers for breast cancer. The genes that appear most commonly among the 25,000 clones that were sequenced encode proteins known to be highly expressed in breast cancer, such as erbB2, MUC1, and keratins 18, 8, and 20 *(29)*. Using this approach, we have identified many new candidate genes, but these candidates need to be verified experimentally as breast cancer-specific. The following is an example of one candidate that we have characterized.

### 2.3.1. *BASE* (Breast Cancer and Salivary Gland Expression)

*BASE* is a gene that appears four times in the subtracted MAPcL; however, no ESTs in the database align with *BASE*. The full-length sequence of *BASE* reveals that the RNA encodes a 19.5-kDa protein with a secretion sequence at the N-terminus. The RNA is detected only in the normal salivary gland and in 13 of 20 breast cancer samples examined. *BASE* was highly expressed in one of the breast cancer cell lines used to make the cDNA library and weakly expressed in two others *(29)*. Breast and salivary gland have a common embryological origin, which could account for this common expression pattern. The function of BASE is unknown. It does not have disulfide bonds or have a structure like a growth factor. It is distantly related to a protein found in horse sweat termed Latherin. If BASE is secreted into the blood of breast cancer patients, it could potentially be used as a diagnostic marker for breast cancer.

The results with *BASE* indicate the subtracted MAPcL contains new and interesting genes, which for some unknown reason, possibly technical, are not yet in the EST database.

## 3. DISCUSSION

Our effort to identify new molecular targets for the treatment of breast and prostate cancer has produced many promising candidates. Our strategy of identifying new genes is not as time-consuming as the conventional approaches. In addition to identifying several therapeutically important targets, we also identified several noncoding prostate- and breast-specific genes, which could have regulatory roles in gene expression. The overall success rate of identifying tissue-specific targets from the computer-generated cluster was about 20%, that is, only about 20% of the candidates identified by EST database screening are "prostate or breast cancer"-specific. We believe that is the result of the incompleteness of the EST database.

## ACKNOWLEDGMENTS

We acknowledge the former and present members of the Gene Discovery Group from the Pastan and Lee sections of the Laboratory of Molecular Biology, NCI for their contributions in different aspects of this project.

## REFERENCES

1. Jemal A, Murray T, Samuels A, Ghafoor A, Ward E, Thun MJ. Cancer statistics, 2003. CA—Cancer J Clin 2003; 53:5–26.
2. Liang P, Pardee AB. Differential display of eukaryotic messenger RNA by means of the polymerase chain reaction. Science 1992; 257:967–971.
3. Hara T, Harada N, Mitsui H, Miura T, Ishizaka T, Miyajima A. Characterization of cell phenotype by a novel cDNA library subtraction system: expression of CD8 alpha in a mast cell-derived interleukin-4-dependent cell line. Blood 1994; 84:189–199.
4. Velculescu VE, Zhang L, Vogelstein B, Kinzler KW. Serial analysis of gene expression. Science 1995; 276:1268–1272.
5. Schena M, Shalon D, Davis RW, Brown PO. Quantitative monitoring of gene expression patterns with a complementary DNA microarray. Science 1995; 270:467–470.
6. International Human Sequencing Consortium. Initial sequencing and analysis of the human genome. Nature 2001; 409:860–920.
7. Vasmatzis G, Essand M, Brinkmann U, Lee B, Pastan I. Discovery of three genes specifically expressed in human prostate by expressed sequence tag database analysis. Proc Natl Acad Sci USA 1998; 95: 300–304.
8. Bera TK, Das S, Maeda H, Beers R, Wolfgang C, Kumar V, et al. NGEP, a gene encoding a membrane protein only detected in prostate cancer and normal prostate. Proc Natl Acad Sci USA 2004; 101:3059–3064.
9. Bera TK, Popescu N, Zimonjic D, Sathyanarayana B, Kumar V, Lee BK, Pastan I. POTE, a highly homologous gene family located on numerous chromosomes and expressed in prostate, ovary, testis, placenta and prostate cancer. Proc Natl Acad Sci USA 2002; 99:16,975–16,980.
10. Essand M, Vasmatzis G, Brinkmann U, Duray P, Lee B, Pastan I. High expression of a specific T-cell receptor γ transcript in epithelial cells of the prostate. Proc Natl Acad Sci USA 1999; 96:9287–9292.
11. Wolfgang CD, Essand M, Vincent JJ, Lee B, Pastan I. TARP: a novel protein expressed in prostate and breast cancer cells derived from an alternate reading frame of the TCRγ locus. Proc Natl Acad Sci USA 2000; 97:9437–9442.

12. Oh S, Terabe M, Pendleton CD, Bhattacharyya A, Bera TK, Epel M, et al. Human CTL to wild type and enhanced epitopes of a novel prostate and breast tumor-associated protein, TARP, lyse human breast cancer cells. Cancer Res 2004; 64:2610–2618.

13. Olsson P, Bera TK, Essand M, Kumar V, Duray P, Vincent J, et al. GDEP, a new gene differentially expressed in normal prostate and prostate cancer. Prostate 2001; 48:231–241.

14. Bera TK, Maitra R, Iavarone C, Salvatore G, Kumar V, Vincent JJ, et al. PATE, a new gene expressed in prostate cancer, normal prostate and testis identified by a functional genomic approach. Proc Natl Acad Sci USA 2002; 99:3058–3063.

15. Greenwald J, Fischer WH, Vale WW, Choe S. Three-finger toxin fold for the extracellular ligand-binding domain of the type II activin receptor serine kinase. Nature Struct Biol 1999; 6:18–22.

16. Kieffer B, Driscoll PC, Campbell ID, Willis AC, Vandermerwe PA, Davis SJ. Three-dimensional solution structure of the extracellular region of the complement regulatory protein CD59, a new cell-surface protein domain related to snake-venom neurotoxins. Biochemistry 1994; 33:4471–4482.

17. Liu XF, Olsson P, Wolfgang CD, Bera TK, Durey P, Lee BK, et al. PRAC: a novel small nuclear protein that is specifically expressed in human prostate and colon. Prostate 2001; 47:125–131.

18. Zeltser L, Desplan C, Heinz N. Hoxb-13: a new Hox gene in a distant region of the HOXB cluster maintains colinearity. Development 1996; 122:2475–2484.

19. Economides KD, Capecchi MR. Hoxb-13 is required for normal differentiation and secretory function of the ventral prostate. Development 2003; 130:2061–2069.

20. Olsson P, Motegi A, Bera TK, Lee BK, Pastan I. PRAC2: a novel small nuclear protein that is expressed in human prostate and prostate cancer. Prostate 2003; 56:123–130.

21. Bera TK, Hahn YS, Lee BK, Pastan I. TEPP a new gene specifically expressed in testis, prostate, and placenta and well conserved in chordates. Biochem Biophys Res Commun 2003; 312:1209–1215.

22. Brinkmann U, Vasmatzis G, Lee B, Yerushalmi N, Essand M, Pastan I. PAGE-1, an X chromosome-linked GAGE-like gene that is expressed in normal and neoplastic prostate, testis, and uterus. Proc Natl Acad Sci USA 1998; 95:10,757–10,762.

23. Iavarone C, Wolfgang C, Kumar V, Duray P, Willingham M, Pastan I, et al. PAGE4 is a cytoplasmic protein that is expressed in normal prostate and prostate cancer. Mol Cancer Ther 2002; 1:329–335.

24. Brinkmann U, Vasmatzis G, Lee B, Pastan I. Novel genes in the PAGE and GAGE family of tumor antigens found by homology walking in the dbEST database. Cancer Res 1999; 59:1445–1448.

25. Liu XF, Helman LJ, Yeung C, Bera TK, Lee BK, Pastan I. XAGE-1, a new gene that is frequently expressed in Ewing's sarcoma. Cancer Res 2000; 60:4752–4755.

26. Egland KA, Kumar V, Duray P, Pastan I. Characterization of overlapping XAGE-1 transcripts encoding a cancer testis antigen expressed in lung, breast, and other types of cancers. Mol Cancer Ther 2002; 1: 441–450.

27. Bera TK, Lee S, Salvatore G, Lee BK, Pastan I. MRP8, a new member of ABC transporter superfamily, identified by EST database mining and gene prediction program, is highly expressed in breast cancer. Mol Med 2001; 7:509–516.

28. Bera TK, Lee S, Iavarone C, Lee BK, Pastan I. MRP9, an unusual truncated member of the ABC transporter superfamily, is highly expressed in breast cancer. Proc Natl Acad Sci USA 2002; 99:6997–7002.

29. Egland KA, Vincent JJ, Strausberg R, Lee BK, Pastan, I. Discovery of the breast cancer gene BASE using a molecular approach to enrich for genes encoding membrane and secreted proteins. Proc Natl Acad Sci USA 2003; 100:1099–1104.

# 4

# Tree-Based Cancer Classification and Diagnosis Using Gene Expression Data

*Heping Zhang, PhD*

## CONTENTS

## SUMMARY

The microarray gene expression profile has led to a promising technology for cell, tumor, and cancer classification. Despite some noted pitfalls, many authors have explored and demonstrated the value of this technology in cancer diagnosis. Better diagnosis beyond the standard pathology is regarded as critical to cancer treatment. In this chapter, we review some applications of microarray gene expression profiles for cancer diagnosis and tumor classification. In particular, we describe the recursive partitioning technique and tree-based methodology and demonstrate its use in cancer diagnosis based on gene expression.

**Key Words:** Recursive partitioning; decision trees; forests; gene expression; microarray.

## 1. INTRODUCTION

DNA microarray technology enables us to measure the expression of tens of thousands of genes simultaneously. As a technological intersection between biology and computer and statistical sciences, this revolutionary technology has the potential to be extremely valuable for the study of the genetic basis of complex diseases (*1*). Ramaswamy and Golub (*2*) reviewed clinical applications of DNA microarray technology by identifying promising avenues of research in this emerging field of study and discussing the likely impact that expression profiling will have on clinical oncology.

From: *Cancer Drug Discovery and Development: The Oncogenomics Handbook*
Edited by: W. J. LaRochelle and R. A. Shimkets © Humana Press Inc., Totowa, NJ

One of the applications of this technology is to develop more precise diagnostic procedures to predict and classify tumor and cancer cells using gene expression profiles. Classical approaches to cancer diagnosis do not discriminate among tumors with similar histopathologic features, even if they might vary in clinical course and/or in response to treatment *(3)*. In contrast, classification and diagnosis based on gene expression profiles can identify tumor types that are indistinguishable through a microscope but are biologically different at the gene expression level *(4)*.

Nutt et al. *(5)* pointed out that in modern clinical neuro-oncology, histopathological diagnosis affects therapeutic decisions and prognostic estimation more than any other variable. Among high-grade gliomas, histologically classic glioblastomas and anaplastic oligodendrogliomas follow markedly different clinical courses. It is challenging, however, to distinguish many malignant gliomas because these nonclassic lesions are difficult to classify by histological features, and diagnostic reproducibility is limited. Using the expression levels of 12,000 genes in a set of 50 gliomas, 28 glioblastomas, and 22 anaplastic oligodendrogliomas, Nutt et al. *(5)* suggested that class-prediction models, based on defined molecular profiles, classify diagnostically challenging malignant gliomas in a manner that better correlates with clinical outcome than does standard pathology. Rifkin et al. *(6)* also demonstrated that accurate gene-expression-based multiclass cancer diagnosis is possible using DNA microarray expression profiles.

Despite the potential pitfalls *(1,7,8)* and analytic challenges *(9)* of using microarray data for this purpose, cancer diagnosis is an important area of genomic applications, because targeting specific therapies to pathogenetically distinct tumor types is important for cancer treatment *(5)* and it maximizes efficacy and minimizes toxicity *(10)*. For example, Bertucci et al. *(11)* demonstrated that the systematic use of cDNA array testing holds great promise to improve the classification of breast cancer in terms of prognosis and chemosensitivity and by providing new potential therapeutic targets.

To explore the enormous potential of gene expression profiling in cancer diagnosis, many authors have investigated and compared a variety of classification methods *(4,10, 12–22)*. Commonly used approaches include discriminant analysis and support vector machine. Linear discriminant analysis is a classic statistical method. The support vector machine is a popular supervised learning method in machine learning literature. It can take advantage of prior knowledge by beginning with a set of genes that have a common function, and what is learned from the known genes will be used to discriminate new genes. For example, Golub et al. *(10)* used discriminant analysis to predict human acute leukemias. Brown et al. *(12)* applied the support vector machine to classify genes and to predict the functional roles of 2,467 uncharacterized genes from yeast *Saccharomyces cerevisiae* using the expression data. However, they did not provide a procedure for selecting the threshold of prediction strength, an essential ingredient for classification. Heuristic rules for selection of the threshold of prediction strength can be used, but with a certain unavoidable level of subjectivity. Ramaswamy et al. *(23)* used the support vector machine to classify 218 tumor samples, spanning 14 common tumor types, and 90 normal tissue samples using oligonucleotide microarrays of 16,063 genes and expressed sequence tags.

The objective of this chapter is to review one of the analytic methods and to demonstrate its applications in classifying various cancers. Specifically, we will describe classification trees and forests that make use of the recursive partitioning technique *(24,25)*. This approach is commonly referred to as supervised learning in the machine learning

Table 1
Illustrative Data Structure for Colon Cancer Classification

| Tissue Sample (i.e., unit) | Class Label (i.e., response) | Genes (i.e., Features or Predictors) | | | |
|---|---|---|---|---|---|
| | | H55933 | R39465 | R39465 | ... |
| 1 | Normal | 2,510.325 | 7,823.5341 | 5,955.835 | ... |
| 2 | Normal | 6,246.4487 | 1,960.6545 | 1,566.315 | ... |
| 3 | Normal | 4,028.71 | 3,156.1591 | 2,870.255 | |
| ⋮ | ⋮ | ⋮ | ⋮ | ⋮ | ⋮ |
| 61 | Cancer | 6,234.6225 | 4,005.3 | 3,093.675 | ... |
| 62 | Cancer | 14,876.407 | 3,201.9045 | 2,327.6263 | ... |

Data are extracted from Alon et al. *(28)*. The second column is the class label, and the entries in the third column through the end are expression levels of genes (by column) for different tissue samples (by row).

literature, because we make use of a training set of observations that contain vectors of gene expressions as well as the labeled (normal or tumor) tissues. These observations are used to develop a classification model, which is, in turn, applied to predict the class label (normal or tumor) in new tissue samples.

Constructions of trees and forests are based on the recursive partitioning technique *(24–27)*. This technique has some major advantages over other commonly used methods such as discriminant analysis, logistic regression, and the support vector machine *(4,24–27)*. It has an embedded variable selection process and is very efficient for dealing with a large number of genes.

## 2. RECURSIVE PARTITIONING

The recursive partitioning technique is the foundation for tree and forest construction. We will use a genomic application to explain the recursive partitioning process. Suppose that we have data from $n$ units of observations. In microarray data, the unit is usually a tissue sample. Each unit contains a vector of feature measurements or covariates (e.g., expression profiles from a particular gene) and a class label (a normal or tumor tissue). Table 1 illustrates the data structure for classifying cancer tissues based on gene expression profiles.

The basic idea of recursive partitioning is to extract homogeneous strata of the tissue samples that are defined by expression profiles, such as a downregulated or upregulated expression levels for a particular gene. The strata are selected according to their homogeneity in the distribution of the response in the learning sample. The recursive partitioning process divides the study sample into smaller and smaller nested strata (every strata is called a node in decision trees), according to whether a particular selected predictor is above a chosen cutoff value. The choices of the selected predictor and its corresponding cutoff value are designed to purify the distribution of the response, namely separating the normal tissues from the cancer tissues in the present context.

Let us use the dataset from Alon et al. *(28)* for illustration. This dataset contains the expression profiles of 2000 genes in 22 normal and 40 colon cancer tissues. As displayed in Table 1, the sample size (or the number of units of observations), $n$ is 62. If we use this entire sample to construct a tree, these 62 samples are called a learning sample. In tree

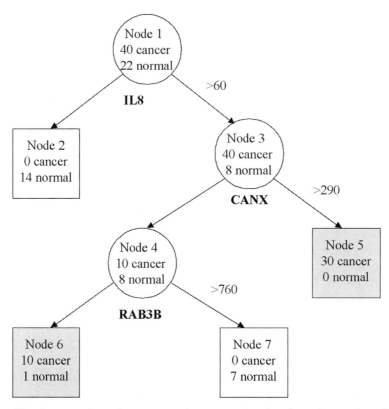

**Fig. 1.** Classification trees for colon cancer using expression data from three selected genes (IL8, CANX, RAB3B). The circles represent internal nodes that are subsequently divided into daughter nodes. The boxes are terminal nodes that do not have further partition and determine the tissue class membership; the shaded ones contain a total of 40 cancer tissues and 1 normal issue and the blank ones contain 21 normal tissues. Beneath each internal node is the gene whose expression level is used to split the node, and the cutoff is displayed on the arrow next to the right. Adapted from ref. *4*.

terminology, these 62 samples form the root node. It is also labeled as node 1 in Fig. 1. How homogenous (or pure) is this root node? In other words, how impure is it? A common measure of node impurity is the entropy function, which is defined as $i_t = -p_t \log(p_t) - (1 - p_t) \log(1 - p_t)$, where $p_t$ is the proportion of cancer tissue in node $t$. At the moment, node $t$ is the root node and $p_t = 40/62$, thus $i_t = 0.65$ for the root node. To have a sense as to how impure the root node is, we should note that $i_t$ reaches its minimum of 0 when $p_t = 0$ or 1 and its maximum of about 0.69 when $p_t = 0.5$. In other words, if all tissues are of the same type within a node, the impurity is at its lowest level. If we have a balanced mix of normal and cancer tissues in a node, the impurity is at its worst level. We can see that the root node is far from being pure, and not too far from the worst scenario. This is not surprising because we have not even begun the recursive partitioning process, and our hope is that this process will improve the situation.

The first step of the recursive partitioning process is to divide the root of 62 samples in Fig. 1 into two nodes, namely nodes 2 and 3. There are many ways of partitioning, and our goal is to reduce both $i_2$ in node 2 and $i_3$ in node 3 simultaneously. Mathematically, we want to minimize the weighted impurity $r_2 i_2 + r_3 i_3$, where $r_2$ and $r_3$ are the proportions of tissue samples in nodes 2 and 3, respectively. For example, for a gene labeled as H55933 in Table 1, we can divide the 62 tissues into two nodes according to whether or not the expression level of H55933 is greater than a certain level $c$. By moving $c$ in the range of the 62 observed levels of H55933, we can find a value of $c$ that gives rise to the lowest $r_2 i_2 + r_3 i_3$. Then, we can perform a similar search for the second, the third, and, eventually, the last gene in Table 1. It turns out that the interleukin 8 (IL8) gene and its threshold of 60 (the best $c$) yield the smallest $r_2 i_2 + r_3 i_3$ among the 2000 genes and their associated thresholds. This is why node 1 is divided into nodes 3 and 2 according to whether or not the expression level of gene IL8 is greater than 60 in Fig. 1. This split assigns 48 tissues (40 cancer and 8 normal tissues) into node 3, whose IL8 levels are beyond 60, and the remaining 14 tissues (all normal tissues) into node 2, whose IL8 levels are below 60. We can easily obtain that and $i_2 = 0$ and $i_3 = 0.45$, and hence $r_2 i_2 + r_3 i_3 = 0.35$. Thus, this one step reduces the impurity from $i_1 = 0.65$ (of the root node) to $r_2 i_2 + r_3 i_3 = 0.35$ (of the two daughter nodes).

Although the improvement is evident in terms of the impurity, further improvement is possible. Because node 2 is already pure, no further partitioning is warranted. However, node 3 is not pure and can be divided further. We can repeat the same partitioning process for node 3 as for the root node, and this recursive algorithm finds the *CANX* gene and its threshold 290 to be the best choice to split node 3 into nodes 4 and 5 as displayed in Fig. 1. Analogously, node 4 is further partitioned into nodes 6 and 7. This concludes our recursive partitioning process for this sample because further partitioning is not necessary.

Through 3 splits involving 3 genes, we partitioned the 62 samples into 4 (terminal) nodes, namely nodes 2, 5, 6, and 7 in Fig. 1. Two of them (nodes 2 and 7) contain purely 21 normal tissues. The other two nodes (nodes 5 and 6) contain 40 cancer tissues and one normal tissue. If we predict the tissue type according to its membership in the terminal node, we misclassify 1 normal tissue out of the total 62 tissues (error rate = 1.6%). This is far more precise than the classification rules using linear discriminant analysis or the support vector machine. The combined impurity of the four terminal nodes is 0.05, as opposed to 0.65 before we began the recursive partitioning process.

## 3. TREE INTERPRETATION

First, we note that nodes 5 and 6 are either purely or predominately cancer. However, these two nodes have different profiles, particularly in terms of CANX. In the existing literature, the expression of the molecular chaperone CANX was found to be decreased in HT-29 human colon adenocarcinoma cells *(29)* and to be involved in apoptosis in human prostate epithelial tumor cells *(30)*. Although a tree-based analysis *per se* cannot determine whether the selected genes are in the pathways to cancer, Fig. 1 suggests different genetic mechanisms of colon cancer if the role of the three selected genes is confirmed. There exists preliminary evidence in the literature that associates the three selected genes with colon cancer *(4)*, but further investigation is warranted.

Second, caution is warranted in reporting the precision of a decision tree. So far, the construction and quality of the tree in Fig. 1 are based on the same 62 samples. Because this tree was constructed to minimize the number of misclassifications, its quality, if without adjustments, tends to look better than the reality. A commonly used statistical approach is cross-validation when no other independent sample exists to validate the tree quality. The idea is to divide the 62 tissues into a learning sample and a test sample. The learning sample is used to construct a tree and the test sample is used to validate the tree. Because we have a limited number of samples to begin with, Zhang et al. *(4)* proposed a localized procedure to balance the needs of validating the results and retaining as many as observations as possible in the learning step. Specifically, one normal and one cancer tissue are saved for the test sample. In tree construction, the basic tree structure is fixed as in Fig. 1, except that the threshold levels for the three genes can be rechosen according to the newly defined learning sample. Through this localized cross-validation, Zhang et al. *(4)* reassured the high predictive quality of the tree and reported an adjusted error rate of between 6% and 8%. This is still much lower than that obtained by other analyses.

We have cautioned earlier that the three genes identified in Fig. 1 are not necessarily involved in the etiology of colon cancer. Even if they were, they would not necessarily be the only ones. This is because many genes manifest highly correlated expression profiles. In fact, there are many triplets of genes that produce trees of equivalent quality to Fig. 1, suggesting that there could be multiple pathways to colon cancer. To identify the other competitive trees, Zhang et al. *(22)* proposed constructing a deterministic forest by collecting all trees of a certain structure and of similar quality. We will elaborate on this idea next.

## 4. CONSTRUCTION OF FORESTS

In the machine learning literature, the chief motivation for constructing forests is to improve the predictive precision of classification rules. This is also an important consideration in genomic analysis. As discussed earlier, another important aspect of constructing forests is to explore and understand multiple, potential pathways to the outcome of interest, such as cancer. We have this luxury because we have a large number of gene expressions and many of them are highly correlated *(22)*.

The most common approach to constructing forests is to perturb the data randomly, form a tree from the perturbed data, repeat this process to form a series of trees—which is called a random forest—and then aggregate information from the forest. One of such schemes, called bagging (bootstrapping and aggregating), is to generate a bootstrap sample from the original sample. The final classification is then based on the majority vote of all trees in the forest *(31)*.

After observing the uncertainty in the random forest and the fact that there are typically many trees that are of equally high predictive quality in analyzing genomic data, Zhang et al. *(22)* proposed a method to construct forests in a deterministic manner. Empirically, the deterministic forests appear to perform similarly to the random forests in terms of prediction error based on several public microarray datasets. The idea is straightforward. For example, in many microarray datasets, a tree with three to four splits provides a high-quality classification. We can search and collect all distinct trees that have a nearly perfect classification. In some applications where there are not many trees with a perfect classification, we can set a threshold for the classification quality and then cumulate all trees with quality at or above the prespecified level. This process is not only reproducible but also displays an extensive array of potential, alternative pathways that might underlie the disease of interest.

From a methodological point of view, forests also provide a way to select important variables. Many data mining techniques including support vector machine do not have a built-in feature selection. As we discussed earlier, tree-based methods select variables while forming a classification rule. A limitation for a single tree is that it contains a very limited amount of information for genomic data. In contrast, forests reveal much more information. After a forest is constructed, we can examine the frequency of genes as they appear in the forest. Frequent and prominent genes can then be used and analyzed by any method; they are not restricted to tree constructions. In other words, forest construction offers a mechanism to select important variables even though some of them are highly correlated. To illustrate this, Zhang et al. *(22)* analyzed two datasets.

The first dataset is on leukemia *(10)*. It includes 25 mRNA samples with acute myeloid leukemia (AML), 38 samples with B-cell acute lymphoblastic leukemia (B-ALL), and 9 samples with T-cell acute lymphoblastic leukemia (T-ALL). Expression profiles were assessed for 7129 genes for each sample. Thirty-five genes appeared frequently in a deterministic forest of about 100 trees.

The second dataset is on lymphoma *(32)*. Data are available on the three most prevalent adult lymphoma malignancies: B-cell chronic lymphocytic leukemia (B-CLL), follicular lymphoma (FL), and diffuse large B-cell lymphoma (DLBCL). There are a total of 84 samples (29 B-CLL, 9 FL, and 46 DLBCL) with expressions from 4026 genes. Forty-nine genes appeared frequently in a deterministic forest of about 100 trees.

CD33 is the most frequent gene in the forest for the leukemia dataset. Zhang et al. *(22)* highlighted some treatment studies *(33,34)* that have shown significant anticancer activity of an agent that targets the CD33 antigen on malignant myeloid cells. CD33 is expressed by ALL cells in >80% of patients but not by normal hematopoietic stem cells, suggesting that elimination of CD33(+) cells could be therapeutically beneficial. More recently, several authors have reported diagnostic and treatment implications of CD33 on leukemia *(35–38)*. For example, Mulford and Jurcic *(37)* reported that the humanized anti-CD33 monoclonal antibody HuM195 can eliminate minimal residual disease detectable by reverse transcription–polymerase chain reaction (RT-PCR) in acute promyelocytic leukemia. Furthermore, targeted chemotherapy with the anti-CD33–calicheamicin construct gemtuzumab ozogamicin has produced remissions as a single agent in patients with relapsed AML and appears promising when used in combination with standard chemotherapy in the treatment of newly diagnosed AML.

For the lymphoma dataset, several human cyclin genes (CCNB1, CCND2, CCNA2) are among the most frequent genes in the forest. It is known that cyclins play an important role in cell cycle regulation *(39)*. Some of the human cyclin genes have been found to be a target gene of mature B-cell malignancies *(40)* and are downregulated when dexamethasone is added to P1798 murine T lymphoma cells *(41)*. An antibody to cyclin B1 is also found to be discriminative of a node for gastric and lung cancers, as well as for hepatocellular carcinoma *(14)*. In summary, there are abundant scientific studies that support the biological relevance of the top genes revealed by the forests.

Another alternative is to cluster similar genes together and construct a summary index using methods such as principal component analysis. It would be interesting to compare this approach with forests.

## 5. FINAL REMARKS

The technology of microarray gene expression profiling is evolving rapidly, and more and more genes can be simultaneously monitored on a single chip. Although the quality such as the reproducibility of the expression level of microarray data remains to be an important issue, numerous applications have demonstrated the great potential of this technology in biomedical studies that include cancer diagnosis. It is hopeful that cancer classification and diagnosis based on gene expression levels will not only be more precise than the classic approaches, but it will also lead to a better understanding of cancer in terms of its heterogeneity and multiple pathways.

Exploring and understanding the data structures in large genomic databases are important and challenging. Many analytic approaches are available, but it remains to be seen which one(s) will be truly effective. Clearly, the tree- and forest-based approaches have some appealing features, as we discussed. It is not yet obvious as to how the results discovered from such analyses can be systematically placed into the relevant biological context. We have explored the use of frequencies as genes appear in forests, but other than through empirical validation, it is not clear as to how much confidence we have in those highly frequent genes. In conclusion, these important analytic issues warrant serious investigation.

## ACKNOWLEDGMENT

This research was supported in part by NIH grants DA012468, DA017713, and DA016750.

## REFERENCES

1. King HC, Sinha AA. Gene expression profile analysis by DNA microarrays—promise and pitfalls. JAMA 2001; 286:2280–2288.
2. Ramaswamy S, Golub TR. DNA microarrays in clinical oncology. J Clin Oncol 2002; 20:1932–1941.
3. Stephenson J. Human genome studies expected to revolutionize cancer classification. JAMA 1999; 282: 927–928.
4. Zhang HP, Yu CY, Singer B, Xiong M. Recursive partitioning for tumor classification with gene expression microarray data. Proc Natl Acad Sci USA 2001; 98:6730–6735.
5. Nutt CL, Mani DR, Betensky RA, Tamayo P, Cairncross JG, Ladd C, et al. Gene expression-based classification of malignant gliomas correlates better with survival than histological classification. Cancer Res 2003; 63:1602–1607.
6. Rifkin R, Mukherjee S, Tamayo P, Ramaswamy S, Yeang CH, Angelo M, et al. An analytical method for multiclass molecular cancer classification. SIAM Rev 2003; 45:706–723.
7. Simon R. Diagnostic and prognostic prediction using gene expression profiles in high-dimensional microarray data. Br J Cancer 2003; 89:1599–1604.
8. Simon R, Radmacher MD, Dobbin K, McShane LM. Pitfalls in the use of DNA microarray data for diagnostic and prognostic classification. J Nat Canc Inst 2003; 95:14–18.
9. Ambroise C, McLachlan GJ. Selection bias in gene extraction on the basis of microarray gene-expression data. Proc Natl Acad Sci USA 2002; 99:6562–6566.
10. Golub TR, Slonim DK, Tamayo P, Huard C, Gaasenbeek M, Mesirov JP, et al. Molecular classification of cancer: class discovery and class prediction by gene expression monitoring. Science 1999; 286: 531–537.
11. Bertucci F, Houlgatte R, Benziane A, Granjeaud S, Adelaide J, Tagett R, et al. Gene expression profiling of primary breast carcinomas using arrays of candidate genes. Hum Mol Genet 2000; 9:2981–2991.
12. Brown MPS, Grundy WN, Lin D, Cristianini N, Sugnet CW, Furey TS, et al. Knowledge-based analysis of microarray gene expression data by using support vector machines. Proc Natl Acad Sci USA 2000; 97:262–267.
13. Ishibashi Y, Hanyu N, Nakada K, Suzuki Y, Yamamoto T, Yanaga K, et al. Profiling gene expression ratios of paired cancerous and normal tissue predicts relapse of esophageal squamous cell carcinoma. Cancer Res 2003; 63:5159–5164.
14. Koziol JA, Zhang JY, Casiano CA, Peng XX, Shi FD, Feng AC, et al. Recursive partitioning as an approach to selection of immune markers for tumor diagnosis. Clin Cancer Res 2003; 9:5120–5126.
15. Lu Y, Han JW. Cancer classification using gene expression data. Inform Syst 2003; 28:243–268.

16. Lyons-Weiler J, Patel S, Bhattacharya S. A classification-based machine learning approach for the analysis of genome-wide expression data. Genome Res 2003; 13:503–512.

17. Moler EJ, Chow ML, Mian IS. Analysis of molecular profile data using generative and discriminative methods. Physiol Genom 2000; 4:109–126.

18. Romualdi C, Campanaro S, Campagna D, Celegato B, Cannata N, Toppo S, et al. Pattern recognition in gene expression profiling using DNA array: a comparative study of different statistical methods applied to cancer classification. Hum Mol Genet 2003; 12:823–836.

19. Tibshirani R, Hastie T, Narasimhan B, Chu G. Diagnosis of multiple cancer types by shrunken centroids of gene expression. Proc Natl Acad Sci USA 2002; 99:6567–6572.

20. Xiong MM, Jin L, Li W, Boerwinkle E. Computational methods for gene expression-based tumor classification. Biotechniques 2000; 29:1264–1270.

21. Zhang HP, Yu CY. Tree-based analysis of microarray data for classifying breast cancer. Front Biosci 2002; 7:c63–c67.

22. Zhang HP, Yu CY, Singer B. Cell and tumor classification using gene expression data: construction of forests. Proc Natl Acad Sci USA 2003; 100:4168–4172.

23. Ramaswamy S, Tamayo P, Rifkin R, Mukherjee S, Yeang CH, Angelo M, et al. Multiclass cancer diagnosis using tumor gene expression signatures. Proc Natl Acad Sci USA 2001; 98:15,149–15,154.

24. Breiman L, Friedman J, Stone C, Olshen R. Classification and regression trees. San Francisco: Wadsworth, 1984.

25. Zhang HP, Bracken MB. Tree-based risk factor analysis of preterm delivery and small-for-gestational-age birth. Am J Epidemiol 1995; 141:70–78.

26. Zhang HP, Holford T, Bracken MB. A tree-based method in prospective studies. Statist Med 1996; 15:37–50.

27. Zhang HP, Singer B. Recursive partitioning in the health sciences. New York: Springer-Verlag, 1999.

28. Alon U, Barkai U, Notterman DA, Gish K, Ybarra S, Mack D, et al. Broad patterns of gene expression revealed by clustering analysis of tumor and normal colon tissues probed by oligonucleotide arrays. Proc Natl Acad Sci USA 1999; 96:6745–6750.

29. Yeates LC, Powis G. The expression of the molecular chaperone calnexin is decreased in cancer cells grown as colonies compared to monolayer. Biochem Biophys Res Commun 1997; 238:66–70.

30. Nagata K, Okano Y, Nozawa Y. Differential expression of low Mr GTP-binding proteins in human megakaryoblastic leukemia cell line, MEG-01, and their possible involvement in the differentiation process. Thromb Haemostas 1997; 77:368–375.

31. Breiman L. Random forests. Mach Learn 2001; 45:5–32.

32. Alizadeh AA, Eisen MB, Davis RE, Ma C, Lossos IS, Rosenwald A, et al. Distinct types of diffuse large B-cell lymphoma identified by gene expression profiling. Nature 2000; 403:503–511.

33. Hamann PR, Hinman LM, Hollander I, Beyer CF, Lindh D, Holcomb R, et al. Gemtuzumab ozogamicin, a potent and selective anti-CD33 antibody–calicheamicin conjugate for treatment of acute myeloid leukaemia. Bioconjug Chem 2002; 13:47–58.

34. Parisi E, Draznin J, Stoopler E, Schuster SJ, Porter D, Sollecito TP. Acute myelogenous leukaemia: advances and limitations of treatment. Oral Surg Oral Med Oral Pathol Oral Radiol Endodont 2002; 93: 257–263.

35. Gokbuget N, Hoelzer D. Treatment with monoclonal antibodies in acute lymphoblastic leukemia: current knowledge and future prospects. Ann Hematol 2003; 83:201–205.

36. Khoury H, Dalal BI, Nevill TJ, Horsman DE, Barnett MJ, Shepherd JD, et al. Acute myelogenous leukaemia with t(8;21)—identification of a specific immunophenotype. Leuk Lymphoma 2003; 44:1713–1718.

37. Mulford DA, Jurcic JG. Antibody-based treatment of acute myeloid leukaemia. Expert Opin Biol Ther 2004; 4:95–105.

38. Xavier L, Cunha M, Goncalves C, Teixeira Mdos A, Coutinho J, Ribeiro AC, et al. Hematological remission and long term hematological control of acute myeloblastic leukaemia induced and maintained by granulocyte–colony stimulating factor (G-CSF) therapy. Leuk Lymphoma 2003; 44:2137–2142.

39. Milatovich A, Francke U. Human cyclin B1 gene (CCNB1) assigned to chromosome 5 (q13-qter). Somat Cell Mol Genet 1992; 18:303–307.

40. Sonoki T, Harder L, Horsman DE, Karran L, Taniguchi I, Willis TG, et al. Cyclin D3 is a target gene of t(6;14)(p21.1;q32.3) of mature B-cell malignancies. Blood 2001; 98:2837–2844.

41. Krissansen GW, Owen MJ, Verbi W, Crumpton MJ. Primary structure of the t3-gamma subunit of the t3/t cell antigen receptor complex deduced from cDNA sequences—evolution of the t3-gamma and t3-delta subunits. EMBO J 1986; 5:1799–1808.

# 5

# From FISH to Proteomics

*A Molecular Brush*
*to Define Antitumor Drug Action*

*Balanehru Subramanian, PhD,*
*Alexander Nakeff, PhD,*
*and Frederick Valeriote, PhD*

## CONTENTS

## SUMMARY

Technological milestones in genomics have initiated a new approach in the development of novel anticancer drugs to specific genes. However, the heterogeneity of cancer involving multigene complexity calls upon a complementary approach to effectively develop novel anticancer drugs either to specific tumors or with broad range of antitumor activity. Among various techniques, fluorescence *in situ* hybridization (FISH) provides the opportunity to identify mRNA sequences at the subcellular level and has, therefore, become an important tool in gene expression studies. In our drug discovery and development program, we adopt a new hypothesis focusing on the whole cancer cell as a single target. A component of our unique developmental paradigm includes a drug-action profile paradigm defining the drug-specific antiproliferative effects of newly discovered investigational agents, at the molecular level using a genomic–proteomic

From: *Cancer Drug Discovery and Development: The Oncogenomics Handbook*
Edited by: W. J. LaRochelle and R. A. Shimkets © Humana Press Inc., Totowa, NJ

interface. Such an approach using multicolor fluorescence hybridization on cDNA microarray and two-dimensional gel electrophoresis called, Painting with a Molecular Brush, has been successfully adopted to unravel the mechanism of action of a new anticancer agent, XK469.

**Key Words:** FISH; drug action profile; proteomics; molecular brush; microarray; XK469; drug development.

# 1. INTRODUCTION

Understanding the complexity of the polygenic disease, cancer, has remained and continues to remain one of the greatest challenges to mankind's health. Technological milestones in genomics have initiated a new approach in the development of novel anticancer drugs to specific genes selectively targeting cancer cells while sparing normal cells *(1)*. Although this approach is promising, the heterogeneity of the disease involving multigene complexity calls upon a complementary approach to effectively develop novel anticancer drugs either to specific tumors or with broad range of antitumor activity.

# 2. *IN SITU* HYBRIDIZATION

Advances in RNA expression measurements combined with improved detection methods allow the genetic complexity and its response, following exposure to anticancer agents, to be investigated simultaneously. Among various techniques, *in situ* hybridization (ISH) provides the opportunity to identify mRNA sequences at the subcellular level and has, therefore, become an important tool in gene expression studies *(2)*. Application-based evolution in the methodology has resulted in variants of ISH with advanced detection capabilities, sensitivity, and the ease of use *(3)*. These include fluorescence *in situ* hybridization (FISH), cDNA arrays, and comparative genomic hybridization (CGH).

# 3. FLUORESCENCE *IN SITU* HYBRIDIZATION

Over the past two decades, FISH has evolved into a key technology for the localization and detection of nucleic acid sequences in this genomic era *(4)*. FISH is based on the principle that a single-stranded DNA will bind to its complementary DNA sequence. mRNA from tissues or cells are used to generate single-strand DNA by reverse transcription while simultaneously labeling them with fluorescent markers. These single-stranded DNAs (or specific sequences/regions of the DNA), referred to as DNA probes, are then hybridized to the target DNA to reanneal in double-stranded form. After hybridization, the probe DNA is located or detected by fluorescence identifying the complementary target DNA sequence of interest.

Fluorescence *in situ* hybridization offers many advantages over conventional radioactive and chromogenic methods. These include its ease, speed, precision, and ability to simultaneously analyze multiple probes that may be spatially overlapping *(5–8)*. Probes fall under different categories, including chromosome painting, telomeric, centromeric, and gene-specific probes that target whole chromosomes, the repetitive sequence TTA GGG, centromeric region, and specific nucleic acid sequences, respectively. Since its first report in 1980 *(9)*, the basic principles of FISH have remained unchanged. Nevertheless, high-sensitivity detection, simultaneous assay of multiple species, and automated data collection and analysis have advanced the field significantly in detecting RNAs in living cells *(10,11)*. Under different contexts, detection can be achieved by epifluorescence or confocal laser scanning microscopy or by flow cytometry *(12–14)*. The milestones in the development of multitarget FISH have been reviewed by Levsky and Singer *(15)*.

## 4. FISH IN GENOMICS

Fluorescence *in situ* hybridization is widely used as a cytogenetic technique in chromosome mapping, detection of chromosomal rearrangements in interphase/metaphase nuclei or abnormalities such as deletions, and additions or translocations that are frequent in common cancers such as breast, colorectal, and ovarian carcinoma *(16–19)*. Depending on the probes used, whole-chromosome and chromosome-arm painting identifies specific chromosomes and chromosome arms in metaphase and interphase cells *(20)*. In reverse chromosome painting, chromosome paints are prepared from abnormal chromosomes and used to paint normal metaphase chromosomes to reveal complex chromosomal derangements *(21,22)*. These applications have been expanded by the applications of FISH to formalin-fixed or paraffin-wax-embedded tissues, thus providing an opportunity to retrieve the library of archived samples for retrospective cytogenetic analysis *(23,24)*. Yet, several limitations, such as poor probe penetration, excessive probe requirement, and background in addition to autofluorescence, have led to modifications *(25–28)*. To overcome such limitations, Schurter et al. *(29)* described an improved technique for FISH analysis of isolated nuclei from archival, B5, or formalin-fixed, paraffin-wax-embedded tissue.

The multicolor FISH (mFISH) or spectral karyotyping (SKY) uses various fluorescent dyes to represent different probes at the same time. This has found extensive use in detecting chromosome abnormalities *(30)* and karyotyping of all human chromosomes with a single hybridization made possible by the flexibility of the fluorescence detection systems *(31)*. Multiexcitation wavelength is one of the shortcomings of mFISH. König et al. *(32)* have addressed this issue with a new technique called two-photon multicolor FISH that allows excitation of a variety of conventional fluorophores and DNA counterstains within a subfemtoliter excitation volume with a single near-infrared wavelength. Signal amplification protocols have improved the use of FISH in detecting the expression of low-abundance genes, which are limited by detection sensitivity and interference of background signals. Van de Corput et al. *(33)* have used horseradish peroxidase directly conjugated to oligodeoxynucleotides in combination with peroxidase-driven tyramide signal amplification *(34,35)* to detect low-abundance cytokine mRNAs by FISH.

The applicability of FISH as a routine investigative tool both at diagnosis and subsequent monitoring has been reported in conjunction with other cytogenetic analyses *(36–38)*. Differential diagnosis of germ cell tumors by chromosome painting has revealed abnormalities of 12p *(39)*. Its potential as a prognostic tool has gained increasing clinical application following determination of oncogene amplifications in the tumor; for example, *Her2/neu*, *c-myc*, and *cyclin D1* gene amplification in human breast cancers *(40)*. The use of FISH as an efficient protocol for mapping genes, expressed sequence tags (ESTs), and other DNA sequences *(41–43)* has led to the identification of ribosomal DNA gene clusters and telomore sequences using both single probes and multiple probes simultaneously *(44)*. These methods have great potential for performing comparative genomics between different species or samples. However, exploring thousands of genes at a time is beyond the limits of these techniques. Advances in genomic information and the necessity for high-throughput methods set the stage for the development of array-based fluorescence hybridization techniques providing the means to analyze thousands of genes at a time following a single hybridization *(45,46)*. Multicolor fluorescence hybridization on microarray (cDNA or oligonucleotide array) is a powerful tool for investigating the mechanism of drug action *(47,48)*.

In our drug discovery and development program, we adopt a new hypothesis focusing on the whole cancer cell as a single target using drugs with demonstrated in vivo activity, the antithesis of the drug target approach for development of new drugs. A component of our unique developmental paradigm includes a drug-action profile paradigm defining the drug-specific antiproliferative effects of newly discovered investigational agents, at the molecular level using a genomic–proteomic interface. Such an approach, called Painting with a Molecular Brush, has been successfully adopted to unravel the mechanism of action of a new anticancer agent, XK469 *(49–51)*.

## 5. DRUG-ACTION PROFILING

Each gene is expressed in the cell under specific conditions. An altered expression, either increased or decreased, reflects the specific conditions under which it is expressed. This directly elicits an mRNA expression, the detection and quantitation of which would corroborate the effect. Exposure of cells to drugs generate a response that can be deciphered at the genetic level and, on a genomic scale, can identify the regulatory biopathways involved. This phenomenon defined as "drug-action profiling" *(49)* is the first step toward deconvoluting the response.

The information obtained from the profile of transcripts can be used to construct a dynamic molecular picture of the cell at any given time following drug exposure. Comparative reading of the differential molecular alterations obtained by comparing untreated to drug-treated cells can help delineate the regulatory association of genes and the biochemical pathways modulated by the drug. Drug-action profiling at this stage can help predict the mechanism of the drug under investigation. However, the lack of a perfect correlation between gene expression and the translation rate of genes to proteins, degree of posttranslational modifications, or the protein–protein interactions necessitates further investigation to establish the functional role(s) of the genes. In our studies, conventional two-dimensional (2D) gel electrophoresis was applied to generate the proteomic profile. A simultaneous proteomic analysis will bridge and interface the gene expression pattern to the ultimate functional units in the cell, providing a valuable tool to paint with so-called Molecular Brush, the drug-action profile of drugs. This approach provides a powerful platform for expediting the development of novel drugs at a relatively lower cost compared to target-based approach. There are, however, certain limitations, such as the number and selection of key genes arrayed and the availability of their protein counterparts in addition to technical limitations (e.g., low-abundance transcriptional regulators are mostly undetected by 2D gel electrophoresis). The impressive technological growth since we published this platform has made other options to address such limitations available *(52)*.

We used this genomic/proteomic platform to elucidate the drug-action profile of a novel solid tumor-selective anticancer agent, XK469 *(49)*. XK469 is an investigational agent in preclinical development that exhibits active antiproliferative activity against a variety of syngenic murine solid tumors, including adriamycin-resistant mammary tumors *(53,*

*54)*. Topoisomerase IIβ has been proposed as the sole target responsible for this activity *(55)*, although in vitro HCT-116 human colon adenocarcinoma clonogenic cell kill data did not support this conclusion *(56)*. To further understand how XK469 acts at the molecular level, genomic and proteomic analyses were conducted.

## 6. ARRAY-BASED FLUORESCENCE HYBRIDIZATION

HCT-116 cells in log-phase growth (d 3, approx $7 \times 10^6$ cells per T75 flask) were either exposed to 100 µg/mL of XK469 for 24 h or left untreated. Cells were collected at the end of incubation for RNA extraction for genomic analysis. High-quality RNA is crucial for successful microarray experiments and different standard protocols are available. We used the TRIzol protocol as recommended by the manufacturer (Gibco-BRL). The yield and purity of RNA was determined by gel electrophoresis. RNA isolated from XK469-treated cells was used to synthesize cDNA by reverse transcription using the Superscript II RNAse RT reverse transcriptase kit (Gibco-BRL). cDNA synthesis was performed in 50 µL reaction volume at 42°C with Superscript II RT, 0.5 µg of anchored oligo $(dT)_{12,18}$ primer, and a minimum of 50 µg total RNA per reaction.

Two different fluorescent labels, Cy3 and Cy5, was used as dNTP-Cy3 and dNTP-Cy5 to label RNA isolated from untreated control HCT-116 cells and XK469-treated HCT-116 cells, respectively. Cy3 and Cy5 are preferentially used because they are readily incorporated by reverse transcription, exhibit good photostability, and are widely separated in terms of their excitation and emission spectra. The DNA probes were purified using Centricon spin columns and incorporation of fluorescent label confirmed by running aliquots on 1% agarose gel electrophoresis.

The fluorescent-labeled cDNA of the two samples were then hybridized onto a single microarray in an automated GeneTAC Hybridization Station (Genomic Solutions, Inc., Ann Arbor, MI). The desired amount of probe in 1X hybridization buffer (Ambion, Austin, TX) was pipetted onto silanated slides, spotted previously with the template DNA of the 1152 cancer genes (Human Cancerarray, Genomic Solutions, Ann Arbor, MI). This custom-manufactured cDNA microarray comprised of a total of 1152 defined human cancer genes (spotted in duplicate) that were subdivided into 17 functional categories. Hybridization was carried out for 1 h at 65°C and then increased to 14–24 h over a 3-d period at 55°C with probe agitation. Starting the hybridization at high temperature and then stepping down to the desired hybridization temperature increased its specificity and decreased levels of cross-hybridization. To minimize background/cross-hybridization as a result of nonspecific binding of the probe, slides were washed gently in Low Stringency Wash Solution (Genomics Solutions) for 10 min at room temperature and repeated twice. The same wash step was repeated twice for 10 min at 30–40°C. After subsequent brief washings in 100% ethanol, slides were dried at room temperature.

The amount of fluorescent signal was quantified by scanning on the GeneTAC 1000 Biochip Analyzer (Genomic Solutions) and the images analyzed using GeneTAC integrator software (Genomic Solutions) for rapid spot detection, quantification, and calculation of the ratio of spots to determine gene expression changes. The raw data represented a normalized ratio of Cy3 : Cy5 that represents the difference in mRNA expression between the two samples. Ratios were normalized to correct for differences in fluorescent probe incorporation either by using landmark samples that had been spiked into each probe at known concentration or by determining the mean for 80% of the population. All ratios were then multiplied by this normalization factor to correct for differences in labeling efficiency between probes and to remove aberrant samples that could distort the population distribution. Those clearly significant (>twofold) and reproducible changes that reflected either loss of expression or overexpression were listed, and mismatched spots were discarded (typically <1% of the genes).

## 7. FUNCTIONAL GENE CLUSTERING PROFILE ANALYSIS

Gene expression changes >twofold that were reproduced in duplicate spots on at least one of the cancer arrays and that also had appeared on the other were chosen for further analysis following a subsequent visual confirmation of the digital images of cancer array (digitally color coded such that red represented genes upregulated in treated versus control, green represented downregulated, and yellow represented those genes that exhibit no difference); all other unduplicated expression changes were discarded. Table 1 lists those genes, within each of the 17 functional categories, whose expression levels were ranked in descending order of change for each of the altered expression levels.

Gene accession number and the gene name were used to compose a coherent biological map on a gene-by-gene basis (Fig. 1). Public databases available over the Internet like Unigene, Locuslink, and OMIM (Online Mendelian Inheritance in Man) were used to relate altered genes to each other and within molecular pathways for correlation with HCT-116 antiproliferative activity. It should be remembered that no single database covers all of the information about the gene and that an interdatabase reference minimizes the challenges.

Using a discriminator of >twofold change in expression (comprising 0.2% of genes detected in duplicate control Cancerarrays) in drug-treated as compared with untreated control HCT-116 cells, a total of 314 of 1152 genes (28.8% of the total Cancerarray) were identified as potential targets on either of the two microarrays. To validate key genes, the analysis of gene expression was restricted to those genes whose signals were duplicated on both Cancerarrays. The resulting 71 of 1152 potential target genes clustered in 12 of the 17 functional gene categories comprising the FGCP (Table 1).

There was a predominance of decreased over increased expression of the 71 specific genes in the FGCP. Of these, 54 out of 71 genes exhibited a >twofold decrease in expression in 12 functional gene categories whereas 17 out of 71 genes increased their expression >twofold in 7 of the 12 categories composing the FGCP. The preponderance was a decrease in expression (10 out of 11 genes), of which the largest (3.86-fold) was observed for the dual-specificity mitogen-activated protein kinase 2 (MEK) gene. This decrease was superceded only by the 4.09-fold decrease in expression of the vasopressin V1A receptor gene whose product constitutes one of the four major upstream regulators of MEK (Fig. 1). Five functional gene categories that contained no genes with a >twofold change in their expression contained a total of 119 genes (10.3% of the total Cancerarray). They included cell-to-cell interactions (33 genes), DNA damage response, damage repair or recombination (34 genes), stress response proteins (15 genes), initiation, translation, or elongation (12 genes), and ribosomal proteins or subunits (25 genes).

## 8. PROTEOMIC ANALYSIS

Proteomic analysis of total cellular proteins from untreated and XK469-treated HCT-116 cells were performed by conventional 2D gel electrophoresis and Western blotting as described (49–51). Gels were compared for differences in protein spot intensity, in

Table 1
FGCP of >Twofold Gene Expression Levels
of XK469-Treated HCT-116 Cells over Control in Two Cancerarrays

| Gene Function | No. | % Change ↓ | % Change ↑ | N-Fold | Gene Name |
|---|---|---|---|---|---|
| Receptors | 93 | 5.4 | 1.1 | 2.37 | CD63 antigen (melanoma 1 antigen) |
| | | | | −4.09 | Vasopressin V1A receptor |
| | | | | −2.60 | Neurotrophic tyrosine kinase, receptor |
| | | | | −2.63 | Thyroid hormone receptor, alpha |
| | | | | −2.30 | Endothelin receptor |
| | | | | −2.29 | T-Cell receptor, alpha-chain |
| Modulators/ effectors/ transducers | 65 | 10.8 | 0 | −3.67 | Protein kinase, cAMP-dependent, regulatory type 1 |
| | | | | −2.56 | Human sodium phosphate transporter (NPT3) mRNA |
| | | | | −2.32 | Human mRNA for cerebroside sulfotransferase |
| | | | | −2.29 | LIM domain kinase 1 (H51404) |
| | | | | −2.21 | RYK receptor-like tyrosine kinase (T77810) |
| | | | | −2.18 | AXL receptor tyrosine kinase (H15718) |
| | | | | −2.09 | Human protein kinase (MLK-3 mRNA) |
| Oncogenes/ tumor suppressors | 123 | 6.5 | 3.3 | 2.82 | Wilm's tumor 1 (AA130187) |
| | | | | 2.70 | AF-9 protein (AA443284) |
| | | | | 2.55 | ELK1, ETS oncogene family |
| | | | | 2.45 | Myeloid leukemia differentiation protein MCL1 |
| | | | | −3.62 | Ewing sarcoma breakpoint region 1 (R32756) |
| | | | | −2.92 | Thrombopoietin (AA479058) |
| | | | | −2.88 | JUN B proto-oncogene (T99236) |
| | | | | −2.62 | B-cell translocation gene, anti-proliferative (N70463) |
| | | | | −2.47 | V-ets avian erythroblastosis virus E26 |
| | | | | −2.35 | Met proto-oncogene (hepatocye growth factor recep) |
| | | | | −2.31 | Tumor protein p53 (Li–Fraumani syndrome) (R39356) |
| | | | | −2.25 | B cell CLL/lymphoma 3 (AA496678) |
| DNA binding/ transcription factors | 242 | 3.7 | 2.9 | 3.18 | Zinc-finger protein 74 (cos52) (AA629838) |
| | | | | 2.86 | Zinc-finger protein 137 (clone PZH-30) |
| | | | | 2.42 | DAX-1 (AHC) (A1027742) |
| | | | | 2.41 | Human TF11D subunit TAF20 and TAF15 mRNA |
| | | | | 2.26 | Zinc-finger protein 9 |
| | | | | 2.14 | Zinc-finger protein 174 ((AA700196) |
| | | | | 2.09 | Zinc-finger protein 131 (clone PZH-10) |
| | | | | −3.18 | Zinc-finger protein HRX (W16724) |
| | | | | −2.74 | Transcription factor 11 (basic leucine zipper type) |
| | | | | −2.58 | Homeo box B2 (AA911661) |
| | | | | −2.55 | ESTs, highly similar to homeobox gene DLX5 protein |
| | | | | −2.34 | Transcription factor 7 (T-cell-specific) (AA480071) |

(continued)

## Table 1 (Continued)

| Gene Function | No. | % Change ↓ | % Change ↑ | N-Fold | Gene Name |
|---|---|---|---|---|---|
| DNA binding/ transcription factors (continued) | | | | −2.20 | Human HOX4C mRNA |
| | | | | −2.16 | Nuclear factor I/X (CCAAT-binding transcription factor) |
| | | | | −2.13 | Transcription elongation factor S-11 (H27379) |
| | | | | −2.09 | TERC (RNA component Telomerase) (A1825849) |
| Cell Fate/ development regulators | 18 | 11 | 0 | −2.89 | Wingless-type MMTV intergration site 2 |
| | | | | −2.79 | *H. sapiens* jagged 2 mRNA, complete cd (R72432) |
| Housekeeping | 196 | 5.1 | 0.5 | 2.80 | gal-8 (A1651369) |
| | | | | −3.86 | Dual-specificity mitogen-activated protein kinase kinase 2 |
| | | | | −2.85 | Myoinositol-1(or 4) monophosphatase (H90219) |
| | | | | −2.62 | Aldolase B, fructose bisphosphate (H72098) |
| | | | | −2.54 | Aminoacylase-1 (AA402915) |
| | | | | −2.40 | Aspartoacylase (aminoacylase 2, Canavan disease) |
| | | | | −2.34 | Dihydropteridine reductase (R38198) |
| | | | | −2.33 | Human metallothionein 1-B gene (H72722) |
| | | | | −2.31 | Cytochrome P450, subfamily XXVII (steroid 21-hydolase) |
| | | | | −2.31 | ATPase, $Cu^{2+}$ transporting, β polypeptide |
| | | | | −2.09 | AMP deaminase (AA485376) |
| Growth factors/ cytokines | 65 | 7.7 | 0 | −2.95 | Transforming growth factor, β receptor III |
| | | | | −2.40 | IL-(7) (AA626701) |
| | | | | −2.29 | Transforming growth factor, β 3 (AA040617) |
| | | | | −2.21 | Insulin-like growth factor binding protein 2 (36kD) |
| | | | | −2.12 | TGFβ1 precursor (R36467) |
| Cell adhesion/ motility/ invasion | 69 | 5.8 | 2.9 | 2.84 | Neurofibromin 2 (bilateral acoustic neuroma) |
| | | | | 2.70 | Human Sec7p-like protein mRNA |
| | | | | −2.64 | Axonin-1 precursor (R40446) |
| | | | | −2.60 | Integrin, α 2 (CD49B, α 2 subunit VLA-2 receptor) |
| | | | | −2.58 | T-Cell surface glycoprotein CD8 β.3 chain precursor |
| | | | | −2.46 | Actin, α 2 smooth muscle, aorta (AA634006) |
| Cell cycle regulation | 71 | 2.8 | 0 | −2.42 | *H. sapiens* apoptosis-related protein TFAR15 (TFAR15) |
| | | | | −2.42 | *H. sapiens*, growth inhibitor p33ING1 (ING1) mRNA |
| Invasion regulator | 28 | 0 | 3.6 | 2.16 | Human metastasis associated mta1 mRNA |
| Intermediate filament | 18 | 5.5 | 0 | −2.83 | Keratin 13 (W23757) |
| Miscellaneous | 45 | 2.2 | 2.2 | 2.46 | EST, pregnant uterus cDNA (AA099138) |
| | | | | −2.53 | *S*-Adenosylmethionine synthetase, gamma form (T59286) |

Modified from ref. *49*, with permission.

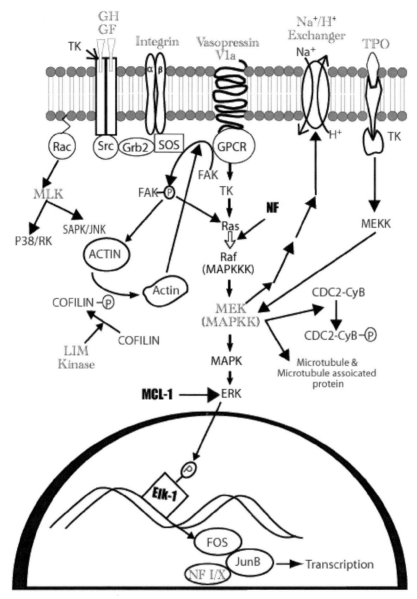

**Fig. 1.** Gene expression pathway of XK469 antiproliferative activity through the MAPK cascade. Open font denotes decreased (>twofold), closed font denotes increased (>twofold), and the regular (remaining) font denotes unaltered (<twofold) changes in gene expression. CDC, cell division control (cyclin-dependent kinase also known as cdk1); Cofilin, a protein that binds to actin filaments; CyB, cyclin B; ERK, extracellular signal-related kinase; FAK, focal adhesion kinase; GF, growth factor; GH, growth hormone; GPCR, G protein-coupled receptor; LIM, the LIM domain was first identified in three developmentally regulated transcription factors Lin-1, Isl-1, and Mec-3; MAPKK, mitogen-activated protein kinase kinase; MAPKKK, mitogen-activated protein kinase kinase kinase; MEK, MAPK/ERK kinase; MAPK, mitogen-activated protein kinase; NF, neurofibromin; P, phosphate; Rac, member of a family of proteins called Rho GTPases; Raf, a serine-threonine kinase; Ras, GTP-binding small protein; SOS, son of sevenless protein (Ras guanine-nucleotide exchange factor); Src, protein tyrosine kinase of the src family; TK, tyrosine kinase; TPO, thrombopoietin. (Modified from ref. *49*, copyright 2002, Wiley. Used with permission of Wiley-Liss, Inc., a subsidiary of John Wiley & Sons, Inc.)

Table 2
List of Proteins Identified by MALDI-TOF and Database Matching

| MALDI-TOF (Molecular Weight/pI–Protein Name) | Database Matching (Protein Name) |
|---|---|
| 83264.6/4.97–90 KD heat shock protein | > 10× Increase |
| 41635.6/5.44–Actin | Ubiquitin carboxyl terminal hydrolase 6 |
| 28750.9/4.57–Human PCNA, chain E | Anion exchange transmembrane protein |
| 29804.2/5.57–Proinhibitin | Ubiquitin carboxyl terminal hydrolase 5 |
| 56560.2/5.26–ATP synthase β | E-Cadherin |
| 16832.4/5.08–eIF-5A | NF-ATC transcription factor |
| 38570.7/4.74–Similar to beta tubulin | Calreticulin |
| 57104.6/4.82–Thyroid hormone binding | 7–10× Increase |
| 36638.7/5.71–Lactate dehydrogenase B | Guanine nucleotide-binding protein |
| 23208.8/5.44–Glutathione S-transferase | 7–10× Decrease |
| 50151.9/4.94–α-Tubulin | Actin-associated protein |
| 43171.4/4.79–XP-C repair complementing protein | Retinoblastoma-binding protein |
| | 5–7× Increase |
| | N-Arginine convertase |
| | Glycoprotein in basement membrane |
| | Cytoplasmic leucine rich protein |
| | Metalloproteinase-like protein |
| | 5–7× Decrease |
| | Putative transcription factor |
| | Keratin type I |

addition to molecular weight, pI identity, and intensity ratio using visually selected anchor points. A total of 782 protein spots were separated from the total cell lysate of untreated control HCT-116 cells. By matching these spots with those from XK469-treated cells, we identified 188 protein spots that were differentially expressed >twofold compared with untreated controls, of which 125 showed increased spot intensity and 63 showed decreased spot intensity. The initial identification of the proteins spots was carried out by database matching to the Swiss-Prot/TrEMBL protein database available over the Internet (http://us.expasy.org/sprot/). Using molecular weight and pI, 15 proteins were closely matched to the known protein database and tentatively identified (Table 2). We then identified 12 additional proteins by matrix-assisted laser desorption ionization–time-of-flight mass spectrometry (MALDI-TOF MS) analysis.

## 9. MOLECULAR BRUSHING

Cellular responses to antiproliferative agents involve modulation of complex pathways that ultimately determine whether a cell survives or dies. One such pathway is the MAPK signal transduction cascade (57) that is constitutively activated in colon tumors (58). Analysis of changes in the expression of specific genes in the FGCP revealed a central role for the MAPK cascade in the manifestation of the antiproliferative activity of

XK469 in vitro. Within the gene pathway, a substantial (3.86-fold) decrease in expression of the MEK gene was observed. Because specific MEK inhibitors, such as PD98059, are not active in vivo in contrast to XK469 *(53,54)*, the potential involvement of this gene pathway in the in vivo activity of XK469 might constitute a unique mode of drug action. MEK protein is a convergence point in numerous receptor-mediated events controlled by four major upstream regulators of MEK (specifically, TGF, vasopressin V1A, neurotrophic tyrosine kinase receptor, and α-integrin). Their expressions are negatively regulated by MEK, and the decrease in their gene expression constituted among the most substantial measured (2.95-, 4.09-, 2.6-, and 2.6-fold, respectively) (Fig. 1).

XK469-induced suppression of the ERK gene pathway is supported by the absence of any effect at the mRNA level on the expression of p38-MAPK and JNK/SAPKs. Nevertheless, the direct antiproliferative effect of XK469 on inhibition of the ERK gene pathway can be amplified by a secondary suppression of gene expression in these latter two signaling pathways through the 2.09-fold decrease in expression of the MLK-3 gene whose product, a GTP-binding kinase, is critical in activating both the p38–MAPK and SAPK–JNK pathways *(59)*. Similarly, although we were unable to detect a direct effect of XK469 on RAS gene expression in the MAPK cascade, XK469 exposure resulted in a substantial 2.84-fold increase in the expression of the neurofibromin gene whose product interferes with the interaction between RAS and RAF *(60)*. In summary, we suggest that the antiproliferative activity of XK469 can be mediated through the RAS/MEK/ERK gene pathway.

The MAPK cascade also regulates microtubule dynamics and other cytoskeletal changes that accompany growth through phosphorylation of microtubule-associated proteins *(61)*. Furthermore, $G_2M$ transition is triggered by the activation of the cdc2–cyclin B kinase complex *(62)* and MEK activity is required both for the activation of cdc2 at the $G_2M$ transition *(63)* and phosphorylation/dephosphorylation of the cdc2–cyclin B complex *(64)*. Having generated a gene expression biological pathway of XK469 antiproliferative activity through the MAPK cascade, it was essential to study the effect of XK469 at the proteome level.

Western blot analysis of the phosphorylated MEK (active form) revealed a time-dependent decrease in the enzyme activity that supported the effect of XK469 being upstream of cdc–cyclin B. Taken together, these data support the conclusion that the MAPK pathway could play a central role in XK469-induced cell cycle arrest.

Although exposure of HCT-116 cells to 100 µg/mL of XK469 for 24 h resulted in the arrest of 90% of the cells in $G_2M$ phase of the cell cycle with increase levels of cyclin B1 *(56)*, we observed no increase in the expression of either the cyclin B1 or cdc2 genes on the Cancerarray. The cellular accumulation of cyclin B1 also could be a consequence of an XK469-induced inhibition of the ubiquitin-mediated breakdown of cyclin B1. Further studies using specific antibodies confirmed this hypothesis correlating the accumulation of cyclin B1 in XK469-treated cells with the inhibition of cyclin B1 ubiquitination, a metabolic process mandatory for proteasome-mediated protein turnover *(51)*. Using immunoblot analysis, we have also reported that the antiproliferative effect of XK469 is mediated by inhibiting the MEK–MAPK signaling pathways in U-937 human leukemia cells *(50)*.

Conclusions drawn based on in vitro studies provide a basis for further extension to in vivo studies that has clinical use. Also, both the genomic and proteomic approachs applied either separately or together are valuable tools in pointing to the pathways involved and, thereby, the targets modulated by a given anticancer agent. However, the link between gene expression, proteins, and drug-action profile is only correlative when it can aid in testing the hypothesis of the mechanism. Finally, although the number of genes (and their respective proteins) represented on the array platform is limited, it, nevertheless, permits the identification of drug-modulated genes and proteins of interest.

## 10. CONCLUSION

The use of array-based fluorescence hybridization techniques such as cDNA microarrays, comparative genomic hybridization, and other alternative techniques such as differential display *(65)* and serial analysis of gene expression *(66)* have been reported to effectively determine transcriptional profiles as a means of defining downstream signaling pathways and mechanisms of action of novel targeted anticancer drugs *(67–69)*. Using the molecular brushing platform, we have generated evidence that XK469 acts via the MAPK signaling pathway with downstream involvement of ubiquitin proteins. As such, the platform provides a valuable paradigm to generate information on the mechanism of action of novel anticancer drugs and could prove useful in understanding drug resistance and pharmacogenomics. This approach is also equally important at a time when single-target theory is being superceded by the involvement of multiple targets on different molecular regulatory pathways to better define the basis of antiproliferative activity/selectivity.

## ACKNOWLEDGMENTS

The authors acknowledge Wiley–Liss, Inc., a subsidiary of John Wiley & Sons, Inc., for their permission to reprint our work published in ref *49* and Dr. Prem Reddy and Dr. Narendar Sivvasamy for their critical review of this manuscript.

## REFERENCES

1. Pegram M, Hsu S, Lewis G, Pietras R, et al. Inhibitory effects of combinations of HER-2/new antibody and chemotherapeutic agents used for treatment of human breast cancer. Oncogene 1999; 18:2241–2251.
2. Singer RH, Lawrence JB, Villanave CA. Optimization of *in situ* hybridization using isotopic and non-isotopic detection methods. Biotechniques 1986; 4:230–250.
3. Going JJ, Gusterson BA. Molecular pathology and future developments. Eur J Cancer 1999; 35:1895–1904.
4. Carter NP. Fluorescence *in situ* hybridization—state of the art. Bioimaging 1996; 4:41–51.
5. Dirks RW, van Gijlswijk RPM, Vooijs MA, et al. 3-End fluorochromized and haptenized oligonucleotides as *in situ* hybridization probes for multiple, simultaneous RNA detection. Exp Cell Res 1991; 194: 310–315.
6. Wiegant J, Ried T, Nederlof PM, van der Ploeg M, Tanke HJ, Raap AK. *In situ* hybridization with fluoresceinated DNA. Nucleic Acids Res 1991; 19:3237–3241.
7. Dirks RW, van Gijlswijk RP, Tullis RH, et al. Simultaneous detection of different mRNA sequences coding for neuropeptide hormones by double *in situ* hybridization using FITC- and biotin-labeled oligonucleotides J Histochem Cytochem 1990; 38:467–473.
8. Lichter P, Tang CC, Call K, Hermanson G, Evans GA, Housman D, et al. High resolution mapping of human chromosome 11 by *in situ* hybridization with cosmid clones. Science 1990; 247:64–69.
9. Bauman JG, Wiegant J, Borst P, van Duijn P. A new method for fluorescence microscopical localization of specific DNA sequences by *in situ* hybridization of fluorochromelabelled RNA. Exp Cell Res 1980; 128:485–490.
10. Raap AK. Advances in fluorescence *in situ* hybridization. Mutat Res 1998; 400:287–298.
11. Boulon S, Basyuk E, Blanchard JM, Bertrand E, Verheggen C. Intra-nuclear RNA trafficking: insights from live cell imaging. Biochimie 2002; 84:805–813.

12. Gygi MP, Ferguson M, Mefford HC, et al. Use of fluorescent sequence-specific polyamides to discriminate human chromosomes by microscopy and flow cytometry. Nucleic Acids Res 2002; 31:2790–2799.

13. Amann RI, Binder BJ, Olson RJ, Chisholm SW, Devereux R, Stahl DA. Combination of 16S rRNA-targeted oligonucleotide probes with flow cytometry for analyzing mixed microbial populations. Appl Environ Microbiol 1990; 56:1919–1925.

14. Giovannoni SJ, DeLong EF, Olsen GJ, Pace NR. Phylogenetic group-specific oligonucleotide probes for identification of single microbial cells. J Bacteriol 1988; 170:720–726.

15. Levsky JM, Singer RH. Fluorescence *in situ* hybridization: past, present and future. J Cell Sci 2003; 116: 2833–2838.

16. Trask BJ. Human genetics and disease: human cytogenetics: 46 chromosomes, 46 years and counting. Nature Rev Genet 2002; 3:769–778.

17. Blancato JK. Fluorescence *in situ* hybridization. In: Gersen S, Keagle M, eds. The principles of clinical cytogenetics. Totowa, NJ: Humana, 1999;443–471.

18. Abdel-Rahman WM, Katsura K, Rens W, et al. Spectral karyotyping suggests new subsets of colorectal cancers characterized by pattern of chromosome rearrangement. Proc Natl Acad Sci USA 2001; 98: 2538–2543.

19. Courtay-Cahen C, Morris JS, Edwards PAW. Chromosome translocations in breast cancer with breakpoints at 8p12. Genomics 2000; 66:15–25.

20. Ried T, Schrock E, Ning Y, Wienberg J. Chromosome painting: a useful art. Hum Mol Genet 1998; 7: 1619–1626.

21. Morris JS, Carter NP, Ferguson-Smith MA, Edwards PAW. Cytogenetic analysis of three breast carcinoma cell lines using reverse chromosome painting. Genes Chromosome Cancer 1997; 20:120–139.

22. Arkesteijn G, Jumelet E, Hagenbeek A, Smit E, Slater R, Martens A. Reverse chromosome painting of the identification of marker chromosomes and complex translocations in leukaemia. Cytometry 1999; 35: 117–124.

23. Hedley DW, Friedlander ML, Taylor IW, et al. Method for analysis of cellular DNA content of paraffin-embedded pathological material using flow cytometry. J Histochem Cytochem 1983; 31:1333–1335.

24. Thompson CT, LeBoit PE, Nederlof PM, et al. Thick section fluorescence *in situ* hybridization on formalin-fixed paraffin-embedded archival tissue provides a histogenic profile. Am J Pathol 1994; 144: 237–243.

25. Hyytinen E, Visakorpi T, Kallioniemi A, et al. Improved technique for analysis of formalin-fixed, paraffin-embedded tumours by fluorescence *in situ* hybridization. Cytometry 1994; 16:93–99.

26. DiFrancesco LM, Murthy SK, Luider J, et al. Laser-capture microdissection-guided fluorescence *in situ* hybridization and flow cytometric cell cycle analysis of purified nuclei from paraffin sections. Mod Pathol 2000; 13:705–711.

27. McKay JA, Murray GI, Keith WN, et al. Amplification of fluorescent *in situ* hybridisation signals in formalin fixed paraffin wax embedded sections of colon tumor using biotinylated tyramide. J Clin Pathol Mol Pathol 1997; 50:322–325.

28. Chin SF, Daigo Y, Huang HE, et al. A simple and reliable pretreatment protocol facilitates fluorescence *in situ* hybridization on tissue microarrays of paraffin wax embedded tumour samples. J Clin Pathol Mol Pathol 2003; 56:275–279.

29. Schurter MK, LeBrun DP, Harrison KJ. Improved technique for fluorescence *in situ* hybridization analysis of isolated nuclei from archival, B5 or formalin fixed, paraffin wax embedded tissue. J Clin Pathol Mol Pathol 2002; 55:121–124.

30. Coco-Martin JM, Lolkus M, Ottenheim CPE, Oomen LCJM, Blommestijn GJF, Begg AC. Automatic detection of stable and unstable chromosome aberrations visualized by three color imaging after fluorescence *in situ* hybridization with a painting and a pancentromeric DNA probe. Cytometry 1998; 32: 327–336.

31. Speicher MR, Ballard SG, Ward DC. Karyotyping human chromosomes by combinatorial multi-fluor-FISH. Nature Genet 1996; 12:368–375.

32. König K, Göhlert A, Liehr T, Loncarevic IF, Riemann I. Two-photon multicolor FISH: a versatile technique to detect specific sequences within single DNA molecules in cells and tissues. Single Mol 2000; 1:41–51.

33. Van de Corput MPC, Dirks RW, van Gijlswijk RPM, et al. Sensitive mRNA detection by fluorescence *in situ* hybridization using horseradish peroxidase-labeled oligodeoxynucleotides and tyramide signal amplification. J Histochem Cytochem 1998; 46:1249–1259.

34. Kerstens HMJ, Poddighe PJ, Hanselaar AGJM. A novel *in situ* hybridization signal amplification method based on the deposition of biotinylated tyramine. J Hitochem Cytochem 1995; 43:347–350.

35. van Gijlswijk RPM, Zijlmans HJMAA, Wiegant J, et al. Fluorochrome-labeled tyramides: use in immunohistochemsitry and fluorescence *in situ* hybridization. J Histochem Cytochem 1997; 45:375–382.

36. Wan TSK, Ma SK, AU WY, Chan LC. Derivative chromosome 9 deletions in chronic myeloid leukemia: interpretation of atypical D-FISH pattern. J Clin Pathol 2003; 56:471–474.

37. Buno I, Wyatt W, Zinsmeister AR, et al. A special fluorescent *in situ* hybridization technique to study peripheral blood and assess the effectiveness of interferon therapy in chronic myeloid leukemia. Blood 1998; 92:2315–2321.

38. Forus A, Hoifodt HK, Overli GET, Myklebost O, Fodstad O. Sensitive fluorescent *in situ* hybridization method for the characterization of breast cancer cells in bone marrow aspirates. Br Med J 1999; 52: 68–74.

39. Blough RI, Heerema NA, Ulbricht TM, Smolarek TA, Roth LM, Einhorn LH. Interphase chromosome painting of paraffin-embedded tissue in the differential diagnosis of possible germ-cell tumors. Mod Pathol 1998; 11:634–641.

40. Janocko LE, Brown KA, Smith CA, et al. Distinctive patterns of Her2/neu, c-myc and cyclin D1 gene amplification by fluorescence *in situ* hybridization in primary human breast cancers. Cytometry 2001; 46: 136–149.

41. Horelli-Kuitunen N, Aaltonen J, Yaspo ML, et al. Mapping ESTs by fiber-FISH. Genomic Res 1999; 9:62–71.

42. Fan YS, Davis LM, Shiws TB. Mapping small DNA sequences by fluorescence *in situ* hybridization directly on banded metaphase chromosomes. Proc Natl Acad Sci USA 1990; 87:6223–6227.

43. Florijn RJ, van de Rijke FM, Vrolijk H, et al. Exon mapping by fiber-FISH or LR-PCR. Genomics 1996; 38:277–282.

44. Castro LFC, Holland PWH. Fluorescence *in situ* hybridization to amphioxus chromosome. Zool Sci 2002; 19:1349–1353.

45. Schulze A, Downward J. Navigating gene expression using microarrays—a technology review. Nature Cell Biol 2001; 3:E190–E195.

46. Bertucci F, Viens P, Rebecca T, Catherine Nguyen, Houlgatte R, Birnbaum D. DNA arrays in clinical oncology: promises and challenges. Lab Invest 2003; 83:305–316.

47. Debouck C, Goodfellow PN. DNA microarrays in drug discovery and development. Nature Genet 1999; 21(Suppl):48–50.

48. Marton MJ, DeRisi JL, Bennet HA, et al. Drug target validation and identification of secondary drug target effects using DNA microarrays. Nature Med 1998; 11:1293–1301.

49. Nakeff A, Sahay N, Pisano M, Subramanian B. Painting with a molecular brush: genomic/proteomic interfacing to define the drug action profile of novel solid-tumor selective anticancer agents. Cytometry 2002; 47:72–79.

50. Lin H, Subramanian B, Nakeff A, Chen B. XK469, a novel antitumor agent, inhibits signaling by the MEK/MAPK signaling pathway. Cancer Chemother Pharmacol 2002; 49:281–286.

51. Lin H, Liu XY, Subramanian B, Nakeff A, Valeriote F, Chen B. Mitotic arrest induced by XK469, a novel antitumor agent, is correlated with the inhibition of cyclin B1 ubiquitination. Int J Cancer 2002; 97:121–128.

52. Yan F, Subramanian B, Nakeff A, et al. A comparison of drug-treated and untreated HCT-116 human colon adenocarcinoma cells using a 2D liquid separation mapping method based upon chromatofocusing pI fractionation. Anal Chem 2003; 75:2299–2308.

53. Corbett TH, LoRusso P, Demchick I, et al. Preclinical antitumor efficacy of analogs of XK469: sodium-(2[4-(7-chloro-2-quinoxalinoxy)phenoxy]propionate. Invest New Drugs 1998; 16:129–139.

54. LoRusso PM, Parchment R, Demchik I, et al. Preclinical antitumor activity of XK469 (NSC 656889). Invest New Drugs 1999; 16:287–296.

55. Gao H, Huang KC, Yamasaki EF, Chan KK, Chohan I, Snapka RM. XK469, a selective toposiomerase IIβ poison. Proc Natl Acad Sci USA 1999; 96:12,168–12,173.

56. Subramanian B, Nakeff A, Media J, Wentland M, Valeriote FA. Cellular drug action profile paradigm applied to XK469. J Exp Ther Oncol 2001; 2:253–263.

57. Gutkind JS. The pathways connecting G protein coupled receptors to the nucleus through divergent mitogen-activated protein kinase cascades. J Biol Chem 1998; 273:1839–1842.

58. Hoshino R, Chatani Y, Yamori T, et al. Constitute activation of the 41-/43-kDa mitogen activated kinase signaling pathway in human tumors. Oncogene 1999; 21:813–822.

59. Tibbles LA, Ing YL, Kiefer F, et al. MLK-3 activates the SAPK/JNK and p38/RK pathways via SEK1 and MKK3/6. EMBO J 1996; 15:7026–7035.
60. Li Y, White R. Suppression of a human colon cancer cell line by introduction of an exogenous NF1 gene. Cancer Res 1996; 56:2872–2876.
61. Reszka AA, Serger R, Diltz CD, Krebs EG, Fischer EH. Association of mitogen-activated protein kinase with the microtubule cytoskeleton. Proc Natl Acad Sci USA 1995; 92:8881–8885.
62. Riabowol K, Draaetta G, Brizuela L, Vandre D, Beach D. The cdc2 kinase is a nuclear protein that is essential for mitosis in mammalian cells. Cell 1989; 57:393–401.
63. Wright JH, Munar E, Jameson D, et al. Mitogen activated protein kinase kinase activity is required for the G(2)/M transition of the cell cycle in mammalian fibroblasts. Proc Natl Sci USA 1996; 96:11,335–11,340.
64. Morgon DO. Principles of CDK regulation. Nature 1995; 374:131–134.
65. Tanaka H, Arakawa H, Yamaguchi T, et al. A ribonucleotide reductase gene involved in a p53-dependent cell-cycle checkpoint for DNA damage. Nature 2000; 404:42–49.
66. Yu J, Zhang L, Hwang PM, et al. Identification and classification of p53-regulated genes. Proc Natl Acad Sci USA 1999; 96:14,517–14,522.
67. Harkin DP. Uncovering functionally relevant signaling pathways using microarray-based expression profiling. Oncologist 2000; 5:501–507.
68. Macgregor PF, Squire JA. Application of microarrays to the analysis of gene expression in cancer. Clin Chem 2002; 48:1170–1177.
69. Clarke PA, George NL, Easdale S, et al. Molecular pharmacology of cancer therapy in human colorectal cancer by gene expression profiling. Cancer Res 2003; 63:6855–6863.

# 6

# Gene Program Signatures for Papillomavirus E2-Mediated Senescence in Cervical Cancer Cells

## Finding the Points of No Return

*Sarah S. Williams, Bruce J. Aronow, PhD, and Susanne I. Wells, PhD*

### CONTENTS

### SUMMARY

Infection with the high-risk types of human papillomavirus is strongly linked to the development of cancers of the uterine cervix. Carcinogenesis depends on the continuous expression of the viral E6 and E7 oncogenes in the affected individual. Transcription of these oncogenes can be negatively regulated by the viral E2 protein. Carcinogenic progression of human papillomavirus (HPV)-positive lesions is accompanied by the integration of the viral DNA into the cellular genome and the disruption of the viral E2 open reading frame. When reintroduced into HPV-positive cancer cells, E2 proteins suppress cellular growth through senescence induction. E2 repression of E6/E7 is necessary and sufficient for this process, indicating that important senescence mediators must be inhibited by the viral oncoproteins for both the initiation and maintenance of HPV-associated carcinogenesis. We describe in this chapter the use of an E2-based inducible senescence system to determine the transcriptome of HPV-positive cells during an early, yet irreversibly committed senescence state. Insights into the regulation of specific genes and gene groups during E2 senescence compared to their regulation during E6/E7 immortalization

From: *Cancer Drug Discovery and Development: The Oncogenomics Handbook*
Edited by: W. J. LaRochelle and R. A. Shimkets © Humana Press Inc., Totowa, NJ

might elucidate mechanisms of senescence inhibition by the HPV oncogenes. We will discuss how future studies of bona fide regulators of the balance between senescence and carcinogenesis might ultimately lead to novel drug targets, diagnostic markers, and more refined approaches for cancer treatment both within and outside of the HPV context.

**Key Words:** Human papillomavirus; cervical cancer; viral oncogenes; immortality; senescence; transcriptional profiling.

## 1. PAPILLOMAVIRUS INFECTION AND CERVICAL CANCER

Papillomaviruses are a group of small DNA tumor viruses that are known to induce a broad range of benign and malignant epithelial lesions in the infected host (for a review, see ref. *1*). Of the over 100 human papillomavirus types (HPVs) that have been identified to date, approx 25–30 are associated with lesions of the anogenital tract. Depending on the likelihood of associated lesions to progress to malignancy or to remain benign, genital-tract-associated HPVs are further classified as high- vs low-risk HPVs. High-risk HPVs such as HPV16 or HPV18 are strongly associated with cervical cancer irrespective of other risk factors and geographic location *(2)*. Cervical cancer is the second most common cancer in women worldwide, causing 15% of female cancer mortality *(3)*. Approximately 400,000 new cases of invasive cancer are diagnosed each year with 5-yr survival ranging from 44% to 66% for all clinical stages *(4)*. Over 97% of cervical cancers contain high-risk HPV DNA and express the viral oncogenes E6 and E7. Expression of these oncogenes is detected in all cells of the primary tumor and metastases thereof, supporting a direct link between HPV infection and carcinogenesis *(5,6)*. This link is further emphasized by the documented in vitro immortalizing and transforming activities of the two oncoproteins. Almost all HPV-positive human cancers have lost expression of the viral E2 protein, a negative regulator of E6 and E7 under certain circumstances. Investigation of the concequences of the re-expression of E2 in cervical cancer cells, as described in Section 2, might have clinical implications for future treatment options.

Infection with high-risk HPV types has clearly been implicated in the development of cytological abnormalities. The role of high-risk HPVs in human tumorigenesis might be reflected in their ability to immortalize primary human keratinocytes in contrast to the low-risk HPVs *(8–11)*. Such immortalized cells are nontumorigenic at low passage, but induce tumors in nude mice upon the coexpression of activated oncogenes *(12)* or after extended passaging in tissue culture *(13,14)*. Therefore, neither individual nor the combined effects of the two viral oncogenes are sufficient for cellular transformation. Thus, transformation requires additional mutations within cellular genes *(15)*. These in vitro experiments likely reflect the need for HPV-positive human tumors in vivo to aquire specific mutations within cellular genes for the progression to malignant stages over time. Despite the fact that E6/E7 expression is clearly not sufficient, their sustained expression is a necessary requirement for malignant progression and maintenance of the malignant phenotype once attained *(16)*. Inhibiting E6 and E7 activities is, therefore, an attractive goal for the treatment of HPV-associated cancers. Various experimental approaches to inhibit E6/E7 expression in malignant cervical carcinoma cells including an inducible viral oncogene expression system, antisense oligonucleotides, specific ribozymes or the overexpression of E2 have, indeed, resulted in cellular growth arrest *(17–24)*.

Targeted expression of E6 and/or E7 in the basal cells of squamous mouse epithelium supports different, but complementary, functions for the two oncogenes in the process of carcinogenesis (25–30). The viral E6 and E7 proteins have been shown to bind a number of cellular proteins and to possess a variety of activities that could contribute to carcinogenic progression (see ref. 31 for a for review). E6 actions include (1) formation of a trimeric complex with p53 and the E6AP ubiquitin ligase that leads to the targeted degradation of both p53 and E6AP (32,33), (2) interactions with a protein E6TP1 (now known as SIPA1L1) exhibiting homology to Rap1–GTPase-activating proteins (GAPs) (34,35), (3) interactions with proapoptotic proteins Bak and c-myc (36–38), (4) binding of a number of PDZ proteins, including the human homolog of the *Drosophila* tumor suppressor Dlg and MAGI I (39–41), and (5) interactions with the cellular transcriptional co-activators CBP/p300 (42,43) and human ADA3 (44). Importantly, E6 has also been shown to activate the transcription of the human telomerase catalytic subunit, an enzyme whose activation is a hallmark of many human tumors (45). With regard to E7, most of the interactions can be roughly categorized into those that (1) inhibit Rb-related pocket proteins and their activating cyclin-dependent cdk kinase inhibitors (46–50), (2) regulate specific transcription and chromatin remodeling factors with key functions in cellular proliferation (51–54), (3) induce directly fundamental changes in the cellular energy metabolism (55–57), and (4) uncouple centrosome duplication from cellular replication to promote early genomic instability (58–60). Taken together, it is likely that a multiplicity of individual interactions between the HPV oncoproteins and cellular proteins are responsible for a myriad of downstream oncogenic transcriptional responses.

## 2. E2 INHIBITION OF CELLULAR GROWTH

Exploiting the functions of E2 represents one possibility for the treatment of HPV-associated cancers. A number of reports have shown that whereas HPV DNA is maintained episomally in benign, precancerous lesions, it is generally found integrated into the cellular genome in malignant carcinomas and cell lines derived from them (6,16). One frequent characteristic of HPV integration is the disruption of the viral E2 open reading frame and accompanying high expression levels of the E6 and E7 oncoproteins (61–66). This observation has led to the hypothesis that disruption of the regulatory activities of E2 and deregulated E6/E7 expression are important steps in the development of malignancy. Implicit in this hypothesis is the possibility for treatments of HPV-positive carcinomas based on E2 re-expression via gene delivery approaches or based on small-molecule approaches which mimic E2 function.

The papillomavirus E2 protein is a regulatory factor with multiple roles in the transcription and replication of the viral DNA (67,68). E2 proteins resemble prototypical transcription factors, with an N-terminal transcriptional activation domain and a C-terminal DNA binding domain, separated from each other by a less conserved hinge region. E2 proteins from all viral strains form dimers and interact sequence-specifically with a palindromic motif $ACC\underline{G}(N)_4\underline{C}GGT$, where the affinity of the natural E2-binding sites is modulated by the nature of the $(N)_4$ spacer and where the underlined nucleotides are preferred (69–73). The bovine papillomavirus (BPV) E2 proteins have been studied most extensively. Distinct BPV E2 proteins have been detected in BPV-transformed C127 cells. The largest 48-kDa form, E2-TA, represents the product of the complete open reading frame. A short internally initiated 30-kDa form of BPV E2, known as E2-TR, is devoid of most of the transactivation domain, but contains the C-terminal DNA binding/dimerization domain *(7)*. E2 proteins can either activate or repress transcription depending on the promoter context and the arrangement of E2-binding sites within a given promoter *(74–81)*. This flexible transcriptional behavior is in accordance with the reported ability of full-length BPV E2 proteins to interact with a multitude of basal and activated transcription factors, including TBP, TFIIB, and AMF1, as well as the cellular coactivators CBP/ p300 and P/CAF *(82–86)*.

Several experimental observations suggest that the loss of E2 protein expression aids in the progression of HPV-associated carcinogenesis. First, E2 is known to directly repress the viral E6/ E7 promoter of high-risk HPVs *(81,87–89)*. Second, inactivating mutations within the E2 gene increase the immortalization efficiency of viral genomic DNA *(90)*. Third, the re-expression of E2 in HPV-positive cancer lines results in either a G1 growth arrest followed by senescence or in apoptotic cell death *(18,19,21,91–97)*. This chapter will focus on BPV1 E2-mediated senescence in HPV-positive cervical cancer cells, although this is by no means intended to downplay the importance of apoptosis induction in response to E2.

## 3. CELLULAR SENESCENCE

The term "cellular" or "replicative senescence" defines the finite replicative capacity of most somatic cells in culture, which eventually results in terminal cessation of cellular division. (see refs. *98* and *99*). Markers of senescence in vitro include an irreversible arrest in the G1-phase of the cell cycle, enlarged cellular morphology, positive staining for senescence-associated $\beta$-galactosidase activity (SA-$\beta$Gal) *(100)*, lipofuscin accumulation *(101)*, and upregulation of growth regulatory molecules such as p53, p21$^{\text{CIP}}$, and p16$^{\text{INK4a}}$. Several experimental conditions can induce cellular senescence in vitro. Senescence by replicative exhaustion results from the gradual loss of telomeres from chromosome ends with each replicative cycle. Critically shortened telomeres lose their protective conformation and trigger senescence initiation *(102)*. Aside from replicative exhaustion, various forms of stress such as DNA damage or oncogene expression trigger senescence *(103)*. Cultured cell senescence limits our ability to expand and manipulate somatic cells for replacement therapies ex vivo. Approaches to inhibit senescence pathways (without supporting cellular transformation) can therefore, be desirable for a large number of clinical applications such as replacement therapies.

In limiting the number of times that a given cell can divide in response to intrinsic or extrinsic signals, cellular senescence is thought to represent a natural barrier to cancer development in vivo. This notion is further emphasized by the fact that tumor suppressors such as p53 or pRB, which are frequently inactivated in human cancers in vivo, play important roles during cellular senescence in vitro *(104,105)*. Findings by Schmitt et al. emphasized an antagonistic relationship between cellular senescence and carcinogenesis in vivo and positively correlated intact senescence pathways with tumor regression following chemotherapy *(106)*. In addition, senescence has been suggested to underlie aspects of the organismal aging process *(107,108)*. Interesting in this regard is the fact that molecules involved in senescence such as telomerase, p53, and BRCA1 can cause aging phenotypes when deleted or mutated in mice *(109–111)*. Despite the intriguing physiological implications of these observations—and the possibility that senescence might be a double-edged sword in the organismal context—this process remains a poorly understood phenomenon. Both underlying and contributing to this lack of knowledge is the absence of molecular markers for the senescence process. A thorough understanding of the regulatory and executive senescence machinery will be critical for the development of novel approaches to the treatment of carcinogenesis and the loss of functional and proliferative homeostasis associated with aging.

## 4. E2 EXPRESSION AND SENESCENCE IN HPV-POSITIVE CERVICAL CANCER CELLS

Expression of BPV1 or HPV16 full-length E2 protein in HPV-positive cervical cancer cells results in either apoptotic cell death or senescence. Apoptosis and senescence take place in different subsets of E2-expressing cells and are controlled by distinct pathways. Apoptosis is observed within 24 h after E2 expression and requires neither E2 DNA-binding nor E2 transcriptional activity (91,92,94). Apoptosis is independent of E6/E7 promoter repression, as it occurs in HPV-positive and HPV-negative cell lines and is mediated at least, in part, via direct interactions between specific residues in the E2 transcriptional activation domain and cellular apoptotic regulators (91–94). In contrast to the timing and mechanism of E2 apoptosis, senescence induction occurs at later times in HPV-positive cell lines such as HPV18-positive HeLa and HPV16-positive Caski cells as well as human keratinocytes immortalized with HPV16 genomic DNA (96,112,113). Senescence is not observed in HPV-negative U$_2$OS osteosarcoma or C33A cervical carcinoma cells (96). This specificity for HPV-positive cells is in accordance with the fact that E2-mediated repression of the E6/E7 promoter is required for G1 growth arrest and senescence induction (97,114,115). Future therapeutic approaches that target the E2-based pathways can involve the use of E2 proteins that exhibit maximal ability to target HPV-positive cancer cells via senescence, yet lead to minimal nonspecific toxicity through apoptosis induction. The fact that oncogene repression in cervical cancer cells results in senescence underscores the fact that relevant pathways have remained intact and must be continuously inhibited by the viral oncoproteins. Interference with this inhibition and the orderly reactivation of senescence mediators such as p53 and pRB (115) can then be exploited for approaches to treat HPV carcinogenesis. It should be added that senescent cells not only secrete growth inhibitory but also growth stimulatory molecules, in the latter case reminiscent of a tumor supporting stromal environment (116). Together with the ability of these cells to survive for months to years in tissue culture and possibly also in the tumor environment, it is critical to improve our understanding of such paracrine pro-carcinogenic effects and potentially incorporate this into the design of therapeutic approaches to arrest cancer cell growth via senescence. The promise and dangers of using senescence induction in the treatment of cancer are the subject of an elegant recent review (117).

## 5. TRANSCRIPTIONAL PROFILING OF SENESCING CERVICAL CANCER CELLS

In an effort to explore in detail the molecular consequences of E2 expression in HeLa cells and to identify regulators and markers of senescence in this system, we have monitored global transcriptional changes associated with sensescence in HPV-positive, E2-expressing HeLa cells using high-density oligonucleotide microarrays (118). An early timepoint was chosen to examine transcriptional changes in initial stages of the senescence phenotype with the goal of identifying regulators of the process rather than genes whose expression is altered later as a consequence of senescence. Because a defining, early event during cellular senescence is the establishment of irreversibility, we targeted entrance into this phase as potentially the most revealing. Adenoviral delivery of a temperature-sensitive E2 protein was used in conjunction with temperature-shift experiments to determine the point of irreversibility in the HeLa cell system *(118)*. The E2ts protein is functional at the permissive temperature of 32°C, but not at the restrictive temperature of 39.5°C *(119)*. Infection of HeLa cells with the E2ts-expressing virus (AdE2ts) at 32°C, but not at 39.5°C, resulted in cellular senescence using the typical morphological changes as well as SA-βGal activity as a readout. Temperature-shift experiments revealed that cells had traversed into the irreversible phase of senescence by d 3. Induced levels of p53 and its transcriptional target p21$^{CIP}$ were observed at this timepoint, as well as hypophosphorylation of retinoblastoma pRB protein, all of which represent cell growth arrest mediators and all of which have been implicated functionally in the observed E2 senescence phenotype *(96,118)*. Transcriptional profiling experiments were performed on d 3 after definitive senescence commitment to identify genes that either reflect or contribute directly to the senescence phenotype.

The experimental strategy for the profiling of senescence-associated genes was as follows. HeLa cells were infected with E2ts-expressing adenovirus (Ad) at the permissive temperature for synchronized senescence induction and at the restrictive temperature as a control. Empty Ad-infected cells were treated in the same fashion in order to account for any transcriptional changes that might be associated with temperature shift alone in the presence of various expressed adenoviral gene products. Each experiment group, therefore, contained four samples and was carried out in triplicate. Total RNA was harvested on d 3 after senescence induction and was used to generate targets for the Affymetrix HG-U95Av2 GeneChip® probe array representing approx 12,651 gene elements and somewhat less than 10,000 unique full-length human genes. GeneChip® arrays are high-density oligonucleotide arrays manufactured using photolithography and combinatorial chemistry technology, where, in the case of the U95Av2, approx 16 pairs of 25-mer probes are used to measure the transcript level of each of the sequences represented on the array. The biotin-labeled RNA target was hybridized to the HG-U95Av2 array, washed, stained, and scanned. The amount of light emitted at 570 nm is proportional to the bound target at each location on the probe array. The Microarray Suite 5.0 software (MAS 5.0; Affymetrix Inc., Santa Clara, CA) was used to compute the intensity for each cell, as well as Absent/Present calls. Subsequent analyses were performed with GeneSpring software (Silicon Genetics Inc., Redwood City, CA).

In order to optimize analysis of E2 effects at the permissive temperature, a two-step normalization procedure was performed. First, a global per-chip normalization was applied, where the signal intensity for each gene was divided by the median signal intensity of all genes not flagged as "Absent" on the corresponding GeneChip. A per-gene normalization was then applied to the three trials independently, where each gene's signal intensity was divided by the average signal intensity of the corresponding Ad- and AdE2ts-infected samples that were incubated at 39.5°C. The per-chip normalization controls for interarray variations in intensity as a result of a variety of factors (e.g., inconsistent sample preparation, labeling efficiency, array defects), whereas the per-gene normalization accounts for differences in detection efficiencies between probes, some degree of interexperimental trial-specific variation, and enables comparison of relative change in gene expression levels across each of the conditions across each trial. The resulting normalized data were filtered for genes that were flagged as "Present" in two or more arrays, generating an initial pool of 6475 genes from which all subsequent analyses where generated. Three statistical group comparisons were then used to find differentially expressed genes between Ad and AdE2ts at 32°C: Student's two-sample $t$-test identified 193 genes ($p = 0.025$), Welch's $t$-test identified 266 genes ($p = 0.05$), and a nonparametric (Wilcoxon/Mann–Whitney $U$) test identified 703 genes ($p = 0.0215$). Because all of the genes identified by the Student's $t$-test and Welch's $t$-test were also contained in the nonparametric gene list, the nonparametric list (703 genes) was used to perform two types of clustering to identify groups of genes exhibiting similar expression patterns across the four experimental groups. Hierarchical clustering of the 703-gene list using a Pearson correlation produced the gene tree shown in Fig. 1A (*see* Color Plate 3 following p. 78). Triplicate experiments are indicated as a, b, and c for the four experimental conditions. Repressed genes are represented in blue, induced genes are represented in red, and the branch length is an indicator of expression similarity between genes. The 12 samples were also clustered into a condition tree using a Pearson correlation, where the replicate experiments clustered together as expected (not shown). The fully annotated dataset is available at http://genet.cchmc.org in the U95Av2 genome under Experiments/Wells_Howley (login as guest).

Examples of four relevant types of expression pattern are boxed in Fig. 1A (I–IV). These correspond to the four plots (I–IV) in Fig. 1B, which illustrate ideally expected transcriptional patterns for the above experiment. The indicated four regulatory groups were considered relevant for subsequent studies of E2 senescence and represented: genes that were specifically induced by E2 and heat shock (I) or by E2 alone (II) and genes that were specifically repressed by E2 alone (III) or by E2 and heat shock (IV). Inclusion of genes that were heat shock and E2 responsive was important because known components of the E2 regulatory circuit, such as p21$^{CIP}$, were also temperature sensitive in this system *(118)*.

In order to identify the top regulators in AdE2ts, the 703 genes were additionally filtered for those whose mean expression was either upregulated or downregulated by greater than 1.7-fold in the AdE2ts relative to the empty Ad at 32°C. The resulting subset of 283 genes were subjected to K-means clustering using a Pearson correlation where genes were divided into 9 sets based on similar expression profiles across all samples (Fig. 2, unpublished data; *see* Color Plate 4 following p. 78). This allowed distinction between gene regulation by E2 alone and regulation by both E2 and temperature. Examples of gene regulation by temperature and/or E2 (groups I–IV) as illustrated in Fig. 1 are indicated.

As expected, p21$^{CIP}$ is contained in set 2, where gene behavior is induced by both E2 and temperature. Included in set 2 are other known p53 responsive (underlined) and G1 growth arrest (pink) genes. An example of the inverse gene expression behavior, namely gene repression by both E2 and high temperature, is observed in set 8. In correlation with the growth arrest phenotype, this set reveals the repression of several genes (green) that have been associated with G2/M-phase progression. Genes that are specifically upregulated by E2 and that are not responsive to temperature shift are contained in set 5. Because gene upregulation in this set directly correlates with senescence induction, individual genes might be of functional importance for the senescence phenotype. In agreement with a reversal of immortality via senescence, three genes—tissue inhibitor of metalloproteinase 4 (TIMP4), T-cell leukemia translocation associated gene (TCTA), and the reversion-inducing cysteine-rich protein with kazal motifs (RECK)—are induced, which have been linked to tumor suppression *(120–122)*. Upregulation of RECK is especially interesting

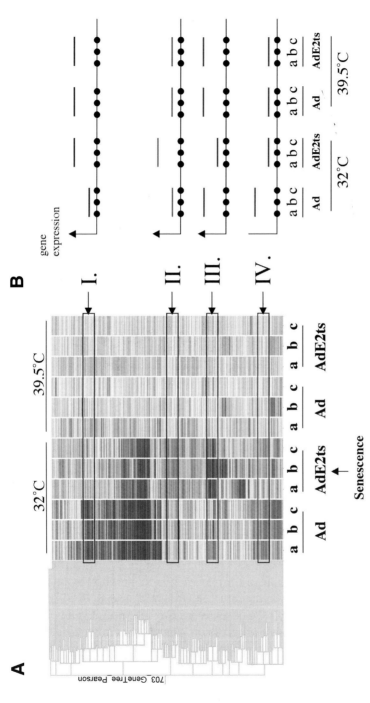

**Fig. 1.** A hierarchical tree of senescence-associated transcriptionally regulated genes. (**A**) Results from clustering three independent experiments (a, b, c) within the four treatment groups are depicted as a gene tree. Pearson correlation was applied to the sample measurements using the 703-gene list derived from statistical group comparisons. Transcriptionally induced genes are indicated in red; repressed genes are indicated in blue. (Adapted from ref. *118.*) (**B**) Anticipated expression patterns in the E2ts HeLa cell system. Graphs I–IV correspond to boxed examples in (A). Three experiments (a, b, c) are shown for the four treatment groups I: induced by E2; II: induced by heat shock, induced by E2; III: repressed by E2; IV: repressed by heat shock, repressed by E2. (*See* Color Plate 3 following p. 78.)

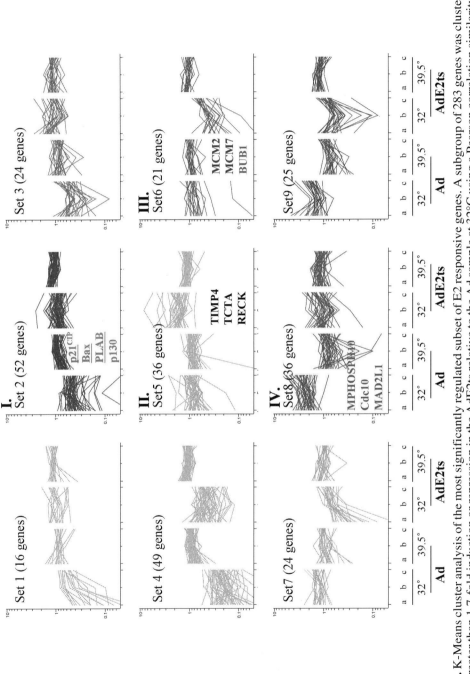

**Fig. 2.** K-Means cluster analysis of the most significantly regulated subset of E2 responsive genes. A subgroup of 283 genes was clustered based on a greater than 1.7-fold induction or repression in the AdE2ts relative to the Ad sample at 32°C using a Pearson correlation similarity measure (Wells laboratory, unpublished data). Signal intensities are shown on a log scale for three independent experiments (a, b, c). Samples were from empty Ad-infected cells at 32°C and 39.5°C and from AdE2ts-infected cells at 32°C and 39.5°C as depicted below the graphs. Select examples of E2-responsive genes are indicated by name, underlined genes are known p53 targets, genes in pink are associated with G1 growth arrest, genes in blue are associated with DNA replication, and genes in green are associated with G2/M-phase promotion. (*See* Color Plate 4 following p. 78.)

with respect to the senescent cell morphology because it was originally identified as a mediator of the reversion of round cancer cell morphology to a flattened appearance. Finally, genes that are specifically downregulated during E2 senescence, yet not affected by temperature, are contained in set 6 and include a number of S- and G2/M-phase promoting molecules. It is important to recognize that an optimally controlled temperature-shift experiment such as the one described here does not provide a simple on–off situation. Each of the experimental steps introduces variability and, consequently, differences in the signal intensities between experiments. Variability was observed for a number of genes across the three experiments (see Fig. 2 for illustration). Each experiment was monitored in parallel for successful senescence induction with AdE2ts at the permissive temperature compared to the controls to rule out the possibility that data variations might result from phenotypical variability. Consistent differences that were observed for specific genes in this experimental setting can, therefore, represent stringently, perhaps obligatorily, regulated players in the senescent cell system.

Our working model for E2ts senescence induction is depicted in Fig. 3 *(118)*. E2ts function is compromised at the restrictive temperature, where high levels of the viral oncogenes maintain cellular immortality. Upon shift to the permissive temperature, E2ts represses oncogene expression, followed by cell cycle arrest, traversal through the point of irreversibility, and senescence execution. Gene profiling was performed after the point of no return from senescence. A list of several gene groups is shown below the model, where an asterisk indicates gene induction; all others are repressed genes.

# 6. ANTAGONISTIC ASPECTS OF SENESCENCE AND IMMORTALITY

The upregulation of known mediators of G1 cell growth arrest (p21$^{CIP}$, p57$^{KIP}$, the retinoblastoma p130 family member, and cyclin G2) was in line with the reported G1 arrest. In addition, the S-phase mediator E2F1, several replication proteins, and a large number of genes associated with G2/M progression were found repressed in this system in correlation with the growth-arrested cellular phenotype. Although in some respects pro-carcinogenic (*see* Section 4), cellular senescence is often viewed as a barrier and, thus, functionally opposite to carcinogenesis. Supporting this view is the observed regulation of a number of replication and G2/M-phase progression, which is opposite to their reported expression during E6/E7 oncogene immortalization. These include cyclin F, BUB1, Cdc2, 10, and 20, Polo-like kinase, and TTK protein kinase *(123)*. Inverse expression patterns in the immortalized vs senescent cell system can reflect the ability of E2 to repress E6/E7 expression and, thus, release downstream targets from oncogene control. It will be interesting to determine which of these molecules might have functional roles in cellular immortalization via the suppression of cellular senescence pathways. In this way, novel mediators of cancer initiation or progression and, thus, novel targets for cancer therapy might be identified in the future. Along the same lines, coordinated repression of a group of tumor-associated antigens (GAGE 1, 2, 4, 5, and 6) by E2 was noted. GAGE genes belong to a group of tumor-specific antigens that are presented by human leukocyte antigen (HLA) class I molecules and recognized by cytolytic T-lymphocytes. Because of their tumor-specific expression, GAGE antigens are promising targets for cancer immunotherapy. The downregulation of GAGE genes by E2 not only correlates well with a reversal of the tumorigenic phenotype through E2 senescence but also suggests prospects for GAGE-specific immunotherapy in cervical cancer treatment.

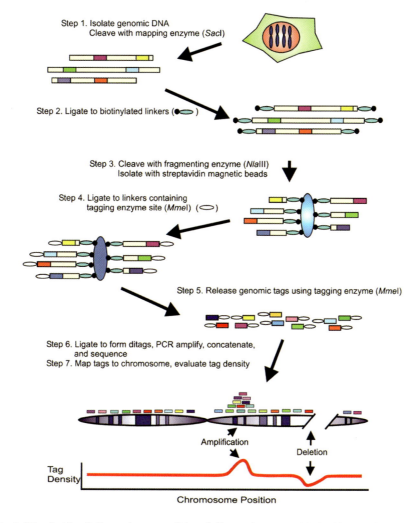

**Color Plate 1, Fig. 2.** (*See* full caption on p. 24 and discussion on p. 23. in Ch. 2. With permission from *PNAS*.) Summary of the Digital Karyotyping procedure.

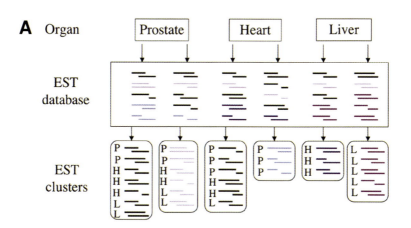

**Color Plate 1, Fig. 1A.** (*See* full caption on p. 34 and discussion on p. 32. in Ch. 3) Schematic description of ESTs from different tissue libraries and their corresponding clusters.

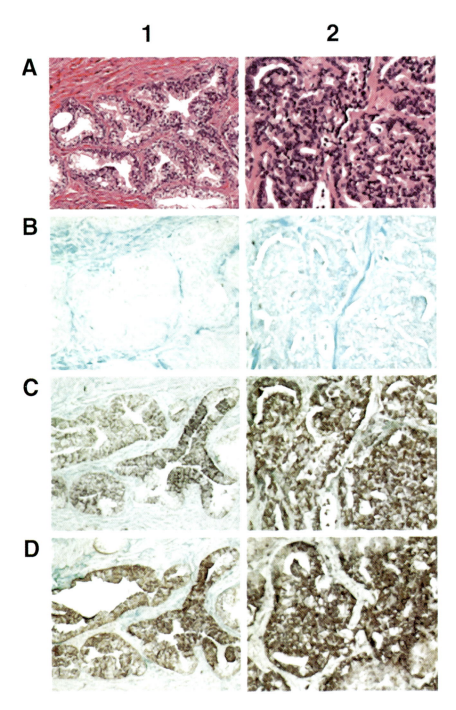

**Color Plate 2, Fig. 3.** (*See* complete caption on p. 36 and discussion on pp. 34–35 in Ch. 3.) Localization of *NGEP* mRNA in epithelial cells of prostate tissues.

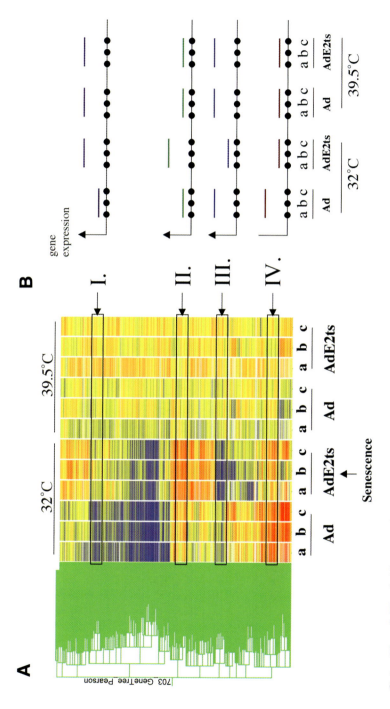

**Color Plate 3, Fig. 1.** (*See* complete caption on p. 76 and discussion on p. 75 in Ch. 6.) A hierarchical tree of senescence-associated transcriptionally regulated genes.

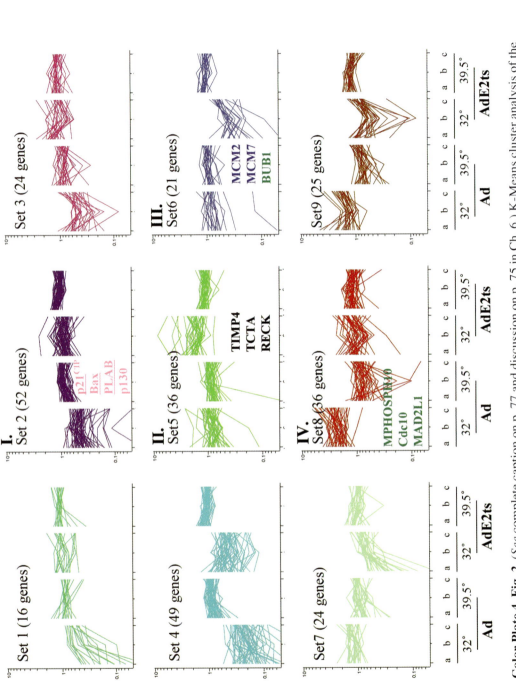

**Color Plate 4, Fig. 2.** (*See* complete caption on p. 77 and discussion on p. 75 in Ch. 6.) K-Means cluster analysis of the most significantly regulated subset of E2 responsive genes.

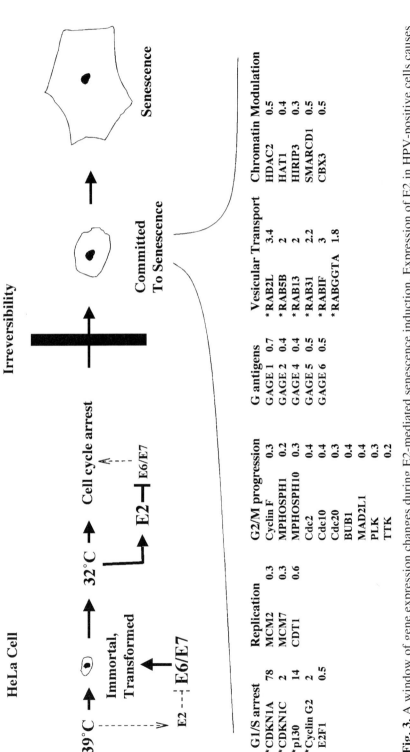

**Fig. 3.** A window of gene expression changes during E2-mediated senescence induction. Expression of E2 in HPV-positive cells causes senescence via the repression of the viral E6/E7 oncogenes. Several gene groups that are regulated during senescence induction were categorized according to biological processes that they are known to regulate. An asterisk marks induced genes. All others are repressed genes. (Modified from ref. *118*.)

## 7. NOVEL PATHWAYS
## REGULATED DURING E2 SENESCENCE

Little is known about the molecular machinery triggering the cellular senescence decision and execution, but a multitude of cellular pathways is likely involved. The above analysis revealed a number of novel candidate gene groups, two of which are depicted in Fig. 3 and discussed here. Coordinate induction of six members and regulators of the Ras-related RAB family of small GTPases, RAB2, 5B, 13, 31, RAB interacting factor and the RAB geranylgeranyltransferase α-subunit might reflect or perhaps even functionally relate to the senescence phenotype. RAB GTPases are highly conserved regulators of fluid-phase and receptor-mediated endocytosis, transport between intracellular compartments, and exocytosis (for review, see ref. *124*). Membrane association of RAB proteins is mediated by C-terminal geranylgeranyl anchors, and RAB protein function is exerted through interactions with specific effectors at individual transport steps. Consistent with the specific localization of RABs, such as RAB2 at pre-Golgi intermediates *(125)*, RAB5B at the plasma membrane *(126)* and RAB13 at epithelial tight junctions *(127)*, different RAB proteins could be required to regulate vesicular trafficking at specific subcellular compartments. Coordinate transcriptional regulation of members and regulators of the RAB GTPase family in senescent cells could stimulate vesicular transport in the HeLa cell system, perhaps with a role in the generally highly vesicularized cytoplasmic appearance of senescent cells. Alternatively, individual aspects of protein trafficking might be causally or consequentially related to senescence. What might be the significance of RAB upregulation during senescence? Considering that HeLa cells were originally derived from an HPV-positive adenocarcinoma of the cervix, the observed vesicular regulation might recapitulate aspects of the glandular differentiation process. It has been argued that senescence might represent a specialized form of differentiation based on known similarities between the two processes. These include a permanent cell cycle arrest, induction of cyclin/cdk kinase inhibitors like p21[CIP], and distinct morphological changes. Existing similarities between the two processes might be further supported by the upregulated expression of the differentiation-specific cyclin G during E2 senescence. An alternative hypothesis relates to the secretion of defined molecules by senescent cells, which might be influenced by RAB GTPase activities in addition to expression levels of the relevant molecules. Because paracrine factors can stimulate the growth of precarcinogenic or carcinogenic neighboring cells *(116)*, the inhibition of RAB-dependent vesicular transport systems might ultimately be useful in the treatment of cancer via senescence. Whether RAB protein regulation lies downstream from the HPV oncogenes, thus perhaps linking HPV-driven transformation and cellular trafficking, remains to be determined. It is not known how and why members and regulators of the RAB protein family might be coordinately induced in the above system and whether such regulation also exists in a normal cellular context. Continued studies of coordinate RAB regulation might therefore, elucidate new aspects of basic transcriptional regulatory networks, perhaps via the identification of common transcriptional cis and trans elements within RAB promoter/enhancer regions. Ultimately, manipulation of these regulatory components might then help define the biological significance for the observed regulation with respect to senescence and cancer.

The field of epigenetics has in recent years greatly expanded our view of chromatin remodeling in cellular senescence, cancer, and aging and has provided important links among these processes (reviewed in refs. *128* and *129*). Defects in the maintenance of repressive heterochromatin accumulate progressively with increased cellular life span and have been hypothesized to ultimately trigger an irreversible exit from the cell cycle and senescence *(130)*. Five chromatin regulatory genes (HDAC2, HAT1, HIRIP3, SMARCD1, and CBX3) were identified within the transcriptome signature of senescent HeLa cells, and each was found to be repressed (Fig. 3). Chemical HDAC inhibitors have been reported to induce senescence in human diploid fibroblasts *(131)* and HPV-positive cervical cancer cells *(132)*, suggesting that repression of the histone deacetylase HDAC2 in the above system might be functionally relevant. However, histone acetylase 1 (HAT1), a functional opposite of HDACs, was also found to be repressed during E2 senescence. This seemingly paradoxical finding might indicate that rather than a defined level of deacetylation, a critical balance between acetylated and deacetylated chromatin is required for cellular proliferation. Disturbing the balance between hypoacetylated and hyperacetylated chromatin domains by either excessive histone acetyltransferase or deacetylase activities might then lead to senescence or apoptosis *(133)* induction depending on additional internal or external parameters. This hypothesis was recently supported in human melanocytes by the finding that levels of histone acetylases p300/CBP decrease with increasing population doublings and that interference with p300–CBP histone acetylase activities can serve as a senescence trigger *(134)*. Repression of three additional components of major chromatin remodeling complexes might play a similar role in the senescence phenotype. The actin-dependent chromatin regulator SMARCD1 is a component of the mammalian SWI/SNF complex, a highly conserved, tumor-suppressive enzyme complex involved in chromatin remodeling and transcription (reviewed in ref. *135*) The chromobox CBX3 protein is a homolog of the Drosophila HP1 family involved in chromatin silencing, nuclear localization, and assembly (reviewed in ref. *136*) The histone-associated HIRIP3 protein was identified on the basis of its interaction with the mammalian HIRA homolog of the *S. cerevisiae* Hir corepressors, which have recently been implicated in the gene-specific targeting of SWI/SNF complexes *(137)*. The fact that several chromatin modifiers are repressed in response to E2 might indicate reduced epigenetic activity and accumulating chromatin defects accompanying or perhaps actively involved in the cellular senescence phenotype.

As described earlier, cervical carcinogenesis depends on the continuous expression of the viral E6 and E7 oncogenes in the affected individual. Transcription of E6/E7 is negatively regulated by E2 and this repression is both necessary and sufficient for a reversal of transformation via senescence *(114,138)*. This argues, in turn, that important senescence mediators must be inhibited by the viral oncoproteins at the onset and during maintenance of HPV-positive carcinogenesis. Regulation of specific genes during E2 senescence might, thus, help elucidate how HPV oncoproteins target important senescence regulators and might uncover basic molecular relationships between HPV carcinogenesis and senescence. Immortalization of human primary foreskin keratinocytes by E6 and E7 reflects certain aspects of carcinogenesis in vivo and, indeed, a number of senescence-associated genes as identified earlier have already turned out to be novel transcriptional targets of HPV oncogenes in this model system (unpublished data). Functional studies of such molecules in senescence and cervical cancer should be interfaced with an assessment of the clinical potential that E2 (and other repressors of E6/E7 activities) might have for cancer treatment. Similarities exist between E2-induced senescence in cervical cancer cells and doxorubicin-induced senescence in human colon carcinoma cells *(139)*. These include the induction of intracellular and secreted growth inhibitory molecules such as p21$^{CIP}$, BTG2, IGFBP-6, Maspin, and MIC-1 in both systems, as well as repression of regulators of mitotic progression PLK1, MAD2, CDC2, and survivin. Emphasis on the role of such common denominators in various senescence systems might ultimately allow for adaptation and application of senescence induction in the treatment of human cancer in general. Interestingly, the above studies of doxorubicin-induced senescence in human colon carcinoma cells have implicated p21$^{CIP}$ in the enhanced expression of clinically undesirable mitogenic and anti-apoptotic paracrine factors, thus emphasizing cancer treatment strategies that might rely on p21$^{CIP}$-independent senescence. Whether similar adjustments might be possible and useful for the treatment of cervical cancer via E6/E7 repression will require clarification of the somewhat controversial role and regulatory consequences of p21$^{CIP}$ activities (97, 118). As mentioned earlier, progress in the field of senescence has been severely hampered by the scarcity of bona fide in vivo senescence markers. Apart from the identification of molecules with roles in the senescence process, upregulated markers might be identifiable in systematic comparisons between senescence vs growth arrest and differentiation models in vitro and in vivo. In summary, continued analyses of genes that are transcriptionally regulated during E2-mediated cellular senescence should aid in the identification of novel markers and regulators of senescence and will yield new insights into cellular senescence mediators that are transcriptionally targeted by viral oncoproteins. We hope that a more detailed understanding of senescence pathways will result in novel diagnostic and therapeutic tools for the treatment of cervical cancer and perhaps other human malignancies in the future.

## REFERENCES

1. Howley PM, Lowy DR. Papillomavirinae: the viruses and their replication. In: Howley PM, Knipe DM, eds. Fields virology. Vol. 2. Philadelphia: Lippincott Williams and Wilkins, 2001:2197–2229.
2. Group IW. Human papillomaviruses. IARC monograph on the evaluation of carcinogenic risks to humans. Lyon, France: International Agency for Research on Cancer, 1995.
3. Ferenczy A, Franco E. Persistent human papillomavirus infection and cervical neoplasia. Lancet 2002; 3:11–16.
4. Parkin DM, Pisani P, Ferlay J. Estimates of the worldwide incidence of 25 major cancers in 1990. Int J Cancer 1999; 80:827–841.
5. Franco EL, Rohan TE, Villa LL. Epidemiologic evidence and human papillomavirus infection as a necessary cause of cervical cancer. J Natl Cancer Inst 1999; 91:506–511.
6. Walboomers JM, Jacobs MV, Manos MM, et al. Human papillomavirus is a necessary cause of invasive cervical cancer worldwide. J Pathol 1999; 189:12–19.
7. Khleif SN, DeGregori J, Yee CL, et al. Inhibition of cyclin D-CDK4/CDK6 activity is associated with an E2F-mediated induction of cyclin kinase inhibitor activity. Proc Natl Acad Sci USA 1996; 93: 4350–4354.
8. Münger K, Phelps WC, Bubb V, Howley PM, Schlegel R. The E6 and E7 genes of the human papillomavirus type 16 together are necessary and sufficient for transformation of primary human keratinocytes. J Virol 1989; 63:4417–4421.
9. Hawley-Nelson P, Vousden KH, Hubbert NL, Lowy DR, Schiller JT. HPV16 E6 and E7 proteins cooperate to immortalize human foreskin keratinocytes. EMBO J 1989; 8:3905–3910.
10. Pecoraro G, Morgan D, Defendi V. Differential effects of human papillomavirus type 6, 16 and 18 DNAs on immortalization and transformation of human cervical epithelial cells. Proc Natl Acad Sci USA 1989, 563–567.
11. Woodworth CD, Doninger J, DiPaolo JA. Immortalization of human foreskin keratinocytes by various human papillomavirus DNAs corresponds to their association with cervical carcinoma. J Virol 1989; 63:159–164.

12. DiPaolo JA, Woodworth CD, Popescu NC, Notario V, Doniger J. Induction of human cervical squa-mous cell carcinoma by sequential transfection with human papillomavirus 16 DNA and viral Harvey ras. Oncogene 1989; 4:395–399.
13. Durst M, Gallahan D, Jay G, Rhim JS. Glucocorticoid-enhanced neoplastic transformation of human keratinocytes by human papillomavirus type 16 and an activated ras oncogene. Virology 1989; 173: 767-771.
14. Hurlin PJ, Kaur P, Smith PP, Perez-Reyes N, Blanton RA, McDougall JK. Progression of human papil-lomavirus type 18-immortalized human keratinocytes to a malignant phenotype. Proc Natl Acad Sci USA 1991; 88:570–574.
15. Chen TM, Pecoraro G, Defendi V. Genetic analysis of in vitro progression of human papillomavirus-transfected human cervical cells. Cancer Res 1993; 53:1167–1171.
16. Schwarz E, Freese UK, Gissman L, et al. Structure and transcription of human papillomavirus sequences in cervical carcinoma cells. Nature 1985; 314:111–114.
17. Alvarez-Salas LM, Cullinan AE, Siwkowski A, Hampel A, DiPaolo JA. Inhibition of HPV-16 E6/E7 immortalization of normal keratinocytes by hairpin ribozymes. Proc Natl Acad Sci USA 1998; 95: 1189–1194.
18. Dowhanick JJ, McBride AA, Howley PM. Suppression of cellular proliferation by the papillomavirus E2 protein. J Virol 1995; 69:7791–7799.
19. Goodwin EC, Naeger LK, Breiding DE, Androphy EJ, DiMaio D. Transactivation-competent bovine papillomavirus E2 protein is specifically required for efficient repression of human papillomavirus oncogene expression and for acute growth inhibition of cervical carcinoma cell lines. J Virol 1998; 72: 3925–3934.
20. Hu G, Liu W, Hanania EG, Fu S, Wang T, Deisseroth AB. Suppression of tumorigenesis by transcrip-tion units expressing the antisense E6 and E7 messenger RNA (mRNA) for the transforming proteins of the human papilloma virus and the sense mRNA for the retinoblastoma gene in cervical carcinoma cells. Cancer Gene Ther 1995; 2:19–32.
21. Hwang ES, Riese DJ, Settleman J, et al. Inhibition of cervical carcinoma cell line proliferation by the introduction of a bovine papillomavirus regulatory gene. J Virol 1993; 67:3720–3729.
22. Venturini F, Braspenning J, Homann M, Gissmann L, Sczakiel G. Kinetic selection of HPV 16 E6/E7-directed antisense nucleic acids: anti-proliferative effects on HPV 16-transformed cells. Nucleic Acids Res 1999; 27:1585–1592.
23. von Knebel Doeberitz M, Rittmuller C, zur Hausen H, Durst M. Inhibition of tumorigenicity of cervical cancer cells in nude mice by HPV E6-E7 anti-sense RNA. Int J Cancer 1992; 51:831–834.
24. Watanabe S, Kanda T, Yoshiike K. Growth dependence of human papillomavirus 16 DNA-positive cervical cancer cell lines and human papillomavirus 16-transformed human and rat cells on the viral oncoproteins. Jpn J Cancer Res 1993; 84:1043–1049.
25. Griep AE, Herber R, Jeon S, Lohse JK, Dubielzig RR, Lambert PF. Tumorigenicity by human papil-lomavirus type 16 E6 and E7 in transgenic mice correlates with alterations in epithelial cell growth and differentiation. J Virol 1993; 67:1373–1384.
26. Comerford SA, Maika SD, Laimins LA, Messing A, Elsasser HP, Hammer RE. E6 and E7 expression from the HPV 18 LCR: development of genital hyperplasia and neoplasia in transgenic mice. Oncogene 1995; 10:587–597.
27. Arbeit JM, Munger K, Howley PM, Hanahan D. Neuroepithelial carcinomas in mice transgenic with human papillomavirus type 16 E6/E7 ORFs. Am J Pathology 1993; 142:1187–1197.
28. Herber R, Liem A, Pitot H, Lambert PF. Squamous epithelial hyperplasia and carcinoma in mice trans-genic for the human papillomavirus type 16 E7 oncogene. J Virol 1996; 70:1873–1881.
29. Song S, Pitot HC, Lambert PF. The human papillomavirus type 16 E6 gene alone is sufficient to induce carcinomas in transgenic animals. J Virol 1999; 73:5887–5893.
30. Riley RR, Duensing S, Brake T, Munger K, Lambert PF, Arbeit JM. Dissection of human papillo-mavirus E6 and E7 function in transgenic mouse models of cervical carcinogenesis. Cancer Res 2003; 63:4862–4871.
31. Munger K, Howley PM. Human papillomavirus immortalization and transformation functions. Virus Res 2002; 89:213–228.
32. Kao WH, Beaudenon SL, Talis AL, Huibregtse JM, Howley PM. Human papillomavirus type 16 E6 induces self-ubiquitination of the E6AP ubiquitin-protein ligase. J Virol 2000; 74:6408–6417.
33. Scheffner M, Werness BA, Huibregtse JM, Levine AJ, Howley PM. The E6 oncoprotein encoded by human papillomavirus types 16 and 18 promotes the degradation of p53. Cell 1990; 63:1129–1136.

34. Gao Q, Singh L, Kumar A, Srinivasan S, Wazer DE, Band V. Human papillomavirus type 16 E6-induced degradation of E6TP1 correlates with its ability to immortalize human mammary epithelial cells. J Virol 2001; 75:4459–4466.

35. Gao Q, Srinivasan S, Boyer SN, Wazer DE, Band V. The E6 oncoproteins of high-risk papillomaviruses bind to a novel putative GAP protein, E6TP1, and target it for degradation. Mol Cell Biol 1999; 19: 733–744.

36. Gross-Mesilaty S, Reinstein E, Bercovich B, et al. Basal and human papillomavirus E6 oncoprotein-induced degradation of Myc proteins by the ubiquitin pathway. Proc Natl Acad Sci USA 1998; 95: 8058–8063.

37. Thomas M, Banks L. Human papillomavirus (HPV) E6 interactions with Bak are conserved amongst E6 proteins from high and low risk HPV types. J Gen Virol 1999; 80(Pt 6):1513–1517.

38. Jackson S, Harwood C, Thomas M, Banks L, Storey A. Role of Bak in UV-induced apoptosis in skin cancer and abrogation by HPV E6 proteins. Genes Dev 2000; 14:3065–3073.

39. Glaunsinger BA, Lee SS, Thomas M, Banks L, Javier R. Interactions of the PDZ-protein MAGI-1 with adenovirus E4-ORF1 and high-risk papillomavirus E6 oncoproteins. Oncogene 2000; 19:5270–5280.

40. Kiyono T, Hiraiwa A, Fujita M, Hayashi Y, Akiyama T, Ishibashi M. Binding of high-risk human papillomavirus E6 oncoproteins to the human homologue of the *Drosophila* discs large tumor suppressor protein. Proc Natl Acad Sci USA 1997; 94:11,612–11,616.

41. Lee SS, Weiss RS, Javier RT. Binding of human virus oncoproteins to hDlg/SAP97, a mammalian homolog of the Drosophila discs large tumor suppressor protein. Proc Natl Acad Sci USA 1997; 94: 6670–6675.

42. Patel D, Huang SM, Baglia LA, McCance DJ. The E6 protein of human papillomavirus type 16 binds to and inhibits co-activation by CBP and p300. EMBO J 1999; 18:5061–5072.

43. Zimmermann H, Degenkolbe R, Bernard HU, O'Connor MJ. The human papillomavirus type 16 E6 oncoprotein can down-regulate p53 activity by targeting the transcriptional coactivator CBP/p300. J Virol 1999; 73:6209–6219.

44. Kumar A, Zhao Y, Meng G, et al. Human papillomavirus oncoprotein E6 inactivates the transcriptional coactivator human ADA3. Mol Cell Biol 2002; 22:5801–5812.

45. Klingelhutz AJ, Foster SA, McDougall JK. Telomerase activation by the E6 gene product of human papillomavirus type 16. Nature 1996; 380:79–81.

46. Dyson N, Howley PM, Munger K, Harlow E. The human papillomavirus-16 E7 oncoprotein is able to bind the retinoblastoma gene product. Science 1989; 243:934–937.

47. Dyson N, Guida P, Munger K, Harlow E. Homologous sequences in adenovirus E1A and human papillomavirus E7 proteins mediate interaction with the same set of cellular proteins. J Virol 1992; 66: 6893–6902.

48. Funk JO, Waga S, Harry JB, Espling E, Stillman B, Galloway DA. Inhibition of CDK activity and PCNA-dependent DNA replication by p21 is blocked by interaction with the HPV-16 E7 oncoprotein. Genes Dev 1997; 11:2090–2100.

49. Jones DL, Alani RM, Munger K. The human papillomavirus E7 oncoprotein can uncouple cellular differentiation and proliferation in human keratinocytes by abrogating p21Cip1-mediated inhibition of cdk2. Genes Dev 1997; 11:2101–2111.

50. Zerfass-Thome K, Zwerschke W, Mannhardt B, Tindle R, Botz JW, Jansen-Durr P. Inactivation of the cdk inhibitor p27KIP1 by the human papillomavirus type 16 E7 oncoprotein. Oncogene 1996; 13: 2323–2330.

51. Massimi P, Pim D, Banks L. Human papillomavirus type 16 E7 binds to the conserved carboxy-terminal region of the TATA box binding protein and this contributes to E7 transforming activity. J Gen Virol 1997; 78(Pt 10):2607–2613.

52. Brehm A, Nielsen SJ, Miska EA, et al. The E7 oncoprotein associates with Mi2 and histone deacetylase activity to promote cell growth. EMBO J 1999; 18:2449–2458.

53. Antinore MJ, Birrer MJ, Patel D, Nader L, McCance DJ. The human papillomavirus type 16 E7 gene product interacts with and trans-activates the AP1 family of transcription factors. EMBO J 1996; 15: 1950–1960.

54. Nead MA, Baglia LA, Antinore MJ, Ludlow JW, McCance DJ. Rb binds c-Jun and activates transcription. EMBO J 1998; 17:2342–2352.

55. Zwerschke W, Mannhardt B, Massimi P, et al. Allosteric activation of acid alpha-glucosidase by the human papillomavirus E7 protein. J Biol Chem 2000; 275:9534–9541.

56. Zwerschke W, Mazurek S, Massimi P, Banks L, Eigenbrodt E, Jansen-Durr P. Modulation of type M2 pyruvate kinase activity by the human papillomavirus type 16 E7 oncoprotein. Proc Natl Acad Sci USA 1999; 96:1291–1296.

57. Mazurek S, Zwerschke W, Jansen-Durr P, Eigenbrodt E. Effects of the human papilloma virus HPV-16 E7 oncoprotein on glycolysis and glutaminolysis: role of pyruvate kinase type M2 and the glycolytic-enzyme complex. Biochem J 2001; 356:247–256.

58. Duensing S, Duensing A, Crum CP, Munger K. Human papillomavirus type 16 E7 oncoprotein-induced abnormal centrosome synthesis is an early event in the evolving malignant phenotype. Cancer Res 2001; 61:2356–2360.

59. Duensing S, Lee LY, Duensing A, et al. The human papillomavirus type 16 E6 and E7 oncoproteins cooperate to induce mitotic defects and genomic instability by uncoupling centrosome duplication from the cell division cycle. Proc Natl Acad Sci USA 2000; 97:10,002–10,007.

60. Duensing S, Munger K. Human papillomavirus type 16 E7 oncoprotein can induce abnormal centrosome duplication through a mechanism independent of inactivation of retinoblastoma protein family members. J Virol 2003; 77:12,331–12,335.

61. Baker CC, Phelps WC, Lindgren V, Braun MJ, Gonda MA, Howley PM. Structural and transcriptional analysis of human papillomavirus type 16 sequences in cervical carcinoma cell lines. J Virol 1987; 61: 962–971.

62. Durst M, Kleinheinz A, Hotz M, Gissmann L. The physical state of human papillomavirus type 16 DNA in benign and malignant genital tumours. J Gen Virol 1985; 66:1515–1522.

63. Jeon S, Lambert PF. Integration of human papillomavirus type 16 into the human genome correlates with a selective growth advantage of cells. J Virol 1995; 69:2989–2997.

64. Park T-W, Fujiwara H, Wright TC. Molecular biology of cervical cancer and its precursors. Cancer 1995; 76:1902–1913.

65. Southern SA, Herrington CS. Disruption of cell cycle control by human papillomaviruses with special reference to cervical carcinoma. Int J Gynecol Cancer 2000; 10:263–274.

66. zur Hausen H. Papillomavirus causing cancer: evasion from host-cell control in early events in carcinogenesis. J Natl Cancer Inst 2000; 92:690–698.

67. Desaintes C, Demeret C. Control of papillomavirus DNA replication and transcription. Semin Cancer Biol 1996; 7:339–347.

68. McBride AA, Romanczuk H, Howley PM. The papillomavirus E2 regulatory proteins. J Biol Chem 1991; 266:18,411–18,414.

69. Hines CS, Meghoo C, Shetty S, Biburger M, Brenowitz M, Hegde RS. DNA structure and flexibility in the sequence-specific binding of papillomavirus E2 proteins. J Mol Biol 1998; 276:809–818.

70. Hedge RS, Rossman SR, Laimins LA, Sigler PB. Crystal structure at 1.7A of the bovine papillomavirus-1 E2 DNA-binding domain bound to its DNA target. Nature 1992; 359:505–512.

71. Hegde RS, Wang A-F, Kim S-S, Schapira M. Subunit rearrangement accompanies sequence-specific DNA binding by the bovine papillomavirus-1 E2 protein. J Mol Biol 1998; 276:797–908.

72. Li R, Knight J, Bream G, Stenlund A, Botchan M. Specific recognition nucleotides and their context determine the affinity of E2 protein for 17 binding sites in the BPV-1 genome. Genes Dev 1989; 3: 510–526.

73. Kim S-S, Tam JK, Wang A-F, Hegde RS. The structural basis of DNA target discrimination by papillomavirus E2 proteins. J Biol Chem 2000; 275:31,245–31,254.

74. Chin MT, Hirochika R, Hirochika H, Broker TR, Chow LT. Regulation of human papillomavirus type 11 enhancer and E6 promoter by activating and repressing proteins from the E2 open reading frame: functional and biochemical studies. J Virol 1988; 62:2994–3002.

75. Cripe TP, Haugen TH, Turk JP, et al. Transcriptional regulation of the human papillomavirus-16 E6-E7 promoter by a keratinocyte-dependent enhancer, and by viral E2 trans-activator and repressor gene products: Implications for cervical carcinogenesis. EMBO J 1987; 6:3745–3753.

76. Dostatni N, Lambert PF, Sousa R, Ham J, Howley PM, Yaniv M. The functional BPV-1 E2 transactiving protein can act as a repressor by preventing formulation of the initiation complex. Genes Dev 1991; 5:1657–1671.

77. Hermonat PL, Spalholz BA, Howley PM. The bovine papillomavirus $P_{2443}$ promoter is E2 *trans*-responsive: evidence for E2 autoregulation. EMBO J 1988; 7:2815–2822.

78. Hirochika H, Broker TR, Chow LT. Enhancers and trans-acting E2 transcriptional factors of papillomaviruses. J Virol 1987; 61:2599–2606.

79. Hirochika H, Hirochika R, Broker TR, Chow LT. Functional mapping of the human papillomavirus type 11 transcriptional enhancer and its interaction with the trans-acting E2 proteins. Genes Dev 1988; 2:54–67.

80. Phelps WC, Howley PM. Transcriptional trans-activation by the human papillomavirus type 16 E2 gene product. J Virol 1987; 61:1630–1638.

81. Thierry F, Howley PM. Functional analysis of E2 mediated repression of the HPV-18 $P_{105}$ promoter. New Biol 1991; 3:90–100.

82. Lee D, Lee B, Kim J, Kim DW, Choe J. cAMP response element-binding protein-binding protein binds to human papillomavirus E2 protein and activates E2-dependent transcription. J Biol Chem 2000; 275: 7045–7051.

83. Lee D, Hwang SG, Kim J, Choe J. Functional Interaction between p/CAF and human papillomavirus E2 protein. J Biol Chem 2002; 277:6483–6489.

84. Breiding DE, Sverdrup F, Grossel MJ, Moscufo N, Boonchai W, Androphy E. Functional interaction of a novel cellular protein with the papillomavirus E2 transactivation domain. Mol Cell Biol 1997; 17: 7208–7219.

85. Benson JD, Lawande R, Howley PM. Conserved interaction of the papillomavirus E2 transcriptional activator proteins with human and yeast TFIIB proteins. J Virol 1997; 71:8041–8047.

86. Rank NM, Lambert PF. Bovine papillomavirus type 1 E2 transcriptional regulators directly bind two cellular transcription factors, TFIID and TFIIB. J Virol 1995; 69:6323–6334.

87. Demeret C, Desaintes C, Yaniv M, Thierry F. Different mechanisms contribute to the E2-mediated transcriptional repression of human papillomavirus type 18 viral oncogenes. J Virol 1997; 71:9343–9349.

88. Romanczuk H, Thierry F, Howley PM. Mutational analysis of *cis*-elements involved in E2 modulation of human papillomavirus type 16 $P_{97}$ and Type 18 $P_{105}$ promoters. J Virol 1990; 64:2849–2859.

89. Tan S-H, Gloss B, Bernard H-U. During negative regulation of the human papillomavirus-16 E6 promoter, the viral E2 protein can displace Sp1 from a proximal promoter element. Nucleic Acids Res 1992; 20:251–256.

90. Romanczuk H, Howley PM. Disruption of either the E1 or the E2 regulatory gene of human papillomavirus type 16 increases viral immortalization capacity. Proc Natl Acad Sci USA 1992; 89:3159–3163.

91. Webster K, Parish J, Pandya M, Stern PL, Clarke AR, Gaston K. The human papillomavirus (HPV) 16 E2 protein induces apoptosis in the absence of other HPV proteins and via a p53-dependent pathway. J Biol Chem 2000; 275:87–94.

92. Desaintes C, Demeret C, Goyat S, Yaniv M, Thierry F. Expression of the papillomavirus E2 protein in HeLa cells leads to apoptosis. EMBO J 1997; 16:504–514.

93. Desaintes C, Goyat S, Garbay S, Yaniv M, Thierry F. Papillomavirus E2 induces p53-independent apoptosis in HeLa cells. Oncogene 1999; 18:4538–4545.

94. Demeret C, Garcia-Carranca A, Thierry F. Transcription-independent triggering of the extrinsic pathway of apoptosis by human papillomavirus 18 E2 protein. Oncogene 2003; 22:168–175.

95. Goodwin EC, Yang E, Lee C-J, Lee H-W, DiMaio D, Hwang E-S. Rapid induction of senescence in human cervical carcinoma cells. Proc Natl Acad Sci USA 2000; 97:10,978–10,983.

96. Wells SI, Francis DA, Karpova AY, Dowhanick JJ, Benson JD, Howley PM. Papillomavirus E2 induces senescence in HPV-positive cells via pRB- and p21$^{CIP}$-dependent pathways. EMBO J 2000; 19:5762–5771.

97. DeFilippis RA, Goodwin EC, Wu L, DiMaio D. Endogenous human papillomavirus E6 and E7 proteins differentially regulate proliferation, senescence, and apoptosis in HeLa cervical carcinoma cells. J Virol 2003; 77:1551–1563.

98. Campisi J. Cancer, aging and cellular senescence. In Vivo 2000; 14:183–188.

99. Lloyd AC. Limits to lifespan. Nature Cell Biol 2002; 4:E25–E27.

100. Dimri GP, Lee X, Basile G, et al. A biomarker that identifies senescent human cells in culture and in aging skin in vivo. Proc Natl Acad Sci USA 1995; 92:9363–9367.

101. von Zglinicki T, Nilsson E, Docke WD, Brunk UT. Lipofuscin accumulation and ageing of fibroblasts. Gerontology 1995; 41(Suppl 2):95–108.

102. Karlseder J, Smogorzewska A, de Lange T. Senescence induced by altered telomere state, not telomere loss. Science 2002; 295:2446–2449.

103. Serrano M, Blasco MA. Putting the stress on senescence. Curr Opin Cell Biol 2001; 13:748–753.

104. Campisi J. Cellular senescence as a tumor-suppressor mechanism. Trends Cell Biol 2001; 11:S27–S31.

105. Lundberg AS, Hahn WC, Gupta P, Weinberg RA. Genes involved in senescence and immortalization. Curr Opin Cell Biol 2000; 12:705–709.

106. Schmitt CA, Fridman JS, Yang M, et al. A senescence program controlled by p53 and p16INK4a contributes to the outcome of cancer therapy. Cell 2002; 109:335–346.

107. Smith JR, Pereira-Smith OM. Replicative senescence: implications for in vivo aging and tumor suppression. Science 1996; 273:63–67.

108. Campisi J, Kim SH, Lim CS, Rubio M. Cellular senescence, cancer and aging: the telomere connection. Exp Gerontol 2001; 36:1619–1637.

109. Cao L, Li W, Kim S, Brodie SG, Deng CX. Senescence, aging, and malignant transformation mediated by p53 in mice lacking the Brca1 full-length isoform. Genes Dev 2003; 17:201–213.

110. Rudolph KL, Chang S, Lee HW, et al. Longevity, stress response, and cancer in aging telomerase-deficient mice. Cell 1999; 96:701–712.

111. Tyner SD, Venkatachalam S, Choi J, et al. p53 mutant mice that display early ageing-associated phenotypes. Nature 2002; 415:45–53.

112. Goodwin EC, DiMaio D. Induced senescence in HeLa cervical carcinoma cells containing elevated telomerase activity and extended telomeres. Cell Growth Differ 2001; 12:525–534.

113. Lee CJ, Suh EJ, Kang HT, et al. Induction of senescence-like state and suppression of telomerase activity through inhibition of HPV E6/E7 gene expression in cells immortalized by HPV16 DNA. Exp Cell Res 2002; 277:173–182.

114. Francis DA, Schmid SI, Howley PM. Repression of the integrated papillomavirus E6/E7 promoter is required for growth suppression of cervical cancer cells. J Virol 2000; 74:2679–2686.

115. Goodwin EC, DiMaio D. Repression of human papillomavirus oncogenes in HeLa cervical carcinoma cells causes the orderly reactivation of dormant tumor suppressor pathways. Proc Natl Acad Sci USA 2000; 97:12,513–12,518.

116. Krtolica A, Parrinello S, Lockett S, Desprez P-Y, Campisi J. Senescent fibroblasts promote epithelial cell growth and tumorigenesis: a link between cancer and aging. Proc Natl Acad Sci USA 2001; 98: 12,072–12,077.

117. Roninson IB. Tumor cell senescence in cancer treatment. Cancer Res 2003; 63:2705–2715.

118. Wells SI, Aronow BJ, Wise TM, Williams SS, Couget JA, Howley PM. Transcriptome signature of irreversible senescence in human papillomavirus-positive cervical cancer cells. Proc Natl Acad Sci USA 2003; 100:7093–7098.

119. DiMaio D, Settleman J. Bovine papillomavirus mutant temperature defective for transformation, replication and transactivation. EMBO J 1988; 7:1197–1204.

120. Aplan PD, Johnson BE, Russell E, Chervinsky DS, Kirsch IR. Cloning and characterization of TCTA, a gene located at the site of a t(1;3) translocation. Cancer Res 1995; 55:1917–1921.

121. Takahashi C, Sheng Z, Horan TP, et al. Regulation of matrix metalloproteinase-9 and inhibition of tumor invasion by the membrane-anchored glycoprotein RECK. Proc Natl Acad Sci USA 1998; 95: 13,221–13,226.

122. Wang M, Liu YE, Greene J, et al. Inhibition of tumor growth and metastasis of human breast cancer cells transfected with tissue inhibitor of metalloproteinase 4. Oncogene 1997; 14:2767–2774.

123. Nees M, Geoghegan JM, Hyman T, Frank S, Miller L, Woodworth CD. Papillomavirus type 16 oncogenes downregulate expression of interferon-responsive genes and upregulate proliferation-associated and NF-kappaB-responsive genes in cervical keratinocytes. J Virol 2001; 75:4283–4296.

124. Segev N. Ypt/rab gtpases: regulators of protein trafficking. Sci STKE 2001; 2001:RE11.

125. Tisdale EJ, Balch WE. Rab2 is essential for the maturation of pre-Golgi intermediates. J Biol Chem 1996; 271:29,372–29,379.

126. Wilson DB, Wilson MP. Identification and subcellular localization of human rab5b, a new member of the ras-related superfamily of GTPases. J Clin Invest 1992; 89:996–1005.

127. Zahraoui A, Joberty G, Arpin M, et al. A small rab GTPase is distributed in cytoplasmic vesicles in nonpolarized cells but colocalizes with the tight junction marker ZO-1 in polarized epithelial cells. J Cell Biol 1994; 124:101–115.

128. Bandyopadhyay D, Medrano EE. The emerging role of epigenetics in cellular and organismal aging. Exp Gerontol 2003; 38:1299–1307.

129. Hasty P, Campisi J, Hoeijmakers J, van Steeg H, Vijg J. Aging and genome maintenance: lessons from the mouse? Science 2003; 299:1355–1359.

130. Howard BH. Replicative senescence: considerations relating to the stability of heterochromatin domains. Exp Gerontol 1996; 31:281–293.

131. Ogryzko VV, Hirai TH, Russanova VR, Barbie DA, Howard BH. Human fibroblast commitment to a senescence-like state in response to histone deacetylase inhibitors is cell cycle dependent. Mol Cell Biol 1996; 16:5210–5218.
132. Terao Y, Nishida J, Horiuchi S, et al. Sodium butyrate induces growth arrest and senescence-like phenotypes in gynecologic cancer cells. Int J Cancer 2001; 94:257–267.
133. Finzer P, Kuntzen C, Soto U, zur Hausen H, Rosl F. Inhibitors of histone deacetylase arrest cell cycle and induce apoptosis in cervical carcinoma cells circumventing human papillomavirus oncogene expression. Oncogene 2001; 20:4768–4776.
134. Bandyopadhyay D, Okan NA, Bales E, Nascimento L, Cole PA, Medrano EE. Down-regulation of p300/CBP histone acetyltransferase activates a senescence checkpoint in human melanocytes. Cancer Res 2002; 62:6231–6239.
135. Klochendler-Yeivin A, Muchardt C, Yaniv M. SWI/SNF chromatin remodeling and cancer. Curr Opin Genet Dev 2002; 12:73–79.
136. Eissenberg JC, Elgin SC. The HP1 protein family: getting a grip on chromatin. Curr Opin Genet Dev 2000; 10:204–210.
137. Dimova D, Nackerdien Z, Furgeson S, Eguchi S, Osley MA. A role for transcriptional repressors in targeting the yeast Swi/Snf complex. Mol Cell 1999; 4:75–83.
138. Hall AH, Alexander KA. RNA Interference of human papillomavirus Type 18 E6 and E7 induces senescence in HeLa cells. J Virol 2003; 77:6066–6069.
139. Chang BD, Swift ME, Shen M, Fang J, Broude EV, Roninson IB. Molecular determinants of terminal growth arrest induced in tumor cells by a chemotherapeutic agent. Proc Natl Acad Sci USA 2002; 99: 389–394.

# II ADVANCES IN PROTEOMIC AND ENZYMATIC CANCER-PROFILING TECHNOLOGIES

# 7

# Mass-Spectrometry-Based Proteomics for Cancer Biology

*Chen Xu, PhD and John R. Yates III, PhD*

## SUMMARY

Proteomic technology has accelerated the discovery of protein function in biological systems. To achieve these advances, mass spectrometry methods have been developed for facile identification of proteins separated by gel electrophoresis or separated by liquid chromatography. A detailed description of proteomic methods to discover new elements of biological systems and to understand protein function is presented. Current use of these techniques in cancer research is described.

**Key Words:** Mass-spectrometry; protein identification; quantitation; electrospray ionization; MALDI; MudPIT; 2-DGE.

## 1. INTRODUCTION

Preceding the introduction of proteomics technology, genomic techniques were used to understand disease mechanisms in cancer research. After the completion of the Human Genome Project, the characterization of the proteins encoded by the genome became a more feasible undertaking to extend the knowledge obtained through genetic and genomic study of cancer disease mechanisms. A synergistic relationship developed between mass-spectrometry-based proteomic technologies and the sequence infrastructures produced through large-scale whole-genome sequencing. The study of the gene products will be essential to discover new biomarkers and therapeutic targets for the diagnosis and treatment of cancer and generally increase our mechanistic understanding of tumorigenesis.

From: *Cancer Drug Discovery and Development: The Oncogenomics Handbook*
Edited by: W. J. LaRochelle and R. A. Shimkets © Humana Press Inc., Totowa, NJ

This chapter gives an overview of mass-spectrometry-based proteomics, followed by a brief discussion of applications in drug target identification, biomarker discovery, and cancer treatments.

## 2. OVERVIEW OF MASS-SPECTROMETRY-BASED PROTEOMICS TECHNOLOGY (FIG. 1)

### *2.1. Mass Spectrometry*

Mass spectrometers consist of three elements: an ion source that converts molecules into gas-phase ions, a mass analyzer that separates individual mass-to-charge ratios ($m/z$) of the ionized analytes, and an ion detector that registers the number of ions at each $m/z$ value *(1–3)*. The invention of electrospray ionization (ESI) and matrix-assisted laser desorption/ionization (MALDI) techniques has revolutionized the field of biological mass spectrometry *(4,5)*. The capability of ESI and MALDI to create intact gas-phase ions from polar or charged molecules is the principle force driving the extension of mass range of molecules amenable to mass spectrometry and the resolution of the ions detected, making them the two most commonly used ionization methods for large-scale proteomics research. These soft ionization techniques have stimulated technological developments in mass spectrometers to further extend its power through increases in sensitivity, resolution, mass accuracy, dynamic range, and throughput.

#### 2.1.1. IONIZATION

Electrospray ionization operates at atmospheric pressure and produces a fine mist of charged droplets through an electric potential placed between a capillary and the inlet to a mass spectrometer *(4)*. By applying a drying gas or heat, the solvent evaporates and the droplet shrinks, eventually resulting in the formation of desolvated ions. A characteristic of ESI is the formation of intact multiply-charged ions that lowers the $m/z$ values for high-molecular-weight biomolecules to a range easily measured by many different types of mass spectrometer. Once the charge state of the ions is determined, an accurate molecular weight can be calculated. Another feature of ESI is continuous ionization, which makes it readily adaptable to tandem MS instruments, including time-of-flight (TOF), ion trap (ITMS), and quadrupole mass spectrometers.

MALDI creates ions from polar or charged biomolecules embedded in a dry, crystalline ultraviolet (UV)-absorbing matrix *(5)*. After the energy of the nitrogen laser (generally 337 nm) is absorbed by the matrix crystals, emission of the absorbed energy causes rapid thermal expansion of matrix and analyte into the gas phase. MALDI produces primarily singly-charged ions resulting from proton transfer from analyte to matrix. MALDI is also less sensitive to common components of biological buffers than ESI. However, as a pulsed ionization technique, MALDI can only interface to mass analyzers capable of collecting ions for subsequent $m/z$ separation (ITMS and Fourier transform mass spectrometry [FTMS]) or be capable of measuring a complete mass spectrum for each ionization event (TOF).

#### 2.1.2. MASS ANALYZERS

Mass analyzers use electric or magnetic fields to manipulate ions in a mass-dependent manner. There are three basic types of mass analyzer currently used in proteomics research. These are the ion trap, time-of-flight (TOF), and quadrupole analyzers. They are very different in design and performance, each with its own strengths and weakness. These analyzers

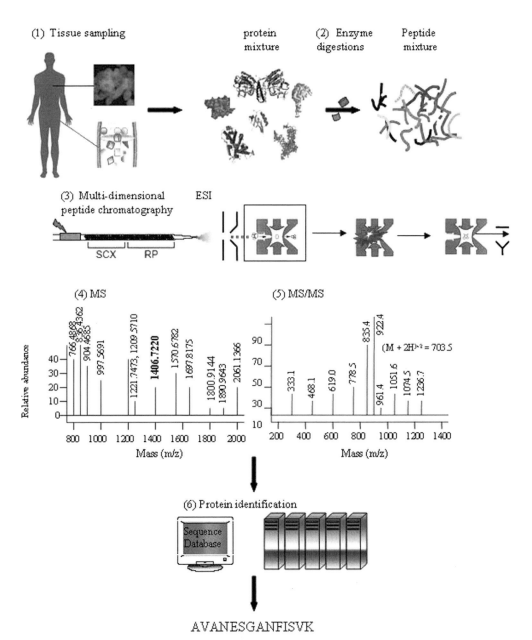

**Fig. 1.** Schematic illustrating six general procedures involved in mass-spectrometry-based proteomics analysis. Step 1: protein mixtures are extracted and fractionated from tissue samples; step 2: enzymatic digestion, to produce a complex peptide mixture; step 3: separate the peptides by multidimensional capillary LC and directly eluted them off from the column into an electrospray ion source. The multiply protonated peptides then enters a mass spectrometer in step 4 for generating MS spectrum. Step 5: a series of tandem mass spectra (MS/MS) are performed on selected ions. These MS and MS/MS spectra are used for identify proteins using computer algorithm to search against protein databases for the best matches (step 6).

can be stand-alone or, in some cases, put together in tandem to take advantage of the strengths of each (Fig. 2).

Ion-trap (IT) analyzers create three-dimensional radio-frequency (RF) fields to trap ions in the center of a ring electrode for a certain time interval (6,7). The field can be manipulated to selectively eject ions of a particular $m/z$ value to a detector to record the $m/z$ ratios or to selectively retain a particular $m/z$ value for collision-activated dissociation (CAD), which is used to fragment ions by exciting the trapped ions to increase their motion, causing hundreds to thousands of ion-molecular collisions with the helium bath gas. Thus, additional structural information is obtained about the selected precursor ion. This represents the primary advantage of tandem mass spectrometry in selecting a particular precursor ion from a mixture of ions, thereby creating a powerful tool for peptide mixture analysis (7). Ion traps are robust, sensitive, and relatively inexpensive, and so have produced much of the proteomics data reported in the literature. However, relatively low mass accuracy (±0.3 amu) is a disadvantage of the ion trap. Space-charging arises when the accumulated number of ions exceeds the capacity of the ion trap, which negatively affects the accuracy of mass measurement by perturbing the ideal motion of ions in electric field. The linear or two-dimensional ion trap is an exciting recent development where ions are stored in a cylindrical volume that is considerably larger than that of the traditional three-dimensional (3D) ion traps, allowing more efficient ion trapping and greater ion-trapping capacity with increased sensitivity, dynamic range, resolution, and mass accuracy (8–11).

A mainstay of research and applications in mass spectrometry over the last 15 yr has been the triple-quadrupole mass spectrometers (12). Quadrupole (Q) mass spectrometers use a RF voltage applied to four metal rods, the quadrupoles, with RF voltage of alternate polarity placed on opposite rods. A direct (DC) voltage is overlayed on the rods. The time-varying electric fields maintained by the ratio of RF to DC voltage permit a stable trajectory only for ions of a particular desired $m/z$ value as they pass through the analyzer. Ions of a particular $m/z$ are selected in a first section (Q1), fragmented within a collision cell (Q2), and the fragments then separated in Q3 (5,13–15). The resulting fragment ion current is recorded at a detector as ions exit the analyzer.

Reflector time-of-flight (TOF) mass analyzers accelerate a packet of ions with a set of electric potentials to high kinetic energy and separate them by the time they take to traverse a flight tube. The ions are reflected in an ion mirror, which compensates for slight differences in kinetic energy, and then impinge on a detector that amplifies and counts arriving ions. An $m/z$ value can be determined by measuring the time required for an ion to move from the ion source to the detector (16). More recently, TOF mass analyzers have been combined to incorporate a collision cell between two TOF sections, thus creating tandem mass spectrometers (TOF-TOF) (17–19). Ions of one $m/z$ ratio are selected in the first TOF section, fragmented in the collision cell, and the masses of the fragments are separated in the second TOF section.

Hybrid mass spectrometers such as quadrupole TOF instrument that combine quadrupole with TOF mass analyzers have been constructed to produce unique capabilities (20, 21). In a quadrupole TOF instrument, the collision cell is placed between a quadrupole mass filter and a TOF analyzer. Ions of a particular $m/z$ are selected in the first mass analyzer (quadrupole), and fragmented in a collision cell, and the fragment ion masses are recorded by a TOF analyzer. Q-TOF hybrids produce mass spectra with 5,000–10,000 resolution and 10–50 ppm mass accuracy.

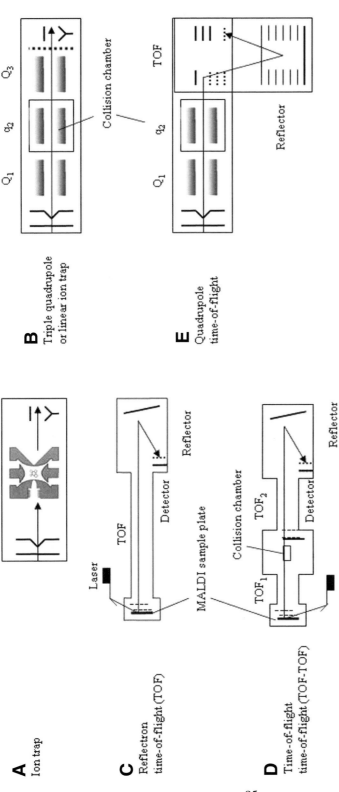

**Fig. 2.** Schematic of the five mass spectrometers most often used in proteome research. (**A**) Quadrupole ion trap mass spectrometer; the 3D, as well as the linear ion trap, captures and isolates a precursor ion by ejecting all other ions from the trap. The isolated ion then fragments by multiple low-energy collisions resulting from the application of a resonance voltage. The fragmented ions are scanned out to generate the tandem mass spectrum. (**B**) Triple quadrupole mass spectrometer. Ions are selected in the first section (Q1) and fragmented in a collision chamber (Q2); the fragmented ions are separated in the last mass analyzer (Q3). (**C**) Reflectron TOF mass spectrometer. Ions are accelerated from the ion source into the field-free region, then turned around in a reflector. Ions are separated based on kinetic energy difference, with the lighter fragment ions exiting earlier. A particular $m/z$ value can be selected by timing the arrival of ions at an electronic gate. (**D**) TOF-TOF tandem mass spectrometer. A collision cell is incorporated between two TOF sections for collision-induced dissociation (CID). Ions are selected in the first TOF section based on mass-to-charge ratio and passed into the collision cell for activation. The fragments are subsequently separated in the second TOF section. (**E**) Quadrupole TOF mass spectrometer. In this hybrid instrument, the third quadrupole section is replaced by a TOF analyzer, where the Q1 mass-selected and Q2 dissociated ions are pulsed into the reflector and then impinge onto the detector for recording ions.

95

### 2.1.3. ESI-MS/MS

Electrospray ionization has mostly been coupled with ion traps and triple-quadrupole instruments that are able to perform two-stage (or multistage) mass analysis of selected precursor ions to generate fragment ion spectra (CID spectra).

Although ESI is generally tolerant of low levels of buffers, salts, and detergents, these substances can either suppress the formation of analyte ions or form adducts with the analyte interfering with molecular mass determination. ESI ionizes the analytes out of a solution; thus, it is readily interfaced with high-performance liquid chromatography (HPLC) to eliminate contaminated substances from the analytes prior to ionization *(3)*. High sensitivity can also be achieved with ESI when flow rates are reduced to 100 nL/min or less *(3)*. Furthermore, multiple protonation of proteins and peptides make amide bonds more prone to fragmentation during collision-induced dissociation (CID), thereby promoting the generation of tandem mass spectrum for protein identification.

### 2.1.4. MALDI-TOF AND MALDI-TOF-TOF

Matrix-assisted laser desorption/ionization is usually coupled to TOF analyzers that measure the collection of ions created by the laser pulse without scanning the mass range. More recently, new configurations of ion sources and mass analyzers have found wide application for protein analysis *(22)*. The use of higher-repetition-rate lasers yielded MS/MS rates comparable with, and potentially greater than, liquid chromatography (LC)-ESI-MS/MS. To allow the fragmentation of MALDI-generated precursor ions, MALDI ion sources have recently been coupled to quadrupole ion-trap mass spectrometers and two types of TOF instrument (TOF-TOF and Q-TOF). The quadrupole TOF instrument can be used interchangeably with an ESI ionization source *(23)*. The resulting fragment ion spectra are often more extensive and informative than those generated in trapping instruments.

### 2.1.5. SELDI-TOF

Surface-enhanced laser desorption/ionization time-of-flight mass spectrometry (SELDI-TOF MS) extends MALDI-TOF's capability by incorporating an element of chromatography-based selection to isolate different sets of proteins based on their biophysical properties *(24,25)*. By combining protein capture on chromatographic surfaces with MS and artificial intelligence, SELDI is capability of generating protein profiles reproducibly from crude biological fluids with relative high throughput. The ease and speed of screening samples have made SELDI a popular method for biomarker discovery *(26)*. Ion signatures generated by cluster analysis has achieved high specificity and sensitivity for ovarian, prostate, and breast cancer diagnosis *(27–32)*. Despite these impressive results, a different view argues against the commonly held idea that biomolecules or fragments of biomolecules constituting the diagnostic pattern are derived from the tumor itself, thus casting doubt on the value of using the signature pattern for diagnosis *(33)*. Validation will need to rely on extensive clinical trials. SELDI has limitations in the ability to detect large ions and, thus, implementing the strategy with higher performance mass analyzers and tandem mass spectrometers to further characterize those unknown molecules are warranted. Better interpretation of the diagnostic patterns for a better understanding of cancer disease mechanism would be useful.

The contribution of laser capture microdissection (LCM) to SELDI's success in biomarker discovery cannot be overstated *(34,35)*. Cancer proteomics has long been hampered by limited sample material and tissue heterogeneity. The capability of LCM to enrich cells of interest from tissue sections overcame the problem of tissue heterogeneity, thus becoming an indispensable component of the SELDI-TOF technique in cancer biomarker discovery.

## 2.2. Large-Scale Separation Methods in Proteomics

Cells are complicated entities containing a variety of different proteins. Therefore, pre-fractionation of protein mixtures before mass spectrometry analysis is often desirable. Separations can be conducted either before protease digestion to resolve intact protein mixtures into individual component or after protease digestion to reduce the complexity of peptide mixtures to the extent that can be analyzed by a mass spectrometer in maximum capacity (36–38). Both strategies could also incorporate affinity capture to isolate groups of proteins or peptides with specific functionality or modification for subproteome analysis (39).

### 2.2.1. MULTIDIMENSIONAL SEPARATIONS OF PROTEINS

Two-dimensional polyacrylamide gel electrophoresis (2D-PAGE) is the most familiar multidimensional separation method in proteomics. The power of 2D-PAGE resides in its orthogonal separation format: separating proteins in the first dimension according to their isoelectric point and in the second dimension by denaturing gel electrophoresis based on molecular weight (40). The use of 2D-PAGE for large-scale protein profiling can be traced back more than 25 yr, even preceding genomic profiling (41). 2D-PAGE separations gained increased relevance when MALDI TOF mass spectrometers and ESI tandem mass spectrometers allowed proteins to be readily identified (42–45). The capability of using mass spectra of peptides for sequence database searches made rapid identification of proteins a reality. Software for differential 2D-PAGE analysis allows the identification of proteins in diseases with altered expression so that critical proteins in diseases and relevant for drug discovery can be profiled and quantitatively mapped. However, 2D-PAGE is not amenable to high-throughput automation and has difficulty detecting proteins at the extreme of both molecular weight and isoelectric point. More importantly, 2D-PAGE has limitations in its sensitivity and dynamic range, leading to difficulty in detecting low-abundance proteins (46). The separation of integral membrane, membrane-associated, and other hydrophobic proteins by 2D-PAGE remains a significant challenge as well (47–50).

Because of these limitations, other multidimensional methods for the fractionation of protein mixtures have been developed. Opiteck et al. attempted the coupling of strong cation-exchange (SCX) or size-exclusion chromatography (SEC) with reversed-phase (RP) HPLC for *Escherichia coli* whole-cell lysates (51,52). Results showed a limited resolution. A recent study by Wagner reported a more impressive result in terms of peak capacity and short analysis time for small proteins and peptides from a human hemofiltrate (53). However, the multipump and valve configuration for the combination of ion-exchange (IEX) with RP chromatography made it a somewhat cumbersome practice. Other multi-dimensional formats such as liquid-phase isoelectric focusing (IEF) with fast RP-HPLC, and either continuous-tube gel electrophoresis or continuous-elution gel electrophoresis with RP-HPLC have been explored to resolve proteins from whole-cell lysates (54). These methods have made some improvement in identifying basic and low-molecular-weight proteins compared to 2D gel electrophoresis (37); however, their peak capacity still lags behind that of 2D gel electrophoresis. Furthermore, the inability to rapidly identify unknown proteins by molecular weight alone remains the intrinsic weakness for applying these multidimensional protein separation methods for proteome analysis.

### 2.2.2. Multidimensional Separations of Peptides

Early multidimensional peptides separations based on the combination of IEX or SEC with RP-HPLC, capillary electrophoresis (CE) with RP-HPLC, and SEC, RP with CE have been proof-of-principle in the context of mapping peptides from known proteins. Of the various LC-based multi-dimensional peptide separation strategies, the most prevalent method is the multidimensional protein identification technology (MudPIT). MudPIT was introduced by Yates' Laboratory (38,55,56). This technique uses one or more proteases to digest proteins extracted from the biological material of interest to form a more complex peptide mixture. This peptide mixture is then fractionated by a specially packed biphasic LC column composed of a strong cation exchange (SCX) support as the initial phase and a RP material as the second phase. Peptides are eluted from the SCX phase onto the RP phase in a series of salt steps that increase in concentration. A subsequent RP gradient separates the peptides and delivers the peptides into the mass spectrometer through a nanoelectrospray source to generate tandem mass spectra for each individual peptide. These MS/MS spectra can then be searched using the SEQUEST algorithm against a protein database to identify various proteins extracted from the cell. MudPIT can identify proteins over a wide range of p$I$'s and molecular weights (55). Because of the increased sensitivity and dynamic range of sophisticated mass spectrometer, MudPIT is also capable of detecting low-abundance proteins such as transcription factors and protein kinases (55), which has significant applications in cancer research. Furthermore, MudPIT has shown improved confidence in comprehensive mapping of posttranslationally modified sites in complex protein mixtures (57). The most impressive aspect of MudPIT is its success in identifying membrane proteins (58,59). The surface membrane is a rich source of growth factor receptors that regulating signal transduction pathways critical in oncogenesis. Anticancer therapies have been developed targeting growth factor receptors itself such as HER2 (Herceptin) or specific components of the receptor mediated signal transduction pathway such as EGFR (Erbitux) (60,61). The restricted expression pattern of HER2 in breast cancer has also be used successfully as a biomarker to select effective therapy and to predict therapeutic response and prognosis (62). In viewing the importance of membrane proteins in cancer treatment and diagnosis, it is natural to envision that MudPIT, with its unique strength in membrane protein identification, will play a significant role in anticancer drug target and cancer diagnosis biomarker discovery.

### 2.2.3. Affinity-Based Multidimensional Separation

Affinity-based separation methods have been used in conjunction with RP-HPLC for the specific enrichment and fractionation of proteins and peptides with defined functionality or modification that constitute subproteomes. Two biologically important subproteomes are the phosphoproteome and glycoproteome. Preliminary experiments using $Fe^{3+}$ or $Ga^{3+}$ immobilized metal-affinity chromatography (IMAC) has shown specific enrichment of phosphorylated peptides from a protein digest or synthetic peptide mixture (63,64). These captured phosphopeptides were then separated by a second dimension, CE or RP-HPLC (65,66). More recently, Ficarro et al. reported a significant improvement of the specificity of IMAC-$Fe^{3+}$ by minimizing column interaction with free carboxylate groups via methyl ester derivatization. Coupling with RP-HPLC and a automated tandem mass spectrometry, they were able to identify 216 phosphopeptides out of the total of number of over 1000 from whole-cell lysate. Tyrosine phosphorylation on rare and low-abundance proteins has also been detected *(67)*.

The same affinity concept can be applied to the analysis of glycosylated peptides by using specific lectins. Regnier's group has coupled lectin affinity chromatography with RP chromatography for identifying whole proteins in a complex mixture through the proposed signature peptide approach *(68)*. A more recent study also shows that mannose-binding proteins can be identified by coupling $\alpha$-D-mannose-based affinity chromatography with 1D electrophoresis (1DE) followed by HPLC tandem mass spectrometry *(69)*.

Another application of affinity-based multidimensional separation is using avidin affinity chromatography to capture peptides containing biotinylated cysteine from a complex peptide mixture followed by the second-dimension RP-HPLC separation *(70)*. Taken together, multidimensional affinity chromatography has shown increasing power to identify and characterize specific classes of peptides and proteins in subproteomes.

## *2.3. Quantitation*

The ability to quantify protein expression in normal vs diseased tissue is important for discovering biomarker and therapeutic targets. Mass spectrometry can be used for quantification but requires the use of internal standards. This is because different peptides ionize with different efficiencies, depending on the precise chemical properties of the polypeptide, and it is impractical to include a control peptide for every possible protein present within a proteomics sample. Quantitative methods based on isotope tagging of peptides have since been developed. Washburn et al. has incorporated a quantitative component to MudPIT by metabolic labeling cell cultures in $^{14}N$ vs $^{15}N$. The subsequent ratio of $^{14}N : ^{15}N$ was determined to quantify >800 proteins with a dynamic range of at least 10 : 1 *(71)*. A second method uses proteolytic digestion in the presence of $^{18}O$ or $^{16}O$ water *(72,73)*. A useful labeling method is the isotope-coded affinity tag (ICAT) developed by Gygi et al. *(74)*. Briefly, samples to be compared are each labeled at cysteine residues with either a d0 or deuterated d8 ICAT$^{TM}$ agent. The samples are then combined and enzymatically digested to generate peptide fragments. Cysteine-tagged peptides are then captured by the avidin affinity of the biotin moiety of ICAT reagent. Affinity-captured peptides are subsequently separated by RP-HPLC and analyzed by mass spectrometry. Because the mass spectrometer responds similarly to both tags, which only differ by 8 amu, yet give a slight spacing of the *m/z* peaks in the spectrum, the relative abundance of peptides from each sample can be determined from the ratio of peak intensities. ICAT has shown impressive results in the systematic identification and quantification of 491 proteins contained in the microsomal fractions of naive and in vitro differentiated human myeloid leukemia (HL-60) cells *(75)*.

The drawback of ICAT is that only cysteine-containing peptides can be analyzed. Approaches such as the global internal standard strategy (GIST) has since been introduced to overcome this problem *(76–78)*. ICAT still cannot accurately measure the expression levels of all proteins because the orders of magnitude difference in the proteome might not coincide with the dynamic range of the chemical tag. In addition, ICAT might not be sufficient to label minute amounts of sample because of unfavorable kinetics. This can be overcome by either labeling with up to 55 *M* concentration of large excess of $^{18}O$

or $^{16}O$ water to favor the reaction kinetics or using newly developed chemical agent that can achieve 100% alkylation of all –SH residues in complex proteins *(79)*.

It is worth noting that the concept of isotope metabolic labeling for cultured cells has been extended to label a whole animal. Preliminary results show that the $^{15}N$ isotope can be successfully incorporated into proteins from various tissues within the animal *(86)*. The subtractive proteomics approach is a more sophisticated variation of MudPIT. It provides an elegant approach to discover novel disease-related proteins using animal model systems of disease.

## 2.4. Identifying Proteins With Mass Spectrometry

An essential feature of global proteomic is high-throughput analysis. Mass spectrometry when coupled with algorithm-based database searching can meet this requirement by quickly generating data and simplifying data analysis. The two main protein identification approaches—peptide mass mapping and peptide tandem mass spectrometry—are performed on peptides of the protein because of their more uniform size and chemistry. Peptide molecular-weight measurements are predictive of amino acid composition, and peptide fragmentation information relates to amino acid sequence. Both types of information can be correlated to protein sequences in the database.

### 2.4.1. PEPTIDE MASS FINGERPRINTING

A widely used approach to identify a protein is to first digest the unknown protein with a protease of known specificity such as trypsin. By measuring the masses of this resulting peptide set, a mass fingerprint can be readily derived. This mass map is then compared against the theoretical one generated by the same protease of each protein in a database *(3,81)*. When more than three peptide masses match (depending on the accuracy of the molecular-weight measurement), a unique protein is generally considered to be identified. The identification of heavily modified proteins can be more difficult because some peptide molecular weights might not match because of the difficulty of predicting sites of posttranslational modification. In this case, as long as a statistically significant number of other peptides from the protein can be matched to a protein in the database, this problem can be overcome.

Although peptide mass fingerprinting has become the primary technology for large-scale proteomics analysis when coupled with 2D-GE (gel electrophoresis) and MALDI-TOF, there are several important limitations. One is that the database must contain enough of the protein sequence to compare with experimentally derived mass maps for the identification of variants derived from alternative splicing or transcript editing. The most significant limitation of MALDI-TOF peptide mass mapping is the inability to correctly identify proteins from mixtures containing three or more proteins. It becomes more and more difficult for protein identification when the number of proteins and/or their degree of modification increases. Proteins in complex mixtures are unlikely to be identified.

### 2.4.2. PEPTIDE SEQUENCING

These problems can be circumvented by a second approach to identify proteins in mixtures through the use of tandem mass spectra of peptides derived from proteins in the mixtures *(82,83)*. In this method, peptide mixtures derived from enzyme digestion of intact proteins is separated by HPLC and introduced into a mass spectrometer for MS/MS spectra acquisition. In the collision-induced dissociation (CID) process, peptides fragmentation occurs in a predictable manner. Although tandem mass spectra contain information that is specific to the amino acid sequence of peptides, manual evaluation of peptide MS/MS spectra is tedious. Therefore, a rapid and accurate automated peptide sequence interpretation method has been developed by comparing experimental MS/MS data with predicted MS/MS spectra generated from database sequence. This can either be done by partial sequence interpretation to generate sequence tags followed by a database query *(84)* or by an uninterrupted comparison of the experimental spectrum to predicted spectra from the database. Using the latter method, the SEQUEST program has proven to be quite robust and sensitive in identifying the peptide from which a given MS/MS spectrum was formed.

An advantage of this approach is that each peptide tandem mass spectrum represents a unique piece of information; consequently, matching one or more tandem mass spectra to sequences in the same protein provides a high level of confidence in the identification. Another advantage is the ability of tandem mass spectrometry to rapidly and precisely isolate and fragment peptides so that identification of proteins, even if they exist in a mixture, is achievable *(85)*.

## 3. MASS-SPECTROMETRY-BASED PROTEOMICS: APPLICATIONS IN CANCER DRUG TARGETS DISCOVERY, DIAGNOSIS, AND TREATMENT

### *3.1. Cancer Drug Targets Identification*

Membrane proteins are common drug and antibody targets *(86)*. The three postgenomics mechanism-based cancer drugs and antibody, Gleevec, Herceptin, and Iressa, are all targeted against membrane proteins *(87–89)*. These therapeutic successes have led to efforts to adopt cutting-edge technology such as mass-spectrometry-based proteomics to speed up the traditional one-molecule-at-a-time-based approach for cancer therapeutic targets discovery. The most recent achievement is potential therapeutic targets identification by a comprehensive proteomic analysis using the breast cancer cell membrane *(90)*. In this study, tandem mass spectra were searched against a comprehensive database using the SEQUEST search program, resulting in the identification of tumor-cell-specific plasma-membrane-associated novel proteins. Among them are many highly abundant proteins such as her2/neu and rare unique proteins such as BCMP101, showing a wide dynamic range of breast cancer membrane proteins. Three unique proteins, BCMP11/hAG3, BCMP101, and BCMP84, were characterized further and found significant expression in clinical breast tumor tissues. Among them, BCMP11/hAG3 was found to have potential localization in secretory organelles, interacts with C4.4A, and represents a potential autocrine receptor for BCMP11. BCMP101 has highly restricted expression in breast cancer with localization in the plasma membrane and interaction with $\alpha$-1-catenin, through which its potential role of blocking tumor suppression can be achieved. BCMP84 is particularly interesting in terms of tumor-specific translocation from cytosol to plasma membrane in breast cancer. This translocation of BCMP84 is regulated in a calcium-dependent manner through interaction with nucleobindin, which has strong association with Ga proteins. These findings suggests a possible role for BCMP84 in G-protein-coupled signal transduction events and further showcase the strength of mass-spectrometry-based proteomic in detecting cancer-associated protein translocation, an event that cannot be detected at the level of transcriptome.

Stathmin (Op18), a major tubulin regulatory protein in leukemia, has been discovered by 2D electrophoresis (2DE) mass-spectrometry-based proteomics as a potential target to inhibit the proliferation of leukemia cell *(91,92)*. Stathmin is a substrate of several kinase families; thus, it is a phosphorylation-responsive regulator of multiple signal transduction pathways in microtubule dynamics. The study showed a significant overexpression of the phosphorylated form of Stathmin in childhood leukemia *(93)*. The important role of Stathmin in regulating leukemia cell proliferation and differentiation was further confirmed by an in vivo functional study *(92)*. This study emphasized the unsurpassed power of mass-spectrometry-based proteomics to identify posttranslational modified proteins as a cancer therapeutic target because genomics lack the ability to detect protein posttranslational modifications.

These studies suggest that application of more advanced methodologies such as multidimensional protein identification technology or isotope-coded affinity tagging as well as new MS technologies, including linear ion trap and TOF-TOF instruments, could enable the direct identification of proteins of lower abundance and posttranslational modifications for the discovery of potential targets for cancer therapy.

### 3.2. Proteomics for Cancer Diagnosis, Cancer Recurrence Prediction, and Personalized Cancer Therapy Monitoring

Early diagnosis of ovarian cancer has been shown to yield cure rates of 95%, whereas late-stage discovery results in a cure rate of only 35% *(94,95)*. A novel biomarker for early diagnosis of ovarian cancer is critical because the conventional biomarker CA-125 is relatively insensitive for early-stage detection of ovarian cancer *(96)*. Using mass-spectrometry-based proteomics approach, Petricoin et al. has achieved a breakthrough in identifying distinctive serum protein pattern "fingerprints" to discriminate ovarian cancer patient from normal with 100% sensitivity and 95% specificity, which was improved to 100% sensitivity and 100% specificity, respectively, by a more sophisticated bioinformatic approach *(27,97)*. This result showed the emergence of an accurate yet cost-effective, real-time, noninvasiveness proteomic method for early-stage detection of ovarian cancer. Similar proteomic techniques have also been developed for other cancers, including prostate, breast, lung, and colon cancers *(29–32,98–100)*.

Clinical trials sponsored by the National Cancer Institute (NCI) are ongoing for further assessment and validation of proteomic technology in diagnosing and staging ovarian cancer for regulatory approval *(101,102)*. In parallel, pilot studies are underway to evaluate proteomic technology for predicting the recurrence of epithelial ovarian cancer after first remission, selecting appropriate therapy regimens, and identifying patient subpopulations that will respond to therapy.

Proteomics can also be used as a tool to understand cancer drug function. Gleevec (imatinib mesylate) is a targeted therapy, designed to interfere with the function of two tyrosine kinases, c-kit and the PDGF (platelet-derived growth factor) receptor, suggesting Gleevec as a potential therapy for patients with ovarian cancer *(103)*. In the much anticipated phase II trial to evaluate the effectiveness of Gleevec and determine whether it affects the predicted pathways in cancer cells, biopsies of patients' tumors will be taken prior to and after treatment. The proteomic pattern will then be measured and correlated to clinical response to treatment for a better understanding of the specific ways that Gleevec affects tumor cells. The result of this study can also be used to help physicians determine early in treatment whether Gleevec is working effectively for an individual cancer patient, suggesting an approach to tailor treatment to individual patients. Similar studies are under-going at NCI to use the proteomic approach for the monitoring of key pathways influenced by the molecularly targeted drugs Herceptin® and Iressa®.

## 4. CONCLUDING REMARKS

As mass-spectrometry-based methods for protein analysis have begun to mature, their use is rapidly expanding throughout biology. It is only natural for proteomic methods to find increasing utility in cancer research. Initial applications in studies to understand or discover the functions of proteins involved in cellular processes have evolved into efforts to discover biomarkers representative of disease status. As both mass spectrometry tech-nology and proteomic applications will continue to evolve at high rates, these applications are only the tip of the iceberg.

## REFERENCES

1. Aebersold R, Mann M. Mass spectrometry-based proteomics. Nature 2003; 422:198–207.
2. Lin D, Tabb DL, Yates JR III. Large-scale protein identification using mass spectrometry. Biochim Biophys Acta 2003; 1646:1–10.
3. Yates JR III. Mass spectrometry and the age of the proteome. J Mass Spectrom 1998; 33:1–19.
4. Fenn JB, Mann M, Meng CK, Wong SF, Whitehouse CM. Electrospray ionization for the mass spec-trometry of large biomolecules. Science 1989; 246:64–71.
5. Karas M, Hillenkamp F. Laser desorption ionization of proteins with molecular mass exceeding 10000 daltons. Anal Chem 1988; 60:2299–2301.
6. Busch K, Glish SA, McLuckey SA. Mass Spectrometry/Mass Spectrometry: techniques and applica-tions of tandem mass spectrometry. New York: VCH, 1988.
7. Jonscher KR, Yates JR III. The quadrupole ion trap mass spectrometer—a small solution to a big chal-lenge. Anal Biochem 1997; 244:1–15.
8. Hager JW. A new linear ion trap mass spectrometer. Rapid Commun Mass Spectrom 2002; 16:512–526.
9. Schwartz JC, Senko MW, Syka JEP. A two-dimensional quadrupole ion trap mass spectrometer. J Am Soc Mass Spectrom 2002; 13:659–669.
10. Wells JM, Badman ER, Cooks RG. A quadrupole ion trap with cylindrical geometry operated in the mass-selective instability mode. Anal Chem 1998; 70:438–444.
11. Tabert AM, Griep-Raming J, Guymon AJ, Cooks RG. High-throughput miniature cylindrical ion trap array mass spectrometer. Anal Chem 2003; 75:5656–5664.
12. Yates JR III. Protein structure analysis by mass spectrometry. Methods Enzymol 1996; 271:351–377.
13. McLafferty FW. Tandem mass spectrometry. New York: Wiley–Interscience, 1983.
14. Dongre AR, Somogyi A, Wysocki VH. Surface-induced dissociation: an effective tool to probe struc-ture, energetics and fragmentation mechanisms of protonated peptides. J Mass Spectrom 1996; 31:339–350.
15. Schwartz JC, Wade AP, Enke CG, Cooks RG. Systematic delineation of scan modes in multidimen-sional mass spectrometry. Anal Chem 1990; 62:1809–1818.
16. Cotter RJ. Time-of-flight mass spectrometry: an increasing role in the life sciences. Biomed Environ Mass Spectrom 1989; 18:513–532.
17. Cornish TJ, Cotter RJ. Tandem time-of-flight mass spectrometry. Anal Chem 1993; 65:1043–1047.
18. Cordero MM, Cornish TJ, Lys IA, Cotter RJ. Sequencing peptides without scanning the reflectron: post-source decay with a curved-field reflectron time-of-flight mass spectrometer. Rapid Commun Mass Spectrom 1995; 9:1356–1361.
19. Medzihradszky KF, Campbell JM, Baldwin MA, Falick PJ, Vestal ML, Burlingame AL. The character-istics of peptide collision-induced dissociation using a high-performance MALDI-TOF/TOF tandem mass spectrometer. Anal Chem 2000; 72:552–558.
20. Morris HR, Paxton T, Dell A, Langhorne J, Berg M, Bordoli RS, et al. (1996) High sensitivity col-lisionally-activated decomposition tandem mass spectrometry on a novel quadrupole/orthogonal-accel-eration time-of-flight mass spectrometer. Rapid Commun Mass Spectrom 1996; 10:889–896.

21. Loboda AV, Krutchinsky AN, Bromirski M, Ens W, Standing KG. A tandem quadrupole/time-of-flight mass spectrometer with a matrix-assisted laser desorption/ionization source: design and performance. Rapid Commun Mass Spectrom 2000; 14:1047–1057.

22. Mo W, Karger BL. Analytical aspects of mass spectrometry and proteomics. Curr Opin Chem Biol 2002; 6:666–675.

23. Krutchinsky AN, Zhang W, Chait BT. Rapidly switchable matrix-assisted laser desorption/ionization and electrospray quadrupole-time-of-flight mass spectrometry for protein identification. J Am Soc Mass Spectrom 2000; 11:493–504.

24. Hutchens TW, Yip TT. New desorption strategies for the mass-spectrometric analysis of macromolecules. Rapid Commun Mass Spectrom 1993; 7:576–580.

25. Tang N, Tomatore P, Weinberger SR. Current developments in SELDI affinity technology. Mass Spectrom Rev 2004; 23:34–44.

26. Issaq HJ, Veenstra TD, Conrads TP, Felschow D. The SELDI-TOF MS approach to proteomics: protein profiling and biomarker identification. Biochem Biophys Res Commun 2002; 292:587–592.

27. Petricoin EF, Ardekani AM, Hitt BA, Levine PJ, Fusaro VA, Steinberg SM, et al. Use of proteomic patterns in serum to identify ovarian cancer. Lancet 2002; 359:572–577.

28. Ardekani AM, Liotta LA, Petricoin EF III. Clinical potential of proteomics in the diagnosis of ovarian cancer. Expert Rev Mol Diagn 2002; 2:312–320.

29. Grubb RL, Calvert VS, Wulkuhle JD, Paweletz CP, Linehan WM, Phillips JL, et al. Signal pathway profiling of prostate cancer using reverse phase protein arrays. Proteomics 2003; 3:2142–2146.

30. Cazares LH, Adam B-L, Ward MD, Nasim S, Schellhammer PF, Semmes OJ, et al. Normal, benign, preoplastic, and malignant prostate cells have distinct protein expression profiles resolved by surface enhanced laser desorption/ionization mass spectrometry. Clin Cancer Res 2002; 8:2541–2552.

31. Paweletz CP, Trock B, Pennanen M, Tsangaris T, Magnant C, Liotta LA. Proteomic patterns of nipple aspirate fluids obtained by SELDI-TOF: potential for new biomarkers to aid in the diagnosis of breast cancer. Dis Markers 2001; 17:301–307.

32. Zhang LJ, Rosenzweig J, Wang YY, Chan DW. Proteomic and bioinformatics approaches for identification of serum biomarkers to detect breast cancer. Clin Chem 2002; 48:1296–1304.

33. Diamandis EP. Point: proteomics patterns in biological fluids: do they represent the future of cancer diagnostics? Clin Chem 2003; 49:1272–1275.

34. Simone N, Paweletz CP, Charboneau L, Petricoin EF III, Liotta LA. Laser capture microdissection: beyond functional genomics to proteomics. Mol Diag 2000; 5:301–307.

35. Craven RA, Banks RE. Laser capture microdissection and proteomics: possibilities and limitation. Proteomics 2001; 1:1200–1204.

36. Ong SE, Pandey A. An evaluation of the use of two-dimensional gel electrophoresis in proteomics. Biomol Eng 2001; 18:195–205.

37. Wall DB, Kachman MT, Gong S, Hinderer R, Parus S, Misek DE, et al. Isoelectric focusing nonporous RP HPLC: a two-dimensional liquid-phase separation method for mapping of cellular proteins with identification using MALDI-TOF mass spectrometry. Anal Chem 2000; 72:1099–1111.

38. Link AJ, Eng J, Schieltz DM, Carmack E, Mize GJ, Morris DR, et al. Direct analysis of protein complexes using mass spectrometry. Nature Biotechnol 1999; 17:676–682.

39. Link A. Multidimensional peptide separations in proteomics. Trends Biotechnol 2002; 20:S8–S13.

40. Klose J, Kobalz U. Two-dimensional electrophoresis of proteins: an updated protocol and implications for a functional analysis of the genome. Electrophoresis 1995; 16:1034–1059.

41. O'Farrell PH. High resolution two-dimensional electrophoresis of proteins. J Biol Chem 1975; 250: 4007–4021.

42. Cottrell JS. Protein identification by peptide mass fingerprinting. Pept Res 1994; 7:115–124.

43. Wilm M, Shevchenko A, Houthaeve T, Breit S, Schweigerer L, Fotsis T, et al. Femtomole sequencing of proteins from polyacrylamide gels by nano-electrospray mass spectrometry. Nature 1996; 379: 466–469.

44. Henzel WJ, Billeci TM, Stults JT, Wong SC, Grimley C, Watanabe C. Identifying proteins from two-dimensional gels by molecular mass searching of peptide fragments in protein sequence databases. Proc Natl Acad Sci USA 1993; 90:5011–5015.

45. Rosenfeld J, Capdevielle J, Guillemot JC, Ferrara P. In-gel digestion of proteins for internal sequence analysis after one- or two-dimensional gel electrophoresis. Anal Biochem 1992; 203:173–179.

46. Gygi SP, Corthals GL, Zhang Y, Rochon Y, Aebersold R. Evaluation of two-dimensional gel electrophoresis-based proteome analysis technology. Proc Natl Acad Sci USA 2000; 97:9390–9395.

47. Vuillard L, Marret N, Rabilloud T. Enhancing protein solubilization with nondetergent sulfobetaines. Electrophoresis 1995; 16:295–297.

48. Rabilloud T. Solubilization of proteins for electrophoretic analyses. Electrophoresis 1996; 17:813–829.

49. Rabilloud T, Adessi C, Giraudel A, Lunardi J. Improvement of the solubilization of proteins in two-dimensional electrophoresis with immobilized pH gradients. Electrophoresis 1997; 18:307–316.

50. Galeva N, Altermann M. Comparison of one-diemnsional and two-dimensional gel electrophoresis as a separation tool for proteomic analysis of rat liver microsomes: cytochromes P450 and other membrane proteins. Proteomics 2002; 2:713–722.

51. Opiteck GJ, Lewis KC, Jorgenson JW, Anderegg RJ. Comprehensive on-line LC/LC/MS of proteins. Anal Chem 1997; 69:1518–1524.

52. Opiteck GJ, Ramirez SM, Jorgenson JW, Moseley MA III. Comprehensive two-dimensional high-performance liquid chromatography for the isolation of overexpressed proteins and proteome mapping. Anal Biochem 1998; 258:349–361.

53. Wagner K, Miliotis T, Marko-Varga G, Bischoff R, Unger KK. An automated on-line multidimensional HPLC system for protein and peptide mapping with integrated sample preparation. Anal Chem 2002; 74:809–820.

54. Meng F, Cargile BJ, Patrie SM, Johnson JR, McLoughlin SM, Kelleher NL. Processing complex mixtures of intact proteins for direct analysis by mass spectrometry. Anal Chem 2002; 74:2923–2929.

55. Washburn MP, Wolters D, Yates JR III. Large-scale analysis of the yeast proteome by multidimensional protein identification technology. Nat Biotechnol 2001; 19:242–247.

56. Wolters DA, Washburn MP, Yates JR III. An automated multidimensional protein identification technology for shotgun proteomics. Anal Chem 2001; 73:5683–5690.

57. MacCoss MJ, McDonald WH, Saraf A, Sadygov R, Clark JM, Tasto JJ, et al. Shotgun identification of protein modifications from protein complexes and lens tissue. Proc Natl Acad Sci USA 2002; 99: 7900–7905.

58. Wu CC, MacCoss MJ, Howell KE, Yates JR III. A method for the comprehensive proteomic analysis of membrane proteins. Nature Biotechnol 2003; 21:532–538.

59. Wu CC, Yates JR III. The application of mass spectrometry to membrane proteomics. Nature Biotechnol 2003; 21:262–267.

60. Goldenberg MM. (1999) Trastuzumab, a recombinant DNA-derived humanized monoclonal antibody, a novel agent for the treatment of metastatic breast cancer. Clin Ther 1999; 21:309–318.

61. Ciardiello F, De VF, Orditura M, De PS, Tortora G. Epidermal growth factor receptor tyrosine kinase inhibitors in late stage clinical trials. Expert Opin Emerg Drugs 2003; 8:501–514.

62. Ross JS, Gray GS. Targeted therapy for cancer: the HER-2/neu and Herceptin story. Clin Leadersh Manag Rev 2003; 17:333–340.

63. Andersson L, Porath J. Isolation of phosphoproteins by immobilized metal ($Fe^{3+}$) affinity chromatography. Anal Biochem 1986; 154:250–254.

64. Posewitz MC, Tempst P. Immobilized gallium (III) affinity chromatography of phosphopeptides. Anal Chem 1999; 71:2883–2892.

65. Cao P, Stults JT. Mapping the phosphorylation sites of proteins using on-line immobilized metal affinity chromatography/capillary electrophoresis/electrospray ionization multiple stage tandem mass spectrometry. Rapid Commun Mass Spectrom 2000; 14:1600–1606.

66. Watts JD, Affolter M, Krebs DL, Wange RL, Samelson LE, Aebersold R. Identification by electrospray ionization mass spectrometry of the sites of tyrosine phosphorylation induced in activated Jurkat T cells on the protein tyrosine kinase ZAP-70. J Biol Chem 1994; 269:29,520–29,529.

67. Ficarro SB, Mccleland ML, Stukenberg PT, Burke DJ, Ross MM, Shabanowitz J, et al. Phosphoproteome analysis by mass spectrometry and its application to *Saccaromyces cerevisiae*. Nature Biotechnol 2002; 20:301–305.

68. Geng M, Ji J, Regnier FE. Signature-peptide approach to detecting proteins in complex mixtures. J Chromatogr A 2000; 870:295–313.

69. Andon NL, Eckert D, Yates JR 3rd, Haynes PA. High-throughput functional affinity purification of mannose binding proteins from *Oryza sativa*. Proteomics 2003; 3:1270–1278.

70. Gygi SP, Rist B, Griffin TJ, Eng J, Aebersold R. Proteome analysis of low-abundance proteins using multidimensional chromatography and isotope-coded affinity tags. J Proteome Res 2002; 1:47–54.

71. Washburn MP, Ulaszek R, Deciu C, Schieltz DM, Yates JR III. Analysis of quantitative proteomic data generated via multidimensional protein identification technology. Anal Chem 2002; 74:1650–1657.

72. Stewart II, Thomson T, Figeys D. 18O labeling: a tool for proteomics. Rapid Commun Mass Spectrom 2001; 15:2456–2465.

73. Mirgorodskaya OA, Kozmgin YP, Titov MI, Korner R, Sonksem CP, Roepstorff P. Quantitation of peptides and proteins by matrix-assisted laser desorption/ionization mass spectrometry using (18)O-labeled internal standards. Rapid Commun Mass Spectrom 2000; 14:1226–1232.

74. Gygi SP, Rist B, Gerber SA, Turecek F, Gelb MH, Aebersold R. Quantitative analysis of complex protein mixtures using isotope-coded affinity tags. Nature Biotechnol 1999; 17:994–999.

75. Han DK, Eng J, Zhou H, Aebersold R. Quantitative profiling of differentiation-induced microsomal proteins using isotope-coded affinity tags and mass spectrometry. Nature Biotechnol 2001; 19:946–951.

76. Ji J, Chakraborty A, Geng M, Zhang X, Amini A, Bina M, et al. Strategy for qualitative and quantitative analysis in proteomics based on signature peptides. J Chromatogr B Biomed Sci Appl 2000; 745: 197–210.

77. Chakraborty A, Regnier FE. Global internal standard technology for comparative proteomics. J Chromatogr A 2002; 949:173–184.

78. Hamdan M, Righetti PG. Assessment of protein expression by means of 2-D gel electrophoresis with and without mass spectrometry. Mass Spectrom Rev 2003; 22:272–284.

79. Sebastiano R, Citterio A, Lapadula M, Righetti PG. A new deuterated alkylating agent for quantitative proteomics. Rapid Commun Mass Spectrom 2003; 17:2380–2386.

80. Schirmer EC, Florens L, Guan T, Yates JR III, Gerace L. Nuclear membrane proteins with potential disease links found by subtractive proteomics. Science 2003; 301:1380–1382.

81. Yates JR III, McCormack AL, Eng J. Mining genomes with mass spectrometry. Anal Chem 1996; 68: 534A–540A.

82. Eng JK, McCormack AL, Yates JR III. An approach to correlate tandem mass spectral data of peptides with amino acid sequences in a protein database. J Am Soc Mass Spectrom 1994; 5:976–989.

83. Yates JR III. Mass spectrometry from genomics to proteomics. Trends Genet 2000; 16:5–8.

84. Mann M, Wilm M. Error-tolerant identification of peptides in sequence databases by peptides in sequence databases by peptide sequence tags. Anal Chem 1994; 66:4390–4399.

85. McCormack AL, Schieltz DM, Goode B, Yang S, Barnes G, Drubin D, et al. Direct analysis and identification of proteins in mixtures by LC/MS/MS and database searching at the low-femtomole level. Anal Chem 1997; 69:767–776.

86. Hopkins AL, Groom CR. The druggable genome. Nature Rev Drug Discov 2003; 1:727–730.

87. O'Dwyer ME, Mauro MJ, Druker BJ. STI571 as a targeted therapy for CML. Cancer Invest 2003; 21: 429–438.

88. Brenner TL, Adams VR. First Mab approved for treatment of metastatic breast cancer. J Am Pharm Assoc 1999; 39:236–238.

89. Ranson M, Mansor W, Jayson G. ZD1839 (IRESSA): a selective EGFR-TK inhibitor. Expert Rev Anticancer Ther 2002; 2:161–168.

90. Adam PJ, Boyd R, Tyson KL, Fletcher GC, Stamps A, Hudson L, et al. Comprehensive proteomic analysis of breast cancer cell membranes reveals unique proteins with potential roles in clinical cancer. J Biol Chem 2003; 278:6482–6489.

91. Hanash SM, Baier LJ, McCurry L, Schwartz S. Lineage related polypeptide markers in acute lymphoblastic leukemia detected by two-dimensional electrophoresis. Proc Natl Acad Sci USA 1986; 83: 807–811.

92. Hanash SM, Madoz-Gurpide J, Misek DE. Identification of novel targets for cancer therapy using expression proteomics. Leukemia 2002; 16:478–485.

93. Melhem R, Hailat N, Kuick R, Hanash SM. (1997) Quantitative analysis of Op18 phosphorylation in childhood acute leukemia. Leukemia 1997; 11:1690–1695.

94. Friedlander ML. Prognostic factors in ovarian cancer. Semin Oncol 1998; 25:305–314.

95. McGuire V, Jesser CA, Whittemore AS. (2002) Survival among U.S. women with invasive epithelial ovarian cancer. Gynecol Oncol 2002; 84:399–403.

96. Bast RG, Klug TL, St. John E, Jennison E. A radioimmunoassay using a monoclonal antibody to monitor the course of epithelial ovarian cancer. N Engl J Med 1983; 309:883–887.

97. Zhu W, Wang X, Ma Y, Rao M, Glimm J, Kovach JS. Detection of cancer-specific markers amid massive mass spectral data. Proc Natl Acad Sci USA 2003; 100:14,666–14,671.

98. Zhukov TA, Johanson RA, Cantor AB, Clark RA, Tockman MS. Discovery of distinct protein profiles specific for lung tumors and pre-malignant lung lesions by SELDI mass spectrometry. Lung Cancer 2003; 40:267–279.

99. Yanagisawa K, Shyr Y, Xu BJX, Massion PP, Larsen PH, White BC, et al. Proteomics patterns of tumour subsets in non-small-cell lung cancer. Lancet 2003; 362:433–439.

100. Satoshi N, Sing-Tsung C, Fuad GG. Diagnostic markers that distinguish colon and ovarian adeno-carcinomas: identification by genomic, proteomic, and tissue array profiling. Cancer Res 2003; 63: 5243–5250.

101. Espina V, Dettloff KA, Cowherd S, Petricoin EF III, Liotta LA. Use of proteomic analysis to monitor responses to biological therapies. Expert Opin Biol Ther 2004; 4:83–93.

102. Reynolds T. Validating biomarkers: early detection research network launches first phase III study. J Natl Cancer Inst 2003; 95:422–423.

103. Schmandt RE, Broaddus R, Lu KH, Shvartsman H, Thornton A, Malpica A, et al. Expression of c-ABL, c-KIT, and platelet-derived growth factor receptor-beta in ovarian serous carcinoma and normal ovarian surface epithelium. Cancer 2003; 98:758–764.

# 8

# Chemical Proteomics in Drug Development

*Douglas A. Jeffery, PhD, Amos Baruch, PhD, and Matthew Bogyo, PhD*

## Contents

## Summary

Small-molecule activity-based probes (ABPs) can be applied to several stages in the drug discovery process. These biochemical tools bind irreversibly to target enzymes and can be used to monitor enzyme activity in complex protein mixtures, live cells, or whole organisms. Chemical probes have been used to identify and validate drug targets and to assess enzyme inhibitor potency and selectivity. In addition, they can be used to validate animal models of disease and measure drug pharmacodynamics in both preclinical and clinical studies. Most of the work with chemical probes has focused on the study of cysteine proteases and serine hydrolases/proteases, but recent work has expanded the repertoire of enzyme families that can be targeted by ABPs. This chapter will focus both on recent applications of chemical probes to drug discovery as well as potential future applications of this powerful technology.

**Key Words:** Activity-based probes; affinity probes; chemical proteomics; drug discovery and development; cysteine proteases; serine proteases; oncology.

From: *Cancer Drug Discovery and Development: The Oncogenomics Handbook*
Edited by: W. J. LaRochelle and R. A. Shimkets © Humana Press Inc., Totowa, NJ

# 1. INTRODUCTION

The process of drug discovery and development has changed dramatically in the last 5 yr, particularly with respect to anticancer therapeutics. The newest generations of drugs are designed to target specific proteins in critical metabolic and regulatory pathways rather than function via generally cytotoxic mechanisms. With the approval of Herceptin *(1)*, Glivec *(2)*, Velcade *(3)*, and Iressa *(4)*, there is now support for the idea that cancer can be treated by targeting a single molecule or enzyme in a single defined pathway. Such "rational" therapies are likely to lead to a reduction in the commonly observed side effects associated with general cytotoxic agents. Discovery of targeted cancer drugs requires a molecular understanding of the pathways that control cell growth. Now that the human genome has been sequenced *(5,6)* and the total complement of human proteins can be at least partially predicted, it is hoped that, with time, all of the pathways involved in cell growth and survival will be mapped out. Such an understanding of global cellular pathways could lead to the identification of new drug targets and the development of targeted therapies to treat many different diseases.

Large-scale bioanalytical technologies have recently begun to emerge with the goal of understanding signaling pathways through the elucidation of the complement of protein interactions, modifications, activities, structures, and subcellular localizations in cells. Such techniques can be used to define the global networks involved in the complex regulation of cell physiology. Some of the more commonly used techniques include 2D gel electrophoresis *(7)*, mass-spectrometry-based protein quantitation *(8)*, protein–protein "interactome" mapping *(9)*, posttranslational modification identification *(10)*, chemical proteomics *(11,12)*, proteomic subcellular localization *(13)*, high-throughput protein crystallization *(14,15)*, and systems biology *(16)*. This chapter will focus on the multidisciplinary field of chemical proteomics and how its application to the drug discovery process can speed the development of new anticancer drugs.

The central component of the chemical proteomic technology is the synthetic activity-based probe (ABP). This reactive small molecule covalently modifies the active site of an enzyme and can be subsequently visualized using a reporter group (Fig. 1). Because enzyme modification is activity dependent, it allows identification of active targets and provides a quantifiable readout of target activity under defined physiological conditions. Application of ABPs to complex proteomes at various stages of disease progression therefore provides information regarding the identity of enzymes whose regulated activity is likely to be required for establishment of disease pathology. Furthermore, an ABP serves as a direct link to the active site of an enzyme, thereby allowing direct screening for lead compounds to validate their potential as drug targets. Thus, chemical proteomics can be implemented to accelerate the drug discovery and development process at multiple stages (Fig. 2).

# 2. THE CHEMICAL PROBE

The ABP has three functional elements: the reactive group or warhead; a reporter group or attachment site for a reporter group; and a linker region connecting these two elements (Fig. 1A). The design and synthesis of class-specific probes that covalently attach to the active sites of enzymes is the first and foremost challenge. Probes must be designed such that they are specifically reactive toward the enzyme(s) of interest yet not reactive toward other molecules present in the complex milieu of the cell or cell extract. A detailed under-

**A**

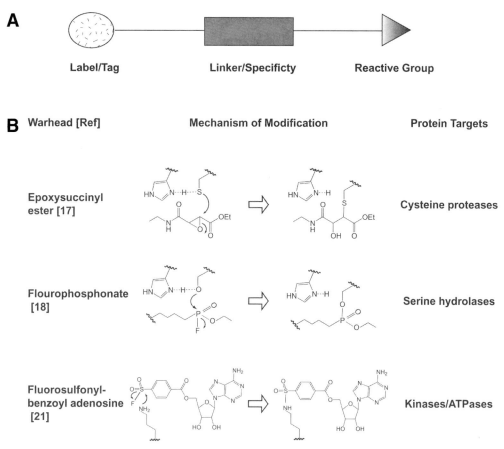

**B**

Fig. 1. (A) Schematic of the general structure of a chemical probe. The probe consists of three parts: a warhead that reacts covalently with the enzyme(s) of interest, a linker that promotes solubility and infers specificity, and a tag (e.g., biotin or fluorophore) that is used to visualize the labeled enzyme, normally by sodium dodecyl sulfate–polyacrylamide gel electrophoresis. (B) Three examples of chemical probes, their mechanism of action, and target enzymes. The epoxysuccinyl ester probe, typi-fied by DCG04 *(17)*, and based on the natural product E-64 *(18)*, is very specific for the papain family of cysteine proteases and reacts covalently with the active-site cysteine. A ring-opening event at the epoxide group is the irreversible chemical reaction. The flourophosphonate warhead is very specific for serine hydrolases *(19)*, and reacts with the active-site serine nucleophile. This results in the loss of fluoride ion and covalent bond formation. FSBA (5'-*O*-[4-fluorosulfonylbenzoyl]-ester of ade-nosine) is an ATP mimetic that reacts covalently with a number of ATP-binding enzymes, most nota-bly protein kinases *(20)*. For protein kinases, an active-site lysine residue binds covalently to the sulfone *(21)* with the subsequent release of fluoride ion.

standing of the enzyme reaction mechanism, substrate(s), and kinetics is often, but not always, critical to the design of such a specific probe. The second challenge is the syn-thesis of the probe itself, which can often be complicated by complex chemistries. Several reviews have been recently published regarding the design of chemical probes and their structures *(11,12)*, therefore, we will only briefly touch on issues of probe design in this chapter.

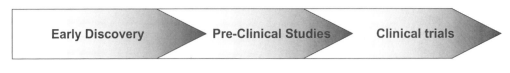

**Early Discovery**          **Pre-Clinical Studies**          **Clinical trials**

Target Identification                Model Selection                      *In vivo* Imaging
 - Enzyme activity profiling          - Target localization                 - Target inhibition
Lead Optimization                    *In vivo* Pharmacodynamics          *Ex vivo* Pharmacodynamics
 - Off-target identification           - Target inhibition                   - Target inhibition
 - Measurement of inhibitor          Toxicology                          Biomarkers
   potency and selectivity            - Off-target identification           - Efficacy readout, disease
                                                                              progression

**Fig. 2.** List of the areas of the drug development pipeline where chemical probes can provide value. Chemical probes can be applied at all of the stages of drug discovery and development. *See* text for details.

## 3. THE REACTIVE GROUP

Small-molecule ABPs forms covalent, irreversible bonds with target enzymes. It is the reactive group, or warhead, that controls the selectivity of this reactivity (Fig. 1B). The use of small-molecule covalent modifiers of proteins and enzymes is not a new concept in biological research, but their use in chemical probes has increased in recent years. The majority of warheads contain an electrophilic group that reacts with a nucleophilic amino acid side chain that is essential for the catalytic mechanism of the enzyme or that is present in the vicinity of the active site. This class of probe is simply a mechanism-based inhibitor that binds to the active site of an enzyme, thereby facilitating direct attack by the active-site nucleophile. Covalent attachment of this warhead to an enzyme requires an active enzyme conformation, thereby allowing probe modification to serve as a readout of enzyme activity. Examples of this type of reactive group include the epoxide present in the natural product E-64 that targets cysteine proteases *(18)*, and the fluorophosphonate that broadly targets serine hydrolyases *(19)*.

A second class of reactive warheads, often referred to as suicide substrates, behave as pseudosubstrates that expose a reactive electrophile only after processing by the target enzyme. This is exemplified by difluoromethyl phenylphosphate (DFPP), a compound that contains a warhead designed to covalently modify protein phosphatases *(22,23)*. In this case, dephosphorylation of the probe results in the formation of a reactive quinone methide that can then rapidly alkylate nucleophiles in the active site.

A third class of warheads does not directly rely on modification of a key active-site residue but, rather, reacts with strong nucleophiles in the active site through a proximity-enhanced reaction. This class of probes requires an optimized scaffold that confers selectivity by directing binding only to a "privileged" set of target proteins. An example of this type of probe is 5'-fluorosulfonylbenzoyl adenosine (5'-FSBA), which mimics the ligand for ATP-binding enzymes but contains a reactive electrophile that covalently modifies the enzyme after binding *(20)*.

## 4. THE REPORTER GROUP

The application of chemical probes to biological research requires that labeled enzymes be visualized after formation of the covalent bond. The most frequently used method for detection of modified proteins involves a 1D or 2D gel separation followed by detection of the reporter group. These reporter groups are fluorescent, radioactive, and biotin tags. These tags can be easily visualized and quantitated with a flatbed fluorescent/radioactive scanner or by streptavidin-affinity blotting. Biotin has the advantage that it can be used to purify labeled enzymes for identification; however, it can decrease cell permeability and solubility of the probe. Fluorescent tags are the easiest to use, most sensitive, and can be easily quantitated but can significantly increase the cost of developing probes.

To circumvent some of the pitfalls associated with the standard tagging methods, several research groups have developed methods that allow labeling of targets with a reporter group that can be chemically coupled to the probe after reaction with the target enzyme(s) in a complex proteome *(24,25)*. These methods take advantage of selective reactive groups that can undergo specific chemistry with one another in an aqueous environment. Because the chemistry that is used to facilitate the linkage of the tag to the probe is selective, the reaction can be performed directly within cells or cell extracts. In a typical experiment, the warhead is attached to one of the reactive species and the reporter group is attached to the other reactive group. After labeling of target proteins, chemical ligation is used to attach a range of labels to the probe, and enzymes are visualized by standard methods. This method has the advantage of making the probe containing the warhead smaller and potentially more cell permeable, allowing for easier labeling of enzymes in live cells or live animals.

## 5. THE LINKER REGION

The final component of a chemical probe is a linker region that is used to connect the warhead to the reporter group. The linker serves three primary purposes: First, it provides distance between the warhead and the reporter such that there is no interference between their separate and critical activities; second, it can control the hydrophobicity of the probe (and, therefore, its solubility and cell permeability) based on the type of backbone used (e.g., an alkyl chain for a hydrophobic probe or a polyethylene glycol chain for a hydrophilic probe); third, it provides some level of specificity for the desired protein target by making use of structural elements such as amino acids.

However, in some cases the linker might not be required for recognition purposes *(19)*, whereas in others, it plays a critical role in target recognition *(17)*. Adding specificity elements to the linker region, usually in the form of amino acids, can dramatically change both the specificity and reactivity of the probe toward enzyme families and subsets of enzyme families. Although there has not been a detailed analysis of the effect of peptide scaffolds on probes themselves, there is empirical evidence that the specificity of probe-like inhibitors (i.e., irreversible inhibitors) is dramatically affected by peptide elements in the linker region. This is particularly true of cysteine, serine, and threonine proteases and there is extensive literature on this topic *(26)*.

Steric hindrance can be a problem for targets that bind the probe within shallow or restricted binding pockets. Therefore, there is a clear need to be able to separate the warhead from the reporting group. Additionally, some fluorescent reporting groups can be quenched by close proximity to polypeptides, again suggesting a need for flexible linkers.

The hydrophobicity of a probe is a critical parameter, mostly because the probe must be soluble under physiological conditions of enzyme labeling. Although cell permeability is essential for labeling live cells or animals, it is likely that properties of the bulky warhead and reporter groups or the overall high molecular weight of a probe will prevent it from crossing cell membranes.

In summary, the three components of a chemical probe (the warhead, the reporter group, and the linker) must be coupled together synthetically to generate probes that are reactive against distinct families or subfamily of enzymes in complex proteomes. The optimal type and structure of probe must be determined empirically through a process of chemical synthesis and biological testing, followed by modifications and improvements before the final probe is ready for use.

## 6. APPLICATIONS OF CHEMICAL PROTEOMICS TO DRUG DISCOVERY

The broad range of applications for chemical probes makes them ideally suited to accelerate the process of drug discovery. Probes can be applied to several stages in the drug discovery process, leading to a decrease in overall timelines and an increase in the efficiency of the entire process (Fig. 2). Perhaps the greatest advantage of using chemical probes stems from the fact that they can be used to directly report the activity of a specific subset of enzymes within a complex proteome. By sampling proteomes from diseased vs normal conditions, it is possible to identify enzymes that are selected both by their ability to bind to the small-molecule probe and by a change in their activity during disease progression. Such enzymes have the potential to be promising drug targets that can be readily targeted by small-molecule inhibitors. It also becomes possible to distill a complex mixture of proteins from cells or tissues into a manageable number of discernible data points in a single step. In early discovery applications, these data can establish which targets are present and active (target identification) as well as the potency and selectivity of lead drug candidates (lead optimization). Furthermore, in preclinical stages, chemical probes can be used for model selection to determine if a desired drug target is present and active in the model of choice for initial screening of lead compounds. Probes can also be used for in vivo biochemical imaging to determine whether the drug candidate is, indeed, modulating target activity in cell or animal models of disease (i.e., pharmacodynamics). Probes can assist toxicology studies to determine effects of crossreactivity of lead drug candidates with undesired targets allowing lead candidates to be redesigned to minimize adverse side effects. Finally, in clinical trials, chemical probes have the potential to be used as in vivo imaging tools to obtain pharmacodynamic profiles in subjects treated with a drug candidate as well as for the identification of biomarkers in blood or other bodily fluids to provide a measure of drug efficacy. Such information provides a powerful link between drug action and observed clinical outcomes.

## 7. EARLY-STAGE DRUG DISCOVERY

### 7.1. Target Identification and Validation

The majority of reported applications for chemical probes impact the early stages of the drug discovery process. Probes have been used most recently to discover enzyme activities that are regulated during disease-associated events. The hope is that discovery of such regulated enzymes will lead to a better understanding of the disease processes while also identifying new small-molecule drug targets. One of the earliest and most critical steps for a new drug discovery program is picking an optimal target. Typically, a good small-molecule drug target is an enzyme whose activity can be modulated by binding of an inhibitor to a defined active site on the protein. Inhibition of the drug target should also have positive clinical outcome. The best drug targets, therefore, are proteins that have been validated through studies linking biological function to disease and that can be inhibited with small molecules, resulting in therapeutic benefits. Chemical probes provide a means to address both of these criteria simultaneously. Enzymes that are labeled by chemical probes have an increased activity in the biological system(s) being probed and are druggable with small-molecule inhibitors because they are proven to interact with druglike probes. In this section, we discuss recent efforts to identify enzymes involved in disease processes using chemical probes.

The most well-characterized chemical probes target cysteine proteases and serine hydrolases (for review, see refs. *11* and *12*).There are a range of reactive groups that can be used to selectively target cysteine proteases because the cysteine nucleophile is fairly promiscuous in terms of its ability to alkylate a wide variety of electrophiles *(26)*. The probes that have shown the most promise contain halomethylketones, epoxides (Fig. 1B), or vinyl sulfone warheads. The halomethylketone probes have been used to label caspases and, therefore, can be used for direct measurement of apoptosis *(27)*. The caspases make up a small family of enzymes whose functions are well defined in disease processes such as cancer *(28)*. The papain family cysteine proteases are emerging as important regulators of cell physiology and, as such, represent potentially important new drug targets *(29, 30)*. Although this family of enzymes is also relatively small (11 lysosomal cathepsins and 15 calpains currently in humans), their roles in specific physiological processes are poorly understood. In addition to being responsible for protein degradation in the lysosome, it is becoming increasingly clear that cathepsins can play critical roles in bone remodeling, antigen presentation, and potentially in cancer *(30–33)*. Using chemical probes, papain family proteases have also been implicated in cataract formation *(34)*, parasitic infection *(35)*, and, most recently, angiogenesis and tumor invasion *(36)*. For several of these processes, chemical probes have played a key role in defining function of specific family members.

Using an epoxide-based probe that reacts specifically with the papain family of proteases *(17)*, Joyce and colleagues addressed the role of cathepsin cysteine proteases in tumor progression in the RIP1-Tag2 *(36,37)* transgenic mouse model of pancreatic cancer. In this model, animals develop pancreatic β-islet tumors in defined stages beginning with hyperproliferation of islets that undergo angiogenic switching and finally form benign, encapsulated, and invasive tumors. A general papain family probe was used to demonstrate a dramatic upregulation of the enzymatic activity of multiple cathepsins during the progression from normal to tumor tissues. Interestingly, labeling with the probe in sorted cell populations from solid tumors indicated that the majority of cathepsin activity was contributed by immune cells that had infiltrated tumors. Furthermore, fluorescently labeled probes provided a means to visualize cathepsin activity in vivo through direct intravenous injection of the probes. These imaging studies further confirmed that cathepsin activity is elevated in developing and mature tumors and is specifically localized at the leading edge of invasive tumors. Finally, extended treatment of animals with a general papain family protease inhibitor resulted in a decrease in angiogenesis, tumor growth, and invasiveness. This work highlights the utility of chemical probes and provides an example of the uses of these tools to identify new drug targets.

A second family of cysteine proteases that has been targeted with chemical probes is the ubiquitin (Ub) and ubiquitinlike (Ubl) protease family. Ubiquitin and ubiquitinlike proteins are tags that are enzymatically conjugated to target proteins to affect a change in their stability, subcellular localization, and interactions with other proteins (38). There is a large family of cysteine proteases responsible for the processing of Ub and Ubl precursors and for facilitating the removal of Ub and Ubl proteins from target substrates. Several groups have devised elegant methods to conjugate reactive electrophiles to the C-terminus of the intact Ub or Ubl proteins. Derivatives in which a vinyl sulfone is fused to Ub and Ubl proteins have been used to screen for the presence of active Ub and Ubl proteases in complex proteomes (39–41). These probes have opened the door for studies aimed at validating the Ub and Ubl proteases as important new drug targets in a variety of diseases.

In addition to cysteine proteases, the serine hydrolase family of enzymes has been targeted with small-molecule ABPs. This family is large and includes proteases, esterases, lipases, amidases, and transacylases. Serine hydrolases show selective reactivity with a number of electrophiles, including halomethylketones, aza-peptide esters, carbamates, sulfonyl flourides, and phosphonates (26). The fluorophosphonate warhead (Fig. 1B) is specific for serine hydrolases and has been used extensively by Cravatt and co-workers to characterize serine hydrolases in a range of biological samples (19,42,43). In one particularly exciting application, a general serine hydrolyase probe was used to profile the activity of membrane-bound and secreted serine hydrolases in a range of cancer cells. These studies showed that serine hydrolyase activity could be correlated with properties of the tumor cells such as tissue origin and invasiveness.

Within the serine hydrolase family, serine proteases represent the most attractive drug targets, as there is evidence that inhibition of specific serine protease targets is an effective means to treat a variety of human diseases (19,44). A more directed approach is required to use probes to specifically target serine proteases. This could be accomplished by incorporating peptide structure into the backbone of phosphonate chemical probes. Peptide phosphonate inhibitors of serine proteases have been developed (26), but there is only one example of their use in chemical probes (45).

In addition to the directed approaches to develop probes that react with enzyme targets through well-defined mechanisms of action, efforts have been made to explore general electrophiles and natural products as probes. A broad range of enzymes, including epoxide hydrolase, aldehyde dehydrogenase, thiolase, and hydratase, can be labeled using a simple sulfonate ester reactive group fused to a linker and tag (46,47). Interestingly, there is no general mechanism to describe how these enzymes are labeled by the probe. In a separate approach, a chemical proteomic approach was used to identify carboxyl esterase-1 (CE-1) as a covalently bound target of the natural product FR182877 (48). Because this natural product has been shown to have antitumor effects, discovering its mechanism of action could lead to the validation of new anticancer drug targets. This approach using natural product scaffolds for probe design represents a promising new direction for chemical proteomics, as there are a large number of natural products with interesting pharmacological properties whose mechanism of action are still not clear.

The success using both nondirected and natural-product-based probes also highlights the need for the development of an increasing number of diverse probe families to broaden the scope of enzymes that can be studied using chemical proteomic methods. Already, some limited success has been achieved in the development of ABPs for phosphatases (22,23,49) and the potential exists to develop probes for protein/lipid kinases using covalent inhibitors such as 5'-FSBA (Fig. 1B) (20) and natural products such as wortmannin (50).

## 7.2. Lead Compound Discovery

Perhaps the most critical and time-consuming step in early-stage drug discovery is the process of designing and screening for selective inhibitors of a target enzyme. This is a long and arduous process that can take years to accomplish and is often very resource-intensive. The process usually begins by expressing and purifying large quantities of the target enzyme to be used for high-throughput enzymatic assays. Enzymes that have similar structure and activity are also expressed and purified as part of an off-target panel that must be screened to determine selectivity of potential leads. In most cases, this process is not comprehensive, as it is usually unclear which are the most relevant antitargets to use in counterscreening. Using chemical probes, it is possible to screen drug leads in a complex proteome to determine potency and selectivity against a desired target (Fig. 3). The benefit of this approach is that compounds can be screened in more physiologically relevant systems in which key targets and antitargets are all present. Furthermore, screening can be accomplished in crude samples, thereby circumventing the need to express and purify a series of enzymes for individual screening. Finally, the tissue or cell homogenate can be chosen based on knowledge of expression patterns of the drug target as well as expression of related enzymes.

Several specific examples of inhibitor screens using ABPs as a readout have been reported. A papain family cysteine protease-specific probe was used to identify selective inhibitors of cathepsin B in rat liver homogenates from a small peptide library containing an irreversible epoxide warhead (52). In a similar approach, a small synthetic library was screened to identify potent, selective, reversible inhibitors of three enzymes in mouse tissue homogenates (53). In both of these examples, inhibitors were identified in a short period of time by screening small amounts of crude protein material. These assays are easily quantified by comparing the labeling intensity of each target in the presence and absence of the small-molecule inhibitor. By titrating in the inhibitors, it is possible to use the relative competition values to obtain $IC_{50}$ values for each compound. In most cases, these values can be correlated with $K_i$ values obtained through standard enzymology assays. With the advent of high-throughput protein and peptide separation techniques such as capillary electrophoresis (54), these assays have the potential to be developed into high-throughput screens for large libraries of inhibitors.

## 8. PRECLINICAL STUDIES

After targets have been selected and lead compounds developed, the process of preclinical development begins. These studies are typically carried out to determine pharmacokinetic properties, efficacy in animal models of disease, and toxic side effects of lead compounds. Chemical probes have the potential to aid in multiple aspects of the preclinical process.

Animal models of disease are used as surrogates for human clinical trials because they are easier to manage and less expensive. In spite of this, they can be poor predictors of efficacy in humans, especially if a poor model system is chosen. Many animal models have been established for different disease indications; however, many of them are not fully characterized genetically or biochemically. An animal model is only useful if the drug target being investigated is present, active, and contributes to a measurable disease phenotype.

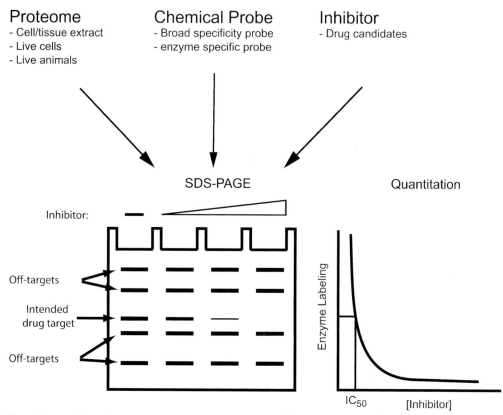

**Fig. 3.** Use of chemical probes in a competition assay. The most powerful application of chemical probes is in the determination of enzyme activity in the presence of a specific inhibitor (e.g., a drug candidate). By premixing the inhibitor with the proteome of interest and then incubating with a chemical probe, it is possible to get a quantitative readout of enzyme activity that measures inhibitor potency and selectivity. This competition assay can be done in crude protein extracts or in live cells or animals if the probe is cell and tissue permeable. Using a fluorescent or radioactive tag, it is straightforward to quantitate the decrease in enzyme labeling and, therefore, the decrease in enzyme activity that occurs with an increase in drug concentration. Potency is determined as an $IC_{50}$ value. Selectivity can be determined by the inhibition of off-targets that are present in the same proteome, and $IC_{50}$ values for those enzymes can be determined similarly. For details on the competition assay, see ref. *51*.

Using chemical probes, it is possible to validate an animal model of disease. This can be done in vitro by profiling of homogenates from the diseased animal tissue(s) and determining if the target is present and active. Alternatively, probes can be directly administered to the animal, allowing visualization of labeled enzymes using in vivo imaging or ex vivo biochemical analysis. The prospect of direct in vivo labeling using the chemical probe is particularly exciting, as it provides a method to assay enzyme activity in a physiologically relevant environment. However, this is also a challenging procedure, as it is often difficult to develop probes with optimal biological distribution. Probes could be cell or tissue impermeable or might be rapidly inactivated by metabolic pathways and/or excretion mechanisms. For these reasons, extensive development will be required for each probe family in order to generate probes that can be used for in vivo imaging applications.

Several examples have been reported for the use chemical probes *in situ* and in vivo. The papain family of cysteine proteases were labeled *in situ* using tissue culture cells treated with a fluorescent probe *(52)*. This same probe was used to visualize cathepsin activity in tissues from mice that had been labeled in vivo by intravenous injection of the probe *(36)*. Another recent example used a sulfonate ester probe to label enoyl CoA hydratase in mouse heart tissue by intravenous injection into the live animal *(24)*. In the first two examples, an untagged inhibitor could be used to effectively block labeling with the chemical probe, demonstrating the utility of these probes for monitoring inhibitor activity in living cells or animals *(see* Fig. 3). It is this last point that is the most critical, because a powerful application of chemical probes to drug discovery is to measure pharmacodynamics. Chemical probes can be used to directly measure inhibition of the drug target, correlating inhibitor potency with efficacy. A more straightforward way to measure pharmacodynamics with chemical probes would be to use them for whole-body imaging in the live animal. Several methods have been developed to measure enzyme activity in vivo *(55)*, but none so far have used chemical probes.

Toxicology studies are a critical step in preclinical drug development. Federal guidelines dictate that toxicology studies must be carried out for a drug candidate before it can be approved for testing in humans. Toxicity can be the result of inhibition of the drug target (mechanistic toxicity) or of related targets (off-target toxicity), or more general mechanisms such as perturbation of organ function. Mechanistic toxicity can sometimes be overcome by attempting to alter the pharmacokinetic and bioavailability parameters of a drug candidate, but it can also lead to early failure of a preclinical candidate. In some cases, off-target toxicity can be overcome if the enzyme responsible for the adverse side effects can be identified. Using chemical probes early in the drug discovery process, it is possible to obtain information regarding target selectivity, thereby providing a method to minimize side effects through early-stage optimization of compound selectivity. In most cases, off-targets can be labeled by a chemical probe, either in vivo or ex vivo, purified and identified by mass spectrometry. This off-target profiling can be accomplished in tissues from preclinical animal models in which toxicity has been identified.

## 9. CLINICAL STUDIES

Because the cost of late-stage drug development is so high, increasing the efficiency and success rates of clinical trials is a major issue of concern for drug companies. Drugs most often fail because of toxicity or lack of efficacy. In addition to the application of chemical probes to eliminate off-target toxicity, they also have the potential to be used for pharmacodynamic studies in humans. Although there are no specific examples demonstrating this application for chemical probes, several probes have been used for in vivo applications supporting a potential role for this technology in late-stage clinical trials. Furthermore, when a drug fails in clinical trials, it is critical to determine if the compound reached its target enzyme. In the case where a drug inhibited its target but no therapeutic outcome was observed, then the wrong target was chosen and the drug program should be altered or dropped. However, if lack of efficacy was the result of the inability of the drug to inhibit its target, then there is the potential to further refine the lead candidate. As mentioned earlier, chemical probes can be used to give a direct and quantifiable read-out of target activity and could, therefore, be useful in pharmacodynamics studies in clinical trials.

Protein or nucleic acid biomarkers are very important as surrogate markers for target inhibition. These markers are discovered and validated in the preclinical stages of the drug discovery process. Protein biomarker discovery is complicated by the large concentration of a small number of proteins present in serum. Current methods for serum-based biomarker discovery depend on depletion of major serum proteins (e.g., albumin, IgG) as well as several time-consuming and resource-intensive separation steps (chromatography, precipitation, 2D gel electrophoresis) before low abundance serum markers can be visualized, quantitated, and identified. Chemical probes have the potential to dramatically simplify this process by allowing rapid isolation of a small subset of the serum enzymes. Thus, the complex mixture of serum proteins, dominated by a handful of highly concentrated proteins, can be distilled into just a few probe-reactive markers.

## 10. CONCLUSIONS

Chemical proteomics is the fusion of synthetic organic chemistry, enzymology, biochemistry, cell biology, pharmacology, and peptide chemistry. This multidisciplinary field has the potential to increase the speed and efficiency of drug discovery through application of chemical probes to various stages of the process. Chemical probes have been shown to be useful in the identification of new drug targets and in the measurement of potency and selectivity of drug candidates. Future applications are likely to include robust screening methods for identification of antitargets responsible for drug toxicity, and whole-body imaging for monitoring pharmacodynamics during disease progression. As the applications of chemical probes become more widespread, there will be a need for a greater diversity of probes that target a range of enzyme families. Although recent work has expanded the repertoire of available probes, there remains a need for probes that target other major families of drug targets, including protein kinases and G protein-coupled receptors (GPCRs). As the quality and quantity of chemical probes increases, so will the number of applications in drug discovery and development.

## REFERENCES

1. Slamon DJ, Leyland-Jones B, Shak S, et al. Use of chemotherapy plus a monoclonal antibody against HER2 for metastatic breast cancer that overexpresses HER2. N Engl J Med 2001; 344:783–792.
2. Capdeville R, Buchdunger E, Zimmermann J, Matter A. Glivec (STI571, imatinib), a rationally developed, targeted anticancer drug. Nat Rev Drug Discov 2002; 1:493–502.
3. Paramore A, Frantz S. Bortezomib. Nat Rev Drug Discov 2003; 2:611–612.
4. Muhsin M, Graham J, Kirkpatrick P. Gefitinib. Nat Rev Drug Discov 2003; 2:515–516.
5. Lander ES, Linton LM, Birren B, et al. Initial sequencing and analysis of the human genome. Nature 2001; 409:860–921.
6. Venter JC, Adams MD, Myers EW, et al. The sequence of the human genome. Science 2001; 291:1304–1351.
7. Corthals GL, Wasinger VC, Hochstrasser DF, Sanchez JC. The dynamic range of protein expression: a challenge for proteomic research. Electrophoresis 2000; 21:1104–1115.
8. Goshe MB, Smith RD. Stable isotope-coded proteomic mass spectrometry. Curr Opin Biotechnol 2003; 14:101–109.
9. Drewes G, Bouwmeester T. Global approaches to protein-protein interactions. Curr Opin Cell Biol 2003; 15:199–205.
10. Kalume DE, Molina H, Pandey A. Tackling the phosphoproteome: tools and strategies. Curr Opin Chem Biol 2003; 7:64–69.
11. Campbell DA, Szardenings AK. Functional profiling of the proteome with affinity labels. Curr Opin Chem Biol 2003; 7:296–303.

12. Jeffery DA, Bogyo M. Chemical proteomics and its application to drug discovery. Curr Opin Biotechnol 2003; 14:87–95.
13. Huh WK, Falvo JV, Gerke LC, et al. Global analysis of protein localization in budding yeast. Nature 2003; 425:686–691.
14. Kuhn P, Wilson K, Patch MG, Stevens RC. The genesis of high-throughput structure-based drug discovery using protein crystallography. Curr Opin Chem Biol 2002; 6:704–710.
15. Hosfield D, Palan J, Hilgers M, Scheibe D, McRee DE, Stevens RC. A fully integrated protein crystallization platform for small-molecule drug discovery. J Struct Biol 2003; 142:207–217.
16. Ehrenberg M, Elf J, Aurell E, Sandberg R, Tegner J. Systems biology is taking off. Genome Res 2003; 13:2377–2380.
17. Greenbaum D, Medzihradszky KF, Burlingame A, Bogyo M. Epoxide electrophiles as activity-dependent cysteine protease profiling and discovery tools. Chem Biol 2000; 7:569–581.
18. Barrett AJ, Kembhavi AA, Brown MA, et al. L-*trans*-Epoxysuccinyl-leucylamido(4-guanidino)butane (E-64) and its analogues as inhibitors of cysteine proteinases including cathepsins B, H and L. Biochem J 1982; 201:189–198.
19. Liu Y, Patricelli MP, Cravatt BF. Activity-based protein profiling: the serine hydrolases. Proc Natl Acad Sci USA 1999; 96:14,694–14,699.
20. Colman RF. Affinity labeling of purine nucleotide sites in proteins. Annu Rev Biochem 1983; 52:67–91.
21. Zoller MJ, Nelson NC, Taylor SS. Affinity labeling of cAMP-dependent protein kinase with *p*-fluorosulfonylbenzoyl adenosine. Covalent modification of lysine 71. J Biol Chem 1981; 256:10,837–10,842.
22. Betley JR, Cesaro-Tadic S, Mekhalfia A, et al. Direct screening for phosphatase activity by turnover-based capture of protein catalysts. Angew Chem Int Ed 2002; 41:775–777.
23. Wang Q, Dechert U, Jirik F, Withers SG. Suicide inactivation of human prostatic acid phosphatase and a phosphotyrosine phosphatase. Biochem Biophys Res Commun 1994; 200:577–583.
24. Speers AE, Adam GC, Cravatt BF. Activity-based protein profiling in vivo using a copper(i)-catalyzed azide-alkyne [3 + 2] cycloaddition. J Am Chem Soc 2003; 125:4686–4687.
25. Ovaa H, Van Swieten PF, Kessler BM, et al. Chemistry in living cells: detection of active proteasomes by a two-step labeling strategy. Angew Chem Int Ed Engl 2003; 42:3626–3629.
26. Powers JC, Asgian JL, Ekici OD, James KE. Irreversible inhibitors of serine, cysteine, and threonine proteases. Chem Rev 2002; 102:4639–4750.
27. Garcia-Calvo M, Peterson EP, Leiting B, Ruel R, Nicholson DW, Thornberry NA. Inhibition of human caspases by peptide-based and macromolecular inhibitors. J Biol Chem 1998; 273:32608–2613.
28. Hanahan D, Weinberg RA. The hallmarks of cancer. Cell 2000; 100:57–70.
29. Turk V, Turk B, Turk D. Lysosomal cysteine proteases: facts and opportunities. EMBO J 2001; 20: 4629–4633.
30. Turk V, Turk B, Guncar G, Turk D, Kos J. Lysosomal cathepsins: structure, role in antigen processing and presentation, and cancer. Adv Enzyme Regul 2002; 42:285–303.
31. Yan S, Sameni M, Sloane BF. Cathepsin B and human tumor progression. Biol Chem 1998; 379:113–123.
32. Rao JS. Molecular mechanisms of glioma invasiveness: the role of proteases. Nature Rev Cancer 2003; 3:489–501.
33. Lah TT, Kos J. Cysteine proteinases in cancer progression and their clinical relevance for prognosis. Biol Chem 1998; 379:125–130.
34. Baruch A, Greenbaum D, Levy ET, et al. Defining a link between gap junction communication, proteolysis, and cataract formation. J Biol Chem 2001; 276:28,999–29,006.
35. Greenbaum DC, Baruch A, Grainger M, et al. A role for the protease falcipain 1 in host cell invasion by the human malaria parasite. Science 2002; 298:2002–2006.
36. Joyce JA, Baruch A, Chehade K, et al. Cathepsin cysteine proteases are effectors of angiogenesis and invasion during multistage tumorigenesis. Cancer Cell 2004; 5:443–453.
37. Hanahan D. Heritable formation of pancreatic beta-cell tumours in transgenic mice expressing recombinant insulin/simian virus 40 oncogenes. Nature 1985; 315:115–122.
38. Schwartz DC, Hochstrasser M. A superfamily of protein tags: ubiquitin, SUMO and related modifiers. Trends Biochem Sci 2003; 28:321–328.
39. Gan-Erdene T, Nagamalleswari K, Yin L, Wu K, Pan ZQ, Wilkinson KD. Identification and characterization of DEN1, a deneddylase of the ULP family. J Biol Chem 2003; 278:28,892–28,900.
40. Borodovsky A, Ovaa H, Nagamalleswari K, et al. Chemistry-based functional proteomics reveals novel members of the deubiquitinating enzyme family. Chem Biol 2002; 10:495–507.

41. Hemelaar J, Borodovsky A, Kessler BM, et al. Specific and covalent targeting of conjugating and deconjugating enzymes of ubiquitin-like proteins. Mol Cell Biol 2004; 24:84–95.
42. Kidd D, Liu Y, Cravatt BF. Profiling serine hydrolase activities in complex proteomes. Biochemistry 2001; 40:4005–4015.
43. Jessani N, Liu Y, Humphrey M, Cravatt BF. Enzyme activity profiles of the secreted and membrane proteome that depict cancer cell invasiveness. Proc Natl Acad Sci USA 2002; 99:10,335–10,340.
44. Rosenblum JS, Kozarich JW. Prolyl peptidases: a serine protease subfamily with high potential for drug discovery. Curr Opin Chem Biol 2003; 7:496–504.
45. Hawthorne S, Hamilton R, Walker BJ, Walker B. Utilization of biotinylated diphenyl phosphonates for disclosure of serine proteases. Anal Biochem 2004; 326:273–275.
46. Adam GC, Cravatt BF, Sorensen EJ. Profiling the specific reactivity of the proteome with non-directed activity-based probes. Chem Biol 2001; 8:81–95.
47. Adam GC, Sorensen EJ, Cravatt BF. Proteomic profiling of mechanistically distinct enzyme classes using a common chemotype. Nat Biotechnol 2002; 20:805–809.
48. Adam GC, Vanderwal CD, Sorensen EJ, Cravatt BF. (–)-FR182877 is a potent and selective inhibitor of carboxylesterase-1. Angew Chem Int Ed Engl 2003; 42:5480–5484.
49. Arabcai G, Guo X, Beebe KD, Coggeshall KM, Pei D. Alpha-haloacetophenone derivatives as photo-reversible covalent inhibitors of protein tyrosine phosphatases. J Am Chem Soc 1999; 121:5085–5086.
50. Wymann MP, Bulgarelli-Leva G, Zvelebil MJ, et al. Wortmannin inactivates phosphoinositide 3-kinase by covalent modification of Lys-802, a residue involved in the phosphate transfer reaction. Mol Cell Biol 1996; 16:1722–1733.
51. Baruch A, Jeffery DA, Greenbaum D, et al. Applications for chemical probes of proteolytic activity. In: Ploegh HL, Speicher DW, Wingfield PT, eds. Current protocols in protein science. New York: Wiley, 2004.
52. Greenbaum D, Baruch A, Hayrapetian L, et al. Chemical approaches for functionally probing the proteome. Mol Cell Proteomics 2002; 1:60–68.
53. Leung D, Hardouin C, Boger DL, Cravatt BF. Discovering potent and selective reversible inhibitors of enzymes in complex proteomes. Nat Biotechnol 2003; 21:687–691.
54. Watzig H, Gunter S. Capillary electrophoresis-a high performance analytical separation technique. Clin Chem Lab Med 2003; 41:724–738.
55. Baruch A, Jeffery DA, Bogyo M. Enzyme activity—it's all about image. Trends Cell Biol 2004; 14: 29–35.

# 9

# Proteomics-Based Anticancer Drug Discovery

## *K. K. Jain, MD, FRACS, FFPM*

**SUMMARY**

Proteomic technologies are being used in an effort to correct some of the deficiencies in traditional drug discovery. Proteins are important targets for drug discovery, particularly for cancer as well because there is a defect in the protein machinery of the cell in malignancy. Because proteome analysis can produce comprehensive molecular description of the differences between normal and diseased states, it can be used to compare the effect of candidate drugs on the disease process. The trend now is to integrate oncoproteomics with oncogenomics for drug discovery and target validation in oncology. Among the large number of proteomic technologies available for this purpose, the most important ones are three-dimensional protein structure determination, protein biochips, laser capture microdissection, and study of protein–protein and protein–drug interactions. Cancer biomarkers and signaling pathways involved in malignancy are important drug targets. The wealth of new information in proteomics databases, along with microarrays and bioinformatics, provides unlimited possibilities for designing new therapeutic agents for cancer. Proteomic approaches will also play an important role in the discovery and development of personalized medicines.

**Key Words:** Anticancer drugs; biomarkers; cancer; drug discovery; drug targets; oncoproteomics; proteomics; target validation.

From: *Cancer Drug Discovery and Development: The Oncogenomics Handbook*
Edited by: W. J. LaRochelle and R. A. Shimkets © Humana Press Inc., Totowa, NJ

# 1. INTRODUCTION

The term "proteomics" indicates PROTEins expressed by a genOME and is the systematic analysis of protein profiles of tissues. The emphasis during the last decade was on genomics, but proteomic technologies are now being incorporated in oncology in the postgenomic era and play an important role in drug discovery *(1)*. Parallel to genomics, proteomics research can be categorized as structural and functional. Structural proteomics, or protein expression, measures the number and types of protein present in normal and diseased cells. This approach is useful in defining the structure of proteins in a cell. Some of these proteins might be targets for drug discovery. Functional proteomics is the study of the proteins' biological activities. An important function of proteins is the transmission of signals using intricate pathways populated by proteins, which interact with one another. In cancer, the malignant transformation is associated with several changes at the genome level that cause a defect in the protein machinery of the cell. Proteins are targets for most drugs and drug discovery for cancer shares the basic problems with drug discovery for other diseases.

## 1.1. Conventional Drug Discovery for Cancer

Traditionally, drugs were discovered by associating disease with specific proteins in a nonsystemic manner. The usual duration of traditional drug discovery is 5–6 yr, which is half of the total development time (10–12 yr) taken from target identification to marketing of a drug. All of these steps involve distinct protein, protein–protein, or protein–ligand interactions, each involving disparate assay methods and data complexity. The traditional drug discovery process also involves testing or screening of compounds in disease models. Researchers often engage in the process with little knowledge of the intracellular processes underlying the disease or the specific drug target within the cell. Thus, companies must screen a very large number of arbitrarily selected compounds to obtain a desired change in a disease model. Although this approach sometimes produces drugs successfully, it has the following limitations:

- Inefficiency: It is capital-intensive and time-consuming in identifying and validating targets.
- Low productivity: It yields relatively few new drug candidates.
- Lack of information: It provides little information about the intracellular processes or targets, to guide target selection and subsequent drug development.
- Risk of side effects: It often results in drug candidates with a risk of serious side effects.
- Very expensive: Current estimates of bringing a drug to the market range from $600–$800 million.

## 1.2. Innovative Approaches to Drug Discovery

Functional genomics and proteomics have provided a large number of new drug targets. High-throughput (HT) screening and compound libraries produced by combinatorial chemistry have increased the number of new lead compounds, creating a bottleneck in the drug discovery pipeline. The challenge now is to increase the efficiency of testing lead efficacy and toxicity. The traditional methods of toxicity testing in laboratory animals using hematological, clinical chemistry, and histological parameters are inadequate to cope with this challenge. Gene and protein expression studies following treatment with drugs have shown that it is possible to identify changes in biochemical pathways that are related to a drug's efficacy and toxicity and precede tissue changes. The patterns of these changes can be used as efficacy or toxicity markers in HT screening assays.

### 1.3. Oncogenomics/Oncoproteomics for Drug Discovery

In an effort to overcome some of the difficulties associated with traditional drug discovery, scientists have turned to genomics as a means of better understanding the pathomechanism of disease. The hope was that a comprehensive knowledge of an organism's genetic makeup would lead to more efficient drug discovery. Although useful, DNA sequence analysis alone does not lead efficiently to new target identification, because one cannot easily infer the functions of gene products, or proteins, and protein pathways from the DNA sequence. It is important to understand how the protein function gets deranged in order to design molecules that will correct the aberrant protein.

Advantages of the proteomic approach over the genomic approach are that it can identify the most promising protein targets (tumor marker proteins) and it a more accurate characterization of molecular pathology of tumors. The limitation of this approach is that promising protein targets are only found in tissue and not in the blood. Expression profiling in cancer can be done by genomics and/or proteomics approaches. Studies of gene expression using DNA microarrays provide distinct patterns of gene expression among related tumors, whereas proteomics-based profiling uniquely allows delineation of global changes in protein expression. Expression profiles obtained using genomics and proteomics are highly complementary. A combined approach to profiling might well uncover expression patterns that could not be predicted using a single approach. For drug discovery, oncogenomics for the study of cancer is now integrated with the use of oncoproteomics, the term used for the application of proteomic technologies in cancer. Aims of the integration are the molecular classification of tumors and the identification of tumor biomarkers. Important features of the combined approach are as follows:

- Microdissected tissues are simultaneously investigated for genomic, transcriptomic, and proteomic changes.
- Genomic alterations in tumor cells are noted.
- Expression analysis is done at the RNA level by cDNA microarrays.
- Large-scale identification and quantitative analysis of tumor proteins is done in whole-cell lysates plus protein compartments.

### 1.4. Proteins as Drug Targets

The majority of drug targets are proteins that are encoded by genes expressed within tissues affected by a disease. It is estimated that there are approx 10,000 different enzymes, 2000 different G protein-coupled receptors, 200 different ion channels, and 100 different nuclear hormone receptors encoded in the human genome. These proteins are key components of the pathways involved in malignant transformation and, therefore, are likely to be a rich source of new drug targets. Even the most useful cancer markers such as prostate-specific antigen are proteins. Two-dimensional polyacrylamide gel electrophoresis (2D PAGE) and mass spectrometry (MS) can identify proteins showing increased expression in lung adenocarcinoma. The association of specific isoforms of these proteins with clinical variables and understanding the regulation of their expression will aid in the determination of their potential use as biomarkers in this cancer *(2)*. Important biomarkers have also been discovered in ovarian carcinoma. These biomarkers can be used as drug targets.

Proven drug targets share certain other characteristics that can only be identified by understanding their expression levels in cells and cannot be determined by their gene sequences alone. Proteomic technologies enable delineation of global changes in protein expression patterns resulting from transcriptional and posttranscriptional control, posttranslational modifications, and shifts in proteins between different cellular compartments *(3)*.

Drug targets are often expressed primarily in specific tissues, allowing for selectivity of pharmacological action and reducing the potential for adverse side effects, but they are generally expressed at low abundance in the cells of the relevant organ. Low-abundance protein can be enriched by purification of primary tissue by microdissection *(4)*. An effective target discovery system would, therefore, enable the detection of genes that encode for proteins expressed in specific tissues at low abundance, thereby permitting the rapid identification of proteins, which are likely to be targets for therapeutic and diagnostic development.

Advances in the understanding of molecular mechanisms of cancer have opened several doors to the discovery of new drugs and anticancer strategies. Application of proteomic technologies has enabled the prediction of all possible protein-coding regions and the choosing of the best candidates among novel drug targets. In relation to cancer, their use includes the following:

- Detection of cancer biomarkers and disease diagnosis
- Drug discovery/development for cancer

## 2. PROTEOMIC TECHNOLOGIES

Traditional treatments of cancer are less than satisfactory. There are few new rational and targeted cancer therapies. Advances in the understanding of molecular mechanism of cancer have opening several new doors to discovery of new drugs. Proteomics-based technologies that can be used for cancer drug discovery are listed in Table 1. They are described in detail elsewhere *(5)*. The role of some of these is described in the following text.

### *2.1. Laser Capture Microdissection*

Laser capture microdissection (LCM) provides an ideal method for extraction of cells from specimens in which the exact morphologies of both the captured cells and the surrounding tissue are preserved. The PixCell II LCM system (Arcturus, Mountain View, CA) enables scientists to localize, extract, and analyze specific single cells or groups of cells microdissected from solid tissue samples, cytological smears, and cell cultures. Selected cells are retrieved by activation of a transfer film placed in contact with a tissue section and use of a laser beam that is focused on a selected area of tissue through an inverted microscope. The laser bonds the film to the tissue beneath it and these cells are then lifted free of surrounding tissue. LCM is established to be compatible with subsequent nucleic acid analysis of tissues and is important for the comprehensive molecular characterization of normal, precancerous, and malignant cells by means of DNA-array technology.

Many changes in gene expression recorded between benign and malignant human tumors are the result of posttranslational modifications, not detected by analyses of RNA. Proteome analyses have also yielded information about tumor heterogeneity and the degree of relatedness between primary tumors and their metastases. Such information has been used to create artificial learning models for tumor classification. The following proteomics technologies, which are relevant to drug discovery, can be combined with LCM *(6)*:

Table 1
**Proteomics-Based Technologies Useful for Cancer Drug Discovery and Development**

2D gel electrophoresis
Antibody microarrays
Bioinformatic tools for evaluation of proteomic data
Biosensors for detection of small molecule–protein interactions
Chemical proteomics
Combination of RNA and protein profiling
Drug design based on 3D structural proteomics
Drug discovery through protein–protein interaction studies
Gene knockout for validating protein targets
*In silico* proteomic approach
Laser capture microdissection
Liquid-chromatography-based proteomics
Mass spectrometry
Molecular beacon aptamers
Phage antibody libraries for target discovery
Protein biochips for drug discovery
Tools for identifying protein kinases
Toxicoproteomics for preclinical drug safety

*Source:* Jain PharmaBiotech, reproduced by permission.

- Two-dimensional polyacrylamide gel electrophoresis (PAGE)
- Mass spectrometry
- Matrix-assisted laser desorption—mass spectrometry
- High-performance liquid chromatography
- ProteinChip: surface-enhanced laser desorption/ionization

Arrays using LCM-procured cancer epithelial cells can test the functional status of the pathways of interest and can be used for rapid identification of targets for pharmacological intervention as well as for assessment of the therapy in correcting the deranged pathways. The impact of proteomics on human cancer and diseases will not be limited to the identification of new biomarkers for early detection and new targets. These tools will be used to design rational drugs tailored according to the molecular profile of the protein circuitry of the diseased cell.

The introduction of LCM has greatly improved the specificity of 2D PAGE for biomarker discovery, as it provides a means of rapidly procuring pure cell populations from the surrounding heterogeneous tissue and also markedly enriches the proteomes of interest. High-density protein arrays, antibody arrays, and small molecular arrays, coupled with LCM, could have a substantial impact on proteomic profiling of human malignancies *(7)*. In combination with techniques like expression library construction, cDNA array hybridization, and differential display, LCM enables the establishment of "genetic fingerprints" of specific pathological lesions, especially malignant neoplasms *(8)*. Tissue Proteomics uses involves study of proteins in microdissected tissue using existing technologies, such as 2D gel electrophoresis and surface-enhanced laser desorption/ionization (SELDI), and developing new technologies along the way to generate protein fingerprints. Tissue Proteomics hopes to find its ultimate impact in the drug development process.

## 2.2. Application of Protein Biochips in Oncoproteomics

Protein biochip technology has excellent future prospects for the drug development process. Profiling proteins will be invaluable, for example, in distinguishing the proteins of normal cells from early-stage cancer cells and from malignant or metastatic cancer. Protein microarrays have the potential of development for a rapid global analysis of the entire proteome. The microarrays can also be used to screen protein–drug interactions and to detect posttranslational modifications. Comparison of proteomic maps of healthy and diseased cells could provide an insight into cell signaling and metabolic pathways and will form a novel base for pharmaceutical companies to develop future therapeutics much more rapidly.

There are numerous biochip/microarray technologies available, with over 50 companies working in this area. One example of biochip technology for oncology is ProteinChip (Ciphergen), which is comparable to GeneChip (Affymetrix) for genomics. It is based on the SELDI process. The ProteinChip Biomarker System enables biomarker pattern recognition analysis. One example of its use is in the discovery of prostate cancer biomarkers. SELDI time-of-flight (TOF) MS is an important tool for the rapid identification of cancer-specific biomarkers and proteomic patterns in the proteomes of both tissues and body fluids. It is useful in high-throughput proteomic fingerprinting of cell lysates and body fluids that uses on-chip protein fractionation coupled to TOF separation. Within minutes, subproteomes of a complex milieu such as serum can be visualized as a proteomic fingerprint or "bar code." SELDI technology has significant advantages over other proteomic technologies in that the amounts of input material required for analysis to identify single disease-related biomarkers for cancer are miniscule compared with more traditional 2D-PAGE approaches *(9)*.

Protein biochip technology is advancing rapidly. Some of the notable advances that are applicable in cancer are as follows:

- Use of protein chip platform for analysis of multiple blood proteins as markers for drug action in oncology clinical trials
- Reverse-phase protein arrays
- Ultraminiaturization of protein biochips, nanoarrays, for analysis of cancer biomarker profiles
- Atomic force microscopy combined with antibody microarrays for biomarker screening using LCM cell samples

Reverse-phase protein array technology is used to study the fluctuating state of the proteome in minute quantities of cells. Changes in pathway activation that occur between early-stage epithelial lesions and the extracellular matrix in cancer can be analyzed by obtaining pure populations of cell types by LCM. The relative states of several key phosphorylation points within the cellular circuitry can be analyzed. This technology can be used to study specific molecular pathways believed to be important in cell survival and progression from normal epithelium to invasive carcinoma directly from human tissue specimens *(10)*.

## 2.3. Molecular Beacon Aptamers

Molecular beacons, biosensors for the detection of nucleic acids, were developed as an extension of the concept of fluorescently labeled oligonucleotides. Aptamers (derived from the Latin word *aptus* = fitting) are short DNA or RNA oligomers, which can bind to a given ligand with high affinity and specificity because of their particular 3D structure and thereby antagonize the biological function of the ligand. A molecular beacon aptamer (MBA) is developed by combining the molecular beacon's excellent signal transduction and the aptamer's protein affinity for real-time and homogeneous protein recognition with specificity. Molecular photonic probes have been engineered for functional imaging of mRNA inside living cells and for the recognition of cancer proteins in homogeneous solutions. MBA provides a novel approach for achieving rapid, ultrasensitive, selective, and multiplex protein determination with a single-step homogeneous assay *(11)*.

## 2.4. ZeptoMARK™ Protein Profiling System

ZeptoMARK CeLyA (Zeptosens AG*, Witterswil, Switzerland) is a microarray-based, high-performance protein profiling system for mapping of signaling pathways. It enables ultrasensitive, multiparallel analysis of a set of proteins and protein modifications with high assay precision in combination with specific detection antibodies. Unlike traditional Western blotting or microtiter plate assays, it allows detection of 60 molecules per cell equivalent and provides the precision necessary to quantify changes of 10–20% in protein expression or activation. The outstanding performance of the systems enables considerable savings in sample and reagent consumption as well as in labor and assay time. The system comprises ZeptoMARK Hydrophobic Chips, ZeptoREADER Microarray Analyzer, and ZeptoVIEW Pro Microarray Analysis Software. It also includes the reagents and protocols for lysing and spotting cells or tissue sections. The system offers a great degree of flexibility in assay design and optimal use of sample material and reagents in a broad range of expression/activation profiling applications relevant to genomics based-research and drug development. Applications are the following:

- Signaling pathway mapping to profile pathway activation by correlating the modifications of multiple proteins
- Profiling of drug candidates in early drug discovery to obtain information on efficacy and toxicity of drug candidates upon treatment of disease related model cell systems
- Biomarker discovery and monitoring to identify and validate biomarkers for specific pathological effects or drug response
- Cell-specific protein expression/activation analysis to find correlations between phenotypic changes (e.g., in pre, early, and advanced metastatic cancer cells and specific biological events)

## 2.5. Proteomic Analysis of Cancer Cell Mitochondria

Because mitochondrial dysfunction has been implicated in cancer, it is probable that the identification of the majority of mitochondrial proteins will be a beneficial tool for developing drug and diagnostic targets for cancer. Mutations in mitochondrial DNA have also been frequently reported in cancer cells. Significance of gene expression patterns is not established yet, but identification of abnormally expressed mitochondrial proteins in cancer cells is possible by mitochondrial functional proteomics. Proteomics can identify new markers for early detection and risk assessment, as well as targets for therapeutic intervention *(12)*.

---

*In November 2004, the company filed for bankruptcy, and at time of publication, it is not known who will acquire this technology.

## 3. USE OF CANCER BIOMARKERS FOR DRUG DISCOVERY

Any measurable specific molecular alteration of a cancer cell either on a DNA, RNA, or protein level can be referred to as a biomarker. The expression of a distinct gene can enable its identification in a tissue with none of the surrounding cells expressing the specific marker. Proteomics approach has been used to identify novel biomarkers. The ideal marker for cancer would have applications in determining predisposition, early detection, assessment of prognosis, and drug response. It would be an additional advantage if the marker could also serve as a target for drug development as well.

Genetic alterations in tumor cells often lead to the emergence of growth-stimulatory autocrine and paracrine signals, involving overexpression of secreted peptide growth factors, cytokines, and hormones. Increased levels of these soluble proteins could be exploited as markers for cancer diagnosis and management or as points of therapeutic intervention. The combination of annotation/protein sequence analysis, transcript profiling, immuno-histochemistry, and immunoassay is a powerful approach for delineating candidate biomarkers with potential clinical significance *(13)*.

## 4. TARGET IDENTIFICATION

### *4.1. Signaling Pathways and Cancer Drug Discovery*

The role of proteomic technologies in studying cell signaling pathways is well recognized. Characterization of intracellular signaling pathways should lead to a better understanding of ovarian epithelial carcinogenesis and provide an opportunity to interfere with signal transduction targets involved in ovarian tumor cell growth, survival, and progression. Challenges to such an effort are significant because many of these signals are a part of cascades within an intricate and likely redundant intracellular signaling network. For instance, a given signal might activate a dual intracellular pathway (i.e., mitogen extracellular signal-regulated kinase 1 [MEK1]–mitogen-activated protein kinase [MAPK] and phosphatidylinositol 3-kinase [PI3K]/Akt required for fibronectin-dependent activation of matrix metalloproteinase *(14)*. A single pathway also might transduce more than one biologic or oncogenic signal (i.e., PI3K signaling in epithelial and endothelial cell growth and sprouting of neovessels). Despite these challenges, evidence for therapeutic targeting of signal transduction pathways is accumulating in human cancer. For instance, the epidermal growth factor-specific tyrosine kinase inhibitor ZD 1839 (Iressa) has a beneficial therapeutic effect on ovarian epithelial cancer.

Some of the most advanced and targeted agents in development for the treatment of cancer involve the epidermal growth factor protein–tyrosine kinase receptor family, such as the epidermal growth factor receptor (EGFR), and their downstream effects on cellular signaling. Cytogen Corporation has assembled a proprietary collection of cellular signaling information that can be utilized to discover novel pathways associated with a number of therapeutically important classes of molecule. Cytogen has produced data revealing novel links between ErbB-4 (a member of the epidermal growth factor protein–tyrosine kinase receptor family), WW-domain containing protein YAP (Yes-associated protein), tumor suppressor protein P73, and a member of the membrane-associated guanylate kinase (MAGUK) family in a signaling pathway regulating several cellular functions important to both the proliferation and survival of cancer cells. The data represent in vivo validation of the company's in vitro drug discovery platform.

## *4.2. Screening of Proteases*

Some of the anticancer strategies are directed against proteases that facilitate several steps in cancer progression. The major proteases are matrix metalloproteases, cathepsins, and the mast cell serine proteases. Assay of actual enzyme activity, and not messenger RNA levels or immunoassay of protein, is ideal for identifying proteases most suitable for drug targeting. Proteases are particularly suitable for functional proteomic screening. This has been achieved by an automated microtiter plate assay format that was modified to allow for the detection of major classes of proteases in tissue samples *(15)*. The results show that matrix metalloproteases are localized to the tumor cells themselves, whereas cathepsin B is predominantly expressed by macrophages at the leading edge of invading tumors. Such an analysis serves to identify proteases whose activity is not completely balanced by endogenous inhibitors and that might be essential for tumor progression. These proteases are logical targets for efforts to produce low-molecular-weight protease inhibitors as potential chemotherapy. The proteasome, a multicatalytic protease, plays a central role in most of the regulatory pathways such as cell cycle regulation, differentiation, and apoptosis. It is a target for anticancer drugs.

## *4.3. Identification of Protein Kinases*

Protein kinases are coded by more than 2000 genes and thus constitute the largest single enzyme family in the human genome. Most cellular processes are, in fact, regulated by the reversible phosphorylation of proteins on serine, threonine, and tyrosine residues. At least 30% of all proteins are thought to contain covalently bound phosphate. A novel method determines if drugs and drug targets are effective in combating disease by identifying the key regulatory protein "switches" (phosphorylation sites) inside human cells *(16)*. This will enable an accurate distinction between healthy and diseased cells to uncover the key protein targets against which new drugs will be made. This technology represents a new way to accelerate the drug development process.

It is important to identify protein kinases that are important in the signaling pathways associated with cancer, as they are rational therapeutic targets. Receptor tyrosine kinases (RTK) and Ras oncoprotein are examples of critical signaling proteins that mediate the processes of cellular growth and differentiation. Gene amplification and/or overexpression of RTK proteins or functional alterations caused by mutations in the corresponding genes or abnormal autocrine–paracrine growth factor loops contribute to constitutive RTK signaling, ultimately resulting in the manifestation of dysregulated cell growth and cancer.

The mechanism of uncontrolled RTK signaling that leads to cancer has provided the rationale for anti-RTK drug development. Drugs being investigated as inhibitors of signal transduction include small-molecule inhibitors, immunotoxins, monoclonal antibodies, and antisense oligonucleotides. Preclinical studies of compounds, which inhibit RTK and Ras, have shown that these targets can be blocked, whereas side effects in animal models are minimal. Early clinical trials reveal that treatment with these compounds is both feasible and tolerable, but many issues remain unresolved, including how to optimize schedule, how long to continue treatment, specific mechanisms of action, and how to optimize combinations of signal transduction inhibitors with standard therapeutic modalities. Addressing these issues could require a shift in the traditional paradigm of drug development, as conventional end points might not adequately capture the potential benefits from agents believed to act in a cytostatic vs cytotoxic manner *(17)*. An example of the success of this approach is Herceptin, a monoclonal antibody against the Her2/neu receptor tyrosine kinase, which has prolonged the survival of women with Her-2/neu-positive metastatic breast cancer when combined with chemotherapy.

### 4.4. Use of Protein Structural Information for Anticancer Drug Discovery

The 3D structure of a protein determines its biological function and is an important basis of drug discovery. Conventional methods for the determination of protein structure include X-rays crystallography. This information can be used to select compounds that might bind to the target site. An X-ray crystallography-driven screening technique that combines the steps of lead identification, structural assessment, and optimization is rapid, efficient, and high throughput, and it results in detailed crystallographic structure information. The process has become increasingly automated and nearly 20,000 protein structures are available in the Protein Data Bank *(18)*. Parallel progress in genomics will result in a great expansion of validated targets for cancer therapy.

Nuclear magnetic resonance (NMR) determines the physical structure of proteins by identifying and locating different atoms within a molecule and elucidating their spatial relationships. Traditionally, NMR is considered complementary to X-ray crystallography. Researchers tend to use X-ray crystallography to investigate the surfaces and surroundings of large proteins in their crystalline state, whereas NMR is more suitable for studying the dynamics of the structure of smaller proteins that are difficult to crystallize. Electron spin resonance (ESR), a sister technique to NMR, has been used for studying basic molecular mechanisms in membranes and proteins by use of nitroxide spin labels *(19)*. In drug discovery, structural data are critical for determining how a new pharmaceutical molecule will bind with a target molecule as illustrated by the following example.

Bcl-2 belongs to a growing family of proteins that regulates programmed cell death (apoptosis). Overexpression of Bcl-2 has been observed in breast cancer, prostate cancer, B-cell lymphomas, colorectal adenocarcinomas, and many other forms of cancer. Therefore, Bcl-2 is an attractive anticancer target. Discovery of novel classes of small-molecule inhibitors targeted at the BH3-binding pocket in Bcl-2 has been reported *(20)*. The 3D structure of Bcl-2 has been modeled on the basis of a high-resolution NMR solution structure of Bcl-X(L), which shares a high sequence homology with Bcl-2. A structure-based computer screening approach was been employed to search the National Cancer Institute 3D database of organic compounds. The results suggest that the structure-based computer screening strategy employed in the study is effective for identifying novel, structurally diverse, nonpeptide small-molecule inhibitors that target the BH3 binding site of Bcl-2.

## 5. TARGET VALIDATION

After a lead molecule is identified, one needs to confirm the efficacy of the drug through the expected mechanism. Target discovery, which involves the identification and early validation of disease-modifying targets, is an essential first step in the drug discovery pipeline. The drive to determine protein function has been stimulated, both in industry and academia, by the completion of the Human Genome Project *(21)*.

Proteomics can be used to study the mode of action of drugs by comparing the proteome of the cells in which the drug target has been eliminated by molecular knockout techniques or with small-molecule inhibitors believed to act specifically on the same target. Proteomic techniques enable the study of protein expression levels, modifications, location, and function in high-throughput automated systems. Because proteome analysis can produce comprehensive molecular description of the differences between normal and diseased states, it can be used to compare the effect of candidate drugs on the disease process. Proteomics can be integrated into the drug discovery process along with the genomic and chemical drug discovery. Proteomics might emerge as a powerful approach for directly identifying highly predictive pharmacogenomic markers in the blood or other body tissues. Definition and validation of drug targets by proteomics will have the following advantages for the pharmaceutical industry:

- Fewer dropout compounds in the developmental pipeline
- Rational drug design of compounds with fewer side effects

## 6. APPLICATION OF PROTEOMICS TO THE DEVELOPMENT OF PERSONALIZED CANCER THERAPY

Normal cells, precancerous cells, and tumor cells from an individual can be isolated using tools that maintain the original protein pattern of the cells. Analysis of the protein patterns of tumor cells taken from a patient after treatment shows how a particular therapy affects the protein pattern of a cell. This approach will help to develop individualized therapies that are optimal for a particular patient rather than to a population and to determine the effects, both toxic and beneficial, of a therapy before using it in patients (22).

Another approach to develop personalized therapy for cancer is to study signal pathway activation within a patient's tumor. Protein signaling can be analyzed by reverse-phase protein microarrays from biopsy tissues. The effect of treatment on the pathway in which the target is located can be studied before, during, and after therapy.

## 7. CONCLUSIONS

Proteomic techniques are uniquely capable of detecting tumor-specific alterations in proteins and will also accelerate the anticancer drug target discovery and validation. Furthermore, proteomic technologies can be used to design rational drugs according to the molecular profile of the protein circuitry of the cancer cell and have the potential to aid the development of personalized cancer therapy. Several technologies are in use both in the academic as well as the industrial sectors and the results in cancer drug discovery are encouraging. The wealth of new information in proteomics databases, along with microarrays and bioinformatics, provides unlimited possibilities for designing new therapeutic agents for cancer. However, the utility of proteomics in target discovery has so far been limited for a number of reasons that are being remedied:

- Membrane-associated, positively charged and hydrophobic, are often difficult to separate using 2D gels. New developments in membrane protein microarrays will facilitate the drug discovery process. Corning Inc. has demonstrated direct pin printing of membrane proteins and ligand-binding assays on biochips (23).
- The lack of an amplification step, such as the polymerase chain reaction used in genomic studies, means that the detection of low-abundance proteins is problematic. With sensitive methods of detection such as the ZeptoMARK CeLyA Protein Profiling System, amplification may not be necessary.
- The separation characteristics of proteins are also affected by posttranslational modifications, including phosphorylation, glycosylation, lipidation, acetylation, and nitration.

# REFERENCES

1. Jain KK. Recent advances in oncoproteomics. Curr Opin Mol Ther 2002; 4:203–209.
2. Chen G, Gharib TG, Huang CC, et al. Proteomic analysis of lung adenocarcinoma: identification of a highly expressed set of proteins in tumors. Clin Cancer Res 2002; 8:2298–2305.
3. Hanash SM, Madoz-Gurpide J, Misek DE. Identification of novel targets for cancer therapy using expression proteomics. Leukemia 2002; 16:478–485.
4. Emmert-Buck MR, Gillespie JW, Paweletz CP, et al. An approach to proteomic analysis of human tumors. Mol Carcinog 2000; 27:158–165.
5. Jain KK. Proteomics: technologies, markets and companies. Basel: Jain PharmaBiotech, 2004.
6. Jain KK. Application of laser capture microdissection to proteomics. Methods Enzymol 2002; 356: 157–167.
7. Bichsel VE, Liotta LA, Petricoin EF 3rd. Cancer proteomics: from biomarker discovery to signal pathway profiling. Cancer J 2001; 7:69–78.
8. Fend F, Raffeld M. Laser capture microdissection in pathology. J Clin Pathol 2000; 53:666–672.
9. Wulfkuhle JD, Liotta LA, Petricoin EF. Proteomic applications for the early detection of cancer. Nat Rev Cancer 2003; 3:267–275.
10. Grubb RL, Calvert VS, Wulkuhle JD, et al. Signal pathway profiling of prostate cancer using reverse phase protein arrays. Proteomics 2003; 3:2142–2146.
11. Li JJ, Fang X, Tan W. Molecular aptamer beacons for real-time protein recognition. Biochem Biophys Res Commun 2002; 292:31–40.
12. Verma M, Kagan J, Sidransky D, Srivastava S. Proteomic analysis of cancer-cell mitochondria. Nat Rev Cancer 2003; 3:789–795.
13. Welsh JB, Sapinoso LM, Kern SG, et al. Large-scale delineation of secreted protein biomarkers overexpressed in cancer tissue and serum. PNAS 2003; 100:3410–3415.
14. Nicosia SV, Bai W, Cheng JQ, et al. Oncogenic pathways implicated in ovarian epithelial cancer. Hematol Oncol Clin North Am 2003; 17:927–943.
15. McKerrow JH, Bhargava V, Hansell E, et al. A functional proteomics screen of proteases in colorectal carcinoma. Mol Med 2000; 6:450–460.
16. Ficarro SB, McCleland ML, Stukenberg PT, et al. Phosphoproteome analysis by mass spectrometry and its application to *Saccharomyces cerevisiae*. Nat Biotechnol 2002; 20:301–305.
17. Hao D, Rowinsky EK. Inhibiting signal transduction: recent advances in the development of receptor tyrosine kinase and Ras inhibitors. Cancer Invest 2002; 20:387–404.
18. Glen RC, Allen SC. Ligand–protein docking: cancer research at the interface between biology and chemistry. Curr Med Chem 2003; 10:763–767.
19. Borbat PP, Costa-Filho AJ, Earle KA, et al. Electron spin resonance in studies of membranes and proteins. Science 2001; 291:266–269.
20. Enyedy IJ, Ling Y, Nacro K, et al. Discovery of small-molecule inhibitors of Bcl-2 through structure-based computer screening. J Med Chem 2001; 44:4313–4324.
21. Lindsay MA. Target discovery. Nat Rev Drug Discov 2003; 2:831–838.
22. Jain KK. Role of oncoproteomics in the personalized management of cancer. Expert Rev Proteomics 2004; 1:49–55.
23. Fang Y, Frutos AG, Lahiri J. Membrane protein microarrays. J Am Chem Soc 2002; 124:2394–2395.

# 10 Cancer Metabolic Phenotype

## Exploiting the Cancer Metabolome in Drug Discovery

*John R. Griffiths, MB BS, DPhil*
*and Marion Stubbs, DPhil*

## Contents

## Summary

Cancer cells exhibit surprisingly uniform metabolic abnormalities, termed the cancer metabolic phenotype. We define six classes of mechanism giving rise to this phenotype: mechanisms associated with (1) oncogenesis; (2) rapid reproduction; (3) stress responses; (4) invasiveness and metastasis; (5) resistance to host immune surveillance; (6) resistance to therapy. Classes 1 and 2 are constitutive mechanisms, involved in the process of oncogenesis, whereas classes 4–6 mainly involve selection for features responsive to the tumor's environment. We next analyze some well-known features of the tumor metabolic phenotype: the Warburg effect, aerobic glycolysis, and tumor pH. Contrary to accepted wisdom, tumors do not rely on glycolysis for their energy needs and their intracellular pH is not acidic.

The concept of the metabolome—the totality of small-molecule metabolites in a cell—has had little attention in cancer. We discuss ways in which the cancer metabolome could be investigated, by metabolic profiling, illustrated by studies on the HIF-1 pathway. Finally, we consider ways in which tumor metabolic profiling could be used in drug discovery programs: to help chose targets from functional genomic data, to refine results from conventional screens or to provide end points for focused screens and medicinal chemistry, to predict cellular and whole-organism toxicity, and to help elucidate drug mechanisms.

**Key Words:** Cancer; metabolic phenotype; metabolomics; NMR; drug discovery.

From: *Cancer Drug Discovery and Development: The Oncogenomics Handbook*
Edited by: W. J. LaRochelle and R. A. Shimkets © Humana Press Inc., Totowa, NJ

# 1. INTRODUCTION

The distinctive metabolic abnormalities of cancer cells are among the most widely recognized features of the cancer phenotype, and many pharmacological and other therapies depend on them. The new science of metabolomics has opened up a novel way of looking at the tumor metabolic phenotype, one that will be exploitable in drug development. This chapter will begin by considering the basic mechanisms underlying metabolic aspects of the tumor phenotype, followed by an analysis of some of its better known features. Contrary to accepted wisdom, for instance, tumors do not rely on glycolysis for their energy needs and their intracellular pH is not acidic. We will next consider the concept of the "cancer metabolome" and ways in which it could be investigated, both in general and in a more limited way by metabolic profiling as illustrated by studies on the HIF-1 pathway. Finally, we will try to predict ways in which tumor metabolic profiling could be used to assist drug discovery.

# 2. THE ORIGINS OF THE CANCER CELL METABOLIC PHENOTYPE

Why do cancer cells have an abnormal metabolic phenotype? Why, indeed, should there be a characteristic cancer cell phenotype, in view of the hundred or so types of cancer, arising from malignant transformation of most types of differentiated cell? There are many reasons why the development of cancer cells channels their metabolism into characteristic phenotypic patterns. They can be loosely grouped into six classes (*see* Fig. 1).

## 2.1. Class 1: Constitutive Mechanisms Associated With Oncogenesis

Many processes have been proposed as causes of malignant transformation, but in the principal current theory, the formation of a cancer cell requires a series of mutations in the DNA sequences of its ancestral cells, either giving rise to oncogenes or impairing the action of tumor suppressor genes. The protein products of oncogenes and tumor suppressor genes tend to fall into characteristic groups. For instance, many oncogenes are growth factors, receptors, or transcription factors or are otherwise concerned in the signaling pathways involved in cell replication. The net effect of such mutations is to produce cells that continue to reproduce in the absence of external mitogenic stimulation. Other tumor suppression factors that are commonly mutated in cancer cells would normally be involved in the culling, by apoptosis, of abnormal cells. Thus, as most of these mutations are clustered in a few pathways, the resulting abnormal metabolic phenotypes will tend to be to be similar.

Genomic instability is another common, constitutive feature of cancer cells, and it results in rapid generation of a large variety of clones that are then subject to natural selection. Genomic instability (as well as aneuploidy, another putative cause of oncogenesis

---

**Fig. 1.** *(Opposite page)*   Illustrative examples from the six classes of mechanism that give rise to the tumor metabolic phenotype. *Class 1, oncogenesis*: One or more mutations cause malignant transformation of a single cell. *Class 2, rapid reproduction*: Clones with metabolic phenotypes characteristic of rapid division predominate. *Class 3, expression of stress response mechanisms*: Stress response pathways such as HIF are activated both constitutively by oncogenic mechanisms in class 1 and in response to the environment. The figure shows the development of a glycolytic phenotype in cells too far from the nearest blood vessel to receive adequate oxygen. *Class 4, invasion and metastasis*:

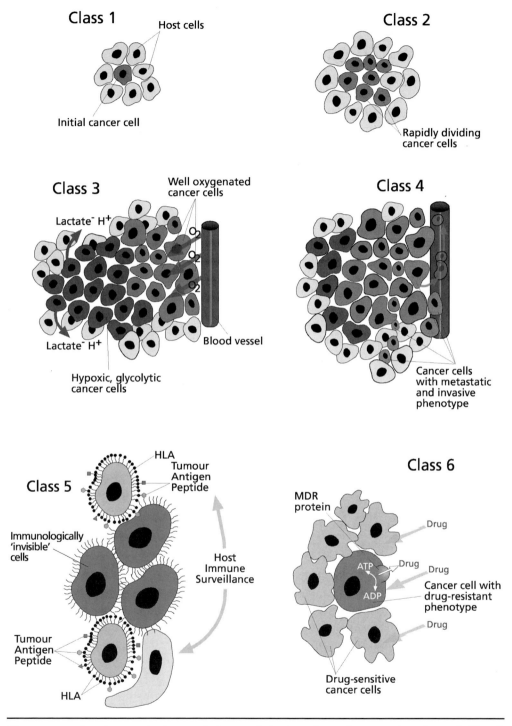

Clones expressing phenotypic characteristics permitting invasion and metastasis are favored. *Class 5, resistance to the host:* Clones with, for example, defective tumor antigen display mechanisms escape the host's immunological surveillance. *Class 6, resistance to therapy:* Acquisition of phenotypic characteristics favoring resistance to therapy, for example, selection of clones overexpressing the multidrug resistance (MDR) protein, which enables them to pump out anticancer drugs.

[reviewed by Duesberg et al. *(1)*] would tend to arise from mutations in the genes and proteins that normally detect and repair DNA damage or those involved in processes (notably apoptosis) that eliminate cells with damaged DNA *(2)*. Once again, certain constitutive features in the metabolic phenotype of cancer-prone cells lead to oncogenesis, and this reinforces the tendency to a standard cancer phenotype.

## 2.2. Class 2: Selection for Rapid Reproduction

All cancer cells, by definition, reproduce inappropriately, and this constitutive effect is enhanced because the more rapidly dividing clones win out over the slower growing ones. Thus, the metabolic phenotype will tend to have features characteristic of rapidly dividing cells.

## 2.3. Class 3: Expression of Stress Response Mechanisms

A growing mass of tumor cells rapidly exhausts the oxygen that can diffuse to it through the host extracellular fluid, and the hypoxic cells then tend to respire anaerobically, producing lactic acid. Although, as will be shown, tumors rely less on glycolysis than is generally believed, there is no doubt that they produce lactic acid and that their extracellular fluids are abnormally acidic. Second, normal cells have a set of ancient, highly conserved stress response mechanisms for surviving in hypoxic, acidic environments, so all cancer cells tend to utilize these mechanisms in order to grow and reproduce in the stressful environments they create for themselves, further unifying the cancer phenotype. Another characteristic feature of tumors arises here: spatial heterogeneity. Because the environmental stresses on some cells are more severe, they will tend to express different stress response factors. Clonal selection might intensify this effect and result in cell types in different parts of the tumor having different variants of the classical phenotype.

## 2.4. Class 4: Selection for Invasiveness and Metastasis

All of the other common features of cancers—invasiveness, metastasis, and so on—will require selection of cells for certain phenotypic characteristics. Thus, as the growing mass of cancer cells matures into a malignant tumor, it will be led down a number of common pathways, so that the progeny cells will tend to conform to a standard phenotype.

An aspect of the metabolic phenotype that may be associated with successful metastasis is illustrated in Fig. 2. This shows the mean (dotted lines) and standard deviation (± SD) plots of $^1$H-MRS (magnetic resonance spectroscopy) spectra taken noninvasively from different classes of human brain tumors. The pattern of peaks in an MR spectrum is derived from the high-concentration metabolites within the region of interest, so the spectrum can be used as a metabolic profile. As can be seen, there are reproducible chemical characteristics in the spectra of these tumor types that allow them to be distinguished, and, indeed, it has been possible to devise pattern-recognition algorithms that will do so without human intervention *(3)*. Figures 2A, 2B, and 2D show the mean ± SD spectra for two primary cancers originating from different cell types: Fig. 2A is from meningiomas and Figs. 2B and 2D are from astrocytomas. Figure 2B and 2D illustrate the remarkable difference in the metabolic phenotypes of astrocytomas with different grades of malignancy: Grade II astrocytomas (Fig. 2B) are relatively benign, whereas glioblastomas (Fig. 2D) are extremely aggressive astrocytomas. The most unexpected feature in this series of spectra is illustrated in Fig. 2C, however, which shows mean ± SD spectra from six cerebral metastases derived from primary tumors elsewhere in the body (three from lung tumors, one

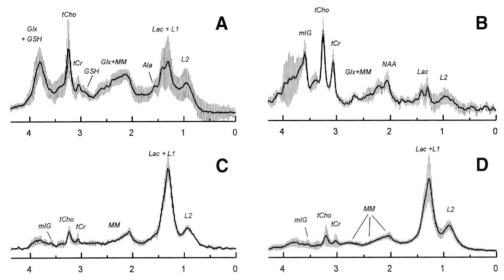

**Fig. 2.** $^1$H-MRS (magnetic resonance spectroscopy) spectra of brain tumors in patients obtained using the STEAM pulse sequence, TE 30 ms, in a 1.5-T GE Signa instrument. **(A)** Meningioma, $n = 8$; **(B)** astrocytoma grade II, $n = 5$; **(C)** cerebral metastases, $n = 6$ (three lung, one stomach, one breast, and one unknown primary); **(D)** glioblastoma, $n = 13$. Ala, alanine; tCho, cholines; tCr, creatines; Glx, glutamate + glutamine; GSH, glutathione; L1, L2, lipids; Lac, lactate; MM, macromolecules; mIG, myo-Inositol + glycine; NAA, $N$-acetyl aspartate.

from a breast tumor, one from a stomach tumor, and one from an unknown primary). What is surprising is that the spectra of all these metastatic brain tumors were almost indistinguishable, regardless of the cell of origin, as can be seen from the low standard deviation on this plot. Larger and more varied series of cerebral metastasis spectra also show marked similarities *(4)*. Perhaps, the fact that these metastases had been "selected" for their ability to spread through the blood system and invade another tissue caused them to develop a common metabolic phenotype. An alternative explanation, based on the similarity of this metastasis metabolic phenotype to that of the highly malignant glioblastomas, both of which tend to have large volumes of necrosis, could be that all of these spectra are dominated by the metabolites present in necrotic tissue.

### 2.5. Class 5: Selection for Resistance to Host Immune Surveillance

Next, the cancer cells will tend to be selected for features that enable them to escape the host's immunological surveillance mechanisms. Many mechanisms have been proposed, particularly in the area of loss or downregulation of the human leukocyte antigen (HLA) class I antigens and other elements in the pathways involved in processing tumor antigens (this mechanism is shown in Fig. 1). Tumor cells might also develop mechanisms allowing them to "counterattack" and kill infiltrating T-cells *(5)*.

### 2.6. Class 6: Selection for Resistance to Therapy

Finally, cells in a malignant tumor find ways to overcome the therapies that physicians use against them, constraining their development into certain characteristic phenotypes. A

Table 1
Characteristics of the Tumor Metabolic Phenotype

| Metabolic Characteristic | Compared to Normal Tissue | Method |
|---|---|---|
| $pO_2$ | Low | Oxylite, Eppendorf |
| ATP/Pi | Low | MRS |
| Intracellular pH | Similar | MRS |
| Extracellular pH | Acidic | pH electrodes, MRS |
| Lactate | High | Enzymatic assay, MRS |
| Cytosolic $NAD^+/NADH$ | Low | Calculated |
| Total $Ca^{2+}$ | High | Assay |
| Glucose consumption | High | PET |
| Glycolytic enzyme activity | High to very high | Enzymatic assay, Western blots for expression |

*Abbreviations:* MRS: magnetic resonance spectroscopy; PET: positron-emission tomography.
Data from ref. 7.

typical example (shown in Fig. 1) would be selection of cells overexpressing the multidrug resistance (MDR) protein, which enables them to pump out chemotherapeutic agents.

All of the factors in these six classes will tend to operate on all cancer cells, so there will be a tendency for them to resemble each other—hence the characteristic cancer phenotype. The mechanisms in classes 1 and 2 are constitutive, whereas those in classes 3–6 involve responses to the tumor's environment.

## 3. THE WARBURG EFFECT

Some key features of the cancer metabolic phenotype were recognized by Warburg in the 1920s *(6)*. He found that, unlike most normal tissues, tumors tended to metabolize glycolytically even in the presence of adequate oxygen—"aerobic glycolysis." The best characterized features of the cancer metabolic phenotype (often termed the "Warburg effect") are shown in Table 1. Several of these characteristics (low $pO_2$, high glucose consumption, and high lactate) are at least, in part, the result of the well-known hypoxia of tumors that is commonly believed to be the result of poor perfusion (an aspect of class 3 of the metabolic phenotype). More recent genomic studies have indicated that some stress responses that are triggered in class 3 by hypoxia (e.g., HIF-1) might also be constitutively switched on *(8)* during the tumor transforming process (class 1). The characteristically low extracellular pH in tumors *(9,10)* has been considered as an essential aid to growth and metastasis (class 4) *(11,12)*.

### 3.1. Tumor Lactate Production

Most studies on the Warburg effect have used either tissue slices (as employed by Warburg himself) or cultured cells. It is very difficult to monitor the flow of metabolites in an undisturbed tumor, growing in a host, so the extent to which solid tumors perform aerobic glycolysis in natural conditions in vivo has been unclear until recently. There are, however, two articles in the literature reporting metabolic balance studies on tumors in vivo. In one, human tumor xenografts had been grown as transplants in nude rats *(13)*, while in the other *(14)*, the balance studies were performed on bowel tumors in human patients during surgery. We have analysed the data in these two articles *(15)* and derived values both for the proportion of glucose taken up from the host that was metabolized to lactate and for the proportion of the tumor's ATP production that was supported by this glycolytic lactate production. The results were surprising: Even in the transplanted tumors, which would be expected to be poorly vascularized and therefore to rely on glycolysis rather than oxidative metabolism, almost one-third of the glucose was oxidized (115 nmol/g/min glucose oxidized from 370 nmol/g/min consumed). Because oxidative metabolism is a much more efficient way of phosphorylating ATP, only 11% of the ATP turnover was derived from glycolysis (510 nmol/g/min from glycolysis compared with 4400 nmol/g/min total ATP synthesis) *(13,15)*. In the human tumors studied during operations, the results were even more striking. More than two-thirds of the glucose consumed was oxidized (220 nmol/g/min oxidized from 320 nmol/g/min consumed) and glycolysis contributed only 2.4% of the ATP that was phosphorylated *(14,15)*.

Although these calculations refute the accepted wisdom that tumors rely almost exclusively on aerobic glycolysis for their energy production, it is still true that they utilize this pathway more than normal tissues and that they produce much more lactate than normal. Holm et al. *(14)* found that the tumors they studied produced lactate 43 times more rapidly than the adjacent normal colon. In summary, it is still true that the characteristic metabolic phenotype of cancers involves excessive lactic acid production, although this pathway generates only a small proportion of the ATP required to meet the tumor's energy needs.

### 3.2. Tumor pH

Another dogma, widely accepted since the time of Warburg, was that that the interior of cancer cells must be acidic because of the excessive amounts of lactic acid that they produce. Our understanding of this and several other aspects of the tumor metabolic phenotype has been strengthened by the use of MR imaging (MRI) and spectroscopy (MRS) two methods that can be used noninvasively on the living tumor in an animal or patient. MRS studies *(16)* have shown that the tumor *intracellular* pH is usually near neutrality, like that of normal cells; it is the *extracellular* pH that is acidic. Presumably, this feature of the cancer phenotype arises because malignant cells are able to pump out the extra lactic acid they produce, but it then accumulates in the extracellular space—perhaps because of the long distances it must diffuse to a blood vessel. This hypothesis is supported by modeling studies *(15)* and by experimental measurements of pH distribution in relation to blood vessels *(17)*. Recently, MRI methods have been developed for monitoring the spatial distribution of extracellular pH *(10)*.

## 4. THE CANCER METABOLOME

In recent years, building on our new understanding of the human genome, it has become possible to monitor the tumor phenotype as a whole, either by following mRNA expression (transcriptomics) or by monitoring the proteins translated from these mRNA molecules (proteomics). However, metabolism takes place at a still lower level than this, by variation in the rates of production of thousands of small-molecule metabolites. By analogy with the genome, the transcriptome, and the proteome, the totality of small-molecule metabolites in an organism is now termed "the metabolome," and methods for studying it are called "metabolomics." There has already been research on the metabolomics of plants and micro-organisms, but little systematic work has been done on the human metabolome (or, indeed, that of any mammalian species), and hardly anything on the metabolomics of cancer. To complete our understanding of the large-scale molecular architecture of human cells, we urgently need automated methods for metabolomics that can be used to investigate thousands of small-molecule metabolites, in the same way that transcriptomics can investigate the expression of thousands of genes. There are no current methods for studying the complete metabolome, but metabolic profiles of groups of metabolites can be obtained with methods that are presently available and they could be used to investigate the cancer metabolome.

## 5. A METHOD FOR METABOLOMIC SCREENING

A recent article by Raamsdonk et al. *(18)* describes a "proof-of-principle" demonstration of a metabolomic screening method. The aim is to predict the functions of the genes in yeast that are said to be "silent" because their deletion causes no obvious effect (approx 85% of the yeast genome). They argue that in such cases, other metabolic pathways must have taken over the function of the protein product of the deleted gene, so there should be widespread changes in the concentrations of small-molecule metabolites. It should be possible, therefore, to deduce the role of any gene by deleting it and then comparing the pattern of changes in the concentrations of metabolites to the patterns caused by deletion of genes with known functions. In their proof-of-principle experiment (termed "FANCY" —Functional Analysis of Co-responses in Yeast), they used $^1$H-NMR (nuclear magnetic resonance) to simultaneously measure the concentrations of large numbers of metabolites in yeasts (i.e., to obtain a metabolic profile). Different strains were used with knockouts of genes coding for various enzymes in the glycolytic and respiratory pathways. They then used statistical clustering algorithms to indicate the pattern of metabolic changes corresponding to deletions of genes in each metabolic pathway. It turned out that the two cell lines with knockouts of (different) enzymes involved in the control of the glycolytic enzyme phosphofructokinase had patterns of altered metabolite concentrations that clustered together. Cell lines with knockouts of enzymes associated with the respiratory chain had patterns of altered metabolite concentrations that did not cluster with the glycolytic ones.

To put this approach into practice, it will be necessary to find the patterns of metabolic derangement associated with knockouts of a substantial number of the genes in an organism. Systematic attempts to do this are beginning with micro-organisms such as yeast, and if successful, they should provide an interpretive framework for metabolic profiles obtained from higher organisms. The FANCY method lends itself to automation: No human interpretation of the spectra is required, and after standardization, they are entered directly into a pattern-recognition algorithm. It should, therefore, be possible to set up a screening program that could handle hundreds or even thousands of mutant organisms. A great attraction is that one does not need to know the chemical identity of the metabolites that give rise to the changes: The clustering algorithm simply recognizes a pattern of NMR peaks. Once enough of the patterns associated with the known genes have been identified, it should be possible to identify the metabolic function of the unknown genes. Furthermore, the pattern of metabolic derangement does not have to be restricted to the pathway in which the gene is situated, provided it is always the same for the gene products in a particular area of metabolism. Finally, a complete knockout of the gene is probably not necessary: antisense DNA, or any other specific method, could be used to inhibit the functioning of the gene in question.

It is likely to be some time, however, before the human metabolome is "solved" in this way; clearly, one cannot knock out genes in humans, although some deductions could be made from studies on the metabolomes of cells in patients with genetic diseases. In principle, one could attempt a systematic study of gene silencing in human cultured cells, comparing their metabolic profiles with those of the corresponding control, "wild-type" cells. Even this would be more difficult than in yeast—the human genome is larger, and the metabolomes of cultured cells are inevitably going to be adapted to a highly abnormal environment. Another problem is that the metabolomes of different cell types in a multicellular organism are likely to differ markedly and will even vary with time and changes in the environment. For instance, when genes acting in a parallel pathway compensate for a knockout (the basis of the FANCY method), it has recently been found that this effect might be mouse-strain dependent in vivo *(19)*, offering two different phenotypes for the same gene knockout. Metabolomics itself might eventually offer a way of distinguishing such subtle differences in genetic background. In the meantime, though, it should be possible to deduce much from knocking out or otherwise silencing genes in individual human cells.

## 6. METABOLIC PROFILE
## BY NMR AFTER GENE MODIFICATION

As Raamsdonk et al. *(18)* have shown, it is already possible to use classical high-resolution NMR methods to measure metabolic profiles in cells or organisms with altered gene expression. This method could be used to monitor metabolomic changes in cells from animals or humans, whether the result of gene knockouts, overexpression, or inhibition (e.g., by RNAi molecules), by comparing the abnormal metabolic profile with that from the corresponding control tissue or cell line in each case. Significant and reproducible alterations in the metabolic profile are often found in such studies. It is, in fact, a little surprising that the NMR method works as well as it does, because the number of metabolites that can be routinely quantified by NMR is quite small in comparison to the metabolome. Brindle *(20,21)* has offered two key insights into this unexpected success. The first is that the metabolites in the metabolome are densely interconnected, so that a modification of any pathway is likely to alter the concentrations of some of those metabolites we can measure by NMR *(20)*. The second is that in NMR assays, all of the metabolites are measured simultaneously in a single extract or in the intact tissue. This removes a major source of error in any quantitative analytical procedure—the sample preparation—and thus preserves any relationships between the concentrations of metabolites *(21)*.

## 7. METABOLIC PROFILE STUDIES ON HIF-1-MODIFIED TUMORS

The HIF-1 pathway, which enables cells to sense and respond to hypoxia, is crucial to numerous aspects of the tumor phenotype, and HIF-1 is overexpressed in many cancer cells. HIF-1 is a dimeric transcription factor that upregulates numerous genes involved in processes such as glucose uptake, glycolytic metabolism, pH regulation (through carbonic anhydrase), cellular proliferation, differentiation, viability, apoptosis, matrix metabolism, iron metabolism, and the formation and regulation of blood vessels *(22,23)*. Which of these myriad of functions is critical to the tumor? Cancer cells are available in which HIF-1 activity is blocked because one or other of the two subunits ($\alpha$ or $\beta$) are deficient, and a number of studies have been performed that have demonstrated changes in the tumor phenotype *(24–26)*. Griffiths et al. *(27,28)* used the [1]H-NMR/perchloric acid extract method outlined earlier, as well as [31]P-MRS in vivo, to compare the metabolic profile of HIF-1$\beta$-deficient tumors (grown as xenografts in nude mice) with that of the wild-type HEPA-1 tumors. The most obvious difference was that the HIF-1$\beta$-deficient tumors had only 20% of the normal ATP [interestingly, Seagroves et al. *(25)* also found low ATP in studies on cultured HIF-1$\alpha$-deficient tumor cells, but only when they were made hypoxic]. The NMR studies showed a number of other statistically significant abnormalities in the metabolic profile: low betaine (36%), phosphocholine (32%), choline (40%), and glycine (49%), but elevated (275%) phosphodiester compounds *(27)*.

The hypothesis we have put forward to explain these findings is outlined in Fig. 3. One of the effects of HIF-1 in the "normal" HEPA-1 cells is increased glucose uptake and glycolysis. This upregulated pathway is shown in heavy arrows in Fig. 3A. One consequence of this increased glycolytic flux is that intermediates can be "bled off" for anabolic synthesis of metabolites required in cell replication *(29)*; Fig. 3A shows an increased formation of glycine, via serine, an essential intermediate in synthesis of new ATP molecules. Figure 3B illustrates the differences in the HIF-1$\beta$-deficient HEPA c4 cells. In these cells, glucose uptake and glycolysis are not upregulated, because of the absence of HIF-1. Perhaps, as a consequence of this (but see later in this section for further discussion), glycine synthesis cannot be upregulated and glycine levels fall. An alternative pathway for glycine synthesis is from phosphocholine and choline, via betaine. All of these metabolites are depleted, consistent with the hypothesis that they are being used to synthesize glycine as an intermediate in ATP synthesis, so this pathway is shown with heavy arrows in Fig. 3B. One class of metabolites present at abnormally high concentrations in the HIF-1$\beta$-deficient HEPA-1 c4 cells is the phosphodiesters (glycerophosphocholine and glycerophosphoethanolamine), which are breakdown products of membrane phosphatidylcholine and phosphatidylethanolamines (pathway shown with a heavy arrow). Perhaps, membrane phospholipids are destabilized by the draining of choline metabolites into glycine synthesis, causing phosphatidylcholine and phosphatidylethanolamine degradation to phosphodiesters.

Can the failure to upregulate glycolytic flux in the HIF-1$\beta$-deficient HEPA c4 cells account for their inadequate formation of glycine and, hence, of ATP? Using the data from Kallinowski et al. *(13)* already discussed, we were able to calculate the rate of tumor ATP synthesis and, thus, the amount of the glycolytic flux that would have to be bled off to make the necessary glycine. It turned out to be only 0.003% *(28)*. Even allowing for the carbon required to synthesize the rest of the nucleotide molecule, it seems unlikely that the HIF-1$\alpha$-deficient cells could not have bled off sufficient glycolytic intermediates for ATP synthesis, despite their inability to upregulate glycolysis. Another possibility would be a failure to upregulate one of the enzymes in the pathway from the glycolytic intermediate 3-phosphoglycerate via serine to glycine. A likely candidate would be serine hydroxymethyltransferase, the enzyme that catalyzes formation of glycine from serine. This enzyme is known to be a target of the Myc oncogene product *(30)*, and Myc expression occurs in HEPA-1 cells *(31,32)*. Furthermore, Matteucci et al. *(32)* also speculated that HIF-1$\beta$-deficient HEPA c4 cells might have less expression of the c-Myc oncogene, which would be consistent with our hypothesis.

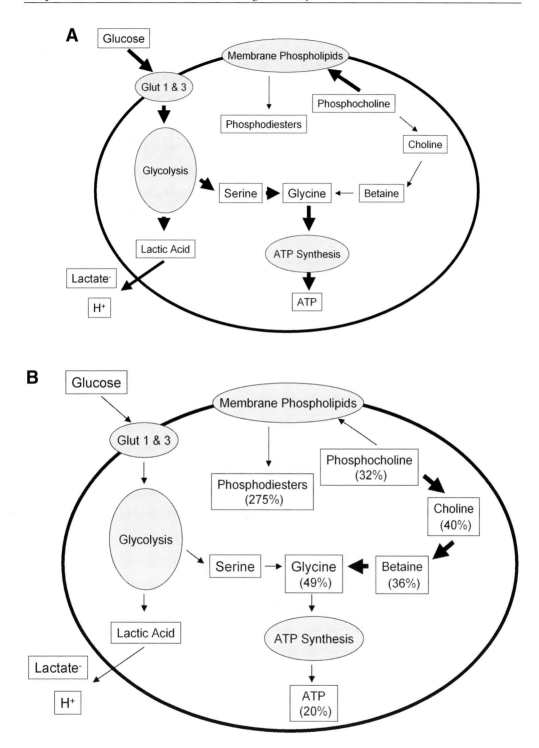

**Fig. 3.** Metabolic pathways contributing to the metabolic profiles found in wild-type HEPA-1 cells (**A**) and HIF-1β-deficient HEPA c4 cells (**B**). Heavy arrows indicate pathways likely to be upregulated. The percentages in parentheses indicate significantly abnormal metabolite concentrations.

Because of the crucial role of HIF-1 and its link with the metabolic phenotype in tumors *(7)*, HIF-1 presents an attractive target for drug therapy, and a number of studies have already been reported *(33,34)*.

## 8. METABOLOMICS TO ASSIST DRUG DISCOVERY PROGRAMS

There is a clear analogy between metabolomic screening and drug screening, and it seems very likely that the methods used for metabolomics will be directly transferable into several aspects of drug discovery programs. Candidate drugs are usually selected in screening programs because they inhibit the function of a gene product, or the gene itself. Thus, they will tend to cause a similar change in the organism's metabolism to that seen when the gene concerned is knocked out or otherwise inhibited. Thus, in the simplest case, one could screen candidate drugs against a suitable cell line (or other preparation) and compare the pattern of metabolic derangement produced by each candidate drug with the metabolomic patterns produced by gene knockouts. This should give useful information about the area of metabolism targeted by each candidate. The method is more powerful than that, however, and a combination of general metabolomic data with specific information from individual studies on candidate drugs could be of assistance in many stages of drug discovery programs and other areas of drug development.

A method similar to FANCY *(18)* should be suitable for screening quite large sets of samples. The cells would be treated with acid to extract the soluble metabolites, a method that could, in principle, be automated. The extracts would then be subjected to conventional high-resolution NMR. A one-dimensional $^1$H-NMR spectrum can be obtained in a few minutes and is routinely performed by automation, so quite large numbers of candidate drug molecules could be screened (hundreds per week) in the same way as unknown genes. Alternatively, magic-angle NMR *(35)* could probably be used to scan the intact cells and data from methods such as mass spectroscopy, fourier transform infrared spectrometry, or liquid chromatography *(36)* could be used instead of, or in addition to, NMR.

### 8.1. Choice of Targets

Information from metabolomics will augment the functional genomic data currently available. Knowing the general area of metabolism that would be affected by inhibition of a gene's product will help in choosing targets to be screened.

### 8.2. Refining Results of a Conventional Screen

High-throughput screening commonly produces large numbers of candidate drugs, many of which could be eliminated from consideration if their action on metabolism were known. It would be possible to perform metabolomic screening on large numbers of candidate compounds in a reasonably short time and to compare the resulting metabolic patterns to the library of patterns characteristic of known genes or known drugs.

### 8.3. Focused Screening

In cases where the desired pattern of metabolic perturbation was very characteristic (e.g., if all existing drugs of a particular class caused similar metabolic effects), it would be possible to perform a tightly focused metabolomic screen using the pattern itself as the end point. In principle, about 1000 compounds a week could probably be screened with a single NMR instrument using current methods.

## *8.4. Medicinal Chemistry*

It will be possible to perform metabolomic studies on large numbers of candidate compounds with systematic structural alterations. Using these data, it should be possible to develop new molecules in which drug actions have been improved or side effects "designed out."

## *8.5. Detection of Unwanted Side Effects*

Few drugs are entirely specific to their intended targets, and many candidates are eliminated because of unwanted side effects, often after prolonged and expensive development. Metabolomic methods might be used to detect side effects at the screening stage, because the pattern of metabolic derangement would often include metabolites in pathways other than the target one.

## *8.6. Whole-Organism Drug Safety and Toxicology*

As we have already seen, toxicity mechanisms manifested in the target cell would often be detectable in the course of metabolomic screening. However, toxicity to another cell type or another organ would not be apparent. A related whole-organism method called "metabonomics" has already been developed to deduce drug toxicity mechanisms from measurements of the small-molecule constituents of body fluids *(37)*.*

## *8.7. Metabolism*

Metabolomic methods, as presently conceived, would not always give clear-cut indications as to the metabolic function of a candidate drug. A characteristic pattern of perturbed metabolism might include secondary or tertiary consequences in other pathways, in addition to the direct effects of inhibition of a target protein for instance. If this pattern was always produced when genes coding for proteins in a particular area of metabolism were deleted, one would be able to make the empirical deduction that a candidate drug acted in this area, but one would not know exactly what it did. However, once such an empirical indication was available, conventional metabolic studies could be used to study the chosen candidate in depth.

## 9. CONCLUSION

Metabolomics, the next step in the paradigm of genomics, transcriptomics, and proteomics that has revolutionized drug discovery, could well be the most fruitful concept of all. Even the first simple methods proposed for metabolomic screening are likely to have a substantial impact on every level of drug discovery and development. Furthermore, the basic methods involved are familiar to the drug industry and are relatively easy to automate, so a rapid take-up can be anticipated.

---

*More recently, the same group has used the term "metabonomics" to refer to studies on cellular metabolites, gene function, and so forth *(38,39)*. For a review of the confusing and evolving nomenclature in this field, *see* ref. *40*.

# REFERENCES

1. Duesberg P, Li R, Rasnick D, Rausch C, Willer A, Kraemer A, Yerganian G, et al. Aneuploidy precedes and segregates with chemical carcinogenesis. Cancer Genet Cytogenet 2000; 119(2):83–93.
2. Hahn WC, Weinberg RA. Rules for making human tumor cells. N Engl J Med 2002; 347(20):1593–1603.
3. Underwood J, Tate AR, Luckin R, Majos C, Capdevila A, Howe F, et al. A prototype decision support system for MR spectroscopy-assisted diagnosis of brain tumours. Medinfo 2001; 10:561–565.
4. Opstad K, Howe FA. Personal communication, 2004.
5. Khong HT, Restifo NP. Natural selection of tumour variants in the generation of "tumour escape" phenotypes. Nature Immunol 2002; 3:999–1005.
6. Warburg O. The metabolism of tumours. London: Arnold Constable, 1930.
7. Stubbs M, Bashford CL, Griffiths JR. Understanding the tumor metabolic phenotype in the genomic era. Curr Mol Med 2003; 3(1):49–59.
8. Semenza GL. HIF-1: using two hands to flip the angiogenic switch. Cancer Metastasis Rev 2000; 19 (1–2):59–65.
9. Stubbs M, Rodrigues LM, Howe FA, Wang J, Jeong K, Veech RL, et al. Metabolic consequences of a reversed pH gradient in rat tumours. Cancer Res 1994; 54:4011–4016.
10. Gillies RJ, Raghunand N, Karczmar GS, Bhujwalla ZM. MRI of the tumor microenvironment. J Magn Reson Imag 2002; 16(4):430–450.
11. Gatenby RA, Gawlinski ET. The glycolytic phenotype in carcinogenesis and tumor invasion: insights through mathematical models. Cancer Res 2003; 63(14):3847–3854.
12. Ivanov S, Liao SY, Ivanova A, Danilkovitch-Miagkova A, Tarasova N, Weirich G, et al. Expression of hypoxia-inducible cell surface transmembrane carbonic anhydrases in human cancer Am J Pathol 2001; 158:905–919.
13. Kallinowski F, Schlenger KH, Runkel S, Kloes M, Stohrer M, Okunieff P, et al. Blood flow, metabolism, cellular microenvironment, and growth rate of human tumour xenografts. Cancer Res 1989; 49: 3759–3764.
14. Holm E, Hagmuller E, Staedt U, Schlickeiser G, Gunther H-J, Leweling H, et al. Substrate balance across colonic carcinomas in humans. Cancer Res 1995; 55:1373–1378.
15. Griffiths JR, McIntyre DJO, Howe FA, Stubbs M. Why are cancers acidic? A carrier-mediated diffusion model for H+ transport in the interstitial fluid. In: Goode JA, Chadwick DJ, eds. The tumour microenvironment: causes and consequences of hypoxia and acidity. Novartis Foundation Symposium Vol. 240. Chichester: Wiley, 2001:46–67.
16. Stubbs M, McSheehy PMJ, Griffiths JR. Causes and consequences of acidic pH in tumours: a magnetic resonance study. Adv Enzyme Regul 1999; 39:13–30.
17. Martin GR, Jain RK. Noninvasive meaurement of interstitial pH profiles in normal and neoplastic tissue using fluorescence ratio imaging microscopy. Cancer Res 1994; 54:5670–5674.
18. Raamsdonk LM, Teusink B, Broadhurst D, Zhang N, Hayes A, Walsh MC, et al. A functional genomics strategy that uses metabolome data to reveal the phenotype of silent mutations. Nature Biotechnol 2001; 19(1):45–50.
19. Pearson H. Surviving a knockout blow. Nature 2002; 415(6867):8–9.
20. Brindle K. Metabolomics; Pandora's box or Aladdin's cave? Biochemist 2003; 25:15–17.
21. Brindle K. Personal communication, 2004.
22. Maxwell PH, Pugh CW, Ratcliffe PJ. Activation of the HIF pathway in cancer. Curr Opin Genet Dev 2001; 11:293–299.
23. Semenza GL. Hypoxia-inducible factor 1: oxygen homeostasis and disease pathophysiology. Trends Mol Med 2001; 7(8):345–350.
24. Maxwell PH, Dachs GU, Gleadle JM, Nicholls LG, Harris AL, Stratford IJ, et al. Hypoxia-inducible factor-1 modulates gene expression in solid tumors and influences both angiogenesis and tumor growth. Proc Natl Acad Sci USA 1997; 94(15):8104–8109.
25. Seagroves TN, Ryan HE, Lu H, Wouters BG, Knapp M, Thibault P, et al. Transcription factor HIF-1 is a necessary mediator of the pasteur effect in mammalian cells. Mol Cell Biol 2001; 21(10):3436–3444.
26. Ryan HE, Poloni M, McNulty W, Elson D, Gassmann M, Arbeit JM, et al. Hypoxia-inducible factor-1alpha is a positive factor in solid tumor growth. Cancer Res 2000; 60(15):4010–4015.
27. Griffiths JR, McSheehy PM, Robinson SP, Troy H, Chung YL, Leek RD, et al. Metabolic changes detected by in vivo magnetic resonance studies of HEPA-1 wild-type tumors and tumors deficient in

hypoxia-inducible factor-1beta (HIF-1beta): evidence of an anabolic role for the HIF-1 pathway. Cancer Res 2002; 62(3):688–695.

28. Griffiths JR, Stubbs M. Opportunties for studying cancer by metabolomics: preliminary observations on tumors deficient in hypoxia-inducible factor 1. Adv Enzyme Regul 2003; 43:67–76.

29. Eigenbrodt E, Reinacher M, Scheefers-Borchel U, Scheefers H, Friis R. Double role for pyruvate kinase type M2 in the expansion of phosphometabolite pools found in tumor cells. Crit Rev Oncog 1992; 3 (1–2):91–115.

30. Nikiforov MA, Chandriani S, O'Connell B, Petrenko O, Kotenko I, Beavis A, et al. A functional screen for Myc-responsive genes reveals serine hydroxymethyltransferase, a major source of the one-carbon unit for cell metabolism. Mol Cell Biol 2002; 22(16):5793–5800.

31. Boulares HA, Giardina C, Navarro CL, Khairallah EA, Cohen SD. Modulation of serum growth factor signal transduction in Hepa 1-6 cells by acetaminophen: an inhibition of c-myc expression, NF-kappaB activation, and Raf-1 kinase activity. Toxicol Sci 1999; 48(2):264–274.

32. Matteucci E, Modora S, Simone M, Desiderio MA. Hepatocyte growth factor induces apoptosis through the extrinsic pathway in hepatoma cells: favouring role of hypoxia-inducible factor-1 deficiency. Oncogene 2003; 22(26):4062–4073.

33. Semenza GL. Targeting HIF-1 for cancer therapy. Nature Rev Cancer 2003; 3(10):721–732.

34. Giaccia A, Siim BG, Johnson RS. HIF-1 as a target for drug development. Nature Rev Drug Discov 2003; 2(10):803–811.

35. Griffin JL, Bollard M, Nicholson JK, Bhakoo K. Spectral profiles of cultured neuronal and glial cells derived from HRMAS $^1$H NMR spectroscopy. NMR Biomed 2002; 15(6):375–384.

36. Kaddourah-Douk R, Beecher C, Kristal BS, Matson WR, Bogdanov M, Asa D. Bioanalytical advances for metabolomics and metabolic profiling. Pharmagenomics 2004; 4:46–52.

37. Waters NJ, Holmes E, Williams A, Waterfield CJ, Farrant RD, Nicholson JK. NMR and pattern recognition studies on the time-related metabolic effects of alpha-naphthylisothiocyanate on liver, urine, and plasma in the rat: an integrative metabonomic approach. Chem Res Toxicol 2001; 14(10):1401–1412.

38. Nicholson JK, Connelly J, Lindon JC, Holmes E. Metabonomics: a platform for studying drug toxicity and gene function. Nature Rev Drug Discov 2002; 1(2):153–161.

39. Nicholson JK, Wilson ID. Opinion: understanding "global" systems biology: metabonomics and the continuum of metabolism. Nature Rev Drug Discov 2003; 2(8):668–676.

40. Harrigan GC, Goodacre, R. Introduction. In: Harrigan GC, Goodacre R, eds. Metabolic profiling. Its role in biomarker discovery and gene function analysis. London: Kluwer Academic, 2003:1–8.

# 11

# Focusing Target Discovery and Validation Through Proteogenomics and Molecular Imaging

*Lucy A. Carver, PhD and Jan E. Schnitzer, MD*

## CONTENTS

## SUMMARY

The analytical power and throughput of current genomic and proteomic techniques is unparalleled in the history of medical research. Yet, directly and specifically targeting solid tumors in vivo remains a long-sought yet elusive goal of molecular medicine that should benefit both therapy and diagnostic imaging of cancer. The staggering molecular complexity of solid tumors and other tissues of the body as well as the in vivo inaccessibility of tumor cells inside the neoplastic tissue limits the ability of global genomic and proteomic analysis to discover key targets for directing tumor-specific delivery of many therapies and imaging agents in vivo. The dilemma in target discovery today has become identifying which few of the many potential targets identified by high-throughput screening are the most meaningful in targeting, imaging, and treating disease. Thus, reducing data complexity to a manageable subset of candidate targets is clearly desired but requires new analytical paradigms for discovery and validation that define and utilize key biological questions to focus the power of global identification technologies. Here, the utility and pitfalls of new technologies developed to address these problems are discussed.

**Key Words:** Immunotargeting; vascular targeting; caveolae; vascular proteomics; imaging.

From: *Cancer Drug Discovery and Development: The Oncogenomics Handbook*
Edited by: W. J. LaRochelle and R. A. Shimkets © Humana Press Inc., Totowa, NJ

# 1. INTRODUCTION

The field of molecular medicine seeks new targets for detecting solid tumors through molecular imaging *(1–4)* and for treatment through directed delivery in vivo *(5–9)*. New imaging probes are needed to more readily permit the noninvasive detection and diagnosis of primary and metastatic cancer as well as to measure patient response to treatment (e.g., level of tumor cell apoptosis after chemotherapy) *(1,2)*. The small-molecule chemotherapeutics in use today to treat solid tumors are problematic because they have nearly universal access to all tissues of the body, which can greatly dilute local concentrations below effective levels, thereby requiring increased dosages leading to serious systemic toxicities.

A desired approach to imaging and therapy of solid tumors has been to create antibody probes directed to tumor cells to deliver diagnostic or therapeutic agents selectively to the tumor while bypassing other tissues. Such immunotargeting to specific antigens, expressed on neoplastic cells inside solid tumors, show excellent specific activity in vitro by binding and, when coupled to toxic agents, killing only tumor cells and not cocultured normal cells. Yet, when injected intravenously, these same agents exhibit limited bioefficacy primarily in vivo because of poor penetration into the neoplastic tissue and, thus, poor access to the intended target—the tumor cells *(10–12)*.

The vascular endothelium creates a significant barrier in most organs and solid tumors that restricts to varying degrees the exchange of many endogenous molecules as well as exogenous agents from the circulating blood to cells inside the tissue or tumor. This barrier function along with physical forces such as high tumor interstitial pressures contributes to the inability of many imaging, drug, and gene vectors to reach their intended target cells inside the tissue and, thus, to be pharmacologically effective in vivo. Consistent with this, many immunotherapies investigated over the last two decades that have centered on tumor cell surface antigens have been less successful when injected into the circulation because of their inability to reach target cells. Typically, antibody uptake as measured in tumor biopsies obtained from patients 3–10 d postinjection has been about 0.001–0.026% of injected dose per gram of tumor tissue *(13,14)*. Clearly, tumor-specific proteins accessible enough to be targeted in the clinic for specific delivery of chemotherapeutic or imaging agents to solid tumors in vivo are currently lacking. Discovering new, accessible, tumor-specific targets to improve molecular imaging and pharmacodelivery will require new analytical strategies that cut through the cumbersome overabundance of molecular information to permit rapid discovery and validation of potential targets in vivo.

# 2. PRESENT STATE OF TARGET DISCOVERY

It was widely expected that tumor-specific target discovery would be greatly accelerated by technological innovations in DNA sequencing, proteomic and genomic analyses, combinatorial chemistry, and cell-based assays that allow automated high-throughput screening to identify potential drug targets. In the past, tumor-associated proteins were identified and validated in a piecemeal fashion by labs each working independently on individual biological questions. These new techniques promised to speed up discovery enabling thousands of genes and gene products to be examined in a single experiment.

One widely used and well-developed approach to molecular profiling of tissues and tumors is through large-scale, high-throughput analysis of gene expression through the use of DNA microarrays *(15,16)*. A DNA array consists of a silicon chip or glass slide onto which up to approx 20,000 oligonucleotides or cDNAs can be immobilized. RNA that has been extracted from a tissue or tumor, amplified, and fluorophore labeled is hybridized to the array. Appropriate pattern-recognition software permits an accurate measurement of the relative abundance of any given transcript between two tissues. These arrays allow the examination of the expression patterns across many tissues of thousands of genes at once and can be used to discover new genes involved in tumorigenesis that might be targetable or provide a system to monitor clinical response. Typically, the putative tumor markers identified by this method are validated in a high-throughput manner using tissue arrays consisting of approx 1000 cylindrical tissue biopsies from different patients mounted on a glass slide *(17)*. These arrays are then subjected to *in situ* hybridization or immuno-histochemistry to compare expression of potential targets across multiple tumor types.

Other methods currently in use for genomic analysis include subtractive hybridization *(18,19)*, differential display *(20,21)*, and serial analysis of gene expression (SAGE) *(22)*. In subtractive hybridization, RNA is extracted from tumor cells, reverse transcribed into single-stranded (ss) cDNAs, radioactively or fluorescently labeled, then mixed with mRNA from the normal cells to which it is being compared. mRNAs expressed in both cell types will hybridize to form double-stranded (ds) duplexes, which can then be separated from ss-cDNAs representing mRNAs uniquely expressed in the tumor cells. In differential display, mRNA isolated from normal and tumor cells are amplified by reverse transcription–polymerase chain reaction (RT-PCR) using oligo-dT primers (to hybridize at the 3' end) and random primers each recognizing a set of 50–100 mRNAs to yield a library of 3' mRNA ends. The resulting cDNA patterns of the two cell types can be compared by electrophoresis to detect differentially expressed bands. For SAGE, mRNA isolated from normal and tumor cells are reversed transcribed to cDNA, then converted to ds-cDNA. The ds-cDNAs are restriction digested, ligated to a linker, concatamerized (25–75 cDNA tags), inserted into a cloning vector, and sequenced. Computer analysis of multiple concatemer sequences reveals the expression level of each mRNA represented by a cDNA tag.

Other approaches to tumor molecular profiling use proteomic technologies to assess expression at the protein level. Two-dimensional (2D) gels have a long history of use in comparing protein expression across tissues but require large amounts of starting material and are both time-consuming and labor-intensive *(23,24)*. In addition, separation of hydrophobic, highly charged, or transmembrane proteins as well as intergel reproducibility can be problematic. For rapid and reproducible profiling, protein arrays are being developed that lend themselves well to high-throughput screening *(25)*. Protein arrays are analogous to DNA arrays in that antibodies, small molecules, phage, or protein baits are immobilized on a slide are then incubated with tagged sample proteins to estimate the concentration of specific proteins in the original sample. Unfortunately, the success of these arrays is wholly dependent on the affinity and specificity of the antibody or protein probes used. In addition, the reactivity of the probe to the target protein might be decreased or abolished if the protein underwent a conformational change or aggregated during the immobilization process.

In recent years, effective mass spectrometric (MS)-based approaches to protein identification have been developed *(26)*. This technology can be coupled to 1D or 2D gel electrophoresis to rapidly identify tumor-specific protein bands or spots excised from the gel. High-throughput analysis using this approach is achieved through the use of robotic gel analysis and spot-picking coupled to automated sample preparation and MS loading technology, which reduces error and radically decreases the amount of hands-on time for technical personnel. In addition, multidimentional protein identification technology (MudPIT) *(27)* coupled to database searching has been developed to analyze whole-protein preparations and could greatly speed the discovery process by obviating the need for 2D gel-based separation.

Attempts have been made to establish an effective analytical paradigm by combining these robust technologies to systematize the identification and validation of potential new targets and result in more rapid development of diagnostic and therapeutic compound directed against the validated targets *(28,29)*. High-throughput screening approaches can be considered successful in that, with the completion of the Human Genome Project, the identification of a potentially useful target pool has been completed. Many of these approaches have been successful in identifying various tumor-associated molecules [e.g., p21 (WAF1) *(30)*, heparin-binding epidermal growth factor (HB-EGF) *(31)*, and p53 upregulated modulator of apoptosis (PUMA) *(32,33)*. However, the overall usefulness of this approach has been limited by technical problems that make them prone to high background noise leading to high error rates that could cause an important gene to be overlooked or complicate the validation process by making it necessary to waste resources eliminating false positives.

## 3. NEED FOR NEW APPROACHES/TECHNOLOGY

The application of high-throughput global genomic and proteomic techniques has resulted in the identification of large numbers of potential targets but few sufficiently validated leads worthy of further development. Apart from the technical problems described in the last section, other related factors negatively affect the ultimate success of the global approach. We are now in the ironic position of going from the relatively piecemeal process of discovery that slowly generated too little data to having the opposite problem with so much more data being generated than can be rapidly and accurately validated. A decade ago, a typical scientist may spend his whole career discovering and studying a single molecule. Although genome-based technologies can provide a catalog of expressed genes (i.e., identify all mRNAs present in a given cell), this information is not always helpful in determining the level of actual protein expression, localization, and accessibility of potential targets. The human genome is estimated to encode 40,000 genes, but the pool of actual targets is far greater in number. At the protein level, this pool expands to several hundred thousand possible targets because of extensive RNA processing, posttranslational modification, and the formation of functional protein complexes *(34)*. This greatly complicates new research efforts using proteomic analysis to identify differentially expressed proteins that might have utility as drug targets.

This overwhelming abundance of potential targets also relates, in part, to the molecular complexity of solid tumors, which limits the ability of global genomic and proteomic analysis to discover key targets in vivo. Often, the tissue samples used as the starting material for analysis are highly heterogeneous, consisting of many different cell populations. For example, solid tumors consist of not only the tumor cells themselves but also stromal cells, perivascular and endothelial cells, inflammatory cells, and, in some cases, adjacent normal tissue cells. Unfortunately, the clinical utility of most of the potential targets on any of these tumor constituents is limited because they reside in compartments that are not readily accessible to the circulating blood. Thus, global survey techniques applied to whole tumors might not be the best approach to identifying useful targets. It could instead be more promising to focus on meaningful subsets of cell types or parts of cells to enrich the starting samples in *bona fide* targetable molecules prior to applying high-throughput, global identification strategies.

Genomic and proteomic analysis of normal and diseased tissue and cell samples have already yielded thousands of genes and gene products as candidate targets for diagnostic and tissue assignment as well as potential therapeutic targeting *(5–8,34,35)*. The development bottleneck occurs when each of these thousands of potential targets must undergo a laborious validation process to evaluate its specificity for the cell type in question and, importantly, but often overlooked at least initially, the accessibility of the target to the targeting drug (biologic composite such as immunotoxin). It is becoming clear that the shear number of candidates discovered via high-throughput, global analytical techniques is overwhelming the required but time-consuming in vivo validation process. These issues have led some to question the ultimate impact these global genomic- and proteomic-based analytical technologies will have on speeding up target discovery *(6,7,34)*.

## 4. NEW STRATEGIES
## FOR DISCOVERY OF ACCESSIBLE TUMOR TARGETS

It is clear that reducing tissue complexity to a manageable subpopulation of the cell types of interest is necessary. Already, much work has been done to develop computer software and statistical approaches to analyze and reduce the complexity of the data generated by global genomic and proteomic experiments. Another approach that might be more successful is, rather than attempt to slog through the mountains of data produced at the end of typical experiments, to reduce tissue sample complexity at the beginning, before high-throughput analyses are applied. This will require new analytical paradigms to focus the power of global, high-throughput identification technologies.

One widely used approach to reducing sample complexity has been to study tumor cells that have been isolated and grown in culture. Unfortunately, both enzymatic/mechanical tissue disassembly and growth in culture contribute to phenotypic changes that alter native cellular function and protein expression *(36)*. Direct comparisons of protein expression have revealed <25% similarity between primary tumor cell biopsies vs cultured, clonally selected prostate tumor cell lines vs patient-matched microdissected cell-populations-derived biopsy specimens *(37)*. For example, in vitro caveolin-1 expression is downregulated in transformed cell lines and in various cultured human cancer cell lines, and induced expression greatly retards tumor cell growth *(38–44)*. Yet, in vivo, caveolin-1 can be highly expressed in tumors and is associated with increased tumor cell survival, aggressiveness, metastatic potential, suppression of apoptosis, acquisition of multidrug resistance, and resistance to chemotherapy *(42,45–52)*. Thus, using cultured tumor cell lines exclusively for discovering tumor markers may cause potentially useful markers to remain undetected.

In response to these difficulties, new technologies, such as laser capture microdissection, have been developed and optimized to isolate specific cell types. By permitting the selection of specific cells from a tissue, laser capture microdissection has the advantage of allowing researchers to focus directly on the cell subpopulation of interest in the absence of contaminating cells so that different cell types can be compared directly. However, the complexity within a single cell is still considerable enough to confound attempts at target discovery. Moreover, even with the discovery of cell-type-specific targets, those targets might not be suitable for selectively targeting a single organ or diseased tissue such as solid tumors in vivo. Most tissue- and disease-associated gene products are expressed by the cells primarily constituting the tissue (e.g., tumor cells) and, as such, these potential targets remain inside tissue compartments that usually are not readily accessible to biological agents, such as antibodies injected into the circulation. This inaccessibility prevents the development of site-directed therapies (5–7,53,54) as well as hinders many molecular imaging agents from revealing important structural and functional information in vivo (1–4). A notable exception has been hematological tumors, such as lymphomas and leukemias, where antibodies can access and, in fact, target the tumor cells in vivo, thereby rendering such immunotherapies quite effective (55,56). However, in solid tumors, multiple barriers to delivery prevent similarly effective treatment in vivo, although many immunotherapies work quite effectively and specifically in vitro (10,53–57).

Because of these accessibility issues, one meaningful subset of the tumor tissue that might inherently be worth pursuing comprises the cells constituting the critical tissue–blood interface immediately accessible to agents absorbed or injected into the circulating blood. Endothelial cells line the blood vessels of all tissues to form an interface as an attenuated cell monolayer that plays a significant role in controlling the passage of blood molecules and cells into the tissue and in many physiological functions, including vasoregulation, coagulation, and imflammation, as well as tissue nutrition, growth, survival, repair, and overall organ homeostasis and function (58). Disruption of the vascular endothelium and its normal barrier function can lead rapidly to tissue edema, hypoxia, pathology, and even organ death (59). Thus, the endothelium forms one in vivo barrier that prevents many current imaging agents, drugs, and gene vectors from optimal access to target cells within organs (10,60–63).

The endothelia of blood vessels are heterogeneous and might express potential tissue and/or disease-specific targets. Yet most of the endothelial cell is again not inherently and fully accessible to agents circulating in the blood. Only the luminal endothelial cell surface is directly in contact with the circulating blood and thus appears to be ideally suited for tissue- and tumor-specific targeting. Yet, discovering useful targets on this surface has not been readily achieved, primarily for technical reasons. The endothelium constitutes a very minor component of the tissue that makes it difficult to study in vivo using genomic or proteomic analytical techniques because the relatively small amount of a potentially useful target protein associated with the endothelial cell surface might be obscured by "molecular noise" from highly abundant, unrelated material originating from other much more abundant cell types within the tissue and, thereby, escape detection.

Multiple advantages for targeting tumor endothelium relative to tumor cells are evident in theory. All tissues in the body and especially tumors rely on the bloodstream to supply critical nutrition. The endothelial cell surface is freely and immediately accessible through the blood circulation, whereas tissue and tumor cells reside inside the tissue on the other side of the vascular wall and are, for the most part, inaccessible (10,54,64). The endothelium elaborates specific mechanisms for selecting molecules to overcome its natural barrier function, which can be usurped to deliver drugs and gene vectors inside the tumor tissue. For example, caveolae are specialized invaginations abundant at the surface of the vascular endothelium that can mediate transport into the cell (endocytosis) and transport across the cell monolayer (transcytosis) (11). Antibodies that target tissue-specific endothelial cell proteins in caveolae can rapidly penetrate the endothelial cell barrier to reach underlying tissue cells (65). In addition, endothelial cells have a stable genome, so that, unlike tumor cells, they are unlikely to undergo substantial mutation to permit the outgrowth of drug- and targeting-resistant cells. Finally, because each microvessel provides oxygen and nutrients for large numbers of underlying tissue cells, there is an inherent amplification mechanism that comes even from the destruction of one endothelial cell, which naturally initiates local coagulation to occlude vessels serving the hundreds and even thousands of tumor cells.

There is growing evidence that tumor-induced molecular targets might exist on the endothelial cell surface of blood vessels feeding tumors. The microenvironment of the tissue surrounding the blood vessels can greatly influence the phenotype of the endothelial cells *(36,66–72)*. Although the degree to which normal and neoplastic tissues can modulate endothelial cell surface protein expression in vivo is unknown, indirect evidence of molecular heterogeneity of endothelial cells in different organs and even solid tumors comes from the reported ability of select cells and even bacteriophage displaying select peptide sequences to home to specific tissues after intravenous injection *(73,74)*. Genomic analysis of human endothelial cells isolated from enzymatically digested neoplastic tissue has provided several angiogenic markers of unknown subcellular localization *(75)*.

Neither global protein nor genomic analysis of whole tissue is likely to discover endothelial cell targets in large part because the endothelial cells are such minor components of the tissue. Subcellular fractionation of the tissue is critical to unveil the protein concentrated in the endothelial cell surface caveolae that otherwise are beyond the dynamic range of detection, effectively "swamped out" by the much stronger signals from nearly 100,000 other, more abundant, proteins. Moreover, endothelial cells become more difficult to analyze because of their exquisite sensitivity to their natural environment in tissue. Endothelial cell responsiveness to a changing tissue microenvironment (e.g., during tumorigenesis) is actually the underlying basis of their tissue-specific qualities and the targets being sought. Past approaches that attempted to define the molecular topography of the vascular endothelium have relied primarily on analyzing endothelial cells isolated from the tissue through enzymatic digestions that disassemble the tissue sufficiently to release single cells that are then usually sorted using endothelial cell markers *(75–77)*. The study of isolated endothelial cells has yielded much functional and molecular information; however, both the significant perturbation of the tissue and the growth in culture contribute to morphologically obvious phenotypic drift that can translate rapidly into loss of native function and protein expression *(36,66)*.

Lastly, another important stumbling block to effectively identifying potential intravenously accessible target molecules at the critical blood–tissue interface is the methodological difficulty in examining endothelium in vivo. Even in highly vascularized tissue, the endothelium represents only a very small percentage of the cells constituting the tissue, and the proteins of the endothelial cell membrane exposed directly to the blood represent only a small fraction of the total proteins of this cell type and even more so of the total tissue. Classic techniques for the isolation of plasma membranes from tissues will yield a membrane fraction that will contain endothelial cell membranes, but only as a small percentage of the total membrane isolated. This makes detection and identification of endothelial-specific proteins very difficult and comparisons between normal and neoplastic tissues nearly impossible.

We have developed a new approach that facilitates the isolation of the luminal cell surface as it exists in its native state in the tissue in vivo by purifying the luminal endothelial cell plasma membranes directly from tissue *(78)*. We perfuse the tissue microvasculature *in situ* with a positively charged, colloidal silica solution that selectively coats the luminal endothelial cell membrane normally exposed to the circulating blood and creates a stable adherent silica pellicle marking this specific membrane of interest *(66,79–81)*. Such a coating increases the plasma membrane's density and is so strongly attached to the plasma membrane that after tissue homogenization, large sheets of silica-coated endothelial cell plasma membrane can be readily isolated away from other cellular membranes and debris by centrifugation through a high-density medium. This technique provides endothelial cell plasma membranes isolated with little contamination from intracellular components or even the plasma membranes of other lung tissue cells *(66,79–82)*. As such, it is a reasonably ideal starting material for proteomic analysis,

## 5. HOW TO VALIDATE TARGETS AND TARGETING OBJECTIVELY IN VIVO

A critical aspect of target discovery is the design and implementation of a validation process robust enough to readily filter out the ineffective molecules. A significant part of in vivo validation in target discovery normally requires ascertaining appropriate protein or mRNA expression in tissue, cell, and/or disease usually by immunohistochemistry or *in situ* hybridization, respectively *(6)*. These techniques are advantageous for examining tissues that are small, nonperfusable, or difficult to dissect, but they have serious limitations that diminish their overall utility. Tissue staining can suffer from sensitivity issues in that certain antigens can be difficult to detect and the quality of the data depends almost entirely on having a highly specific, high-affinity antibody against the potential target, which is not always easy or even possible to obtain. Moreover, neither technique provides information on whether a potential target epitope is accessible via the bloodstream or provide definitive data regarding tissue penetration. Fortunately, many of these problems can be readily overcome by using molecular imaging to assess the specificity of expression of potential targets by ascertaining the tissue selectivity and tissue processing of potential targeting vectors.

Molecular imaging can yield information beyond structure and organ function, by providing an in vivo means to assess receptors and enzymes within normal and diseased tissues without the need of more invasive procedures such as biopsies or exploratory surgery. In addition, molecular imaging is fast emerging as the standard for assessing targeting and specificity *(1–4)*, although we believe, so far, that it has been underutilized in such target validation. It offers many advantages over classic biodistribution technologies by being relatively noninvasive, global, highly sensitive, and easy to use to quickly screen multiple compounds using fewer animals. Moreover, specificity of the molecular probe and accessibility of the protein target can be accurately, objectively, and quickly assessed, and target uptake and accumulation of probe conjugates can be readily quantified. The rather laborious process of imaging antigen expression using light, fluorescence, and electron microscopy might best be performed, as a follow-up on the most relevant targets, in order to provide important additional localization data at the cellular and subcellular levels.

In vivo imaging provides a continuous viewing of tissue uptake, eliminates the need for single animal per data point to reduce the number of test animals, and greatly increases the quality and quantity of data collected. It is invaluable to have the capability to measure noninvasively the distributions of different targeting antibodies within the same animal or monitor the response to our vascular targeting therapy agents with time within the same animal. The ability to observe the true continuous distribution of the compound (as a function of space and time) allows a clearer picture of the efficiency of our targeting strategies in various organs and tissues. Finally, only relative quantification of the targeting accuracy is available. We would like to have more accurate measures of binding rates of the compounds of interest to monitor the efficiency of the delivery system and perhaps also have a measure of the rates of tumor blood vessel development, tumor growth, and subsequent regression after therapy.

## 6. NEW PARADIGM

We have developed a hypothesis-driven, multistep analytical strategy to identify the few specific, inherently targetable proteins from the vast number of proteins expressed in the tissue of interest (83). To reduce the complexity of molecular information and increase its specificity for inherently accessible proteins induced in the normal or diseased tissue, we first fractionate the tissue utilizing the silica-coating method to eliminate >99% of the tissue proteins by focusing on the tissue–blood interface and enrich for proteins that are exposed to the circulating blood and, thus, inherently accessible to specific targeting vectors. This prefractionation step in tissue preparation reduces the number of protein candidates from the >100,000 proteins probably expressed in each tissue (34) to <1000 proteins identified in the subfraction of each sample. To reduce complexity further by another approximately two to three orders of magnitude, we use *in silico* (via the AVATAR database) or differential gel electrophoretic analysis to focus only on those proteins appearing to be differentially expressed. Then, bioinformatic interrogation of this data subset for primary structure and membrane orientation yields those few tissue- or tumor-induced proteins likely to be exposed on the outside of the endothelial cell and, thus, directly accessible to intravenously injected antibodies. Finally, Western analysis and tissue immunostaining provide detailed expression profiling to yield only a few apparent endothelial cell surface proteins exhibiting specificity for a single normal or diseased tissue. Monoclonal antibodies to these proteins are then injected intravenously for biodistribution analysis and SPECT whole-body imaging to provide the final test that validates the intravenous accessibility and tissue specificity of the targets.

Using this approach, we have analyzed the proteins expressed at the endothelial cell surface and generated many new antibodies to interesting target proteins. We performed subcellular fractionation to isolate luminal endothelial cell plasma membranes and caveolae directly from endothelial cells from normal rat lungs and lungs bearing breast adenocarcinomas in vivo (35,36). Two-dimensional gel analysis detected multiple protein spots in tumor endothelial cell plasma membranes but not normal. Prominent spots easily detected in the tumor isolates were not detected in the homogenates, consistent with the small percentage of endothelial cell plasma membranes in the tumors. Tissue subfractionation appeared necessary to unmask differentially expressed tumor vascular proteins obscured by the molecular complexity of the total tumor. We then utilized mass spectrometry (MS) and database searching as well as immunoblotting to analyze these membrane isolates (35,36). We identified 15 differentially expressed proteins, including proteins already implicated in tumor angiogenesis, plus 8 new tumor-induced vascular proteins. Whole-body imaging using [125]I-labeled monoclonal antibodies rapidly validated one promising candidate as a tumor-specific target that is readily accessible to antibody injected intravenously for tumor targeting and imaging in vivo. It rapidly targets tumors with 34% injected dose (ID)/g of tissue accumulating at 2 h. Survival studies showed that a single injection of this $^{125}$I-labeled antibody caused significant remission, even in advanced disease. Thus, our novel multistep analytical approach could effectively identify specific, inherently targetable proteins on the tumor endothelium.

## 7. CONCLUSION

A proteomics-based analysis offers important advantages over DNA microarray or other genome technology. Although genome-based technologies can provide a catalog of expressed genes (i.e., identify all mRNAs expressed in the cell), this information is not always helpful in determining the level of actual protein expression, localization, and accessibility of the potential targets. On the other hand, proteomic analysis is more directly focused on expressed proteins, the actual targets for therapies. For example, our proteomic-based strategy narrows our target discovery to a subset of proteins that are actually expressed at the luminal endothelial cell surface directly exposed to the blood circulation and thus inherently accessible to specific targeting vectors. Isolating starting material directly from the tissue where the endothelium normally resides is imperative to finding "real" targets because the endothelium is exquisitely sensitive to its microenvironment and undergoes significant phenotypic drift when removed from its in vivo environment and grown in culture. Lastly, tissue subfractionation to isolate the key endothelial membranes pertinent to the objective of tumor target accessibility coupled with proteomic technology can promote the unmasking of the small subset of proteins that can be targeted by intravenous injection in vivo.

## REFERENCES

1. Massoud TF, Gambhir SS. Molecular imaging in living subjects: seeing fundamental biological processes in a new light. Genes Dev 2003; 17:545–580.
2. Herschman HR. Molecular imaging: looking at problems, seeing solutions. Science 2003; 302:605–608.
3. Rudin M, Weissleder R. Molecular imaging in drug discovery and development. Nat Rev Drug Discov 2003; 2:123–131.
4. Weissleder R. Scaling down imaging: molecular mapping of cancer in mice. Nat Rev Cancer 2002; 2: 11–18.
5. Drews J. Drug discovery: a historical perspective. Science 2000; 287:1960–1964.
6. Lindsay MA. Target discovery. Nat Rev Drug Discov 2003; 2:831–838.
7. Workman P. New drug targets for genomic cancer therapy: successes, limitations, opportunities and future challenges. Curr Cancer Drug Targets 2001; 1:33–47.
8. Anzick SL, Trent JM. Role of genomics in identifying new targets for cancer therapy. Oncology (Huntingt) 2002; 16:7–13.
9. Cavenee WK. Genetics and new approaches to cancer therapy. Carcinogenesis 2002; 23:683–686.
10. Schnitzer JE. Vascular targeting as a strategy for cancer therapy. N Engl J Med 1998; 339:472–474.
11. Schnitzer JE. Caveolae: from basic trafficking mechanisms to targeting transcytosis for tissue-specific drug and gene delivery in vivo. Adv Drug Deliv Rev 2001; 49:265–280.
12. Burrows FJ, Thorpe PE. Vascular targeting—a new approach to the therapy of solid tumors. Pharmacol Ther 1994; 64:155–174.
13. Chaudhry A, Carrasquillo JA, Avis IL, et al. Phase I and imaging trial of a monoclonal antibody directed against gastrin-releasing peptide in patients with lung cancer. Clin Cancer Res 1999; 5:3385–3393.
14. Scott AM, Lee FT, Hopkins W, et al. Specific targeting, biodistribution, and lack of immunogenicity of chimeric anti-GD3 monoclonal antibody KM871 in patients with metastatic melanoma: results of a phase I trial. J Clin Oncol 2001; 19:3976–3987.

15. Schena M, Shalon D, Davis RW, Brown PO. Quantitative monitoring of gene expression patterns with a complementary DNA microarray. Science 1995; 270:467–470.
16. Chee M, Yang R, Hubbell E, et al. Accessing genetic information with high-density DNA arrays. Science 1996; 274:610–614.
17. Kononen J, Bubendorf L, Kallioniemi A, et al. Tissue microarrays for high-throughput molecular profiling of tumor specimens. Nat Med 1998; 4:844–847.
18. Ermolaeva OD, Sverdlov ED. Subtractive hybridization, a technique for extraction of DNA sequences distinguishing two closely related genomes: critical analysis. Genet Anal 1996; 13:49–58.
19. Zimmermann CR, Orr WC, Leclerc RF, Barnard EC, Timberlake WE. Molecular cloning and selection of genes regulated in Aspergillus development. Cell 1980; 21:709–715.
20. Liang P, Averboukh L, Keyomarsi K, Sager R, Pardee AB. Differential display and cloning of messenger RNAs from human breast cancer versus mammary epithelial cells. Cancer Res 1992; 52:6966–6968.
21. Welsh J, Chada K, Dalal SS, Cheng R, Ralph D, McClelland M. Arbitrarily primed PCR fingerprinting of RNA. Nucleic Acids Res 1992; 20:4965–4970.
22. Velculescu VE, Zhang L, Vogelstein B, Kinzler KW. Serial analysis of gene expression. Science 1995; 270:484–487.
23. O'Farrell PH. High resolution two-dimensional electrophoresis of proteins. J Biol Chem 1975; 250: 4007–4021.
24. Ong SE, Pandey A. An evaluation of the use of two-dimensional gel electrophoresis in proteomics. Biomol Eng 2001; 18:195–205.
25. Templin MF, Stoll D, Schrenk M, Traub PC, Vohringer CF, Joos TO. Protein microarray technology. Drug Discov Today 2002; 7:815–822.
26. Aebersold R, Mann M. Mass spectrometry-based proteomics. Nature 2003; 422:198–207.
27. Washburn MP, Wolters D, Yates JR 3rd. Large-scale analysis of the yeast proteome by multidimensional protein identification technology. Nature Biotechnol 2001; 19:242–247.
28. Liotta L, Petricoin E. Molecular profiling of human cancer. Nat Rev Genet 2000; 1:48–56.
29. Petricoin EF, Zoon KC, Kohn EC, Barrett JC, Liotta LA. Clinical proteomics: translating benchside promise into bedside reality. Nat Rev Drug Discov 2002; 1:683–695.
30. el-Deiry WS, Tokino T, Velculescu VE, et al. WAF1, a potential mediator of p53 tumor suppression. Cell 1993; 75:817–825.
31. McCarthy SA, Samuels ML, Pritchard CA, Abraham JA, McMahon M. Rapid induction of heparin-binding epidermal growth factor/diphtheria toxin receptor expression by Raf and Ras oncogenes. Genes Dev 1995; 9:1953–1964.
32. Nakano K, Vousden KH. PUMA, a novel proapoptotic gene, is induced by p53. Mol Cell 2001; 7:683–694.
33. Yu J, Zhang L, Hwang PM, Kinzler KW, Vogelstein B. PUMA induces the rapid apoptosis of colorectal cancer cells. Mol Cell 2001; 7:673–682.
34. Huber LA. Is proteomics heading in the wrong direction? Nat Rev Mol Cell Biol 2003; 4:74–80.
35. Perou CM, Sorlie T, Eisen MB, et al. Molecular portraits of human breast tumours. Nature 2000; 406: 747–752.
36. Madri JA, Williams SK. Capillary endothelial cell culture: phenotype modulation by matrix components. J Cell Biol 1983; 97:153–165.
37. Ornstein DK, Gillespie JW, Paweletz CP, et al. Proteomic analysis of laser capture microdissected human prostate cancer and in vitro prostate cell lines. Electrophoresis 2000; 21:2235–2242.
38. Koleske AJ, Baltimore D, Lisanti MP. Reduction of caveolin and caveolae in oncogenically transformed cells. Proc Natl Acad Sci USA 1995; 92:1381–1385.
39. Lee SW, Reimer CL, Oh P, Campbell DB, Schnitzer JE. Tumor cell growth inhibition by caveolin re-expression in human breast cancer cells. Oncogene 1998; 16:1391–1397.
40. Engelman JA, Wykoff CC, Yasuhara S, Song KS, Okamoto T, Lisanti MP. Recombinant expression of caveolin-1 in oncogenically transformed cells abrogates anchorage-independent growth. J Biol Chem 1997; 272:16,374–16,381.
41. Engelman JA, Lee RJ, Karnezis A, et al. Reciprocal regulation of neu tyrosine kinase activity and caveolin-1 protein expression in vitro and in vivo. Implications for human breast cancer. J Biol Chem 1998; 273:20,448–20,455.
42. Bender FC, Reymond MA, Bron C, Quest AF. Caveolin-1 levels are down-regulated in human colon tumors, and ectopic expression of caveolin-1 in colon carcinoma cell lines reduces cell tumorigenicity. Cancer Res 2000; 60:5870–5878.

43. Wiechen K, Diatchenko L, Agoulnik A, et al. Caveolin-1 is down-regulated in human ovarian carcinoma and acts as a candidate tumor suppressor gene. Am J Pathol 2001; 159:1635–1643.

44. Wiechen K, Sers C, Agoulnik A, et al. Down-regulation of caveolin-1, a candidate tumor suppressor gene, in sarcomas. Am J Pathol 2001; 158:833–839.

45. Lavie Y, Fiucci G, Liscovitch M. Up-regulation of caveolae and caveolar constituents in multidrug-resistant cancer cells. J Biol Chem 1998; 273:32,380–32,383.

46. Mouraviev V, Li L, Tahir SA, et al. The role of caveolin-1 in androgen insensitive prostate cancer. J Urol 2002; 168:1589–1596.

47. Tahir SA, Yang G, Ebara S, et al. Secreted caveolin-1 stimulates cell survival/clonal growth and contributes to metastasis in androgen-insensitive prostate cancer. Cancer Res 2001; 61:3882–3885.

48. Nasu Y, Timme TL, Yang G, et al. Suppression of caveolin expression induces androgen sensitivity in metastatic androgen-insensitive mouse prostate cancer cells. Nat Med 1998; 4:1062–1064.

49. Timme TL, Goltsov A, Tahir S, et al. Caveolin-1 is regulated by c-myc and suppresses c-myc-induced apoptosis. Oncogene 2000; 19:3256–3265.

50. Li L, Yang G, Ebara S, et al. Caveolin-1 mediates testosterone-stimulated survival/clonal growth and promotes metastatic activities in prostate cancer cells. Cancer Res 2001; 61:4386–4392.

51. Rajjayabun PH, Garg S, Durkan GC, Charlton R, Robinson MC, Mellon JK. Caveolin-1 expression is associated with high-grade bladder cancer. Urology 2001; 58:811–814.

52. Kato K, Hida Y, Miyamoto M, et al. Overexpression of caveolin-1 in esophageal squamous cell carcinoma correlates with lymph node metastasis and pathologic stage. Cancer 2002; 94:929–933.

53. Jain RK. The next frontier of molecular medicine: delivery of therapeutics. Nat Med 1998; 4:655–657.

54. Dvorak HF, Nagy JA, Dvorak AM. Structure of solid tumors and their vasculature: implications for therapy with monoclonal antibodies. Cancer Cells 1991; 3:77–85.

55. von Mehren M, Adams GP, Weiner LM. Monoclonal antibody therapy for cancer. Annu Rev Med 2003; 54:343–369.

56. Farah RA, Clinchy B, Herrera L, Vitetta ES. The development of monoclonal antibodies for the therapy of cancer. Crit Rev Eukaryot Gene Expr 1998; 8:321–356.

57. Carver LA, Schnitzer JE. Caveolae: mining little caves for new cancer targets. Nature Rev Cancer 2003; 3:571–581.

58. Schnitzer JE, Bravo J. High affinity binding, endocytosis, and degradation of conformationally modified albumins. Potential role of gp30 and gp18 as novel scavenger receptors. J Biol Chem 1993; 268: 7562–7570.

59. Michiels C. Endothelial cell functions. J Cell Physiol 2003; 196:430–443.

60. Miller N, Vile R. Targeted vectors for gene therapy. FASEB J 1995; 9:190–199.

61. Thrush GR, Lark LA, Clinchy BC, Vitetta ES. Immunotoxins: an update. Annu Rev Immunol 1996; 14:49–71.

62. Tomlinson E. Theory and practice of site-specific drug delivery. Adv Drug Deliv Rev 1987; 1:87–198.

63. Carver LA, Schnitzer JE. Tissue-specific pharmacodelivery and overcoming key cell barriers in vivo: vascular targeting of caveolae. In: Muzykantov V, Torchilin B, eds. Biomedical aspects of drug targeting. Boston: Kluwer Academic, 2002:107–128.

64. Burrows FJ, Thorpe PE. Eradication of large solid tumors in mice with an immunotoxin directed against tumor vasculature. Proc Natl Acad Sci USA 1993; 90:8996–9000.

65. McIntosh DP, Tan X-Y, Oh P, Schnitzer JE. Targeting endothelium and its dynamic caveolae for tissue-specific transcytosis in vivo: a pathway to overcome cell barriers to drug and gene delivery. Proc Natl Acad Sci USA 2002; 99:1996–2001.

66. Schnitzer JE. The endothelial cell surface and caveolae in health and disease. In: Born GVR, Schwartz CJ, eds. Vascular endothelium: physiology, pathology, and therapeutic opportunities. Stuttgart: Schattauer, 1997:77–95.

67. Goerdt S, Steckel F, Schulze-Osthoff K, Hagemeier HH, Macher E, Sorg C. Characterization and differential expression of an endothelial cell-specific surface antigen in continuous and sinusoidal endothelial, in skin vascular lesions and in vitro. Exp Cell Biol 1989; 57:185–192.

68. Gumkowski F, Kaminska G, Kaminski M, Morrissey LW, Auerbach R. Heterogeneity of mouse vascular endothelium. Blood Vessels 1987; 24:11–23.

69. Hagemeier H-H, Vollmer E, Goerdt S, Schulze-Osthoff K, Sorg C. A monoclonal antibody reacting with endothelial cells of budding vessels in tumors and inflammatory tissues, and non-reactive with normal adult tissues. Int J Cancer 1986; 38:481–488.

70. Aird WC, Edelberg JM, Weiler-Guettler H, Simmons WW, Smith TW, Rosenberg RD. Vascular bed-specific expression of an endothelial cell gene is programmed by the tissue microenvironment. J Cell Biol 1997; 138:1117–1124.

71. Janzer RC, Raff MC. Astrocytes induce blood-brain barrier properties in endothelial cells. Nature 1987; 325:253–257.

72. Stewart PA, Wiley MJ. Developing nervous tissue induces formation of blood–brain barrier characteristics in invading endothelial cells: a study using quail-chick transplantation chimeras. Dev Biol 1981; 84:183–192.

73. Pasqualini R, Ruoslahti E. Organ targeting *in vivo* using phage display peptide libraries. Nature 1996; 380: 364–366.

74. Rajotte D, Arap W, Hagedorn M, Koivunen E, Pasqualini R, Ruoslahti E. Molecular heterogeneity of the vascular endothelium revealed by in vivo phage display. J Clin Invest 1998; 102:430–437.

75. St Croix B, Rago C, Velculescu V, et al. Genes expressed in human tumor endothelium. Science 2000; 289:1197–1202.

76. Auerbach R, Alby L, Morrissey LW, Tu M, Joseph J. Expression of organ-specific antigens on capillary endothelial cells. Microvasc Res 1985; 29:401–411.

77. Belloni PN, Nicolson GL. Differential expression of cell surface glycoproteins on various organ-derived microvascular endothelia and endothelial cell cultures. J Cell Physiol 1988; 136:398–410.

78. Oh P, Li Y, Yu J, et al. Subtractive proteomic mapping of the endothelial surface in lung and solid tumours for tissue-specific therapy. Nature 2004; 10:629–635.

79. Magnet AD, Schnitzer JE. Purification of luminal endothelial membrane with plasmalemmal vesicles from tissues in situ. FASEB J 1992; 6:A1033.

80. Schnitzer JE, McIntosh DP, Dvorak AM, Liu J, Oh P. Separation of caveolae from associated microdomains of GPI-anchored proteins [see comments]. Science 1995; 269:1435–1439.

81. Oh P, Schnitzer JE. Isolation and subfractionation of plasma membranes to purify caveolae separately from glycosyl-phosphatidylinositol-anchored protein microdomain. In: Celis J, ed. Cell biology: a laboratory handbook. Vol. 2. Orlando, FL: Academic, 1998:34–36.

82. Schnitzer JE, Liu J, Oh P. Endothelial caveolae have the molecular transport machinery for vesicle budding, docking, and fusion including VAMP, NSF, SNAP, annexins, and GTPases. J Biol Chem 1995; 270:14,399–14,404.

83. Oh P, Li Y, Yu J, et al. Subtractive proteomic mapping of the endothelial surface in lung and solid tumours for tissue-specific therapy. Nature 2004; 429:629–635.

84. Durr E, Yu J, Krasinska KM, et al. Direct proteomic mapping of the lung microvascular endothelial cell surface in vivo and in cell culture. Nat Biotechnol 2004; 22:985–992.

# III CANCER TARGET VALIDATION: *CELLULAR APPROACHES*

# 12 RNA Interference

*RNAid for Future Therapeutics?*

## Mustapha Diallo, DIPL BIOL, Katja Schmitz, PhD, and Ute Schepers, PhD

### CONTENTS

### SUMMARY

RNA interference (RNAi) is an evolutionarily conserved phenomenon of double-stranded (ds)RNA-mediated mRNA degradation that leads to the posttranscriptional silencing of the corresponding gene. First reports on RNAi emerged in 1998, and since then, it has become one of the most fascinating fields of molecular biology. RNAi has provided important insights about the diversity of RNA molecules and their implication in many biological processes such as the regulation of developmental genes in eukaryotic organisms. Furthermore, RNAi has rapidly developed into a powerful instrument with a great potential for functional genomics and therapeutic applications by silencing normal and disease-related gene functions. To date, the use of RNAi for genetic-based therapies is widely studied, especially in viral infections, cancers, and inherited genetic disorders. Despite the many unanswered questions on how this technology can be efficiently applied to humans, the development of novel approaches, such as vaccines or novel delivery agents, is certainly one of the major goals in RNAi research.

**Key Words:** RNA interference; RNAi; cancer; gene therapy; siRNA; knockout; viral infections; functional genomics.

From: *Cancer Drug Discovery and Development: The Oncogenomics Handbook*
Edited by: W. J. LaRochelle and R. A. Shimkets © Humana Press Inc., Totowa, NJ

# 1. INTRODUCTION

Discovered only a few years ago, RNA interference (RNAi) has already gained access to almost all biomedical and even some chemical laboratories as a technique that allows the suppression of gene function in a very effective way. RNAi is a specific form of RNA silencing that is induced by double-stranded (ds) RNA and results in sequence-specific cleavage of the homologous mRNA *(1)*. RNAi has been first observed in the nematode *Caenorhabditis elegans* by Guo and Kemphues *(2)* during antisense experiments.

However, the decisive discovery was made by Fire and Mello, who tried to explain the silencing activity of sense control RNA found in the Guo and Kemphues experiment *(1,2)*. By simultaneous injection of sense and antisense RNA strands in *C. elegans*, they obtained a 10-fold stronger effect on the silencing of homologous mRNA than with antisense RNA alone. This led to the conclusion that dsRNA triggers an efficient silencing mechanism in which exogenous dsRNA significantly reduces the overall level of target mRNA *(1,3)*.

During further investigations of the phenomenon, a number of features were discovered that made RNAi an exiting new tool for molecular biology *(4)*. RNAi is highly selective in mRNA degradation if the exogenously added dsRNA shares sequences of perfect homology with the target. Because the translation of the protein is inhibited by specific degradation of its encoding mRNA, the transcription of the gene remains unaffected. Because dsRNA homologous to intron sequences or promoters comprised by the DNA sequence showed no effect at all, the silencing appears to take place at the posttranscriptional level *(1,5,6)*. Substoichiometric amounts of dsRNA are sufficient to decrease mRNA levels within 2–3 h, and the RNAi phenotype can progress systemically (distribution between different organs) in a variety of organisms *(7,8)*. Moreover, cultured cells transfected with dsRNA maintain the loss-of-function phenotype for up to nine cell divisions *(9)*.

We know today that RNAi is related to a well-known form of posttranscriptional gene silencing (PTGS), which, until recently, was believed to occur exclusively in plants, *Drosophila* (cosuppression), and in *Neurospora crassa* (quelling) as a response to retroviral and transposable element invasion *(10–13)*. The trigger for this cellular defense mechanism is dsRNA, which occurs during replication of those elements but never from tightly regulated endogenous genes. Intermediate dsRNA will be recognized and degraded. Moreover, the RNAi machinery is presumed to carry out numerous additional functions. There is evidence that it eliminates defective mRNAs by degradation *(14)*, as there are genes that function simultaneously in RNAi and nonsense-mediated mRNA decay (NMD) *(15)*. RNAi is further assumed to tightly regulate protein levels in response to various environmental stimuli, although the extent to which this mechanism is employed by specific cell types remains to be estimated *(16)*. This suggests that RNAi is evolutionarily conserved among all eukaryotes occurring in response to the presence of dsRNA.

In the last few years, intensive molecular and biochemical studies have been undertaken to identify and characterize the participating players of the RNAi pathway. Furthermore, researchers have developed RNAi into a standard tool for in vivo reverse genetic studies in many eukaryotic systems.

This chapter will give an overview about the discovery and the current state of RNAi research and what is known about the mechanism and its implication in functional genomic studies and in designing therapeutic approaches against diseases.

## 2. MECHANISM OF RNAi

Soon after the discovery of RNAi, questions on the mechanism arose. Many laboratories directed their research toward the identification of the proteins implicated in the RNAi pathway and their molecular and biochemical characterization. Even though the RNAi pathway is still not fully understood, many of the main players are already well characterized and many more will follow for sure in the near future.

A first success was the correlation of RNAi with long known RNA silencing phenomena such as cosuppression and quelling. All these phenomena are now referred to as RNA silencing. Indeed, genetic studies in RNA-silencing-deficient mutants of *Arabidopsis (17)*, *N. crassa (18,19)*, and *C. elegans (20,21)* revealed several genes that are conserved throughout all three phenomena, including members of the helicase family, RNase III-related nucleases, members of the Argonaute family, and RNA-dependent RNA polymerases (RdRp).

## 3. DICER

Among the first proteins to be identified and thoroughly investigated was Dicer, a member of the RNase III family. Its discovery was based on the observation that dsRNA is processed to smaller fragments comprising a length of 21–25 nucleotides (nt), depending on the organism in which they are generated *(22,23)*. Such small dsRNAs, complementary to both strands of the silenced gene, were initially observed in plants undergoing transgene- or virus-induced posttranscriptional gene silencing or cosuppression *(22)*. Later, Zamore and co-workers identified the same small RNA species after the incubation of *Drosophila* S2-cell extracts with long dsRNA *(23,24)*. To date, they are known as the active dsRNA species in the RNAi pathway and are referred to as small interfering RNAs (siRNAs). They exhibit the characteristic features of dsRNA fragments originating from the cleavage of long exogenous dsRNA by a dsRNA-specific RNase III.

In addition to the already characterized members of the RNase III family such as the regular canonical RNase III and Drosha, localized to the nucleus *(25)*, homology screens of genomic data from *Drosophila* revealed new candidate genes with RNase III-like domains *(26)*. Among those candidates was a nuclease of 2249 amino acids predicted from *Drosophila* sequence data *(27)*. It contains two RNase III domains *(28,29)*, a dsRNA-binding motif (DSRM) *(30)*, an amino-terminal DexH/DEAH RNA helicase/ATPase domain, and a so-called "PAZ domain" *(31)*. All of these properties characterize members of the ribonucleases (RNase) III family. With reference to its ability to generate equally sized fragments from long dsRNA, this enzyme was called Dicer *(27,32)*.

Catalysis of the "initiator" step in the RNAi pathway by recognition and degradation of dsRNA into siRNAs has been confirmed *(27)* (Fig. 1). Although some organisms only encode one (human, mouse, *C. elegans*, and *Schizosaccharomyces pombe*) or two (*Drosophilia melanogaster*) homologs, some plants like *Arabidopsis* encode at least four Dicer-like enzymes (DCL1–4) *(33)*. The evolutionarily conserved PAZ domain *(27)* is assumed to function as a nucleic-acid-binding motif *(27,34)*. By this means, the multiplication of parasitic elements is prevented and their integration into the host genome inhibited *(23)*.

Furthermore, Dicer plays a dominant role in the processing of another small RNA species, the micro-RNAs (Fig. 1). miRNAs that also resemble a length of 21–22 nt have been recently identified in eukaryotic organisms, including plants, *C. elegans*, and humans

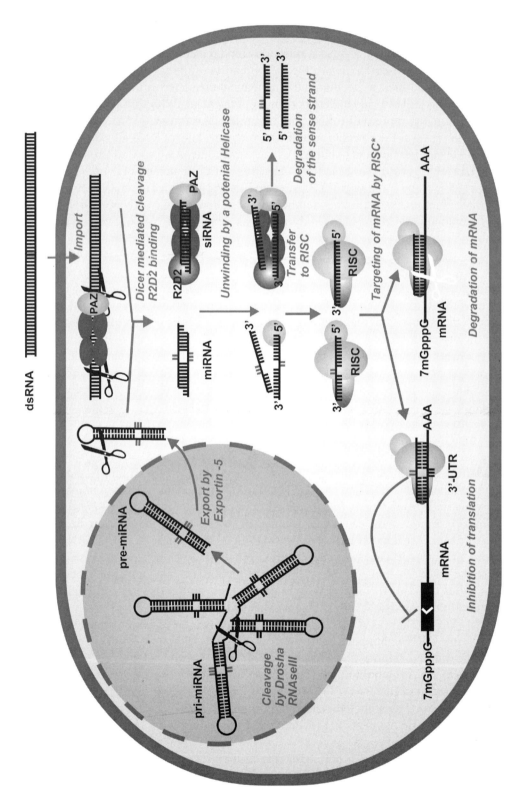

**Fig. 1.** Proposed mechanism of RNAi. (Modified from ref. 260.)

*(35–40).* miRNAs are processed from long stem loop precursors encoded by evolution-arily conserved and nonprotein coding genes and are very heterogeneous in their struc-ture. They have been shown to be *bona fide* regulators of gene expression by repressing transcription. Like all RNase III cleavage products, siRNAs and miRNAs bear a 5'-phos-phate and a 3'-hydroxyl-group and a two-nucleotide overhang at both 3' ends. These struc-tural features are indispensable for their capacity to exhibit their silencing activity *(41).* In accordance with the structure of bacterial RNaseIII, in which two active centers embrace a cleft that can accommodate a dsRNA substrate, Dicer has been proposed to function as an antiparallel dimer *(42).* Dicer contains two catalytic domains and it is suggested that in the dimer, only two of the four centers remain active to process the dsRNA into siRNAs of appropriate size *(27,43).*

Another working model proposes a monomeric action of Dicer cleaving the dsRNA during translocation of the enzyme along its substrate *(27).* This process would require the partial unwinding of the dsRNA, probably by the helicase domain, and an energy-con-suming step to drive the translocation of the enzyme along the dsRNA in an ATP-depen-dent manner *(27,32,44–47).* This mode of action might occur in *Drosophila* and other invertebrates but not in mammals, where Dicer is acting in an ATP-independent way *(45).*

In vivo, Dicer is part of a protein complex. Even though the molecular mechanism of Dicer-mediated dsRNA cleavage is partially unraveled, it is still not fully clarified how the "initiator step" is connected to the "effector" step, because Dicer is not directly involved in the cleavage of the target mRNA *(48).* During the last 2 yr, several proteins were iden-tified that seem to play a role as interaction partners or even RNAi signal transporters.

The siRNAs are not moving freely throughout the cytoplasm *(49).* To ensure a specific target recognition by siRNAs, they are bound by Dicer-associated proteins and, thus, transferred to the "effector" complex, also known as the RNA-induced silencing com-plex (RISC). The interaction might occur between the two PAZ domains of Argonaute-2 and Dicer, facilitating the transfer of siRNAs *(50).*

The recently discovered protein R2D2 *(51)* harbors a tandem dsRNA-binding domain (R2) and a *Drosophila* Dicer-2-binding domain (D2), both required for the transfer of siRNAs. It assures the stabilization of the Dicer cleavage products by forming a stable complex with the nascent siRNAs and serves as the transfer shuttle for siRNA from Dicer to RISC *(51).* Although Dicer alone is sufficient to cleave dsRNA, R2D2 is required to bind not only the nascent siRNAs but also synthetic siRNAs. It appears that newly generated symmetric siRNAs are not released from the complex but, rather, retained by DCR-2/R2D2 in a fixed orientation, which might determine the guiding strand for target cleavage *(51).*

## 4. RNA-INDUCED SILENCING COMPLEX

The siRNAs serve as templates for the sequence-specific cleavage of the endogenous target mRNA. This was proven by the identification of siRNAs associated to RISC *(52).* So far, *Drosophila* RISC was first proposed to be an approx 500-kDa complex bound to ribosomes in cell-free extracts *(49).* Closer studies identified it as a multifunctional ribonucleotide protein complex (RNP) containing a DEAD-box helicase and a nuclease, which both seem to be conserved in *Drosophila, C. elegans,* and mammals, although the overlap is not complete *(53).* Unwinding of the siRNA mediated by an ATP-dependent helicase converts RISC into its active form RISC*. The antisense siRNA strand remains bound to RISC* and serves as a guiding strand for the recognition of the target mRNA.

Target binding occurs via conventional Watson–Crick base-pairing. Perfect homology promotes the cleavage by the nuclease activity of the RISC* *(52)*.

Recent studies have shown that antisense RNA ranging from 19 to 29 nt can also enter the RNAi pathway, albeit less efficiently *(48,54)*. Because of the lack of information about the correct strand orientation, siRNA sense strands may enter the RNAi pathway. Even if the siRNAs are bound by Dicer/R2D2, they are not transferred to RISC in a predetermined orientation. On the other hand, separated antisense and sense strands of a distinct siRNA can reveal similar intrinsic efficacy in targeting their specific mRNA but show different activities when hybridized to a duplex siRNA. The stability of the 5' end determines which strand enters into RISC and which one is released for degradation *(55)*. Because 5' ends starting with a less stable A-U base-pairing are preferred over those beginning with the more stable G-C, it is suggested that the RISC helicase preferably acts from the less stable 5' end, leading to a preferential incorporation of the respective strand by RISC *(55)*. This preference is even enhanced by G:U wobble basepairs at the respective 5' end. Statistical analysis of the internal thermodynamic stability of hundreds of synthetic siRNAs has recently confirmed that a decreased stability at the 5' ends of the functional duplexes referring to the antisense strand *(55,56)* facilitates the incorporation of the antisense strand into RISC. Thus, sense strands with instable 5' ends might be incorporated by RISC, presumably leading to off-target effects *(57)*.

The siRNA single strand eventually resides in the RISC together with homologs of Argonaute proteins Ago-2, eIF2C1, and/or eIF2C2 *(48)*, which all contain a PIWI and a PAZ domain. Screening of Argonaute mutants in plants, *C. elegans*, and *N. Crassa*, established a link between this gene family and RNAi *(31)*. Even though the binding affinity for nucleic acids usually is low, PAZ domains exhibit enhanced affinity for siRNA binding *(58,59)*, recently underlined by the molecular structure of the PAZ domain *(58–60)*.

Across the examined species, mutants for genes of the Argonaute family and their homologs not only exhibit severe defects in RNA silencing but also in developmental timing.

The current research on RISC is now focusing on the antisense RNA guided degradation of the target mRNA. Target cleavage occurs between the ninth and tenth basepair from the 5 end of the guiding antisense RNA strand. Recently, a novel protein comprising five repeats of a nuclease domain known from staphylococcus bacteria could be purified in association with RISC *(61–63)*. One of the nuclease domains is fused to a Tudor domain, leading to the name Tudor–staphylococcal nuclease (Tudor-SN) *(63)*. Despite its conservation in many species, this nuclease is unlikely to be responsible for the siRNA-mediated mRNA cleavage *(63)*. Other nucleases remain to be identified.

## 5. RNAi IN REVERSE GENETIC STUDIES

Traditionally, the function of a gene was determined by forward genetic experiments that start with a mutant phenotype and the analysis of the protein defect and end with the conversion of the protein sequence into genetic information. Mutant phenotypes were found in patients with inherited diseases or knockout animals *(64)*. Today, most gene functions are determined by reverse genetics, which work in the opposite direction. This approach was made possible by huge progress in recombinant DNA technology and the sequencing of a variety of genomes *(65,66)*. Reverse genetic studies, sometimes also referred to as functional genomics, meet the challenge of deciphering the steadily accumulating genetic data into functional information. Meanwhile, the genetic information of several organisms has been deciphered, including *C. elegans*, *D. melanogaster*, and humans *(65,66)*. So far, many methods have been developed to manipulate the expression of genetic information at different levels.

Gene silencing at the genomic level mainly proceeds by subjecting the isolated wild-type gene to in vitro mutagenesis by nucleotide substitution, deletion, or insertion. The mutated gene is then placed back into cultured cells or into the organism of interest, where it replaces the functional gene after homologous recombination. This method has been especially exploited to silence genes in animals such as mice and flies. Many practical approaches have been published, including inducible systems that enable the spatial, tissue-specific, and temporal inhibition of gene expression *(67–69)*. Many of these methods are very time-consuming and laborious.

Other common methods act at the posttranslational level, such as the depletion of proteins by antibodies masking the protein, inhibitors that block protein function by imitating substrates, or docking sites for other interaction partners, as well as RNA-based aptamers and intramers *(70,71)*. With the discovery of RNAi, posttranscriptional silencing is receiving more and more interest.

In antisense technology the target mRNA is bound by homologous strands of antisense DNA, modified DNA, or PNA (peptide nucleic acids) to prevent the binding of the ribosome and, thus, translation. Many modifications have been introduced to stabilize the antisense binding partner and a few systems have made their way to clinical trials. Yet, antisense technology has never quite met its high expectations, whereas RNAi with its catalytic nature seems to create a real hype.

In the generation of loss-of-function phenotypes, RNAi procedures are much faster and straightforward than traditional genetic approaches *(64)*, certainly displaying the method for initial and high-throughput experiments.

In addition, it offers many advantages over other methods comprising specificity and efficiency. Only mRNA sharing perfect homology with catalytic amounts of exogenously applied dsRNA is cleaved, whereas other mRNAs, even those with point mutations, remain unaffected *(1,72,73)*. It further offers a very simple handling. In *C. elegans*, RNAi can be induced by simply injecting adult worms with dsRNA, by soaking the animals in the dsRNA, by electroporation of dsRNA, or by engineering *Escherichia coli* to produce the appropriate dsRNA and feeding the bacteria to the worms *(3,9,74–76)*. Soaking also functions in *Drosophila* S2 cell culture *(77)*. Moreover, in plants and worms, the RNAi effect can diffuse across tissue boundaries and can be transmitted to the progeny *(78,79)*. Moreover, RNAi can be used to simultaneously silence several genes.

Many techniques have already been established by a variety of laboratories, as described earlier. In *C. elegans*, RNAi has already yielded impressive results in investigating the functions of the whole genome *(80)*, including genes implicated in cell division *(81,82)*—fat regulatory genes *(83)*.

Genomewide RNAi screens became feasible with the generation of a library of bacterial strains that each produce dsRNA for an individual nematode gene. The current library contains 16,757 bacterial strains targeting approx 86% of the 19,427 currently predicted genes of the *C. elegans* genome. The loss-of-function phenotype when performing systemic RNAi on a genomewide scale is estimated to be approx 65% *(75,84)* (For review, see refs. *83* and *85–87*). These investigations revealed not only a detailed knowledge about the function of the targeted genes, but also allowed to estimate its relationship to conserved homologs in other species.

Like *C. elegans*, *Drosophila* is a prominent organism for genomewide functional RNAi studies. A huge number of *Drosophila* genes have been silenced since the early days of RNAi research, starting with frizzled-2 and wingless, which are involved in wing development *(88)*. Recently, a genomewide RNAi screen in *Drosophila* Schneider cells (S2 cells) has been reported for the study of phenotypes affecting cell morphology *(89,90)*. Moreover, RNAi has been used to successfully dissect mitosis and cytokinesis and to unravel cell signaling pathways in *Drosophila* tissue culture and cell lines *(91,92)*. All *Drosophila* kinesins and cytoplasmic dynein have been targeted for mitotic phenotypes in S2 cells. For the analysis of functional redundancy and coordinated activity, RNAi was subsequently performed to simultaneously target multiple kinesin genes, an approach that was made feasible only by the RNAi technique *(93)*.

## 6. RNAi IN MAMMALS

Although RNAi constitutes a very powerful tool for studying gene functions in plants and invertebrates, its application in mammalian systems turned out to be a major problem because mammals have evolved a different and more elaborate response to dsRNA. In mammals, dsRNA longer than 30 bp mediates an interferon response, which leads to the simultaneous activation of RNase H, which unspecifically degrades all mRNA transcripts, and protein kinase R (PKR). The latter phosphorylates and, thus, inactivates transcription factor eIF2α leading to a global shutdown of protein biosynthesis and as a result to apoptosis *(94,95)*.

Despite the first impression that RNAi would not work in mammalian cells, several independent groups proved the existence of mammalian RNAi pathways by the introduction of dsRNA or vectors producing dsRNA into cell lines lacking the interferon machinery, like mice oocytes or mice embryonic cancer cell lines *(96,97)*. The most important experiment that established RNAi as the same powerful tool in mammals has been performed by Tuschl and co-workers *(98)*, who used synthetic 21-nt duplexes (siRNAs) to trigger the RNAi pathway. They achieved the knocking down of the activity of transfected and endogenous genes without induction of the interferon response. Obviously, the siRNAs, which act as the active intermediate of RNAi, are too short for the activation of PKR. dsRNAs shorter than 21 bp and longer than 25 bp are inefficient in initiating RNAi as well as siRNAs with blunt ends *(41)*. Only short dsRNAs with a two-nucleotide 3-overhang resembling the naturally active products of Dicer are efficient mediators of RNAi. With this technology, even somatic primary neurons have been successfully treated to produce knock-down RNAi phenotypes *(99)*.

Investigation of the minimal chemical requirements for siRNAs and a detailed mutation scan suggest that the 3'-end modification of the antisense strand usually reduces activity, and mispairing is more crucial for the first 10 nucleotides from the 5'-end of the sense strand. The 10th nucleotide seems to be important for RISC-mediated cleavage of the target mRNA *(41,48,54,100,101)*. Further, the 5'-phosphate residue is essential for siRNAs to direct target–RNA cleavage, but nonphosphorylated siRNAs have been shown to be phosphorylated in vivo by a cytosolic kinase prior to their entrance into the RNAi pathway *(54)*. Shortly after the discovery of siRNA-mediated RNAi in mammals, empirical rules were put up for the design of efficient synthetic siRNAs that are now often referred to as the Tuschl rules *(56)*.

The recent finding that only one strand of the siRNAs enters the RISC depending on thermodynamic properties will help to design siRNAs displaying an even higher efficacy *(55)*.

Novel rules for the design of siRNAs and algorithms, which are based on those rules and consider the accessibility of siRNA binding sites on the secondary structure of the target mRNA, are currently being developed and refined *(55,56,102)*. They also circumvent off-target effects by evaluating the antisense sequence in a Smith–Waterman or BLAST search for possible targets.

To date, the use of siRNAs has become a state-of-the-art tool for the study of gene function in mammals and in cultured mammalian cells. Depending on the type of cells, different chemical and physical methods are used to deliver siRNAs, such as liposom-mediated transfection *(98,103–105)*, electroporation *(106)*, and microinjection. The most common delivery method so far is the regular transfection as described for DNA. Even though electroporation has come into focus lately, transfection is still the most reliable technique, especially for the delivery into adherent cells, such as HeLa, NIH3T3, or 293T cells. It should be mentioned that transfection by calcium phosphate is not as efficient for siRNA as it is for DNA *(107,108)*. Following the use of calcium phosphate and polybrene, various cationic liposomal formulations were developed to increase transfection efficiency to up to 90%, depending on the cell type.

Electroporation is an alternative, which should be considered for nondividing cells or cells resistant to chemical transfection reagents *(109–112)*. Other approaches are exploiting peptides such as the short MPG that forms stable noncovalent complexes with nucleic acids. MPG is a chimeric protein composed of gp41 (the human immunodeficiency virus [HIV-1] fusion peptide domain) and the nuclear localization sequence (NLS) of SV40 large T antigen. Using the MPG bearing a mutation in its NLS prevents nuclear entry and distributes the siRNAs throughout the cytosol *(113)*. Other approaches use the great versatility of cell-penetrating peptides (CPPs) *(114–118)* with respect to cargo and cell type as a valuable tool for the introduction of siRNAs into mammalian cells and even fully grown organisms. The covalent coupling of CPPs with siRNAs yields the so-called pepsiRNAs (peptide-coupled siRNAs) *(119,120)*.

The use of siRNAs has already helped to screen a large number of mammalian genes for their function and to unravel the molecular basis of several important biochemical processes like signal transduction, cell cycle regulation, development, cell motility, cell death, and many more.

The number of targeted mRNAs is constantly increasing together with the validation of a vast number of siRNAs. The field is constantly growing and the first genomewide studies have already been carried out but have just been published in part *(121)*.

Until now, many gene functions responsible for embryogenesis or stem cell differentiation remain to be determined. Although these systems have hardly been accessible by traditional methods, RNAi appears as a practical approach that has already contributed to the characterization of many developmental genes and, thus, constitutes a promising tool for the elucidation of mechanisms involved in development and disease.

The siRNA-mediated silencing of a single isoform of shcA in HeLa cells predicted a crucial role of this protein in regulating cell proliferation *(122)*. Likewise, siRNA-mediated silencing of the phosphatidylinositol 3-kinase causes a drastic decrease in growth and tissue invasiveness of tumor cells *(123)*. By RNAi, the IP3 receptor-1 in germinal vesicle-intact oocytes was found to be responsible for intracellular calcium oscillations, the first steps of development after insemination *(124)*. RNA interference was also used to silence several molecular players of the cell cycle and DNA replication *(125–128)*. The identification and characterization of novel proteins intervening in embryonic *(129,130)* and neuronal development *(99)* are further examples of insights made possible by this new technique.

Its versatily, its high specificity, and the minute amounts required to inhibit gene function render RNAi a highly promising technique to combat diseases. Because RNA silencing serves as a defense against retroviruses in plants and invertebrates it appears only challenging to reintroduce RNAi to fight viruses in mammals and humans. Many studies have been performed to treat HIV-1, herpes simplex virus, and hepatitis B and C by dsRNA-based approaches. Moreover, the high sensitivity toward point mutations qualifies RNAi as a potential tool for the cure of cancers and inherited diseases. In a study of the Ras oncogene, it was possible to target mutated Ras without affecting unmutated Ras, demonstrating the exquisite specificity of RNAi as a therapeutic tool. However, the same specificity could pose problems for therapeutics against viral infection. Viral escape from RNAi selection in poliovirus by mutation of the target sequence has already been demonstrated. The high specificity is already put into doubt by recent findings that the RNAi mechanism can tolerate some sequence mismatches, particularly away from the middle cleavage site. In fact, a recent in vitro study showed that some genes with incomplete homology could be partially silenced, an effect that was more pronounced at higher concentrations of siRNA.

Site-specific delivery of siRNAs broadens the list of genes that can be silenced without inducing toxicity. To target mutated sequences in inherited diseases, the individual gene mutation needs to be determined in order to synthesize appropriate siRNAs. This patient-specific approach would be much more costly and difficult to execute. Therefore, the in vitro studies of RNAi carried out to date focus mainly on viral infection and cancer, which are likely to be the areas in which siRNAs make their way to clinical studies.

The siRNAs are further being studied as therapeutic treatment against genes involved in autoimmuninty, neurodegenerative diseases like Alzheimer's disease, infectious diseases, and inflammatory response and many more.

To date, many prerequisites still need to be fulfilled and obstacles overcome before RNAi can make its way into clinical studies. First of all, silencing is often incomplete—a knockdown rather than a knockout—and residual gene expression might be sufficient to maintain the present phenotype, especially if only low amounts of protein are required to fulfill their cellular function.

Some residual gene expression might be attributed to untransfected cells or to a low affinity of the selected siRNAs toward the target mRNA. In rapidly dividing transformed cells, the silencing effect is rather short-lived, as the transfected siRNAs are rapidly diluted.

Further obstacles of the clinical application of RNAi often are insufficient transfection efficiency and the limited persistence of the transient RNAi phenotype. To obtain persistent RNA silencing in cells and organisms, different plasmid and viral vectors were developed to express short hairpin RNAs under the control of RNA polymerase III (Pol III) and RNAse polymerase II (Pol II) promoters. Upon transfection of these vectors, siRNAs can be constitutively and endogenously expressed.

The currently used vectors employ short hairpin RNA (shRNA) expression cassettes that resemble pre-miRNAs and undergo processing by Dicer *(131–136)*. They are designed according to the same rules as synthetic siRNAas to match perfectly with the target mRNA and, thus, trigger its degradation. To achieve a constitutive silencing effect, the shRNA transcript must translocate from the nucleus to the cytoplasm, where it has to be recognized by Dicer and transferred to RISC. siRNA hairpin-expressing plasmids can specifically suppress gene expression in a transient or persistent manner depending on their design. Thus, loss-of-function phenotypes can be generated if longer periods of time are required to fully deplete the cytosol of residual target protein. The potency of shRNAs to trigger RNAi in mammalian cells is comparable to synthetic siRNA duplexes.

In many cases, strong RNA polymerase III promoters, such as the human H1 and the murine U6, are employed to control the expression of the shRNAs. *(131–136)*. In vivo, RNA polymerase III is responsible for the transcription of a limited number of genes, including 5S RNA, tRNA, 7SL RNA, U6 snRNA, and a number of other small stable RNAs that are involved in RNA processing *(137)*.

It is assumed that long dsRNAs are a more effective trigger because they are more efficiently processed into siRNAs *(49)*. This can be the result of a highly cooperative binding of long dsRNA strands or additional features of cleavage by Dicer, such as incorporation of the nascent siRNAs into transfer protein complexes *(138)*.

Despite some concerns, which are discussed within the field of RNAi, it was recently shown that endogenously expressed long hairpin dsRNAs (lhRNAs) are capable of inducing RNAi in mammalian somatic cells including human primary fibroblasts, melanocytes, HeLa cells *(139,140)*, and even whole mice *(141)*.

To be taken up by cells or tissues, those expression vectors require classical methods like electroporation, microinjection, or liposomal transfer of the DNA precursor vector. Most cell lines are easy to transfect and recombinant cell clones permanently expressing RNAi phenotypes can be selected. However, without cell division, the shRNA (DNA) construct cannot enter the nucleus as required for DNA transcription and it passively resides in cytosol. Therefore, most nondividing cells are not susceptible to transfection, as are primary cells and stem cells. A number of important cell types have been resistant to the introduction of both siRNAs and shRNAs because of the lack of an appropriate delivery system.

Even more problematic is the delivery of siRNAs directly to entire vertebrate animals. High toxicity of most cationic transfection reagents prohibits whole-body application of siRNAs aided by liposomal or chemical approaches, whereas physical techniques like the hydrodynamic transfection method was shown to be successful in mice. Naked siRNAs applied to mice via tail-vein injection caused the knock down of a reporter gene by 80–90% in the liver, kidney, spleen, lung, and pancreas *(142,143)*. Yet, the effect is rather short-lived, lasting only a few days, and not all organs and cell types are accessible.

Another method to circumvent many of those difficulties makes use of viral vectors to infect cells with the dsRNA expression construct. Retroviral vectors *(144)*, like adenoviral vectors, and predominantly lentiviral vectors *(145,146)* are currently being used as viral delivery systems. By this approach, almost every cell or tissue, including stem cells and neurons, can be treated with shRNA-producing vectors.

The advantages of the lentiviral approach lies in the possiblity of systematically testing a gene function in the context of the entire organism. Further animal models can be generated in a straigthforward manner to determine which genes are important to the function of different tissues and organs and which might be effective therapeutic targets in diseases.

Even though Tuschl and co-workers *(98)* observed that siRNAs shorter than 30 nt do not trigger an interferon response, recent reports are concerned about nonspecific effects induced by endogenously expressed shRNAs. Both transfection of siRNAs and transcription of shRNAs leads to an interferon (IFN)-mediated activation of the Jak–Stat pathway and global upregulation of interferon-stimulated genes within the nucleus (147–149). It was found that the dsRNA-dependent protein kinase (PKR) is activated by the intracellular presence of 21-bp siRNAs and triggers the upregulation of IFN and possibly other, cellular signaling molecules. Comparative studies on interferon induction by siRNAs and their shRNA counterparts showed a significantly stronger interferon response after the application of shRNA (149), so that these side effects need to be studied more closely to settle the current controversy. It has to be kept in mind that almost all plasmid vectors can induce interferon response upon transfection independent of the type of insert they are bearing (150).

## 7. RNAi AND GENE THERAPEUTIC SETTINGS

Therapeutic strategies for siRNA are based on silencing of disease-related genes without altering the expression of other essential genes. At the beginning of RNAi research, it was assumed that targeting mRNAs with homologous siRNAs or dsRNA does not influence the expression of other mRNAs. To date, we know that a single knockdown of a gene can induce a variety of changes in the overall gene expression. As long as we cannot distinguish the changes resulting from the silencing of a single gene from those caused by unspecific effects, the approach resembles all of the benefits and drawbacks that were already described for gene therapy.

### 7.1. Infectious Diseases

The first approach aiming at the use of RNAi in therapeutic applications was the silencing of viral genes. With regard to the number of outbreaks and people infected worldwide, several groups of viruses are currently recognized as the most important human pathogens. Among those, aquired immunodeficiency syndrome (AIDS), hepatitis, and influenza are viral diseases of global dimension, bringing along high morbidity and mortality. Influenza even occurs in annual epidemics and in pandemics of infrequent occurrence but very high attack rates (151). Although RNAi is an ancient antiviral defense in plants and invertebrates, it does not play an important role in mammals. Nevertheless, the RNAi machinery is present in mammals and might be exploited to inhibit viral infections upon triggering by siRNAs.

So far, many groups have been successful in activating the pathway against viral targets with diverse replication strategies, including HIV (136,152–162), hepatitis B and C (HBV/ HCV) (163–170), human papilloma virus (HPV) (171–173), polio virus (174,175), herpes virus (176), human T-cell leukemia virus-1 (177), respiratory syncytial virus (178), influenza (179), Epstein–Barr virus (180), and, finally, corona viruses such as SARS (181–185).

At the beginning, mostly genes of the respective virus were targeted. Bitko and Barik were the first to observe specific antiviral effects of siRNA against the respiratory syncytial virus. Shortly after that, the same effects were reported for poliovirus in infected human cells (174) and HIV-1 using siRNAs directed against different regions of the HIV-1 genome, including its long terminal repeat and the genes encoding for the highly conserved genes vif and nef (152). siRNA-treated cells were particularly immune to subsequent HIV-1 infection in short-term experiments. Novina and co-workers used a contrary approach that notably reduced the ability of the HIV-1 to enter cells by targeting the CD-4 receptor, which is responsible for HIV-1 entry into the host cells. This indicates that the viral infectivity can also be stopped if host genes involved in the viral life cycle are targeted (162).

These studies clearly show that RNAi will hold its promise to become an efficient tool in the treatment of viral and other infectious diseases in human. However, before RNAi can make its way to therapeutic applications, an appropriate siRNA delivery system is required to guide the active species to the target organs. Interestingly, siRNA delivery to mice by hydrodynamic injection into the tail vein has led to a gene downregulation of 90% in the majority of liver cells. However, this technique requires high pressure and large volumes of siRNA solutions, making it inappropriate for application in humans *(142,143)*. On the other hand, after the coinjection of luciferase-targeting siRNA and plasmid-luciferase into the tail vein of mice, gene silencing was observed in several organs, including the liver, spleen, kidney and lung. Mice have been also healed for 10 d from Fas-induced fulminant hepatitis by the injection of the appropriate siRNAs *(168)*.

More striking results were obtained on HBV. RNAi could inhibit the production of HBV replicative intermediates in cell culture and in immunocompetent and immunodeficient mice transfected with an HBV plasmid *(186)*. Upon siRNA treatment, substantially reduced levels of HBV RNAs and replicated HBV genomes were found in mouse liver. In these studies, most of the targets are genes that are relatively conserved between different viral strains and exhibit a low mutation activity, as found for the genes essential for replication. Likewise, host genes required for viral entry or playing an essential role in the viral life cycle are also potential targets *(187)*.

In spite of the great excitement created by those studies, it has to be kept in mind that most of the experiments were performed in cell culture or model animals using laboratory strains of viruses that are well characterized.

Some recent studies indicated that a therapeutic treatment of viral infection does not stand up to its expectations *(188,189)*. In the long term, siRNA directed against the highly conserved *Nef* gene (siRNA-Nef) confers resistance to HIV-1 replication. However, the inhibition of replication is not complete. After several weeks of culture, HIV-1 escape variants appeared that were no longer inhibited by siRNA-Nef because of nucleotide substitutions or deletions in the *Nef* gene that altered the homology to the siRNA-Nef sequence *(188,189)*. To minimize the risk of viral escape, several viral and host genes must be targeted simultaneously.

Other infectious diseases such as those spread by parasites are also the subject to therapeutical RNAi approaches *(190–195)*. Protozoan parasites and pathogenic fungi often resist manipulation by standard molecular genetic approaches. The discovery of RNAi in *Trypanosoma brucei* provides a convenient method for generating knockout phenotypes of the parasite *(196)*. Further, erythrocyte-infecting stages of the malaria parasite *Plasmodium falciparum* were successfully treated with dsRNA encoding the dihydroorotate dehydrogenase (DHODH) *(192)*.

The application of RNAi to fight diseases reaches its limit when it comes to bacterial infections, because prokaryotes are not amenable to silencing by siRNA. Yet, the manipulation of the host genes involved in bacterial invasion or in immune response might help to immunize cells and tissues against bacterial infections *(197)*. The recent discovery of the DNA or RNA editing roles of prokaryotic PIN domains, which are strikingly numerous in thermophiles and in organisms such as *Mycobacterium tuberculosis* now supports the idea that, similar to their eukaryotic counterparts, bacterial PIN domains participate in a related RNA silencing mechanism and nonsense-mediated RNA degradation *(198)*. After an initial flood of mainly descriptive reports about the effects of bacterial infection, transcriptome and proteome studies are now becoming more refined in their approach and are shedding light on the role of pathogen–host interactions, which eventually can be targeted by RNAi *(199)*. First, RNAi experiments targeting pro-inflammatory cytokines (interleukin-1 [IL-1], or tumor necrosis factor α [TNF-α]) successfully reduced the sepsis triggered by lipopolysaccharide (LPS) in mice *(200)*. The intervention with the peroxisome proliferation-activated receptor (PPAR)-γ-dependent anti-inflammatory mechanism for the treatment of chronic inflammation is only one of many further possibilities *(201)*.

## 7.2. Cancer

Several in vitro studies have already demonstrated the potential use of RNAi in cancer treatment. Cancer cells usually differ from normal cells by their uncontrolled growth and the ability to escape programmed cell death (apoptosis). For nutrition supply, they assemble a network of blood vessels around tumors, and to evade chemotherapy, they might change surface composition. Therefore, targets for a possible RNAi treatment are genes that are either involved in cell division and proliferation such as growth factors, tumor suppressor genes, transcription factors, and apoptosis inhibitors *(106,171,202–217)* or proto-oncogenes that take part in many regulatory events and signaling cascades such as Ras and Bcl-2 *(208)*, as well as viral oncogenes, such as from human papilloma virus (HPV). Impaired apoptosis signaling is associated with tumor development and confers resistance to chemotherapy and apoptosis triggered by the death receptor pathway *(204)*. In many tumors, antiapoptotic proto-oncogenes are overexpressed and inhibition of their expression has potential to facilitate tumor necrosis factor-related apoptosis inducing ligand (TRAIL)-induced apoptosis *(218–220)*. Multidrug resistance proteins that pump chemotherapeutic drugs out of tumors and factors that stimulate angiogenesis to connect the tumor to nutrition resources are also potential RNAi targets *(221–235)*.

A selection of targets is listed in Table 1. Well-known targets are Bcr-Abl, mutated Ras, human papilloma virus (HPV) E6 and E7, and proto-oncogenes like bcl-2 and c-myb.

Bcl-2 (B-cell lymphoma protein 2) targeting by RNAi is a promising example of how apoptosis can be triggered in tumor cells *(106,210,214,218,236)*. Bcl-2 is an important regulator of programmed cell death, and its overexpression has been implicated in the pathogenesis of some lymphomas. Resistance to chemotherapy, at least in vitro, might also be related to *Bcl-2* overexpression. In a comparative study, single siRNAs or combinations of siRNAs were successfully transfected into HeLa cells, lung adenocarcinoma cells, hepatoma cells, ovarian carcinoma cells, and melanoma cells with cationic lipid complexes. Downregulation of other proto-oncogenes and apopotosis inhibitors, such as cdk-2, mdm-2, pkc-alpha, tgf-beta1, h-Ras, and vegf, effectively suppressed the proliferation of cancer cells to different extents, leading to the conclusion that chemically synthesized and vector-driven siRNAs can inhibit the growth and proliferation of cancer cells *(219)*.

Ras is a powerful regulator of several interconnected receptor-signaling pathways. In its mutated form, it is constitutively active and acts as an oncogene. This process is thought to contribute to malignant transformation in many cell types, which makes elements of this signaling pathway attractive targets for inhibition by RNAi *(237)*. Previous attempts to silence the Ras oncogene with phosphorothioate oligonucleotides succeeded in stabilizing the disease. Silencing of crucial effectors in Ras signaling like the Raf-c kinase by oligonucleotides shows low to moderate effects in vitro and in an in vivo tumor–xenograft model, whereas treatment with siRNAs can specifically silence expression of oncogenic K-Ras in tumor cells *(238,239)*. A tumor suppressor that is often genetically altered is Bcr-Abl. However, targeting the Abl sequence in Bcr-Abl by RNAi might be a therapy for

Table 1
Selection of Cancer-Related Genes Subjected to si/shRNA Treatment

| Gene | Cancer Types | Cell Types | RNA Species | Mode of Action | Ref. |
|---|---|---|---|---|---|
| k-Ras | Most tumors | HeLa cells, lung adenocarcinoma cells, hepatoma cells, ovarian carcinoma cells, melanoma cells, etc. | shRNA/lentivirus siRNAs | Proliferation, cell division Apoptosis inhibitor, chemotherapy resistance | 219,238,239 204,210,214, 218,219 |
| Bcl-2 | Colorectal carcinoma cells, cervix carcinoma, leukemia | | | | |
| VEGF | Most cancer types | HeLa cells, lung adenocarcinoma cells, hepatoma cells, ovarian carcinoma cells, and melanoma cells, K562 | siRNAs, shRNas/vector | Angiogenesis | 219,223 |
| Bcr-Abl | Chronic myeloid leukemia | Leukemic cells | siRNAs, shRNAs / lentivirus | Chemotherapy resistance | 211,261 |
| MDR1 | Human pancreatic carcinoma, gastric carcinoma | EPP85-181RDB EPG85-257RDB | siRNAs | Chemotherapy resistance | 262 |
| HPV-E6/E7 | HPV-positive tumors | HeLa | siRNAs shRNA/vector | Apoptosis inhibitor | 173,263 |
| CXCR4 | Breast cancer, tumors | Breast cancer cells | siRNAs | Cell migration | 264 |
| Wee1 Chk1 Myt1 Cdc2 | | HeLa cells, lung adenocarcinoma cells, hepatoma cells, ovarian carcinoma cells, melanoma cells, etc. | siRNAs | Apoptosis inhibitor, cell cycle control | 203,219 |
| Eph2 receptor | Pancreatic adenocarcinoma | PANC1, MIAPaCa2, BxPC3,Capan2 | siRNAs | Growth factor, tumor invasiveness, metastasis | 202 |
| FASE | Prostate cancer | HeLa | siRNas | Proliferation, apoptosis inhibitor | 265 |
| Tie-2 | Tumors | Endothelial cells | siRNAs | Angiogenesis | 187,225 |

chronic myeloid leukemia. This is only a selection of commonly studied target genes that is supplemented by Table 1. However, the major drawback for the application in therapy so far remains the issue of delivery. Despite the specific targeting of proto-oncogenes that leaves the expression of the wild-type gene unaltered, many of the other target proteins also play their role in nonproliferating cells and healthy organs. Downregulation of those targets requires methods that allow direct delivery to the tumor without affecting other cells. Those delivery agents need to be tailor-made to each tumor and the different organs from which the tumor is derived. So far, many approaches have been made with either modified dendrimers and liposomes or modified lentiviruses and adenoviruses. To date, no reliable results have been obtained.

### 7.3. Cardiovascular and Neurodegenerative Diseases

Apart from cancer and infectious diseases, cardiovascular diseases cause the highest mortality in the Western world. The development of strategies for the prevention of those diseases is, therefore, of high priority. RNAi is currently used to elucidate the underlying mechanisms of cardiovascular diseases *(230,240,241)*; however, therapy is still way out of reach. Likewise, the number of patients with neurodegenerative diseases such as Alzheimer's disease, Parkinson's disease, or amyotrophic lateral sclerosis is growing with the increasing life-span of humans.

Many studies support the therapeutic potential of RNAi-based methods for the treatment of diseases like myotrophic lateral sclerosis *(242–244)*. The search for possible candidate genes responsible for Alzheimer's disease *(245–251)* and Parkinson's disease *(252–254)* is proceeding at a rapid pace. However, delivery is even more a problem when the trespassing of the blood–brain barrier is involved.

Neurones in culture are very sensitive, and transfection efficiencies by conventional methods are poor. In vivo, the blood–brain barrier prevents the uptake of substances from the remaining vascular system with the exception of small (less than 500 Da) and lipid-soluble molecules and, consequently, reduces the bioavailability of intravenously applied oligonucleotides in the brain to virtually zero *(255)*.

Even though it is already possible to treat primary neurons and other neuronal cell lines with siRNAs *(99,256,257)*, in vivo studies in mice are just at their beginning, and many of methods published so far bear their drawbacks. Nonetheless, it could be shown that adenoviral vectors successfully passed the blood–brain barrier after intravenous application and were expressed in the brain *(258)*. Others injected siRNA expressing adenoviral vectors directly into the brain and observed a decent RNAi phenotype *(259)*.

### 8. PERSPECTIVES ON THE FUTURE

In a time when biologists are facing the enormous challenge of decrypting genetic messages encoded by whole genomes, the RNAi technique represents a precious tool. The use of either synthetic or stably expressed siRNAs will greatly facilitate and accelerate genomewide functional screening in model organisms and navigation within the decrypted genetic landscape. Also, siRNA-mediated gene silencing will be one standard method in the studying of specific roles of proteins in integrated cellular pathways. However, although RNAi has turned out to be an efficient approach to downregulate viral activity in cultured mammalian cells, its application as a therapeutic approach in humans will only be feasible if all risks of unspecific responses and other side effects have been eliminated. This demands a better understanding of the RNAi-related processes, particularly the correlation between structural features of the natural miRNAs and their strictly specific mode of action. This, in turn, will provide a basic reference design of siRNAs to be used for therapeutic purposes. At last, an appropriate system of siRNA delivery in vivo still needs to be developed.

RNAi is now one of the largest growing fields in biology, pharmacology, medicine, and even chemistry. Although the mechanism by which dsRNA modulates gene expression is not at all clarified, the development of novel approaches to cure diseases related to gene expression has proceeded to the point at which in vivo experiments in animal models are afoot. The recent development of leukemia cells and other cancer cells resistant to the well-known small-molecule inhibitors is calling for novel treatments. Even though a cell might be able to evolve mutated proteins that evade a small-molecule protein inhibitors, this does not happen if the encoding mRNA is degraded. RNAi might have held many promises, as yet, there is no experience in patients. Without doubt, the time to celebrate significant achievements in the clinical trials will be forthcoming soon.

## REFERENCES

1. Fire A, Xu SQ, Montgomery MK, Kostas SA, Driver SE, Mello CC. Potent and specific genetic interference by double-stranded RNA in *Caenorhabditis elegans*. Nature 1998; 391(6669):806–811.
2. Guo S, Kemphues KJ. Par-1, a gene required for establishing polarity in *C. elegans* embryos, encodes a putative Ser/Thr kinase that is asymmetrically distributed. Cell 1995; 81(4):611–620.
3. Timmons L, Fire A. Specific interference by ingested dsRNA. Nature 1998; 395(6705):854.
4. Schmitz K, Schepers U. Silencio: RNA interference, the tool of the new millennium. Biol Chem 2004; in press.
5. Montgomery MK, Xu SQ, Fire A. RNA as a target of double-stranded RNA-mediated genetic interference in *Caenorhabditis elegans*. Proc Natl Acad Sci USA 1998; 95(26):15,502–15,507.
6. Montgomery MK, Fire A. Double-stranded RNA as a mediator in sequence specific genetic silencing and co-suppression. Trends Genet 1998; 14(7):255–258.
7. Timmons L, Tabara H, Mello CC, Fire AZ. Inducible systemic RNA silencing in *Caenorhabditis elegans*. Mol Biol Cell 2003; 14(7):2972–2983.
8. Winston WM, Molodowitch C, Hunter CP. Systemic RNAi in *C. elegans* requires the putative transmembrane protein SID-1. Science 2002; 295(5564):2456–2459.
9. Tabara H, Grishok A, Mello CC. RNAi in *C. elegans*: soaking in the genome sequence. Science 1998; 282(5388):430–431.
10. Voinnet O. RNA silencing as a plant immune system against viruses. Trends Genet 2001; 17(8):449–459.
11. Ruiz MT, Voinnet O, Baulcombe DC. Initiation and maintenance of virus-induced gene silencing. Plant Cell 1998; 10(6):937–946.
12. Ketting RF, Haverkamp TH, van Luenen HG, Plasterk RH. Mut-7 of *C. elegans*, required for transposon silencing and RNA interference, is a homolog of Werner syndrome helicase and RNaseD. Cell 1999; 99(2):133–141.
13. Tabara H, Sarkissian M, Kelly WG, et al. The rde-1 gene, RNA interference, and transposon silencing in *C. elegans*. Cell 1999; 99(2):123–132.
14. Plasterk RHA. RNA silencing: the genome's immune system. Science 2002; 296(5571):1263–1265.
15. Domeier ME, Morse DP, Knight SW, Portereiko M, Bass BL, Mango SE. A link between RNA interference and nonsense-mediated decay in *Caenorhabditis elegans*. Science 2000; 289(5486):1928–1930.
16. McManus MT, Petersen CP, Haines BB, Chen J, Sharp PA. Gene silencing using micro-RNA designed hairpins. RNA 2002; 8(6):842–850.
17. Mourrain P, Beclin C, Elmayan T, et al. Arabidopsis SGS2 and SGS3 genes are required for posttranscriptional gene silencing and natural virus resistance. Cell 2000; 101(5):533–542.
18. Cogoni C, Macino G. Gene silencing in *Neurospora crassa* requires a protein homologous to RNA-dependent RNA polymerase. Nature 1999; 399(6732):166–169.

19. Cogoni C, Macino G. Isolation of quelling defective (QDE) mutants impaired in posttranscriptional transgene-induced gene silencing in neurospora crassa. Proc Natl Acad Sci USA 1997; 94(19):10,233–10,238.

20. Smardon A, Spoerke JM, Stacey SC, Klein ME, Mackin N, Maine EM. EGO-1 is related to RNA-directed RNA polymerase and functions in germ-line development and RNA interference in *C. elegans*. Curr Biol 2000; 10(4):169–178.

21. Qiao L, Lissemore JL, Shu P, Smardon A, Gelber MB, Maine EM. Enhancers of glp-1, a gene required for cell-signaling in *Caenorhabditis elegans*, define a set of genes required for germline development. Genetics 1995; 141(2):551–569.

22. Hamilton AJ, Baulcombe DC. A species of small antisense RNA in posttranscriptional gene silencing in plants. Science 1999; 286(5441):950–952.

23. Zamore PD, Tuschl T, Sharp PA, Bartel DP. RNAi: double-stranded RNA directs the ATP-dependent cleavage of mRNA at 21 to 23 nucleotide intervals. Cell 2000; 101(1):25–33.

24. Yang D, Lu H, Erickson JW. Evidence that processed small dsRNAs may mediate sequence-specific mRNA degradation during RNAi in *Drosophila* embryos. Curr Biol 2000; 10(19):1191–1200.

25. Wu H, Xu H, Miraglia LJ, Crooke ST. Human RNase III is a 160-kDa protein involved in preribosomal RNA processing. J Biol Chem 2000; 275(47):36,957–36,965.

26. Filippov V, Solovyev V, Filippova M, Gill SS. A novel type of RNase III family proteins in eukaryotes. Gene 2000; 245(1):213–221.

27. Bernstein E, Caudy AA, Hammond SM, Hannon GJ. Role for a bidentate ribonuclease in the initiation step of RNA interference. Nature 2001; 409(6818):363–366.

28. Rotondo G, Frendewey D. Purification and characterization of the Pac1 ribonuclease of *schizosaccharomyces pombe*. Nucleic Acids Res 1996; 24(12):2377–2386.

29. Mian IS. Comparative sequence analysis of ribonucleases Hii, Iii, Ii Ph and D. Nucleic Acids Res 1997; 25(16):3187–3195.

30. Aravind L, Koonin EV. A natural classification of ribonucleases. Methods Enzymol 2001; 341:3–28.

31. Cerutti L, Mian N, Bateman A. Domains in gene silencing and cell differentiation proteins: the novel PAZ domain and redefinition of the Piwi domain. Trends Biochem Sci 2000; 25(10):481–482.

32. Ketting RF, Fischer SEJ, Bernstein E, Sijen T, Hannon GJ, Plasterk RHA. Dicer functions in RNA interference and in synthesis of small RNA involved in developmental timing in *C. elegans*. Genes Dev 2001; 15(20):2654–2659.

33. Schauer SE, Jacobsen SE, Meinke DW, Ray A. DICER-LIKE1: blind men and elephants in Arabidopsis development. Trends Plant Sci 2002; 7(11):487–491.

34. Ketting RF, Plasterk RHA. A genetic link between co-suppression and RNA interference in *C. elegans*. Nature 2000; 404(6775):296–298.

35. Lau NC, Lim LP, Weinstein EG, Bartel DP. An abundant class of tiny RNAs with probable regulatory roles in *Caenorhabditis elegans*. Science 2001; 294(5543):858–862.

36. Lee RC, Ambros V. An extensive class of small RNAs in *Caenorhabditis elegans*. Science 2001; 294 (5543):862–864.

37. Lagos-Quintana M, Rauhut R, Yalcin A, Meyer J, Lendeckel W, Tuschl T. Identification of tissue-specific microRNAs from mouse. Curr Biol 2002; 12(9):735–739.

38. Lee Y, Jeon K, Lee JT, Kim S, Kim VN. MicroRNA maturation: stepwise processing and subcellular localization. EMBO J 2002; 21(17):4663–4670.

39. Reinhart BJ, Weinstein EG, Rhoades MW, Bartel B, Bartel DP. MicroRNAs in plants. Genes Dev 2002; 16(13):1616–1626.

40. Lagos-Quintana M, Rauhut R, Meyer J, Borkhardt A, Tuschl T. New microRNAs from mouse and human. RNA 2003; 9(2):175–179.

41. Elbashir SM, Martinez J, Patkaniowska A, Lendeckel W, Tuschl T. Functional anatomy of siRNAs for mediating efficient RNAi in *Drosophila melanogaster* embryo lysate. EMBO J 2001; 20(23):6877–6888.

42. Blaszczyk J, Tropea JE, Bubunenko M, et al. Crystallographic and modeling studies of RNase III suggest a mechanism for double-stranded RNA cleavage. Structure 2001; 9(12):1225–1236.

43. Hannon GJ. RNA interference. Nature 2002; 418(6894):244–251.

44. Hutvagner G, McLachlan J, Pasquinelli AE, Balint E, Tuschl T, Zamore PD. A cellular function for the RNA-interference enzyme Dicer in the maturation of the let-7 small temporal RNA. Science 2001; 293(5531):834–838.

45. Myers JW, Jones JT, Meyer T, Ferrell JE Jr. Recombinant Dicer efficiently converts large dsRNAs into siRNAs suitable for gene silencing. Nature Biotechnol 2003; 21(3):324–328.

46. Provost P, Dishart D, Doucet J, Frendewey D, Samuelsson B, Radmark O. Ribonuclease activity and RNA binding of recombinant human Dicer. EMBO J 2002; 21(21):5864–5874.

47. Zhang H, Kolb FA, Brondani V, Billy E, Filipowicz W. Human Dicer preferentially cleaves dsRNAs at their termini without a requirement for ATP. EMBO J 2002; 21(21):5875–5885.

48. Martinez J, Patkaniowska A, Urlaub H, Luhrmann R, Tuschl T. Single-stranded antisense siRNAs guide target RNA cleavage in RNAi. Cell 2002; 110(5):563–574.

49. Nykänen A, Haley B, Zamore PD. ATP requirements and small interfering RNA structure in the RNA interference pathway. Cell 2001; 107(3):309–321.

50. Hammond SM, Boettcher S, Caudy AA, Kobayashi R, Hannon GJ. Argonaute2, a link between genetic and biochemical analyses of RNAi. Science 2001; 293(5532):1146–1150.

51. Liu Q, Rand TA, Kalidas S, et al. R2D2, a bridge between the initiation and effector steps of the *Drosophila* RNAi pathway. Science 2003; 301(5641):1921–1925.

52. Hammond SM, Bernstein E, Beach D, Hannon GJ. An RNA-directed nuclease mediates post-transcriptional gene silencing in *Drosophila* cells. Nature 2000; 404(6775):293–296.

53. Carmell MA, Xuan Z, Zhang MQ, Hannon GJ. The Argonaute family: tentacles that reach into RNAi, developmental control, stem cell maintenance, and tumorigenesis. Genes Dev 2002; 16(21):2733–2742.

54. Schwarz DS, Hutvagner G, Haley B, Zamore PD. Evidence that siRNAs function as guides, not primers, in the *Drosophila* and human RNAi pathways. Mol Cell 2002; 10(3):537–548.

55. Schwarz DS, Hutvagner G, Du T, Xu Z, Aronin N, Zamore PD. Asymmetry in the assembly of the RNAi enzyme complex. Cell 2003; 115(2):199–208.

56. Khvorova A, Reynolds A, Jayasena SD. Functional siRNAs and miRNAs exhibit strand bias. Cell 2003; 115(2):209–216.

57. Jackson AL, Bartz SR, Schelter J, et al. Expression profiling reveals off-target gene regulation by RNAi. Nature Biotechnol 2003; 21(6):635–637.

58. Song JJ, Liu J, Tolia NH, et al. The crystal structure of the Argonaute2 PAZ domain reveals an RNA binding motif in RNAi effector complexes. Nature Struct Biol 2003; 10(12):1026–1032.

59. Yan KS, Yan S, Farooq A, Han A, Zeng L, Zhou MM. Structure and conserved RNA binding of the PAZ domain. Nature 2003; 26:468–474.

60. Lingel A, Simon B, Izaurralde E, Sattler M. Structure and nucleic-acid binding of the *Drosophila* Argonaute 2 PAZ domain. Nature 2003; 426:465–469.

61. Ponting CP. Evidence for PDZ domains in bacteria, yeast, and plants. Protein Sci 1997; 6(2):464–468.

62. Callebaut I, Mornon JP. The human EBNA-2 coactivator p100: multidomain organization and relationship to the staphylococcal nuclease fold and to the tudor protein involved in *Drosophila melanogaster* development. Biochem J 1997; 321(Pt 1):125–132.

63. Caudy AA, Ketting RF, Hammond SM, et al. A micrococcal nuclease homologue in RNAi effector complexes. Nature 2003; 425(6956):411–414.

64. Arenz C, Schepers U. RNA interference: from an ancient mechanism to a state of the art therapeutic application? Naturwissenschaften 2003; 90(8):345–359.

65. Venter JC, Adams MD, Myers EW, et al. The sequence of the human genome. Science 2001; 291 (5507):1304–1351.

66. Lander ES, Linton LM, Birren B, et al. Initial sequencing and analysis of the human genome. Nature 2001; 409(6822):860–921.

67. Nagy A, Perrimon N, Sandmeyer S, Plasterk R. Tailoring the genome: the power of genetic approaches. Nature Genet 2003; 33(Suppl):276–284.

68. Rajewsky K, Gu H, Kuhn R, et al. Conditional gene targeting. J Clin Invest 1996; 98(3):600–603.

69. Nagy A. Cre recombinase: the universal reagent for genome tailoring [review]. Genesis 2000; 26(2): 99–109.

70. Famulok M. Oligonucleotide aptamers that recognize small molecules. Curr Opin Struct Biol 1999; 9(3):324–329.

71. Sullenger BA, Gallardo HF, Ungers GE, Gilboa E. Overexpression of TAR sequences renders cells resistant to human immunodeficiency virus replication. Cell 1990; 63(3):601–608.

72. Bosher JM, Labouesse M. RNA interference: genetic wand and genetic watchdog. Nature Cell Biol 2000; 2(2):E31–E36.

73. Hunter CP. Genetics: a touch of elegance with RNAi. Curr Biol 1999; 9(12):R440–R442.

74. Feinberg EH, Hunter CP. Transport of dsRNA into cells by the transmembrane protein SID-1. Science 2003; 301(5639):1545–1547.

75. Kamath RS, Ahringer J. Genome-wide RNAi screening in *Caenorhabditis elegans*. Methods 2003; 30(4):313–321.

76. Montgomery MK. The use of double-stranded RNA to knock down specific gene activity. Methods Mol Biol 2004; 260:129–144.

77. Clemens JC, Worby CA, Simonson-Leff N, et al. Use of double-stranded RNA interference in *Drosophila* cell lines to dissect signal transduction pathways. Proc Natl Acad Sci USA 2000; 97(12):6499–6503.

78. Grishok A, Mello CC. RNAi (Nematodes: *Caenorhabditis elegans*). Adv Genet 2002; 46:339–360.

79. Grishok A, Tabara H, Mello CC. Genetic requirements for inheritance of RNAi in *C. elegans*. Science 2000; 287(5462):2494–2497.

80. Maeda I, Kohara Y, Yamamoto M, Sugimoto A. Large-scale analysis of gene function in *Caenorhabditis elegans* by high-throughput RNAi. Curr Biol 2001; 11(3):171–176.

81. Schumacher JM, Golden A, Donovan PJ. AIR-2: an Aurora/Ip11-related protein kinase associated with chromosomes and midbody microtubules is required for polar body extrusion and cytokinesis in *Caenorhabditis elegans* embryos. J Cell Biol 1998; 143(6):1635–1646.

82. Chase D, Serafinas C, Ashcroft N, et al. The polo-like kinase PLK-1 is required for nuclear envelope breakdown and the completion of meiosis in *Caenorhabditis elegans*. Genesis 2000; 26(1):26–41.

83. Ashrafi K, Chang FY, Watts JL, et al. Genome-wide RNAi analysis of *Caenorhabditis elegans* fat regulatory genes. Nature 2003; 421(6920):268–272.

84. Fraser AG, Kamath RS, Zipperlen P, Martinez-Campos M, Sohrmann M, Ahringer J. Functional genomic analysis of *C. elegans* chromosome I by systematic RNA interference. Nature 2000; 408(6810): 325–330.

85. Castillo-Davis CI, Hartl DL. Conservation, relocation and duplication in genome evolution. Trends Genet 2003; 19(11):593–597.

86. Gonczy P, Echeverri C, Oegema K, et al. Functional genomic analysis of cell division in *C. elegans* using RNAi of genes on chromosome III. Nature 2000; 408(6810):331–336.

87. Lee SS, Lee RY, Fraser AG, Kamath RS, Ahringer J, Ruvkun G. A systematic RNAi screen identifies a critical role for mitochondria in *C. elegans* longevity. Nature Genet 2003; 33(1):40–48.

88. Kennerdell JR, Carthew RW. Use of dsRNA-mediated genetic interference to demonstrate that frizzled and frizzled 2 act in the wingless pathway. Cell 1998; 95(7):1017–1026.

89. Kiger A, Baum B, Jones S, et al. A functional genomic analysis of cell morphology using RNA interference. J Biol 2003; 2(4):27.

90. Boutros M, Kiger AA, Armknecht S, et al. Genome-wide RNAi analysis of growth and viability in *Drosophila* cells. Science 2004; 303(5659):832–835.

91. Somma MP, Fasulo B, Cenci G, Cundari E, Gatti M. Molecular dissection of cytokinesis by RNA interference in *Drosophila* cultured cells. Mol Biol Cell 2002; 13(7):2448–2460.

92. Maiato H, Sunkel CE, Earnshaw WC. Dissecting mitosis by RNAi in *Drosophila* tissue culture cells. Biol Proc Online 2003; 5:153–161.

93. Goshima G, Vale RD. The roles of microtubule-based motor proteins in mitosis: comprehensive RNAi analysis in the *Drosophila* S2 cell line. J Cell Biol 2003; 162(6):1003–1016.

94. Clemens MJ, Elia A. The double-stranded RNA-dependent protein kinase PKR-structure and function [review]. J Interferon Cytokine Res 1997; 17(9):503–524.

95. Clemens MJ. Pkr—a protein kinase regulated by double-stranded RNA. Int J Biochem Cell Biol 1997; 29(7):945–949.

96. Wianny F, Zernicka-Goetz M. Specific interference with gene function by double-stranded RNA in early mouse development. Nature Cell Biol 2000; 2(2):70–75.

97. Billy E, Brondani V, Zhang H, Muller U, Filipowicz W. Specific interference with gene expression induced by long, double- stranded RNA in mouse embryonal teratocarcinoma cell lines. Proc Natl Acad Sci USA 2001; 98(25):14,428–14,433.

98. Elbashir SM, Harborth J, Lendeckel W, Yalcin A, Weber K, Tuschl T. Duplexes of 21-nucleotide RNAs mediate RNA interference in cultured mammalian cells. Nature 2001; 411(6836):494–498.

99. Krichevsky AM, Kosik KS. RNAi functions in cultured mammalian neurons. Proc Natl Acad Sci USA 2002; 99(18):11,926–11,929.

100. Chiu YL, Rana TM. siRNA function in RNAi: a chemical modification analysis. RNA 2003; 9(9):1034–1048.

101. Chiu YL, Rana TM. RNAi in human cells: basic structural and functional features of small interfering RNA. Mol Cell 2002; 10(3):549–561.

102. Reynolds A, Leake D, Boese Q, Scaringe S, Marshall WS, Khvorova A. Rational siRNA design for RNA interference. Nat Biotechnol 2004; 22:326–330.

103. Caplen NJ, Parrish S, Imani F, Fire A, Morgan RA. Specific inhibition of gene expression by small double-stranded RNAs in invertebrate and vertebrate systems. Proc Natl Acad Sci USA 2001; 98(17): 9742–9747.

104. Gitlin L, Andino R. Nucleic acid-based immune system: the antiviral potential of mammalian RNA silencing. J Virol 2003; 77(13):7159–7165.

105. Martins LM, Iaccarino I, Tenev T, et al. The serine protease Omi/HtrA2 regulates apoptosis by binding XIAP through a reaper-like motif. J Biol Chem 2002; 277(1):439–444.

106. Cioca DP, Aoki Y, Kiyosawa K. RNA interference is a functional pathway with therapeutic potential in human myeloid leukemia cell lines. Cancer Gene Therapy 2003; 10(2):125–133.

107. Donze O, Picard D. RNA interference in mammalian cells using siRNAs synthesized with T7 RNA polymerase. Nucleic Acids Res 2002; 30(10):e46.

108. Weil A, Garcon L, Harper M, Dumenil D, Dautry R, Kress M. Targeting the kinesin Eg5 to monitor siRNA transfection in mammalian cells. Biotechniques 2002; 33(6):1244–1248.

109. Dunne J, Drescher B, Riehle H, et al. The apparent uptake of fluorescently labeled siRNAs by elec-troporated cells depends on the fluorochrome. Oligonucleotides 2003; 13(5):375–380.

110. Walters DK, Jelinek DF. The effectiveness of double-stranded short inhibitory RNAs (siRNAs) may depend on the method of transfection. Antisense Nucleic Acid Drug Dev 2002; 12(6):411–418.

111. Scherr M, Morgan MA, Eder M. Gene silencing mediated by small interfering RNAs in mammalian cells. Curr Med Chem 2003; 10(3):245–256.

112. Heidenreich O, Krauter J, Riehle H, et al. AML1/MTG8 oncogene suppression by small interfering RNAs supports myeloid differentiation of t(8; 21)-positive leukemic cells. Blood 2003; 101(8):3157–3163.

113. Simeoni F, Morris MC, Heitz F, Divita G. Insight into the mechanism of the peptide-based gene delivery system MPG: implications for delivery of siRNA into mammalian cells. Nucleic Acids Res 2003; 31(11):2717–2724.

114. Prochiantz A. Getting hydrophilic compounds into cells—lessons from homeopeptides (Commentary). Curr Opin Neurobiol 1996; 6(5):629–634.

115. Schwarze SR, Ho A, Vocero-Akbani A, Dowdy SF. In vivo protein transduction: delivery of a biologi-cally active protein into the mouse [comment]. Science 1999; 285(5433):1569–1572.

116. Schwarze SR, Dowdy SF. In vivo protein transduction: intracellular delivery of biologically active proteins, compounds and DNA. Trends Pharmacol Sci 2000; 21(2):45–48.

117. Derossi D, Joliot AH, Chassaing G, Prochiantz A. The third helix of the Antennapedia homeodomain translocates through biological membranes. J Biol Chem 1994; 269(14):10,444–10,450.

118. Derossi D, Chassaing G, Prochiantz A. Trojan peptides—the penetratin system for intracellular delivery. Trends Cell Biol 1998; 8(2):84–87.

119. Schmitz K, Schepers U. Cell penetrating peptides in siRNA delivery. Expert Opin Biol Ther 2004; in press.

120. Schmitz K, Diallo M, Mundegar R, Schepers U. pepsiRNAs for RNAi in mammals. Submitted.

121. Berns K, Hijmans EM, Mullenders J, et al. A large-scale RNAi screen in human cells identifies new components of the p53 pathway. Nature 2004; 428(6981):431–437.

122. Kisielow M, Kleiner S, Nagasawa M, Faisal A, Nagamine Y. Isoform-specific knockdown and expres-sion of adaptor protein ShcA using small interfering RNA. Biochem J 2002; 363(1):1–5.

123. Czauderna F, Fechtner M, Aygun H, et al. Functional studies of the PI(3)-kinase signalling pathway employing synthetic and expressed siRNA. Nucleic Acids Res 2003; 31(2):670–682.

124. Xu Z, Williams CJ, Kopf GS, Schultz RM. Maturation-associated increase in IP3 receptor type 1: role in conferring increased IP3 sensitivity and $Ca^{2+}$ oscillatory behavior in mouse eggs. Dev Biol 2003; 254(2):163–171.

125. Stucke VM, Sillje HH, Arnaud L, Nigg EA. Human Mps1 kinase is required for the spindle assembly checkpoint but not for centrosome duplication. EMBO J 2002; 21(7):1723–1732.

126. Ohta T, Essner R, Ryu JH, Palazzo RE, Uetake Y, Kuriyama R. Characterization of Cep135, a novel coiled-coil centrosomal protein involved in microtubule organization in mammalian cells. J Cell Biol 2002; 156(1):87–99.

127. Salisbury JL, Suino KM, Busby R, Springett M. Centrin-2 is required for centriole duplication in mam-malian cells. Curr Biol 2002; 12(15):1287–1292.

128. Prasanth KV, Sacco-Bubulya PA, Prasanth SG, Spector DL. Sequential entry of components of the gene expression machinery into daughter nuclei. Mol Biol Cell 2003; 14(3):1043–1057.

129. Cabot RA, Prather RS. Cleavage stage porcine embryos may have differing developmental requirements for karyopherins alpha2 and alpha3. Mol Reprod Dev 2003; 64(3):292–301.

130. Kim VN. RNA interference in functional genomics and medicine [review]. J Korean Med Sci 2003; 18(3):309–318.

131. Paddison PJ, Caudy AA, Bernstein E, Hannon GJ, Conklin DS. Short hairpin RNAs (shRNAs) induce sequence-specific silencing in mammalian cells. Genes Dev 2002; 16(8):948–958.

132. Brummelkamp TR, Bernards R, Agami R. A system for stable expression of short interfering RNAs in mammalian cells. Science 2002; 296(5567):550–553.

133. Sui G, Soohoo C, El Affar B, Gay F, Shi Y, Forrester WC. A DNA vector-based RNAi technology to suppress gene expression in mammalian cells. Proc Natl Acad Sci USA 2002; 99(8):5515–5520.

134. Miyagishi M, Taira K. U6 promoter driven siRNAs with four uridine 3' overhangs efficiently suppress targeted gene expression in mammalian cells. Nature Biotechnol 2002; 20(5):497–500.

135. Paul CP, Good PD, Winer I, Engelke DR. Effective expression of small interfering RNA in human cells. Nature Biotechnol 2002; 20(5):505–508.

136. Lee NS, Dohjima T, Bauer G, et al. Expression of small interfering RNAs targeted against HIV-1 rev transcripts in human cells. Nature Biotechnol 2002; 20(5):500–505.

137. Paule MR, White RJ. Survey and summary: transcription by RNA polymerases I and III. Nucleic Acids Res 2000; 28(6):1283–1298.

138. Zamore PD. RNA interference: listening to the sound of silence. Nature Struct Biol 2001; 8(9):746–750.

139. Diallo M, Arenz C, Schmitz K, Sandhoff K, Schepers U. RNA Interference: a new method to analyze the function of glycoproteins and glycosylating proteins in mammalian cells. Knockout experiments with UDP-glucose/ceramide-glucosyltransferase. Methods Enzymol 2003; 363:173–190.

140. Diallo M, Arenz C, Schmitz K, Sandhoff K, Schepers U. Long endogenous dsRNAs can induce a complete gene silencing in mammalian cells and primary cultures. Oligonucleotides 2003; 13(5):381–392.

141. Shinagawa T, Ishii S. Generation of Ski-knockdown mice by expressing a long double-strand RNA from an RNA polymerase II promoter. Genes Dev 2003; 17(11):1340–1345.

142. Lewis DL, Hagstrom JE, Loomis AG, Wolff JA, Herweijer H. Efficient delivery of siRNA for inhibition of gene expression in postnatal mice. Nature Genet 2002; 32(1):107–108.

143. McCaffrey AP, Meuse L, Pham TTT, Conklin DS, Hannon GJ, Kay MA. Gene expression—RNA interference in adult mice. Nature 2002; 418(6893):38–39.

144. Hemann MT, Fridman JS, Zilfou JT, et al. An epi-allelic series of p53 hypomorphs created by stable RNAi produces distinct tumor phenotypes in vivo. Nature Genet 2003; 33(3):396–400.

145. Tiscornia G, Singer O, Ikawa M, Verma IM. A general method for gene knockdown in mice by using lentiviral vectors expressing small interfering RNA. Proc Natl Acad Sci USA 2003; 100(4):1844–1848.

146. Rubinson DA, Dillon CP, Kwiatkowski AV, et al. A lentivirus-based system to functionally silence genes in primary mammalian cells, stem cells and transgenic mice by RNA interference. Nature Genet 2003; 33(3):401–406.

147. Sledz CA, Holko M, de Veer MJ, Silverman RH, Williams BR. Activation of the interferon system by short-interfering RNAs. Nature Cell Biol 2003; 5(9):834–839.

148. Stark GR, Kerr IM, Williams BR, Silverman RH, Schreiber RD. How cells respond to interferons. Annu Rev Biochem 1998; 67:227–264.

149. Bridge AJ, Pebernard S, Ducraux A, Nicoulaz AL, Iggo R. Induction of an interferon response by RNAi vectors in mammalian cells. Nature Genet 2003; 34(3):263–264.

150. Akusjarvi G, Svensson C, Nygard O. A mechanism by which adenovirus virus-associated RNAI controls translation in a transient expression assay. Mol Cell Biol 1987; 7(1):549–551.

151. Koopmans M, Duizer E. Foodborne viruses: an emerging problem. Int J Food Microbiol 2004; 90(1): 23–41.

152. Jacque JM, Triques K, Stevenson M. Modulation of HIV-1 replication by RNA interference. Nature 2002; 418(6896):435–438.

153. Martinez MA, Clotet B, Este JA. RNA interference of HIV replication. Trends Immunol 2002; 23(12): 559–561.

154. Yamamoto T, Omoto S, Mizuguchi M, et al. Double-stranded nef RNA interferes with human immunodeficiency virus type 1 replication. Microbiol Immunol 2002; 46(11):809–817.

155. Anderson J, Banerjea A, Akkina R. Bispecific short hairpin siRNA constructs targeted to CD4, CXCR4, and CCR5 confer HIV-1 resistance. Oligonucleotides 2003; 13(5):303–312.

156. Anderson J, Banerjea A, Planelles V, Akkina R. Potent suppression of HIV type 1 infection by a short hairpin anti-CXCR4 siRNA. AIDS Res Hum Retroviruses 2003; 19(8):699–706.

157. Boden D, Pusch O, Lee F, Tucker L, Shank PR, Ramratnam B. Promoter choice affects the potency of HIV-1 specific RNA interference. Nucleic Acids Res 2003; 31(17):5033–5038.

158. Pusch O, Boden D, Silbermann R, Lee F, Tucker L, Ramratnam B. Nucleotide sequence homology requirements of HIV-1-specific short hairpin RNA. Nucleic Acids Res 2003; 31(22):6444–6449.

159. Michienzi A, Castanotto D, Lee N, Li S, Zaia JA, Rossi JJ. RNA-mediated inhibition of HIV in a gene therapy setting. Ann NY Acad Sci 2003; 1002:63–71.

160. Boden D, Pusch O, Silbermann R, Lee F, Tucker L, Ramratnam B. Enhanced gene silencing of HIV-1 specific siRNA using microRNA designed hairpins. Nucleic Acids Res 2004; 32(3):1154–1158.

161. Dunn SJ, Khan IH, Chan UA, et al. Identification of cell surface targets for HIV-1 therapeutics using genetic screens. Virology 2004; 321(2):260–273.

162. Novina CD, Murray MF, Dykxhoorn DM, et al. siRNA-directed inhibition of HIV-1 infection. Nature Med 2002; 8(7):681–686.

163. Andino R. RNAi puts a lid on virus replication. Nature Biotechnol 2003; 21(6):629–630.

164. Hamasaki K, Nakao K, Matsumoto K, Ichikawa T, Ishikawa H, Eguchi K. Short interfering RNA-directed inhibition of hepatitis B virus replication. FEBS Lett 2003; 543(1-3):51–54.

165. McCaffrey AP, Meuse L, Karimi M, Contag CH, Kay MA. A potent and specific morpholino antisense inhibitor of hepatitis C translation in mice. Hepatology 2003; 38(2):503–508.

166. Sen A, Steele R, Ghosh AK, Basu A, Ray R, Ray RB. Inhibition of hepatitis C virus protein expression by RNA interference. Virus Res 2003; 96(1-2):27–35.

167. Shlomai A, Shaul Y. Inhibition of hepatitis B virus expression and replication by RNA interference. Hepatology 2003; 37(4):764–770.

168. Song E, Lee SK, Wang J, et al. RNA interference targeting Fas protects mice from fulminant hepatitis. Nature Med 2003; 9(3):347–351.

169. Wilson JA, Jayasena S, Khvorova A, et al. RNA interference blocks gene expression and RNA synthesis from hepatitis C replicons propagated in human liver cells. Proc Natl Acad Sci USA 2003; 100(5): 2783–2788.

170. Yokota T, Sakamoto N, Enomoto N, et al. Inhibition of intracellular hepatitis C virus replication by synthetic and vector-derived small interfering RNAs. EMBO Rep 2003; 4(6):602–608.

171. Milner J. RNA interference for treating cancers caused by viral infection. Expert Opin Biol Ther 2003; 3(3):459–467.

172. Butz K, Ristriani T, Hengstermann A, Denk C, Scheffner M, Hoppe-Seyler F. siRNA targeting of the viral E6 oncogene efficiently kills human papillomavirus-positive cancer cells. Oncogene 2003; 22(38): 5938–5945.

173. Hall AH, Alexander KA. RNA interference of human papillomavirus type 18 E6 and E7 induces senescence in HeLa cells. J Virol 2003; 77(10):6066–6069.

174. Gitlin L, Karelsky S, Andino R. Short interfering RNA confers intracellular antiviral immunity in human cells. Nature 2002; 418(6896):430–434.

175. Wang QC, Nie QH, Feng ZH. RNA interference: antiviral weapon and beyond. World J Gastroenterol 2003; 9(8):1657–1661.

176. Godfrey A, Laman H, Boshoff C. RNA interference: a potential tool against Kaposi's sarcoma-associated herpesvirus. Curr Opin Infect Dis 2003; 16(6):593–600.

177. Stewart SA, Dykxhoorn DM, Palliser D, et al. Lentivirus-delivered stable gene silencing by RNAi in primary cells. RNA 2003; 9(4):493–501.

178. Bitko V, Barik S. Phenotypic silencing of cytoplasmic genes using sequence-specific double-stranded short interfering RNA and its application in the reverse genetics of wild type negative-strand RNA viruses. BMC Microbiol 2001; 1(1):34.

179. Ge Q, McManus MT, Nguyen T, et al. RNA interference of influenza virus production by directly targeting mRNA for degradation and indirectly inhibiting all viral RNA transcription. Proc Natl Acad Sci USA 2003; 100(5):2718–2723.

180. Li XP, Li G, Peng Y, Kung HF, Lin MC. Suppression of Epstein–Barr virus-encoded latent membrane protein-1 by RNA interference inhibits the metastatic potential of nasopharyngeal carcinoma cells. Biochem Biophys Res Commun 2004; 315(1):212–218.

181. Zhang J, Hua ZC. Targeted gene silencing by small interfering RNA-based knock-down technology. Curr Pharm Biotechnol 2004; 5(1):1–7.
182. Zhang Y, Li T, Fu L, et al. Silencing SARS-CoV Spike protein expression in cultured cells by RNA interference. FEBS Lett 2004; 560(1-3):141–146.
183. He ML, Zheng B, Peng Y, et al. Inhibition of SARS-associated coronavirus infection and replication by RNA interference. JAMA 2003; 290(20):2665–2666.
184. Qin L, Xiong B, Luo C, et al. Identification of probable genomic packaging signal sequence from SARS-CoV genome by bioinformatics analysis. Acta Pharmacol Sin 2003; 24(6):489–496.
185. Wu HY, Guy JS, Yoo D, Vlasak R, Urbach E, Brian DA. Common RNA replication signals exist among group 2 coronaviruses: evidence for in vivo recombination between animal and human coronavirus molecules. Virology 2003; 315(1):174–183.
186. McCaffrey AP, Nakai H, Pandey K, et al. Inhibition of hepatitis B virus in mice by RNA interference. Nature Biotechnol 2003; 21(6):639–644.
187. Lieberman J, Song E, Lee SK, Shankar P. Interfering with disease: opportunities and roadblocks to harnessing RNA interference. Trends Mol Med 2003; 9(9):397–403.
188. Das AT, Brummelkamp TR, Westerhout EM, et al. Human immunodeficiency virus type 1 escapes from RNA interference-mediated inhibition. J Virol 2004; 78(5):2601–2605.
189. Boden D, Pusch O, Lee F, Tucker L, Ramratnam B. Human immunodeficiency virus type 1 escape from RNA interference. J Virol 2003; 77(21):11,531–11,535.
190. Bastin P, Ellis K, Kohl L, Gull K. Flagellum ontogeny in trypanosomes studied via an inherited and regulated RNA interference system. J Cell Sci 2000; 113(18):3321–3328.
191. LaCount DJ, Bruse S, Hill KL, Donelson JE. Double-stranded RNA interference in *Trypanosoma brucei* using head-to-head promoters. Mol Biochem Parasitol 2000; 111(1):67–76.
192. McRobert L, McConkey GA. RNA interference (RNAi) inhibits growth of *Plasmodium falciparum*. Mol Biochem Parasitol 2002; 119(2):273–278.
193. Lillico S, Field MC, Blundell P, Coombs GH, Mottram JC. Essential roles for GPI-anchored proteins in African trypanosomes revealed using mutants deficient in GP18. Mol Biol Cell 2003; 14(3):1182–1194.
194. Mohmmed A, Dasaradhi PV, Bhatnagar RK, Chauhan VS, Malhotra P. In vivo gene silencing in *Plasmodium berghei*—a mouse malaria model. Biochem Biophys Res Commun 2003; 309(3):506–511.
195. Blackman MJ. RNAi in protozoan parasites: what hope for the Apicomplexa? Protist 2003; 154(2):177–180.
196. Ngo H, Tschudi C, Gull K, Ullu E. Double-stranded RNA induces mRNA degradation in *Trypanosoma brucei*. PNAS 1998; 95(25):14,687–14,692.
197. Aballay A, Drenkard E, Hilbun LR, Ausubel FM. *Caenorhabditis elegans* innate immune response triggered by *Salmonella enterica* requires intact LPS and is mediated by a MAPK signaling pathway. Curr Biol 2003; 13(1):47–52.
198. Arcus VL, Backbro K, Roos A, Daniel EL, Baker EN. Distant structural homology leads to the functional characterisation of an archaeal PIN-domain as an exonuclease. J Biol Chem 2004; 279:16,471–16,478.
199. Walduck A, Rudel T, Meyer TF. Proteomic and gene profiling approaches to study host responses to bacterial infection. Curr Opin Microbiol 2004; 7(1):33–38.
200. Sorensen DR, Leirdal M, Sioud M. Gene silencing by systemic delivery of synthetic siRNAs in adult mice. J Mol Biol 2003; 327(4):761–766.
201. Kelly D, Campbell JI, King TP, et al. Commensal anaerobic gut bacteria attenuate inflammation by regulating nuclear-cytoplasmic shuttling of PPAR-gamma and RelA. Nature Immunol 2004; 5(1):104–112.
202. Duxbury MS, Ito H, Benoit E, Zinner MJ, Ashley SW, Whang EE. RNA interference targeting focal adhesion kinase enhances pancreatic adenocarcinoma gemcitabine chemosensitivity. Biochem Biophys Res Commun 2003; 311(3):786–792.
203. Wang Y, Decker SJ, Sebolt-Leopold J. Knockdown of Chk1, Wee1 and Myt1 by RNA interference abrogates G(2) checkpoint and induces apoptosis. Cancer Biol Ther 2004; 3:305–313.
204. Zangemeister-Wittke U. Antisense to apoptosis inhibitors facilitates chemotherapy and TRAIL-induced death signaling. Ann NY Acad Sci 2003; 1002:90–94.
205. Chatterjee B. The role of the androgen receptor in the development of prostatic hyperplasia and prostate cancer. Mol Cell Biochem 2003; 253(1-2):89–101.

206. Wall NR, Shi Y. Small RNA: can RNA interference be exploited for therapy? Lancet 2003; 362(9393): 1401–1403.
207. Brummelkamp TR, Nijman SM, Dirac AM, Bernards R. Loss of the cylindromatosis tumour suppressor inhibits apoptosis by activating NF-kappaB. Nature 2003; 424(6950):797–801.
208. Tanaka Y, Gavrielides MV, Mitsuuchi Y, Fujii T, Kazanietz MG. Protein kinase C promotes apoptosis in LNCaP prostate cancer cells through activation of p38 MAPK and inhibition of the Akt survival pathway. J Biol Chem 2003; 278(36):33,753–33,762.
209. Milner J. RNA interference for treating cancers caused by viral infection [review]. Expert Opin Biol Ther 2003; 3(3):459–467.
210. Jiang M, Milner J. Bcl-2 constitutively suppresses p53-dependent apoptosis in colorectal cancer cells. Genes Dev 2003; 17(7):832–837.
211. Wilda M, Fuchs U, Wossmann W, Borkhardt A. Killing of leukemic cells with a BCR/ABL fusion gene by RNA interference (RNAi). Oncogene 2002; 21(37):5716–5724.
212. Lin SL, Chuong CM, Ying SY. A novel mRNA–cDNA interference phenomenon for silencing bcl-2 expression in human LNCaP cells. Biochem Biophys Res Commun 2001; 281(3):639–644.
213. Chen YG, Lui HM, Lin SL, Lee JM, Ying SY. Regulation of cell proliferation, apoptosis, and carcinogenesis by activin. Exp Biol Med (Maywood) 2002; 227(2):75–87.
214. Subramanian T, Chinnadurai G. Pro-apoptotic activity of transiently expressed BCL-2 occurs independent of BAX and BAK. J Cell Biochem 2003; 89(6):1102–1114.
215. Grzmil M, Thelen P, Hemmerlein B, et al. Bax inhibitor-1 is overexpressed in prostate cancer and its specific down-regulation by RNA interference leads to cell death in human prostate carcinoma cells. Am J Pathol 2003; 163(2):543–552.
216. Dzitoyeva S, Dimitrijevic N, Manev H. Gamma-aminobutyric acid B receptor 1 mediates behavior-impairing actions of alcohol in *Drosophila*: adult RNA interference and pharmacological evidence. Proc Natl Acad Sci USA 2003; 100(9):5485–5490.
217. Aza-Blanc P, Cooper CL, Wagner K, Batalov S, Deveraux QL, Cooke MP. Identification of modulators of TRAIL-induced apoptosis via RNAi-based phenotypic screening. Mol Cell 2003; 12(3):627–637.
218. Lima RT, Martins LM, Guimaraes JE, Sambade C, Vasconcelos MH. Specific downregulation of bcl-2 and xIAP by RNAi enhances the effects of chemotherapeutic agents in MCF-7 human breast cancer cells. Cancer Gene Ther 2004; 11:309–316.
219. Yin JQ, Gao J, Shao R, Tian WN, Wang J, Wan Y. siRNA agents inhibit oncogene expression and attenuate human tumor cell growth. J Exp Ther Oncol 2003; 3(4):194–204.
220. Konnikova L, Kotecki M, Kruger MM, Cochran BH. Knockdown of STAT3 expression by RNAi induces apoptosis in astrocytoma cells. BMC Cancer 2003; 3(1):23.
221. Sun B, Nishihira J, Suzuki M, et al. Induction of macrophage migration inhibitory factor by lysophosphatidic acid: relevance to tumor growth and angiogenesis. Int J Mol Med 2003; 12(4):633–641.
222. Liu LT, Chang HC, Chiang LC, Hung WC. Histone deacetylase inhibitor up-regulates RECK to inhibit MMP-2 activation and cancer cell invasion. Cancer Res 2003; 63(12):3069–3072.
223. Zhang L, Yang N, Mohamed-Hadley A, Rubin SC, Coukos G. Vector-based RNAi, a novel tool for isoform-specific knock-down of VEGF and anti-angiogenesis gene therapy of cancer. Biochem Biophys Res Commun 2003; 303(4):1169–1178.
224. Ameri K, Lewis CE, Raida M, Sowter H, Hai T, Harris AL. Anoxic induction of ATF-4 through HIF-1-independent pathways of protein stabilization in human cancer cells. Blood 2004; 103(5):1876–1882.
225. Niu Q, Perruzzi C, Voskas D, Lawler J, Dumont DJ, Benjamin LE. Inhibition of Tie-2 signaling induces endothelial cell apoptosis, decreases akt signaling, and induces endothelial cell expression of the endogenous anti-angiogenic molecule, thrombospondin-1. Cancer Biol Ther 2004; 3:402–405.
226. Tien ES, Davis JW, Vanden Heuvel JP. Identification of the CBP/p300 interacting protein CITED2 as a PPARalpha coregulator. J Biol Chem 2004; 279:24,053–24,063.
227. Zippo A, De Robertis A, Bardelli M, Galvagni F, Oliviero S. Identification of Flk-1-target genes in vasculogenesis: Pim-1 is required for endothelial and mural cell differentiation in vitro. Blood 2004; 103:4536–4544.
228. Bachelder RE, Lipscomb EA, Lin X, et al. Competing autocrine pathways involving alternative neuropilin-1 ligands regulate chemotaxis of carcinoma cells. Cancer Res 2003; 63(17):5230–5233.
229. Sun Y, Mochizuki Y, Majerus PW. Inositol 1,3,4-trisphosphate 5/6-kinase inhibits tumor necrosis factor-induced apoptosis. J Biol Chem 2003; 278(44):43,645–43,653.

230. Schafer R, Abraham D, Paulus P, et al. Impaired VE–cadherin/beta–catenin expression mediates endothelial cell degeneration in dilated cardiomyopathy. Circulation 2003; 108(13):1585–1591.
231. Liu Y, Lashuel HA, Choi S, et al. Discovery of inhibitors that elucidate the role of UCH-L1 activity in the H1299 lung cancer cell line. Chem Biol 2003; 10(9):837–846.
232. Riss D, Jin L, Qian X, et al. Differential expression of galectin-3 in pituitary tumors. Cancer Res 2003; 63(9):2251–2255.
233. Deroanne C, Vouret-Craviari V, Wang B, Pouyssegur J. EphrinA1 inactivates integrin-mediated vascular smooth muscle cell spreading via the Rac/PAK pathway. J Cell Sci 2003; 116(Pt 7):1367–1376.
234. Nagashima K, Endo A, Ogita H, et al. Adaptor protein Crk is required for ephrin-B1-induced membrane ruffling and focal complex assembly of human aortic endothelial cells. Mol Biol Cell 2002; 13 (12):4231–4242.
235. Jarad G, Wang B, Khan S, et al. Fas activation induces renal tubular epithelial cell beta 8 integrin expression and function in the absence of apoptosis. J Biol Chem 2002; 277(49):47,826–47,833.
236. Futami T, Miyagishi M, Seki M, Taira K. Induction of apoptosis in HeLa cells with siRNA expression vector targeted against bcl-2. Nucleic Acids Res Supplement 2002; (Suppl 2):251–252.
237. Cunningham JM, Weinberg RA. Ras oncogenes in human tumours: identification, mechanism of activation and cooperative role in transformation. IARC Sci Publ 1985(60):359–364.
238. Duursma AM, Agami R. Ras interference as cancer therapy. Sem Cancer Biol 2003; 13(4):267–273.
239. Brummelkamp TR, Bernards R, Agami R. Stable suppression of tumorigenicity by virus-mediated RNA interference. Cancer Cell 2002; 2(3):243–247.
240. Wolff JA, Herweijer H. Nonviral vectors for cardiovascular gene delivery. Ernst Schering Res Found Workshop 2003(43):41–59.
241. Lorenz K, Lohse MJ, Quitterer U. Protein kinase C switches the Raf kinase inhibitor from Raf-1 to GRK-2. Nature 2003; 426(6966):574–579.
242. Maxwell MM, Pasinelli P, Kazantsev AG, Brown RH Jr. RNA interference-mediated silencing of mutant superoxide dismutase rescues cyclosporin A-induced death in cultured neuroblastoma cells. Proc Natl Acad Sci USA 2004; 101(9):3178–3183.
243. Ding H, Schwarz DS, Keene A, et al. Selective silencing by RNAi of a dominant allele that causes amyotrophic lateral sclerosis. Aging Cell 2003; 2(4):209–217.
244. Xia XG, Zhou H, Ding H, Affar el B, Shi Y, Xu Z. An enhanced U6 promoter for synthesis of short hairpin RNA. Nucleic Acids Res 2003; 31(17):e100.
245. Miller VM, Xia H, Marrs GL, et al. Allele-specific silencing of dominant disease genes. Proc Natl Acad Sci USA 2003; 100(12):7195–7200.
246. Francis R, McGrath G, Zhang J, et al. aph-1 and pen-2 are required for Notch pathway signaling, gamma-secretase cleavage of betaAPP, and presenilin protein accumulation. Dev Cell 2002; 3(1): 85–97.
247. Asai M, Hattori C, Szabo B, et al. Putative function of ADAM9, ADAM10, and ADAM17 as APP alpha-secretase. Biochem Biophys Res Commun 2003; 301(1):231–235.
248. Mattson MP. Neurobiology: ballads of a protein quartet. Nature 2003; 422(6930):385–387.
249. Takasugi N, Tomita T, Hayashi I, et al. The role of presenilin cofactors in the gamma-secretase complex. Nature 2003; 422(6930):438–441.
250. Marlow L, Canet RM, Haugabook SJ, Hardy JA, Lahiri DK, Sambamurti K. APH1, PEN2, and Nicastrin increase Abeta levels and gamma-secretase activity [erratum Biochem Biophys Res Commun 2003 Aug 1; 307(3):756]. Biochem Biophys Res Commun 2003; 305(3):502–509.
251. Kao SC, Krichevsky AM, Kosik KS, Tsai LH. BACE1 suppression by RNA interference in primary cortical neurons. J Biol Chem 2004; 279(3):1942–1949.
252. Kiehl TR, Shibata H, Pulst SM. The ortholog of human ataxin-2 is essential for early embryonic patterning in C. elegans. J Mol Neurosci 2000; 15(3):231–241.
253. Yang Y, Nishimura I, Imai Y, Takahashi R, Lu B. Parkin suppresses dopaminergic neuron-selective neurotoxicity induced by Pael-R in Drosophila. Neuron 2003; 37(6):911–924.
254. Love R. First disease model created by RNA interference. Lancet Neurol 2004; 3(1):7.
255. Trulzsch B, Wood M. Applications of nucleic acid technology in the CNS. J Neurochem 2004; 88(2): 257–265.
256. Omi K, Tokunaga K, Hohjoh H. Long-lasting RNAi activity in mammalian neurons. FEBS Lett 2004; 558(1-3):89–95.
257. Trulzsch B, Davies K, Wood M. Survival of motor neuron gene downregulation by RNAi: towards a cell culture model of spinal muscular atrophy. Brain Res Mol Brain Res 2004; 120(2):145–150.

258. Moon C, Kang WS, Jeong DC, Jin JY. Distribution of adenoviral vector in brain after intravenous administration. J Korean Med Sci 2003; 18(1):108–111.

259. Xia H, Mao Q, Paulson HL, Davidson BL. siRNA-mediated gene silencing in vitro and in vivo. Nature Biotechnol 2002; 20(10):1006–1010.

260. Schepers U. Die Wiederentdeckung der RNA. Nachr Chem 2004; 52:302–305.

261. Wohlbold L, van der Kuip H, Miething C, et al. Inhibition of bcr-abl gene expression by small interfering RNA sensitizes for imatinib mesylate (STI571). Blood 2003; 102(6):2236–2239.

262. Nieth C, Priebsch A, Stege A, Lage H. Modulation of the classical multidrug resistance (MDR) phenotype by RNA interference (RNAi). FEBS Lett 2003; 545(2-3):144–150.

263. Crnkovic-Mertens I, Hoppe-Seyler F, Butz K. Induction of apoptosis in tumor cells by siRNA-mediated silencing of the livin/ML-IAP/KIAP gene. Oncogene 2003; 22(51):8330–8336.

264. Chen Y, Stamatoyannopoulos G, Song CZ. Down-regulation of CXCR4 by inducible small interfering RNA inhibits breast cancer cell invasion in vitro. Cancer Res 2003; 63(16):4801–4804.

265. Zha S, Ferdinandusse S, Denis S, et al. Alpha-methylacyl-CoA racemase as an androgen-independent growth modifier in prostate cancer. Cancer Res 2003; 63(21):7365–7376.

# 13

# Image-Based Assays of Cellular Phenotype for Drug Target Discovery and Validation

*Kris F. Sachsenmeier, PhD*
*and Jonathan A. Terrett, PhD*

#### Contents

### Summary

The application of Automated Cell Inc. (ACI) image-based assays of cellular phenotype for target discovery and validation is presented. The need for functional cellular assays as complementary to target discovery strategies that infer a link with disease without demonstrating a cellular phenotype for candidates is discussed. ACI cellular phenotypic assays are shown being used early in the target discovery process for primary screening, as well as later in target validation or pathway dissection studies. Examples include data supporting MEK as a target in HT1080 cells expressing an activated *ras* oncogene as well as a case study demonstrating the utility of Automated Cell assays in validating a novel breast cancer target.

**Key Words:** Target validation; cell based assays; phenotypic assays; functional genomics; proteomics; breast cancer; NSE-2; image based.

## 1. INTRODUCTION

In the postgenomic land-grab of drug target discovery and validation, most strategies infer disease-linked function by methods such as protein–protein association (e.g., two hybrid systems or immunoprecipitation), disease-linked expression profiling (e.g., two-dimensional [2D] gel electrophoresis or various nucleic acid or protein chip technologies),

From: *Cancer Drug Discovery and Development: The Oncogenomics Handbook*
Edited by: W. J. LaRochelle and R. A. Shimkets © Humana Press Inc., Totowa, NJ

or genetic association. The challenge of demonstrating functional relevance and target-ability remains an inevitable downstream step in the development of promising candidates. Whether performing target discovery or validation, screening for novel protein therapeutics, lead optimization, or determining a mechanism of action, the successful candidate must affect some aspect of the disease phenotype. Often, the return on any investment in screening efforts is lost when a candidate eventually fails to show a functional role in a disease-relevant system. This situation underscores the need for discerning functional roles and relevant responses early in the discovery process.

Despite these drawbacks, inference-based target discovery has been the mode of choice for many drug discovery programs. This choice for inferred rather than direct functional screens is typically made because of the high-throughput capacity of inference-based methods as compared with the relatively low throughput of various cellular and animal functional assay systems. An efficient balance between throughput and function-linked bioinformation remains a biotechnological challenge.

Automated Cell, Inc. (ACI) has met this challenge by developing a unique combination of multi-end-point image-based cellular assay systems that maximize throughput efficiency while establishing a functional role for every hit. By screening at the level of function, any loss of time and investment as a result of subsequent failure in a functional assay is minimized. Putative protein targets and therapeutics are discovered, prioritized, and prevalidated at the screening step.

Automated Cell leverages this assay system in developing a pipeline of therapeutic antibodies in cancer and immune disease. The ACI approach offers at least two distinct advantages over conventional drug discovery strategies. First, a functionally active antibody–antigen combination represents both a novel potential therapeutic agent (the antibody) as well as a potential novel target (the antigen). Targets discovered in this way are "pre-validated" candidates for nonantibody-mediated therapies as well as likely links to potentially expanded target discovery through novel molecular disease pathways; that is, the cellular moiety targeted by the antibody during a primary screen as well as all associated cellular proteins become immediately implicated as potential drug targets on the basis of the cellular phenotype detected during the primary screen. A second advantage lies in the fact that therapeutically active antibodies are discovered independent of prior knowledge of target identity. Following such a "target-independent" approach to primary screening, various requisite aspects of preclinical drug development (antibody isolation, optimization, and scale-up) are addressed *in parallel* with target identification and validation. This is in contrast with the more conventional pattern of target identification prior to validation and drug discovery. Applications of ACI image-based cellular assays are illustrated in this chapter, with examples in both primary and secondary screening assays. The successful application of these assays in the validation of a novel breast cancer target is also described.

## 2. CELLULAR PHENOTYPE IN PRIMARY SCREENING

In collaboration with the American Red Cross, ACI has expanded a bead-based method of screening plasma-derived immunoglobulins for cytotoxic activity against melanoma cell lines. Using this method, thousands of antibodies are isolated and screened daily in an image-based assay that measures both cell number and propidium iodide (PI) fluorescence as an index of antibody-mediated phenotypic change.

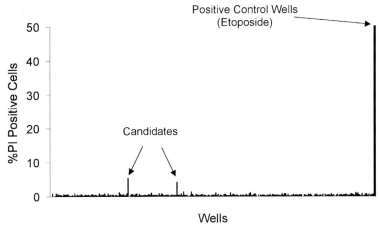

**Fig. 1.** Five hundred WM266-4 human melanoma cells were plated to individual wells of a 384-well microculture plate. Beads conjugated with a random library of hexapeptides were incubated with patient plasma immunoglobulins and placed into the melanoma cell cultures at an average density of 30 beads per well. Culture medium included propidium iodide (PI) as an indicator of cell death. Visible and fluorescent red images of each entire well at ×40 magnification were taken after 72 h. The percentage of PI-positive cells is plotted for each well. Two wells were treated with 50 μ*M* etoposide as a positive control for cell death.

Briefly, randomly generated libraries of six-member amino acid chains are synthesized on individual polystyrene beads, with each bead containing multiple copies of a single hexamer. These beads are incubated with human plasma to allow binding of plasma antibodies in an antibody–hexamer-specific manner. Plasma is obtained from patients in various stages of melanoma disease progression. In this reaction, antibodies are effectively purified by affinity interactions with the bead-linked hexapeptide. Beads are then rinsed and multiple beads are placed into 384-well microplate cultures of target cells. Bead-bound antibodies dissociate into the culture medium over time, forming an equilibrium between free and bound antibody.

Free antibody can bind to cellular targets, and cellular responses to antibody effects are detected by time-lapse digital imaging and quantified using image analysis. In this way, each well of the culture plate becomes a microbioassay system in which many antibodies are tested directly from plasma in a relatively purified form. Plates include control wells with antibody-free beads, and beads from wells showing statistically significant effects are removed from the well. At this point, one or more of this group of "hit well" beads is known to be loaded with an antibody already demonstrated to have a functional role in a disease-related bioassay.

Sample data from a single 384-well microculture plate assay are shown in Fig. 1. Melanoma cells were cultured with beads that had been incubated with melanoma patient plasma immunoglobulins for 3 d. Cells in more than 300 wells containing an average of 30 beads per well were imaged for visible and red fluorescent light. The total number of cells present as well as those that fluoresced red because of PI incorporation was determined using image analysis software. Wells showing increased levels of cell death when compared with wells containing unloaded, antibody-free beads are clearly identifiable.

Beads in positive primary assay wells are deconvoluted into separate wells, at a density of one bead per well, containing the same target cell line used in the multibead well. In this manner, the peptide–antibody combination responsible for the original functional response is both identified and confirmed in identical bioassays. The hexamer responsible for isolating the active antibody might or might not represent an actual linear portion of the B-cell epitope specific for the antibody. However, the peptide is a proven affinity ligand for the isolation of the antibody. Peptides from positive beads are sequenced by standard methods, and large-scale preparations of beads containing this peptide are synthesized. These scaled-up beads are, in turn, used to isolate large-scale preparations of antibody from plasma for secondary screening, in vivo studies, and monoclonal antibody sequencing to enable identification and cloning.

The value of an image-based cell death assay is apparent when considering that some drug candidates might cause cytostasis, only reducing cell proliferation without actually causing cells to die. Commonly used single-readout assays, such as annexin staining or caspase activation, fail to detect cytostasis if not coupled with a means of measuring absolute cell number. A simple comparison of cell numbers at the beginning and end of an assay period, such as that afforded through image analysis, is less likely to yield false negatives arising from candidates that act through annexin (1,2) or caspase-independent pathways (reviewed in refs. 3 and 4). The importance of simply observing cell cultures cannot be underestimated. With various cell/compound combinations, Automated Cell scientists have detected dividing cells that stained positive for either PI or annexin (unpublished observations and reviewed in ref. 5). The automated nature of the ACI platform allows for screening of millions of antibody–bead combinations at the phenotypic level on a weekly basis. Thus, the sensitivity of image-based cellular assays does not compromise the efficiency of the discovery engine for target discovery and validation.

## 3. CELLULAR PHENOTYPE IN SECONDARY SCREENING

Data in Fig. 1 were obtained from a single phenotypic readout—that of cell death—at a single time-point. The ACI platform is not limited to single-readout assays, however. Certain steps in the drug development process require a more in-depth look at cellular behavior. Such "secondary" steps include the stack ranking of primary screen hits, cellular pathway dissection, or studies aimed at determining mechanism of action. The efficiency and automation of ACI assays also enables their use in such downstream applications as quality assurance and control of candidate therapeutics during scale-up for clinical trials.

A key strength of ACI phenotypic assays is the capacity for concurrent observation of multiple assay readouts with a high degree of quantitative sophistication—all from each well of a 384-well microculture plate. Because each assay is nondestructive, a single assay well yields kinetic information about target-related behavior of a given set of cells over assay periods of hours to weeks. Subtle cellular phenotypes over time are detected and quantified at high temporal resolution. In addition to nonspecific cell death and growth, phenotypic readouts include changes in cell morphology and migration as well as cell–cell interactions in mixed-cell bioassays.

These analyses are performed within the same well, on the same set of cells at a single cell resolution. Sophisticated proprietary image analysis algorithms make the quantification of individual cell behavior possible. This means that each cell in an assay is being observed individually for its response to an exogenously added or transfected protein or protein combination. Quantification at single-cell resolution eliminates the masking of subpopulation effects because of averaging. This highly sensitive quantitative resolution, combined with the capacity for extended kinetic assays, ensures that subtle or short-lived cellular responses to proteins are not overlooked. Each cell's behavior at each second of the assay is recorded and can be precisely correlated with other phenotypic changes. Examples of in-depth, phenotypic assays are presented in Figs. 2–4. In these examples, the phenotypic effects of targeting the *ras* oncogene pathway at the cellular level are demonstrated. The HT1080 fibrosarcoma cell line expresses a constitutively activated ras oncoprotein *(6)*. Activated *ras* is known to yield classical features of the transformed phenotype in vitro in these cells *(7,8)*. Among others, these include accelerated proliferation *(9)*, a rounded, phase-refractile morphology *(10,11)*, and increased cell motility *(12)*.

Although a common means of assaying cellular proliferation, tritiated thymidine incorporation offers only a populationwide measure of general DNA synthesis rather than a direct measure of cellular proliferation. Results can be influenced by any subpopulation of rapidly dividing cells. The ability to detect subpopulation effects is crucial to discerning target effects upon cellular phenotype, especially when targets might be transiently transfected or expressed at less than 100% efficiency in a given population of cells. Image-based proliferation assays solve this dilemma. By counting each cell in a culture well at a series of time-points, the behavior of subpopulations can be quantified within the context of the entire culture. Figure 2A shows cell counts over a 48-h time period from culture of HT1080 cells treated with or without the MEK inhibitor U0126 and Raf kinase Inhibitor-1. These data indicate a significant decrease in cell numbers after only 24 h. Similar data for *ras*-targeted inhibition of HT1080 cell division from cell counts required as many as 6 d of trypsinization and manual cell counting *(9)*. Raf kinase inhibitor-1 and MEK inhibitor U0126 appear to have similar effects upon HT1080 culture proliferation when viewed with a single readout: cell number. However, these cells were also observed for incorporation of PI by taking both visible and fluorescent images during the assay period. Phenotypic differences between the two *ras* pathway inhibitors are clearly discerned by plotting the fraction of dead cells present under each treatment condition at a single time-point (Fig. 2B). These data show that although both inhibitors reduce the number of live cells, HT1080 cultures incubated with Raf kinase inhibitor-1 show approximately fourfold more PI-positive cells. These data reveal the differing phenotypic consequences of targeting these two components of the *ras* pathway.

As the data in Fig. 2 were being gathered, additional phenotypic information was being gathered from the same set of images. A role for MEK as a target in HT1080 transformation was confirmed by changes in HT1080 morphology. Images in Fig. 3 were taken during the assay, yielding the data shown in Fig. 2. Cells were left untreated (Fig. 3A) or incubated with U0126 (Fig. 3B). U0126 caused a "flat reversion" (Fig. 3B) from the more rounded morphology typical of transformed cells. The effect of targeting MEK upon cellular morphology was quantified by ACI image analysis software by measuring the area of HT1080 cultures as shown in Fig. 3C. Because MEK inhibition led to the flat revertant phenotype, the image analysis settings required to distinguish individual cells within a colony change. By maintaining settings suitable for distinguishing untreated cells, the area of cells perceived by the software increases as individual cells flatten and stretch out. Eventually, individual, flat revertant cells are indistinguishable at these settings

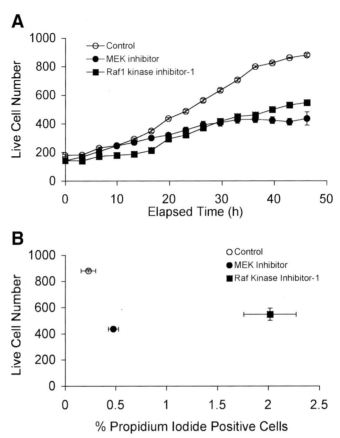

**Fig. 2.** Seven hundred fifty HT1080 human fibrosarcoma cells were plated to individual wells of a 384-well microculture plate. Culture medium included PI as an indicator of cell death. Cells were left untreated (open circles) or incubated with 20 $\mu M$ MEK Inhibitor U0126 (closed circles) or 20 $\mu M$ Raf kinase Inhibitor-1 (squares) in triplicate wells. Visible and fluorescent red images of each well at ×100 magnification were taken every 20 min for 48 h. The total number of PI-positive and PI-negative cells was calculated using proprietary ACI image analysis software. Total live (i.e., PI-negative) cell numbers are plotted for each 3 h interval in (**A**). At the 48-h time-point, both the live cell numbers ($y$-axis) and the percentage of PI-positive cells ($x$-axis) are plotted in (**B**). Error bars represent the standard error of triplicate wells for each time period.

and are recognized as large colonies. Figure 3C shows a frequency histogram of cell/colony area after categorizing cell and flattened colony areas into four equal bins. Bins are numbered 1 to 4 based on order of increasing size and in units of pixels. This histogram indicates what portion of cells in each treatment condition fell into each size category. Consistent with what can be seen by eye in Figs. 3A and 3B, greater than 90% of the untreated, activated *ras*-containing HT1080 cells are clearly discernable as single cells. Fewer than 40% of the U0126-treated cells remained in an area category similar to that of untreated cells with greater than 30% forming large flattened aggregates. This effect is statistically significant ($p < 0.0001$), as determined by performing model-based cluster analysis and provides quantitative validation of MEK as a target with functional relevance to the transformed phenotype in vitro.

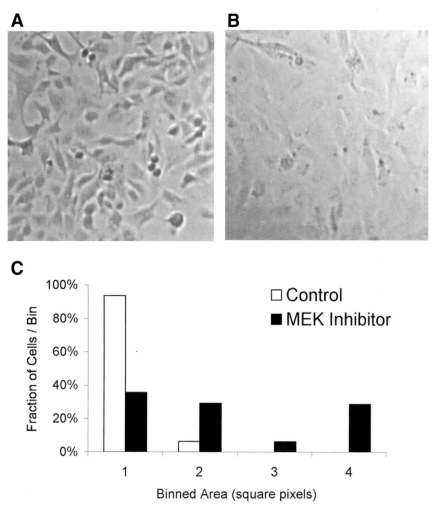

**Fig. 3.** Seven hundred fifty HT1080 human fibrosarcoma cells were plated to individual wells of a 384-well microculture plate. Culture medium included PI as an indicator of cell death. Cells were left untreated (**A**) or incubated with 20 µ*M* MEK inhibitor U0126 (**B**). Visible and fluorescent red images of each well at ×100 magnification were taken at 20-min intervals. Image analysis settings designed for the detection of individual untreated HT1080 cells were used for images from both treatment conditions. (A) and (B) show images (×100 magnification) of control and U0126-treated cell morphology after 5 d of incubation. (**C**) shows a frequency histogram after dividing cell and flattened colony areas into four equal bins, numbered 1 to 4 based on size in units of pixels. These data indicate what portion of all of the cells in each treatment condition (control: open bars; U0126: closed bars) fell into each size category. Data for (C) were obtained at a preconfluent culture density following 36 h of culture from a single representative replicate well for each treatment condition.

In a further phenotypic dimension, the images yielding data for cell growth and morphology also showed changes in cell motility. As seen with other cells (reviewed in refs. *13–16*), a correlation exists for HT1080 cells between motility and metastatic potential *(17,18)*. Consistent with growth inhibition and a flat revertant morphology, MEK inhibition by U0126 reduced the motility of HT1080 cells (Fig. 4). In a two-dimensional plot

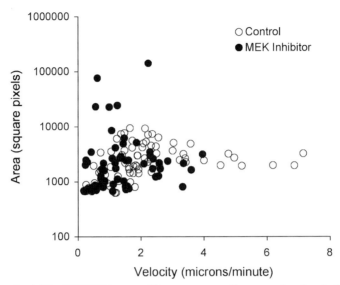

**Fig. 4.** Seven hundred fifty HT1080 human fibrosarcoma cells were plated to individual wells of a 384-well microculture plate. Culture medium included PI as an indicator of cell death. Cells were left untreated (open circles) or incubated with 20 μ$M$ MEK Inhibitor U0126 (closed circles). Image analysis settings designed for the detection of individual untreated HT1080 cells were used for images from both treatment conditions. Visible and fluorescent red images of each well at ×100 magnification were taken at 20-min intervals. The area of each cell or flattened colony is plotted (*y*-axis) along with its corresponding velocity (*x*-axis). Data were obtained at a preconfluent culture density following 36 h of culture from a single representative replicate well for each treatment condition. Note: Data were obtained from the same cultures shown in Figs. 2 and 3.

directly analogous to light scatter and fluorescence measurements in fluorescence activated cell sorting (FACS) analysis of suspended cells, two readouts of cellular phenotype—velocity and flat reversion—are shown to correlate in Fig. 4. The cellular velocity, calculated using the distance traveled by each cell in successive time-lapse images, is plotted against the area of each cell. As might be expected of flattened, adherent cells in which the oncogenic *ras* pathway has been targeted, HT1080 cells treated with U0126 showed fewer rapidly moving cells. Untreated controls showed a number of very rapidly moving cells and a higher mean population velocity. Combined data in Figs. 2–4 provide four different phenotypic readouts; each contributing a means of cellular validation for MEK as a target in ras-pathway-mediated cancers.

## 4. EXAMPLE OF TARGET VALIDATION
## USING IMAGE-BASED CELLULAR PHENOTYPIC ASSAYS

### 4.1. Selection of Target Candidates

One of the issues facing users of high-throughput inference-based methods is deciding which of the many genes and proteins that appear to change significantly are actually causative and targetable with drugs. This applies to mRNA and protein differential analyses as well as genetic association studies. Adam et al. *(19)* showed a path to generate a subset of targetable proteins from a larger list. In this case, the "long list" was of plasma-membrane-associated proteins from breast cancer cell lines identified by proteomics. The aim was to identify targets for small-molecule or antibody therapeutics. Although the initial proteomic studies were not differential in nature (i.e., the membrane components of the cancer cell lines were cataloged with no initial comparison to normal tissues), the validation work required is similar for all inference-based experiments.

As an initial step for cancer targets, some specificity over normal tissues is required. A subset of candidates fulfilling this criteria was generated using bioinformatics tools such as expressed sequence tag (EST) coverage per tissue for each protein (National Center for Biotechnology Information, Bethesda, MD). These candidates were then examined more comprehensively on normal and cancer clinical samples using both quantitative reverse transcription–polymerase chain reaction (RT-PCR) and immunohistochemistry. Although this process appeared to narrow down the candidate target list to three proteins, additional factors prevented the transition to high-throughput screens (HTSs). These factors included the fact that none of these candidate targets were readily screenable by classic HTS methods, that some of the membrane-bound proteins were not obviously targetable with antibodies, and that the company originally performing this work (Oxford Glycosciences, UK) had data from previous studies on other cancer types, suggesting candidates additional to those under consideration from 2D differential proteomic studies. The resources and time required by HTS demanded that the most relevant targets be selected.

### 4.2. Selection of Phenotypic Assays

In oncology, a number of phenotypes relevant to disease process can be readily examined in vitro (reviewed in ref. *20*). Such phenotypes include increased proliferation, morphological changes, and resistance to changes in the culture environment such as the presence of cytotoxic agents or reduced nutrients and changes in morphology. A number of the candidate targets were engineered to be overexpressed in different cell lines to be examined using image-based cellular phenotypic assays. Using a single 384-well plate format, 3 candidate target proteins were examined in 2 cell lines over 5 d under 8 different culture conditions, including 4 doses of etoposide as well as normal to very low serum culture conditions. Data from phenotypic assays using these cells are presented in Fig. 5 in the form of a "phenotypic fingerprint" (*see* Color Plate 5 following p. 302).

### 4.3. Using a Phenotypic Fingerprint

For each phenotypic readout in an assay, the average value for replicate wells over a user-specified time period is compared with a control set of replicates using a Student's *t*-test. For each comparison and its corresponding *p*-value, a square in the fingerprint is assigned a color according the magnitude of the value used to make the comparison. If the *p*-value arising from the compound-control comparison *t*-test is greater than 0.05, the square is colored green. Thus, all nongreen squares represent compound effects that are statistically significant at $p = 0.05$. If the compound reduced the value of a given readout (e.g., live cell number) relative to control at a given time-point, the square is colored blue at that time-point. If the compound increased the value at a given time-point relative to control, then the square is colored red. Time-points at which there was insufficient data for a valid *t*-test comparison are colored black. The intensity of red or blue indicates the magnitude of the distance of each value from the control value. Viewing all phenotypic

**A**

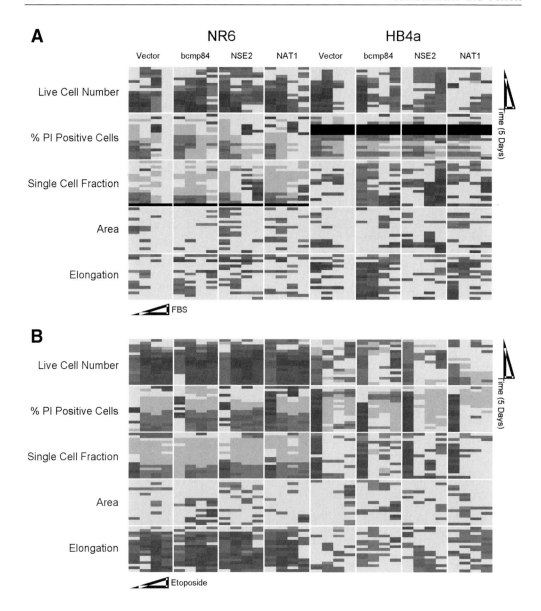

**Fig. 5.** For each phenotypic readout in an assay, the average value for replicate wells over a user-specified time period is compared with a control set of replicates using a Student's *t*-test. For each comparison and its corresponding *p*-value, a square in the phenotypic fingerprint is assigned a color according the magnitude of the value used to make the comparison. If the *p*-value arising from the compound-control comparison *t*-test is greater than 0.05, the square is colored green. Thus, all nongreen squares represent compound effects which are statistically significant at *p* = 0.05. If the compound reduced the value of a given readout (e.g., live cell number) relative to control at a given time-point, the square is colored blue at that time-point. If the compound increased the value at a given time-point relative to control, then the square is colored red. Time-points at which there was insufficient data for a valid *t*-test comparison are colored black. The intensity of red or blue indicates the magnitude of the distance of each value from the control value. (*See* Color Plate 5 following p. 302.)

For phenotypic assays, mouse fibroblast-derived cell line NR6 and human mammary epithelial cell line HB4a were stably transfected with target candidate cDNAs expressing bcmp84, NSE2, and NAT1 or empty plasmid vector. Cells were incubated in culture medium containing PI in addition to data at once, cell- and compound-specific trends can be readily discerned. Observations can be used to make decisions regarding candidate targets that match the desirable phenotypic fingerprints (e.g., high tissue specificity) of known and effective targets, on one hand, or those that show phenotypic profiles similar to undesirable target candidates. Phenotypic fingerprints can also be used to design therapeutics with a view toward pursuing or avoiding effective or failed drugs, respectively.

## 4.4. Prioritizing Targets Using Phenotypic Fingerprints

Although various phenotypic readouts were performed concurrently in these assays, discussion here will focus on cell proliferation and death as measured by "Live Cell Number" and "%PI-Positive Cells." The greatest changes in the transformed phenotype (i.e., increased growth rates and ability to resist apoptosis) were induced by NSE2 as shown by the red (greater than control) squares at the two highest serum conditions in both NR6 and HB4a cells. NAT-1 showed more consistent resistance to etoposide when compared with NSE2 by combining data from both cell lines and treatment conditions; that is, NAT1 increased live cell number in HB4a cells in addition to reduced PI uptake in NR6 cells. These data supported a decision to focus on NSE2 and NAT-1 as reported by Craggs et al. *(21)* and Adam et al. *(22)*. Ultimately, different screening mechanisms are likely to be required for these two proteins. NSE2 is a protein of unknown function and, at present, can only be screened by affinity ligand selection as offered by companies such as Neogenesis (Cambridge, MA). NAT-1 is an enzyme with known function and assay systems, allowing for the development of conventional HTS methods. This situation highlights an additional benefit to automated phenotypic screening. Because the targets have been selected for screening based on the disease-relevant phenotypes, the same cellular models and assays can be used to test candidate drugs for reversion to a nononcogenic phenotype.

## 5. OVERVIEW

With or without image-based technology, the value of cellular phenotypic assays is gaining recognition, giving rise to the coining of a new term: "phenomics" *(23)*. Companies such as Rigel Pharmaceuticals (San Francisco, CA), Galapagos Genomics (Mechelen, Belgium), and Xantos (Martinsried, Germany) use functional cellular assays at the primary screening stage of their discovery processes. These companies screen for function by assaying cellular phenotype following exogenous addition of target candidate genes at relatively high efficiencies. Rigel Pharmaceuticals has reported a series of functionally validated novel drug targets *(24–26)*. Whereas Rigel makes use of the high efficiency

---

**Fig. 5.** *(Continued)* a range of fetal bovine serum (FBS) concentrations (0.5%, 1%, 2.5%, and 10%; **A**) or various doses of etoposide (0.01, 10, 30, and 100 µ*M*; **B**). Visible and fluorescent red images were taken every 30 min for 5 d. *t*-Test comparisons were made at 6-h intervals using 10% FBS or dimethyl sulfoxide (DMSO) vehicle controls in (**A**) and (**B**), respectively. Statistical comparisons are depicted in panels with dimensions of time (top to bottom) and treatment dose (left to right). Live Cell Number is the number of PI-negative cells per image. %PI -Positive Cells is the proportion of cells in an image incorporating PI as an indicator of cell death. The Single Cell Fraction is the percentage of live cells in an image with no contact with any other cells. The area (square pixels) and elongation (dimensionless ratio of length to breadth) of cells is calculated for individual live cells only.

offered by flow cytometric phenotypic assays, the image-based assays of Automated Cell offer a range of phenotypic readouts that encompass both suspended and adherent cellular models of disease. The wealth of information to be had from image-based observation of cellular behavior has led to an increase in the number of companies offering platform technologies for use within established drug discovery programs. Image-based cellular assay systems include those offered by Cellomics (Pittsburgh, PA), Universal Imaging (Sunnyvale, CA) and Perkin-Elmer (Boston, MA), among others. Image-based platform technologies such as these promise an increase in the quality and quantity of validated targets available for drug discovery programs. This promise is currently being fulfilled as Automated Cell Inc. combines the value and predictive relevance of cellular phenotypic readouts with the efficiency of image-based assays.

# REFERENCES

1. Li J, Kleeff J, Guo J, et al. Effects of STI571 (gleevec) on pancreatic cancer cell growth. Mol Cancer 2003; 2:32.
2. Devitt A, Pierce S, Oldreive C, Shingler WH, Gregory CD. CD14-dependent clearance of apoptotic cells by human macrophages: the role of phosphatidylserine. Cell Death Differ 2003; 10:371–382.
3. Lockshin RA, Zakeri Z. Caspase-independent cell deaths. Curr Opin Cell Biol 2002; 14:727–733.
4. Jaattela M, Tschopp J. Caspase-independent cell death in T lymphocytes. Nature Immunol 2003; 4: 416–423.
5. Watanabe M, Hitomi M, van der Wee K, et al. The pros and cons of apoptosis assays for use in the study of cells, tissues, and organs. Microsc Microanal 2002; 8:375–391.
6. Paterson H, Reeves B, Brown R, et al. Activated N-ras controls the transformed phenotype of HT1080 human fibrosarcoma cells. Cell 1987; 51:803–812.
7. Kato-Stankiewicz J, Hakimi I, Zhi G, et al. Inhibitors of Ras/Raf-1 interaction identified by two-hybrid screening revert Ras-dependent transformation phenotypes in human cancer cells. Proc Natl Acad Sci USA 2002; 99:14,398–14,403.
8. Plattner R, Gupta S, Khosravi-Far R, et al. Differential contribution of the ERK and JNK mitogen-activated protein kinase cascades to Ras transformation of HT1080 fibrosarcoma and DLD-1 colon carcinoma cells. Oncogene 1999; 18:1807–1817.
9. Gupta S, Plattner R, Der CJ, Stanbridge EJ. Dissection of Ras-dependent signaling pathways controlling aggressive tumor growth of human fibrosarcoma cells: evidence for a potential novel pathway. Mol Cell Biol 2000; 20:9294–9306.
10. Takeoka M, Ehara T, Sagara J, Hashimoto S, Taniguchi S. Calponin h1 induced a flattened morphology and suppressed the growth of human fibrosarcoma HT1080 cells. Eur J Cancer 2002; 38:436–442.
11. Plattner R, Anderson MJ, Sato KY, Fasching CL, Der CJ, Stanbridge EJ. Loss of oncogenic ras expression does not correlate with loss of tumorigenicity in human cells. Proc Natl Acad Sci USA 1996; 93: 6665–6670.
12. Kohno M, Hasegawa H, Miyake M, Yamamoto T, Fujita S. CD151 enhances cell motility and metastasis of cancer cells in the presence of focal adhesion kinase. Int J Cancer 2002; 97:336–343.
13. Quaranta V, Giannelli G. Cancer invasion: watch your neighbourhood! Tumori 2003; 89:343–348.
14. Giese A, Bjerkvig R, Berens ME, Westphal M. Cost of migration: invasion of malignant gliomas and implications for treatment. J Clin Oncol 2003; 21:1624–1636.
15. Salerno M, Ouatas T, Palmieri D, Steeg PS. Inhibition of signal transduction by the nm23 metastasis suppressor: possible mechanisms. Clin Exp Metastasis 2003; 20:3–10.
16. Quaranta V. Motility cues in the tumor microenvironment. Differentiation 2002; 70:590–598.
17. Laug WE, Cao XR, Yu YB, Shimada H, Kruithof EK. Inhibition of invasion of HT1080 sarcoma cells expressing recombinant plasminogen activator inhibitor 2. Cancer Res 1993; 53:6051–6057.
18. Nakajima M, Katayama K, Tamechika I, et al. WF-536 inhibits metastatic invasion by enhancing the host cell barrier and inhibiting tumour cell motiltiy. Clin Exp Pharmacol Physiol 2003; 30:457–463.
19. Adam PJ, Boyd R, Tyson KL, et al. Comprehensive proteomic analysis of breast cancer cell membranes reveals unique proteins with potential roles in clinical cancer. J Biol Chem 2003; 278:6482–6489.
20. Hanahan D, Weinberg RA. The hallmarks of cancer. Cell 2000; 100:57–70.

21. Craggs G, Berry J, Tyson KL, et al. NSE2, a protein up-regulated in breast cancer, exhibits multiple oncogenic properties. Appl Genomics Proteomics 2003; 2:101–111.

22. Adam PJ, Berry J, Loader JA, et al. Arylamine *N*-acetyltransferase-1 is highly expressed in breast cancers and conveys enhanced growth and resistance to etoposide in vitro. Mol Cancer Res 2003; 1:826–835.

23. Gerlai R. Phenomics: fiction or the future? Trends Neurosci 2002; 25:506–509.

24. Hitoshi Y, Gururaja T, Pearsall DM, et al. Cellular localization and antiproliferative effect of peptides discovered from a functional screen of a retrovirally delivered random peptide library. Chem Biol 2003; 10:975–987.

25. Chu P, Pardo J, Zhao H, et al. Systematic identification of regulatory proteins critical for T-cell activation. J Biol 2003; 2:21.

26. Gururaja TL, Li W, Payan DG, Anderson DC. Utility of peptide-protein affinity complexes in proteomics: identification of interaction partners of a tumor suppressor peptide. J Pept Res 2003; 61:163–176.

# 14 Targeting Inducible Chemotherapy Resistance Mechanisms in Colon Cancer

*David Ljungman, MD*
*and James C. Cusack, Jr., MD*

## CONTENTS

## SUMMARY

Resistance toward chemotherapy remains one of the principle obstacles to the effective treatment of malignancies. As our knowledge of mechanisms involved in cancer biology expands, new molecular targets emerge. This chapter aims to overview the major resistance mechanisms, in order to identify potential targets appropriate for developmental therapeutics. An emphasis on the role of transcription factor NF-κB in colorectal cancer is presented as an example of how targeted therapies may advance from the bench to the bedside.

**Key Words:** Chemotherapy resistance; apoptosis; transcription factors; NF-κB; proteasome inhibition; combination chemotherapy.

## 1. INTRODUCTION

The majority of solid tumor malignancies including colon cancer will inevitably exhibit resistance to chemotherapy and/or radiation therapy (1–4). In some cases, tumors might exhibit resistance to therapy from the outset of treatment. Examples of this type

From: *Cancer Drug Discovery and Development: The Oncogenomics Handbook*
Edited by: W. J. LaRochelle and R. A. Shimkets © Humana Press Inc., Totowa, NJ

of *intrinsic* drug resistance include the overexpression of proteins that export chemotherapy agents from tumor cells *(4)* and genetic-based errors that result in loss of tumor suppressor gene function *(1–3)*. Resistance to drug therapy might also arise as a result of exposure to the chemotherapy agents. The most commonly depicted example of this form of *acquired* resistance is the emergence of drug-resistant subclones of cancer cells that result from the selection pressures of drug treatment. However, another form of *inducible* resistance has recently been described: In this form of *transient* chemotherapy resistance, mechanisms involved in drug resistance are induced directly as a response to chemotherapy exposure. One well-described mechanism of *transient* chemotherapy resistance is mediated by the activation of the transcription factor NF-κB. In this case, the cellular response to drug exposure leads to the expression of a variety of genes involved in the suppression of the apoptotic response to treatment, thereby rescuing the cells from cell death *(5–8)*. Once drug exposure is terminated, levels of activated (nuclear) NF-κB return to baseline, and the expression of the protective antiapoptotic genes subsides. As many chemotherapy agents such as irinotecan and oxaliplatin function by actually inducing apoptosis *(1–3,9)*, the ability of cancer cells to be rescued from apoptosis via the activation of NF-κB represents a potentially challenging obstacle to effective treatment. An in-depth understanding of the mechanisms responsible for NF-κB activation in response to chemotherapy has yielded the development of targeted molecular therapies that suppress the activation of this transcription factor. The use of NF-κB inhibitors in combination with cytotoxic chemotherapy agents has resulted in dramatic augmentation of chemotherapy response in preclinical animal models *(6,8)* and is currently undergoing further evaluation in clinical trials.

In this chapter, we will discuss how targeting chemotherapy resistance mechanisms might promote the efficacy of some anticancer therapies. To facilitate this discussion, we will distinguish *inducible* chemotherapy resistance from the more commonly described forms of *intrinsic* and *acquired* mechanisms of resistance, and we will regard apoptosis as the desired therapeutic end point of cancer treatment. Our discussion will focus particular attention on the mechanisms involving NF-κB-mediated chemotherapy resistance.

## 2. CHEMOTHERAPY RESISTANCE TAKES ON MANY FORMS

Until recently, the mainstay of treatment for metastatic colorectal cancer has been fluorouracil-based therapy with no demonstrable survival benefit *(10)*. The recent emergence of more effective poly-chemotherapy regimens for colon cancer has resulted from combining conventional 5-fluorouracil (5-FU)-based therapy with relatively new compounds that exert their effects through unrelated mechanisms of action. This improvement in treatment response is evidenced by the results from phase III clinical trials that combine 5-FU and leucovorin with the cytotoxic agents irinotecan *(11,12)* or oxaliplatin *(13,14)*. These advances have correlated with improvements in survival of patients with metastatic colorectal cancer from less than 12 mo *(15)* up to between 17 and 22 mo *(16)*. Further progress in improved treatment response has resulted by combining these poly-chemotherapy regimens with targeted therapeutics such as epidermal growth factor (EGF) inhibitors (cetuximab) or vascular endothelial growth factor (VEGF) inhibitors (bevacizumab) *(16)*. Despite these advances, failure to respond to these agents at some time-point during the treatment course results in progression of disease and prompts the call for new drugs and more effective treatment strategies. The mechanisms of resistance to these new therapies are multiple and frequently involve a variety of cellular processes that affect drug transport, drug metabolism, and changes in genes regulating cell cycle or DNA repair. Identification and targeting of the mechanisms responsible for drug resistance provides opportunities to extend effective treatment response and might facilitate the incorporation of existing drugs into poly-chemotherapy regimens.

## 2.1. Alterations in Drug Transport and Metabolism

One common type of resistance involves actively pumping out cytotoxic compounds from cancer cells. Notable substrates for this mechanism include anthracyclines, vinca alkaloids, and taxanes. Increased drug efflux might be mediated by the ATP-binding cassette (ABC) transporter proteins including P-glycoprotein (Pgp), multidrug resistance (MDR) protein (MRP-1), and breast cancer resistance protein (BCRP) (17). MDR1 has been found to be overexpressed in many resistant cancer cells (18), whereas high levels of Pgp expression in chemotherapy naïve cancer cells has been found to negatively impact patient survival (19). Expression of BCRP leads to a reduction in the intracellular accumulation of adriamycin/doxorubicin and CPT-11 (20,21). Interestingly, expression of BCRP is actually induced by CPT-11 exposure (20). Circumvention of BCRP-mediated resistance to camptothecins in vitro has been demonstrated using nonsubstrate drugs or the BCRP inhibitor GF120918 (22). MDR 1 is only one of many genes that might be upregulated in drug-resistant colorectal cancer. Resistance in colon cancer has also been associated with overexpression of adenine phosphoribosyltransferase and the breast cancer-specific gene 1 (BCSG 1) (23).

Although the overexpression of some proteins increases drug transport out of the cancer cells, overexpression of proteins involved in drug metabolism might increase the degradation of chemotherapy agents. For example, the increased expression of thymidylate synthase (TS) and the decreased expression of folylpolyglutamate synthetase have been linked to 5-FU resistance (24). Many of these mechanisms of resistance have provided new targets for drug development. For example, the potent TS inhibitor ZD9331 is currently under evaluation in phase II clinical studies in a range of solid tumors, including colorectal and ovarian carcinomas (25). Another new compound, CB300638, has been evaluated in murine xenograft models and demonstrated higher tumor specificity than ZD9331 (26).

Resistance resulting from increased drug metabolism might also involve detoxification systems such as the glutation-S-transferase (GST) enzyme system. It has recently been proposed that GSTs may serve two distinct roles in the development of drug resistance. This dual effect involves upregulation and thereby increased conjugation of the cytotoxic substance as the first step in elimination by the mercapturic acid pathway, and, at the same time, inhibition of the mitogen-activated protein (MAP) kinase pathway (27). The establishment of this link between GSTs and the MAP kinase pathway provides a rationale as to why, in many cases, the drugs used to select for resistance are neither subject to conjugation with GSH nor substrates for GSTs. Because specific GST isozymes are overexpressed in a wide variety of tumors, GSTs have emerged as a promising therapeutic target (27). The cytochrome P450 family of drug metabolism enzymes is another important metabolic factor that might alter drug sensitivity. In particular, the CYP3A subfamily plays a role in the metabolism of epipodophyllotoxins, ifosfamide, tamoxifen, paclitaxel, and vinca alkaloids. Subtle alterations in these enzymes could account for interindividual variations affecting toxicity and tumor response (28).

## 2.2. Genetic Basis
## of Chemotherapy Resistance in Colorectal Cancer

In addition to the overexpression of genes involved in drug metabolism and transport, resistance to therapy might also result from the lack of expression of genes involved in cell cycle and stress response mechanisms. One such example involves the tumor suppressor gene *TP53*—one of the most frequently mutated genes in human cancers. The wild-type protein encoded by *TP53* has been found to be mutated or underexpressed in more than half of human tumors analyzed so far. Following genotoxic injury p53 typically functions to induce cell cycle arrest to repair DNA damage or, under certain conditions, induce apoptosis (through the G1–G2 DNA-damage checkpoint). When mutated, the lack of functional p53 might contribute to drug resistance by making the cell unable to undergo apoptosis in response to DNA damage. Some authors have even speculated that p53 might actually play a dual role after exposure to cytotoxic drug treatment, activating either mechanisms that lead to apoptosis or launching processes that direct DNA repair and survival of the cell *(29)*.

There are a few examples of successful targeting of defective tumor suppressor gene function in colorectal cancer. One is the transfer of the wild-type p53 into cancer cells, with mutated p53 leading to enhanced chemosensitivity and increased apoptosis *(30–33)*; Other studies have examined whether the activity of certain p53 mutants can be restored by second-site suppressor mutations that introduce an additional DNA contact and thereby correct the local structural distortion or increase the stability of the core domain structure *(34)*. Small molecules have been developed to stabilize the wild-type and mutant p53 core domain, presumably by binding specifically to the native protein. Correction of mutant folding restores p53 function to cancer cells and inhibits tumor growth in mice *(34)*. In one such example, a drug prototype CP-31398 achieves a 75% suppression of growth in colorectal carcinoma xenograft models *(35,36)*. The compound is thought to increase the thermostability of p53 through its expected binding in a bivalent manner to hydrophobic and acidic sites. However, despite these promising early results cellular concentrations are not maintained high enough for practical treatment and further investigation is warranted.

## 3. ALTERED REGULATION OF APOPTOSIS PROVIDES
## POTENTIAL MECHANISM FOR CHEMOTHERAPY RESISTANCE

There are two principal modes of action by which chemotherapy agents affect the cell: either direct blockage of a vital cellular process or induction of programmed cell death (apoptosis) *(37)*. Recently, it has also been shown that some chemotherapy agents induce a permanent cell cycle arrest that resembles the replicative senescence seen in the aging of normal cells; this represents a more cytostatic rather than tumoricidal approach *(38–40)*. It is not clear to what extent the three are, separately or together, responsible for the cytotoxicity effects of chemotherapy; however, increasing data suggest that apoptosis is one of the principle tumoricidal mechanisms of response *(41–44)*. It follows that interference with the apoptotic response to drug therapy provides a viable defense against the damaging effects of cancer therapies *(45,46)*. As a result, over the past decade, increasing attention has focused on the development of new therapeutic targets that either singly or in conjunction with existing treatments promote apoptosis. To better understand the variety of mechanisms by which apoptosis can be positively or negatively regulated in cancer cells, we will review some of the key features of the apoptotic response to therapy.

### 3.1. Role of Apoptosis in Chemotherapy Response and Resistance

Apoptosis plays an important role in the equilibrium of normal tissue homeostasis. This equilibrium is often disturbed in cancer cells through inactivation or inhibition of the apoptotic response pathways and an upregulation of mitotic activity. Suppression of apoptosis via a variety of mechanisms represents a means by which cancer cells might be rescued from the killing effects of chemotherapy. In the process of apoptosis, the fate of cells is dependent on the intracellular response involving sensors and an extensive network of transmitters regulated by positive and negative factors. Central to this response is the role of a series of apoptotic executors called cysteine-aspartyl-specific proteases (caspases) *(47)*. Two principle pathways are involved in apoptosis: the *extrinsic or death receptor-mediated pathway* and the *intrinsic or mitochondrial pathway (see* Fig. 1). The "extrinsic" pathway functions via activation of membrane-linked death receptors and is initiated by the binding of cytokines such as FasL, TRAIL, and tumor necrosis factor (TNF-$\alpha$) *(48)*. A multimeric death-inducing signaling complex (DISC) is formed by the combination of FADD and procaspase-8/10. Caspase-8 or caspase-10 is subsequently activated through a process of autoproteolysis and, in turn, cleaves and activates effector caspase-3, caspase-6 or caspase-7 through induction of the proteolytic cascade *(48,49)*. The "intrinsic" mitochondrial pathway can be activated by oncogenes, hypoxia, cell–cell detachment (anoikis), or the withdrawal of growth factors. As a response to stimuli, the mitochondrial membrane potential ($\Delta\psi$) is altered, resulting in the release of cytochrome-c (cyt c) from the mitochondria *(50)* to the cytoplasm, where it binds the apoptotic activator 1 (Apaf-1) to form the apoptosome *(51)*. The apoptosome binds and activates caspase-9, which is responsible for the initiation of the proteolytic cascade.

### 3.2. Regulation of Apoptosis: the Bcl-2 and IAP Protein Families

The Bcl-2 family of proteins regulates the mitochondrial pathway of apoptosis and consists of antiapoptotic members (Bcl-2, Bcl-$X_L$, and Boo) and pro-apoptotic members (Bid, Bad, Bax, Bag, Bak, Bok, and others). These proteins contribute to the regulation of the homeostatic balance, wherein the pro-apoptotic members facilitate the release of factors such as cyt c, AIF (apoptosis-inducing factor), endonuclease G, and Smac/DIABLO from the mitochondria. The antiapoptotic members of the Bcl-2 family counteract this process by binding and inhibiting the activity of the pro-apoptotic family members following a survival stimulus trigger *(52)*. One example of a pro-apoptotic family member is Bid, which is activated by caspase-8 and works as a link between the extrinsic and the intrinsic pathways in certain cells. This happens when the apoptotic stimulus is not enough to induce a death receptor-mediated cell death response *(53,54)*. In other cells, however, no involvement of the mitochondrial pathway is needed and the apoptotic process is mainly death receptor mediated. Once the apoptotic factors are released by the mitochondria, they exert downstream effects to achieve apoptosis *(55)*. As an example, Smac/DIABLO binds members of the inhibition of apoptosis proteins (IAP) family such as IAP-1 and IAP-2, XIAP, ML-IAP, Livin, Survivin, and others *(56,57)*. Uninhibited, these are capable of blocking apoptosis at the level of activated caspases.

### 3.3. Therapeutic Approaches Involving Regulatory Proteins of Apoptosis

Several interesting therapeutic approaches that target antiapoptotic regulators are noteworthy. The first is the antiapoptotic factor Bcl-2 that has been administered as an antisense

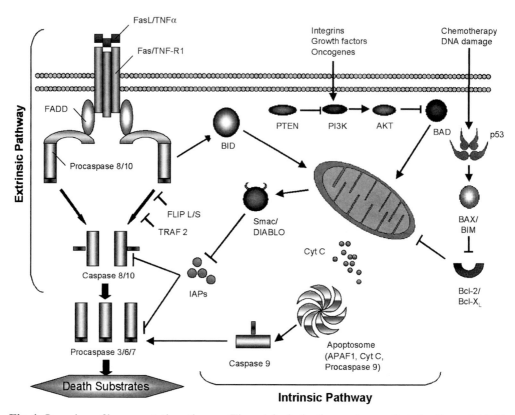

**Fig. 1.** Overview of key apoptotic pathways. The extrinsic death receptor-mediated pathway (at left) is activated by ligand–receptor interaction. Examples known to induce apoptosis are the Fas-ligand (FasL) binding the membrane-bound Fas receptor or the tumor necrosis factor-α (TNF-α) binding a TNF receptor (i.e., TNF-R1). A death-inducing signaling complex (DISC) is formed on the cytoplasmic side of the membrane consisting of the intracellular end of the receptor called the "death domain," a series of adaptor proteins (i.e., Fas [TNFRSF6]-associated via death domain [FADD]) and the inactive precursor of a cysteine-aspartyl-protease (caspase) procaspase-8 or -10. This triggers a proteolytic cascade involving conversion of procaspase-3, -6, or -7 into active caspases. These effector caspases act on various death substrates to induce apoptosis. In some cells, the stimulus is too weak to result in a cascade this way and the pro-apoptotic protein Bid communicate the signal to the mitochondria, which as a response to stress (i.e., Bid, oncogenes, hypoxia, growth factor deprivation, cell–cell detachment or chemotherapy) releases apoptotic factors such as cytochrome-$c$ (cyt c) and Smac/DIABLO. Cyt c merges with the apoptotic activator 1 (APAF1) and procaspase-9 to form an apoptosome that activates caspase-9 and downstream effector caspase-3, -6, and -7. Smac/DIABLO inhibits inhibitors of apoptosis proteins (IAPs). The tumor suppressor p53 can upregulate expression of Bax or Bim in response to stress and inhibit Bcl-2 or Bcl-XL inhibition of the mitochondria and thereby promote apoptosis. Illustrating the complex homeostasis, activation of the transcription factor pathway PTEN/PI3K/AKT inhibits the proapoptotic Bad protein in a survival response to multiple mitogens, thereby inhibiting mitochondria-mediated apoptosis.

infusion. In a human melanoma xenograft model using SCID mice, a marked reduction in tumor growth was noted following treatment with antisense Bcl-2 *(58)*. A phase I clinical trial on non-Hodgkin's lymphoma (NHL) has similarly demonstrated potential for antitumor activity using this method *(59)*. In this particular study, 21 patients with

Bcl-2-positive relapsed NHL were treated through subcutaneous infusion with G3139, an 18-mer oligonucleotide complementary to the first 6 codons of the Bcl-2 reading frame. Response assessed by computerized tomography and using standard response criteria demonstrated one complete response, two minor responses, nine cases of stable disease, and nine cases of progressive disease. Another clinical trial using Bcl-2 antisense therapy showed promising outcome on malignant melanoma *(60)*. Bcl-XL, which belongs to the same family of proteins, has also been downregulated in vitro in A549 and HeLa cells using an antisense approach that induced higher levels of apoptosis in cells treated with ultraviolet radiation and cisplatinum *(61)*. This was based on the knowledge that alternate splicing of the Bcl-X pre-mRNA gives rise to two transcripts, coding for either a long (Bcl-XL) or a short (Bcl-XS) form of the protein. Because Bcl-XL is antiapoptotic and Bcl-XS is proapoptotic and functions by antagonizing antiapoptotic proteins like Bcl-XL, a shift toward Bcl-XS expression should increase sensitivity and facilitate apoptosis. This objective was achieved by inhibiting the 5' splice site in exon II of the Bcl-XL RNA, thereby redirecting the splicing machinery to the 5' Bcl-XS splice site.

The enhancement of apoptosis through the manipulation of members of the IAP family has also been demonstrated. For example, Grossman et al. demonstrated that expression of a dominant negative mutant of surviving-triggered apoptosis in several human melanoma cell lines inhibited tumor growth in xenografts and enhanced sensitivity to cisplatin in vitro *(62)*. This study supports the manipulation of the antiapoptotic pathway maintained by survivin as a potentially useful therapeutic intervention. A new and attractive tool is the RNAi *(63,64)* where genes can be targeted with perfectly matching synthetic 21-mer oligonucleotide RNA fragments resulting in silencing of the expression of the targeted genes. Silencing of the *livin* gene through this technique strongly increased apoptotic rate in HeLa cervical carcinoma cells in response to doxorubicin, ultraviolet (UV) irradiation, and TNF-α *(65)*. Indirect targeting of the IAP family and induction of apoptosis has also been accomplished through administration of Smac/DIABLO peptides in T-cells potentiating the antimicrotubule agent epothilone *(66)*. Similarly, neuroblastoma xenografts could be successfully sensitized to death receptor ligation or cytotoxic drugs by the addition of Smac/DIABLO agonists and completely eliminated when combined with Apo2L/TRAIL *(67)*. Furthermore, these agonists were able to enhance apoptosis of MCF-7 and other breast carcinoma cell lines to the chemotherapeutic drugs etoposide, paclitaxel, camptotecin, and doxorubicin by inhibitory binding to XIAP and cIAP1 *in situ (68)*.

## 4. TARGETING TRANSCRIPTION FACTORS TO ENHANCE CHEMOTHERAPY SENSITIVITY

Highly attractive targets for drug design are the transcription factors, which are upregulated in a large variety of human cancers. In addition, there are only a few transcription factors reported (compared to the number of oncogenes, for example) *(69)*. The potential advantages of targeting a transcription factor in cancer cells are as follows: (1) A variety of dysregulated signal transduction pathways might be effected by targeting a single transcription factor and (2) targeted therapy effective in one form of malignancy might be equally effective in many types of malignancy. There are three major groups of transcription factors: the steroid receptors, the resident nuclear proteins, and the latent cytoplasmic factors *(70)*. Exemplified in the steroid receptor group, one finds the estrogen receptors in breast cancer and the androgen receptors in prostate cancer. Drugs targeting these steroid receptors such as tamoxifen, bicalutamide, and glucocorticoids have been explored in clinical trials for many years *(71–73)*. Perhaps, the most well known of the resident proteins is c-JUN. As is characteristic of this group, c-JUN is activated by a serine kinase cascade to induce transcription. The last group, the latent cytoplasmic factors, is usually activated by receptor–ligand interactions at the cell surface *(70)*. This latter group represents an area of promising drug development and has been the field of interest for our laboratory. Our subsequent discussion will focus on the third group of transcription factors (the latent cytoplasmic factors) and will include a discussion of the STATs pathway, the AKT signaling pathway, the β-catenin-signaling pathway, and the NF-κB activation pathway.

### 4.1. The Signal Transducers and Activators of Transcription Pathway

The signal transducers and activators of transcription (STATs) transcription factors are positioned latently in the cytoplasm and activated by a variety of receptors *(74,75)*. To activate the transcription of chromosomal genes, the STATs (and other transcription factors) need to recruit the coactivators CREB-binding protein (CBP) and p300 or other histone acetyl-transferases (HATs) through the carboxy-terminal STAT domain *(75)*. There are many different negative regulators for STATs, including SOCS (suppressors of cytokine signaling) and at least two members of the PIAS protein family that decrease STAT transcription in vivo and block DNA binding in vitro *(76,77)*. Failure in this regulation might be one reason for uninhibited transcription. Persistently activated STATs have been reported in many tumor models; one example is STAT5 in leukemia and lymphomas *(78)*. In one type of lymphoma, STAT5 is chromosomally translocated; treatment of these cells with dominant-negative STAT results in apoptosis *(79,80)*. STAT3 has been reported to be persistently activated in most head and neck cancers as a result of a dysregulation of the EGF pathway *(81)*. In one series, all multiple myeloma specimens tested had persistently activated STAT3, and in some cases, this was associated with an interleukin (IL)-6 overproduction *(78,82)*. In these cases, introduction of dominant-negative STAT also resulted in induction of apoptosis *(78)*. Possible molecular targets for inhibition of persistently active STAT3 include homodimer–homodimer interaction (tetramer formation) on DNA and interactions between STAT3 and c-JUN, CBP/p300, or the glucocorticoid receptor. All of these are required for maximal transcriptional activation by STAT3 *(75)*.

### 4.2. The AKT Signaling Pathway

Growth factors, oncogenic Ras, and integrins could activate this survival pathway. Once activated, the phosphatidylinositol-3 kinase (PI3K) facilitates the conversion of $PIP_2$ to $PIP_3$, which then activates the transcription factor AKT. This has been shown to promote transcription of antiapoptotic Bcl-XL and inactivate Bad, caspase-9 and FKHRL1 (an inducer of many proapoptotic factors) *(83)*. A tumor suppressor, phosphatase and tensin homolog (PTEN), is regulatory and counteracts AKT by phosphorylating $PIP_3$. AKT is constitutively activated in a wide range of tumors such as prostate, liver, lung, ovary, and breast carcinomas *(84)*. Also, this pathway has been observed to cause resistance to chemotherapy; one example is inhibition of cisplatin-induced apoptosis in ovarian carcinoma through phosphorylation of the proapoptotic Bad. Treatment with either the AKT inhibitor wortmannin or exogenous expression of a dominant-negative AKT sensitized the cells to cisplatin *(85)*. Another successful approach in AKT inhibition is the compound genistein, which potentiates TRAIL-induced apoptosis in breast cancer cells *(86)*. Yet another compound, rapamycin, targets mTOR kinase that is activated by AKT and has demonstrated activity in cancers with mutations in PTEN, such as glioblastoma, prostate, and breast carcinomas *(87,88)*.

### 4.3. The β-Catenin Pathway

WNT are small proteins that are most effective as inducers of signaling when they reside in the extracellular matrix *(89,90)*. They act through the β-catenin, or *canonical*, pathway or, alternatively, through an increase in intracellular $Ca^{2+}$ *(91)*. WNT can act as a ligand binding to a seven-transmembrane receptor of the Frizzled protein family. This results in the activation of an intracellular signaling cascade that results in inhibition of the serine kinase GSK3β that is responsible for the phosphorylation of both the tumor suppressor adenomatous polyposis coli (APC) and any excess β-catenin *(69)*. β-Catenins are cytoplasmic structural proteins bound to either E-cadherins or are included in protein complexes with the tumor suppressor APC *(90,92)*. The inhibited GSK3β leaves β-catenins to enter the nucleus to bind DNA-binding proteins like T-cell factors/lymphocyte-enhancer factors (TCFs/LEFs) that lack a transcription activation domain (TAD) *(89)*. Together, they activate transcription *(93)*. In human cancers, the most common reason for β-catenin overactivity is a mutation or deletion of APC in colonic epithelium *(90,94)*. Overexpression and/or mutation in β-catenin has also been reported in hepatocellular carcinoma *(92)*, and deranged β-catenin metabolism has been found in hepatoblastoma, a nonmalignant brain tumor, and skin growths called desmoids *(94)*. A possible cancer therapeutic target is the interaction between β-catenin and TCF/LEF *(69)*.

### 4.4. NF-κB Activation Pathway

The transcription factor nuclear factor-κB (NF-κB) was the first latent cytoplasmic factor to be discovered and is really "at the crossroads of life and death" in its central role as a modulator of inflammation, angiogenesis, cell cycle regulation, differentiation, adhesion, migration, and survival *(95)*. It is activated by the same stimuli that induce apoptosis, such as ionizing radiation, chemotherapy, and TNF-α, and, in most cases, counteracts this apoptosis through an inhibitory cell survival response (see Fig. 2) *(96–101)*. There is some evidence that NF-κB plays a proapoptotic role in certain scenarios—for instance, in p53-mediated apoptosis *(102)*. However, most data support the antiapoptotic role of NF-κB, particularly in the context of chemotherapy exposure *(6–8,103)*. NF-κB is classically a heterodimer consisting of p65 and p50, but another three, less studied, family members have been identified (c-Rel, Rel B, and p52). When inactive p65 is bound in the cytoplasm by an inhibitor of κB (IκB), stimuli trigger the IKK complex, which consists of the catalytic subunits IKKα and IKKβ and the regulatory IKKγ protein, to phosphorylate IκB, which is thereby ubiquitinated and degraded by the 26S proteasome *(104,105)*. p65 is released during this proteolysis and is bound by p50, which is cleaved from a p100 primary translation product. The free and activated NF-κB translocates to the nucleus, where it binds κB promoter motifs and activates transcription of antiapoptotic genes such as those encoding Bcl-$X_L$, FLICE-inhibitory protein (c-FLIP), TNF receptor-associated protein (TRAF-1 and TRAF-2) and IAPs *(106)*. The transcription of IκB itself is regulated by NF-κB and the initiation of this determines the duration of the active NF-κB cycle *(107)*.

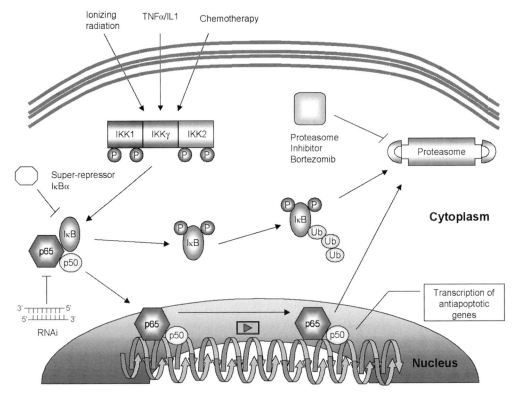

**Fig. 2.** NF-κB activation and therapeutic interventions. As a response to stressors like ionizing radiation, TNF-α or interleukin-1 (IL-1) and chemotherapy, the NF-κB survival pathway is activated. This generally involves phosphorylation of the IκB kinase complex (IKK), which contains the catalytic subunits IKKα and IKKβ and the regulatory IKKγ protein. This leads to downstream phosphorylation and ubiquitination of the inhibitor of κB (IκB). Ubiquitination targets IκBα for degradation by the 26S proteasome and release of the NF-κB heterodimer p65/p50. The activated NF-κB translocates to the nucleus and induces antiapoptotic gene transcription. Various therapeutic approaches such as administration of proteasome inhibitor bortezomib, superrepressor IκBα, or RNAi might interfere with this NF-κB activation and thereby promote the apoptotic response.

A protein called A20 that blocks further NF-κB activation by binding to the IL-1 or TNF-α receptor *(108)* is also regulated by NF-κB-induced transcription. TNF-α is a key cytokine in the regulation of apoptosis. Through its binding of TNF receptors, recruitment of TRAF-2 takes place, leading to NF-κB activation and transcription of FLIP that inhibits caspase-8 and thereby acts in an antiapoptotic manner *(109)*.

Nuclear factor κB might enhance cell survival in other ways other than inducing the transcription of antiapoptotic genes. The NF-κB transcription factor is known to promote cell cycle transition by a direct transcriptional upregulation of the cyclin D1 gene *(110)*. It has been speculated that this might possibly provide the cells with an uncontrolled replicative potential. Another example is the antagonistic role toward p53 that might result in increased genomic instability *(111)*. Furthermore, in a study of IKKα$^{-/-}$IKKβ$^{-/-}$ double knockout mice, IKKβ-mediated activation of NF-κB led to increased Mdm2 levels, destabilization of p53, and resistance to doxorubicin-induced apoptosis *(112)*. It has also been observed that increased expression of the proapoptotic Bcl-2 family member Bax occurs following expression of a dominant-negative inhibitor of NF-κB in breast, colorectal, and ovarian carcinoma, indicating that Bax suppression by NF-κB might contribute to cell survival *(113)*. Finally, NF-κB and IκB have been observed to localize to mitochondria and suppress mitochondrial gene expression. These observations have contributed to the evidence that supports the mitochondria as playing a central role in the apoptotic pathways *(114,115)*.

### 4.4.1. ACTIVATION OF NF-κB IN MALIGNANCIES

The genes encoding NF-κB or IκB are frequently amplified or translocated in human cancers *(116)*. Examples of NF-κB overexpression include a splice variant of *relA* that encodes the p65 subunit in non-small-cell lung carcinomas (NSCLC) *(117)*, the overexpression of *relA* in thyroid carcinoma *(118,119)*, and overexpression of *nfkb1* encoding the p50/p105 subunit in NSCLC *(120)*. Inactivating mutations in the inhibitor protein IκBα might also lead to dysregulated NF-κB activity *(121)*, as has been reported in Hodgkin's lymphoma. The increased activity of NF-κB has been shown in many types of soluble malignancys such as multiple myeloma. In myeloma, accumulation of B-cells results from a defect in the apoptotic pathway and is associated with constitutively activated NF-κB. In this setting, NF-κB is responsible for the expression of cytokines (IL-6 and VEGF), cell adhesion molecules (ICAM-1 and VCAM-1) and cell growth and survival factors (Bcl-2 and IAP family members) *(97,122)*. Inhibition of NF-κB in these cells results in apoptosis of the B-cells *(123)*. All of these factors have been shown to play key roles in cancer cell survival and proliferation. For example, IL-6 is a paracrine growth factor that stimulates DNA synthesis and cell proliferation in myeloma cells *(124,125)* and protects these cells from dexamethasone-induced apoptosis *(126)*. NF-κB activates expression of cell adhesion molecules that facilitates interaction with stromal cells in the bone marrow —another prosurvival stimulus contributing to multiple myeloma proliferation and chemotherapy resistance *(124,127)*. Thus, inhibition of NF-κB interferes with a multitude of survival mechanisms in myeloma cells. The importance of NF-κB activation as a survival factor has also been demonstrated in solid tumors. Downstream NF-κB targets like *c-myc*, cyclin D1, the antiapoptotic factor TRAF-2, the invasion-associated protein Mel-CAM, or the proangiogenic chemokine GRO are frequently upregulated in melanoma *(105)*. Pancreatic ductal adenocarcinoma is known to be highly refractory to treatment. In several chemotherapy-resistant cell lines, NF-κB has been found to be maximally activated *(128)*. Also in breast *(129–132)*, colon *(120,133)*, lung *(134)*, and ovarian *(120,135, 136)* cancer, constitutive NF-κB activity has been found.

### 4.4.2. NF-κB INHIBITION BY IκBα ENHANCES CHEMOTHERAPY SENSITIVITY

The activation of NF-κB in response to some chemotherapy agents results in protection against the cell-killing effects of the therapy (Fig. 3). Several strategies to inhibit this response of NF-κB have evolved in attempts to increase chemosensitivity in various tumor cell lines. When considering the development of antitumor agents, it is particularly attractive to target the cytoplasmic proteases or other upstream factors involved in the activation of NF-κB. Another possible approach is to interfere with nuclear NF-κB interactions directly. In our lab, we initially investigated inhibition of NF-κB using the adenovirus-

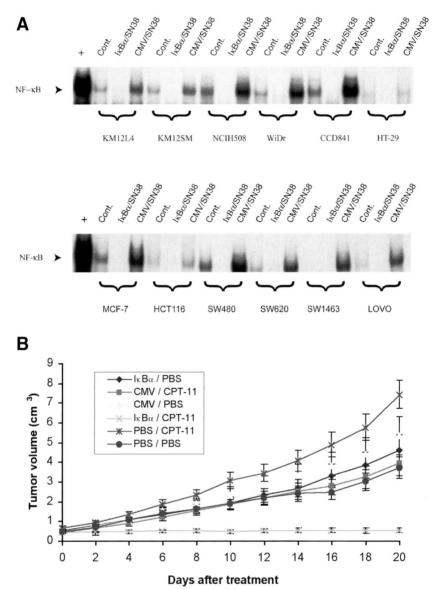

**Fig. 3. (A)** The EMSA was used to evaluate NF-κB activation induced by 1 μg/mL SN38 (active metabolite of irinotecan) in human colorectal and breast (MCF-7) cancer cell lines. Chemotherapy-induced activation of NF-κB was observed in 11 of 12 cancer cell lines tested, suggesting that NF-κB activation is induced by SN38 in most colorectal cancer cell lines. Positive control (+) was KM12L4 cells treated for 2 h with 10 ng/mL TNF-α (a potent activator of NF-κB). The figure is representative of the findings from two experiments. **(B)** Effect of NF-κB inhibition on human cancer cells treated with different concentrations of SN38. Cells were treated with adenovirus control vector (CMV) alone or with SN38 (CMV/SN38), adenovirus vector expressing the superrepressor IκBα alone (IκBα) or with SN38 (IκBα/Sn38), SN38 alone (SN38) or vehicle alone (Cont.) All virus infections were performed 24 h prior to drug treatment. Cell counts obtained at 96 h after drug treatment are reported as the mean of triplicate cultures; bars = SD. [Reprinted with permission from (A) ref. *136a*, copyright Nature Publishing Group and (B) *Cancer Research*, ref. *138*.]

mediated delivery of a modified (Ser 32 and 36) form of IκBα that resists degradation called superrepressor IκBα *(6,8)*. We demonstrated that the superrepressor IκBα sensitized chemoresistant tumors to treatment with SN38 (the active metabolite of the topoisomerase I inhibitor irinotecan) in fibrosarcoma and colorectal cancer xenograft models *(6)*. Similar results were reported by Duffey et al. in studies on head and neck squamous cell carcinoma (HNSCC), where transfection with IκBα showed a 70–90% reduction in cell viability. The cells were also grafted into SCID mice and tumor growth was significantly reduced compared to untreated cells *(137)*. Our studies provided the impetus to search for small-molecule inhibitors of NF-κB that would have the added advantage of systemic distribution requisite for the successful treatment of metastatic disease.

### 4.4.3. PROTEASOME INHIBITION AS SYSTEMIC ALTERNATIVE

One of the many effects of proteasome inhibition is the inhibition of NF-κB activation as a result of the failure of IκBα to be degraded (*see* Fig. 2). We found that using the proteasome inhibitor bortezomib (Velcade®, formerly PS-341) in combination with irinotecan in colorectal cancer cells potently enhanced the apoptotic response to chemotherapy and resulted in a strong tumoricidal response in murine xenografts (Fig. 4) *(138)*. Furthermore, we found that bortezomib or, alternatively, infection with an adenovirus encoding the superrepressor IκBα could reverse radiation-induced activation of NF-κB in colorectal cancer cells and increase apoptotic response in treated cells *(139)*. LeBlanc and colleagues recorded that a strong response to treatment with bortezomib was seen in RPMI 8226 myeloma xenografts with prolonged survival, tumor growth inhibition, and decreased tumor microvessel density. It was also noted that proteasome inhibition was greater in normal tissue than tumor, but the regimen was well tolerated, thus underscoring the heightened sensitivity of tumor cells to proteasome inhibition *(140–143)*. In a phase II clinical trial, it has been shown that bortezomib is active in patients with relapsed multiple myeloma that is refractory to conventional chemotherapy *(144)*. As a result, in May 2003, the Food and Drug Administration (FDA) approved bortezomib for treatment of multiple myeloma. Ongoing phase III clinical trials in patients with either relapsed or refractory multiple myeloma and phase II trials are currently underway for patients with metastatic colorectal cancer and advanced NSCLC.

Proteasome inhibition exerts its role in part by inhibition of induced NF-κB activation; however, other mechanisms should be acknowledged for contribution. When enhancing treatment response to irinotecan (CPT-11), the proteasome degradation of the topoisomerase 1–campthotecin complex is inhibited and, therefore, results in prolongation of the half-life of the active drug CPT-11 *(145,146)*. The proteasome also mediates the degradation of cell cycle regulators and apoptotic factors such as p53 *(147)*, p21 *(148)*, p27 *(149)*, Bcl-2 *(150)*, c-Myc *(151)*, and cyclins A, B, D, and E *(152–154)*. The proteasome degrades p53 after the ubiquitin ligase MDM2 has ubiquitylated the tetrameric p53 *(155)*. This process takes place unless p14$^{ARF}$ sequesters MDM2 in the situation of stress, such as oncogene activation. Proteasome inhibition therefore results in an increase in p53, as in FH109 lung fibroblasts, where it caused an arrest at the G1/S boundary *(156)*. However, bortezomib induces apoptosis also in p53$^{-/-}$ PC-3 prostate cancer cells *(157)* and, therefore, the p53 is not an obligate for the antiproliferative effect. In the pancreatic cancer cells, MIA-PaCa-2, the anti-apoptotic protein Bcl-2, is constitutively expressed, and when treated with bortezomib, this expression was eliminated and resulted in a significantly improved response to gemcitabine in both cell culture and mouse xenograft *(158)*.

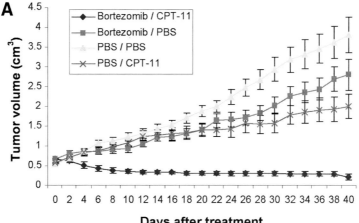

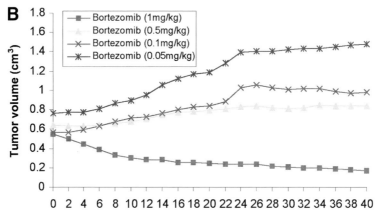

**Fig. 4.** The effects of combination therapy using the proteasome inhibitor bortezomib and irinotecan were assessed in a xenograft model. One-centimeter-diameter LOVO tumors were grown in the flanks of nude mice. The tumoricidal effect of systemic treatment was assessed (**A**) after pretreatment with bortezomib (1 mg/kg iv bolus injection) or vehicle alone, followed by iv bolus administration of irinotecan (33 mg/kg) or vehicle. Treatment was administered biweekly (Monday and Thursday), and tumor diameter along two orthogonal axes was recorded every other day. Tumor volume was calculated by assuming a spherical shape of the tumor, using the formula Volume = $4/3\pi r^3$, where $r$ is ½ (mean diameter of the tumor), and recorded as the means for each treatment group ($n = 8$–10); bars = SE. The dose response to increasing concentrations of bortezomib when used in combination with a fixed dosage of irinotecan (33 mg/kg) was assessed in a LOVO xenograft model (**B**). The tumoricidal response to different concentrations of bortezomib, including the maximum tolerated dose (MTD) (1 mg/kg) in nude mice, was determined by pretreatment with an iv bolus administration of bortezomib, followed by an iv bolus administration of irinotecan. Treatment was administered biweekly, and tumor diameter along two orthogonal axes was recorded every other day ($n = 8$–10). Tumor volume was calculated as described. (Reprinted with permission from *Cancer Research* ref. *138*.)

## 5. FUTURE OUTLOOK

With an exponentially increasing body of knowledge of cellular mechanisms and molecular events involved in tumorigenesis, chemotherapy response, and drug resistance, the development of new approaches to sensitize tumor cells will most likely be rapid. Because the variation of tumoral responses to chemotherapy and resistance patterns is large, the possibility to individualize a combination therapy consisting of drugs enhancing apoptosis and others targeting the resistance response seems promising. Further research and development of a wide repertoire of designed molecular drugs will most likely make this feasible.

## ACKNOWLEDGMENT

The authors thank Rong Liu for assistance in the preparation of the text.

## REFERENCES

1. Kastan MB. Molecular determinants of sensitivity to antitumor agents. Biochim Biophys Acta 1999; 1424(1):R37–R42.
2. Fisher DE. Apoptosis in cancer therapy: crossing the threshold. Cell 1994; 78(4):539–542.
3. Schmitt CA, Lowe SW. Apoptosis and therapy. J Pathol 1999; 187(1):127–137.
4. Baldini N. Multidrug resistance—a multiplex phenomenon. Nature Med 1997; 3(4):378–380.
5. Wang CY, Mayo MW, Baldwin AS Jr. TNF- and cancer therapy-induced apoptosis: potentiation by inhibition of NF-kappaB. Science 1996; 274(5288):784–787.
6. Wang CY, et al. Control of inducible chemoresistance: enhanced anti-tumor therapy through increased apoptosis by inhibition of NF-kappaB. Nature Med 1999; 5(4):412–417.
7. Beg AA, Baltimore D. An essential role for NF-kappaB in preventing TNF-alpha-induced cell death. Science 1996; 274(5288):782–784.
8. Cusack JC Jr, Liu R, Baldwin AS Jr. Inducible chemoresistance to 7-ethyl-10-[4-(1-piperidino)-1-piperidino]- carbonyloxycamptothe cin (CPT-11) in colorectal cancer cells and a xenograft model is overcome by inhibition of nuclear factor-kappaB activation. Cancer Res 2000; 60(9):2323–2330.
9. Fulda S, et al. Molecular ordering of apoptosis induced by anticancer drugs in neuroblastoma cells. Cancer Res 1998; 58(19):4453–4460.
10. Modulation of fluorouracil by leucovorin in patients with advanced colorectal cancer: evidence in terms of response rate. Advanced Colorectal Cancer Meta-Analysis Project. J Clin Oncol 1992; 10(6): 896–903.
11. Saltz LB, et al. Irinotecan plus fluorouracil and leucovorin for metastatic colorectal cancer. Irinotecan Study Group. N Engl J Med 2000; 343(13):905–914.
12. Douillard JY, et al. Irinotecan combined with fluorouracil compared with fluorouracil alone as first-line treatment for metastatic colorectal cancer: a multicentre randomised trial. Lancet 2000; 355(9209): 1041–1047.
13. de Gramont A, et al. Leucovorin and fluorouracil with or without oxaliplatin as first-line treatment in advanced colorectal cancer. J Clin Oncol 2000; 18(16):2938–2947.
14. Tournigand C, et al. FOLFIRI followed by FOLFOX6 or the reverse sequence in advanced colorectal cancer: a randomized GERCOR study. J Clin Oncol 2004; 22(2):229–237.
15. Vincent M, Labianca R, Harper P. Which 5-fluorouracil regimen?—the great debate. Anticancer Drugs 1999; 10(4):337–354.
16. Andre T, Louvet C, de Gramont A. [Colon cancer: what is new in 2004?]. Bull Cancer 2004; 91(1): 75–80.
17. Kern A, et al. Nucleotide and transported substrates modulate different steps of the ATPase catalytic cycle of MRP1 multidrug transporter. Biochem J 2004; 380(Pt. 2):549–560.
18. Baldini N. Multidrug resistance—a multiplex phenomenon. Nature Med 1997; 3(4):378–380.
19. Sikic BI, et al. Modulation and prevention of multidrug resistance by inhibitors of P-glycoprotein. Cancer Chemother Pharmacol 1997; 40(Suppl):S13–S29.
20. Maliepaard M, et al. Overexpression of the BCRP/MXR/ABCP gene in a topotecan-selected ovarian tumor cell line. Cancer Res 1999; 59(18):4559–4563.
21. Sikic BI. New approaches in cancer treatment. Ann Oncol 1999; 10(Suppl 6):149–153.
22. Maliepaard M, et al. Circumvention of breast cancer resistance protein (BCRP)-mediated resistance to camptothecins in vitro using non-substrate drugs or the BCRP inhibitor GF120918. Clin Cancer Res 2001; 7(4):935–941.

23. Sinha P, et al. Search for novel proteins involved in the development of chemoresistance in colorectal cancer and fibrosarcoma cells in vitro using two-dimensional electrophoresis, mass spectrometry and microsequencing. Electrophoresis 1999; 20(14):2961–2969.

24. Mini E, et al. Marked variation of thymidylate synthase and folylpolyglutamate synthetase gene expression in human colorectal tumors. Oncol Res 1999; 11(9):437–445.

25. Plummer R, et al. A phase I trial of ZD9331, a water-soluble, nonpolyglutamatable, thymidylate synthase inhibitor. Clin Cancer Res 2003; 9(4):1313–1322.

26. Gibbs D, Raynaud CP, Valenti M, Jackman AL. CB300638, an alpha-folate receptor (a-FR) targeted antifolate thymidylate synthase (TS) inhibitor that inhibits TS in human tumour xenografts but not in normal tissues. Proc Am Assoc Cancer Res 2003; 2624a.

27. Townsend DM, Tew KD. The role of glutathione-S-transferase in anti-cancer drug resistance. Oncogene 2003; 22(47):7369–7375.

28. Kivisto KT, Kroemer HK, Eichelbaum M. The role of human cytochrome P450 enzymes in the metabolism of anticancer agents: implications for drug interactions. Br J Clin Pharmacol 1995; 40(6):523–530.

29. Ferreira CG, Tolis C, Giaccone G. p53 and chemosensitivity. Ann Oncol 1999; 10(9):1011–1021.

30. Yamamoto M, et al. The p53 tumor suppressor gene in anticancer agent-induced apoptosis and chemosensitivity of human gastrointestinal cancer cell lines. Cancer Chemother Pharmacol 1999; 43(1):43–49.

31. Zheng M, et al. The influence of the p53 gene on the in vitro chemosensitivity of colorectal cancer cells. J Cancer Res Clin Oncol 1999; 125(6):357–360.

32. Fujiwara T, et al. Induction of chemosensitivity in human lung cancer cells in vivo by adenovirus-mediated transfer of the wild-type p53 gene. Cancer Res 1994; 54(9):2287–2291.

33. Spitz FR, et al. In vivo adenovirus-mediated p53 tumor suppressor gene therapy for colorectal cancer. Anticancer Res 1996; 16(6B):3415–3422.

34. Bullock AN, Fersht AR. Rescuing the function of mutant p53. Nature Rev Cancer 2001; 1(1):68–76.

35. Wang W, Rastinejad F, El-Deiry WS. Restoring p53-dependent tumor suppression. Cancer Biol Ther 2003; 2(4 Suppl 1):S55–S63.

36. Foster BA, et al. Pharmacological rescue of mutant p53 conformation and function. Science 1999; 286(5449):2507–2510.

37. Kaufmann SH, Vaux DL. Alterations in the apoptotic machinery and their potential role in anticancer drug resistance. Oncogene 2003; 22(47):7414–7430.

38. te Poele RH, et al. DNA damage is able to induce senescence in tumor cells in vitro and in vivo. Cancer Res 2002; 62(6):1876–1883.

39. Schmitt CA, et al. A senescence program controlled by p53 and p16INK4a contributes to the outcome of cancer therapy. Cell 2002; 109(3):335–346.

40. Chang BD, et al. Molecular determinants of terminal growth arrest induced in tumor cells by a chemotherapeutic agent. Proc Natl Acad Sci USA 2002; 99(1):389–394.

41. Brown JM, Wouters BG. Apoptosis, p53, and tumor cell sensitivity to anticancer agents. Cancer Res 1999; 59(7):1391–1399.

42. Leist M, Jaattela M. Four deaths and a funeral: from caspases to alternative mechanisms. Nature Rev Mol Cell Biol 2001; 2(8):589–598.

43. Kaufmann SH, Gores GJ. Apoptosis in cancer: cause and cure. Bioessays 2000; 22(11):1007–1017.

44. Johnstone RW, Ruefli AA, Lowe SW. Apoptosis: a link between cancer genetics and chemotherapy. Cell 2002; 108(2):153–164.

45. Violette S, et al. Resistance of colon cancer cells to long-term 5-fluorouracil exposure is correlated to the relative level of Bcl-2 and Bcl-X(L) in addition to Bax and p53 status. Int J Cancer 2002; 98(4):498–504.

46. Oliver L, et al. Resistance to apoptosis is increased during metastatic dissemination of colon cancer. Clin Exp Metastasis 2002; 19(2):175–180.

47. Thornberry NA, Lazebnik Y. Caspases: enemies within. Science 1998; 281(5381):1312–1316.

48. Ashkenazi A, Dixit VM. Death receptors: signaling and modulation. Science 1998; 281(5381):1305–1308.

49. Budihardjo I, et al. Biochemical pathways of caspase activation during apoptosis. Annu Rev Cell Dev Biol 1999; 15:269–290.

50. Wang X. The expanding role of mitochondria in apoptosis. Genes Dev 2001; 15(22):2922–2933.

51. Acehan D, et al. Three-dimensional structure of the apoptosome: implications for assembly, procaspase-9 binding, and activation. Mol Cell 2002; 9(2):423–432.

52. Cheng EH, et al. BCL-2, BCL-X(L) sequester BH3 domain-only molecules preventing BAX- and BAK-mediated mitochondrial apoptosis. Mol Cell 2001; 8(3):705–711.

53. Ozoren N, El-Deiry WS. Defining characteristics of Types I and II apoptotic cells in response to TRAIL. Neoplasia 2002; 4(6):551–557.

54. Barnhart BC, Alappat EC, Peter ME. The CD95 type I/type II model. Semin Immunol 2003; 15(3): 185–193.

55. Ravagnan L, Roumier T, Kroemer G. Mitochondria, the killer organelles and their weapons. J Cell Physiol 2002; 192(2):131–137.

56. Srinivasula SM, et al. Molecular determinants of the caspase-promoting activity of Smac/DIABLO and its role in the death receptor pathway. J Biol Chem 2000; 275(46):36,152–36,157.

57. Martins LM, et al. The serine protease Omi/HtrA2 regulates apoptosis by binding XIAP through a reaper-like motif. J Biol Chem 2002; 277(1):439–444.

58. Jansen B, et al. bcl-2 antisense therapy chemosensitizes human melanoma in SCID mice. Nature Med 1998; 4(2):232–234.

59. Waters JS, et al. Phase I clinical and pharmacokinetic study of bcl-2 antisense oligonucleotide therapy in patients with non-Hodgkin's lymphoma. J Clin Oncol 2000; 18(9):1812–1823.

60. Jansen B, et al. Chemosensitisation of malignant melanoma by BCL2 antisense therapy. Lancet 2000; 356(9243):1728–1733.

61. Taylor JK, et al. Induction of endogenous Bcl-xS through the control of Bcl-x pre-mRNA splicing by antisense oligonucleotides. Nature Biotechnol 1999; 17(11):1097–1100.

62. Grossman D, et al. Inhibition of melanoma tumor growth in vivo by survivin targeting. Proc Natl Acad Sci USA 2001; 98(2):635–640.

63. Zamore PD. RNA interference: listening to the sound of silence. Nature Struct Biol 2001; 8(9):746–750.

64. McManus MT, Sharp PA. Gene silencing in mammals by small interfering RNAs. Nature Rev Genet 2002; 3(10):737–747.

65. Crnkovic-Mertens I, Hoppe-Seyler F, Butz K. Induction of apoptosis in tumor cells by siRNA-mediated silencing of the livin/ML-IAP/KIAP gene. Oncogene 2003; 22(51):8330–8336.

66. Guo F, et al. Ectopic overexpression of second mitochondria-derived activator of caspases (Smac/ DIABLO) or cotreatment with N-terminus of Smac/DIABLO peptide potentiates epothilone B derivative-(BMS 247550) and Apo-2L/TRAIL-induced apoptosis. Blood 2002; 99(9):3419–3426.

67. Fulda S, et al. Smac agonists sensitize for Apo2L/TRAIL- or anticancer drug-induced apoptosis and induce regression of malignant glioma in vivo. Nature Med 2002; 8(8):808–815.

68. Arnt CR, et al. Synthetic Smac/DIABLO peptides enhance the effects of chemotherapeutic agents by binding XIAP and cIAP1 in situ. J Biol Chem 2002; 277(46):44,236–44,243. Epub 2002 Sep 5.

69. Darnell JE Jr. Transcription factors as targets for cancer therapy. Nature Rev Cancer 2002; 2(10): 740–749.

70. Brivanlou AH, Darnell JE Jr. Signal transduction and the control of gene expression. Science 2002; 295(5556):813–818.

71. Gibbs JB. Mechanism-based target identification and drug discovery in cancer research. Science 2000; 287(5460):1969–1973.

72. Tilley WD, et al. Hormones and cancer: new insights, new challenges. Trends Endocrinol Metab 2001; 12(5):186–188.

73. Barnes PJ. Anti-inflammatory actions of glucocorticoids: molecular mechanisms. Clin Sci (Lond) 1998; 94(6):557–572.

74. Stark GR, et al. How cells respond to interferons. Annu Rev Biochem 1998; 67:227–264.

75. Levy DE, Darnell JE Jr. Stats: transcriptional control and biological impact. Nature Rev Mol Cell Biol 2002; 3(9):651–662.

76. Starr R, Hilton DJ. Negative regulation of the JAK/STAT pathway. Bioessays 1999; 21(1):47–52.

77. Shuai K. Modulation of STAT signaling by STAT-interacting proteins. Oncogene 2000; 19(21):2638–2644.

78. Bowman T, et al. STATs in oncogenesis. Oncogene 2000; 19(21):2474–2488.

79. Lacronique V, et al. Transforming properties of chimeric TEL–JAK proteins in Ba/F3 cells. Blood 2000; 95(6):2076–2083.

80. Lacronique V, et al. A TEL-JAK2 fusion protein with constitutive kinase activity in human leukemia. Science 1997; 278(5341):1309–1312.

81. Song JI, Grandis JR. STAT signaling in head and neck cancer. Oncogene 2000; 19(21):2489–2495.

82. Catlett-Falcone R, et al. Constitutive activation of Stat3 signaling confers resistance to apoptosis in human U266 myeloma cells. Immunity 1999; 10(1):105–115.

83. Cantley LC. The phosphoinositide 3-kinase pathway. Science 2002; 296(5573):1655–1657.

84. Vivanco I, Sawyers CL. The phosphatidylinositol 3-Kinase AKT pathway in human cancer. Nature Rev Cancer 2002; 2(7):489–501.

85. Hayakawa J, et al. Inhibition of BAD phosphorylation either at serine 112 via extracellular signal-regulated protein kinase cascade or at serine 136 via Akt cascade sensitizes human ovarian cancer cells to cisplatin. Cancer Res 2000; 60(21):5988–5994.

86. Park SY, Seol DW. Regulation of Akt by EGF-R inhibitors, a possible mechanism of EGF-R inhibitor-enhanced TRAIL-induced apoptosis. Biochem Biophys Res Commun 2002; 295(2):515–518.

87. Neshat MS, et al. Enhanced sensitivity of PTEN-deficient tumors to inhibition of FRAP/mTOR. Proc Natl Acad Sci USA 2001; 98(18):10,314–10,319.

88. Guba M, et al. Rapamycin inhibits primary and metastatic tumor growth by antiangiogenesis: involvement of vascular endothelial growth factor. Nature Med 2002; 8(2):128–135.

89. Barish GD, Williams BO. In: Gutkind JS, ed. Signaling networks and cell cycle control: the molecular basis of cancer and other diseases. Humana, Totowa, NJ, 2000:53–82.

90. Taipale J, Beachy PA. The Hedgehog and Wnt signalling pathways in cancer. Nature 2001; 411(6835): 349–354.

91. van Gijn ME, et al. The wnt-frizzled cascade in cardiovascular disease. Cardiovasc Res 2002; 55(1): 16–24.

92. Wong CM, Fan ST, Ng IO. beta-Catenin mutation and overexpression in hepatocellular carcinoma: clinicopathologic and prognostic significance. Cancer 2001; 92(1):136–145.

93. Kramps T, et al. Wnt/wingless signaling requires BCL9/legless-mediated recruitment of pygopus to the nuclear beta-catenin–TCF complex. Cell 2002; 109(1):47–60.

94. Barker N, Clevers H. Catenins, Wnt signaling and cancer. Bioessays 2000; 22(11):961–965.

95. Karin M, Lin A. NF-kappaB at the crossroads of life and death. Nature Immunol 2002; 3(3):221–227.

96. Wang CY, Mayo MW, Baldwin AS Jr. TNF- and cancer therapy-induced apoptosis: potentiation by inhibition of NF-kappaB. Science 1996; 274(5288):784–787.

97. Wang CY, et al. NF-kappaB antiapoptosis: induction of TRAF1 and TRAF2 and c-IAP1 and c-IAP2 to suppress caspase-8 activation. Science 1998; 281(5383):1680–1683.

98. Hsu H, et al. TNF-dependent recruitment of the protein kinase RIP to the TNF receptor-1 signaling complex. Immunity 1996; 4(4):387–396.

99. Hsu H, Xiong J, Goeddel DV. The TNF receptor 1-associated protein TRADD signals cell death and NF-kappa B activation. Cell 1995; 81(4):495–504.

100. Santana P, et al. Acid sphingomyelinase-deficient human lymphoblasts and mice are defective in radiation-induced apoptosis. Cell 1996; 86(2):189–199.

101. Tartaglia LA, Goeddel DV. Two TNF receptors. Immunol Today 1992; 13(5):151–153.

102. Ryan KM, et al. Role of NF-kappaB in p53-mediated programmed cell death. Nature 2000; 404(6780): 892–897.

103. Cusack JC, Liu R, Baldwin AS. NF-kappa B and chemoresistance: potentiation of cancer drugs via inhibition of NF-kappa B. Drug Resist Update 1999; 2(4):271–273.

104. Spencer E, Jiang J, Chen ZJ. Signal-induced ubiquitination of IkappaBalpha by the F-box protein Slimb/beta-TrCP. Genes Dev 1999; 13(3):284–294.

105. Baldwin AS. Control of oncogenesis and cancer therapy resistance by the transcription factor NF-kappaB. J Clin Invest 2001; 107(3):241–246.

106. Soengas MS, Lowe SW. Apoptosis and melanoma chemoresistance. Oncogene 2003; 22(20):3138–3151.

107. Tam WF, Wang W, Sen R. Cell-specific association and shuttling of IkappaBalpha provides a mechanism for nuclear NF-kappaB in B lymphocytes. Mol Cell Biol 2001; 21(14):4837–4846.

108. Song HY, Rothe M, Goeddel DV. The tumor necrosis factor-inducible zinc finger protein A20 interacts with TRAF1/TRAF2 and inhibits NF-kappaB activation. Proc Natl Acad Sci USA 1996; 93(13): 6721–6725.

109. Micheau O, Tschopp J. Induction of TNF receptor I-mediated apoptosis via two sequential signaling complexes. Cell 2003; 114(2):181–190.

110. Joyce D, et al. Integration of Rac-dependent regulation of cyclin D1 transcription through a nuclear factor-kappaB-dependent pathway. J Biol Chem 1999; 274(36):25,245–25,249.

111. Wadgaonkar R, et al. CREB-binding protein is a nuclear integrator of nuclear factor-kappaB and p53 signaling. J Biol Chem 1999; 274(4):1879–1882.

112. Tergaonkar V, et al. p53 stabilization is decreased upon NFkappaB activation: a role for NFkappaB in acquisition of resistance to chemotherapy. Cancer Cell 2002; 1(5):493–503.

113. Bentires-Alj M, et al. Inhibition of the NF-kappa B transcription factor increases Bax expression in cancer cell lines. Oncogene 2001; 20(22):2805–2813.

114. Bottero V, et al. Ikappa b-alpha, the NF-kappa B inhibitory subunit, interacts with ANT, the mitochondrial ATP/ADP translocator. J Biol Chem 2001; 276(24):21,317–21,324.

115. Cogswell PC, et al. NF-kappa B and I kappa B alpha are found in the mitochondria. Evidence for regulation of mitochondrial gene expression by NF-kappa B. J Biol Chem 2003; 278(5):2963–2968.

116. Rayet B, Gelinas C. Aberrant rel/nfkb genes and activity in human cancer. Oncogene 1999; 18(49): 6938–6947.

117. Maxwell SA, Mukhopadhyay T. A novel NF-kappa B p65 spliced transcript lacking exons 6 and 7 in a non-small cell lung carcinoma cell line. Gene 1995; 166(2):339–340.

118. Visconti R, et al. Expression of the neoplastic phenotype by human thyroid carcinoma cell lines requires NFkappaB p65 protein expression. Oncogene 1997; 15(16):1987–1994.

119. Mathew S, et al. Chromosomal localization of genes encoding the transcription factors, c-rel, NF-kappa Bp50, NF-kappa Bp65, and lyt-10 by fluorescence *in situ* hybridization. Oncogene 1993; 8(1): 191–193.

120. Bours V, et al. The NF-kappa B transcription factor and cancer: high expression of NF-kappa B- and I kappa B-related proteins in tumor cell lines. Biochem Pharmacol 1994; 47(1):145–149.

121. Cabannes E, et al. Mutations in the IkBa gene in Hodgkin's disease suggest a tumour suppressor role for IkappaBalpha. Oncogene 1999; 18(20):3063–3070.

122. Chen C, Edelstein LC, Gelinas C. The Rel/NF-kappaB family directly activates expression of the apoptosis inhibitor Bcl-x(L). Mol Cell Biol 2000; 20(8):2687–2695.

123. Ni H, et al. Analysis of expression of nuclear factor kappa B (NF-kappa B) in multiple myeloma: downregulation of NF-kappa B induces apoptosis. Br J Haematol 2001; 115(2):279–286.

124. Hideshima T, et al. The proteasome inhibitor PS-341 inhibits growth, induces apoptosis, and overcomes drug resistance in human multiple myeloma cells. Cancer Res 2001; 61(7):3071–3076.

125. Ogata A, et al. IL-6 triggers cell growth via the Ras-dependent mitogen-activated protein kinase cascade. J Immunol 1997; 159(5):2212–2221.

126. Chauhan D, et al. Dexamethasone induces apoptosis of multiple myeloma cells in a JNK/SAP kinase independent mechanism. Oncogene 1997; 15(7):837–843.

127. Palombella VJ, et al. Role of the proteasome and NF-kappaB in streptococcal cell wall-induced polyarthritis. Proc Natl Acad Sci USA 1998; 95(26):15,671–15,676.

128. Wang W, et al. The nuclear factor-kappa B RelA transcription factor is constitutively activated in human pancreatic adenocarcinoma cells. Clin Cancer Res 1999; 5(1):119–127.

129. Nakshatri H, et al. Constitutive activation of NF-kappaB during progression of breast cancer to hormone-independent growth. Mol Cell Biol 1997; 17(7):3629–3639.

130. Sovak MA, et al. Aberrant nuclear factor-kappaB/Rel expression and the pathogenesis of breast cancer. J Clin Invest 1997; 100(12):2952–2960.

131. Palayoor ST, et al. Constitutive activation of IkappaB kinase alpha and NF-kappaB in prostate cancer cells is inhibited by ibuprofen. Oncogene 1999; 18(51):7389–7394.

132. Patel NM, et al. Paclitaxel sensitivity of breast cancer cells with constitutively active NF-kappaB is enhanced by IkappaBalpha super-repressor and parthenolide. Oncogene 2000; 19(36):4159–4169.

133. Lind DS, et al. Nuclear factor-kappa B is upregulated in colorectal cancer. Surgery 2001; 130(2):363–369.

134. Mukhopadhyay T, Roth JA, Maxwell SA. Altered expression of the p50 subunit of the NF-kappa B transcription factor complex in non-small cell lung carcinoma. Oncogene 1995; 11(5):999–1003.

135. Reuning U, et al. Inhibition of NF-kappa B-Rel A expression by antisense oligodeoxynucleotides suppresses synthesis of urokinase-type plasminogen activator (uPA) but not its inhibitor PAI-1. Nucleic Acids Res 1995; 23(19):3887–3893.

136. Grundker C, et al. Luteinizing hormone-releasing hormone induces nuclear factor kappaB-activation and inhibits apoptosis in ovarian cancer cells. J Clin Endocrinol Metab 2000; 85(10):3815–3820.

136a. Wang CY, Cusack JC Jr, Liu R, Baldwin AS Jr. Control of inducible chemoresistance: enhanced anti-tumor therapy through increased apoptosis by inhibition of NF-kappaB. Nature Med 1999; 5(4): 412–417.

137. Duffey DC, et al. Expression of a dominant-negative mutant inhibitor-kappaBalpha of nuclear factor-kappaB in human head and neck squamous cell carcinoma inhibits survival, proinflammatory cytokine expression, and tumor growth in vivo. Cancer Res 1999; 59(14):3468–3474.

138. Cusack JC Jr, et al. Enhanced chemosensitivity to CPT-11 with proteasome inhibitor PS-341: implications for systemic nuclear factor-kappaB inhibition. Cancer Res 2001; 61(9):3535–3540.

139. Russo SM, et al. Enhancement of radiosensitivity by proteasome inhibition: implications for a role of NF-kappaB. Int J Radiat Oncol Biol Phys 2001; 50(1):183–193.

140. An B, et al. Novel dipeptidyl proteasome inhibitors overcome Bcl-2 protective function and selectively accumulate the cyclin-dependent kinase inhibitor p27 and induce apoptosis in transformed, but not normal, human fibroblasts. Cell Death Differ 1998; 5(12):1062–1075.

141. Masdehors P, et al. Ubiquitin–proteasome system and increased sensitivity of B-CLL lymphocytes to apoptotic death activation. Leuk Lymphoma 2000; 38(5-6):499–504.

142. Delic J, et al. The proteasome inhibitor lactacystin induces apoptosis and sensitizes chemo- and radio-resistant human chronic lymphocytic leukaemia lymphocytes to TNF-alpha-initiated apoptosis. Br J Cancer 1998; 77(7):1103–1107.

143. LeBlanc R, et al. Proteasome inhibitor PS-341 inhibits human myeloma cell growth in vivo and prolongs survival in a murine model. Cancer Res 2002; 62(17):4996–5000.

144. Richardson PG, et al. A phase 2 study of bortezomib in relapsed, refractory myeloma. N Engl J Med 2003; 348(26):2609–2617.

145. Desai SD, et al. Ubiquitin-dependent destruction of topoisomerase I is stimulated by the antitumor drug camptothecin. J Biol Chem 1997; 272(39):24,159–24,164.

146. Cusack JC Jr. Overcoming antiapoptotic responses to promote chemosensitivity in metastatic colorectal cancer to the liver. Ann Surg Oncol 2003; 10(8):852–862.

147. Maki CG, Huibregtse JM, Howley PM. In vivo ubiquitination and proteasome-mediated degradation of p53(1). Cancer Res 1996; 56(11):2649–2654.

148. Cayrol C, Ducommun B. Interaction with cyclin-dependent kinases and PCNA modulates proteasome-dependent degradation of p21. Oncogene 1998; 17(19):2437–2444.

149. Pagano M, et al. Role of the ubiquitin-proteasome pathway in regulating abundance of the cyclin-dependent kinase inhibitor p27. Science 1995; 269(5224):682–685.

150. Chadebech P, et al. Phosphorylation and proteasome-dependent degradation of Bcl-2 in mitotic-arrested cells after microtubule damage. Biochem Biophys Res Commun 1999; 262(3):823–827.

151. Salvat C, et al. Differential directing of c-Fos and c-Jun proteins to the proteasome in serum-stimulated mouse embryo fibroblasts. Oncogene 1998; 17(3):327–337.

152. Clurman BE, et al. Turnover of cyclin E by the ubiquitin-proteasome pathway is regulated by cdk2 binding and cyclin phosphorylation. Genes Dev 1996; 10(16):1979–1990.

153. Diehl JA, Zindy F, Sherr CJ. Inhibition of cyclin D1 phosphorylation on threonine-286 prevents its rapid degradation via the ubiquitin–proteasome pathway. Genes Dev 1997; 11(8):957–972.

154. Sudakin V, et al. The cyclosome, a large complex containing cyclin-selective ubiquitin ligase activity, targets cyclins for destruction at the end of mitosis. Mol Biol Cell 1995; 6(2):185–197.

155. Buschmann T, et al. SUMO-1 modification of Mdm2 prevents its self-ubiquitination and increases Mdm2 ability to ubiquitinate p53. Cell 2000; 101(7):753–762.

156. Dietrich C, et al. p53-dependent cell cycle arrest induced by N-acetyl-L-leucinyl-L-leucinyl-L-nor-leucinal in platelet-derived growth factor-stimulated human fibroblasts. Proc Natl Acad Sci USA 1996; 93(20):10,815–10,819.

157. Adams J, et al. Proteasome inhibitors: a novel class of potent and effective antitumor agents. Cancer Res 1999; 59(11):2615–2622.

158. Bold RJ, Virudachalam S, McConkey DJ. Chemosensitization of pancreatic cancer by inhibition of the 26S proteasome. J Surg Res 2001; 100(1):11–17.

# 15 Targeting Apoptosis Pathways for Cancer Therapy

*Bharvin K. R. Patel, PhD*

## CONTENTS

INTRODUCTION
MOLECULAR MECHANISMS OF APOPTOSIS
APOPTOSIS REGULATORS
FUTURE PROSPECTS
ACKNOWLEDGMENT
REFERENCES

## SUMMARY

Apoptosis, or programmed cell death (PCD), is a highly organized physiologic event that plays an essential role in controlling cell number in many normal processes, ranging from fetal development to adult tissue homeostasis. The process of apoptosis is tightly regulated by a number of gene products that promote or block cell death at different stages of apoptosis. Abnormal regulation of apoptosis has been implicated in the onset of a wide range of diseases, including cancer. Approaches to resensitize cancer cells to apoptosis represent an important future strategy for cancer treatment, which include restoring lost apoptosis intermediates, inactivating antiapoptotic proteins, triggering apoptosis pathways that remain intact in cancer cells, and inducing apoptosis by targeting specific tumorigenic lesions. This chapter discusses recent advances in this field and highlights novel therapeutic approaches exploiting apoptotic pathways for cancer treatment.

**Key Words:** Apoptosis; programmed cell death; caspase; cancer; therapy; TRAIL; FAS; Bcl-2; Bcl-xL; XIAP; survivin; PI3K; NF-κB; AKT.

## 1. INTRODUCTION

The term "apoptosis" (derived from the Greek word for "falling off") was originally coined by Kerr and his colleagues to describe morphological changes associated with cell death *(1)*. Apoptosis, or programmed cell death (PCD), is a highly organized physiologic

From: *Cancer Drug Discovery and Development: The Oncogenomics Handbook*
Edited by: W. J. LaRochelle and R. A. Shimkets © Humana Press Inc., Totowa, NJ

event that plays an essential role in controlling cell number in many normal processes, ranging from fetal development to adult tissue homeostasis *(1–8)*. Morphologically, apoptosis is characterized by chromatin condensation, nuclear fragmentation, and the loss of mitochondrial inner transmembrane potential resulting in plasma membrane blebbing, with cells breaking into small membrane-surrounded fragments (apoptotic bodies). These apoptotic bodies are quickly phagocytosed and digested by neighboring cells or macrophages *(2,5,9–11)*. These morphological changes are believed to be caused by a family of cysteine proteases known as caspases *(12–16)*. The recognition site for caspases is marked by three to four amino acids followed by an aspartic acid residue, with cleavage occurring after the aspartate *(7,14,17)*. Caspases are typically synthesized as inactive zymogens but are activated as a result of their proteolytic processing at conserved internal aspartate through autocatalysis or by another protease *(7,15,18)*. Caspase-3, caspase-6, and caspase-7 are a key downstream effector in the apoptosis pathway, amplifying the signal from initiator caspases such as caspase-8, caspase-9, and caspase-10 *(15,18)*. Caspase-3 has been shown to cleave nuclear lamins, poly(ADP-ribose) polymerase (PARP), DNA-dependent protein kinase (PKC-δ), and gelsolin, leading to the controlled degradation of major cell structures such as the nucleus, actin cytoskeleton, and mitochondria *(7,15,18,19)*. The process of apoptosis is tightly regulated by a number of gene products that promote or block cell death at different stages of apoptosis (Fig. 1). Abnormal regulation of apoptosis has been implicated in the onset of wide range of diseases, including cancer *(20–22)*. Uncontrolled proliferation has traditionally been viewed as the major underlying mechanism for tumor formation *(20,23–25)*. However, cellular changes that lead to inhibition of apoptosis is now recognized as one of the major molecular mechanisms for cancer progression and resistance of cancer to chemotherapeutic drugs and radiation therapy *(26–38)*. Pharmacologic manipulation of this pathway that resensitizes cancer cells to apoptosis represents a novel therapeutic strategy in cancer therapy. This chapter discusses recent advances in this field and highlights novel therapeutic approaches exploiting the apoptotic pathway for cancer treatment.

## 2. MOLECULAR MECHANISMS OF APOPTOSIS

Apoptosis has several common elements regardless of the ultimate molecular pathways utilized *(2,18,39)*. Generically, a cellular sensor (such as death receptors or mitochondria) detects the presence of a death-inducing signal (such as death receptor ligands, stress, DNA damage, or chemotherapeutic agents), which activates a signal transduction pathway. This process initiates the execution reactions involving activation of initiator caspases (caspase-8, caspase-9, and caspase-10) to complete the process of cell death ultimately executed by effector caspases (caspase-3, caspase-6, and caspase-7) *(2,18,39)*. Apoptosis

---

**Fig. 1.** *(Opposite page)*  Two major pathways of apoptosis. Several key players in the extrinsic (death receptor mediated) and intrinsic (mitochondrial mediated) apoptosis pathway are potential targets for cancer therapy. DD, death domain; DED, death effector domain; c-FLIP, cellular FLICE-like inhibitory protein; tBID, truncated Bid; Apaf-1, apoptosis activating factor-1; IAP, inhibitor of apoptosis proteins; XIAP, X-linked IAP; AIF, apoptosis-inducing factor; Smac, second mitochondrial derived activator of caspases; Diablo, direct IAP-binding protein with low pI; Bcl-2, B-cell lymphoma gene-2; Bax, Bcl-2 associated protein-x; Bad, Bcl-2 associated protein-d; PI3K, phosphatidylinositol 3 kinase; I-κB, inhibitor of κB; IKK, inhibitor of κB kinase; NF-κB, nuclear factor-κB; HTRA2, heat-inducible serine protease A2.

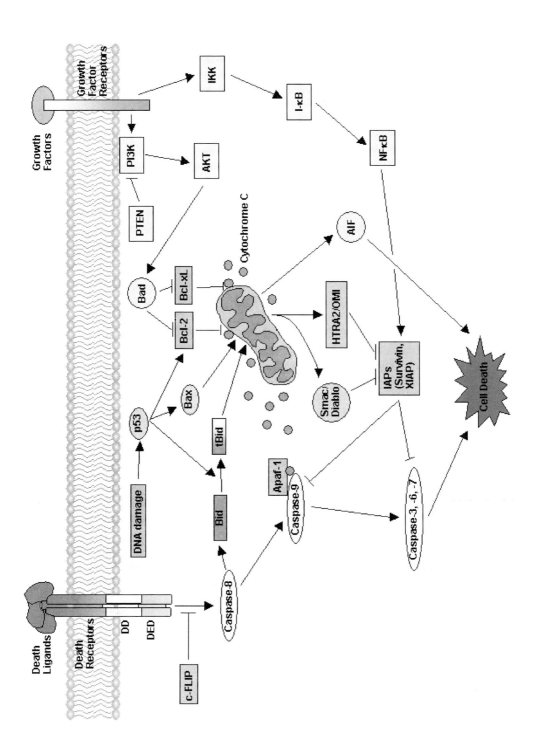

signal transduction can occur by two distinct pathways: extrinsic (receptor mediated) apoptosis pathway or intrinsic (mitochondrial mediated) apoptosis pathway *(18,39–41)*.

## 2.1. Extrinsic (Receptor Mediated) Apoptosis Pathway

The extrinsic apoptosis pathway is triggered by members of the tumor necrosis factor (TNF) receptor superfamily, which contain several cysteine-rich domains (CRDs) in their amino terminal region and death domain (DD) in their cytoplasmic tail *(39,42–47)*. The death-domain-containing receptors, or death receptors (DR), include TNFR1 (TNF receptor)/CD120a, Fas/CD95/Apo1, DR3/Apo2/WSL-1/TRAMP/LARD, DR4/TRAIL (TNF-related apoptosis-inducing ligand)-R1, DR5/TRAIL-R2/TRICK2/KILLER, and DR6 *(18,39,48–51)*. Following the ligation of death receptors by ligand, the death receptor oligomerizes and recruits adapter molecule FADD (Fas-associated death domain protein) and multiple procaspase-8 molecules to a complex, the death-inducing signaling complex (DISC), which results in the activation of initiator caspases *(49–53)*. The protein interactions that lead to the formation of DISC are primarily mediated through two structural motifs *(25,51,54)*. One motif, the DD, facilitates interaction of FADD adapter proteins to the receptors. The other motif, death effector domain (DED), facilitates interaction between pro-caspases and adapter proteins. This pathway is negatively regulated by c-FLIP, a DED-containing antagonists of FADD and pro-caspases *(52,55)*.

## 2.2. Intrinsic (Mitochondria Mediated) Apoptosis Pathway

Mitochondria play a central role in the intrinsic apoptosis pathway. The intrinsic apoptosis pathway is generally triggered in response to number of extracellular stimuli and internal insults, including ultraviolet (UV) radiation, chemotherapeutic agents, growth factor withdrawal, stress molecules, and increased expression of the pore-forming pro-apoptotic protein such as Bax and Bid *(18,42)*. These stimuli induce the release of cytochrome-*c* from mitochondria into cytosol to form the apoptosome complex. Once released, cytochrome-*c* binds to an adapter molecule Apaf-1 (apoptotic protease-activating factor). This binding unfolds and exposes the CARD (caspase recruiting domain)-containing oligomerization domain of Apaf-1, allowing binding and activation of procaspase-9 *(39,56)*. Active caspase-9 then cleaves and activates executioner caspases to induce apoptosis. This pathway is negatively regulated by antiapoptotic Bcl-2 family proteins, which prevent cytochrome-*c* release through a yet unknown mechanism *(57–60)*. The antiapoptotic Bcl-2 family proteins, in turn, are suppressed by BH3-only proteins such as BAD that heterodimerize with a death suppressor such as Bcl-2 and Bcl-xL *(11,35,39,46)*.

Although the extrinsic and intrinsic apoptosis pathways can function independent of each other, there is a crosstalk between the two pathways. The link is provided by caspase-8-mediated cleavage of Bid, a pro-apoptotic member of the Bcl-2 family *(18,58)*. Upon cleavage by caspase-8, truncated Bid (tBid) translocates to the mitochondria, where it promotes the release of cytochrome-*c* and, probably, other apoptotic proteins by activation of Bax and Bak *(61)*. Both pathways converge at the level of caspase-3 activation. Apoptotic activity of caspase-3, caspase-7 and caspase-9 are negatively regulated by IAP (inhibitor of apoptosis protein) family proteins *(62–64)*, which, in turn, are inhibited by Smac (second mitochondria-derived activator of caspases)/DIABLO (direct IAP-binding protein with low pI), a protein that is released from mitochondria *(64,65)*. The PI3K (phosphatidylinositol-3-kinase)-AKT (PKB) pathway and nuclear factor-κB (NF-κB) play an important role in the regulation of growth factor receptor-mediated apoptosis. The activated Akt can inhibit apoptosis by phosphorylation and inactivation of pro-apoptotic protein BAD, as well as caspase-9 *(66,67)* The NF-κB suppresses apoptosis via increased transcription of certain IAP family genes and some antiapoptotic Bcl-2 family genes *(68)*.

In mammalian cells, caspase-independent apoptotic DNA fragmentation and chromatin condensation has been attributed to two proteins (endonuclease G and apoptosis-inducing factor [AIF]) that translocates to the nucleus upon release from mitochondria *(69–73)*. The precise mechanism by which these two proteins induce DNA degradation is not fully understood. Additionally, AIF has been implicated in the regulation of mitochondrial membrane permeability promoting apoptosis *(74)*.

## 3. APOPTOSIS REGULATORS

### *3.1. Fas (APO1; CD95)*

Fas (CD95) and Fas-ligand (FasL/CD95L), like most TNF family members, are trimers *(75)*. Two isoforms of Fas proteins are produced as a result of an alternative mRNA splicing of FAS gene: the full-length Fas and the soluble Fas *(76,77)*. Full-length Fas, possessing the transmembrane domain, is the initiator of the receptor-mediated apoptotic pathway. On the other hand, the soluble form of Fas lacks this transmembrane domain and is secreted in the extracellular environment, where it acts as a decoy and binds FasL, thus acting as an inhibitor of apoptosis. Somatic mutations in the *FAS* gene have been found in multiple myelomas *(78)* and a broad range of lymphomas, including non-Hodgkin's lymphomas *(79)*, which has been implicated in the dominant-negative effect on wild-type Fas. Downregulation of the receptors and defects in the apoptotic signaling pathway have also been implicated as a possible mechanism of apoptosis avoidance in tumors *(80,81)*. Although Fas expression has no correlation with patient survival, increased levels of soluble Fas in serum were associated with reduced patient survival *(82)*. Therapeutic approaches involving use of recombinant TNF or CD95L failed in preclinical studies because of the lethal vascular inflammatory syndrome that resembles septic shock and lethal liver toxicity, respectively, in mice *(83)*.

### *3.2. TNF Receptors and TRAIL (Apo-2L)*

TRAIL is an apoptosis-inducing member of the TNF gene superfamily *(84)*. TRAIL-induced apoptosis is signaled through its interaction with two receptors, DR4/TRAIL-R1 and DR5/TRAIL-R2/Apo2/TRICK2/Killer, which contain cytoplasmic death domains *(85–88)*. However, two decoy receptors, DR1/TRAIL-R3/TRID and DR2/TRAIL-R4/TRUNDD, without a functional death domain can function as a ligand sink to prevent TRAIL-induced apoptosis *(89,90)*. TRAIL and its receptors are broadly expressed in most tissues *(91,92)*. Most of the cancer cell lines derived from breast, colon, lung, brain, skin, and kidney tumors are sensitive to TRAIL, whereas most normal cells are relatively resistant to TRAIL *(93)*. Although the precise mechanism of the differential sensitivity has yet to be elucidated *(94,95)* TRAIL has generated tremendous interest from biotech and pharmaceutical industries to develop a cancer therapeutic that can selectively eliminate cancer cells without affecting normal cells. Several lines of preclinical studies involving human xenograft tumors in mice have reported potent antitumor activity of recombinant TRAIL *(96,97)*. Importantly, in these studies, animals were free from hepatotoxicity or septic shock that has prevented further testing of TNF and CD95. Preclinical safety studies in cynomolgus monkeys also did not show adverse reactions to substantial doses of recombinant human TRAIL (10 mg/kg administered once daily for 7 d) *(97)*. One of the most exciting features of TRAIL therapy is the strong positive interaction effect of TRAIL with chemotherapeutic agents or ionizing radiation. TRAIL treatment has been shown to sensitize tumor cells derived from acute leukemia, breast cancer, lung cancer, colon cancer, prostate cancer, and melanoma to chemotherapeutic agents *(98–105)*. In an in vitro setting, TRAIL has been shown to induce apoptosis in normal primary hepatocytes *(106)*. In light of this observation, it remains to be seen whether TRAIL therapy offers a margin of safety in humans, as is seen in mice and monkeys.

### 3.3. Bcl-2

Bcl-2 (B-cell lymphoma gene-2), the first apoptosis inhibitor to be discovered as a proto-oncogene, is the most studied molecule of the Bcl-2 family of proteins in the apoptotic pathway *(58,107–109)*. The gene was cloned from the breakpoint of the t(14;18) translocation in low-grade B-cell lymphoma, where it is juxtaposed to the immunoglobulin heavy-chain gene *(58,110)*. Bcl-2 is constitutively expressed as a result of the chromosomal translocation and promotes cell survival by inhibiting the induction of apoptosis *(58)*. Although the precise mechanism by which Bcl-2 inhibits apoptosis can be debated in a review of its own, the most prevalent and accepted theory is that the chief function of Bcl-2 is to regulate release of cytochrome-*c* from the mitochondria by affecting the mitochondrial membrane permeability *(58)*. Abnormal expression of Bcl-2 has been reported in number hematological malignancies, including acute myeloid leukemia (AML), acute lymphocytic leukemia (ALL), multiple myeloma (MM), B-cell chronic lymphocytic leukemia (B-CLL), and other hematological malignancies *(111–113)*. Additionally, Bcl-2 is highly expressed in a number of solid tumors, including lung, breast, colon, head and neck, prostate, cervix, skin, and others, making it a widespread aberration in many types of human cancer *(58)*. Several lines of in vitro experiments provide evidence that Bcl-2 protects cells from apoptosis induced by activated oncogenes, transforming viral proteins, chemotherapeutic agents, ionizing radiation, and growth factor withdrawals *(34,107,114–118)*. Considering overexpression of Bcl-2 at a high frequency in a broad range of cancers, correlation of Bcl-2 expression with treatment outcome has proven unpredictable.

In the absence of a precise understanding of how Bcl-2 imparts its antiapoptotic function and inherent difficulties associated with targeting protein–protein interactions, discovery of small molecules targeting the Bcl-2 function has remained a challenging task for the pharmaceutical industries. Approaches utilizing crystallography data to develop lead molecules targeting Bcl-2 function through binding to BH3 domain has been less than fruitful in to developing clinical candidates *(119–124)*.

An alternative approach of inhibiting Bcl-2 expression utilizing antisense has been the logical choice and has made significant progress of possibly making it a first antisense drug for cancer therapy *(125)*. G-3139 (Genasense) is the 18-mer antisense first-generation oligonucleotide with a phosphorothioate backbone and is designed to specifically target mRNA coding for first six amino acids of the human Bcl-2 open reading frame. In a series of preclinical animal studies employing human xenograft tumors, G-3139 significantly inhibited tumor growth when infused either as a single agent or in combination with cyclophosphamide (Cytoxan), docetaxel (Taxotere), or dacarbazine (DTIC). Data emerging from clinical evaluation in phase I/IIa and phase III studies have been encouraging. In a phase I study involving 14-d continuous infusion to 21 patients with relapsed non-Hodgkin's lymphoma, disease stabilization was observed in 43% of patients and improvements were seen in 14%, including 1 complete response *(126,127)*. Clear antitumor response was also seen in 43% of melanoma patients. Tumor biopsies from a few patients had reduced level of Bcl-2 protein and increased apoptosis *(125,128)*. G-3139 has shown good safety profiles in a number of clinical studies, with minor toxicity associated with antisense oligonucleotide chemistry, restricted to <20% of patients *(127,128)*. Several additional clinical trials are ongoing to evaluate efficacy of G-3139 in combination with conventional chemotherapeutics, including cyclophosphamide for lymphomas, mitoxan-trone for hormone-independent prostate cancer, irinotecan for colorectal cancer, paclitaxel for small cell lung cancer, docetaxel for breast cancer, and fludaribine and cytosine arab-inoside for acute leukemia (http://www.genta.com). A recently released analysis of phase III data involving 771 patients with malignant melanoma showed that treatment with G-3139 in combination with dacarbazine resulted in a median survival of 9.1 mo, compared with 7.9 mo for patients treated with dacarbazine alone. Although this was not statistically significant, there was significant increase in median progression-free survival to 78 d and antitumor response rate of 11.7%, compared with 49 d and 6.8%, respectively, for patients treated with dacarbazine alone (http://www.genta.com). The Food and Drug Administration (FDA) under priority review status is reviewing the proposed use of G-3139 in combination with dacarbazine for the treatment of patients with advanced melanoma.

### *3.4. XIAP*

The IAP family proteins consist of apoptosis suppressors that are evolutionary conserved *(62,63)*. Members of the IAP family of proteins contain one to three BIR (baculovirus IAP repeat) domains, which are reported to be important for their antiapoptotic function *(62,129)*. To date, sequencing of the human genome has identified eight IAP-encoding genes, which contains at least one BIR domain *(130)*. Most IAP family proteins inhibit apoptosis through direct interaction of the BIR3 domain and flanking region with caspase-9 and/or of the BIR2 domain and flanking region with active caspase-3 and caspase-7 *(131–134)*. XIAP is the best characterized and most potent of the IAP family members in terms of its caspase-inhibitory mechanism. IAP activity is negatively regulated by mitochondrial protein Smac/DIABLO, a homolog of the *Drosophilae* proteins *Reaper*, *Hid*, and *Grim (65,135)*. Once released from mitochondria, it binds to the BIR domain of XIAP, thus facilitating caspase activation *(70–72)*. Additionally, OMI/HTRA2, a newly discovered mitochondrial protein, also regulates IAP activity. Once released from mitochondria, it interacts with IAPs and relieves caspases from XIAP-mediated inhibition, thus modulating cleavage activity of caspases *(70–72)*. HTRA2 can also provide the pro-apototic function through its serine protease activity *(136)*.

Deregulated expression of XIAP has been reported in many acute and chronic leukemias, prostate cancers, lung cancers, and other types of tumor *(130,137–141)*. Several experimental approaches utilizing antisense oligonucleotides or peptide inhibitors targeting BIR domains have suggested that IAPs are important for maintaining tumor cell survival or for conferring resistance to apoptosis induced by known chemotherapeutic agents *(142–145)*. An antisense molecule targeting XIAP has shown antitumor activity in human xenograft models of the lung, prostate, breast, colon, and ovarian *(146)*. The lead antisense molecule AEG35156/GEM®640 is being evaluated in a phase I clinical trial (http://www.aegera.com). Most recently, Reed and colleagues screened approximately 1 million compounds for their ability to inhibit binding of XIAP to caspases *(147)*. This screening effort identified eight polyphenylurea-based molecules that bind to the

BIR2 domain of XIAP. In an in vitro experimental system, the most active of these compounds induced apoptosis in 60 cell lines and primary AML cells with little toxicity to normal cells. These compounds also sensitized tumor cells to the conventional chemotherapeutic agents, including etoposide (VP16), paclitaxel, and doxorubicine and biologic molecules such as TRAIL. Selected active compounds showed antitumor activity in a human colon and prostate xenograft models in mice while producing little toxicity to normal tissue *(147)*. Discovery of these XIAP antagonists raises the possibility of developing more potent molecules to justify clinical evaluation.

### *3.5. Survivin*

Survivin, a smallest member of the IAP family of proteins with a single BIR domain and carboxyl terminal α-helix, is perhaps one of the most prominent proteins associated with a wide variety of cancers and has attracted significant attention in recent years *(148)*. Survivin expression is cell cycle regulated with peak expression in the G2/M-phase and it localizes to various components of mitotic apparatus *(149–151)*. Immunofluorescence and confocal microscopy techniques demonstrated that survivin localizes to kinetochores and centrosomes (microtubule-organizing centers) during prophase, spindle microtubules during metaphase, central spindle midzone during anaphase, and midbodies during late telophase *(149,151–153)*. One of the most exciting and attractive features of survivin is its abnormal overexpression in a vast majority of cancers, but not in normal, terminally differentiated tissues *(150,152)*. Survivin is strongly and broadly expressed in embryonic and fetal tissues *(148,152,154,155)*; however, it is undetectable in most terminally differentiated tissues *(148)* except in thymus, testis, angiogenic endothelium, and intestinal crypt cells *(148,156)*. Several lines of experimental evidence have elegantly demonstrated the role of survivin in the regulation of apoptosis *(149, 150, 152, 153, 157–160)*. However, the precise mechanism by which survivin inhibits apoptosis is not very clear *(152,158)*. Retrospective analysis of clinical samples has provided strong evidence that survivin expression predicts a reduced apoptotic index in tumors and poor patient survival *(150,152)*. Because of its differential expression in tumors vs normal tissues and its role in apoptosis for maintaining cell viability, survivin represents a promising drug target for cancer therapy. Several in vitro and in vivo studies demonstrated T-cell-mediated cytolytic response against survivin peptides *(161)*. Furthermore, the presence of human leukocyte antigen (HLA) class I-restricted cytolytic T-cells against survivin peptides have been detected in breast cancer, melanoma, and leukemia patients *(162,163)*. Thus, an immunotherapy approach employing use of survivin peptide-specific cytolytic T-cells could offer therapeutic benefits.

Antisense molecules have also been used to inhibit survivin function in cancer cells *(151,164–167)* and perhaps provide the best approach to target survivin. We have identified the potent antisense molecule (LY2181308) against survivin that showed a broad spectrum of activity in multiple tumor cells lines *(167)*. LY2181308 is the second-generation antisense oligonucleotide that contains the phosphorothioate backbone plus the addition of 2'O-methoxyethyl (2' MOE) modification of the ribose. This second-generation chemistry offers significant advantage over all phosphorothioate backbone first-generation chemistry, including increased potency because of increased affinity to mRNA, increased stability, and reduced toxicity. In a sequence-specific and a concentration-dependent manner, LY2181308 induced caspase-3-dependent apoptosis, arrested cells in the G2/M-phase of the cells cycle, and produced multinucleated cells. Importantly, in human xenograft models, LY2181308 inhibited survivin expression in tumors that was associated with significant antitumor activity *(167)*. Based on these promising preclinical results, LY2181308 is being developed for the phase I clinical evaluation.

### 3.6. NF-κB

Nuclear factor-κB represents a family of transcription factors, belonging to the REL gene family. NF-κB exists either as a heterodimers comprising of p50 (NF-κB1) and p65 (RelA) or p52 (NF-κB2), RelB, and c-Rel, or as a homodimers. NFκB is an important transcription factor that directly binds to the promoters and regulates the expression of several antiapoptosis genes, including Bcl-2, Bcl-X, cIAP1, cIAP2, TRAF-1, TRAF-2, and c-FLIP *(168,169)*. In the cytoplasm, NF-κB is in an inactive form through its association with one of several inhibitory molecules, including IκBα, IκBβ, IκBε, p105, and p100. Once activated through external stimuli such as tumor necrosis factor (TNF-α), IκB is phosphorylated at two specific serine residues *(170)* by protein kinase complex consisting of two catalytic subunits IKKα (IKK1) and IKKβ (IKK2) and a regulatory subunit IKKγ (NEMO) *(68,168,171,172)*. This phosphorylation results in a 26S proteosome-mediated complete degradation of IκB *(173)* or partial degradation of the C-termini of p105 and p100 precursors, enabling the translocation of free NF-κB dimers to the nucleus, where it activates the transcription of target genes. Thus inhibition of NF-κB activity by targeting components of NF-κB pathway could restore the apoptosis pathway and provide therapeutic benefits.

### 3.7. PI3K and AKT

Phosphatidylinositol-3 kinases (PI3K) belong to a family of lipid kinase that has the ability to phosphorylate the inositol ring 3'-OH group in inositol phospholipids. Class I PI3Ks are heterodimers composed of a catalytic subunit (p110) and an adaptor/regulatory subunit (p85). This class is further divided into the subclass IA, which is activated by receptor protein tyrosine kinase (RTPK), and subclass IB, which is activated by G protein-coupled receptors *(66,67)*. AKT (PKB) is a cellular homolog of the transforming viral oncogene v-Akt and bears significant homology to PKA and PKC *(174)*. AKT (PKB), a serine/threonine kinase and a cellular homolog of the transforming viral oncogene v-Akt *(175)*, plays a central role in linking growth factor receptors and oncoproteins to apoptosis pathways *(176)*. In humans, there are three *AKT* genes: *AKT1*, *AKT2*, and *AKT3*. AKT family proteins contain an amino-terminus pleckstrin homology (PH) domain, which mediates lipid–protein and/or protein–protein interactions, a central catalytic domain, and a carboxyl terminus hydrophobic and proline-rich regulatory domain *(67,176)*. In cells, AKT is activated upon binding of the membrane phospholipids phosphatidylinositol 3,4,5-trisphosphate [PtdIns $(3,4,5)P_3$] and phosphatidylinositol 3,4 bisphosphate [PtdIns $(3,4)P_2$] that are generated by activated PI3K in response to growth factors stimulation, to its regulatory PH domain *(67,176)*. Binding of this second-messenger lipids results in recruitment of Akt to the inner surface of the plasma membrane, where it becomes activated by phosphorylation on residues Thr[308] and Ser[473] *(177)*. Among the downstream targets of Akt are included, the Forkhead transcription factor, NF-κB, Bad, glycogen synthase kinase-3 (GSK-3), cyclic AMP response element-binding protein (CREB), caspase-9, mammalian target of rapamycin (mTOR), insulin receptor substrate-1 (IRS-1), phospho-diesterase-3B (PDE-3B), and the cyclin-dependent kinase (CDK) inhibitor p21[waf1/cip1] *(67, 176)*. Thus, the PI3K/AKT pathway plays a critical role in cell cycle, cell proliferation, and cell survival. PTEN (phosphatase and tensin homolog deleted on chromosome 10), originally identified as a tumor suppressor, is a phosphatase with dual activity on lipids and proteins. PTEN act as a negative regulator of PI3K-induced signaling by dephosphorylation of PtdIns $(3,4,5)P_3$ at the 3' inositol position. PTEN is frequently mutated in the advance stages of human malignancies, notably glioblastoma, non-Hodgkin's lymphoma, multiple myeloma, and endometrial and prostate cancers *(67,178)*. Thus, loss of PTEN activity results into constitutive activation of the PI3K/Akt pathway. Aberrant Akt expression and activity have been reported in a number of malignancies either through amplification of Akt or PI3K or deregulated signaling of PI3K/Akt *(179)*. Various studies have found Akt, particularly Akt2, gene amplifications in pancreas, ovarian, breast, and stomach malignant tumors *(174,180)*. PI3K gene amplification has been reported in number of malignancies, including ovarian and cervix cancer *(181,182)*. Thus, the PI3K/AKT/PTEN pathway is an attractive target for drug development. An inhibitor of this pathway might inhibit proliferation and reverse the repression of apoptosis and the resistance to cytotoxic therapy in cancer cells.

## 4. FUTURE PROSPECTS

The goal of most traditional cancer therapies, including radiation, chemotherapy, and immunotherapy, is the reduction or elimination of cancer cells—but at the cost of significant toxicity. Approaches to resensitize cancer cells to apoptosis represent an important future strategy for cancer treatment, which include restoring lost apoptosis intermediates, inactivating antiapoptotic proteins, triggering apoptosis pathways that remain intact in cancer cells, and inducing apoptosis by targeting specific tumorigenic lesions. As reviewed here, insight into the molecular mechanisms of apoptosis has already led to a surge in research to identify novel targets and strategies that can be explored to develop cancer therapeutics. Additionally, rational drug design opens the door to highly specific therapies with fewer adverse effects. Although these are still early days in the "Omics" science (genomics, proteomics, pharmacogenomics, etc.), these global efforts will contribute significantly to our understanding of different pathways, including apoptosis and key players involved, and might help determine whether a tumor will benefit from induction of apoptosis. Thus, a molecular understanding of apoptosis and its regulation in both normal and cancer cells might contribute significantly to the discovery of improved cancer therapeutics.

## ACKNOWLEDGMENT

I acknowledge and apologize to all those whose contributions to the field were not directly referenced here.

## REFERENCES

1. Kerr JF, Wyllie AH, Currie AR. Apoptosis: a basic biological phenomenon with wide-ranging implications in tissue kinetics. Br J Cancer 1972; 26:239–257.
2. Danial NN, Korsmeyer SJ. Cell death: critical control points. Cell 2004; 116:205–219.
3. Vaux DL, Flavell RA. Apoptosis genes and autoimmunity. Curr Opin Immunol 2000; 12:719–724.
4. Jacobson MD, Weil M, Raff MC. Programmed cell death in animal development. Cell 1997; 88: 347–354.
5. Steller H. Mechanisms and genes of cellular suicide. Science 1995; 267:1445–1449.
6. Horvitz HR. Nobel lecture. Worms, life and death. Biosci Rep 2003; 23:239–303.
7. Hengartner MO. Programmed cell death in invertebrates. Curr Opin Genet Dev 1996; 6:34–38.

8. White E. Life, death, and the pursuit of apoptosis. Genes Dev 1996; 10:1–15.
9. Majno G, Joris I. Apoptosis, oncosis, and necrosis. An overview of cell death. Am J Pathol 1995; 146: 3–15.
10. Vaux DL, Haecker G, Strasser A. An evolutionary perspective on apoptosis. Cell 1994; 76:777–779.
11. Green DR, Reed JC. Mitochondria and apoptosis. Science 1998; 281:1309–1312.
12. Alnemri ES. Mammalian cell death proteases: a family of highly conserved aspartate specific cysteine proteases. J Cell Biochem 1997; 64:33–42.
13. Patel T, Gores GJ, Kaufmann SH. The role of proteases during apoptosis. FASEB J 1996; 10:587–597.
14. Cryns V, Yuan J. Proteases to die for. Genes Dev 1998; 12:1551–1570.
15. Thornberry NA. Caspases: key mediators of apoptosis. Chem Biol 1998; 5:R97–R103.
16. Thornberry NA, Lazebnik Y. Caspases: enemies within. Science 1998; 281:1312–1316.
17. Salvesen GS, Dixit VM. Caspase activation: the induced-proximity model. Proc Natl Acad Sci USA 1999; 96:10,964–10,967.
18. Reed JC. Mechanisms of apoptosis. Am J Pathol 2000; 157:1415–1430.
19. Villa P, Kaufmann SH, Earnshaw WC. Caspases and caspase inhibitors. Trends Biochem Sci 1997; 22:388–393.
20. Reed JC, Tomaselli KJ. Drug discovery opportunities from apoptosis research. Curr Opin Biotechnol 2000; 11:586–592.
21. Bellamy CO, Malcomson RD, Harrison DJ, Wyllie AH. Cell death in health and disease: the biology and regulation of apoptosis. Semin Cancer Biol 1995; 6:3–16.
22. Thompson CB. Apoptosis in the pathogenesis and treatment of disease. Science 1995; 267:1456–1462.
23. Wyllie AH, Kerr JF, Currie AR. Cell death: the significance of apoptosis. Int Rev Cytol 1980; 68: 251–306.
24. Jaattela M. Escaping cell death: survival proteins in cancer. Exp Cell Res 1999; 248:30–43.
25. Jaattela M. Multiple cell death pathways as regulators of tumour initiation and progression. Oncogene 2004; 23:2746–2756.
26. Sen S, D'Incalci M. Apoptosis. Biochemical events and relevance to cancer chemotherapy. FEBS Lett 1992; 307:122–127.
27. McDonnell TJ, Meyn RE, Robertson LE. Implications of apoptotic cell death regulation in cancer therapy. Semin Cancer Biol 1995; 6:53–60.
28. Kerr JF, Winterford CM, Harmon BV. Apoptosis. Its significance in cancer and cancer therapy. Cancer 1994; 73:2013–2026.
29. Martin DS, Schwartz GK. Chemotherapeutically induced DNA damage, ATP depletion, and the apoptotic biochemical cascade. Oncol Res 1997; 9:1–5.
30. Reed JC, Miyashita T, Takayama S, et al. BCL-2 family proteins: regulators of cell death involved in the pathogenesis of cancer and resistance to therapy. J Cell Biochem 1996; 60:23–32.
31. Meyn RE, Milas L, Stephens LC. Apoptosis in tumor biology and therapy. Adv Exp Med Biol 1997; 400B:657–667.
32. Meyn RE, Stephens LC, Milas L. Programmed cell death and radioresistance. Cancer Metastasis Rev 1996; 15:119–131.
33. Milas L, Stephens LC, Meyn RE. Relation of apoptosis to cancer therapy. In Vivo 1994; 8:665–673.
34. Reed JC. Bcl-2 family proteins: regulators of chemoresistance in cancer. Toxicol Lett 1995; 82–83: 155–158.
35. Reed JC. Regulation of apoptosis by bcl-2 family proteins and its role in cancer and chemoresistance. Curr Opin Oncol 1995; 7:541–546.
36. Reed JC. Bcl-2: prevention of apoptosis as a mechanism of drug resistance. Hematol Oncol Clin North Am 1995; 9:451–473.
37. Hannun YA. Apoptosis and the dilemma of cancer chemotherapy. Blood 1997; 89:1845–1853.
38. Hickman JA. Apoptosis and chemotherapy resistance. Eur J Cancer 1996; 32A:921–926.
39. Hengartner MO. The biochemistry of apoptosis. Nature 2000; 407:770–776.
40. Gupta S. Molecular steps of death receptor and mitochondrial pathways of apoptosis. Life Sci 2001; 69:2957–2964.
41. Gupta S. Molecular signaling in death receptor and mitochondrial pathways of apoptosis [review]. Int J Oncol 2003; 22:15–20.
42. Zamzami N, Kroemer G. The mitochondrion in apoptosis: how Pandora's box opens. Nature Rev Mol Cell Biol 2001; 2:67–71.

43. Green DR, Evan GI. A matter of life and death. Cancer Cell 2002; 1:19–30.
44. Ashkenazi A, Dixit VM. Apoptosis control by death and decoy receptors. Curr Opin Cell Biol 1999; 11:255–260.
45. Ashkenazi A, Dixit VM. Death receptors: signaling and modulation. Science 1998; 281:1305–1308.
46. Kroemer G, Reed JC. Mitochondrial control of cell death. Nature Med 2000; 6:513–519.
47. Martinou JC, Green DR. Breaking the mitochondrial barrier. Nature Rev Mol Cell Biol 2001; 2:63–67.
48. Scaffidi C, Fulda S, Srinivasan A, et al. Two CD95 (APO-1/Fas) signaling pathways. EMBO J 1998; 17:1675–1687.
49. Wallach D. Apoptosis. Placing death under control. Nature 1997; 388:123–126.
50. Wallach D, Boldin M, Varfolomeev E, Beyaert R, Vandenabeele P, Fiers W. Cell death induction by receptors of the TNF family: towards a molecular understanding. FEBS Lett 1997; 410:96–106.
51. Yuan J. Transducing signals of life and death. Curr Opin Cell Biol 1997; 9:247–251.
52. Peter ME, Krammer PH. The CD95(APO-1/Fas) DISC and beyond. Cell Death Differ 2003; 10:26–35.
53. Medema JP, Scaffidi C, Kischkel FC, et al. FLICE is activated by association with the CD95 death-inducing signaling complex (DISC). EMBO J 1997; 16:2794–2804.
54. Jaattela M. Programmed cell death: many ways for cells to die decently. Ann Med 2002; 34:480–488.
55. Park SJ, Kim YY, Ju JW, Han BG, Park SI, Park BJ. Alternative splicing variants of c-FLIP transduce the differential signal through the Raf or TRAF2 in TNF-induced cell proliferation. Biochem Biophys Res Commun 2001; 289:1205–1210.
56. Li P, Nijhawan D, Budihardjo I, et al. Cytochrome c and dATP-dependent formation of Apaf-1/caspase-9 complex initiates an apoptotic protease cascade. Cell 1997; 91:479–489.
57. Kluck RM, Bossy-Wetzel E, Green DR, Newmeyer DD. The release of cytochrome c from mitochondria: a primary site for Bcl-2 regulation of apoptosis. Science 1997; 275:1132–1136.
58. Reed JC. Bcl-2 family proteins. Oncogene 1998; 17:3225–3236.
59. Reed JC, Jurgensmeier JM, Matsuyama S. Bcl-2 family proteins and mitochondria. Biochim Biophys Acta 1998; 1366:127–137.
60. Reed JC. Double identity for proteins of the Bcl-2 family. Nature 1997; 387:773–776.
61. Wei MC, Zong WX, Cheng EH, et al. Proapoptotic BAX and BAK: a requisite gateway to mitochondrial dysfunction and death. Science 2001; 292:727–730.
62. Deveraux QL, Reed JC. IAP family proteins—suppressors of apoptosis. Genes Dev 1999; 13:239–252.
63. Deveraux QL, Stennicke HR, Salvesen GS, Reed JC. Endogenous inhibitors of caspases. J Clin Immunol 1999; 19:388–398.
64. Verhagen AM, Ekert PG, Pakusch M, et al. Identification of DIABLO, a mammalian protein that promotes apoptosis by binding to and antagonizing IAP proteins. Cell 2000; 102:43–53.
65. Du C, Fang M, Li Y, Li L, Wang X. Smac, a mitochondrial protein that promotes cytochrome c-dependent caspase activation by eliminating IAP inhibition. Cell 2000; 102:33–42.
66. Blume-Jensen P, Janknecht R, Hunter T. The kit receptor promotes cell survival via activation of PI 3-kinase and subsequent Akt-mediated phosphorylation of Bad on Ser136. Curr Biol 1998; 8:779–782.
67. Blume-Jensen P, Hunter T. Oncogenic kinase signalling. Nature 2001; 411:355–365.
68. Karin M, Lin A. NF-kappaB at the crossroads of life and death. Nature Immunol 2002; 3:221–227.
69. Srinivasula SM, Gupta S, Datta P, et al. Inhibitor of apoptosis proteins are substrates for the mitochondrial serine protease Omi/HtrA2. J Biol Chem 2003; 278:31,469–31,472.
70. Hegde R, Srinivasula SM, Zhang Z, et al. Identification of Omi/HtrA2 as a mitochondrial apoptotic serine protease that disrupts inhibitor of apoptosis protein-caspase interaction. J Biol Chem 2002; 277: 432–438.
71. Suzuki Y, Takahashi-Niki K, Akagi T, Hashikawa T, Takahashi R. Mitochondrial protease Omi/HtrA2 enhances caspase activation through multiple pathways. Cell Death Differ 2004; 11:208–216.
72. Suzuki Y, Imai Y, Nakayama H, Takahashi K, Takio K, Takahashi R. A serine protease, HtrA2, is released from the mitochondria and interacts with XIAP, inducing cell death. Mol Cell 2001; 8:613–621.
73. Li LY, Luo X, Wang X. Endonuclease G is an apoptotic DNase when released from mitochondria. Nature 2001; 412:95–99.
74. Lipton SA, Bossy-Wetzel E. Dueling activities of AIF in cell death versus survival: DNA binding and redox activity. Cell 2002; 111:147–150.
75. Locksley RM, Killeen N, Lenardo MJ. The TNF and TNF receptor superfamilies: integrating mammalian biology. Cell 2001; 104:487–501.
76. Cheng J, Liu C, Koopman WJ, Mountz JD. Characterization of human Fas gene. Exon/intron organization and promoter region. J Immunol 1995; 154:1239–1245.

77. Cheng J, Zhou T, Liu C, et al. Protection from Fas-mediated apoptosis by a soluble form of the Fas molecule. Science 1994; 263:1759–1762.

78. Landowski TH, Qu N, Buyuksal I, Painter JS, Dalton WS. Mutations in the Fas antigen in patients with multiple myeloma. Blood 1997; 90:4266–4270.

79. Gronbaek K, Straten PT, Ralfkiaer E, et al. Somatic Fas mutations in non-Hodgkin's lymphoma: association with extranodal disease and autoimmunity. Blood 1998; 92:3018–3024.

80. Yanagisawa J, Takahashi M, Kanki H, et al. The molecular interaction of Fas and FAP-1. A tripeptide blocker of human Fas interaction with FAP-1 promotes Fas-induced apoptosis. J Biol Chem 1997; 272: 8539–8545.

81. Hitoshi Y, Lorens J, Kitada SI, et al. Toso, a cell surface, specific regulator of Fas-induced apoptosis in T cells. Immunity 1998; 8:461–471.

82. Kamihira S, Yamada Y, Tomonaga M, Sugahara K, Tsuruda K. Discrepant expression of membrane and soluble isoforms of Fas (CD95/APO-1) in adult T-cell leukaemia: soluble Fas isoform is an independent risk factor for prognosis. Br J Haematol 1999; 107:851–860.

83. Nagata S. Apoptosis by death factor. Cell 1997; 88:355–365.

84. Wiley SR, Schooley K, Smolak PJ, et al. Identification and characterization of a new member of the TNF family that induces apoptosis. Immunity 1995; 3:673–682.

85. Marsters SA, Pitti RA, Sheridan JP, Ashkenazi A. Control of apoptosis signaling by Apo2 ligand. Recent Prog Horm Res 1999; 54:225–234.

86. Marsters SA, Pitti RM, Donahue CJ, Ruppert S, Bauer KD, Ashkenazi A. Activation of apoptosis by Apo-2 ligand is independent of FADD but blocked by CrmA. Curr Biol 1996; 6:750–752.

87. Marsters SA, Sheridan JP, Pitti RM, et al. A novel receptor for Apo2L/TRAIL contains a truncated death domain. Curr Biol 1997; 7:1003–1006.

88. Pitti RM, Marsters SA, Ruppert S, Donahue CJ, Moore A, Ashkenazi A. Induction of apoptosis by Apo-2 ligand, a new member of the tumor necrosis factor cytokine family. J Biol Chem 1996; 271:12,687–12,690.

89. Baetu TM, Hiscott J. On the TRAIL to apoptosis. Cytokine Growth Factor Rev 2002; 13:199–207.

90. LeBlanc HN, Ashkenazi A. Apo2L/TRAIL and its death and decoy receptors. Cell Death Differ 2003; 10:66–75.

91. Screaton GR, Mongkolsapaya J, Xu XN, Cowper AE, McMichael AJ, Bell JI. TRICK2, a new alternatively spliced receptor that transduces the cytotoxic signal from TRAIL. Curr Biol 1997; 7:693–696.

92. Martinez-Lorenzo MJ, Alava MA, Gamen S, et al. Involvement of APO2 ligand/TRAIL in activation-induced death of Jurkat and human peripheral blood T cells. Eur J Immunol 1998; 28:2714–2725.

93. Kim CH, Gupta S. Expression of TRAIL (Apo2L), DR4 (TRAIL receptor 1), DR5 (TRAIL receptor 2) and TRID (TRAIL receptor 3) genes in multidrug resistant human acute myeloid leukemia cell lines that overexpress MDR 1 (HL60/Tax) or MRP (HL60/AR). Int J Oncol 2000; 16:1137–1139.

94. Griffith TS, Chin WA, Jackson GC, Lynch DH, Kubin MZ. Intracellular regulation of TRAIL-induced apoptosis in human melanoma cells. J Immunol 1998; 161:2833–2840.

95. Zhang XD, Nguyen T, Thomas WD, Sanders JE, Hersey P. Mechanisms of resistance of normal cells to TRAIL induced apoptosis vary between different cell types. FEBS Lett 2000; 482:193–199.

96. Walczak H, Miller RE, Ariail K, et al. Tumoricidal activity of tumor necrosis factor-related apoptosis-inducing ligand in vivo. Nature Med 1999; 5:157–163.

97. Ashkenazi A, Pai RC, Fong S, et al. Safety and antitumor activity of recombinant soluble Apo2 ligand. J Clin Invest 1999; 104:155–162.

98. Mori S, Murakami-Mori K, Nakamura S, Ashkenazi A, Bonavida B. Sensitization of AIDS–Kaposi's sarcoma cells to Apo-2 ligand-induced apoptosis by actinomycin D. J Immunol 1999; 162:5616–5623.

99. Wen J, Ramadevi N, Nguyen D, Perkins C, Worthington E, Bhalla K. Antileukemic drugs increase death receptor 5 levels and enhance Apo-2L-induced apoptosis of human acute leukemia cells. Blood 2000; 96:3900–3906.

100. Hernandez A, Wang QD, Schwartz SA, Evers BM. Sensitization of human colon cancer cells to TRAIL-mediated apoptosis. J Gastrointest Surg 2001; 5:56–65.

101. Keane MM, Ettenberg SA, Nau MM, Russell EK, Lipkowitz S. Chemotherapy augments TRAIL-induced apoptosis in breast cell lines. Cancer Res 1999; 59:734–741.

102. Sun SY, Yue P, Hong WK, Lotan R. Augmentation of tumor necrosis factor-related apoptosis-inducing ligand (TRAIL)-induced apoptosis by the synthetic retinoid 6-[3-(1-adamantyl)-4-hydroxyphenyl]-2-naphthalene carboxylic acid (CD437) through up-regulation of TRAIL receptors in human lung cancer cells. Cancer Res 2000; 60:7149–7155.

103. Griffith TS, Lynch DH. TRAIL: a molecule with multiple receptors and control mechanisms. Curr Opin Immunol 1998; 10:559–563.
104. Bradbury J. TRAIL leads to apoptosis in acute promyelocytic leukaemia. Lancet 2001; 357:1770.
105. Sun SY, Yue P, Lotan R. Implication of multiple mechanisms in apoptosis induced by the synthetic retinoid CD437 in human prostate carcinoma cells. Oncogene 2000; 19:4513–4522.
106. Jo M, Kim TH, Seol DW, et al. Apoptosis induced in normal human hepatocytes by tumor necrosis factor-related apoptosis-inducing ligand. Nature Med 2000; 6:564–567.
107. Miyashita T, Reed JC. Bcl-2 oncoprotein blocks chemotherapy-induced apoptosis in a human leukemia cell line. Blood 1993; 81:151–157.
108. Adams JM, Cory S. The Bcl-2 protein family: arbiters of cell survival. Science 1998; 281:1322–1326.
109. McDonnell TJ, Deane N, Platt FM, et al. bcl-2-immunoglobulin transgenic mice demonstrate extended B cell survival and follicular lymphoproliferation. Cell 1989; 57:79–88.
110. Gauwerky CE, Hoxie J, Nowell PC, Croce CM. Pre-B-cell leukemia with a t(8; 14) and a t(14; 18) translocation is preceded by follicular lymphoma. Oncogene 1988; 2:431–435.
111. Campos L, Rouault JP, Sabido O, et al. High expression of bcl-2 protein in acute myeloid leukemia cells is associated with poor response to chemotherapy. Blood 1993; 81:3091–3096.
112. Pepper C, Bentley P, Hoy T. Regulation of clinical chemoresistance by bcl-2 and bax oncoproteins in B-cell chronic lymphocytic leukaemia. Br J Haematol 1996; 95:513–517.
113. Pepper C, Hoy T, Bentley P. Elevated Bcl-2/Bax are a consistent feature of apoptosis resistance in B-cell chronic lymphocytic leukaemia and are correlated with in vivo chemoresistance. Leuk Lymphoma 1998; 28:355–361.
114. Miyashita T, Reed JC. bcl-2 gene transfer increases relative resistance of S49.1 and WEHI7.2 lymphoid cells to cell death and DNA fragmentation induced by glucocorticoids and multiple chemotherapeutic drugs. Cancer Res 1992; 52:5407–5411.
115. Miyashita T, Krajewski S, Krajewska M, et al. Tumor suppressor p53 is a regulator of bcl-2 and bax gene expression in vitro and in vivo. Oncogene 1994; 9:1799–1805.
116. Delia D, Aiello A, Formelli F, et al. Regulation of apoptosis induced by the retinoid N-(4-hydroxyphenyl) retinamide and effect of deregulated bcl-2. Blood 1995; 85:359–367.
117. Reed JC. Bcl-2 and the regulation of programmed cell death. J Cell Biol 1994; 124:1–6.
118. Tang C, Willingham MC, Reed JC, et al. High levels of p26BCL-2 oncoprotein retard taxol-induced apoptosis in human pre-B leukemia cells. Leukemia 1994; 8:1960–1969.
119. Wang JL, Liu D, Zhang ZJ, et al. Structure-based discovery of an organic compound that binds Bcl-2 protein and induces apoptosis of tumor cells. Proc Natl Acad Sci USA 2000; 97:7124–7129.
120. Enyedy IJ, Ling Y, Nacro K, et al. Discovery of small-molecule inhibitors of Bcl-2 through structure-based computer screening. J Med Chem 2001; 44:4313–4324.
121. Degterev A, Lugovskoy A, Cardone M, et al. Identification of small-molecule inhibitors of interaction between the BH3 domain and Bcl-xL. Nature Cell Biol 2001; 3:173–182.
122. Cochran AG. Antagonists of protein-protein interactions. Chem Biol 2000; 7:R85–R94.
123. Cochran AG. Protein–protein interfaces: mimics and inhibitors. Curr Opin Chem Biol 2001; 5:654–659.
124. Tzung SP, Kim KM, Basanez G, et al. Antimycin A mimics a cell-death-inducing Bcl-2 homology domain 3. Nature Cell Biol 2001; 3:183–191.
125. Banerjee D. Genasense (Genta Inc). Curr Opin Investig Drugs 2001; 2:574–580.
126. Cotter FE, Waters J, Cunningham D. Human Bcl-2 antisense therapy for lymphomas. Biochim Biophys Acta 1999; 1489:97–106.
127. Waters JS, Webb A, Cunningham D, et al. Phase I clinical and pharmacokinetic study of bcl-2 antisense oligonucleotide therapy in patients with non-Hodgkin's lymphoma. J Clin Oncol 2000; 18:1812–1823.
128. Jansen B, Wacheck V, Heere-Ress E, et al. Chemosensitisation of malignant melanoma by BCL2 antisense therapy. Lancet 2000; 356:1728–1733.
129. Fesik SW. Insights into programmed cell death through structural biology. Cell 2000; 103:273–282.
130. Tamm I, Kornblau SM, Segall H, et al. Expression and prognostic significance of IAP-family genes in human cancers and myeloid leukemias. Clin Cancer Res 2000; 6:1796–1803.
131. Takahashi R, Deveraux Q, Tamm I, et al. A single BIR domain of XIAP sufficient for inhibiting caspases. J Biol Chem 1998; 273:7787–7790.
132. Sun C, Cai M, Meadows RP, et al. NMR structure and mutagenesis of the third Bir domain of the inhibitor of apoptosis protein XIAP. J Biol Chem 2000; 275:33,777–33,781.

133. Huang Y, Park YC, Rich RL, Segal D, Myszka DG, Wu H. Structural basis of caspase inhibition by XIAP: differential roles of the linker versus the BIR domain. Cell 2001; 104:781–790.

134. Deveraux QL, Leo E, Stennicke HR, Welsh K, Salvesen GS, Reed JC. Cleavage of human inhibitor of apoptosis protein XIAP results in fragments with distinct specificities for caspases. EMBO J 1999; 18:5242–5251.

135. Ekert PG, Silke J, Hawkins CJ, Verhagen AM, Vaux DL. DIABLO promotes apoptosis by removing MIHA/XIAP from processed caspase 9. J Cell Biol 2001; 152:483–490.

136. Verhagen AM, Silke J, Ekert PG, et al. HtrA2 promotes cell death through its serine protease activity and its ability to antagonize inhibitor of apoptosis proteins. J Biol Chem 2002; 277:445–454.

137. Byrd JC, Kitada S, Flinn IW, et al. The mechanism of tumor cell clearance by rituximab in vivo in patients with B-cell chronic lymphocytic leukemia: evidence of caspase activation and apoptosis induction. Blood 2002; 99:1038–1043.

138. Ferreira CG, van der Valk P, Span SW, et al. Assessment of IAP (inhibitor of apoptosis) proteins as predictors of response to chemotherapy in advanced non-small-cell lung cancer patients. Ann Oncol 2001; 12:799–805.

139. Ferreira CG, van der Valk P, Span SW, et al. Expression of X-linked inhibitor of apoptosis as a novel prognostic marker in radically resected non-small cell lung cancer patients. Clin Cancer Res 2001; 7: 2468–2474.

140. Hofmann HS, Simm A, Hammer A, Silber RE, Bartling B. Expression of inhibitors of apoptosis (IAP) proteins in non-small cell human lung cancer. J Cancer Res Clin Oncol 2002; 128:554–560.

141. Krajewska M, Krajewski S, Banares S, et al. Elevated expression of inhibitor of apoptosis proteins in prostate cancer. Clin Cancer Res 2003; 9:4914–4925.

142. Bilim V, Kasahara T, Hara N, Takahashi K, Tomita Y. Role of XIAP in the malignant phenotype of transitional cell cancer (TCC) and therapeutic activity of XIAP antisense oligonucleotides against multidrug-resistant TCC in vitro. Int J Cancer 2003; 103:29–37.

143. Fulda S, Meyer E, Debatin KM. Inhibition of TRAIL-induced apoptosis by Bcl-2 overexpression. Oncogene 2002; 21:2283–2294.

144. Sasaki H, Sheng Y, Kotsuji F, Tsang BK. Down-regulation of X-linked inhibitor of apoptosis protein induces apoptosis in chemoresistant human ovarian cancer cells. Cancer Res 2000; 60:5659–5666.

145. Yang L, Mashima T, Sato S, et al. Predominant suppression of apoptosome by inhibitor of apoptosis protein in non-small cell lung cancer H460 cells: therapeutic effect of a novel polyarginine-conjugated Smac peptide. Cancer Res 2003; 63:831–837.

146. Hu Y, Cherton-Horvat G, Dragowska V, et al. Antisense oligonucleotides targeting XIAP induce apoptosis and enhance chemotherapeutic activity against human lung cancer cells in vitro and in vivo. Clin Cancer Res 2003; 9:2826–2836.

147. Schimmer AD, Welsh K, Pinilla C, et al. Small-molecule antagonists of apoptosis suppressor XIAP exhibit broad antitumor activity. Cancer Cell 2004; 5:25–35.

148. Ambrosini G, Adida C, Altieri DC. A novel anti-apoptosis gene, survivin, expressed in cancer and lymphoma. Nature Med 1997; 3:917–921.

149. Altieri DC. Survivin in apoptosis control and cell cycle regulation in cancer. Prog Cell Cycle Res 2003; 5:447–452.

150. Li F. Survivin study: what is the next wave? J Cell Physiol 2003; 197:8–29.

151. Li F, Ackermann EJ, Bennett CF, et al. Pleiotropic cell-division defects and apoptosis induced by interference with survivin function. Nature Cell Biol 1999; 1:461–466.

152. Altieri DC. Validating survivin as a cancer therapeutic target. Nature Rev Cancer 2003; 3:46–54.

153. Altieri DC. Survivin, versatile modulation of cell division and apoptosis in cancer. Oncogene 2003; 22:8581–8589.

154. Adida C, Crotty PL, McGrath J, Berrebi D, Diebold J, Altieri DC. Developmentally regulated expression of the novel cancer anti-apoptosis gene survivin in human and mouse differentiation. Am J Pathol 1998; 152:43–49.

155. Kobayashi K, Hatano M, Otaki M, Ogasawara T, Tokuhisa T. Expression of a murine homologue of the inhibitor of apoptosis protein is related to cell proliferation. Proc Natl Acad Sci USA 1999; 96: 1457–1462.

156. Gianani R, Jarboe E, Orlicky D, et al. Expression of survivin in normal, hyperplastic, and neoplastic colonic mucosa. Hum Pathol 2001; 32:119–125.

157. Altieri DC, Marchisio PC, Marchisio C. Survivin apoptosis: an interloper between cell death and cell proliferation in cancer. Lab Invest 1999; 79:1327–1333.

158. Altieri DC. Coupling apoptosis resistance to the cellular stress response: the IAP–Hsp90 connection in cancer. Cell Cycle 2004; 3:255–256.

159. Altieri DC. Survivin and apoptosis control. Adv Cancer Res 2003; 88:31–52.

160. Altieri DC. Blocking survivin to kill cancer cells. Methods Mol Biol 2003; 223:533–542.

161. Andersen MH, Thor SP. Survivin—a universal tumor antigen. Histol Histopathol 2002; 17:669–675.

162. Andersen MH, Pedersen LO, Becker JC, Straten PT. Identification of a cytotoxic T lymphocyte response to the apoptosis inhibitor protein survivin in cancer patients. Cancer Res 2001; 61:869–872.

163. Andersen MH, Pedersen LO, Capeller B, Brocker EB, Becker JC, thor Straten P. Spontaneous cytotoxic T-cell responses against survivin-derived MHC class I-restricted T-cell epitopes in situ as well as ex vivo in cancer patients. Cancer Res 2001; 61:5964–5968.

164. Chen J, Wu W, Tahir SK, et al. Down-regulation of survivin by antisense oligonucleotides increases apoptosis, inhibits cytokinesis and anchorage-independent growth. Neoplasia 2000; 2:235–241.

165. Olie RA, Simoes-Wust AP, Baumann B, et al. A novel antisense oligonucleotide targeting survivin expression induces apoptosis and sensitizes lung cancer cells to chemotherapy. Cancer Res 2000; 60: 2805–2809.

166. Ambrosini G, Adida C, Sirugo G, Altieri DC. Induction of apoptosis and inhibition of cell proliferation by survivin gene targeting. J Biol Chem 1998; 273:11,177–11,182.

167. Patel BKR, Carrasco RA, Stamm NB, et al. Antisense inhibition of survivin expression as a cancer therapeutic, AACR–NCI–EORTC International Conference on Molecular Targets and Cancer Therapeutic, 2003.

168. Karin M, Cao Y, Greten FR, Li ZW. NF-kappaB in cancer: from innocent bystander to major culprit. Nature Rev Cancer 2002; 2:301–310.

169. Yamamoto Y, Gaynor RB. Therapeutic potential of inhibition of the NF-kappaB pathway in the treatment of inflammation and cancer. J Clin Invest 2001; 107:135–142.

170. Brown K, Gerstberger S, Carlson L, Franzoso G, Siebenlist U. Control of I kappa B-alpha proteolysis by site-specific, signal-induced phosphorylation. Science 1995; 267:1485–1488.

171. Zandi E, Chen Y, Karin M. Direct phosphorylation of IkappaB by IKKalpha and IKKbeta: discrimination between free and NF-kappaB-bound substrate. Science 1998; 281:1360–1363.

172. Verma UN, Yamamoto Y, Prajapati S, Gaynor RB. Nuclear role of I kappa B Kinase-gamma/NF-kappa B essential modulator (IKK gamma/NEMO) in NF-kappa B-dependent gene expression. J Biol Chem 2004; 279:3509–3515.

173. Pahl HL. Signal transduction from the endoplasmic reticulum to the cell nucleus. Physiol Rev 1999; 79:683–701.

174. Bellacosa A, de Feo D, Godwin AK, et al. Molecular alterations of the AKT2 oncogene in ovarian and breast carcinomas. Int J Cancer 1995; 64:280–285.

175. Bellacosa A, Franke TF, Gonzalez-Portal ME, et al. Structure, expression and chromosomal mapping of c-akt: relationship to v-akt and its implications. Oncogene 1993; 8:745–754.

176. Datta SR, Brunet A, Greenberg ME. Cellular survival: a play in three Akts. Genes Dev 1999; 13:2905–2927.

177. Alessi DR, Caudwell FB, Andjelkovic M, Hemmings BA, Cohen P. Molecular basis for the substrate specificity of protein kinase B; comparison with MAPKAP kinase-1 and p70 S6 kinase. FEBS Lett 1996; 399:333–338.

178. Sakai A, Thieblemont C, Wellmann A, Jaffe ES, Raffeld M. PTEN gene alterations in lymphoid neoplasms. Blood 1998; 92:3410–3415.

179. Stambolic V, Mak TW, Woodgett JR. Modulation of cellular apoptotic potential: contributions to oncogenesis. Oncogene 1999; 18:6094–6103.

180. Cheng JQ, Ruggeri B, Klein WM, et al. Amplification of AKT2 in human pancreatic cells and inhibition of AKT2 expression and tumorigenicity by antisense RNA. Proc Natl Acad Sci USA 1996; 93: 3636–3641.

181. Ma YY, Wei SJ, Lin YC, et al. PIK3CA as an oncogene in cervical cancer. Oncogene 2000; 19:2739–2744.

182. Shayesteh L, Lu Y, Kuo WL, et al. PIK3CA is implicated as an oncogene in ovarian cancer. Nature Genet 1999; 21:99–102.

# IV   CANCER TARGET VALIDATION:
## *ANIMAL APPROACHES*

# 16

# Genetically Engineered Mouse Models of Human Cancer for Drug Discovery and Development

*Rónán C. O'Hagan, Min Wu, PhD,*
*William M. Rideout III, PhD,*
*Yinghui Zhou, PhD, and Joerg Heyer, PhD*

**CONTENTS**

**SUMMARY**

Animal models for cancer research, although not perfect, have traditionally been crucial to the drug discovery and development process. Recent advances in genetically modified mice have created opportunities to model many aspects of cancer biology, which established xenograft models ignore. Selection of the right model will be of increasing importance in the search for efficacious human therapeutics. These improved mouse models also permit a new concept of preclinical trials in which the efficacy of novel drugs can be tested against spontaneous tumors.

**Key Words:** Cancer; engineered mouse model; drug discovery; transgenic; knockout (targeted mutagenesis); tissue reconstitution; imaging.

## 1. INTRODUCTION

Historically, mouse models of human cancer (MMHC) began with spontaneous tumors in inbred mouse strains *(1)*, which were often the result of endogenous tumor viruses *(2)* (e.g., MMTV [originally the "milk factor"] and MuLV) or were induced by radiation or chemical carcinogenesis. These early tumor models approximated human tumorigenesis

From: *Cancer Drug Discovery and Development: The Oncogenomics Handbook*
Edited by: W. J. LaRochelle and R. A. Shimkets © Humana Press Inc., Totowa, NJ

in terms of growth kinetics, physiology, invasion, and metastasis, but they involved generally long latencies and variable penetrance, making drug screening and development difficult, if not impossible, in many of these solid tumor models.

The early in vivo tumor models used in drug development (e.g., P388, murine leukemia) were chosen for their ability to rapidly screen many compounds; however, several studies ultimately revealed a poor correlation between the performance of trial compounds in these preclinical screens and their performance in phase II clinical trials. The National Cancer Institute (NCI) later shifted the initial prescreening of clinical compounds away from the rapidly growing mouse leukemia models to the NCI 60 panel of human tumor cell lines used both in vitro and as xenografts in immunodeficient mice. However, these current preclinical models still preferentially select compounds that directly influence cellular proliferation and leave most other tumor and host interactions unaddressed. In vitro assays combined with xenografts of long established cell lines do not mimic the normal environment of human tumors, in which complex interactions with both the stroma and immune system occur. Human tumors develop *de novo* in a normal tissue background of wild-type cells. Thus, there is a need for models to better encompass these interactions as well as provide an environment to test compounds that interfere in invasion, metastasis, and hypoxia tolerance.

The mouse is the best animal to use in new models for several reasons: its genome sequence is largely complete; it has a short, productive life-span; it is well adapted to the laboratory and its well-understood genetics is easily combined with genetic manipulation. Genetic engineering of the mouse can be used to replicate the common genetic lesions identified in specific human cancers and act as one or more of the mutations in the multistep process of tumorigenesis. Therefore, xenograft models are rapidly being supplanted by genetically engineered mice (GEM) which carry activated oncogenes, inactivated tumor suppressor genes, or both (for a summary, see the Mouse Models of Human Cancer Consortium [MMHCC] website http://emice.nci.nih.gov/mouse_models/).

Inbred genetically susceptible animals have not been widely adopted because of long tumor latency, low penetrance, and variable growth, yet it is these very attributes that mimic spontaneous human tumors. GEM are prone to the development of spontaneous tumors in specific tissues with more predictable penetrance and much shorter latency. The forefront of genetic tumor models combines conditional or traditional knockouts of tumor suppressor genes with inducible-oncogene models, which express the oncogene upon the administration of a drug (e.g., doxycycline). Drug-inducible expression of oncogenes has several advantages: First, it increases the utility of spontaneous tumor models by creating a more uniform timeframe for tumorigenesis; second, it shortens latency; third, it avoids problems caused by deregulated expression of oncogenes during development; and, fourth, it allows characterization of the dependence of the tumor on continued oncogene expression (i.e., is the oncogene required for tumor maintenance?). For example, the doxycycline-inducible melanoma model brings all of these genetic modifications together and creates a regulated system with potential applications in target identification, validation, and drug discovery *(3)*. Thus, the tumors induced in these mice are driven by the same primary genetic events that are thought to induce the same cancer in humans. In fact, in this context, there is mounting evidence that the secondary genetic lesions that occur are also similar to those that arise in the cognate human cancer *(4–7)*. In addition, the histology of tumors that arise in these mouse models closely mimics the histology of equivalent human tumors (www.emice.nci.nih.org).

The current revolution in MMHC stems from the combination of a completed genome sequence, precise and controllable engineering of mouse genetics, and new technologies in high-throughput screening for the analysis of gene expression and compounds. The new models provide an opportunity to stringently validate candidate drugs in the best available models. Better validation and assessment of efficacy will ultimately reduce the number of compounds that fail in costly phase II clinical trials.

## 2. GENETICALLY ENGINEERED MICE

### 2.1. Modeling Tumorigenesis in Transgenic Mice

The ability to stably introduce foreign DNA into the mouse genome through micro-injection is arguably one of the most significant technical breakthroughs in the cancer modeling field. Since the production of the first tumor prone transgenic mice 20 yr ago, hundreds of mouse models have been generated to represent a broad spectrum of human cancerous conditions (8,9). Detailed information about these mice can be found in the Mouse Tumor Biology Database (MTB) at the website http://tumor.informatics.jax.org/. These mice are not only invaluable tools for deciphering the functions of individual genes or signaling pathways during tumorigenesis but are also playing increasingly significant roles in drug discovery.

The most straightforward construct used to generate transgenic mice consists of a promoter/enhancer element driving the expression of a gene of interest. Some promoters/ enhancers can lead to ubiquitous expression (e.g., the *β-actin* or *PGK* promoters). However, using a tissue- or cell-type-specific promoter permits restriction of the expression of the gene of interest to a tissue type in which the gene is known or suspected to be involved in transformation. Examples include *MMTV LTR* for mammary gland specific expression (9), *CCSP* promoter for lung-specific expression (10), rat *Probasin* promoter for prostate-specific expression (11) and *K14* promoter for epithelial-cell-specific expression (12). The gene of interest might be a viral oncogene (e.g., SV40 *large T antigen* and polyoma *middle T [pyMT]) (8)* or a cellular component involved in cell survival and proliferation, such as *MYC*, members of the *RAS* family, and various growth factors and their receptors. For instance, a transgenic mammary tumor model that mimics mutations seen in human cancer was established by overexpressing *Her2/neu* under the control of the MMTV LTR. Female mice carrying this transgene developed mammary adenocarcinomas during their early pregnancies (13). It is worth noting that, in many cases, it is critical to have the relevant oncogenic mutations incorporated, even though sometimes simply overexpressing an oncogene leads to malignancy. For example, in one report, only 50% of the mice overexpressing a wild-type *H-Ras* gene developed tumors by 18 mo. In tumors that did arise, there were invariably mutations in the *H-Ras* transgene (14). In contrast, mice carrying the *H-Ras$^{G12V}$* transgene developed tumors within several weeks to several months, with a much higher penetrance (15,16).

An important improvement over the single transgene system is the introduction of controllable systems. These systems typically have more than one element, providing investigators with more control over when and where the gene of interest is expressed. One of these systems is based on the bacterial TetR gene, which enables the precise control of the timing of transgene expression. This system exploits a modified TetR, called rtTA, which activates RNA polymerase II-dependent transcription from a TetO promoter only in the presence of tetracycline or doxycycline. Therefore, in mice that are doubly transgenic for

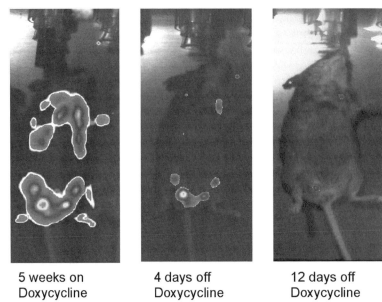

5 weeks on          4 days off          12 days off
Doxycycline         Doxycycline         Doxycycline

**Fig. 1.** Regression of tumors after deinduction. Mammary gland tumors were induced by expressing an oncogene in the mammary gland under the control of a doxycycline-dependent promoter. After 5 wk of induction, the animal was imaged for luciferase activity. Four or 12 d after oncogene withdrawal, the animal was imaged again and a reduced tumor load was detected on d 4 and minimal tumors were detectable after 12 d. (*See* Color Plate 6 following p. 302.)

both rtTA under the control of a tissue-specific promoter and a gene of interest under the control of TetO promoter, one can switch on the expression of the gene of interest in the appropriate tissue by administrating doxycycline to the mice. Using bitransgenic mice harboring both MMTV-rtTA and TetO-*LacZ*, Gunther and Belka elegantly demonstrated that the reporter gene can be quickly induced and deinduced in a highly tissue-specific manner. Furthermore, the level of transgene expression has a linear correlation with the concentration of doxycycline in the water up to 2 mg/mL *(17)*. Tumor models utilizing this strategy include an inducible mammary tumor model generated by D'Cruz et al. *(18)*, a T-cell lymphoma and acute myelogenous leukemia (AML) model generated by Felsher et al. *(19)*, and a B-cell leukemia model generated by Huettner et al. *(20)*. Figure 1 shows the initiation and regression of tumors in an inducible breast tumor model generated at GenPath Pharmaceuticals (*see* Color Plate 6 following p. 302). A less commonly used technique that can achieve the same goal is to create a fusion protein of the gene of interest with the hormone-binding domain of the estrogen receptor, thereby conferring hormone responsiveness *(21)*.

Sometimes, it is desirable to express the oncogene only in a small number of cells within a certain tissue in order to reduce the number of tumors produced. One strategy to accomplish that is to take advantage of the Cre/loxP recombination system. In this case, a stop cassette, flanked by loxP sites, separates the oncogene from the promoter. When these mice are exposed to a Cre expressing virus, the stop cassette is excised in infected cells, thereby activating the gene of interest. By carefully controlling the titer of the virus, one can greatly reduce the number of cells expressing the gene. This strategy has been employed by a number of labs to generate lung tumor models that better mimic the human condition *(22,23)*.

## 2.2. Loss of Function Models/Knockout Technology

With the advent of the gene targeting through homologous recombination (Knockout/ embryonic stem cell [ES] technology), modeling-inherited recessive disease became feasible. One of the first mouse models using ES cells was an attempt to model a metabolic disorder, Lesch–Nyhan syndrome *(24)*. The first generation of tumor-prone knockout mice were models of loss-of-function genetic diseases, which caused familial predisposition to cancer syndromes (e.g., retinoblastoma, Li–Fraumeni syndrome, familiar adenomatous polyposis coli [FAP], hereditary nonpolyposis coli [HNPPC], neurofibromatosis) *(25–27)*. Inactivation of one or both alleles of a tumor suppressor gene in mice leads to a predisposition to cancer. For some tumor suppressor genes, inactivation led to a similar predisposition as the human phenotypic manifestation (*APC, MLH1, MSH2,* and *MSH6*), but for others, the susceptibility phenotype in mice does not mimic the human tumor phenotype (p53, Rb) *(28)*. Such exceptions highlight important differences in the tissue-specific function of these tumor suppressor genes, an issue that might be addressed with complex tumor models (*see* Section 2.3). Exceptions to the tumor prone phenotype in mutant mice include the breast tumor predisposition genes *BRCA1* and *BRCA2*. Only conditional inactivation of these genes in the mammary gland predisposes to tumors with long latency and low penetrance *(29)*. In general, tissue-specific conditional inactivation leads to models closer to human tumor phenotypes.

Genetically engineered mice harboring mutations in tumor suppressor genes are being used increasingly in preclinical settings. These mice are prone to develop spontaneous tumors in which the molecular defects resulting from the absence of the tumor suppressor gene are similar in man and mouse. Additionally, the diversity of secondary mutations in these tumors mimics a "patient pool" for use in preclinical trial settings and can enhance the ability to predict efficacy patterns in human patients. Another important application of GEM is their use in chemoprevention studies as exemplified by Yang et al. *(30,31)*. Thus, it is possible to choose and utilize the appropriate mouse model for understanding aspects of disease that are not accessible in the patient setting.

Recent advances in knockout/ES cell technology have made it possible to further refine modeling efforts. Tumor-relevant point mutations have been introduced into tumor suppressor genes and oncogenes by targeted homologous recombination *(32)*. For example, in a tumor suppressor gene, point mutations were made in the mouse *p53* locus to mimic the mutations found in *p53* in human tumors and led to more relevant tumor development than the corresponding *p53*-null mutation. For the *K-Ras* oncogene locus, a series of targeted knock-in alleles of the *K-Ras* locus were generated *(23,33)*, which harbor silent versions of the activated *K-Ras* gene. After either spontaneous or CRE–mediated recombination, the mutated version of *K-Ras* gets expressed by its own promoter in its original chromosomal setting. The expression of activated oncogenes from their original locus is clearly advantageous to the forced overexpression of wild-type or activated oncogenes off of transgenes. The combination of the knockout and knock-in approaches, thus, offer the potential for introducing precise mutations into the mouse genome and model the mutations found in patient tumor samples.

Table 1
Complex Inducible Models of Human Cancer

| Activator | Oncogene | Tumor Suppressor | Tumor Types | Ref. |
|-----------|----------|------------------|-------------|------|
| Tyr-rtTA | TetO-H-Ras$^{G12V}$ | Ink4a/Arf $^{-/-}$ | Melanomas | 3 |
| CCSP-rtTA | TetO-K-Ras$^{G12D}$ | Wild type or Ink4a/Arf $^{-/-}$ or p53$^{-/-}$ | Lung adenomas and adenocarcinomas | 10 |
| MMTV-rtTA | TetO-Wnt1 | Wild type or p53$^{-/-}$ | Mammary adenocarcinomas and lung metastasis | 34 |
| PDX-Cre | K-Ras$^{G12D}$ | Ink4a/Arf $^{-/-}$ | Pancreatic carcinomas | 35 |

## 2.3. Tumor Models With Complex Genetic Engineering

It is now generally accepted that tumor formation in humans is the result of multiple genetic alterations, including loss of tumor suppressor genes and mutation/amplification/overexpression of oncogenes. Therefore, mouse models carrying multiple relevant mutations are likely to represent human conditions more faithfully. In recent years, an increasing number of mouse models with complex genetic engineering have been produced. These models have greatly enhanced our understanding of several aspects of tumorigenesis that have not been addressed previously.

Chin and colleagues generated mice carrying an activated *H-Ras* transgene under the control of the tyrosinase promoter, which drives expression in melanocytes *(3)*. They discovered that melanomas derived from these mice frequently had lost the *Ink4a* tumor suppressor alleles. By crossing the transgene into an *Ink4a*-null background, they were able to produce tumors with a much shorter latency and higher penetrance. This work established a causal link between *Ink4a* mutation and the development of melanomas. In addition, they also established a Tet-inducible version of this model and showed that melanomas arose in a doxycycline-dependent manner. More interestingly, these tumors regressed upon doxycycline withdrawal, demonstrating that Ras is not only required for tumor induction but remains important for tumor maintenance. These results highlight the strength of models with complex genetic engineering. Examples of complex, inducible models are listed in Table 1.

## 3. RECONSTITUTION MODELS

Transgenic and knockout technologies are powerful tools in generating tumor models. However, both systems have their limitations. Tissue reconstitution is another method to generate primary tumors in mice. Tissue reconstitution has been developed to recapitulate the events leading to cancer development in adult mice. The concept is to reconstitute a tissue from genetically modified cells, thereby allowing the opportunity to study the tumorigenic effects of genetic factors and hormonal factors from various components of the tissue. This approach has been best illustrated by the reconstitution of mammary and prostate glands.

### 3.1. Mammary Gland Reconstitution Models

Mammary gland reconstitution was initially developed by De Ome et al. *(36)*. This method takes advantage of the fact that mouse mammary epithelium develops postna-

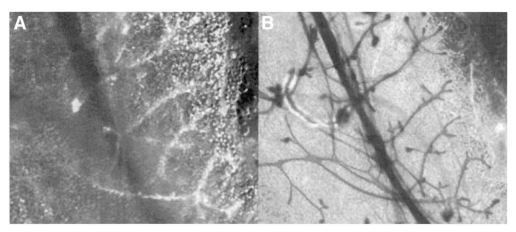

**Fig. 2.** Reconstitution of a mammary gland. Mammary epithelial cells (MECs) were collected from the mammary glands of *EYFP* transgenic mice, and implanted into the cleared fat pad of NOD-SCID mice. The reconstituted mammary gland was collected 6 wk after implantation. (**A**) Visualization of the reconstituted mammary gland under ultraviolet light. The green-fluorescent epithelial cells are derived from the donor *EYFP* transgenic mice. (**B**) Carmine staining of the reconstituted mammary gland. The ductal structures of the mammary gland are stained in pink. Therefore, the ductual structures of the reconstituted mammary glands are derived from the donor MECs. (*See* Color Plate 6 following p. 302.)

tally by extending from the nipple area into the mammary fat pad. By 3 wk of age, the mammary ducts formed by the mammary epithelial cells (MECs) have not progressed far into the fat pad. Therefore, the epithelium component of the mammary gland can be eliminated by removing the portion of the fat pad near the nipple, which leaves a cleared fat pad for reconstitution. Donor MECs can be obtained from other mice and injected into the cleared fat, in which they will form normal ductal structures. The reconstituted mammary glands are normal in terms of histology and hormone responsiveness. Figure 2 presents an example of a reconstituted mammary gland in which *EYFP*-positive mammary epithelium cells were implanted into cleared fat pads of Nonobese Diabetic-Severe Combined Immunodeficiency Disease (NOD-SCID) mice (*see* Color Plate 6 following p. 302).

During the brief culture period, oncogenes can be introduced into the donor MECs by retrovirus infection. Depending on the oncogenes introduced, the reconstituted mammary glands display a wide range of abnormal growth, ranging from *Wnt1-*, *v-myc-*, and *V-Ha-ras*-induced hyperplasias to *erbB2*-induced carcinoma *in situ* and invasive tumors *(37)*. Multistep carcinogenesis has also been achieved by introducing *v-Ha-ras* to mammary epithelium cells from a *v-myc*-induced reconstituted mammary gland and generating a second series of reconstituted mammary glands with the remodified MECs. Most of *v-myc/v-Ha-ras* reconstituted mammary glands developed tumors within 6–8 wk *(38)*.

### 3.2. Prostate Reconstitution Models

Prostate is another tissue in which reconstitution has been successfully established. The prostate develops from the embryonic urogenital sinus (UGS), which is composed of urogenital sinus epithelium (UGE) and urogenital sinus mesenchyme (UGM). When implanted under kidney capsule, dissociated UGS cells or the mixture of UGE and UGM cells can develop into prostate tissue with normal morphogenesis and functional differentiation

*(39)*. If the UGS cells are infected with retroviruses carrying *v-Ha-ras* and/or *Myc* prior to implantation, carcinomas develop from the reconstituted prostate *(40)*.

The reconstitution system also allows the opportunity to explore the interaction between epithelium and stroma during tumorigenesis *(41,42)*. BPH-1 is an immortalized but non-tumorigenic human prostatic epithelium cell line. When mixed with rat UGM, benign, but nontumorigenic, growth developed in the reconstituted prostate. However, if the host mice were treated with testosterone plus estradiol (T+E2), the BPH-1 + UGM recombinants formed invasive carcinomas. In addition, when mixed with carcinoma-associated fibroblasts (CAFs), the BPH-1 + CAF recombinants developed carcinomas. These studies indicate that stromal microenviroment is a critical factor in the malignant transformation of human prostate epithelial cells.

### 3.3. Pros and Cons of Reconstitution Models

There are several advantages to reconstitution models. (1) In the reconstituted tissue, the oncogene expressing cells proliferate in a mixture with normal cells, which mimics tumor growth in humans. (2) The reconstitution procedure itself restricts expression of onco-genes to specific cell types. Therefore, any ubiquitous promoter can be used to drive the expression of the oncogenes, whereas tissue-specific promoters are needed in establishing transgenic models. (3) The stroma environment can be modified by choosing specific mouse strains as recipient mice. (4) Early or mild lesions can be observed and propagated through reconstitution. (5) Mammary or prostate glands can be rescued from mutant mice with a lethal phenotype. (For example, $Brca2^{ASH/ASH}$ mutant mice start to die at around birth, yet, the MECs of those mice can be collected from E15.5 embryos and used in reconstitution.) (6) This system allows the implantation of donor cells into isogenic hosts, thereby retaining the dynamic interaction of the immune system with the tumor.

The disadvantage of this system is that each reconstitution has to be established surgically. Therefore, it is not suitable for the production of large numbers of mice, limiting their utility in the drug discovery process to late-stage preclinical characterization of development candidates. These models are also applicable in testing the efficacy of lead compounds.

## 4. MOUSE MODELS IN DRUG DEVELOPMENT: FROM TARGET DISCOVERY TO PRECLINICAL STUDIES

Mice are the primary preclinical model used in the development of human therapies for cancer. Although rat and dog tumor models exist, their application is limited because of time constraints and lack of manipulable genetics. Consequently, they are used for specific aspects of drug development, primarily toxicological studies. However, the mouse has become the work horse for in vivo studies of compound efficacy and pharmacology. In addition to studying therapeutic efficacy, we propose that mouse models of human cancers can provide ideal settings in which to identify important targets for therapeutic intervention in cancer, and in which to validate the importance of these targets. Moreover, such mouse models provide the ideal setting in which to conduct preclinical studies that will aid in the design of clinical trials and in the selection of patient populations for these trials.

### 4.1. Target Identification

The advent of mouse models of cancer that closely resemble human cancers and contain human disease-relevant genetic lesions facilitates the use of these mice as tools for the identification of novel targets for therapeutic intervention. Genomic and proteomic approaches to identify genes and proteins that are dysregulated in the mouse cancers give valuable insight into possible targets for human disease. Moreover, diagnostic and prognostic biomarkers in serum, urine, or the tumors themselves can be identified in these mouse models and subsequently evaluated as biomarkers in human patients. In addition, the recent use of forward genetic approaches, such as retroviral insertional mutagenesis to identify oncogenic events in mice, suggests that powerful genetic screens similar to those used in yeast, *Drosophilia* and *Caenorhabditis elegans* can now be applied in vivo to mammalian systems *(43–45)*. Significantly, these studies identified different retroviral insertion profiles in tumors arising in mice with different permissive genetic lesions. These results suggest that the genetic background of the mice predisposes them to respond to specific oncogenic events and thus determines the nature of the oncogenes that will be identified. This underlines the need to perform such screens in animals engineered to contain, as near as possible, the appropriate human orthologous genetic lesions. Thus, MMHC may provide distinct opportunities to perform genetic screens and identify functionally important cancer targets.

## 4.2. Target Validation

Mouse models are valuable tools for understanding and validating proposed targets for therapeutic intervention. Deletion of genes encoding such targets in the mouse provides insight into the potential side effects of inhibiting the function of the encoded protein *(46)*. Traditional gene-targeting approaches indicate the requirement for a particular gene for viability. Conditional gene-targeting technology, in conjunction with regulatable systems, enables gene deletion in tissues of interest at specific times and eliminates concerns about potential embryonic lethality. Hence, the requirement for the target gene can be elucidated in adult animals. This analysis can be limited to selected tissues with appropriate engineering of the gene-targeting system. Such knockout models can be interbred with cancer models to determine whether conditional gene deletion prevents tumor formation, inhibits progression, or causes regression of established tumors *(46)*. With the advent of RNA interference (RNAi) technology and the ability to knock down gene expression in vivo in mice, RNAi-based inhibition of candidate targets could also be used to assess the requirement for the target in the oncogenic process *(47–51)*.

Transgenic overexpression of genes of interest, or activated variants thereof, can reveal a role in oncogenesis either through an oncogenic effect of the gene itself or through its ability to potentiate oncogenic signals arising from other genetically engineered events, or from chemical or physical mutagens *(52)*. The use of inducible transgenic technologies *(3,10,17,21,34)* has provided a valuable tool for studying the role of particular cancer-relevant genes in multiple stages of cancer, including initiation, progression, maintenance, regression, and minimal residual disease. In addition, mouse tumors that are dependent on a specific engineered transgene or tumor suppressor deletion can be used to study the effects of compounds that target that gene or the pathway in which it is thought to be involved (e.g., treating *erbB2* transgenic mice with Herceptin, or treating *PTEN*$^{-/-}$ mice with mTOR inhibitors [www.emice.nci.nih.org; *53*]).

Cell lines, or in vivo propagated cells, from tumors that arise as a result of engineered oncogenic events also can be used for target identification and validation. For example, cell lines derived from tumors can be used for cell-based studies to better understand the effects of the engineered genetic alterations on cellular proliferation, survival, anchorage-independent growth, or growth under conditions of stress. Non-tumor-derived cells, such as primary mouse embryonic fibroblasts (MEFs) derived from intercrosses within a particular mouse model also provide valuable tools. Investigation of the events required to transform normal MEFs in the face of engineered genetic alterations facilitates understanding of the mechanism of action for a gene of interest in the oncogenic process.

### 4.3. Preclinical Development

It is clear that mouse models provide valuable tools for the discovery and validation of cancer targets and for studying and understanding the biology of these targets. In addition, the increasing sophistication of these models and the development of medical technologies for application to the study of small animals might provide new opportunities to use mouse models as predictive preclinical models. As such, mouse models of cancer might increasingly aid in validating that compounds act on their proposed target, elucidating their mechanism of action, and identifying target clinical populations.

Mouse models have traditionally been used to determine efficacy of compounds in vivo. Until recently, studies were limited to assessing compound efficacy because the target and mechanism of action of traditional cytotoxic chemotherapeutics were unclear and, therefore, not assayable. The ability to use pharmacodynamic readouts of the effect of compounds on known targets enables the use of xenograft and genetically engineered mouse models to confirm that compounds are inhibiting the appropriate target in the tumor. The same pharmacodynamic parameters can be assayed in parallel in other tissues of the mouse.

Studies of compound efficacy in xenografts have been largely unsuccessful in predicting ultimate clinical efficacy. In fact, a recent study suggests that analysis of compound efficacy in tumor cell lines in culture is a better predictor of clinical effectiveness than xenograft models *(54)*. Historically, xenografts have been the mouse models of choice for preclinical studies for a number of reasons, including short and consistent tumor latencies, ease of measurement, and well-defined tumor source material. However, these models limit analysis to tumors that are derived from established cell lines. The presence of artifacts of long-term culture in these cell lines and the abnormal environment in which the tumors arise confer an unrealistic etiology on the resultant tumors. Hence, it is perhaps not surprising that compound efficacy in xenograft models does not predict success in treating human cancers.

One mechanism to predict patient populations that are most likely to benefit from a particular therapeutic is to identify cytogenetic, gene expression, or proteomic biomarker profiles that are predictive of drug response. This approach is becoming increasingly prevalent in retrospective studies of human cancers *(55–64)*. Predicting the ideal target patient population prior to entering clinical trials would greatly accelerate the discovery of novel cancer therapeutics. Unfortunately, tumors derived from clonal human cell lines do not provide the genetic variation observed in human tumors and spontaneous mouse models, precluding their use in identifying predictive markers of therapeutic response in humans. The more faithful reproduction of human disease in genetically engineered mouse models suggests that these models will be better predictors of clinical response to therapy.

The spontaneous nature of the tumors that arise in mouse models of human cancer means that each tumor exhibits genetic heterogeneity both cytogenetically and in terms of gene and protein expression patterns *(4–6,65,66)*. This heterogeneity resembles the variable cytogenetics and expression profiles found in human cancers. As a result, it might be possible to translate the profiles of responsive and nonresponsive tumors in mouse models into predictive profiles for human cancers. It remains to be proven that the heterogeneity in mouse tumors can be used in this manner. However, promising studies from a number of groups indicate that mouse tumors treated with established therapeutics can be divided into responsive and nonresponsive subpopulations (66–69) and a number of groups have shown that expression and cytogenetic profiles in mouse models closely resemble those found in the cognate human cancers (7,65). Moreover, these profiles can be used to predict tumor etiology (65). As a result, identification of cytogenetic, gene expression or proteomic biomarker profiles that are predictive of drug response in the mouse are likely to aid in developing similar predictors for human patients. This will facilitate the selection of patients that will most benefit from specific therapies.

The use of mice in which tumors have arisen with an etiology similar to the cognate human cancer, in the appropriate stromal and tissue environment, and with equivalent primary oncogenic events adds credence to pharmacodynamic studies performed to identify correlates among pharmacokinetic profiles of the compound, pharmacodynamic markers in the blood, urine, or tumor, and compound efficacy. Thorough characterization of pharmacodynamic readouts in mice can provide the route to identify appropriate pharmacodynamic assays in human patients. With the development of these assays, the pharmacokinetic profile of the compound and the pharmacodynamics associated with the most efficacious dosing regimen in mice can be used as a tool to rapidly identify the most efficacious dosing regimen in humans.

Established tumors in inducible mouse models of human cancers can be regressed by removing the effect of the primary oncogene (3,17,21,34) (Fig. 1). These tumors exhibit complete clinical regression, but often leave microscopic foci that serve as good models of minimal residual disease, a complex problem in human cancer (70). Hence, these mouse models can be used to determine the ability of therapies to affect complex problems in human cancer treatment and to assist in the design of novel therapies targeting aspects of the oncogenic process that are otherwise intractable.

### 4.4. Imaging Tumors in Mice

Characterization of oncogenesis and therapeutic response in the mouse is becoming more tractable in light of new high-resolution imaging technologies available for small animal studies (71,72). These imaging technologies include magnetic resonance imaging (MRI), X-ray computed tomography (CT), ultrasound, positron-emission tomography (PET), single-photon emission computed tomography (SPECT), fluorescence-mediated molecular tomography (FMT), fluorescence reflectance imaging (FRI), and bioluminescent imaging (BLI) (Fig. 1) (72). These approaches can be used to assess both efficacy and pharmacologic properties of therapeutics. For example, quantitative PET can be used to monitor drug biodistribution, and various imaging approaches can be used to determine whether a drug reaches its target, affects function of the target, and exhibits efficacy (72). Importantly, many of these imaging technologies are used in the diagnosis and observation of human cancer patients. As a result, observations made in mouse models can be rapidly translated into an understanding of cellular and molecular events in human cancers.

### 4.5. Considerations for the Use of Mouse Models for Human Cancer

There has been significant progress in the development of mouse models of human cancer. A common concern with genetically engineered mouse models of cancer is the development of multiple tumors from a single tissue. In human patients, it is uncommon to find more than a single tumor arising from a tissue field. In addition, sporadic cancers in humans arise in a field of normal tissue. In the majority of mouse models described to date, the expression of the oncogene and/or deletion of the tumor suppressor of interest occurs throughout the tissue, leading to cancerization of the entire tissue field *(73)*. More recently, a mouse model for lung cancer has avoided this problem by relying on spontaneous recombination events to activate expression of the primary oncogene in a small number of scattered cells in the mouse *(33)*. The increasing sophistication of genetic manipulations such as this will continue to increase the effectiveness of mouse models in the study of cancer.

In general, the spontaneous tumors developed in MMHC arise with a latency that is significantly slower than tumors that develop in xenograft models. In addition, tumors in these genetically engineered models arise with different latencies. Although both of these characteristics are often viewed as liabilities, the underlying cause of these variable and extended latencies in fact enhances the value of mouse models of human cancer. The extended latency is associated with the acquisition of required secondary genetic lesions and establishing a tumor permissive milieu in a normal tissue field *(73)*. The variable secondary tumorigenic genetic events found in these mouse tumors facilitates the discovery of essential processes in tumorigenesis and provides a model in which response to therapeutics will exhibit heterogeneity reminiscent of human tumors.

One area in which mouse models are not well suited to predicting clinical response to therapeutics is toxicology. The P450 gene complement in mice is not well conserved in humans, and tissue distribution of expression patterns of some genes are known to vary between mouse and humans *(74)*. It is not possible to assess the toxic effects of inhibiting a target in a specific mouse tissue if the target is not expressed there. However, information on general tissue toxicity can be obtained from organs in which the target is expressed. Hence, mouse models are currently limited to the identification of mechanism-based toxicity and the ability of a compound to hit the appropriate target. Characterization of metabolism-related toxicity for human patients is not likely to be a strong point of any mouse model, and toxicology of this nature is more readily studied in other systems *(75)*. However, initial attempts have also been made to produce P450 humanized mice *(76)*. Mouse models of cancer generated in this context might eventually allow concomitant studies of drug efficacy and toxicity.

In general, two significant limitations to the use of mouse models in drug development are commonly cited: the slow pace and high cost of mouse experiments other than xenograft models, and the poor clinical predictive power of xenograft models. In short, it is too expensive or it does not work. The development of increasingly more sophisticated mouse models of human cancers, as described herein, will lead to increased understanding of cancer biology and the effects of therapies on tumor initiation, progression, maintenance, and regression and on minimal residual disease. As a result, these models will provide greater power to predict the clinical efficacy of novel therapies in human cancer patients. Although these models are complex, time-consuming to develop, and expensive to maintain, their potential to increase the success rate of drugs in clinical trials negates these arguments. The use of mouse models of human cancers to select the right drugs and the right patients for clinical trials will increase the success rate for drugs in trials, enable pharmaceutical companies to focus resources on drugs with a greater likelihood of success, and ultimately accelerate delivery of effective therapies to cancer patients. Even a small percentage increase in clinical success translates into significant numbers of lives saved.

In fact, in the United States alone, 1500 patients die each day from cancer, highlighting the need to develop and adapt new approaches to accelerate the successful development of new therapeutics (http://www.cancer.org/statistics).

## ACKNOWLEDGMENTS

We thank Geoffrey Boynton, Angela Sullivan, and Rebecca Rancourt for excellent technical support. We also thank Steve Clark and Murray Robinson for helpful comments and criticism.

## REFERENCES

1. Furth J, Seibold HR, Rathbone RR. Experimental studies on lymphomatosis of mice. Am J Cancer 1933; 19:521–526.
2. Bittner JJ. Some possible effects of nursing on the mammary gland tumor incidence in mice. Science 1936; 84:162.
3. Chin L, Tam A, Pomerantz J, et al. Essential role for oncogenic Ras in tumour maintenance. Nature 1999; 400(6743):468–472.
4. Artandi SE, Chang S, Lee SL, et al. Telomere dysfunction promotes non-reciprocal translocations and epithelial cancers in mice. Nature 2000; 406(6796):641–645.
5. O'Hagan RC, Chang S, Maser RS, et al. Telomere dysfunction provokes regional amplification and deletion in cancer genomes. Cancer Cell 2002; 2(2):149–155.
6. You MJ, Castrillon DH, Bastian BC, et al. Genetic analysis of Pten and Ink4a/Arf interactions in the suppression of tumorigenesis in mice. Proc Natl Acad Sci USA 2002; 99(3):1455–1460.
7. Ellwood-Yen K, Graeber TG, Wongvipat J, et al. Myc-driven murine prostate cancer shares molecular features with human prostate tumors. Cancer Cell 2003; 4(3):223–238.
8. Brinster RL, Chen HY, Messing A, van Dyke T, Levine AJ, Palmiter RD. Transgenic mice harboring SV40 T-antigen genes develop characteristic brain tumors. Cell 1984; 37(2):367–379.
9. Stewart TA, Pattengale PK, Leder P. Spontaneous mammary adenocarcinomas in transgenic mice that carry and express MTV/myc fusion genes. Cell 1984; 38(3):627–637.
10. Fisher GH, Wellen SL, Klimstra D, et al. Induction and apoptotic regression of lung adenocarcinomas by regulation of a K-Ras transgene in the presence and absence of tumor suppressor genes. Genes Dev 2001; 15(24):3249–3262.
11. Greenberg NM, DeMayo FJ, Sheppard PC, et al. The rat probasin gene promoter directs hormonally and developmentally regulated expression of a heterologous gene specifically to the prostate in transgenic mice. Mol Endocrinol 1994; 8(2):230–349.
12. Vassar R, Rosenberg M, Ross S, Tyner A, Fuchs E. Tissue-specific and differentiation-specific expression of a human K14 keratin gene in transgenic mice. Proc Natl Acad Sci USA 1989; 86(5):1563–1567.
13. Muller WJ, Sinn E, Pattengale PK, Wallace R, Leder P. Single-step induction of mammary adenocarcinoma in transgenic mice bearing the activated c-neu oncogene. Cell 1988; 54(1):105–115.
14. Saitoh A, Kimura M, Takahashi R, et al. Most tumors in transgenic mice with human c-Ha-ras gene contained somatically activated transgenes. Oncogene 1990; 5(8):1195–1200.
15. Maronpot RR, Palmiter RD, Brinster RL, Sandgren EP. Pulmonary carcinogenesis in transgenic mice. Exp Lung Res 1991; 17(2):305–320.
16. Suda Y, Aizawa S, Hirai S, et al. Driven by the same Ig enhancer and SV40 T promoter ras induced lung adenomatous tumors, myc induced pre-B cell lymphomas and SV40 large T gene a variety of tumors in transgenic mice. EMBO J 1987; 6(13):4055–4065.
17. Gunther EJ, Belka GK, Wertheim GB, et al. A novel doxycycline-inducible system for the transgenic analysis of mammary gland biology. FASEB J 2002; 16(3):283–292.
18. D'Cruz CM, Gunther EJ, Boxer RB, et al. c-MYC induces mammary tumorigenesis by means of a preferred pathway involving spontaneous Kras2 mutations. Nature Med 2001; 7(2):235–359.
19. Felsher DW, Bishop JM. Reversible tumorigenesis by MYC in hematopoietic lineages. Mol Cell 1999; 4(2):199–207.
20. Huettner CS, Zhang P, Van Etten RA, Tenen DG. Reversibility of acute B-cell leukaemia induced by BCR-ABL1. Nature Genet 2000; 24(1):57–60.

21. Pelengaris S, Littlewood T, Khan M, Elia G, Evan G. Reversible activation of c-Myc in skin: induction of a complex neoplastic phenotype by a single oncogenic lesion. Mol Cell 1999; 3(5):565–577.

22. Pao W, Klimstra DS, Fisher GH, Varmus HE. Use of avian retroviral vectors to introduce transcriptional regulators into mammalian cells for analyses of tumor maintenance. Proc Natl Acad Sci USA 2003; 100 (15):8764–8769.

23. Jackson EL, Willis N, Mercer K, et al. Analysis of lung tumor initiation and progression using conditional expression of oncogenic K-ras. Genes Dev 2001; 15(24):3243–3248.

24. Hooper M, Hardy K, Handyside A, Hunter S, Monk M. HPRT-deficient (Lesch–Nyhan) mouse embryos derived from germline colonization by cultured cells. Nature 1987; 326(6110):292–295.

25. Jacks T. Tumor suppressor gene mutations in mice. Annu Rev Genet 1996; 30:603–636.

26. McClatchey AI, Jacks T. Tumor suppressor mutations in mice: the next generation. Curr Opin Genet Dev 1998; 8(3):304–310.

27. Heyer J, Yang K, Lipkin M, Edelmann W, Kucherlapati R. Mouse models for colorectal cancer. Oncogene 1999; 18(38):5325–5333.

28. Rangarajan A, Weinberg RA. Comparative biology of mouse versus human cells: modelling human cancer in mice. Nature Rev Cancer 2003; 3(12):952–959.

29. Van Dyke T, Jacks T. Cancer modeling in the modern era: progress and challenges. Cell 2002; 108(2): 135–144.

30. Yang K, Edelmann W, Fan K, et al. Dietary modulation of carcinoma development in a mouse model for human familial adenomatous polyposis. Cancer Res 1998; 58(24):5713–5717.

31. Lipkin M, Yang K, Edelmann W, et al. Preclinical mouse models for cancer chemoprevention studies. Ann NY Acad Sci 1999; 889:14–19.

32. de Vries A, Flores ER, Miranda B, et al. Targeted point mutations of p53 lead to dominant-negative inhibition of wild-type p53 function. Proc Natl Acad Sci USA 2002; 99(5):2948–2953.

33. Johnson L, Mercer K, Greenbaum D, et al. Somatic activation of the K-ras oncogene causes early onset lung cancer in mice. Nature 2001; 410(6832):1111–1116.

34. Gunther EJ, Moody SE, Belka GK, et al. Impact of p53 loss on reversal and recurrence of conditional Wnt-induced tumorigenesis. Genes Dev 2003; 17(4):488–501.

35. Aguirre AJ, Bardeesy N, Sinha M, et al. Activated Kras and Ink4a/Arf deficiency cooperate to produce metastatic pancreatic ductal adenocarcinoma. Genes Dev 2003; 17(24):3112–3126.

36. De Ome KB FL Jr, Bern H, Blair PB. Development of mammary tumors from hyperplastic alveolar nodules transplanted into gland-free mammary fat pads of female C3H Mice. Cancer Res 1959; 19:515–525.

37. Paul Edwards CA, Bradbury J. Genetic manipulation of mammary epithelium by transplantation. J Mammary Gland Biol Neoplasia 1996; 1(1):75–89.

38. Bradbury JM, Sykes H, Edwards PAC. Induction of mouse mammary tumors in a transplantation system by the sequential introduction of the *MYC* and *RAS* oncogenes. Int J Cancer 1991; 48:908–915.

39. Cunha GR, Donjacour AA, Cooke PS, et al. The endocrinology and developmental biology of the prostate. Endocr Rev 1987; 8(3):338–362.

40. Thompson TC, Southgate J, Kitchener G, Land H. Multistage carcinogenesis induced by ras and myc oncogenes in a reconstituted organ. Cell 1989; 56(6):917–930.

41. Cunha GR, Hayward SW, Wang YZ. Role of stroma in carcinogenesis of the prostate. Differentiation 2002; 70(9–10):473–485.

42. Cunha GR, Hayward SW, Wang YZ, Ricke WA. Role of the stromal microenvironment in carcinogenesis of the prostate. Int J Cancer 2003; 107(1):1–10.

43. Lund AH, Turner G, Trubetskoy A, et al. Genome-wide retroviral insertional tagging of genes involved in cancer in Cdkn2a-deficient mice. Nature Genet 2002; 32(1):160–165.

44. Mikkers H, Allen J, Knipscheer P, et al. High-throughput retroviral tagging to identify components of specific signaling pathways in cancer. Nature Genet 2002; 32(1):153–159.

45. Suzuki T, Shen H, Akagi K, et al. New genes involved in cancer identified by retroviral tagging. Nature Genet 2002; 32(1):166–174.

46. Zambrowicz BP, Sands AT. Knockouts model the 100 best-selling drugs—will they model the next 100? Nature Rev Drug Discov 2003; 2(1):38–51.

47. Hannon GJ. RNA interference. Nature 2002; 418(6894):244–251.

48. Tuschl T. RNA interference and small interfering RNAs. Chembiochemistry 2001; 2(4):239–245.

49. Rubinson DA, Dillon CP, Kwiatkowski AV, et al. A lentivirus-based system to functionally silence genes in primary mammalian cells, stem cells and transgenic mice by RNA interference. Nature Genet 2003; 33(3):401–406.

50. McManus MT, Haines BB, Dillon CP, et al. Small interfering RNA-mediated gene silencing in T lymphocytes. J Immunol 2002; 169(10):5754–5760.
51. Carmell MA, Zhang L, Conklin DS, Hannon GJ, Rosenquist TA. Germline transmission of RNAi in mice. Nature Struct Biol 2003; 10(2):91–92.
52. Noonan FP, Otsuka T, Bang S, Anver MR, Merlino G. Accelerated ultraviolet radiation-induced carcinogenesis in hepatocyte growth factor/scatter factor transgenic mice. Cancer Res 2000; 60(14):3738–3743.
53. Inui A. Targeted therapy in cancer and transgenic animal model. Cancer Invest 2003; 21(5):819–820.
54. Voskoglou-Nomikos T, Pater JL, Seymour L. Clinical predictive value of the in vitro cell line, human xenograft, and mouse allograft preclinical cancer models. Clin Cancer Res 2003; 9(11):4227–4239.
55. Alizadeh AA, Eisen MB, Davis RE, et al. Distinct types of diffuse large B-cell lymphoma identified by gene expression profiling. Nature 2000; 403(6769):503–511.
56. Bhattacharjee A, Richards WG, Staunton J, et al. Classification of human lung carcinomas by mRNA expression profiling reveals distinct adenocarcinoma subclasses. Proc Natl Acad Sci USA 2001; 98(24): 13,790–13,795.
57. DeRisi J, Penland L, Brown PO, et al. Use of a cDNA microarray to analyse gene expression patterns in human cancer. Nature Genet 1996; 14(4):457–460.
58. Golub TR, Slonim DK, Tamayo P, et al. Molecular classification of cancer: class discovery and class prediction by gene expression monitoring. Science 1999; 286(5439):531–537.
59. Hedenfalk I, Duggan D, Chen Y, et al. Gene-expression profiles in hereditary breast cancer. N Engl J Med 2001; 344(8):539–548.
60. Sorlie T, Perou CM, Tibshirani R, et al. Gene expression patterns of breast carcinomas distinguish tumor subclasses with clinical implications. Proc Natl Acad Sci USA 2001; 98(19):10,869–10,874.
61. Takahashi M, Rhodes DR, Furge KA, et al. Gene expression profiling of clear cell renal cell carcinoma: gene identification and prognostic classification. Proc Natl Acad Sci USA 2001; 98(17):9754–9759.
62. van't Veer LJ, Dai H, van de Vijver MJ, et al. Gene expression profiling predicts clinical outcome of breast cancer. Nature 2002; 415(6871):530–536.
63. Su YA, Bittner ML, Chen Y, et al. Identification of tumor-suppressor genes using human melanoma cell lines UACC903, UACC903(+6), and SRS3 by comparison of expression profiles. Mol Carcinog 2000; 28(2):119–127.
64. Clark EA, Golub TR, Lander ES, Hynes RO. Genomic analysis of metastasis reveals an essential role for RhoC. Nature 2000; 406(6795):532–535.
65. O'Hagan RC, Brennan CW, Strahs A, et al. Array comparative genome hybridization for tumor classification and gene discovery in mouse models of malignant melanoma. Cancer Res 2003; 63(17):5352–5356.
66. Green JE, Desai K, Ye Y, Kavanaugh C, Calvo A, Huh JI. Genomic approaches to understanding mammary tumor progression in transgenic mice and responses to therapy. Clin Cancer Res 2004; 10(1 Pt 2): 385S–390S.
67. Desai KV, Xiao N, Wang W, et al. Initiating oncogenic event determines gene-expression patterns of human breast cancer models. Proc Natl Acad Sci USA 2002; 99(10):6967–6972.
68. Renou JP, Bierie B, Miyoshi K, et al. Identification of genes differentially expressed in mouse mammary epithelium transformed by an activated beta-catenin. Oncogene 2003; 22(29):4594–4610.
69. Dillner K, Kindblom J, Flores-Morales A, et al. Gene expression analysis of prostate hyperplasia in mice overexpressing the prolactin gene specifically in the prostate. Endocrinology 2003; 144(11):4955–4966.
70. Kostler WJ, Brodowicz T, Hejna M, Wiltschke C, Zielinski CC. Detection of minimal residual disease in patients with cancer: a review of techniques, clinical implications, and emerging therapeutic consequences. Cancer Detect Prev 2000; 24(4):376–403.
71. Weissleder R. Scaling down imaging: molecular mapping of cancer in mice. Nature Rev Cancer 2002; 2(1):11–18.
72. Rudin M, Weissleder R. Molecular imaging in drug discovery and development. Nature Rev Drug Discov 2003; 2(2):123–131.
73. Berns A. Cancer. Improved mouse models. Nature 2001; 410(6832):1043–1044.
74. Graham J, Mushin M, Kirkpatrick P. Oxaliplatin. Nature Rev Drug Discov 2004; 3(1):11–12.
75. Pritchard JF, Jurima-Romet M, Reimer ML, Mortimer E, Rolfe B, Cayen MN. Making better drugs: decision gates in non-clinical drug development. Nature Rev Drug Discov 2003; 2(7):542–553.
76. Gonzalez FJ. Role of gene knockout and transgenic mice in the study of xenobiotic metabolism. Drug Metab Rev 2003; 35(4):319–335.

# 17

# Unraveling the Complexity of Oncogenesis Through In Vivo Optical Imaging

*Pamela Reilly Contag, PhD*

## CONTENTS

## SUMMARY

The global promise of genomics is undeniable, yet in any given therapeutic area, the immediate value has been variable. From the identification of the molecular mechanisms in normal physiology to the aberrant mechanisms of disease and the subsequent identification of targets and the drugs that bind those targets, genomics has led the way with a virtual avalanche of information on the involvement of specific genes and pathways. The iterative analysis of information that is acquired from the genomic database and the differential transcriptional arrays between diseased and normal tissue has produced a multitude of fascinating leads for the ultimate understanding of disease processes and, thus, potential therapeutic targets. Now, our job as researchers and clinicians in this new era of "functional genomics" is to sort out the vast array of information from our global view of the genome and turn this knowledge into translational research for clinical benefit in both diagnostics and therapeutics. A novel approach to functional genomics, available now to all researchers is noninvasive in vivo bioluminescent imaging using reporters that are molecular tags, directly labeling the gene of interest. In vivo

From: *Cancer Drug Discovery and Development: The Oncogenomics Handbook*
Edited by: W. J. LaRochelle and R. A. Shimkets © Humana Press Inc., Totowa, NJ

imaging using luciferase as a reporter has the sensitivity to allow data collection early in the tumor formation for access to the entire biological process. Several new methods to build predictive animal models that allow determination of gene function providing both spatial and temporal data from living animals will be presented.

**Key Words:** Oncology; bioluminescence; in vivo imaging; gene expression; cell lines; transgenics; mouse models; genomics; drug discovery.

## 1. INTRODUCTION

The technological advances surrounding genomics and the high-throughput systems of array analysis for mRNA and proteins have had a profound affect on the field of oncology. The complexity of oncogenesis lends itself to the many approaches to identify groups of genes and proteins that differ in expression and molecular structure between the normal and diseased states, the field of oncogenomics. There is a tendency to begrudge anyone the use of the suffix "omics" because it is overused and overinterpreted; however, the amazing ability of oncology researchers to mobilize and march in step through the application of new technologies to the complex puzzle of oncogenesis and to the benefit of the patient has earned them the right to the designation "oncogenomics." Now, the challenge is to harvest biological data from the vast amount of genomics data. This requires more sensitive, higher-throughput animal models that reveal information about the biological system at the gene level. Oncology, as a field, has lead the way in developing these animal models, which will be described here.

The complexity of oncogenesis has been defined by the unprecedented expansion in the understanding of the new molecular mechanisms by which cancer develops (1,2). Malignancies are often characterized by abnormal or unregulated cell growth of cells that contain a genetic lesion (3). For many years, the understanding of the disease process revolved around cell cycle deregulation and the subsequent proliferation because of insensitivity to antigrowth signals, evasion of natural killer cell activity, deregulated angiogenesis, and the formation of metastases (1,3).

Conventional molecular biology and other cancer genetic approaches lead to the discovery and study of individual genes involved in these processes (1). Examples of genes identified in these pathways by such approaches include HER2 and HER-2/neu involved in metastatic disease and the target of a novel monoclonal antibody treatment (Herceptin-, Genentech, South San Francisco, CA) and tyrosine kinase enzyme, critical in proliferation, differentiation and survival, a target for a tyrosine kinase inhibitor Glivec (Glivec; Novartis, Basel, Switzerland) (3).

The acknowledgment that the global picture of the disease process still eluded researchers arose from clinical data suggesting that patients with similar disease did not respond equally to the various treatments, very different cancers contained similar biomarkers, and the demonstration that there were multiple mechanisms of disease both genetic and environmental often expressed in the same tumor cell. Genetic changes that result in tumorigenesis can arise from DNA mutations, chromosomal aberrations or allelic imbalance, epigenetic events, including aberrant promoter methylation and other expression alterations, and protein alterations such as microtubule dysfunction and the collapsing response mediator protein (CRMP) family of proteins (3,4). One or more gene defects could give rise to specific tumors and these events have been identified in several tumor types. The patterns of how these events occur and especially the timing for these events overall in tumorigenesis is a direct result of postgenomic technologies that allowed researchers to ask questions well beyond capabilities of typical cytogenetic and chemical mutagenesis studies *(5)*.

The first part of the 1990s was highlighted by large-scale genetic and physical maps of the genome. This was followed by a complete sequence of the human genome to which all researchers had access. Expressed sequence tags (ESTs) allowed the identification of thousands of genes. Bioinformatics made it possible to collect and compare data from these databases and from mRNA expression and protein arrays made from normal and diseased tissues *(6)*.

Following these important scientific milestones, researchers in the field of oncology made the important connection between genetic and epigenetic events as the crucial link that changed the way that researchers thought about postgenomic technologies and experimental design. At this time, it was not intuitive to move away from large-scale gene discovery technologies to study the complex biology in the whole organism *(6)*. For oncology researchers, this change in paradigm to functional and systems biology was "the" approach that would bring together the role of individual genes and the alteration of the sequence and expression of these genes through environmental effects.

Longitudinal study design in the whole animal was beyond the reach of most bench scientists until the advent of in vivo optical imaging, which created a method for identifying and tracking multiple genetic and epigenetic alterations that cause tumorigenesis. Oncology researchers seemed to have embraced the molecular imaging capability to explode the number of target, therapeutic, and diagnostic opportunities. The knowledge of when and where these genetic and epigenetic changes occur during the disease process will bring together researchers and clinicians over diagnosis, treatment, and prognosis of cancer patients.

## 2. ANIMAL MODELS OF CANCER

To validate a hypothesis concerning the effects of a drug on, or the role of a gene or protein in, a biological system, researchers must test the hypothesis in animal models. Animal models, although slower and more expensive than in vitro technologies, provide more relevant information. Much of the uniformity in mouse models arises from the practice of using inbred mice. These models differ from humans in that humans have great biological variability and, therefore, a constant concern is whether or not inbred mouse models are predictive of the response and mechanism of disease in humans *(7)*. In addition, the mouse does not mirror the natural history of the human. It is 2 logs smaller and lives 2 yr instead of 70 yr. This might mean that it does not have a high enough number of cells or live a long enough period of time to accumulate the same type of mutations and environmental exposure that humans do *(8)*. Small-animal models of cancer can be placed on a matrix of types of tumor, whether induced, transplanted, or spontaneous, and strain of mouse whether susceptible, resistant, or immune compromised *(7)*. Mice differ greatly in their susceptibility to cancers because of allelic variations in their cancer susceptibility genes. This results in variations in tumor formation from xenografts even in inbred strains of mice *(7,8)*.

However, the combination of genetically modified animals and molecular imaging has created more reliable models of human cancer. Transgenic mice made either by pronuclear injection or gene targeting (gene knockout animals) have resulted in new models for cancer research. There are over 2000 entries in Medline relating to mouse transgenesis

Table 1
Animal Models: Advantages and Disadvantages

| Typical Animal Models | Description | Advantages | Disadvantages |
|---|---|---|---|
| Conventional animal models | Animals that measure one end point | Lower cost Lower technology requirements | Lack real-time information Low throughput Variability in data impacts predictiveness |
| Knockout animals | Animals that are genetically modified to disable or knock out to express a gene of interest | Ability to observe impact of knocked-out gene on the physical characteristics | Lack real-time information Low throughput Variability in data impacts predictiveness |
| Transgenic animals | Animals that are genetically modified to express a human gene | Ability to observe impact of a new gene on the physical characteristics | Lack real-time information Low throughput Variability in data impacts predictiveness |

and the study of cancer. Nearly 80 different transgenes cause cancer in mice, 25% of which are viral oncogenes (8). Genetically modified animals in combination with small-animal imaging techniques have moved molecular imaging to the forefront of systems biology in oncogenesis. Transgenic animal models developed for in vivo imaging are disease-specific model animals that enable analysis of gene expression, protein activity, and disease progression. In these models, the gene for luciferase is present in every cell in the body of the animal, but only produces light when that gene is turned on in a specific cell type.

A summary of the advantages and disadvantages of animal models is given in Table 1.

## 3. SMALL-ANIMAL IMAGING

Because of the limitations of current in vivo and in vitro assays, researchers have been seeking new technologies that provide physiologically relevant data. Other in vivo imaging modalities that are under investigation for use in the clinical setting and in drug discovery and development generally lack the ease of use of in vitro and conventional animal model assessment. These modalities are not amenable to high throughput and require more expense and skill level in collecting and analyzing the data (9). Table 2 briefly describes what we consider to be the comparative advantages and disadvantages of various in vivo technologies.

## 4. IN VIVO BIOPHOTONIC IMAGING

Bioluminescent or biophotonic imaging is a technology that uses optically active reporters (reporters that emit photons) to access complex biological systems in the form of dynamic functional data (10). Visual capabilities enable researchers to track and monitor

Table 2
Modality Resolution and Most Frequent Applications in Drug Discovery Development

| Modality | Resolution | Application/Advantages | Disadvantages |
|---|---|---|---|
| Magnetic resonance imaging (MRI) | 10–200 nm | Structural imaging | Long scan and analysis time |
| MRI (functional) | 0.8–2 mm | Metabolic/function Gene expression | Contrast-agent chemistry |
| Positron-emission tomography (PET) | 3 mm | Metabolic Gene expression | Synthesis of radionuclide |
| Single-photon emission computed tomography (SPECT) | Lower or similar to PET | Structural Gene expression | Isotopes, limited reporter chemistry |
| General optical imaging | 3–5 mm | Noninvasive localization | Lower resolution |
| Computed tomography (CT) | 100 µm | Structural | X-ray |
| Biophotonic imaging | 3–5 mm | Noninvasive localization Gene expression, function Relative high throughput | Lower resolution |

a diverse range of molecular and cellular activities, such as gene expression and protein activity, tumor growth, and progression of infectious diseases across different tissues or organs within an animal.

Real-time capabilities of noninvasive biophotonic imaging enable observation of mechanisms of action or cascading events within the animal that would not otherwise be detected using conventional animal models. This is particularly important in studies where genes are altered by environmental determinants and in studies in which drugs are delivered and affect biological pathways of whole tissues in a manner that cellular systems or other in vitro systems do not (11).

As it relates to oncology, biophotonic imaging allows longitudinal study design using the same animal and collecting data from time 0 to the end point of the studies to allow the zero time-point to be a relative internal control. Biophotonic imaging is a sensitive method of detecting metastatic disease, visualizing the efficacy and safety of a drug within the same animal, looking earlier in the disease process specifically at early genes, and, in addition, monitoring inducible and controllable systems to determine gene function (11).

The main reporter systems of biophotonic imaging are luciferase, green fluorescent protein (GFP), cyanine dyes, and other fluorescent markers. The key differentiating factors among reporters and markers are whether it is a genetic reporter (luciferase and GFP are genetic reporters), whether the reporter requires excitation light, and the wavelength. Longer-wavelength light is more easily detected through opaque tissues. Most wavelengths used in optical imaging range from 489 to 620 nm. Near-infrared fluorophores are between 700 and 900 nm (10). Luciferase has been reported to be a more sensitive reporter than GFP (10), but each has unique applications. Here, the focus will be on bioluminescent imaging using luciferase as an optical reporter for use in oncology.

## 5. LUCIFERASES

Firefly and other luciferases have been used for decades as the basis of sensitive in vitro and whole-cell assays with a wide dynamic range. The fundamental biochemistry of luciferase reactions has been reviewed frequently and in great detail. Briefly, light production from luciferase gene expression occurs via an enzyme reaction to create a cool light. These enzyme reactions vary according to the structure of the luciferase and enzyme substrates; however, all of the luciferase enzymatic reaction usually involves a heterodimeric enzyme, an energy source, and cofactors *(12)*.

## 6. BIOLUMINESCENT OPTICAL IMAGING

The sensitivity of bioluminescent imaging arises from the fact that mammalian tissues do not emit significant levels of intrinsic bioluminescence, and because photon emission is restricted to cells engineered to express the bioluminescent reporter gene, there is an inherently low background. Thus, virtually no signal can be detected from naive cells or tissues that have not been engineered to express luciferase. Nonetheless, penetration of photons through mammalian tissues, whether from internal or external sources, is limited by both absorption and scatter. The basic principles of photon migration through absorbing and scattering media, such as mammalian tissue, have been the subject of intense investigation and have been reviewed in refs. *11* and *13*. The amount of light that passes through mammalian tissues is determined by the amount of scatter and absorption, which is determined by the tissue depth and type, the number of tissue boundaries that are encountered along the path of the photons, and the concentration of absorbing pigments in the tissues. The interaction of light with biological materials comprises the field of biophotonics and the discoveries in this area have a tremendous impact on the interpretation of optical signals that originate from within the body *(11,13)*.

## 7. IMAGING METHODS

Bioluminescent imaging is performed using a highly sensitive charged coupled device (CCD) camera that is cooled to below 100°C to minimize environmental photon noise. For in vivo imaging of firefly luciferase reporters, animals are given the substrate D-luciferin by intraperitoneal injection at 150 mg/kg and then anesthetized (1–3% isoflurane). Usually, mice are placed on a warmed stage and imaged for 1–5 min. Generally, several mice can be imaged at the same time, which contributes to a higher-throughput experiment. Quantification can be done across the whole body or in specific regions of interest. Photons correlate with cell number, with a correlation coefficient of $r^2 = 0.99$ *(14)*.

## 8. BIOLUMINESCENT ANIMAL MODELS OF CANCER

### *8.1. Xenograft Models Using Cultured Tumor Cells Constitutively Expressing Luciferase*

By far, the most common measure of tumor burden in the mouse model is performed in the subcutaneous xenograft model, which allows monitoring of tumor growth following implantation of cultured tumor cells subcutaneously on the flank of a syngenic mouse strain. Tumor growth is measured in the presence and absence of a therapeutic agent by either caliper measurement or by the weight of the extracted tumor. Limitations with these two methods are the inability to measure the exact number of viable tumor cells and the inclusion of the weight or size increase resulting from edema and the presence of nontumor cell types *(14)*.

Many cultured tumor cell lines have been transfected to express luciferase constitutively, including mouse colon adenocarcinoma line MC38 and human prostate PC-3M C6 and human colon HT-29 D6. These luc-labeled cultured tumor cells have been used in models of tumorigenesis that have increased sensitivity over conventional models and allow for longitudinal study design. Imaging the same group of mice over time also permits the kinetics of drug efficacy to be monitored over time with increased statistical significance *(9,14,15)*.

## 8.2. Metastatic Models of Disease Using Luciferase Reporters

Detection of metastatic disease in conventional animal models depend on ex vivo analysis. Thus, the throughput of the assay would be inversely correlated to the tissue sampling required for histopathology to analyze the extent of the tumor burden. Noninvasive bioluminescent imaging of metastatic disease permits the quantification of total tumor burden in the whole living animal. The value of this has been demonstrated on overcoming two major limitations of conventional models. First, progressive disease can be evaluated both spatially and temporally in the presence and absence of antitumor agents. Second, drug resistance or relapse can be monitored over time as an indicator of the ability of the tumor cell to escape the action of the chemotherapeutic agent. In other words, the tempo of the disease could reveal important information not available in single-end-point studies. This feature has been studied using traditional chemotherapeutic agents and immune cytotherapy in the treatment of metastatic disease and minimum residual disease following surgical intervention *(13,16)*.

## 8.3. Inducible Models of Oncogenesis

The lessons learned from the xenograft and metastatic models have been extended to include inducible promoters involved in oncogenesis. An example of an important inducible gene involved in tumor formation is the *p53* gene, a tumor suppressor protein that is a potent inducer of apoptosis and cell cycle arrest through transactivation of many genes involved in these pathways. Enhancing, restoring, or activating p53 function in cells is one approach to antitumor therapies. More importantly, p53 activity could also be an indicator of tumor response to experimental and clinical therapies *(17)*, Wang and El-Deiry *(17)* stably transfected a HCT116 colon cancer cell line with a p53 inducible firefly luciferase and a constitutively expressed renilla luciferase to track cell viability and then used this dual-labeled cell line for both in vitro and in vivo studies. In Fig. 1, A549/p53RE tumor cells labeled with the p53 promoter controlling the luciferase gene were used in a xenograft model to measure the induction of p53 in the presence of doxorubicin (*see* Color Plate 7 following p. 302). Doxorubicin is a potent inducer of p53 in both normal and tumor cells. This demonstrates the potential usefulness of inducible luciferase reporter in deter-mining gene expression in vivo and as a reporter assay for compound screening.

## 8.4. Transgenic Mice Expressing Luciferase as an Inducible Reporter of Gene Expression

Arguably, whole-cell assays with either constitutive expression of luciferase for cell tracking or inducible expression of luciferase for monitoring gene expression are higher

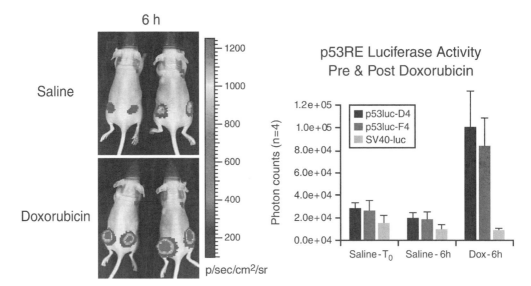

**Fig. 1.** p53-RE luciferase induction with doxorubicin in vivo. (Courtesy of Dr. Lidia Sambuccetti, Xenogen Corporation; *see* Color Plate 7 following p. 302.)

throughput, more simply performed, and easily interpreted because of fewer experimental variables than any in vivo experiment. This deconstructive mode of experimentation has given us a hook into gene function that made sequencing and genomic the technological advance that it represents today. After all, what would be the point of knowing the sequence if pairing that sequence with a gene function or disease state remained a mystery.

However, now is the time to press on and reach though our basic understanding of genomics and animal models and begin to piece together complex biology that surround the process of oncogenesis. One elegant way to approach complex systems biology is to pair in vivo bioluminescent imaging with genetically modified animals and label with a luciferase reporter gene. By building these models, pathways that cross therapeutic areas and the order of genes in these pathways can be determined. By cross-referencing gene function among pathways and therapeutic areas, we can begin to understand gene and protein interactions and their role in disease.

Luciferase has been added to both transgenic mice and rats and knockout or gene-targeted animals. Both endogenous mouse promoter and human promoters and receptors have been labeled with luciferase in these transgenic models (*18–20*). By creating transgenic animals with genes in the same pathway labeled, it is possible to build datasets around time and location of expression of multiple genes in one pathway.

One example of this would be analysis of VegF and VegFR2. The binding of vascular endothelial growth factor (VEGF) to its receptor (VegFR2) on the surface of endothelial cell membrane triggers a mitogenic signal in the endothelial cells and promotes the angiogenesis process to the proliferation/invasion stage (see Fig. 2). At this stage, endothelial cells start to proliferate to form vascular sprouts. Both endothelial cells and stromal cells secrete a broad range of proteolytic enzymes, which degrade the extracellular matrix and allow growth of blood vessels into the tumor mass. The establishment of circulation to the tumor triggers rapid tumor growth. The endothelial cells in the newly

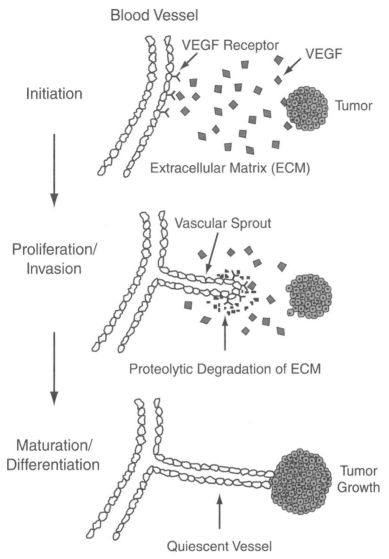

**Fig. 2.** Angiogenesis plays a critical role during tumor development. The tumor angiogenesis process is divided into three stages: initiation, proliferation/invasion, and maturation/differentiation. During the initiation stage, tumor cells secret many growth factors, such as VEGF. (Illustration courtesy of Dr. Ning Zhang, Xenogen Corporation.)

formed blood vessels go through a final stage of maturation/differentiation. Endothelial cells start to differentiate and become quiescence. The new established blood vessels ensure efficient blood flow and nutrient supply to the tumor. This process is an important target of antiagents. (*See* Fig. 3 and Color Plate 7 following p. 302.)

Another of the most promising transgenic models to date is the spontaneous-tumor-forming mouse model. These genetically modified animals allow researchers to address questions of the environmental effects on gene expression (epigenetic changes), changes as a result of mutation, and tissue- or organ-specific tumors.

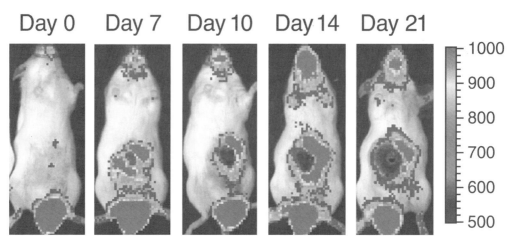

**Fig. 3.** Inducible Vegfr2-luc during tumor development. The Vegfr2-luc transgenic mice were generated in a FVB background. We generated hybrid transgenic mice using FVB Vegfr2-luc and C57 BL/6 albino mice. We implanted Lewis lung carcinoma cells (LL/2) into the hybrid Vegfr2-luc transgenic mice and monitored Vegfr2-luc expression during tumor development using an IVIS™ imaging system (Xenogen, Alameda, CA). We were able to detect tumor-induced Vegfr2-luc expression through imaging. At d 7, the tumor was only a few millimeters in diameter. The Vegfr2-luc expression was ready detectable, indicating that the endothelial cells started to proliferate to form new blood vessels. The signals last through the entire tumor development period because of constant endothelial cell proliferation and growth/reorganization of new formed blood vessels. As the tumor grew larger, the Vegfr2-luc signals started to localize in the tumor periphery, perhaps as a result of necrosis in the center of the tumor mass, especially at the late stage of tumor development. (*See* Color Plate 7 following p. 302.) (Courtesy of Drs. Tony Purchio, Darlene Jenkins, and Ning Zhang, Xenogen Corporation.)

Conditional alleles containing LoxP recombination sites, in conjunction with Cre recombinase (which can be delivered by a variety of means), allow for spatial and temporal control of gene expression in mouse models. Safran et al. *(21)* created a mouse strain in which the LoxP-stop-LoxP (L-S-L) cassette preceded the luciferase gene in the ubiquitously expressed ROSA26 locus. In these animals, when crossed with a mouse in which Cre was under the control of a zygotically expressed promoter (EIIA-Cre) or a liver-specific promoter (Albumin-Cre), luciferase was expressed either diffusely (EIIA-Cre) or in a liver-specific manner (Albumin-Cre). In this model, as the Cre-Recombinase is delivered to the cell containing the promoter/ L-S-L/luciferase construct in the genome, the L-S-L sequence is excised and luciferase is activated.

This idea is the basis for organ-specific spontaneous tumor formation that could be monitored noninvasively by bioluminescent imaging. Vooijs et al. *(20)* used a Cre recombinase system to create a conditional mouse model for retinoblastoma-dependent sporadic cancer. The Rb tumor suppressor gene, if mutated in mice, causes animals to be predisposed to the development of pituitary tumors. Using the Cre/loxP *(20)* or the Flp-mediated system *(21)*, the Rb gene can be conditionally inactivated in the pituitary, causing rapid development of melanotroph tumors. These mice were crossed with a transgenic line that carried a lobe-specific promoter (POMC) controlling both luciferase and the Cre recombinase. Upon the inactivation of the Rb gene, these animals formed pituitary tumors that correlate with the extent that the Rb gene (heterozygous or homozygous inactivation) is inactivated. This method was applied to the generation of a mouse with the potential for the tissue-specific luciferase expression form and luciferase reporter expressed ubiquitously in mice. These authors used the B-actin promoter preceding the luciferase gene in transgenic animals made by pronuclear injection. A Cre-activatable polyadenylated transcription termination site was placed in between the promoter and the luciferase gene. These LucRep animals were then crossed with a conditional oncogenic Kras2 transgenic mouse to demonstrate that the LucRep allele could be used to image spontaneous lung tumor development in vivo *(20)*. In both models, sensitive noninvasive detection facilitated the identification of these genes in the pathway of oncogenesis and the efficacy of therapeutic intervention.

## 9. SUMMARY

Functional genomics will make a significant impact and offer new opportunities to advance our understanding of disease and improve diagnosis. Analysis of high-throughput gene expression data requires creative and computationally intensive approaches, with many challenges remaining *(23)*. Complex diseases like cancer that have as a hallmark multicomponent etiologies lend themselves to those tools that can sort out the functional role of genes and pathways *(24)*. Exciting advances in noninvasive bioluminescent imaging and transgenic technologies will offer a systems biology approach that is necessary to sort out the complicated interaction between genetic pathways and environmental effects that might induce disease. Moreover, it is a technology that all researchers have access to at the benchtop level. It becomes incumbent upon us to take up the challenge of unraveling complex biology for the benefit of therapeutic intervention in oncogenesis, one of the most critical diseases of the human genome.

## ACKNOWLEDGEMENTS

I would like to thank Dr. Ning Zhang, Dr. Darlene Jenkins, and Dr. Lidia Sambuccetti for providing unpublished pictures of biophotonic animal models and Ms. Ro Farrell for help in preparation of the manuscript. Thanks to Dr. Chris Contag and Dr. Scott Lyons for helpful discussions on imaging and transgenic models containing luciferase.

## REFERENCES

1. Strausberg RL, Simpson AJG, Wooster R. Sequence-based cancer genomics: progress, lessons and opportunities. Nature Rev/Genetics 2003; 4:409–418.
2. Chanda SK, Caldwell JS. Fulfilling the promise: drug discovery in the post-genomic era. DDT 2003; 8: 168–174.
3. Balleine RL, Kefford RF. Targeting molecular mechanisms in cancer. ANZ J Surg 2002; 72:760–763.
4. Rosell R, Monzo M, O'Brate A, Taron M. Translational oncogenomics: toward rational therpeutic decision-making. Curr Opin Oncol 2002; 14:171–179.
5. Baak JPA, Path FRC, Hermsen MAJA, Meijer G, Schmidt J, Janssen EAM. Genomics and proteomics in cancer. Eur J Cancer 2003; 39:1199–1215.
6. Strausberg RL, Austin MJF. Functional genomics: technological challenges and opportunities. Physiol Genom 1999; 1:25–32.
7. Strong LC. Genetic nature of the constitutional states of cancer susceptibility and resistance in mice and men. Yale J Biol Med 2000; 73:265–272. (Originally published: 1945; 17:289–299).
8. Largaespada DA. Genetically modified mice in cancer research. In: Hofker LMH, van Deursen J, eds. Transgenic mouse methods and protocols. Totowa, NJ: Humana, 2002:311–332.

9. Choy G, Choyke P, Libutti SK. Current advances in molecular imaging: noninvasive in vivo bioluminescent and fluorescent optical imaging in cancer research. Mol Imaging 2003; 2(4):303–312.

10. Choy G, O'Connor S, Diehn FE, Costouros N, Alexander HR, Choyke P, et al. Comparison of noninvasive fluorescent and bioluminescent small animal optical imaging. BioTechniques 2003; 35:1022–1030.

11. Contag PR. Whole-animal cellular and molecular imaging to accelerate drug development. DDT 2002; 7:10:555–562.

12. McCaffrey A, Kay MA, Contag CH. Advancing molecular therapies through in vivo bioluminescent imaging. Mol Imaging 2003; 2(2):75–86.

13. Contag CH, Jenkins E, Contag PR, Negrin RS. Use of reporter genes for optical measurements of neoplastic disease *in vivo*. Neoplasia 2000; 2(1–2):41–52.

14. Jenkins DE, Oei Y, Hornig YS, Yu S-F, Dusich J, Purchio R, et al. Bioluinescent imaging (BLI) to improve and refine traditional murine models of tumor growth and metastasis. Clin Exp Metastasis 2003; 20:733–744.

15. Jenkins DE, Yu S-F, Hornig YS, Purchio T, Contag PR. *In vivo* monitoring of tumor relapse and metastasis using bioluminescent PC-3M-luc-C6 cells in murine models of human prostate cancer. Clin Exp Metastasis 2003; 20:745–756.

16. Sweeney TJ, Mailander V, Tucker AA, Olomu AB, Zhang W, Cao Y, et al. Visualizing the kinetics of tumor-cell clearance in living animals. PNAS 1999; 96(21):12,044–12,049.

17. Wang W, El-Deiry WS. Bioluminescent molecular imaging of endogenous and exogenous p53-mediated transcription in vitro and in vivo using an HCT116 human colon carcinoma xenograft model. Cancer Biol Ther 2003; 2(2):196–202.

18. Zhang W, Purchio AF, Coffee R, West DB. Differential regulation of the human Cyp3a4 promoter in transgenic mice and rats. Drug Metab Dispos 2004; 32:2:163–167.

19. Zhang N, Fang Z, Contag PR, Purchio AF, West DB. Using a Vegfr2-luciferase transgenic mouse. Blood 2004; 103(2):617–626.

20. Vooijs M, Jonkers J, Lyons S, Berns A. Noninvasive imaging of spontaneous retinoblastoma pathway-dependent tumors in mice. Cancer Res 2002; 62:1862–1867.

21. Safran M, Kim WY, Kung AL, Horner JW, DePinho, Kaelin WG Jr. Mouse reporter strain for non-invasive bioluminescent imaging of cells that have undergone cre-mediated recombination. Mol Imaging 2003; 2:297–302.

22. Lyons SK, Meuwissen R, Krimpenfort P, Berns A. The generation of a conditional reporter that enables bioluminescence imaging of Cre/loxP-dependent tumorigenesis in mice. Cancer Res 2003; 63:7042–7046.

23. Gabrielson E, Berg K, Ramaswamy A. Functional genomics, gene arrays, and the future of pathology. Mod Pathol 2001; 14(12):1294–1299.

24. Weber BL. Cancer genomics. Cancer Cell 2002; 1:37.

# 18 Innovative Strategies for Improving Engineered Mouse Models of Human Cancer for Preclinical Development

*Jeffrey J. Martino and Suzie Chen, PhD*

## CONTENTS

### SUMMARY

Because of the high cost and risk of anticancer drug discovery and development, predictability is highly desirable. Results from a small-animal model system that is highly relevant to a given human tumor are of the highest quality in target identification and validation, in evaluating the efficacy and toxicity, and in targeting the delivery of a therapeutic. Here, we discuss efforts in engineering better mouse model systems of cancer and the promise offered by innovative technologies in further improving them.

**Key Words:** Mouse models; disease models; drug discovery; drug development; imaging; humanized mouse.

## 1. INTRODUCTION

The cost of drug discovery and development is truly staggering—not just in dollars, but in time as well. To ease this ever-increasing burden, investigators continually strive for more predictability in every phase of the process, from identification through postapproval. The attraction of a reductionist approach to address such issues is easy to understand in view of the continuing expansion of knowledge of molecular biology and increasingly high-throughput techniques—particularly in the quest for therapeutic progress against complex and ostensibly intractable diseases such as cancer. Yet, the complexities inherent in human tumor physiology and cancer progression argue against a wholly molecular or even cellular strategy. How can vasculature, neighboring support structures, and local and

From: *Cancer Drug Discovery and Development: The Oncogenomics Handbook*
Edited by: W. J. LaRochelle and R. A. Shimkets © Humana Press Inc., Totowa, NJ

systemic communications be summarily eliminated from the biology of a tumor, for example, or systemwide effects on a person's well-being be ignored? Rather, the micro can inform the macro, and vice versa: There is an increasing need for more and better animal models in drug discovery and development.

In the United States, cancer causes one of every four deaths. In 2004, more than 1.3 million new diagnoses are expected. An inclusive estimate of monetary cost by the National Institutes of Health (NIH), totaled nearly $190 billion in 2003 (1). It is self-evident that research must be directed toward understanding and treating this disease.

## 2. HISTORY OF MOUSE MODELS OF CANCER

### 2.1. The Laboratory Mouse

The laboratory mouse has evolved as the central experimental system to model human disease. For centuries, the importance of selection and breeding to develop or reinforce specific characteristics has been recognized in areas such as animal husbandry. At the start of the 20th century, Mendelian principals began to be applied to studies of inheritance in a variety of animals, beginning with obvious traits like coat color. It soon became evident to pioneers like William E. Castle at Harvard University and his students Sewall Wright and Clarence Cook Little that small mammals might be most useful as model biological systems. Mice were small, hearty, and rapidly prolific, with a source of interesting variants from "fanciers" worldwide. Soon Little and others originated inbred, or isogenic, strains by methodic full-sib matings over many generations to achieve genetic homogeneity at all loci, thus permitting an even finer level of control and consistency of these experimental animals.

Even at this early time, cancer research and the laboratory mouse were linked; the original motivation for such standardization was to determine the genetic contributions to cancer. Little, for example, investigated the susceptibility of Japanese "waltzing" mice to transplanted sarcomas, and later at Cold Spring Harbor, Carleton MacDowell studied the spontaneous leukemia of the C58 strain. In 1929, Little founded the Roscoe B. Jackson Memorial Laboratory in Bar Harbor, ME specifically "for research in cancer and the effects of radiation." A milestone in the history of the Jackson Laboratory was the 1941 release of the first edition of *Biology of the Laboratory Mouse*—much of which dealt with cancer biology. The complex, a National Cancer Institute (NCI)-designated cancer center, still serves as a center for the development, maintenance, and distribution of mouse strains.

Further improvements in methods to manipulate mouse inheritance continued apace. In the 1940s, another former student of Castle, future Nobel Laureate George D. Snell, developed the breeding technique of the congenic strain to address the problem of background effects in studying a mutation established in a noninbred strain. Snell's work on tissue transplantation thus progressed, and with the work of Peter Gorer, it ultimately led to the discovery of the major histocompatibility complex (MHC).

Not all early cancer models were based solely on genetics. J.J. Bittner's studies of inbred strains highly resistant to cancer versus those extremely susceptible found the primary factor in the development of spontaneous mammary tumors in the C3H strain to be transmitted in mother's milk. This marked the first discovery of a tumor virus in mammals.

Of course, the molecular understanding of viral oncogenes and their normal cellular counterparts would await the recognition of DNA as the genetic material and the development of concomitant techniques. Solutions at a "coarse" genetic level of spontaneous and induced mutations, selection, and breeding techniques, however, did continue to yield results.

The laboratory mouse allowed methodical and reproducible studies. Beyond investigations of basic biological mechanisms, researchers were able to examine the effects of various medications, as well as chemotherapy and radiation treatment directed against various cancers. The mouse had been "regularized" and was exceptionally manipulable—except for its molecular genetic structure and the mechanics of its reproduction.

## 2.2. Transgenic Mice

In the following years, the convergence of experimental mouse embryology and reproduction, with recombinant DNA techniques, permitted manipulation of the mouse at previously barred levels, accelerating discovery.

### 2.2.1. PRONUCLEAR INJECTION

Despite the long and rich chronology of mammalian embryology, it was not until the 1950s and 1960s that successful in vitro culture conditions were determined for the mouse gametes and embryo. Even before the maturation of DNA techniques, there were early attempts to more directly manipulate the mouse genome for cancer modeling. For example, in 1974, Rudolf Jaenisch and Beatrice Mintz confirmed the presence of viral sequences in somatic tissues of adult mice derived from preimplantation blastocysts that had been injected with purified SV40 DNA. Jaenisch later showed germline integration and transmission of the Moloney leukemia virus (M-MuLV) after infecting embryos at the 4- to 8-cell stage.

Ralph Brinster's experiments with the injection of globin RNA into fertilized mouse eggs set the stage for the introduction of DNA by similar methods. Using a pronuclear injection technique, a group at Yale, with Jon W. Gordon and Frank Ruddle, showed the presence of introduced foreign DNA in the tissues of resulting mice. In the span of the next few months in 1981, several more groups independently demonstrated integration and expression of the "transgenes" in the animal, and even stable germline transmission. It was thus possible to purposefully alter the mouse germline by the addition of DNA from any source.

### 2.2.2. EMBRYONIC STEM CELLS

Although the integration of a microinjected transgene is essentially random, other mouse embryological studies were the key to a more targeted approach. In the early 1960s, investigators such as Kristof Tarkowski and Beatrice Mintz developed the technique of the aggregation chimera, combining cleaving embryos. The resulting mosaic mice, often exemplified by a pup with a striking patchwork coat color, opened many areas of study such as cell differentiation and migration and even tumor clonality. Richard Gardner extended the technique by injecting dissociated embryonic cells into blastocysts to create chimeras.

Paralleling such embryonic manipulations were studies of spontaneous teratomas displaying a mix of tissue types in the mouse. These mouse models of developmental biology and cancer complemented each other. Derived teratocarcinomas that can grow without limit always contained a population of small, rounded unspecialized cells; those tumors that cease growth show only specialized types. The studies by Leroy Stevens and

Barry Pierce also led to suggestions that cancer could be a disease of delayed or reversed differentiation or might be ameliorated by forcing the differentiation.

This cancer stemmed from undifferentiated cells that were pluripotent, later labeled embryonal carcinoma (EC) cells. The origins of the teratomas were traced back to the genital ridge structure in the prenatal mouse, which is populated by primordial germ cells (PGCs). Grafted into adults, they can generate teratomas. Similar cells from the embryonic inner cell mass (ICM) and other early stages were also implanted into an ectopic location such as the testes of adult mice and, again, some developed into teratomas exhibiting multiple specialized types.

### 2.2.3. Germline Chimeras

Brinster and Mintz and others in the mid-1970s demonstrated that EC cells behave normally if introduced into a normal embryonic milieu and can contribute to normal adult tissues in such a chimeric mouse. In the early 1980s, Martin Evans, Matthew Kaufman, and Gail Martin independently established lines of pluripotent cells directly from the ICM of normal mouse blastocysts. When used to create chimeric mice, these embryonic stem (ES) cells were found to contribute to all tissues, including the germline. Interestingly, PCGs eventually were cultured as cells with similar properties, now known as embryonic germ (EG) cells. Any in vitro modifications to the genomes of the aforementioned embryonic cells would be passed along into new kinds of mice, after the cells are reintegrated into an embryo and contribute to its germline.

In the late 1980s, the ability to manipulate such ES cells in culture converged with in vitro techniques of homologous recombination and selection, permitting the "targeting" of genes and the subsequent derivation of new transgenic mouse strains harboring these precise genetic changes via germline transmission. These now familiar techniques initially demonstrated in the laboratories of Oliver Smithies, Martin Evans, and Mario Capecchi continue to grow in both efficacy and usefulness.

### 2.2.4. Transgenic Technology in Wide Use

Once DNA sequence information for a gene is known, appropriate vectors can be constructed for homologous recombination and selection. The use of both positive and negative selectable markers facilitates the complete disruption, or "knock out" of the function of a particular gene. Other extensions of the gene-targeting methods permit a subtle placement of a target mutation within a gene, a "knock in" of a transgene at a selected locus, or even conditional transgenesis with inducible activation, or tissue- or temporal-specific control of the gene of interest. Unlike the random nature of classical mutagenesis, it is thus possible to purposefully alter the germline, not only to study gene function and development but also to create better disease models.

## 3. GENETICALLY ENGINEERED MOUSE MODELS AND DRUG DISCOVERY AND DEVELOPMENT

### 3.1. Utilization and Cost

Some might contend that genetically engineered mice currently are underutilized for drug discovery and development, with a perception of high cost and low throughput that runs counter to the current paradigm. In recent years, automated in vitro assays and *in silico* analyses have successfully increased throughput and efficiencies for the pharmaceutical industry. It is notable, however, that preclinical animal data are still given more weight by the Food and Drug Administration (FDA) as an indicator of efficacy and safety in humans. As new technology continues to increase the efficiency and accuracy of mouse modeling, the perception for engineered mice might presently be high quality rather than high cost.

With a total cost for a new drug to get to market estimated at over $800 million *(2)* and with identification and preclinical testing, clinical trials, and postclinical trials to file a New Drug or Biologics License Application with the FDA for approval taking more than a decade to complete (The Nation's Investment in Cancer Research, A plan and budget proposal for fiscal year 2005 http://plan.cancer.gov/), it is advisable to invest in early discovery research to focus on the best targets, rather than pay the penalty for attrition in the late stages of development. There is a need for in vivo models *(3)*.

### 3.2. Cancer: A Complex Phenotype

Despite the extraordinarily valuable advances in oncogenomics of the tumor cell, in the end, cancer remains a phenotype. Vasculature, neighboring support structures, and local and systemic communications cannot be eliminated from the biology of a tumor; neither can systemwide effects on a person's well-being be ignored when developing a therapy. Indeed, some consider the basis of malignancy to be mediated by signaling between tumor epithelium and basement membrane and stroma. Recalling the normalization of EC cells in the embryonic environment, they propose to design therapeutics to revert the tumor cell phenotype by correcting only a minimum of signaling defects—even when the cells have suffered multiple genetic and epigenetic lesions—offering the remission of acute promyelocytic leukemia (APL) by retinoic acid-based therapies as an example *(4)*.

### 3.3. Many Targets, Little Biology

With the sequencing and annotation of entire genomes, there comes an overwhelming number of potential targets for preclinical investigation—yet with relatively little knowledge of target biology. Building on the older technologies of mouse reproduction and genetics with new genomic, micromanipulatory, measurement, and informatic techniques, transgenic mouse models can inform the R&D process at many points in the lengthy path. Even the simplest, randomly integrated, transgenic mouse can be considered a model for global overexpression of a target gene; even the crudest knockout mouse is intrinsically a model for testing the effects of downregulating a target.

### 3.4. Disease-Based Target Identification in a Laboratory

Real-world experimental situations can often combine the archetypal transgenic approaches. A transgene introduced by pronuclear injection can cause a randomly targeted mutagenesis at the site of its integration, knocking out or otherwise modulating gene expression. As the phenotypes of transgenic mice are subjected to extensive evaluation, unforeseen effects are generally noted, and in many cases, they have led to the serendipitous identification of new genes and gene functions *(5)*.

An example of the serendipitous identification of a new gene occurred in the study of adipocyte differentiation/melanoma development in our laboratory. Incidence of melanoma is rising at an alarming rate, and on its present course, the lifetime risk will reach 1 in 75 among Caucasians in the United States in the next 10 yr *(6)*. In contrast to most malignancies, melanoma affects a younger population, metastasizes early, and fails to respond to current available therapeutics *(7)*. Despite much clinical and molecular effort directed toward this disease, little is known about the precise genetic lesions leading to melanoma.

Normally, spontaneous malignant melanomas are a rare occurrence in rodents. A model system that intrinsically recapitulates a single type of neoplasm will always be a powerful tool for dissecting the molecular events underlying the initiation, promotion, and progression of that neoplasm.

Several mouse model systems have been engineered that have proved valuable for the definition of susceptibility genes and molecular events leading to the disease *(8–19)*. In contrast to these models, transgenic mice developed in our laboratory display spontaneous melanoma without any known exogenous carcinogenic stimuli or forced expression of viral oncogenes and without involvement of unrelated tissues. These transgenic mice were constructed by pronuclear injection of Clone B DNA—a small fragment of genomic sequence that commits a variety of cells in culture to undergo adipocyte differentiation *(20,21)*. The transgenic mice were expected to display adipocyte-related phenotypes; none of these mice, however, exhibited obesity. The TG-3 transgenic line derived from one of the five independent founder mice, each of which had a different transgene-integration site, displayed raised melanotic lesions detectable in the dermis of the pinnae of the ear and perianal regions as early as 10–14 d of age. These lesions progressed to overt tumors and invaded nearby tissues as they matured into adult mice. About 90% of the animals in this transgenic line, if homozygous at the transgene integration locus, had very large pigmented tumor masses in eyes, ears, snout, and perianal region at 2–5 mo of age. Mice heterozygous for the insertion showed similar tumor phenotypes at 5–7 mo of age. These tumor-bearing animals either died or had to be sacrificed. Animals of the other transgenic lines remain normal even past 2 yr of age *(22,23)*.

Physical mapping determined that with insertion of the transgene into a region of mouse chromosome 10, syntenic to the long arm of human chromosome 6 where rearrangement has been noted in a large number of human nonfamilial malignant melanomas *(24)*, about 70 kb of host sequences were deleted. We identified the deleted host region to be part of intron 3 of the gene encoding for metabotropic glutamate receptor 1 (Grm1). To demonstrate that Grm1 has a direct etiological role in melanoma development in our model system and to distinguish between causes and consequences of elevated levels of Grm1 expression in tumor tissues, we generated a new line of transgenic mice with wild-type mouse Grm1 cDNA under the control of a melanocyte-specific promoter Dct. In one of the founder mice, development of pigmented tumor on the tail was observed by 5–6 mo of age. Subsequent offspring showed pigmented tumors in the ears and tails by 3–4 mo of age. The introduction of Grm1 alone was sufficient to induce melanoma development in our model system *(25)*. Such a result could be considered validation of a role for Grm1 in tumorigenesis or, from a different perspective, a step in the identification, and data possibly supporting validation, of a drug target—a stage of exploratory discovery.

There is additional compelling evidence for the importance of metabotropic glutamate signaling in melanocytic neoplasia: We detected expression of GRM1 in a number of human melanoma biopsies and cell lines but not in benign nevi and melanocytes *(25)*. Again, such data would increase confidence in the validity of a drug target.

Expression of this family of neurotransmitter receptors is usually restricted to neuronal cells; however, the signaling pathways activated by these receptors are widely distributed in both neural and non-neural cells. We hypothesize that the ectopic expression of such a receptor in an unnatural melanocytic cellular environment leads to malignant transformation of normal melanocytes. Grm1, a member of the metabotropic glutamate receptors, belongs to the G protein-coupled seven-transmembrane domain receptor family (GPCRs). GPCRs comprise the largest known family of cell surface receptors and mediate cellular responses to a diverse array of signaling molecules, including hormones, neurotransmitters, and chemokines, as well as autocrine and paracrine factors.

Although a low-throughput process, in target selection and validation strategies, much weight is generally given to linking a gene to a specific disease by molecular genetics and in vivo studies; however, it is considered statistically improbable that any particular disease gene identified will be a member of a family of genes that, by experience, are considered "druggable" targets and are thus given high priority for further validation *(26)*. GPCRs are one of those groups. A review of serendipity in pharmaceutical research has been published *(27)*.

### *3.5. Diverse Uses for Mouse Models of Cancer*

#### 3.5.1. Screening for Autoimmunity: Immune-Based Therapy

Vaccination has been an effective defense against both bacterial and viral diseases. Research to develop vaccine-based cancer immunotherapy targeting tumor-associated antigens (TAAs), although still at an early stage, is proceeding with the assistance of transgenic mouse models. A major concern in the development of such therapeutics is that because TAAs are self-antigens, the benefit of an antitumor effect must not be outweighed by a pathological autoimmunity—particularly with the addition of costimulatory molecules to increase vaccine potency.

Carcinoembryonic antigen (CEA) overexpression, for example, has been associated with a variety of carcinomas, but does exhibit a limited normal tissue expression and is thus considered both a TAA and self-antigen. In a series of studies, a mouse model engineered to correctly express the human CEA has proved useful in evaluating autoimmune reactions. The model permitted a comprehensive evaluation of vaccine effects by biochemical, immunological, and histopathological criteria. Not only was a therapeutic response observed in this system, but it was concluded that vectors for potent vaccines, containing as many as three costimulatory molecules, do not induce autoimmunity or other pathology *(28)*.

#### 3.5.2. Cytotoxic Agents: Targeted Drug Delivery

Many early transgenic models continue to be useful in proving new concepts in the development and delivery of better anticancer drugs. Tumor-directed cytotoxic therapy, for example, attempts to address one of the major problems of chemotherapeutic agents—the lack of selectivity. Whether a gene-, virus-, or antibody-directed enzyme prodrug or a toxin directly conjugated to a monoclonal antibody, the idea is to target the activity of a systemically administered cytotoxic agent specifically to the tumor microenvironment.

The lack of natural animal models for prostate cancer (PCa) was addressed by the generation of a transgenic mouse expressing the SV40 large-T antigen (TAg) under the androgen-regulated prostate-specific rat probasin promoter *(29)*. Later designated the transgenic adenocarcinoma mouse prostate (TRAMP) model, the authors characterized a metastatic disease that closely paralleled the progression of benign, latent, and aggressive stages in the human cancer, yet allowed easy manipulation. Recently, the same model was used to test a gene-directed enzyme prodrug therapy (GDEPT). The prodrug fludarabine phosphate was administered systemically and converted locally to the diffusible toxic metabolite 2-fluoroadenine by the *Escherichia coli* PNP enzyme that had been delivered by a single intraprostatic injection of modified ovine adenovirus. It was found that in this system, a single course of PNP-GDEPT caused a highly significant suppression of PCa *(30)*.

Although the particular metabolite in the aforementioned GDEPT system was designed to, and did, induce a powerful bystander effect, one must always be aware that, currently, in vivo gene transfer is not 100% efficient. Some attempt to use the tumor to target itself.

The efficacy and specificity of chemotherapy for neuroblastoma has been markedly limited. This devastating childhood cancer of the nervous system is marked by high relapse rates, even after intensive therapy. One group set out to rationally design a prodrug for neuroblastoma. Concerned about immunogenicity of the nonhuman protein component of the drug-activating conjugate in eventual human therapy, they selected an endogenous enzyme highly expressed by neuroblastomas—tyrosine hydroxylase—to catalyze activation of the etoposide prodrug. This elegant therapy relies on the natural specificity of the tumor-expressed enzyme and the design of the prodrug as a substrate for it. Having proved cytotoxicity of the drug against neuroblastoma cells in vitro, it is proposed to next test antitumor effects and the therapeutic window in vivo *(31)*.

A transgenic neuroblastoma mouse model will offer a useful system to further evaluate this neuroblastoma-directed enzyme prodrug therapy (NDEPT). As in many other early mouse models, SV40 TAg, when placed under the control of the tissue-specific promoter, was reported to recapitulate metastasizing human infant neuroblastoma. A later model, designed to explore the suspected role of the human proto-oncogene MYCN in the disease, targeted overexpression of the transgene to cells of the mouse neural crest, where neuroblasts are located in normal development *(32)*. Tumors developed several months after birth, and comparative genomic hybridization (CGH) analysis showed that chromosomal changes in the mouse neuroblastomas were in regions syntenic to those in human tumors. Either of these models should prove useful.

### 3.5.3. DELIVERY OF NEW THERAPEUTICS

There are many reviews of developments in the relatively new technology for inhibition of mammalian gene expression by small interfering RNAs (sRNAs) *(33)*. In vitro liposome-mediated transfection of siRNA can be quite efficient and the results easily observed. Pharmaceutical delivery of such double-stranded nucleic acids for therapeutic use in vivo offers particular challenges.

Either by introduction of exogenous synthetic RNA or RNA analog or by endogenous gene-therapy expression, some recent studies aim to directly knock down cancer-related genes, whereas others seek to increase the effectiveness of traditional anticancer therapeutics by modulating genes involved in drug resistance. Transgenic mouse models expressing the target of interest, combined with reporters for molecular imaging, might offer a better way to measure and optimize the properties of an siRNA drug under investigation in vivo.

Already, one group has used a transgenic rodent strain that ubiquitously expresses green fluorescent protein (GFP) to demonstrate silencing by transgene-mediated RNA interference (RNAi) in embryos *(34)*. It is likely that transgenic model systems will play an increasing role in the development of siRNA-related therapeutics.

### 3.5.4. SMALL-ANIMAL IMAGING

Reporter genes like GFP have been used for the measurement of gene activity in vitro for some time now, as has β-galactosidase to mark expression in tissues of a transgenic mouse. Imaging techniques now are being extended to whole, live animals. New optical devices with coupled charge device (CCD) cameras that are sensitive enough to detect in vivo expression of fluorescence and bioluminescence through tissues are being developed. Technologies such as magnetic resonance, positron-emission tomography, and ultrasound are being adapted to small-animal imaging as well *(35,36)*. The NCI has helped establish several In Vivo Cellular and Molecular Imaging Centers (ICMICs) to advance the field.

In vivo cellular and molecular imaging combined with transgenic technology might soon provide animal models even more predictive of therapeutic value. As an example, one group engineered a conditional transgenic mouse model for a retinoblastoma-dependent sporadic cancer by Cre-mediated recombination in the pituitary gland. A luciferase reporter cotransgene expressed under a pituitary-specific promoter permitted the sensitive, noninvasive monitoring of tumor onset, development and regression, and quantitative assessment of tumor response to the anticancer drug doxorubicin *(37)*.

The imaging benefits are not unique to this model. Micro metastases and apoptosis can be pinpointed, and it is expected that enzyme catalysis, metabolic levels, protein binding, and even the action of drug at target site or a labeled candidate drug can be continually monitored. The efficiency inherent in studying single animals (self-controls) could dramatically decrease the numbers of needed mice in pharmaceutical development.

To be most useful, the physiopathology of disease models must be finely detailed. Anatomical structure of parental and engineered mice can presently be cataloged and compared at unprecedented resolution. A system for rapid morphological phenotyping by digital three-dimensional magnetic resonance (MR) microscopy was demonstrated to achieve resolutions more than 250,000 times that of clinical MR. This whole-fixed animal technique does not distort tissue as does standard histology, does not dehydrate and thus provides information about water, and, by nature, permits measurements of organ or tumor volume. The authors propose a common "Visible Mouse" reference archive to compare the anatomy of normal and model mice *(38)*.

### 3.5.5. STANDARDIZATION

Every new transgenic model strain should be minutely characterized. With these developing imaging tools, a complete phenotype can be performed, both structurally and functionally, allowing a more precise correlation with a transgenic genotype, as well as offering a more relevant in vivo measurement of response to any chemical or therapeutic challenge under physiologic conditions. Several organizations, such as the EU community's EUMOR-PHIA, are supporting the development of standardized protocols to characterize mouse models of disease, along with informatics to archive and disseminate detailed phenotype data.

### 3.5.6. HUMANIZING TRANSGENIC MODELS

In 1 yr, there were over 2 million hospitalized patients with serious adverse drug reactions (ADRs) and 100,000 fatal ADRs from properly administered drugs—ranking between the fourth and sixth leading cause of death in the United States *(39)*. It is preferable to become aware of potential toxicity early in drug development, especially before human clinical trials.

Most of the known pharmacogenetic variations occur in drug-metabolizing enzyme (DME) genes, many of which are of members of the cytochrome P-450 (CYP) superfamily and are known to process a number of anticancer drugs. Interestingly, no human polymorphisms have been associated with any overt physiological defect, and a decided lack of phenotype to most DME knockout transgenic mice, beyond a change in drug response, indicates no role for these genes in development or maintenance *(40)*.

To clarify and assist the utility of the mouse as a model mammal and as a surrogate for human biology, comparison and cataloging of the complete CYP families extracted from the published mouse and human genomes was undertaken *(41)*. It has been proposed to start engineering mice humanized for drug metabolism by knocking out DM–P-450s, followed by the insertion of the human orthologs into the P-450-null mouse background— perhaps more efficiently by employing a human allele cassette "gene-swapping" technique, all relevant genes can be humanized *(42)*.

Similarly, the regulation of hepatic cytochrome P-450 enzymes is involved in both drug metabolism and drug–drug interactions. Inducibility of CYP genes by xenobiotics shows species specificity. Subsequent to the knock out of the rodent xenosensor for CYP3A, the pregnane X receptor (PXR), and replacement by its human ortholog hPXR, the model displayed a humanized response profile *(43)*.

Despite the extraordinary similarities, a mouse response cannot always be directly extrapolated to human; humanized models are expected to be more valuable in improved predictability in pharmaceutical development and toxicology *(42)*.

The intrinsic humanization, by transgenesis with human oncogenes and tumor suppressors, has enhanced models; it is likely that further improvement might be achieved by humanization of a variety of types genes. Singular members of signaling pathways and, for example, various components of the human immune system already have been introduced into mice to better model rheumatoid arthritis and other autoimmune disease *(44)*.

Although its relevance to engineered cancers might be problematic, one persistent argument against the general suitability of mouse modeling of cancer is that despite a similar lifetime risk of about 30%, the spectrum and cytogenetics of tumors humans develop with age is quite distinct from those in mouse. Mice tend toward mesenchymal tissue tumors such as lymphomas and sarcomas, whereas humans tend toward epithelial carcinomas marked by highly abnormal karyotypes, including aneuploidy and nonreciprocal translocations (NRTs). Even when the exact pathways to a specific neoplasm have been shown to diverge, the particular mouse model always has proved quite informative, so this observation could have limited significance. However, it does illustrate a significant advantage of transgenic mouse modeling: If the model is discordant, it can be improved.

It had been observed that mouse chromosomes exhibit very long telomeres relative to human and that telomerase is active in most mouse cells but not in most adult human cells. In an effort to humanize a mouse cancer model, mice lacking the RNA component of telomerase (mTERC) were engineered on a Trp53-mutant background. With each generation as telomeres were progressively shortened, there was a significant shift to a more human tumor spectrum of breast, colon, and skin carcinomas—which exhibited more human cytogenetic lesions such as NRTs *(45,46)*.

## 4. CONCLUSION

Francis Collins at a press conference for the publication of the sequence of the mouse genome in *Nature* in 2002 remarked that the laboratory mouse is "man's real best friend."

The mouse is already the mammalian model animal of choice because of its innate physiological and genetic correspondence to humans, its uniquely murine physical, behavioral, and reproductive characteristics facilitating experimentation, and the ever-increasing toolkit of available molecular, cellular, genetic, and physical methods for manipulation and analysis.

Even with an estimated 99% of genes having a clear human counterpart, a general objective might be to use genetic techniques to further humanize the molecular and cellular biology, biochemistry, and drug metabolism of the mouse, while maintaining those characteristics inherently useful for research and disease modeling. Then, perhaps, a more particular goal could be set: to use the efficiency of transgenic technology to provide mice tailored to specific projects and disease states, and for in vivo analysis, thus requiring fewer total animals to achieve the desired ends.

In these ways, better mouse models of human cancers should facilitate oncology drug development for use in prevention, as well as treatment, of primary and advanced cancers, and by increasing the standardization, quality, and predictability throughout the process of drug discovery and development, to reduce time, cost, and attrition.

## REFERENCES

1. American Cancer Society. Cancer facts and figures. Atlanta, GA: American Cancer Society, 2004.
2. DiMasi JA, Hansen RW, Grabowski HG. The price of innovation: new estimates of drug development costs. [see comment]. J Health Econ 2003; 22:151–185.
3. Tornell J, Snaith M. Transgenic systems in drug discovery: from target identification to humanized mice. Drug Discov Today 2002; 7:461–470.
4. Kenny PA, Bissell MJ. Tumor reversion: correction of malignant behavior by microenvironmental cues. Int J Cancer 2003; 107:688–695.
5. Rijkers T, Peetz A, Ruther U. Insertional mutagenesis in transgenic mice. Transgen Res 1994; 3:203–215.
6. Rigel DS. Malignant melanoma: perspectives on incidence and its effects on awareness, diagnosis, and treatment. Ca: Cancer J Clin 1996; 46:195–198.
7. Herlyn M. Molecular and cellular biology of melanoma. Austin, TX: Landes, 1993.
8. Bradl M, Klein-Santo A, Porter S, Mintz B. Malignant melanoma in transgenic mice. Proc Natl Acad Sci USA 1991; 88:164–168.
9. Chin L, Pomerantz J, Polsky D, et al. Cooperative effects of INK4a and ras in melanoma susceptibility in vivo. Genes Dev 1997; 11:2822–2834.
10. Iwamoto T, Takahashi M, Ito M, et al. Aberrant melanogenesis and melanocytic tumour development in transgenic mice that carry a metallothionein/ret fusion gene. EMBO J 1991; 10:3167–3175.
11. Kato M, Takahashi M, Akhand AA, et al. Transgenic mouse model for skin malignant melanoma. Oncogene 1998; 17:1885–1888.
12. Mintz B, Silvers WK, Klein-Szanto AJP. Histopathogenesis of malignant skin melanoma induced in genetically susceptible transgenic mice. Proc Natl Acad Sci USA 1993; 90:8822–8826.
13. Klein-Szanto AJ, Silvers WK, Mintz B. Ultraviolet radiation-induced malignant skin melanoma in melanoma-susceptible transgenic mice. Cancer Res 1994; 54:4569–4572.
14. Powell MB, Gause PR, Hyman P, et al. Induction of melanoma in TPras transgenic mice. Carcinogenesis 1999; 20:1747–1753.
15. Otsuka T, Takayama H, Sharp R, et al. c-Met autocrine activation induces development of malignant melanoma and acquisition of the metastatic phenotype. Cancer Res 1998; 58:5157–5167.
16. Takayama H, LaRochelle WJ, Sharp R, et al. Diverse tumorigenesis associated with aberrant development in mice overexpressing hepatocyte growth factor/scatter factor. Proc Natl Acad Sci USA 1997; 94: 701–706.
17. Krimpenfort P, Quon KC, Mooi WJ, Loonstra A, Berns A. Loss of p16Ink4a confers susceptibility to metastatic melanoma in mice. Nature 2001; 413:83–86.
18. Sharpless NE, Bardeesy N, Lee KH, et al. Loss of p16Ink4a with retention of p19Arf predisposes mice to tumorigenesis. Nature 2001; 413:86–91.
19. Bardeesy N, Wong KK, DePinho RA, Chin L. Animal models of melanoma: recent advances and future prospects. Adv Cancer Res 2000; 79:123–156.
20. Chen S, Tiecher L, Kazim D, Pollack R, Wise L. DNA commitment of mouse fibroblasts to adipocyte differentiation by DNA transfection. Science 1989; 244:582–585.

21. Colon-Teicher L, Wise LS, Martino JJ, et al. Genomic sequences capable of committing mouse and rat fibroblasts to adipogenesis. Nucleic Acids Res 1993; 21:2223–2228.
22. Chen S, Zhu H, Wetzel WJ, Philbert MA. Spontaneous melanocytosis in transgenic mice. J Invest Dermatol 1996; 106:1145–1150.
23. Zhu H, Reuhl K, Zhang X, et al. Development of heritable melanoma in transgenic mice. J Invest Dermatol 1998; 110:247–252.
24. Trent J, Stanbridge E, McBride H, et al. Tumorigenicity in human melanoma cell lines controlled by introduction of human chromosome 6. Science 1990; 247:568–571.
25. Pollock PM, Cohen-Solal K, Sood R, et al. Melanoma mouse model implicates metabotropic glutamate signaling in melanocytic neoplasia. Nature Genet 2003; 34:108–112.
26. Harris S. Transgenic knockouts as part of high-throughput, evidence-based target selection and validation strategies. Drug Discov Today 2001; 6:628–636.
27. Kubinyi H. Chance favors the prepared mind—from serendipity to rational drug design. J Receptor Signal Transduct Res 1999; 19:15–39.
28. Hodge JW, Grosenbach DW, Aarts WM, Poole DJ, Schlom J. Vaccine therapy of established tumors in the absence of autoimmunity. Clin Cancer Res 2003; 9:1837–1849.
29. Greenberg NM, DeMayo F, Finegold MJ, et al. Prostate cancer in a transgenic mouse. Proc Natl Acad Sci USA 1995; 92:3439–3943.
30. Martiniello-Wilks R, Dane A, Voeks DJ, et al. Gene-directed enzyme prodrug therapy for prostate cancer in a mouse model that imitates the development of human disease. J Gene Med 2004; 6:43–54.
31. Jikai J, Shamis M, Huebener N, et al. Neuroblastoma directed therapy by a rational prodrug design of etoposide as a substrate for tyrosine hydroxylase. Cancer Lett 2003; 197:219–224.
32. Weiss WA, Aldape K, Mohapatra G, Feuerstein BG, Bishop JM. Targeted expression of MYCN causes neuroblastoma in transgenic mice. EMBO J 1997; 16:2985–2995.
33. Wall NR, Shi Y. Small RNA: can RNA interference be exploited for therapy? Lancet 2003; 362:1401–1403.
34. Hasuwa H, Kaseda K, Einarsdottir T, Okabe M. Small interfering RNA and gene silencing in transgenic mice and rats. FEBS Lett 2002; 532:227–230.
35. Contag PR. Whole-animal cellular and molecular imaging to accelerate drug development. [see comment]. Drug Discov Today 2002; 7:555–562.
36. Herschman HR. Molecular imaging: looking at problems, seeing solutions. Science 2003; 302:605–608.
37. Vooijs M, Jonkers J, Lyons S, Berns A. Noninvasive imaging of spontaneous retinoblastoma pathway-dependent tumors in mice. Cancer Res 2002; 62:1862–1867.
38. Johnson GA, Cofer GP, Gewalt SL, Hedlund LW. Morphologic phenotyping with MR microscopy: the visible mouse. Radiology 2002; 222:789–793.
39. Nebert DW. Pharmacogenetics and pharmacogenomics: why is this relevant to the clinical geneticist? Clin Genet 1999; 56:247–258.
40. Gonzalez FJ, Kimura S. Study of P450 function using gene knockout and transgenic mice. Arch Biochem Biophys 2003; 409:153–158.
41. Nelson DR, Zeldin DC, Hoffman S, Malttais LJ, Wain HM, Nebert DW. Comparison of cytochrome P450 (CYP) genes from the mouse and human genomes, including nomenclature recommendations for genes, pseudogenes and alternative-splice variants. Pharmacogenetics 2004; 14:1–18.
42. Nebert DW, Dalton TP, Stuart GW, Carvan MJ 3rd. "Gene-swap knock-in" cassette in mice to study allelic differences in human genes. Ann NY Acad Sci 2000; 919:148–170.
43. Xie W, Evans RM. Pharmaceutical use of mouse models humanized for the xenobiotic receptor. Drug Discov Today 2002; 7:509–515.
44. Fugger L. Human autoimmunity genes in mice. Curr Opin Immunol 2000; 12:698–703.
45. DePinho RA. The age of cancer. Nature 2000; 408:248–254.
46. Rangarajan A, Weinberg RA. Opinion: comparative biology of mouse versus human cells: modelling human cancer in mice. Nature Reviews. Cancer 2003; 3:952–959.

# 19

## Use of Adenovirus-Mediated Gene Transfer to Facilitate Biological Annotation of Novel Genes

*Jeff L. Ellsworth, PhD, Andrew Feldhaus, PhD, and Steven D. Hughes, PhD*

CONTENTS

SUMMARY

As part of a large program of gene annotation, use of adenovirus-mediated gene transfer facilitated rapid progress in the functional evaluation of more than 100 genes. Localized or systemic exposure to gene products expressed by adenovirus-transduced cells led to the discovery of several novel activities through analysis of resulting physiochemical or histological changes. In this summary of the work, we present examples of two studies in which activities of novel growth factors were initially characterized using this approach. In the first example, intravenous delivery of adenovirus encoding different forms of platelet-derived growth factor (PDGF) allowed us to evaluate effects of systemic exposure to two new members of this family, PDGF-C and PDGF-D, and led to specific new hypotheses regarding their roles in diseases of the liver and kidney, respectively. In the second example, localized delivery of adenovirus encoding fibroblast growth factor (FGF)-18 to mouse pinna led to the discovery that this novel FGF is a trophic factor for mature chondrocytes and their progenitors and might be useful for treating cartilage disease. These examples serve to illustrate the potential of in vivo gene delivery approaches to facilitate functional analysis and focus of secondary investigation in a large screening effort.

**Key Words:** Adenovirus; FGF-18; PDGF; gene transfer; biological annotation; genomics.

From: *Cancer Drug Discovery and Development: The Oncogenomics Handbook*
Edited by: W. J. LaRochelle and R. A. Shimkets © Humana Press Inc., Totowa, NJ

# 1. INTRODUCTION

Biologic or therapeutic annotation of genes encoding novel secretory proteins has been rate limiting in the development of these molecules as therapeutic agents. Often, a combination of approaches, such as literature searches of known family members, gene transfer using transgenic or viral technologies, gene deletion using various "knockout" methodologies, gene expression studies in diseased and normal tissue, and in vitro/in vivo screens for protein activity, has led to a viable therapeutic hypothesis for a novel protein. We have utilized each of these methodologies in varying degrees, for example, to generate preclinical data supporting a therapeutic role for fibroblast growth factor (FGF)-18 both in cartilage repair *(1,2)* and in stroke *(3,4)*. In the present chapter, we review our experience at ZymoGenetics using adenovirus-mediated gene transfer to gain information on the biological activities of a large number of novel genes. Adenovirus has been used extensively as a research tool to assess the effects of exogenous gene expression in a variety of in vivo systems *(5–10)*. Because we have pursued two general approaches for adenoviral-mediated protein expression in vivo, namely systemic and localized delivery of recombinant adenovirus, results will be presented as case studies using each of these approaches.

# 2. GENERAL METHODS

## *2.1. Construction of Recombinant Adenovirus*

Recombinant adenoviruses have been used for transient protein expression both in vitro and in vivo *(11–13)*. Types 2 and 5 adenoviruses, those which cause respiratory disease in humans but are not associated with human cancers, have been developed for gene therapy *(14)*. The adenovirus genome is linear, double-stranded DNA about 36 kb in length. Deletion of the *E1* gene from the adenoviral genome results in a replication defective virus. The *E1* gene product is a transcription factor that regulates expression from the early and late promoters of adenovirus and is required for viral replication. Expression of *E1* in 293 cells complements the deletion and permits replication of recombinant adenoviral stocks. Second-generation recombinant adenoviral vectors also have the nonessential *E3* gene deleted to increase the cloning capacity of the recombinant virus. Several methodologies have been described for generating recombinant adenoviruses, all with advantages and disadvantages *(15)*. Two general approaches have been taken. One is to clone the gene of interest directly into the *E1* (*E3*)-deleted adenoviral genome. However, the large size of the genome makes this cumbersome. A second approach is to clone the cDNA into a shuttle vector that contains a portion of the adenoviral genome and then transfect the shuttle vector along with a plasmid containing the adenoviral genome into 293 cells. Homologous recombination in 293 cells results in a recombinant adenovirus that replicates in 293 cells, producing a viral plaque. Recombination in mammalian cells is very inefficient and production of a homogenous viral stock requires plaque purification. We have been using an alternative method originally developed in the Vogelstein laboratory *(16)* using adenovirus type A5. This method recombines the shuttle vector and adenoviral genome in rec A+ bacterial cells and the resulting recombinant plasmid can be transfected into 293 cells for virus propagation without the need for plaque purification.

The process of generating a recombinant adenovirus starts with cloning the cDNA of interest into the shuttle vector. The pAdTrack-CMV (cytomegalovirus) shuttle vector *(16)* was designed to express both green fluorescent protein (GFP) and a cDNA. The presence of GFP allows for easy monitoring of virus production and transduction efficiency. We modified the pAdTrack-CMV shuttle vector and called the resulting vector ZyTrack. The vector was altered to express GFP from an SV40 promoter and human growth factor (hGH) polyadenylation signal. The gene of interest remains under the control of a CMV promoter and SV40 polyadenylation signal. The polylinker was modified to include *Fse*I, *Asc*I, and *Eco*RV restriction sites. We express secreted proteins using the native leader and have made both carboxy-terminal tagged proteins and untagged proteins. The ZyTrack shuttle vector containing the cDNA of interest is linearized and cotransformed into BJ5183 bacteria along with a vector containing the adenoviral genome (*E1* and *E3* deleted). Recombinants are selected on Luria-Bertani (LB) plates with the drug for the selectable marker present in ZyTrack.

The recombinant adenoviral genome is transfected into 293A cells (Microbix) and transfection efficiency and plaque formation are monitored via GFP. Plaques form within 5–8 d and the cell–media mixture is harvested at that time. The virus present in the supernatant is subject to two rounds of amplification, the last round in a 1.5-L cell factory. The viral particles are banded on CsCl gradients; the viral band is collected and the CsCl removed using a PD-10 desalting column. Glycerol is added to a final concentration of 15% (v/v) and the viral stocks stored at −80°C. Quality control of each viral stock includes determining virus particle number by reading the absorbance at 260 nm. In our experience, about $(2–5) \times 10^{12}$ particles are obtained. A wide variety of titer methods have been described. A convenient kit for determining titer of adenovirus stocks is available from BD Biosciences. The 293A cells are infected with serial dilutions of the virus stock and expression of the coat hexon protein is determined by immunostaining to assess the infection. A control virus prep is included in each titer assay to verify assay results. We have performed assays for replication competent virus (RCA) on nearly 100 viral stocks with no evidence of wild-type virus. This contrasts with a low percentage (approx 2%) of positives when recombination was performed in 293 cells.

## 2.2. Systemic and Localized Delivery of Recombinant Adenovirus

A generalized experimental design using systemic delivery of adenovirus was carried out using groups of 8–10 C57BL6 mice. At least three treatment groups were studied in a given experiment: (1) mice injected with test adenovirus vector (containing the cDNA of the gene to be tested), (2) mice injected with parental adenovirus vector (containing no cDNA insertion, Av-*null*), and (3) untreated mice. Mice were injected in the tail vein with approx $1 \times 10^{11}$ adenovirus particles ($5 \times 10^8$ to $5 \times 10^9$ plaque forming units [PFU]). During a typical 21-d observation period, body weights were measured weekly, and a serum chemistry panel and a complete blood count (CBC) were determined on d 10 and 21. At the end of this period, mice were euthanized, and complete necropsy was performed. A standard set of tissues was collected and analyzed by routine histological methods. This type of experimental design allowed for groupwise comparison of clinical pathology data (e.g., chemistry, hematology) with statistical methods such as analysis of variance (ANOVA). Histology score data were sometimes subjected to nonparametric statistical tests, but data were most often of a descriptive nature and interpreted using any available knowledge of the gene product under evaluation. When necessary, routine histological analysis was followed up with specialized techniques such as histomorphometry or immunohistochemistry (IHC).

Localized protein expression can be achieved by direct injection of adenovirus to the site of interest. Targeted delivery techniques use lower doses of virus and much smaller injection volumes, typically 5–20 µL. For studies in murine pinna, the virus preparations were diluted to a working concentration of $5 \times 10^{10}$ PFU/mL in 5% glycerol containing 1 mg trypan blue/mL *(1)*. Prior to injection of adenovirus, female BALB/C *nu/nu* mice, 7–9 wk of age, were anesthetized and adenovirus was delivered using a 30-gage needle that was inserted subdermally 2–3 mm from the tip of the pinna. Approximately 20 µL of adenovirus solution (containing $10^9$ PFU virus) was delivered. Mice were injected in the left pinna with adenovirus containing the cDNA of interest and were injected in the right pinna with Av-*null*. At 5, 11, and 17 d following adenovirus injections, mice were sacrificed and the pinna were harvested and processed for histology *(1)*. End-point assessment in localized delivery studies is dependent on the specific experimental setting, although generally similar in outline to that in studies using systemic delivery. We have used localized subcutaneous delivery of recombinant adenovirus to monitor the effects of genes on, for example, angiogenesis in the nude mouse ear *(1)* and wound healing. Intracerebroventricular or intrathecal injection have also been used to express genes in various locations of the central nervous system *(10)*. In a more specialized experimental setting, intratracheal infusion *(17)* and retrograde infusion into the common bile pancreatic duct *(5)* were used to examine effects of exogenous gene expression on cell proliferation and inflammatory processes in the lung and pancreas, respectively.

## 3. RESULTS AND DISCUSSION; CASE STUDIES

As described earlier, ZymoGenetics has pursued both systemic and local delivery for adenovirus-mediated protein expression in vivo. Systemic delivery of adenovirus constructs was conducted as part of a comprehensive in vivo functional evaluation program, which also included the production and analysis of transgenic mice. A diverse collection of genes, more than 100 in total, was analyzed in this way. The only common traits among these were homology to gene families of known therapeutic importance and the prediction of encoding a secreted product. Murine homologs of the human genes were frequently analyzed, if deemed necessary by significant divergence between the gene sequences. The strategy of this approach was to produce a condition of gene overexpression in the mouse and secretion of the gene product into systemic or local environments. This exposure might lead to measurable physiological perturbations and/or result in histologically detectable changes in tissues. For each gene analyzed in this program, the scope of evaluation was dependent on its known and hypothesized biological activities. Whereas intravenous administration of adenovirus evaluated effects of gene expression on liver function and systemic exposure to the gene product, targeted delivery methods were used to analyze its effects on specific processes (e.g., angiogenesis) or in specific anatomical locations.

Potentially useful information was obtained for a number of genes using systemic delivery of adenovirus. Experiments often revealed significant changes in serum chemistry and hematology associated with exposure to specific gene products. These were interpreted by correspondence to tissue pathology and findings in transgenic mice, if available. In general, mice tolerated adenovirus treatment very well. No lethal effects of adenovirus-mediated gene expression were encountered, and only in a few cases did mice exhibit obvious clinical signs of altered physiology. Several effects of adenoviral vectors were consistently observed in both test and control adenovirus treatment groups. Within the first two weeks after adenovirus injection, mice exhibited transient hypoglycemia, elevated cholesterol and globulin, and often extremely elevated serum transaminases. Histological changes routinely noted on d 21 evaluation included hepatocellular degeneration and necrosis and inflammatory infiltrate in the liver. A similar transient inflammatory response to adenovirus administration has been noted by others (18). The severity of these background effects of adenovirus was related to the dose of adenovirus given. In all studies using systemic delivery of adenovirus, dosage was based on particle number because this measurement could be obtained with greater precision than infectivity (PFU). However, background vector effects could be quite different when the PFU dosage was significantly different. In attempt to normalize vector background effects in comparisons of test and control adenovirus, PFU/particle ratios were determined for every preparation of adenovirus vector, and these ratios were required to be no greater than threefold different for test and control vector for any given study.

Systemic delivery of a recombinant adenovirus by tail vein injection with subsequent viral infection of the liver leads to exogenous protein expression almost exclusively in the liver. As is shown in Fig. 1, 4 d after injection of adenovirus encoding GFP, the liver is almost entirely green (see Color Plate 8 following p. 302). Protein expression from the recombinant adenovirus can be seen clearly within virtually all of the hepatic lobules. Little or no expression of GFP was observed in any other tissue sites (Fig. 1). High-level hepatic expression of secreted proteins can be obtained for several weeks following tail vein injection. For example, an adenovirus containing the cDNA for human stanniocalcin-2 (a novel mammalian hormone) (19) was injected via the tail vein and serum expression levels tested by antibody capture enzyme-linked immunosorbent assay (ELISA) once a week for 4 wk (Fig. 2). Serum levels of human stanniocalcin-2 were maximal 1–2 wk postinfection and declined thereafter (Fig. 2). Although stanniocalcin-2 levels declined by 28 d after infection, the estimated concentration in serum was still 10- to 100-fold over the assay background at this time. Thus, human stanniocalcin-2 levels could be consistently elevated in mouse serum for at least 1 mo after adenoviral infection. Although the peak of expression appears to vary with the protein expressed, in general, we have observed high-level expression between 1 to 3 wk postinfection.

### 3.1. Case One: Systemic Delivery of Human PDGF-C or PDGF-D by Adenovirus-Mediated Gene Transfer in Mice

Two new members of the platelet-derived growth factor (PDGF) family of growth factors, PDGF-C and PDGF-D, were discovered using a homology-based computer search of expressed sequence tag (EST) databases (20–23). Initial ESTs were identified by sequence homology to vascular endothelium-derived growth factor (VEGF). By utilizing the sequence from the identified ESTs, full-length human clones were obtained by polymerase chain reaction (PCR) screening and found to encode two unique multidomain proteins, subsequently named PDGF-C and PDGF-D, with predicted N-terminal leader sequences suggestive of secreted proteins. Database searches indicated similar homology relationships within the three-part domain structure of these proteins. The N-terminal portion of each protein had significant homology to the complement-binding (CUB) domain of neuropilin-1. Both proteins contained an intermediary bridge region with no homology to other protein domains, and the C-terminal portion of each protein had significant homology to PDGF and VEGF. The amino acid sequence of human PDGF-D is closely related to human

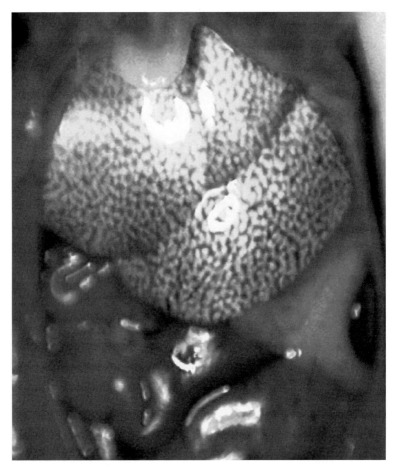

**Fig. 1.** Expression of GFP in mouse liver following infection with Av-*Gfp*. Adenoviral construction and intravenous delivery of Av-*Gfp* was performed as described in Subheading 2. Approximately $1 \times 10^{11}$ Av-*Gfp* particles were injected into the tail vein of a C57Bl6 mouse. Four days postinjection, GFP expression (green staining) was seen exclusively in the liver. The yellow spots and bands are reflections from the camera lighting. (*See* Color Plate 8 following p. 302.)

PDGF-C, demonstrating 50% and 43% identity in the C-terminal (PDGF homology) domain and the full-length structure, respectively.

In contrast to PDGF-A and PDGF-B chains, which are processed intracellularly and secreted as bioactive dimers (i.e., PDGF-AA, PDGF-BB, and PDGF-AB), the PDGF-C and PDGF-D precursor polypeptides are secreted intact from the cell and require extracellular proteolytic cleavage of the receptor interacting domain to produce the active growth factors PDGF-CC or PDGF-DD. Competition binding and immunoprecipitation studies using cells bearing both PDGF receptors (PDGFR) $\alpha$ and $\beta$ revealed high-affinity binding of recombinant PDGF-CC to PDGFR$\alpha$ homodimers and PDGFR$\alpha\beta$ heterodimers *(20)*. In contrast, PDGF-DD bound preferentially to cells expressing PDGFR$\beta$ homodimers *(22)*.

Systemic effects of both PDGF-C and PDGF-D were characterized and compared to those of PDGF-B using adenovirus-mediated gene transfer in mice *(24)* (Hughes et al., unpublished observations). Mice were injected with adenovirus-encoding PDGF-C (Av-

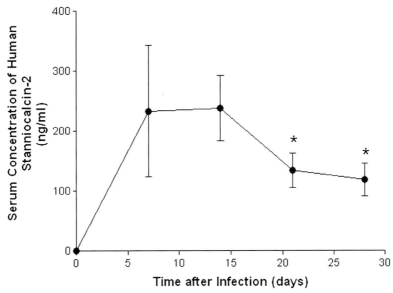

**Fig 2.** Serum levels of recombinant human stanniocalcin-2 (stc-2) following infection with Av-*stc-2*. Mice were injected in the tail vein with approx $1 \times 10^{11}$ Av-*stc-2* particles. Serum levels of stc-2 were measured by ELISA once a week for 4 wk. The 1-, 2-, 3-, and 4-wk points represent the mean ± SD of $n = 15, 14, 9,$ and 5 mice, respectively. Differences were significant compared to d 14; $p < 0.0001$.

*Pdgf-c*), PDGF-D (Av-*Pdgf-d*), PDGF-B (Av-*Pdgf-b*), or with Av-*null*. A 3-wk study was performed with monitoring and histological analysis as described earlier. The total amount of circulating PDGF varied widely among the various isoforms and also between individual mice. Three weeks following administration of virus, Av-*Pdgf-c* mice had circulating PDGF-CC levels averaging 316 ± 93 ng/mL and Av-*Pdgf-d* mice had circulating PDGF-DD levels averaging 216 ± 71 ng/mL. The circulating levels of PDGF-BB observed in Av-*Pdgf-b* mice (average of 20.6 ng/mL) were significantly less than those obtained with the Av-*Pdgf-c* and Av-*Pdgf-d* constructs. In the control mice, serum PDGF levels were generally below the limits of detection.

Mice overexpressing any form of PDGF gained significantly more weight during the experiment compared to mice injected with Av-*null*. Weights of individual organs revealed that the weight gain was largely attributable to increased liver weight, particularly in Av-*Pdgf-c*-treated mice. Mean liver weight in the Av-*Pdgf-c* group was increased greater than twofold over that of Av-*null*-treated mice (2.50 ± 0.07 vs 1.21 ± 0.03 g). Although liver weight was also increased in the Av-*Pdgf-b*- and Av-*Pdgf-d*-treated mice, widespread edema and changes in other organs, particularly the kidney, were additional factors affecting body weight. Mice expressing any form of PDGF also had enlarged spleens, probably as a consequence of extramedullary hematopoiesis.

Microscopic examination of the liver sections from Av-*Pdgf-c*-treated mice revealed a marked increase in perisinusoidal cells. Further analysis was carried out to identify and characterize these cells. IHC staining was performed with a number of antibodies and revealed that the majority of these cells were positive for α smooth muscle actin (α-SMA), suggesting the presence of activated hepatic stellate cells. Activation of these cells, believed to be a key event in the initiation of liver fibrosis, is marked by increased cell proliferation,

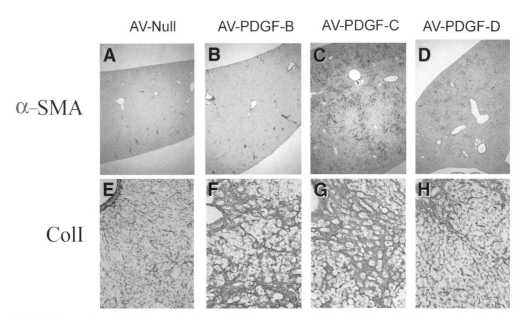

**Fig. 3.** Comparison of cellular activation and collagen accumulation in livers of mice treated with adenovirus encoding different forms of PDGF. (**A–D**) IHC staining for α-SMA revealed abundant, multifocal expression of α-SMA in livers of mice treated with Av-*Pdgf-c* and, to a lesser degree, Av-*Pdgf-d*. In Av-*Pdgf-b*-treated mice, α-SMA staining was restricted to vascular smooth muscle cells, and no staining was observed in mice treated with Av-*null*. (original magnification = ×4). (**E–H**) IHC staining demonstrated marked accumulation of type I collagen in livers of mice treated with Av-*Pdgf-c* or Av-*Pdgf-b*. Lower amounts of type I collagen were observed in mice treated with Av-*Pdgf-d*. In control mice treated with Av-*null*, the normal patterns of type I collagen surrounding the central vein was observed. (Original magnification of all images = ×20.) (*See* Color Plate 8 following p. 302.)

α-SMA expression, and production of extracellular matrix (ECM), including fibrillar (Type I) collagen *(25)*. To evaluate the relative degree to which the newly formed sinusoidal cells produced ECM, adjacent liver sections were analyzed by IHC staining for type I collagen (*see* Fig. 3 and Color Plate 8 following p. 302). Liver sections from mice expressing PDGF-C demonstrated markedly increased amounts of type I collagen, as compared to Av-*null*-treated mice (Fig. 3). Expansion of sinusoidal cells, expression of α-SMA, and increased type I collagen production was also observed in the livers from mice treated with Av-*Pdgf-b* and Av-*Pdgf-d* but were notably less severe than in Av-*Pdgf-c*-treated mice (Fig. 3). Increased deposition of ECM with staining characteristics similar to that shown in Fig. 3 is commonly observed in fibrotic liver of human patients *(26)*. Inflammatory changes were generally more severe in Av-*Pdgf-b*-treated mice, suggesting that PDGF-B has greater chemotactic activity in the liver relative to PDGF-C or PDGF-D. Some of the inflammatory changes might be attributed to the adenovirus vector *(18)*, although at 3 wk after injection, livers of mice injected with Av-*null* had no apparent morphological changes. For transient changes such as inflammation or the expression of cell activation markers (i.e., α-SMA), differences between PDGF forms observed at a single time-point could simply reflect distinct timing of expression or pharmacokinetic properties of the encoded gene product. However, the relative severity of changes in Av-*Pdgf-*

*c*-treated mice, combined with similar observations in *Pdgf-c* transgenic mice, suggested that PDGF-C might play an important role in the development of liver fibrosis.

In addition to changes in liver histopathology, effects on the kidney were noted for mice infected with Av-*Pdgf-d* and Av-*Pdgf-b*. Microscopic examination of the kidney sections from Av-*Pdgf-d*-treated mice revealed severe mesangial proliferative glomerulopathy characterized by a large increase in glomerular size and cellularity, as well as accumulation of extracellular matrix *(24)*. Mice treated with Av-*Pdgf-b* demonstrated a mild response, with slightly enlarged glomeruli and some accumulation of extracellular matrix. Mice treated with Av-*Pdgf-c* construct or Av-*null* showed no apparent kidney pathology.

Proliferative glomerulopathy was consistently observed in mice exposed to exogenous PDGF-D independent of the serum level of PDGF-DD, which showed a relatively high degree of variability. IHC analysis demonstrated accumulation of extracellular matrix, an increase in proliferating cells, and an influx of macrophages in the glomeruli of these mice. These findings suggested that PDGF-DD is a potent mitogen for mesangial cells, but not other cell types in the kidney, and that PDGF-DD can initiate events that lead to a mesangial proliferative glomerulonephritis, including influx of monocyte/macrophages and production of extracellular matrix. A key role for PDGFRβ in mediating mesangial proliferative diseases is indicated by the finding that overexpression of PDGF-D or PDGF-B, but not PDGF-C, produced glomerulopathy in mice.

In addition to the changes in liver and kidney, significant histopathologic changes were also observed in bone and lung of mice treated with Av-*Pdgf-b* and Av-*Pdgf-d*. These changes included endosteal bone proliferation in long bones and perivascular lymphoid cell infiltration in the lung. These changes were not observed in the mice treated with Av-*Pdgf-c* (Topouzis and Hughes, unpublished results).

Thus, adenovirus-mediated gene transfer of members of the *Pdgf* family was instrumental in defining a potential role for several of these factors in human disease. Importantly, these studies allowed us to compare and contrast the effects of overexpression of PDGF-B, PDGF-C, and PDGF-D on metabolic homeostasis and tissue pathology. These studies suggested that PDGF-C might play a role in the development of liver fibrosis, whereas PDGF-D appears to be a potent stimulator of glomerulopathy in mice.

### 3.2. Case 2: Local Delivery of Recombinant Adenovirus Expressing Fibroblast Growth Factor-18

As described earlier, we have used a variety of local delivery modalities to assess the biological effects of novel genes on tissues of interest, including intradermal, subcutaneous, ICV, and intrathecal delivery of recombinant adenovirus. In the specific case described here, we present our findings on fibroblast growth factor-18 (FGF-18) in more detail. *Fgf-18* was initially discovered in the InCyte EST database as a partial sequence from a human lung library. The partial sequence was identified by our group using a text mining approach showing that the new EST was homologous to the N-terminal end of human FGF-8. The *Fgf-18* EST was an InCyte singleton, indicating that it was not commonly observed and, at the time, had little significant homology to any other FGF family member. With additional sequence information, the prototypical FGF motif, CXFXE, was observed at amino acids 100–104 of the final protein sequence, adding further support to the notion that FGF-18 was a novel member of the FGF family. We later showed that *Fgf-18* is located on chromosome 5q34 in humans *(27)*.

The FGF family comprises a group of 23 polypeptides that exert their effects on cells by binding and signaling through cell surface FGF receptors, FGFR-1–FGFR-4 (28,29). In combination with a sulfated proteoglycan, FGFs bind and activate receptor tyrosine kinase activity, a process likely regulated by receptor dimerization (28). Alternative splicing of the third extracellular Ig domain of FGFR-1–FGFR-3 produces the "b" and "c" splice variants that are expressed in epithelial- and mesenchymal-derived tissues, respectively (28). Using BaF3 cells stably expressing the various FGF receptors, we have shown that FGF-18 binds and activates the FGFR-2-(IIIc), FGFR-3-(IIIc), and FGFR-4 (1). It binds neither FGFR-1-(IIIc) nor any of the "b" splice variants of FGFR-1–FGFR-3 (1). Similar results have been reported by other groups (30,31). Thus, relative to FGF-1 or FGF-2, FGF-18 displays a restricted receptor-binding specificity.

Prior to initiating extensive work on the expression and purification of a novel protein, we have often employed gene transfer techniques to acquire biological data on a novel gene. This is particularly important because it is difficult to justify the time and expense of protein production in the absence of such biological information. The chondrogenic activities of FGF-18 were discovered in this manner using adenovirus-mediated transfer of *Fgf18* in an in vivo screen for angiogenic agents (1,32). A rapid, nontraumatic screen for angiogenesis was developed by our group using adenovirus-mediated transfer of genes to the nude mouse pinnae (1). This procedure allowed for daily observations of vascular morphogenesis in the living mouse. Similar screens in mouse ears have recently been reported by others (32). The angiogenic activities of certain members of the FGF family, such as FGF-1 and FGF-2, are well known (33) and are thought to be regulated by FGF binding to the epithelial or "b" splice variants of FGFR (28). Although we observed much later that FGF-18 does not bind to the FGFR "b" splice variants, these data were not in hand prior to initiating the mouse pinna studies, and based on data in the literature, it seemed reasonable to assess the angiogenic activity of FGF-18. Recombinant *Fgf18* adenovirus construction, plaque purification, and amplification were performed as described (1). Left pinna were infected with adenovirus encoding *Fgf18* (Av-*Fgf18*). Pinnal sections (5.0 μm) were stained with hematoxylin and eosin, toluidine blue, anti-type-II collagen, and anti-proliferating cell nuclear antigen (PCNA) antibodies (1).

Although no apparent angiogenic response was observed, pinnae that received Av-*Fgf18* became visibly thicker (1). Thickening of the pinnal tissue was observed 4 d after inoculation and remained localized around the injection site for more than 2 wk. Pinnae that received the Av-*null* (Fig. 4A,C and Color Plates 9, 10 following p. 302) were histologically normal and contained a narrow zone of chondrocytes within the central zone of elastic cartilage. The vacuolated cells in the center of this region are "lipochondrocytes" whose cytoplasmic spaces are swollen by large lipid droplets. The central zone lipochondrocytes were bordered by one or two cell layers of flattened perichondrial cells (Fig. 4C). Infection with Av-*Fgf18* greatly increased the number of basophilic "chondrocytelike" cells observed around the site of inoculation (Fig. 4B,D) and extending outward from the articular zone into the skeletal muscle and subcutis. These cells were actively proliferating as they stained strongly with an antibody to PCNA, as did hair follicles and epithelium (Fig. 4G,H). Importantly, the newly proliferating "chondrocytelike" cells stained with anti-type-II collagen antibodies (Fig. 4F). Enhanced staining was evident by d 5 and was maintained near this level for up to 17 d. No staining was detected with a mouse isotype control antibody (1). The matrix surrounding these cells also showed increased staining with toluidine blue (Fig. 4I,J), demonstrating that accumulation of extracellular matrix was increased by Av-*Fgf18*. Thus, by virtue of their staining for type II collagen and proteoglycans, the proliferating cells appear to be chondrocytes.

It is not yet clear which FGF receptor(s) mediates the Av-*Fgf18*-induced expansion of auricular cartilage. Expressions of *Fgfr-2-(IIIc)*, *Fgfr-3-(IIIc)*, and *Fgfr-4* were detected within the expanded chondrocyte zone in the mouse pinnae treated with Av-*Fgf18* (1). Specific immunostaining of pinnal tissue with antibodies directed against the carboxy-terminal domains of FGFR-1–FGFR-4 was only seen with antibodies directed against FGFR-2 (1). With Av-*Fgf18*, the number of anti-FGFR-2-stained chondrocyte nuclei was greatly increased, with most of the antibody staining observed in the nuclei of the proliferating chondrocytes (1), suggesting that this receptor is involved in the proliferation of these cells in response to FGF-18.

The surprising observation that Av-*Fgf18* stimulated the proliferation of auricular chondrocytes suggested that FGF-18 was a novel growth factor for these cells. These data were extrapolated to primary cultures of adult articular chondrocytes, where FGF-18 produced dose-dependent increases in chondrocyte proliferation and in the production of extracellular matrix (1). These observations suggested that FGF-18 could act as a trophic factor for mature chondrocytes and, moreover, might be useful in promoting the repair of cartilage damaged by injury or disease. To this end, the effects of FGF-18 on repair of cartilage damage in a model of injury-induced osteoarthritis were assessed.

Osteoarthritis (OA) was induced by creating a meniscal tear in the knee joint of rats (34,35). In this model, transection of the medial collateral ligament and damage to the meniscus induces progressive cartilage degeneration and chondrophyte formation that mimic the changes that occur in spontaneous OA. Intra-articular injection of FGF-18 in a carrier matrix induced a dose-dependent increase in cartilage hypertrophy and overgrowth of new cartilage around the damaged areas as well as normal cartilage in the lateral compartment (2). The highest dose of FGF-18 decreased cartilage degeneration scores in the medial tibia plateau (2) and increased medial tibia cartilage thickness, from $243 \pm 21$ to $319 \pm 77$ μm (mean ± SD, $p < 0.05$) (2). Detailed results of these studies will be presented in full elsewhere (2). These data demonstrate that FGF-18, delivered by intra-articular injection, can elicit significant repair of damaged cartilage. The newly proliferated cartilage appeared well integrated with the normal cartilage, thus providing a load-bearing tissue that could withstand any abnormal biomechanics and stresses imposed by damage to the meniscus. The significant cartilage repair induced by FGF-18 in this OA model suggests that this factor might have utility in the treatment of cartilage damaged by OA or cartilage injury. Thus, adenoviral-mediated transfer of *Fgf18* into nude mouse ears was instrumental in defining the chondrocyte biology of FGF-18 and for providing a path toward a potential clinical utility for this novel polypeptide.

## 4. CONCLUSIONS

We have successfully used adenovirus-mediated gene transfer in mice to identify biological activities and potential clinical uses of a large number of genes encoding novel secreted proteins. An important aspect of this work was our use of both systemic and local delivery of recombinant adenovirus to assess the function of these gene products. By designing the experiments with the appropriate viral controls, we were able to differentiate the effects of exogenous protein expression from nonspecific effects that were related to infection with adenovirus. In this way, biological annotation of these genes proceeded

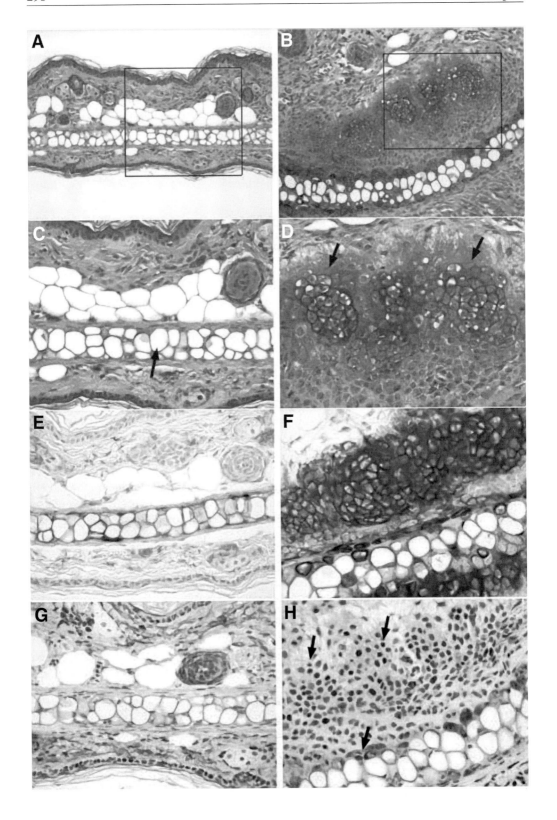

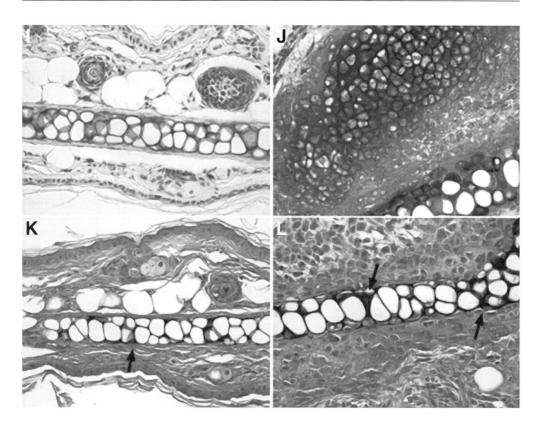

rapidly and provided a rationale for commitment of resources to protein production and further experimentation. Our success using this "gene first" approach to protein drug discovery is exemplified by our discovery that FGF-18 is a potent growth factor for chondrocytes of hyaline cartilage *(1)* and has shown efficacy in a preclinical model of OA *(2)*. Similarly, our findings that PDGF-C and PDGF-D appear to play key roles in liver fibrosis and glomerulopathy *(24)*, respectively, suggests a path for treating hepatic and renal disease by generating therapeutic antagonists of these polypeptides. These examples serve to illustrate the potential of in vivo gene delivery approaches to facilitate functional analysis in a large scale, genomics-driven, biological screening effort.

**Fig. 4.** Histology of mouse pinnae transduced with adenovirus expressing *Fgf18*. Pinnae were harvested on d 5 after infection with either a control adenovirus (left panels) or adenovirus expressing *Fgf18* (right panels). (**A,B**) Hematoxylin and eosin (×10, boxed outlines magnified areas in panels C and D). (**C,D**) Hematoxylin and eosin, ×40, panel c arrow, lipochondrocyte; panel d arrows, newly formed "chondrocyte-like" cells. (**E,F**) Immunoperoxidase, type II collagen, ×40. (**G,H**) Immunoperoxidase, proliferating cell nuclear antigen, ×40, panel h arrow demonstrates PCNA-positive chondrocytes. (**I,J**) Toluidine blue, ×40. (**K,L**) Verhoeff's stain for elastin, ×40, arrows illustrate elastin deposition. (Reprinted from ref. *1,* copyright 2002 with permission from Osteoarthritis Research Society International.) (*See* Color Plates 9, 10 following p. 302.)

# ACKNOWLEDGMENTS

The authors are indebted to many of our colleagues at ZymoGenetics for the work described herein. We would especially like to thank Deb Gilbertson, Stavros Topouzis, PhD, K Waggie, DVM, Tom Palmer, PhD, Emma E. Moore, PhD, Matt Holdren, and Alisa Littau, DVM. We would also like to acknowledge the contributions of Charles Alpers, MD of the Department of Pathology and David R. Eyre, PhD of the Department of Orthropaedics and Sports Medicine at the University of Washington for their work on the PDGF and FGF-18 projects, respectively.

# REFERENCES

1. Ellsworth JL, Berry J, Bukowski T, et al. Fibroblast growth factor-18 is a trophic factor for mature chondrocytes and their progenitors. Osteoarthritis Cartilage 2002; 10:308–320.
2. Moore EE, Bendele A, Thompson DL, et al. Fibroblast growth factor-18 stimulates chondrogenesis and promotes cartilage repair in a rat model of injury-induced osteoarthritis. Trans Orthop Res Soc 2004; 29:199.
3. Ellsworth JL, Garcia R, Yu J, Kindy MS. Fibroblast growth factor-18 reduced infarct volumes and behavioral deficits following occlusion of the middle cerebral artery in rats. Stroke 2003; 34:1507–1512.
4. Ellsworth JL, Garcia R, Yu J, Kindy MS. Time window of fibroblast growth factor-18-mediated neuroprotection after occlusion of the middle cerebral artery in rats. J Cereb Blood Flow Metab 2004; 24: 114–123.
5. Raper SE, DeMatteo RP. Adenovirus-mediated in vivo gene transfer and expression in normal rat pancreas. Pancreas 1996; 12:401–410.
6. Wilson JM. Adenovirus-mediated gene transfer to liver. Adv Drug Deliv Rev 2001; 46:205–209.
7. Panchal RG, Williams DA, Kitchener PD, et al. Gene transfer: manipulating and monitoring function in cells and tissues. Clin Exp Pharmacol Physiol 2001; 28:687–691.
8. Hidaka C, Khan SN, Farmer JC, Sandhu HS. Gene therapy for spinal applications. Orthop Clin North Am 2002; 33:439–446.
9. Goossens PH, Huizinga TW. Adenoviral-mediated gene transfer to the synovial tissue. Clin Exp Rheumatol 2002; 20:415–419.
10. Alisky JM, Davidson BL. Gene transfer to brain and spinal cord using recombinant adenoviral vectors. Methods Mol Biol 2004; 246:91–120.
11. Lai CM, Lai YK, Rakoczy PE. Adenovirus and adeno-associated virus vectors. DNA Cell Biol 2002; 21:895–913.
12. Douglas JT. Adenovirus-mediated gene delivery: an overview. Methods Mol Biol 2004; 246:3–14.
13. Imperiale MJ, Kochanek S. Adenovirus vectors: biology, design, and production. Curr Topics Microbiol Immunol 2004; 273:335–357.
14. Kozarsky KF, Wilson JM. Gene therapy: adenovirus vectors. Curr Opin Genet Dev 1993; 3:499–503.
15. Mizuguchi H, Kay MA, Hayakawa T. Approaches for generating recombinant adenovirus vectors. Adv Drug Deliv Rev 2001; 52:165–176.
16. He TC, Zhou S, da Costa LT, Yu J, Kinzler KW, Vogelstein B. A simplified system for generating recombinant adenoviruses. Proc Natl Acad Sci USA 1998; 95:2509–2514.
17. Sadikot RT, Han W, Everhart MB, et al. Selective I kappa B kinase expression in airway epithelium generates neutrophilic lung inflammation. J Immunol 2003; 170:1091–1098.
18. Liu Q, Muruve DA. Molecular basis of the inflammatory response to adenovirus vectors. Gene Ther 2003; 10:935–940.
19. Moore EE, Kuestner RE, Conklin DC, et al. Stanniocalcin 2: characterization of the protein and its localization to human pancreatic alpha cells. Horm Metab Res 1999; 31:406–414.
20. Gilbertson DG, Duff ME, West JW, et al. Platelet-derived growth factor C (PDGF-C), a novel growth factor that binds to PDGF alpha and beta receptor. J Biol Chem 2001; 276:27,406–27,414.
21. Li X, Ponten A, Aase K, et al. PDGF-C is a new protease-activated ligand for the PDGF alpha-receptor. Nature Cell Biol 2000; 2:302–309.
22. LaRochelle WJ, Jeffers M, McDonald WF, et al. PDGF-D, a new protease-activated growth factor. Nature Cell Biol 2001; 3:517–521.

23. Changsirikulchai S, Hudkins KL, Goodpaster TA, et al. Platelet-derived growth factor-D expression in developing and mature human kidneys. Kidney Int 2002; 62:2043–2054.

24. Hudkins KL, Gilbertson DG, Carling M, et al. Exogenous PDGF-D is a potent mesangial cell mitogen and causes a severe mesangial proliferative glomerulopathy. J Am Soc Nephrol 2004; 15:286–298.

25. Friedman SL. Molecular regulation of hepatic fibrosis, an integrated cellular response to tissue injury. J Biol Chem 2000; 275:2247–2250.

26. Rojkind M, Giambrone MA, Biempica L. Collagen types in normal and cirrhotic liver. Gastroenterology 1979; 76:710–719.

27. Whitmore TE, Maurer MF, Sexson S, Raymond F, Conklin D, Deisher TA. Assignment of fibroblast growth factor 18 (FGF18) to human chromosome 5q34 by use of radiation hybrid mapping and fluorescence in situ hybridization. Cytogenet Cell Genet 2000; 90:231–233.

28. Ornitz DM. FGFs, heparan sulfate and FGFRs: complex interactions essential for development. Bioessays 2000; 22:108–112.

29. Ornitz DM, Itoh N. Fibroblast growth factors. Genome Biol 2001; 2:REVIEWS3005.1–3005.12.

30. Xu J, Liu Z, Ornitz DM. Temporal and spatial gradients of Fgf8 and Fgf17 regulate proliferation and differentiation of midline cerebellar structures. Development 2000; 127:1833–1843.

31. Hoshikawa M, Yonamine A, Konishi M, Itoh N. FGF-18 is a neuron-derived glial cell growth factor expressed in the rat brain during early postnatal development. Brain Res Mol Brain Res 2002; 105:60–66.

32. Pourtier-Manzanedo A, Vercamer C, Van Belle E, Mattot V, Mouquet F, Vandenbunder B. Expression of an Ets-1 dominant-negative mutant perturbs normal and tumor angiogenesis in a mouse ear model. Oncogene 2003; 22:1795–1806.

33. Folkman J, Klagsbrun M. Angiogenic factors. Science 1987; 235:442–447.

34. Janusz MJ, Bendele AM, Brown KK, Taiwo YO, Hsieh L, Heitmeyer SA. Induction of osteoarthritis in the rat by surgical tear of the meniscus: inhibition of joint damage by a matrix metalloproteinase inhibitor. Osteoarthritis Cartilage 2002; 10:785–791.

35. Lozoya KA, Flores JB. A novel rat osteoarthrosis model to assess apoptosis and matrix degradation. Pathol Res Pract 2000; 196:729–745.

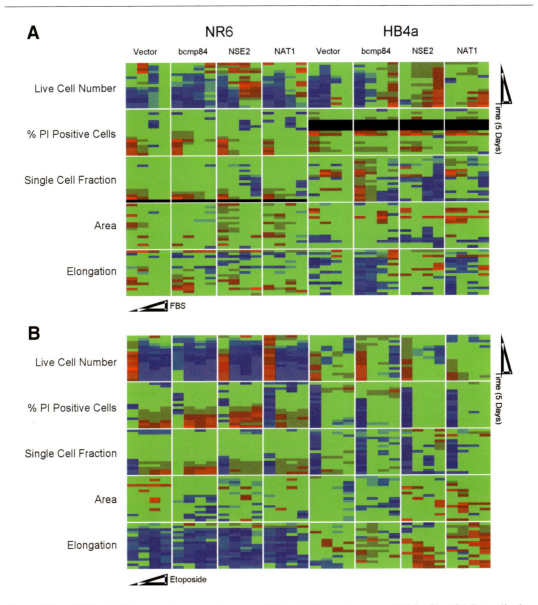

**Color Plate 5, Fig. 5.** (*See* complete caption on p. 204 and discussion on p. 203 in Ch. 13.) Data display from phenotypic assay of candidate drug target.

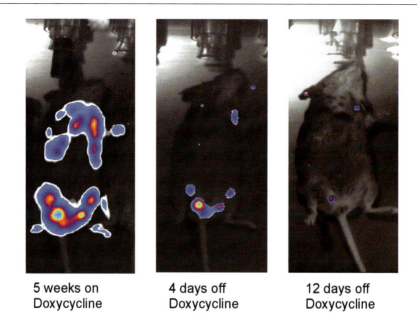

| 5 weeks on | 4 days off | 12 days off |
| Doxycycline | Doxycycline | Doxycycline |

**Color Plate 6, Fig. 1.** (*See* full caption and discussion on p. 250 in Ch. 16.) Regression of tumors after deinduction.

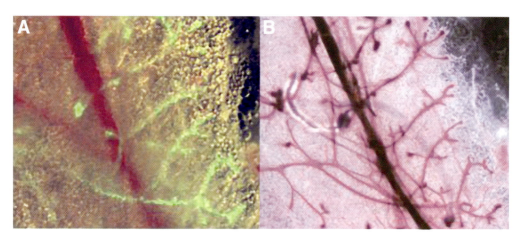

**Color Plate 6, Fig. 2.** (*See* full caption and discussion on p. 253 in Ch. 16.) Reconstitution of mammary gland by implant of epithelium cells.

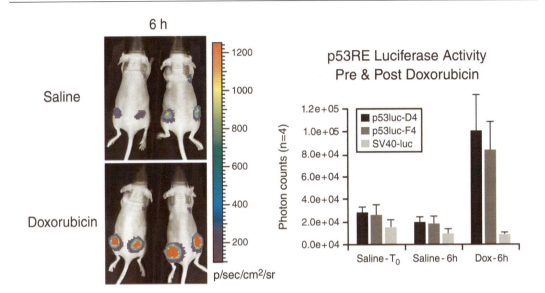

**Color Plate 7, Fig. 1.** (*See* discussion on p. 269 in Ch. 17.) p53-RE luciferase induction with doxorubicin in vivo.

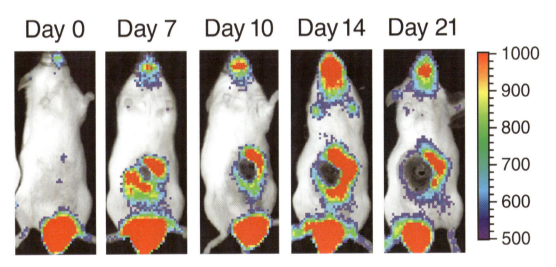

**Color Plate 7, Fig. 3.** (*See* full caption on p. 272 and discussion on pp. 270–271 in Ch. 17.) Inducible Vegfr2-luc during tumor development.

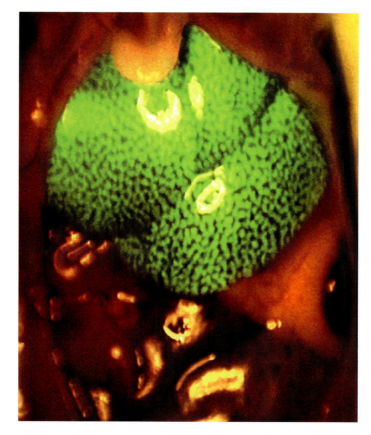

**Color Plate 8, Fig. 1.** (*See* full caption p. 292 and discussion on p. 291 in Ch. 19.) Expression of GFP in mouse liver following infection with Av-*Gfp*.

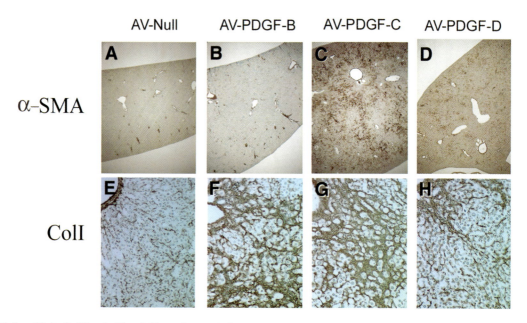

**Color Plate 8, Fig. 3.** (*See* full caption and discussion on p. 294 in Ch. 19.) Cellular change in mouse liver treated with adenovirus encoding different forms of PDGF.

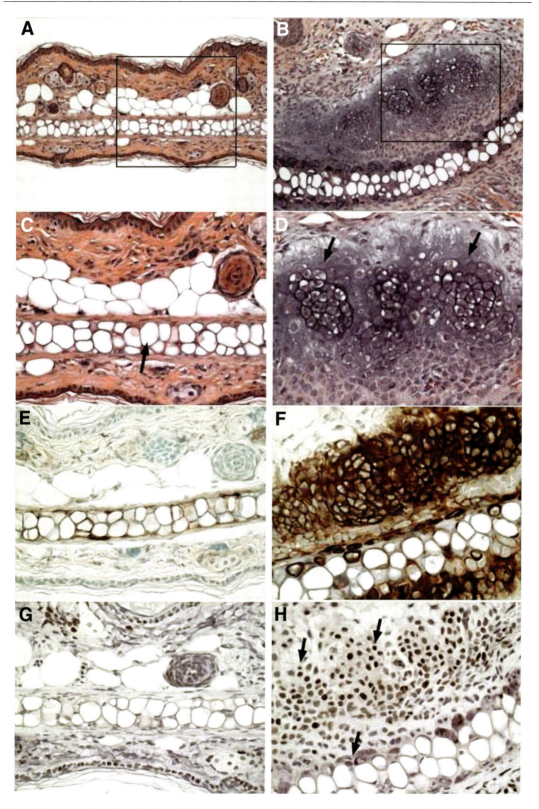

**Color Plate 9, Fig. 4A–H.** (*See* full caption on p. 299 and discussion on pp. 296–297 in Ch. 19.) Histology of mouse pinnae transduced with adenovirus expressing *Fgf18 (continued).*

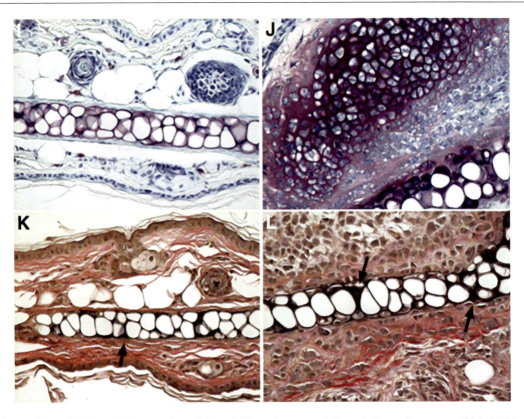

**Color Plate 10, Fig. 4I–L.** *(continued)* (*See* full caption on p. 299 and discussion on pp. 296–297 in Ch. 19.)

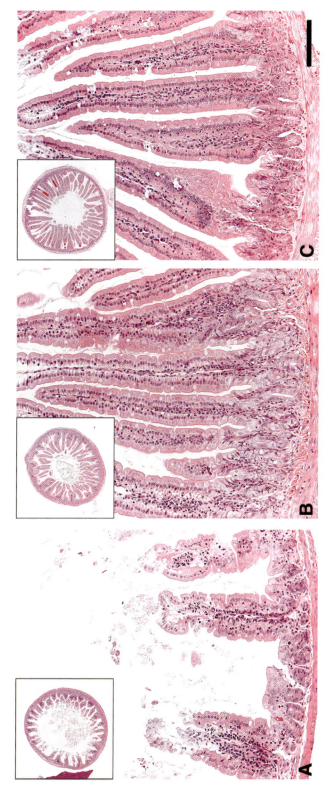

**Color Plate 11, Fig. 2.** (*See* full caption on p. 464 and discussion on pp. 462–463 in Ch. 31.) Effect on KGF on small intestine of 5-FU-treated mice.

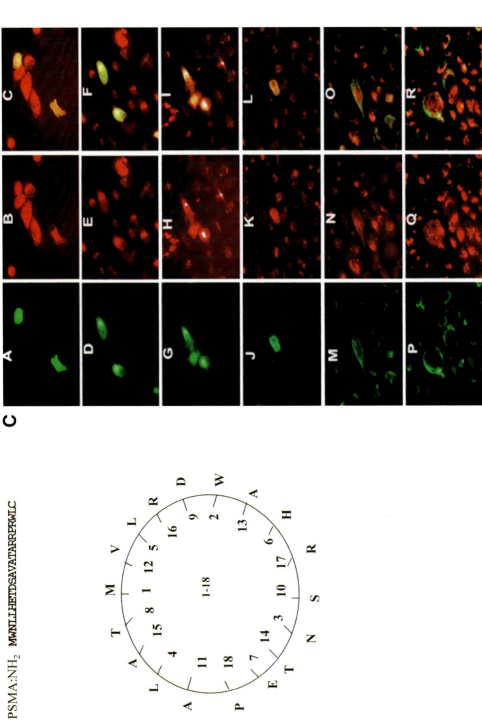

**A**  PSMA:NH₂  MWNLLIHETDSAVATARRPRWLC

**Color Plate 12, Fig. 3.** (*See* full caption on pp. 601–603 and discussion on pp. 605 and discussion on p. 605 in Ch. 38.)

# 20

# Cancer Biology and Transgenic Technology in the Mouse

*Bridging the Functional Gap*

## *Cindy E. McKinney, PhD*
## *and Cooduvalli S. Shashikant, PhD*

**CONTENTS**

**SUMMARY**

Cancer research has benefited from the ability to manipulate the mouse genome. Transgenic technology is being used to produce mice with refined genomic mutations that recapitulate cancer development in the human. Transgenic mice have proven valuable in vivo models to address the biological consequences of mutations found in tumors and interactions of two mutations in the same mouse. Carcinogen screening or therapeutic assessment might be enhanced by conducting 2-yr bioassays in the background of a mutant mouse model. The introduction of transgenic methods to limit mutant gene expression to a single tissue or cell type by Tet-inducible or Cre recombinase-Lox P technology permits genetic models of otherwise lethal phenotypes to be developed. Gene traps in embryonic stem (ES) cells are being used to capture genes and conduct initial screens for gene function in "knockout" mice. Gene "knockdowns" in mouse embryos by lentivirus delivery of small interfering RNA (siRNA) constructs are poised to become valuable tools for studying cancer gene function with some additional technology development. Transgenic mice allow a combinatorial approach utilizing genomic information and physical manipulation of selected genes to dissect pathways altered during tumorigenesis. Finally, although transgenic mouse models are invaluable tools for dissecting cancer and related processes, future goals are to develop "humanized" transgenic mouse models that may more accurately respond to and reflect the human condition.

From: *Cancer Drug Discovery and Development: The Oncogenomics Handbook*
Edited by: W. J. LaRochelle and R. A. Shimkets © Humana Press Inc., Totowa, NJ

**Key Words:** Transgenic mice; cancer; ENU mutagenesis; lentivirus; siRNA; gene "knockouts"; functional genomics; conditional transgenics; Cre-Lox P; tetracycline-inducible transgenics; ES cell gene traps.

## 1. INTRODUCTION

The accumulation of genetic and physiological data on the mouse over the last century linked with the recent completion of the mouse genomic sequence provides opportunities and resources to investigators. The revolution of molecular genetics and transgenic approaches developed in the 1980s and 1990s allows introduction of putative cancer causing mutations directly into the mouse genome. The resulting phenotypes can then be studied in vivo and might more accurately reflect human disease *(1)*. Thus, transgenic methods can be employed to complement genomic sequence information and dissect and map oncological pathways resulting in cancer *(2–4)*.

Cancer is a multistep pathological process. Cancer researchers have taken many different paths to understand the biology of cancer, including developing transgenic mouse models. A subtle DNA alteration in a single cell can trigger tumor development *(5)*. Genomic changes of this type can be introduced into the transgenic mouse and provide valuable insight into pathological progression to cancer *(6)*. Transgenic mouse models of cancer support discovery of the molecular basis of cancer and assist in dissecting oncogenic pathways in cells and tissues *(7)*. For example, transgenic mouse models of mammary cancer used breast epithelial cells to study signaling pathways associated with cancer progression *(8)*. Treating mice with *N*-ethyl-*N*-nitrosourea (ENU), a potent mutagen, permits the use of large-scale genomic screens to identify point mutations that result in either dominant or recessive cancer phenotypes *(9)*. Humans and mice show differential susceptibilities to cancer *(6)*, yet the syntenic relationships between human and mouse chromosomal regions facilitate identifying gene homologs between the two species. Understanding the complex genetic background of human cancers might come from modeling gene–environment interactions in mouse systems. Mouse models of genes involved in carcinogenesis offer enhanced opportunities to develop therapeutic agents targeted to specific cancer types. Newer technologies that produce gene hypomorphs ("knockdowns") can also be used to examine cancer progression in mice. Here, we review transgenic technologies that produce cancer models and provide examples of some strategies employed to investigate cancer in the mouse.

## 2. TRANSGENIC TECHNIQUES

Using transgenic approaches to manipulate genes directly in the mouse has intensified as the technologies mature. Modeling cancer in the mouse continues to be a powerful tool to study the physiology and pathology of the disease (reviewed in ref. *10*). Transgenic mice can also be used to evaluate cancer therapies and to define new proto-oncogenes, tumor suppressors, and cancer modifiers. Transgenic techniques fall broadly into three categories: pronuclear transgene introduction, gene-targeted "knockouts/knockins" and nuclear transplantation (cloning). Essentially, any gene can be mutated and manipulated to gain functional insights into its biological role in cancer or another human disease. Strategic selection of the gene, its transgenic construct, and the mode of genome alteration aid in the analysis of the anticipated phenotype.

Transgenic technologies were developed and refined in several laboratories in the late 1970s and early 1980s *(11–15)*. Advances came from integrating observations in cell culture transfection assays, somatic cell genetics, mouse embryology, and cell virology. Various approaches to transfer DNA to mouse embryos were tried, including retroviral infection *(11)*. The goal of sustained long-term expression of a transferred gene was achieved by introducing a growth hormone gene under the control of the metallothionein promoter *(16)*. This resulted in a phenotype of "giant" mice because of the overproduction of functional growth hormone.

The current use of embryonic stem (ES) cells to transfer altered gene targets to the germline was foreshadowed by observations that embryonal carcinoma (EC) cells could be introduced into blastocysts and contribute to the somatic tissues of chimeras *(15)*. The utility of studying genome alterations in vivo was enhanced by studies that invoked homologous recombination machinery in the cell to integrate a targeted mutant copy of a gene into its endogenous chromosome location. The resultant "knockout" mice have proven useful for modeling monogenic diseases such as Tay–Sachs *(17)*, Gaucher's *(18)*, and cystic fibrosis *(19)*. In time, conditional strategies were developed to limit the "knockout" phenotype to a specific tissue or temporal expression period.

Somatic nuclear transfer, "cloning," was first achieved in sheep *(20)* by exchanging a differentiated nucleus from an udder cell for the nucleus from a fertilized ovine embryo. The cloning of mice also was accomplished *(21)*. This technology holds promise for saving endangered species, bio-"pharming," and xenotransplantation. Animal cloning could also be used in the future to produce cancer models in animals where ES cells are not available.

## *2.1. Pronuclear Microinjection of DNA*

Gain of function (overexpression) of a gene is achieved by microinjecting a DNA construct containing a promoter or other regulatory sequences linked to a gene of interest. The minimal construct might also contain additional gene regulatory elements such as enhancers, insulators, or locus control regions. Transgene size ranges from small cDNA constructs to large genomic inserts from bacterial artificial chromosomes (BACs). There are many laboratory manuals describing the preparations of transgene constructs *(22,23)* for successful microinjections. Founder mice (those carrying the original transgene insertion) are bred with nontransgenic mice of the same strain to establish a line of transgenic mice for which the expression of the transgene can be studied. Analysis of the transgenic phenotype can be done in embryos (transient transgenics) or adult mice (see Fig. 1).

Analysis of transgenic mice can be confounded by several factors: Possibilities include a construct that inserts randomly into the genome but causes lethality or masking of a transgene's phenotype because the insertion site disrupts an essential gene's function. Transgene integration at a random genomic site also might repress expression of the transgene. Mosaic mice contain more than one transgene integration site because of late integration of the transgene into the genome at the two-cell stage or beyond. This situation confounds analysis of the transgene's expression pattern. In practice, several transgenic founders are identified and evaluated for a consistent phenotype.

## *2.2. Embryonic-Stem-Cell-Derived Transgenics*

Loss of function (gene "knockouts") transgenics became available when mouse ES cell lines were produced *(22,24)* from mouse blastocysts. These cells could be cultured in vitro under rigorous conditions and retain the ability to become part of the developing

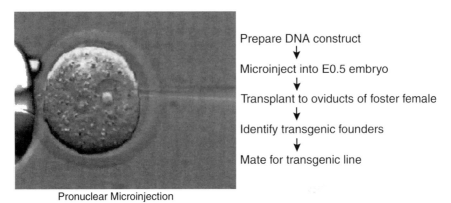

Prepare DNA construct
↓
Microinject into E0.5 embryo
↓
Transplant to oviducts of foster female
↓
Identify transgenic founders
↓
Mate for transgenic line

Pronuclear Microinjection

**Fig. 1.** Pronuclear injection.

mouse embryo when reintroduced into the blastocyst. The first ES cells were isolated from the 129 strain and contained agouti coat color alleles. These ES cells when introduced into C57Bl/6 blastocysts produced agouti and black coat color chimera, yielding an easy visual way of determining potential germline carriers of the introduced ES cell mutations. Today, there are many ES cell lines available from several inbred mouse strains but coat color differences are still used to identify the chimera (22,24).

Embyronic stem cells are derived from the inner cell mass of the blastocyst—those cells that produce the mouse embryo. If cultured under conditions that allow the ES cell to retain its full embryonic potential, they can be used to produce gene "knockouts," "knockins," or "humanized" mice. Gene targeting vectors require specific knowledge of the target gene's sequence and rely on the use of selectable drug cassettes in the final construct. Electroporation of the targeting vector into ES cells results in recombination between homologous regions of the target gene and the 5' and 3' ends of the gene-targeting construct (reviewed in ref. 25). Drug selection in culture permits those ES cells that have incorporated the positive selection cassette into their genome to survive. Those ES clones identified with correctly targeted genes are microinjected into mouse blastocysts to produce chimera. The chimeras are bred to obtain germline transmission of the introduced gene mutation. F1 mutation carriers are bred to obtain "knockout" lines (homozygous for the gene mutation) for study (see Fig. 2).

Analysis of an ES-cell-produced mouse model can be slowed by several factors. The production of a gene "knockout" line is costly and time-consuming. The phenotype of the homozygous mutant is unknown until produced and might be an embryonic lethal. In addition, the phenotype might be subtle as a result of partial compensation by genes with overlapping functions or there might be no overt phenotype from the gene "knockout." When a targeted gene is a member of related family of genes, a phenotype might be discerned only after breeding two targeted lines together. Phenotypes are sometimes only observed in aged mice. These aspects should be considered when designing the "knockout" project. Surprisingly, most single-gene "knockout" models have yielded phenotypes of interest. The gene-targeting techniques can be applied to studying oncogenes and tumor suppressor genes.

Investigators have used "knockout" transgenic mice to examine gene function in many areas. One of these areas is DNA repair genes, where deficiencies in detecting and repair-

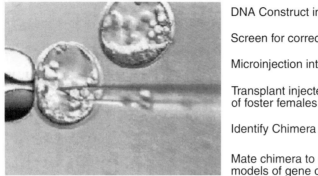

DNA Construct introduced into ES cells
↓
Screen for correct recombinanat allele
↓
Microinjection into E 3.5 blastocysts
↓
Transplant injected blastocysts into uteri
of foster females
↓
Identify Chimera progeny
↓
Mate chimera to obtain germ line mouse
models of gene or disease

Embryonic Stem (ES) Cell Micoinjection

**Fig. 2.** Embryonic stem cell microinjection.

ing DNA base alterations might lead to cancer. For example, DNA repair defects induced by mutation or loss of heterozygosity (LOH) of the complementary allele in humans might be modeled in the mouse *(26)*. The *Xpa* null mouse seems to mimic xeroderma pigmentosum (XP) in humans. Daily ultraviolet B (UVB) exposure produces 100% carcinoma incidence in a short timeframe. Other mouse models of DNA repair deficiencies leading to cancer are reviewed by Wijnhoven and Steeg *(27)*. *H2AX*, whose gene product is a histone variant, is phosphorylated in chromatin with double-stranded DNA (dsDNA) strand breaks *(28)*. Gene targeting produced an H2AX mouse that as a heterozygote showed genomic instability. When the H2AX-deleted mouse was combined with a *P53*-null mouse, the double mutant rapidly developed solid tumors and immature lymphomas in both the T- and B-cell compartments. It appears that H2AX promotes repair of DNA breaks and suppresses tumor formation because of genome instability and this function was defined by using a knockout mouse. Some single-gene "knockouts" not necessarily associated with cancer phenotypes do show spontaneous development of tumors. Two genes encode the enzyme methyl adenosyltransferase (MAT1A and MAT2A), which acts as a methyl donor. The MAT1A-null mouse has low MAT activity and hepatic hyperplasia and eventually develops hepatocellular carcinoma. Microarray analysis of hepatic genes showed that genes involving hepatocyte differentiation and proliferation were altered in the MAT1A-null. These findings suggest that MAT1A might be a suppressor that prevents liver cancer by providing an environment that keeps the hepatocyte functional. These and many other recently published examples of mice carrying single-gene knockouts *(10,29,30)* increase our understanding of how genes act in pathways and the mechanisms that lead to disruption of normal cellular processes and initiate or induce cancer. Used in combinations, gene-engineered tumorigenic mutations allow an integrated in vivo analysis of gene interactions that might lead to promotion and cancer progression.

Although ES cell technology produces complete gene inactivation, these systems must be carefully evaluated. Confounding outcomes are possible when one component of a physiological network is removed. For instance, other genes might compensate for the lost of a gene product because of overlapping functions or a related gene's expression pattern might be altered in the "knockout." The mouse strain used as the source of the ES cells might also have a strain-specific variability in toxicity or carcinogenecity when being used to assess xenobiotic metabolism or drug efficacy *(31)*. Despite these caveats, the phenotypes generated from gene knockouts in mice do enhance our comprehension of cancer and its complex biological interactions.

## 2.3. Cloned Animals

The first report of a cloned sheep was published in 1996 *(20)*. Since then, many species have been produced by somatic nuclear transfer, including cows, pigs, mice, goats, and rats *(32)*. In this approach, somatic nuclei from cells altered in culture are transferred to one-cell fertilized embryos where the embryonic nucleus has been removed. These reconstituted embryos are then transplanted to suitable recipient females and allowed to develop to term. Using nuclei from the same cell source, several presumably "genetically identical" animals can be produced. Although mice have been cloned, this process has seen more application in larger animals like diary cattle, where economic traits such as milk production are important.

Cloning is an inefficient process and is used to produce gene-altered models in animals where no ES cells are currently available. These techniques are labor-intensive and time-consuming and, to date, offer a low percentage of success. Some progeny are born with large-animal syndrome *(33)* and some cloned animals die shortly after birth for no apparent reason. Jaenisch and colleagues have argued that the transferred somatic nuclei must reset itself to an embryonic nuclei (reviewed in ref. *34*). This might be an inefficient process and frequently leaves nuclear methylation and imprinting patterns in disarray. Despite these drawbacks, some laboratories are achieving higher yields of cloned animals that survive. The question remains whether large-animal models with tumor suppressor/onco-gene "knockouts" or other gene alterations derived by cloning are more suitable than mouse models to study the physiology of cancer progression and metastasis *(35)*.

## 3. TRANSGENIC MOUSE MODELS
## AND STRATEGIES FOR CONDITIONAL ANALYSIS

The production of transgenic mice by the standard technologies *(22–25)* has been enhanced by methods developed to limit gene alterations to temporal or spatial domains. This approach offers the possibility of bypassing embryonic lethal phenotypes by limiting transgene expression to adult mice or by transiently turning a gene switch on and off at defined times, creating a pulsatile dose of gene product. Combining the timing of transgene expression with Cre-lox P methods *(36)* offers the opportunity to create defined tissue-specific excisions of target genes. The defined control of gene expression or gene knockout offered by these gene switch systems removes some of the limitations introduced by the standard methods *(37)*. Finally, new transgenic gene delivery systems like the lentivirus-based vectors combined with loss of gene function using short interfering RNAs (siRNA) offer the ability to produce gene hypomorphs of suspected cancer genes. Transgenic mice that mimic cancerous changes in humans and those mice that allow more defined control of tumor suppressor loss or oncogene activation will prove valuable in understanding the initiation and progression of tumorigenesis. The use of several types of transgenic systems is outlined in the following subsections.

## 3.1. Inducible Transgenic Systems

Restriction of the transgene's expression to a specific time or a specific tissue employs inducible systems. These systems give the investigator control over when and where the putative cancer-causing gene's product is expressed. Gossen and Bujard *(38)* described a tetracycline-inducible approach modeled on bacterial operons. These systems have been reviewed *(8,38–40)*. Tetracycline, and later doxcycline, was used to remove the *tet* repressor from a silenced gene, allowing expression. The gene to be activated is placed under the control of a *tet* repressor protein that blocks expression of the gene until the repressor is removed by binding to a small molecule. Alternatively, in the reverse *tet* system, the gene to be expressed is silent until bound by an activator (rTA) protein produced by administration of the inducer. Doxycycline, the inducer in many examples, is injected or placed in the drinking water of the mouse harboring the transgene to be expressed. In the presence of doxycycline, the repressor protein is bound and removed from the gene regulatory sequence by a conformational change, and the transgene becomes active. Depending on the design of the experiment, the transgene can be induced in all tissues or restricted to a single entity such as the mammary epithelium by choice of the transgene's regulatory sequences.

One of the drawbacks of the early systems was "leakiness" from pleiotropic actions of the chemical inducer. Many of the inducer-activated transgene expression systems were not rigorously confined to the tissue of choice. The inducer molecules were active in several tissues or were too similar to natural agonists and produced effects in many tissues. The use of synthetic inducers with no known natural agonists has reduced these problems. Improved systems with better control of dosage and temporal expression has led to more selective and stringent control of gene expression with relatively few nonspecific effects. Lamartina et al. *(8)* recently described a bi-allelic therapeutic *tet* system that has low basal activity and good inducibility when the transgene vector is injected into mouse muscle. The activity of the gene's expression was correlated with doxcycline dose over a prolonged timeframe. Newer systems, like the *Lac*I *(41)*, also offer more specificity. A list of *tet* mice may be found at http://www.zmg.uni-mainz.de/tetmouse/.

In principal, one or several genes can be induced in a mouse using the same inducer by judicious selection of the transgene sequences. This could allow the use of transgenic systems to look at genes with small effects on carcinogenesis in a single mouse paradigm. Baron and Bujard *(40)* reported the use of a tetracycline-based system that was designed to discriminate between two gene promoters (or two alleles of a gene) so that each could be regulated independently in the same mouse. This approach could offer a way to look at cooperativity in cells containing more than one cancer mutation.

Components of the *Wnt* signaling pathway are increasingly implicated in human breast cancer *(42)* and a variety of other tumors. Indeed, *Wnt1* was defined as a proto-oncogene when it was shown that transgenic mice expressing *Wnt1* in their mammary glands had adenocarcinomas of the ductal epithelium. Gunther et al. *(42)* developed a doxycycline-dependent mouse where *Wnt1* expression could be controlled in the mammary epithelium. Using the inducible *Wnt1* model, these investigators were able to experimentally test the effects of *P53* loss and downregulation of *Wnt* pathway intermediates on neoplastic processes and progression using bitransgenic mice and doxycycline induction of *Wnt1*. This experimental design permits the evaluation of more than one cancer mutation in a mouse and, perhaps, is a better model of human disease than single-gene analyses.

### 3.2. Cre-Lox P Conditional Transgenic Systems

The Cre-lox P system is an approach utilized in transgenesis that allows conditional expression of a transgene (see reviews in refs. *36* and *43–45*). The Cre recombinase enzyme from bacteriophage P1 recognizes 34-bp DNA repeats that are used to flank genomic targets to be excised from the genome. The maximum size of the genomic DNA fragment that can be excised has not been defined. Therefore, a single target gene or several linked genes potentially can be altered in a mouse. The directionality of the lox P sites in the target DNA is important, as the lox P sites can be used for other types of genome manipulation (reviewed in refs. *30, 46,* and *47*). Recent reports of double lox P targeting that allow shuttling of different mutants to a genome engineered site both in vitro in the ES cell and possibly in vivo will allow the rapid analysis of multiple mutations in the same target gene *(48,49)*.

Using a Cre strategy to flank the gene to be deleted by lox P sites, a mouse can be made with the gene of interest still functional through development and parturition. This avoids many of the problems associated with early lethals from standard "knockout" technology. Time-specific expression of Cre recombinase is introduced by breeding the mouse containing the lox P-flanked gene ("floxed") to a Cre-deleter strain. Many Cre-deleter strains have been produced and a list is available at http://www.mshri.on.ca/nagy. When Cre is expressed, the DNA between the flanking lox P sites is excised producing a null or "knockout" of the "floxed" gene. Cre recombinase is remarkably efficient and specific in most of the mice tested. Grippo et al. *(50)* reported that less that 4% of the Cre mice investigated in their model were false negatives. However, there are some reports of cryptic lox P sites in the mammalian genome that have produced unwanted results *(51,52)*. Cre-expressing mouse strains combined with the inducible mouse systems previously described provide powerful tools for altering gene expression in the mouse.

The Cre system (or the similar FLP/FRT system from *Saccharomyces (53–55)* might be used to introduce conditional expression of an oncogene or tumor suppressor in a targeted tissue. As an example, the retinoblastoma (Rb) tumor suppressor gene, one of the first tumor suppressor genes identified, regulates cellular differentiation, parts of the cell cycle, and apoptosis. It was demonstrated that a heritable mutation followed by somatic LOH results in ocular tumors in children. In fact, a majority of human tumors might contain *Rb* mutations. In addition to cancer phenotypes observed in heterozygous *Rb*+/– mice, *Rb*-null embryos also exhibit a defect in fetal liver erythropoiesis that results in death at E14.5. A conditional gene-targeting approach *(56)* removed *Rb* from the central nervous system (CNS), peripheral nervous system (PNS), and lens tissue using a Nestin–Cre deletor mouse. Using this approach, it could be shown that the CNS cells of *Rb*-null mice were rescued from apoptosis if the erythroid defect was controlled by using an early Cre-based deletion.

Loss of function of *P53* might be one of the initiating events of neoplastic transformation. Families with heritable mutations of *P53* have a 13% CNS tumor incidence where the majority of the tumors are astrocytomas *(57)*. *P53*-null mice have been generated and characterized and have a very short life-span because of rapid tumor development. There is no apparent increase in CNS tumors in these mice; yet, cells from the *P53*-null mouse are spontaneously immortal. *Rb*, the retinoblastoma gene, helps regulate entry into the cell cycle. *Rb* is mutated in many sporadic and heritable human tumors *(58)* and its protein appears to be required for terminal differentiation and maturation of neural and glial precursors. Neural tumors are reported in adults who as children were treated for inherited retinoblastoma. *Rb*-null mice are embryonic lethals, so the Cre-lox P system was utilized to study the effects of *Rb* on neoplastic transformation in a *P53*-null background. A Cre transgene with a nuclear localizing signal (nls) was linked to the glial fibrillary acidic protein (GFAP) promoter. The GFAP promoter was found to be expressed in mature astrocytes and precursor cells located in the external granular layer of the cerebellum and some other sites using a *LacZ* reporter mouse strain *(57)*. A conditional *Rb* allele was generated resulting in a truncated RB protein when Cre is active. Bitransgenic GFAP-Cre/Rb$^{\text{lox P/loxP}}$ showed no brain histology up to 1 yr of age. Some experimental evidence suggested that loss of *P53* function might act as a tumor initiator; therefore, the conditional GFAP-Rb was introduced into the *P53* transgenic background. Mice with the genotype *GFAP-Cre; Rb$^{loxP/loxP}$;P53$^{+/-}$* were followed for 8 mo with no observable signs of CNS disease, although there were other tumors reported in these mice *(57)*. Mice with the genotype GFAP-Cre; Rb loxP/loxP;*P53–/–* were euthanized at 3–4 mo because of observable CNS pathology in three of seven mice. Upon histological examination, all seven mice showed cerebellar tumors with invasive growth patterns strikingly similar to medulloblastomas seen in children *(57)*. Polymerase chain reaction (PCR) analysis confirmed loss of the Rb allele. These experiments show that the combined loss of two genes, *P53* and *Rb*, involved in human cancer can be modeled in the mouse with informative outcomes. As an ancillary outcome, the GFAP-Cre mouse can now be used to delete other genes designed as conditional constructs.

Lasko et al. *(7)* used a Cre strategy to turn on a loxP-STOP-loxP silenced SV40 T-antigen linked to an α-crystallin promoter. This transgene was expected to produce tumors of the eye when activated by Cre-mediated excision. A mouse with the lox P-flanked STOP signal inserted between the SV40 T-antigen transgene and its crystallin promoter was mated to a transgenic mouse that expressed Cre in early development. When Cre was active, deletion of the STOP signal was achieved, SV40 T-antigen was expressed, and lens tumors developed. The use of bitransgenic mice carrying both a lox P-flanked allele and the transgene driving Cre expression could result in reduced Cre expression because of effects on endogenous promoters. For example, a transgenic mouse using an elastase promoter to drive *c-myc* expression to pancreatic acinar cells produced neoplasms but also resulted in a 95% decline in endogenous elastase expression. The decreased elastase expression might also reduce transgenes linked to that promoter *(5,7)*. Thus, careful consideration must be given to the experimental design of bitransgenic mouse models to avoid such confounding results.

Human patients with multiple endocrine neoplasia type 1 (MEN1) present with primary endocrine tumors in the parathyroid and pancreas because of loss of the MEN1 gene. Mouse MEN1 mapped to a region of chromosome 19 was syntenic with the MEN1 locus on human 11q13 *(59)*. Familial MEN1 cases suggest that 85% or more involve germline mutations. A conditional Cre mutant mouse model of MEN1 was developed by flanking exon 3 with lox P sites *(60)*. Employing the rat insulin promoter (RIP) to drive Cre expression in pancreatic β-cells, transgenic mice with a MEN1 deletion specifically in the pancreas was confirmed by PCR. The incidence of insulinomas reached 100% by age 6 mo in this model. Control mice showed no abnormalities. In another mouse, the mouse homolog of MEN1 was targeted by flanking exons 3–8 with lox P sites. When mice carrying the lox P-flanked MEN1 alleles are mated to the RIP-Cre-deletor strain, the MEN1 gene is inactivated only in the mouse pancreas *(61)*. The pancreas shows formation of adenomas, an increase in insulin, and a decrease in serum blood glucose. Crossing the lox P-flanked MEN1 mice with PTH-Cre mice created a model where the bitransgenic mice showed hyperparathyroidism and hypercalcemia, similar to patients with MEN1. These studies show the utility of targeting one gene with lox P-flanking segments and then using several tissue-specific Cre-deletor strains to remove the gene's activity in selected tissues. Cre conditional models are also advantageous because initiation and progression of tumorigenesis can be studied

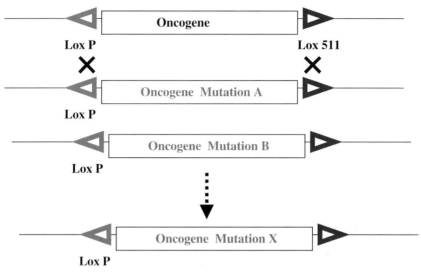

**Fig. 3.** Double lox targeting.

in defined tissue and the deletion does not kill the mouse early, as seen in many models where the homozygous deletion is engineered in all tissues.

Finally, double lox-targeting strategies *(48,49,62)* might allow the introduction of an allelic series of tumor suppressor or oncogene mutations into the endogenous gene's location. This will permit the analysis and the effect on function of mutations found in specific tumors or families. This approach flanks the wild-type gene with a loxP site and a loxP511 site (see Fig. 3). The sequence of these two lox P sites differs enough that excision of DNA between the sites does occur. Instead, recombination happens between like Lox P sites so that a DNA fragment is shuttled into the genomic location. This has been confirmed in ES cells with a neural system *(49)*, however, its utility requires examination in other systems.

### 3.3. Combining Inducible Transgene Systems With Conditional Cre Recombinase Systems

Deleting genes with Cre recombinase during development often precludes studying that gene's loss of expression in the adult animal due to lethality. Temporal control of Cre recombinase expression to delete lox P-flanked genes avoids some of the complications of gene excision during embryogenesis. Thus, it is not surprising that Cre expression was placed under the control of *tet* controlled expression systems *(63)*. Independent and stringent temporal control of Cre recombinase expression are the goals of these approaches *(64,65)*. Several criteria should be met when combining Cre recombinase strategies with inducible systems. These include the following: (1) When the inducer is absent, there is no "leaky" Cre expression; (2) there is no position effect from integration of the transgenes used to construct these systems; and (3) when the inducer is present, Cre excision is complete and occurs in only those tissues where the inducible promoter is expected to be active. When developing a Cre-deletor mouse or a regulated Cre-deletor line, it is usually tested with one of the lox P-flanked reporter *LacZ* or green fluorescent protein (GFP) mouse lines to confirm its tissue specificity prior to using it in an experimental test. Scenarios can be envisioned where two "floxed" genes can be engineered in the same mice and an inducible Cre-activated loss accomplished. This type of combinatorial analysis allows modeling of LOH of more than one gene in a controlled timeframe in the adult mouse.

Several problems do arise in these scenarios and the investigator should be aware of their possibility. First, ectopic expression of Cre might occur that would excise the lox P-flanked gene in an unwanted tissue. Second, an endogenous protein might induce the Cre transgene, introducing premature excision of the gene of interest. Because these combinatorial systems have been refined and the Cre lines tested, these complications have been reduced.

### 3.4. siRNA Transgenic Systems and Viral-Based Delivery

Human immunodeficiency virus-1 (HIV-1)-based lentivirus vectors are classified as retroviruses but are able to infect both active and inactive postmitotic cells. Lentivirus vectors are largely able to evade proviral silencing and thus remain able to express the engineered gene insert. Sequence-specific gene silencing from dsRNA was reported initially in *Caenorhabditis elegans (66)*. The RNA interference (RNAi) effect was also reported for other organisms, raising interest in using this method for examining gene function. RNAi "knockdown" of gene expression potentially permits gene products in a pathway to be studied individually and in combinations. Combining the siRNA systems with *tet*-inducible or Cre systems extends the analytic possibilities.

Experimental evidence shows that the active element of RNAi is a short 21- to 23-nt dsRNA that can be generated as an RNase III cleavage product from a longer dsRNA (reviewed in ref. *67*). The short interfering RNAs (siRNA) are complexed with proteins and require ATP to unwind the dsRNA to a single-stranded sequence-specific "silencer" RNA. Inhibition is achieved by the siRNA complex binding to the complementary mRNA sequence, resulting in degradation of the targeted mRNA. Employing dsRNAs longer than 30 nt evokes a nonspecific interferon-mediated response that causes mRNA degradation by RNase I. The global result of the interferon response is inhibition of RNA translation by secondary activation of PKR protein kinase that inhibits eIF2α translation initiation factor *(67)*. It has also been shown that different sequence siRNAs targeted to the same mRNA are differentially effective at silencing the gene *(68,69)*. Hence, several siRNA constructs need to be evaluated in vitro prior to producing transgenic mice *(92)*. The siRNA sequence should be checked for similarities with other genes to ensure its specificity, avoiding the potential complication of altering expression of another gene entirely.

Xia et al. *(70)* showed in a proof of concept experiment that recombinant adenoviruses could be used to deliver siRNAs. Adenovirus-containing siGFP linked to dsRed, to localize the injection site, was injected into the brain's striatal region of transgenic mice expressing enhanced green fluorescent protein (EGFP). EGFP expression in these mice was reduced and confined to the site of siGFP injection. siRNA directed against β-glucuronidase activity in mouse liver tested whether an endogenously expressed gene product could be reduced. Fluorescent-based assays on liver homogenates showed β-glucuronidase gene silencing in the liver. Reduction of gene expression using liposome-mediated delivery (DOTAP) of siRNA constructs to adult mouse tissues has also been shown by Soreson et al. *(71)*.

Tiscornia et al. *(72)* demonstrated germline transmission of an siGFP after lentivirus delivery to two cell mouse embryos. The zona pellucida was removed from the embryo and transduction was preformed in drops of buffer containing lentivirus siRNA. Some of the resulting progeny showed integrated lentivirus by PCR analysis using siGFP primers. One pup showed "knockdown" of GFP. This animal had two copies/cell of the siGFP, whereas the original GFP-expressing transgenic mice had multiple copies of GFP. This result suggests that even a few copies of expressed siRNA can effectively reduce expression of the target gene. Another study *(73)* employing siRNA against the target gene *Neil1,* a gene involved in DNA repair, introduced *siNeil1* into ES cells by electroporation. Stable *siNeil1* ES integrants showed an 80% reduction in the target's endogenous enzyme activity, correlating with a similar decrease in *Neil1* mRNA. Two ES clones were used to produce chimera that were crossed to obtain F1 germline carriers. siRNA to *Neil1* was found in about 46% of the progeny from each ES cell line. Expression analyses showed a similar 80% reduction in enzyme activity as that demonstrated in the original ES cell clones. Adenovirus-based delivery of *siVEGF* was examined in vivo in a mouse model of age-related macular degeneration *(74)*. The results show that *VEGF* expression in mouse retinal pigment epithelial cells is inhibited by *sihVEGF*. Consequently, neovascularization in the eye was reduced. However, the long-term expression of the siRNA in the retina after a single administration of viral siRNA remains to be determined. All of these examples are encouraging and suggest that siRNA loss of function or production of gene hypomorphs in mice will allow this system to be used to examine the effect of "knockdowns" on oncogenes or tumor suppressor gene activity *(75)*.

The next steps using siRNA approaches will involve producing conditional mice where spatial and temporal control of siRNA expression is achieved. Human prostate carcinoma cells (PC-3) were engineered to contain a *Tet*-inducible siRNA for either the p110α or p110β subunits of phosphatidylinositol 3-kinase (PI-3 kinase) *(76)*. Inhibition of PI-3 kinase was tested and confirmed in vitro. The siRNA containing PC-3 cells were injected into the left dorsolateral prostate gland of male nude mice to develop an orthoptopic prostate tumor/metatasis model. Doxycycline (Dox) was administered in the drinking water for 56 d postimplant. Prostate tumors, local and distant metastases, were evaluated. Mice with the p110β siRNA induced by Dox for 56 d showed a significant decrease in lymph node metastases even though the prostate tumor size in siRNA-treated and mice controls was similar. Results with the p110α siRNA showed no observable reduction in tumor metastases from controls. The existence of siRNA expression was confirmed in tumors by Northern blot. The authors speculate that the reduction of metastatic tumors in p110β subunit siRNA mice might be the result of a specific effect on the ability of treated PC-3 tumor cells to migrate to distant body sites *(76)*.

*TrP53* encodes protein P53 that acts as a tumor suppressor. Normally, the P53 protein induces apoptosis in cells responding to hyperproliferation signals. Inactivation of the *P53* gene enhances tumorigenecity in cells where mitogenic oncogene signals are present *(77)*. A series of *P53* siRNA constructs (A–C) were made and tested in tissue culture. *P53*-C siRNA showed the largest decline in *P53* levels. A nonspecific GFP siRNA used as a control showed no decline in *P53* activity in vitro. A *P53* retroviral construct was used to transduce liver stem cells from Eμ-Myc fetal livers, and these cells were transplanted into lethally irradiated recipient mice. The expectation was that "knockdown" of *P53* in the oncogenic mouse line would decrease the survival time compared to controls that had a normal *P53* suppressor effect. In both the *P53*-B and the *P53*-C siRNA mice, 100% of the mice developed lymphomas and reached a terminal end point much earlier than control mice. Consequently, siRNA suppression of P53 protein accelerates tumorigenesis in this mouse model. In contrast to *P53*-null mice where significant aneuploidy in the tumor tissue is seen upon histological analysis, this was not observed in siRNAB or siRNAC series *P53* mice.

These studies demonstrate sustained reduction in target gene activity and the heritability of some siRNA constructs. These types of study suggest that a variety of target genes are accessible by siRNA strategies and that individual steps in pathways can be targeted independently. They also validate both viral and nonviral delivery systems. This opens the door to using single, stepwise, or combinatorial "knockdowns" to assess the interactions or contributions of multiple genes to the development of cancer and other human diseases. Inducible siRNA systems will permit "dampening" of the oncogene or tumor suppressor target at any stage in the physiological network or pathway. (*See* Chapter 12.)

Finally, lentiviral vectors are reported to have produced transgenic pigs *(78)* that carried a GFP transgene reporter in 65% of the embryos transplanted. GFP expression was confirmed in all tissues and was transmitted through the germline. This achievement might foreshadow the use of siRNA strategies in larger-animal models to evaluate cancer biology.

## 4. USING TRANSGENIC SYSTEMS TO IDENTIFY CARCINOGENS OR DEVELOP THERAPEUTICS

Mutations, induced or spontaneous, historically are one of the best methods for linking gene function to a physical location in the genome. This technique can be applied to carcinogenesis by using large-scale induced mutation/phenotype screens to locate cancer genes (reviewed in ref. *6*). The goal of using transgenic mice to evaluate carcinogenesis is to develop a model where carcinogenesis is accelerated, spontaneous background is low, and a reliable readout relevant to human clinical data is obtained *(79)*. In addition, mouse and other animal models of cancer are important first steps in evaluating potential chemotherapeutics *(9,80)*. These systems can provide bioassays for identifying effective chemical/drug treatments, contribute toward an understanding of the mechanisms of drug action, and evaluate toxicity and dosages. This information leads to better designed clinical trials for drugs to treat human cancers.

Cancer-causing chemicals undergo in vivo long-term risk assessment in the 2-yr rodent assay *(81)*. Transgenic models, such as the *P53* knockout mouse, might be more useful than nontransgenic rodents in this assay if it can be determined that these models are more sensitive to cancer drug actions. The enhanced carcinogen sensitivity of engineered mice could be used to reduce the time and cost of the animal carcinogenesis assay *(82)*. However, rigorous interpretation of results and comprehension of strain background differences need to be considered if transgenic mice are to replace the standard rodent bioassay. Transgenic models are effective (1) in dissecting the biological contribution of mutated genes to cancer, (2) as biological screening systems to evaluate drug toxicity and efficacy for newly developed cancer-preventive pharmaceuticals and (3) to study the mechanism of action of a cancer-preventive drug *(79)*. Of particular interest would be mouse models that are hypomorphs of (1) key oncogenes, (2) tumor suppressor genes, or (3) receptors of endogenous, therapeutic, and environmental ligands. Finally, human clinical trials might be optimized by using transgenic systems to mimic the human cancer before committing to expensive phase I–III drug trials. If evaluated rigorously, transgenic mouse models might allow more cancer therapeutics to move rapidly through the evaluation process and might provide a powerful tool to assess efficacy of cancer preventives using models developed to test mechanisms of action *(31)*.

Pritchard et al. *(81)* reported evaluating three transgenic mouse models (Trp 53 +/–, TgAC, and RasH2) with known carcinogens in a bioassay and comparing the results to the standard rodent bioassay protocol. The transgenic mice did provide correct "readouts" for about 81% of the chemicals tested; yet they gave false-negative results for several known carcinogens. In other studies, mammary cancer has been induced in transgenic mice and used to evaluate chemicals that might effectively inhibit tumor progression (reviewed in ref. 8). Nude mouse models that receive transplantable human tumor cells might not be good predictors of therapeutic outcomes because the tumor cells maintained in culture might have accumulated several mutations (82). Investigators using transgenic mouse models to evaluate risk assessments and evaluate new cancer therapies must show that these models reliably predict human efficacy and toxicity. Consequently, transgenic mice might prove valuable in bioassays, but the models to be used need to be carefully selected and validated. (See Chapter 12.)

### 4.1. ENU Mutagenic Screens

N-Ethyl-N-nitrosourea (ENU) is a chemical carcinogen and mutagen that has been used in several model systems to efficiently produce point mutations. In mice, ENU mutagenesis is combined with phenotype screens to identify genomic changes with disease relevance. These can include both dominant phenotypes and recessive phenotypes that are unmasked by breeding. Like gene trapping, this method is unbiased (ENU can affect any gene) and relies on forward genetic screens to establish the phenotype. Although the large-scale ENU mouse screens do not need genomic sequence, the availability of the mouse genomic databases makes the process of mapping and isolating the mutation more straightforward (83).

Male mice are treated with ENU and bred to normal females. F1 progeny from this mating are evaluated for observable phenotype (dominant mutation). Seemingly unaffected F1 male progeny can be mated to normal females, and the F2 females are then backcrossed to the original ENU-treated male. These F3 progeny are evaluated for recessive phenotypes. Mice with cancer-related phenotypes of interest could be maintained by breeding.

Several drawbacks are inherent in this approach. First, the genomic site of the ENU-induced mutation is random and might not produce a cancer phenotype without screening many mice. Identifying the gene where the mutation exists is demanding. In some cases, the phenotypes produced between studies are from a small pool of alleles, making identification of novel genes more difficult. Finally, a cancer phenotype identified in a large mutagenic screen leaves the investigator with the challenge of linking an ENU mutation with biology (84,85).

### 4.2. Gene Trap Approaches

The completion of the mouse and human genome sequences provides a vast resource of new genetic information to mine for functional associations. Rapidly integrating a gene or gene family with its associated biology will provide a large resource of therapeutic targets. Traditional gene knockout methods are limited to those classes of genes considered valid drug targets such as (1) those including nuclear hormone receptors, (2) cell cycle modulators and apoptotic and/or proliferation processing receptors, (3) channel and transporter proteins, and (4) many different classes of enzymes like kinases and phosphorylases (9,83). Whereas the time and cost required to "knockout" and evaluate the phenotype of each individual gene in the mouse presents a daunting task, high-throughput mutagenesis screens, without a functional bias, might capture active genes that are viable targets for drug development or can be screened for cancer phenotypes. This approach also produces gene-targeted mice that are hypomorphs rather than nulls of the gene activity and has the potential to identify new types of gene interaction.

Gene trap screens use a vector designed to insert and capture transcriptionally active genes (reviewed in refs. *83, 86,* and *87*). Trapping constructs are generally exogenous reporter DNA elements engineered to capture gene activity (such as enhancers, promoters, or polyadenylation signals). The trap vector contains splice acceptor or donor sites linked with *lacZ* or another reporter and a selectable ES marker of integration such as neomycin. Random insertion of these constructs into the ES cells genome produce a fusion transcript between an active gene and the trap vector. The trap acts as a genomic tag that can be used as a starting point for sequence identity from a database. Although gene trapping can be used to capture active genes of unknown function, the task of linking biology with the trapped gene requires cloning the gene, breeding, and analyzing phenotypes. The gene trap approach remains labor-intensive but potentially can produce models of carcinogenic action or of pharmaceutical relevance to cancer.

## 5. CONCLUSIONS

Cancer research has benefited from the ability to manipulate the mouse genome *(88)*. One goal is to produce mice with refined genomic mutations that recapitulate cancer development in the human. Transgenic mice allow these analyses to be carried out in an intact physiological system where the cancer precursor "sees" the cellular environment *(3,4)*. Consequently, transgenic systems, although more expensive than cell-based assays, might be better predictors of human cancer biology.

Transgenic mice provide insights into in vivo gene function, assign biological activity to protein products, and link interacting gene partners. Mouse transgenic technology allows a combinatorial approach utilizing genomic information and physical manipulation of selected genes to dissect pathways altered during tumorigenesis. Genetically altered mouse models are valuable tools for evaluating and validating genes involved in cancer, cell proliferation, tumorigenesis, and metastasis. Some methods demand significant knowledge of the gene sequence and bioinformatics and some require labor-intensive phenotype screens and long-term breeding. Technological advances that can (1) improve or enhance ES cell homologous recombination, (2) deliver gene vectors more efficiently to obtain higher transgenic rates, or (3) produce good large-animal models of cancer will facilitate understanding the gene–environment interactions that lead to cancer in humans. Transgenic systems that can speed the analysis of putative cancer therapeutics will allow more effective drugs to reach the patient sooner and potentially at lower cost. Although most transgenic mouse models are designed to study gene products that promote cancer, several mouse models (reviewed in ref. *79*) have shown cancer-resistant phenotypes, suggesting that therapeutic strategies can be targeted to abrogate cancer development as well *(89)*. Finally, whereas transgenic mouse models have proven to be invaluable tools for studying a variety of cancer-related processes, future goals would be to develop mouse models that might more accurately respond to and reflect the human condition (see reviews in refs. *90* and *91*).

## REFERENCES

1. Hirst GL, Balmain A. Forty years of cancer modelling in the mouse. Eur J Cancer 2004; 40:1794–1780.
2. Hardouin S, Nagy A. Mouse models for human disease. Clin Genet 2000; 57:237–244.

3. Sakatani T, Onyango P. Oncogenomics: prospects for the future. Expert Rev Anticancer Ther 2003; 3: 891–901.

4. Winter SF, Cooper AB, Greenberg NM. Models of metastatic prostate cancer: a transgenic perspective. Prostate Cancer Prostatic Dis 2003; 6:204–211.

5. Sandgren EP, Quaife CJ, Paulovich AG, et al. Pancreatic tumor pathogenesis reflects the causative genetic lesion. Proc Natl Acad Sci USA 1991; 88:93–97.

6. Perkins AS. Functional genomics in the mouse. Funct Integrat Genom 2002; 2:81–91.

7. Lakso M, Sauer B, Mosinger B Jr, et al. Targeted oncogene activation by site specific recombination in transgenic mice. Proc Natl Acad Sci USA 1992; 89:6232–6236.

8. Lamartina S, Silvi L, Roscilli G, et al. Construction of an rtTA2$^S$-M2/tTS$^{kid}$ based transcription regulatory switch that displays no basal activity, good inducibility and high responsiveness to doxycycline in mice and non-human primates. Mol Ther 2003; 7:271–276.

9. Mitsumori K. Evaluation on carcinogenecity of chemicals using transgenic mice. Toxicology 2002; 181–182:241–244.

10. Jackson-Gusby L. Modeling cancer in the mouse. Oncogene 2002; 21:5504–5514.

11. Jaenisch J. Germ line integration and Mendelian transmission of the exogenous Moloney leukemia virus. Proc Natl Acad Sci USA 1976; 73:1260–1264.

12. Gordon J, Ruddle F. Integration and stable germline transmission of genes injected into mouse pronuclei. Science 1981; 214:1244–1246.

13. Doetschman T, Gregg RG, Maeda N, et al. Targeted correction of a mutant HPRT gene in mouse embryonic stem cells. Nature 1987; 330:576–578.

14. Evans M, Kaufman M. Establishment in culture of pluripotent cells from mouse embryos. Nature 1981; 292:154–156.

15. Mintz B, Illmensee K. Normal genetically mosaic mice produced from malignant teratocarcinoma cells. Proc Natl Acad Sci USA 1975; 72:3585–3589.

16. Palmiter RD, Brinster RL, Hammer HE, et al. Dramatic growth of mice that develop from eggs microinjected with metallothionein-growth hormone fusion genes. Biotechnology 1992; 24:429–433.

17. Miklyaeva EL, Dong W, Bureau A, et al. Late onset Tay–Sachs disease in mice with targeted disruption of the Hexa gene: behavioral changes and pathology of the central nervous system. Brain Res 2004; 1001(1–2):37–50.

18. Tybulewicz VL, Tremblay ML, LaMarca ME, et al. Animal model of Gaucher's disease from targeted disruption of the mouse glucocerebrosidase gene. Nature 1992; 357:407–410.

19. Haston CK, McKerlie C, Newbigging S, et al. Detection of modifier loci influencing the lung phenotype of cystic fibrosis knockout mice. Mamm Genome 2002; 13:605–613.

20. Campbell KH, McWhir J, Ritchieet WA, et al. Sheep cloned by nuclear transfer from a cultured cell line. Nature 1996 380:64–66.

21. Wakayama T. Cloned mice and embryonic stem cell lines generated from adult somatic cells by nuclear transfer. Oncol Res 2003; 13:309–314.

22. Nagy A, Perrimon N, Sandmeyer S, et al. Tailoring the genome: the power of genetic approaches. Nat Genet 2003; 33(Suppl):276–284.

23. Houdebine L-M. Animal transgensis and cloning. New York: Wiley, 2003:1–217.

24. Hofker M, van Deursen J. Transgenic mouse: methods and protocols. Totowa, NJ: Humana Press, 2003: 1–374.

25. Joyner A. Gene targeting: a practical approach. Oxford: IRL Press.

26. Hurlin PJ, Zhou ZQ, Toyo-oka K, et al. Deletion of Mnt leads to disrupted cell cycle control and tumorigenesis. EMBO J 2003; 22:4584–4596.

27. Wijnhoven SWP, van Steeg H. Transgenic and lnockout mice for DNA repair functions in carcinogenesis and mutagenesis. Toxicology 2003; 193:171–187.

28. Bassing CH, Suh H, Ferguson DO. Histone H2AX: dosage dependent suppressor of oncogenic translocction and tumors. Cell 2003; 114:359–370.

29. Anisimov VN. Aging and cancer in transgenic mice. Front Biosci 2003; 8:s883–902.

30. Mills AA, Bradley A. From mouse to man: generating megabase chromosome rearrangements. Trends Genet 2001; 17:331–339.

31. Rudmann DG, Durham SK. Utilization of genetically altered animals in the pharmaceutical industry. Toxicol Pathol 1999; 27:111–114.

32. Mullins LJ, Wilmut I, Mullins JJ. Nuclear transfer in rodents. J Physiol 2004; 554(Pt 1):4–12.

33. McEvoy TG, Ashworth CJ, Rooke JA, Sinclair KD. Consequences of manipulating gametes and embryos of ruminant species. Reproduction 2003; 61(Suppl):167–182.

34. Hochedlinger K, Jaenisch R. Nuclear transplantation: lessons from frogs and mice. Curr Opin Cell Biol 2002; 14:741–748.

35. Fan J, Watanabe T. Transgenic rabbits as therapeutic protein bioreactors and human disease models. Pharmacol Ther 2003; 99:261–282.

36. Sauer B. Cre/lox: one more step in taming the genome. Endocrine 2002; 19:221–228.

37. Bockamp E, Maringer M, Spangenberg C, et al. Of mice and models: improved animal models for biomedical research. Physiol Genom 2002; 11:115–132.

38. Gossen M, Bujard H. Studying gene function in eukaryotes by conditional gene inactivation. Annu Rev Genet 2002; 36:153–173.

39. Schonig K, Bujard H. Generating conditional mouse mutants via tetracycline-controlled gene expression. Totowa, NJ: Humana Press, 2003:69–104.

40. Baron U, Bujard H. Tet repressor-based system for regulated gene expression in eukaryotic cells: principles and advances. Methods Enzymol 2000; 327:401–421.

41. Cronin CA, Gluba W, Scrable H et al. The lac operator–repressor system is functional in the mouse. Genes Dev 2001; 15(12):1506–1517.

42. Gunther EJ, Moody SE, Belka GK, et al. Impact of *P53* loss on reversal andrecurrence of conditional Wnt-induced tumorigenesis. Genes Devel 2003; 17:488–501.

43. Le Y, Sauer B. Conditional gene knockout using Cre recombinase. Totowa, NJ: Humana Press, 2000: 477–485.

44. Sauer B. Inducible gene targeting in mice using the Cre/lox system. Methods 1998; 14:381–392.

45. Lewandoski M. Conditional control of gene expression in the mouse. Nature Rev Genet 2001; 2:743–755.

46. Shannon KM, Le Beau MM, Largaespada DA, et al. Modeling myeloid leukemia tumor suppressor gene inactivation in the mouse. Semin Cancer Biol 2001; 11:191–200.

47. Smith AJ, Xian J, Richardson M, et al. Cre-loxP chromosome engineering of a targeted deletion in the mouse corresponding to the 3p21.3 region of homozygous loss in human tumors. Oncogene 2002; 21: 4521–4529.

48. Soukharev S, Miller JL, Sauer B. Segmental genomic replacement in embryonic stem cells by double lox targeting. Nucleic Acids Res 1999; 27:e21.

49. Adams LD, Choi L, Xian HQ, et al. Double lox targeting for neural cell transgenesis. Mol Brain Res 2003; 110:220–233.

50. Grippo PJ, Nowlin PS, Cassaday RD, Sandgren EP. Cell-specific transgene expression from a widely transcribed promoter using Cre/lox mice. Genesis 2002; 32:277–286.

51. Thyagarajan B, Guimaraes MJ, Groth AC, et al. Mammalian genomes contain active recombinase recognition sites. Gene 2000; 244(1–2):47–54.

52. Schmidt EE, Taylor DS, Prigge JR, et al. Illegitimate Cre-dependent chromosome rearrangements in transgenic mouse spermatids. Proc Natl Acad Sci USA 2000; 97:13,702–13,707.

53. Takeuchi T, Nomura T, Tsujita M, et al. Flp recombinase transgenic mice of C57Bl/6 strain for conditional gene targeting. Biochem Biophys Res Commun 2002; 293:953–957.

54. Chen Y, Rice PA. New insights into site specific recombination from FLP recombinase switches. Annu Rev Biophys Biomol Struct 2003; 32:135–159.

55. Vooijs M, van der Valk M, te Riele H, Berns A. Flp mediated tissue specific inactivation of the retinoblastoma tumor suppressor gene in the mouse. Oncogene 1998; 17:1–12.

56. MacPherson D, Sage J, Crowley D, et al. Conditional mutation of Rb causes cell cycle defects without apoptosis in the central nervous system. Mol Cell Biol 2003; 23:1044–1053.

57. Marino S, Vooijs M, van Der Gulden, et al. Induction of medulloblastomas in *P53* null mutant mice by somatic inactivation of Rb in the external granular layer cells of the cerebellum. Genes Devel 2000; 14:994–1004.

58. Weinberg R. The retinoblastoma protein and cell cycle control. Cell 1995; 81:323–330.

59. Biondi C, Gartside M, Tonks I, et al. Targeting and conditional inactivation of the murine MEN1 locus using the Cre recombinase: lox P system. Genesis 2002; 32:150–151.

60. Bertolinin P, Tong W-M, Herrera L, et al. Pancreatic β-cell specific ablation of the multiple endocrine neoplasia type 1 (MEN1) gene causes full penetrance of insulinoma development in mice. Cancer Res 2003; 63:4836–4841.

61. Crabtree JS, Scacheri PC, Ward JM, et al. Of mice and MEN1: insulinomas in a conditional mouse knockout. Mol Cell Biol 2003; 23:6075–6085.

62. Langer SJ, Ghafoori AP, Byrd M, Leinwand L. A genetic screen identifies novel non-compatible lox P sites. Nucleic Acids Res 2002; 30:3067–3077.

63. St-Onge L, Furth PA, Gruss P. Temporal control of Cre recombinase in transgenic mice by a tetracycline responsive promoter. Nucleic Acids Res 1996; 24:3875–3877.

64. Schonig K, Schwenk F, Rajewsky K, Bujard H. Stringent doxycycline dependent control of Cre recombinase in vivo. Nucleic Acids Res 2002; 30:e134.

65. Baron U, Schnappinger D, Helbl V, et al. Generation of conditional mutants in higher eukaryotes by switching between expression of two genes. Proc Natl Acad Sci USA 1999; 96:1013–1018.

66. Kamath R, Ahringer J. Genome-wide RNAi screening in *Caenorhabditis elegans*. Methods 2003; 30: 313–312.

67. Dykxhoorn DM, Novina CD, Sharp PA, et al. Killing the messenger: short RNAs that silence gene expression. Nat Rev Mol Cell Biol 2003; 4:457–467.

68. Torgeir H, Amarzguioui M, Wiiger MT, et al. Positional effects of short interfering targeting human coagulation trigger tissue factor. Nucleic Acids Res 2002; 30:1757–1766.

69. Rubinson DA, Dillon CP, Kwiatkowski AV, et al. A lentivirus-based system to functionally silence genes in primary mammalian cells, stem cells and transgenic mice by RNA interference. Nature Gene 2003; 33:396–400.

70. Xia H, Mao Q, Paulson HL, et al. siRNA-mediated gene silencing in vitro and in vivo. Nature Biotechnol 2002; 20:1006–1010.

71. Sorensen DR, Leirdal M, Sioud M, et al. Gene silencing by systemic delivery of synthetic siRNAs in adult mice. J Mol Biol 2003; 327:761–766.

72. Tiscornia G, Singer O, Ikawa M, et al. A general method for gene knockdown in mice by using lentiviral vectors expressing small interfering RNA. Proc Natl Acad Sci USA 2003; 100:1844–1848.

73. Carmell MA, Zhang L, Conklin DS, et al. Germline transmission of RNAi in mice. Nature Struct Biol 2003; 10:91–92.

74. Reich SJ, Fosnot J, Kuroki A, et al. Small interfering RNA (siRNA) targeting VEGF effectively inhibits ocular neovascularization in a mouse model. Mol Vision 2003; 9:210–216.

75. Matsukura S, et al. Establishment of conditional vectors for hairpin siRNA knockdowns. Nucleic Acids Res 2003; 31:e77.

76. Czauderna F, Santel A, Hinz M, et al. Inducible shRNA expression for application in a prostate cancer model. Nucleic Acids Res 2003; 31:e127.

77. Hemann MT, Fridman JS, Zilfou JT, et al. An epi-allelic series of *P53* hypomorphs created by stable RNAi produces distinct tumor phenotypes *in vivo*. Nature Genet 2003; 33:396–400.

78. Hofmann A, Kessler B, Ewerling S, et al. Efficient transgenesis in farm animals by lentiviral vectors. EMBO Rep 2003; 4:1054–1060.

79. Klatt P, Serrano M. Engineering cancer resistance in mice. Carcinogenesis 2003; 24:817–826.

80. Moser R, Quesniaux V, Ryffel B, et al. Use of transgenics animals to investigate drug hypersensitivity. Toxicology 2001; 158:75–83.

81. Pritchard JB, French JE, Davis BJ, et al. The role of mouse models in carcinogen identification. Environ Health Perspect 2003; 111:444–454.

82. Kerbels RS. What is the optimal rodent model for anti-tumor drug testing? Cancer Metastasis Rev 1998–1999; 17:301–304.

83. Abuin A, Holt KH, Platt KA, et al. Full-speed mammalian genetics: in vivo target validation in the drug discovery process. Trends Biotechnol 2002; 20:36–42.

84. Dirac AM, Bernards R. Reversal of senescence in mouse fibroblasts through suppression of p53. J Biol Chem 2003; 278:11,731–11,734.

85. Rathkolb B, Fuchs E, Kolb HJ, et al. Large scale *N*-ethyl *N*-nitrosurea mutagenesis in mice—from phenotypes to genes. Exp Physiol 2000; 85:635–643.

86. Skarnes WC, Auerbach BA, Joyner AL. A gene trap approach in mouse embryonic stem cells: the Lac Z reported is activated by splicing reflects endogenous gene expression and is mutagenic in mice. Genes Devel 1992; 6:903–918.

87. Wiles MV, Vauti F, Otte J, et al. Establishment of a gene trap sequence tag library to generate mutant mice from embryonic stem cells. Nature Genet 2000; 24:13–24.

88. Demant P. Cancer susceptibility in the mouse:genetics, biology and implications for human cancer. Nature Rev Genet 2003; 4:721–734.
89. Tu SP, Jiang XH, Lin MC, et al. Suppression of survivin expression inhibits in vivo tumorigenecity and angiogenesis in gastric cancer. Cancer Res 2003; 63:7724–7732.
90. Jonkers J, Berns A. Conditional mouse models of sporadic cancer. Nature Rev Cancer 2002; 2:251–265.
91. Rangarajan A, Weinberg RA. Comparative biology of mouse versus human cells: modeling human cancer in mice. Nature Rev Cancer 2003; 3:952–959.
92. Hasuwa H, Kaseda K, Einarsdottir T, et al. Small interfering RNA and gene silencing in transgenic mice and rats. FEBS Lett 2002; 532:227–230.

# 21

# Homology-Based Genomic Mining of Growth Factors Implicated in Neoplasia and Nephritides

## PDGF-D

*Gary C. Starling, PhD,*
*William J. LaRochelle, PhD,*
*and Gulshan Ara, PhD*

### CONTENTS

### SUMMARY

The platelet-derived growth factor (PDGF) family members are molecules that are associated with malignant transformation, neovascularization, and tumor–stromal interactions. Widespread usage of genomic technologies has lead to the identification of a fourth family member, PDGF-D. In this chapter, we focus on the discovery, structure, and function of PDGF-D, a latent, protease-activated growth factor that has recently been implicated in the development of various types of cancer and kidney disease.

**Key Words:** Platelet-derived growth factor (PDGF); PDGF-D; neoplasia; nephritis; receptor; activation; CUB domain; growth factor domain.

## 1. INTRODUCTION

Identification of the platelet-derived growth factor (PDGF) family began with the annotation of functional serum activity and thereafter differentiated among the unique primary structures of PDGF-A and PDGF-B that have been intimately associated with

From: *Cancer Drug Discovery and Development: The Oncogenomics Handbook*
Edited by: W. J. LaRochelle and R. A. Shimkets © Humana Press Inc., Totowa, NJ

malignant transformation, neovascularization, and tumor–stromal interactions. In notable contrast, the widespread use of genomic technologies, including transcript libraries and databases, led to the ability to perform homology-based searches and the discovery of the unique primary sequences of other family members: PDGF-C and PDGF-D. Subsequent functional studies have shown that the new PDGFs are each pleiotropic growth factors for cells expressing PDGF receptors. As ligands for the α and/or β PDGF receptors, these new PDGFs have been associated with several disease states. Here, we will focus on the discovery, structure, and function of PDGF-D, a latent, protease-activated growth factor that has recently been implicated in the development of various types of cancer and kidney disease.

## 2. IDENTIFICATION
## AND CHARACTERIZATION OF PDGF-D

### 2.1. Discovery

Platelet-derived growth factors have a characteristic core domain that encodes a cysteine knot structure also shared by members of the vascular endothelial growth factor (VEGF), transforming growth factor (TGF)-β, and nerve growth factor (NGF) families. Using homology-based searching around core domain nucleotide sequences, three groups published PDGF-D sequences in 2000–2001. From the dbEST database in GenBank (1), Hamada and colleagues identified a molecule with homology to PDGF-C, which they named spinal-cord-derived growth factor-B. Bergsten et al. (2) likewise identified PDGF-D from an expressed sequence tag (EST) database (NCBI) as a gene encoding a molecule with approx 50% homology to PDGF-C. Using a SeqCalling™ database of expressed genes, LaRochelle et al. (3) identified a cDNA with an open reading frame (ORF) that was predicted to encode a new PDGF-D/VEGF family member based on sequence homology. A fourth group also published the PDGF-D sequence identified in an EST from the human iris; however, the group named the molecule iris-expressed growth factor (IRIS) (4).

### 2.2. Structural Comparison to Other PDGFs

Platelet-derived growth factors are structurally characterized by a core domain known as a cysteine knot. PDGF-D is expressed as a polypeptide of 370 amino acids, with a 22-amino-acid signal peptide and a mature secreted protein of 348 amino acids. PDGF-D, like PDGF-C, has a large CUB domain (Complement subcomponents C1r/Cls, Urchin EGF-like protein, and Bone morphogenic protein-1) not observed in PDGF-A and PDGF-B. The role of the CUB domain in PDGF-D appears to constrain the growth factor in a latent state, as proteolytic cleavage of the CUB domain is required for PDGF-D to activate its receptor (2,3). The CUB domain is linked to the core domain by an interdomain region, which except for a dibasic cleavage site has no recognized structural homology. The core domains of the PDGF-A and PDGF-B chains form both homodimers and heterodimers (referred to as PDGF-AA, PDGF-BB, and PDGF-AB). PDGF-D, like PDGF-C, has, to date, only been shown to form homodimers (referred to as PDGF-DD and PDGF-CC) and is expressed as a molecule of approx 84 kDa in its native state. Protease cleavage results in a 35-kDa dimer of core PDGF-D domains (approx 20-kDa monomer under reducing conditions) that is able to bind and activate PDGF receptors. Li and Eriksson (5) have proposed a model where a hemidimer forms from limited proteolysis and removal of one CUB domain, allowing receptor binding but not activation and leading to potential antagonist activity. The ability of PDGF-D to exist in various states of activation allows for both spatial and temporal control of the growth factor activity. Cellular and tissue co-expression of proteases provide control over growth factor activity beyond that which simple variation of PDGF-D expression would otherwise allow.

## 2.3. Genomic Organization

Human *PDGF* genes have somewhat similar structures with either six or seven exons. There are some minor differences reflecting the lack of CUB domains in *PDGFA* and *PDGFB*. The *PDGFD* gene is encoded by seven exons; exon 1 encodes the signal peptide, exons 2 and 3 encodes the CUB domain, the interdomain region is encoded by exons 4 and 5, and exons 6 and 7 encode the core growth factor domain *(6)*. Each *PDGF* gene is situated on a different chromosome, with *PDGFA* found on chromosome 7p22, *PDGFB* found on chromosome 22q12, *PDGFC* found on chromosome 4q32, and *PDGFD* found on chromosome 11q22-23. Although similar in structure, the introns of *PDGFC* and *PDGFD* genes are much larger (approx 10-fold) than those of *PDGFA* and *PDGFB*, spanning approx 200 kb of genomic DNA.

## 2.4. PDGF Receptor Binding, Activation, and Function

### 2.4.1. PDGF-D BINDS TO THE β PDGFR

Platelet-derived growth factors exert a biological effect on cells via binding to and activation of the PDGF receptors α PDGFR and β PDGFR. The signal transducing molecules consist of an extracellular region composed of five Ig-like domains and an intracellular region that contains a split tyrosine kinase domain (reviewed in ref. *7*). The structure of the receptors is similar to other growth factor receptor molecules, including colony-stimulating factor-1 receptor and stem cell factor receptor. α PDGFR and β PDGFR signal via dimerization upon ligand binding; either homodimerization (α–α, β–β) or heterodimerization (α–β) leading to a signaling cascade, the sequelea of which are receptor autophosphorylation and subsequent docking of SH2 domains of various kinases, phosphatases, and adapter proteins.

PDGF-AA is able to activate αα PDGFR homodimers; PDGF-AB activates αα PDGFR homodimers and αβ PDGFR heterodimers. PDGF-BB activates all combinations (αα, αβ, and ββ) of receptor dimers. PDGF-DD competed with PDGF-BB binding to β PDGFR and induced β-receptor phosphorylation in HR5βR cells *(3)*. PDGF-DD was shown to have no effect on the phosphorylation of the α-receptor and was unable to compete with binding of PDGF-AA to α PDGFR-transfected 32D cells *(3)*. Bergsten et al. *(2)* likewise showed that PDGF-DD bound to and activated β PDGFR but not α PDGFR on PAE cells. PDGF-DD phosphorylation of, but not binding to, the α PDGFR in CCD1070 cells was demonstrated by LaRochelle et al. *(3)*, who subsequently showed that α-receptor phosphorylation was the result of ligand-induced heterodimer formation with the β-receptor. In conclusion, PDGF-DD preferentially binds to and activates the β PDGFR homodimer, but might also signal to a lesser extent through PDGFR heterodimers.

### 2.4.2. FUNCTION

The functional consequences of PDGF-DD-binding β-receptor expressing cells include induction of cellular proliferation *(2,3,6)* and transformation of NIH-3T3 cells *(8,9)*. Like *PDGFB*, transfection of NIH-3T3 cells with *PDGFD* induced the loss of normal stress fibers and cells displayed a circular actin structure *(8)*. It is assumed that PDGF-D is able to induce other functions mediated by stimulation of the β-receptor, such as stimulation of $Ca^{2+}$ mobilization and inhibition of apoptosis; however, these have yet to be demonstrated. Ustach et al. have recently shown that PDGF-D enhances both cell motility and induces migration in LNCaP cells *(10)*.

### 2.4.3. Two Ligands for β PDGFR

What is the biological significance of having two β PDGFR ligands? First, the specificity of the molecules for the two PDGF receptors is different. The ability of the PDGF-B chain and the inability of the PDGF-D chain to form both homodimers and heterodimers, along with the ability of PDGF-B chain to bind and activate α PDGFR leads to different receptor activation profiles. Second, differential regulation of β-receptor activation might also be mediated by differential affinities of each of the dimers for receptor binding. It is conceivable that PDGF-BB and PDGF-DD ligation of β PDGFR could result in combinatorial signaling outcomes if the binding affinity for receptor differed significantly between PDGF dimers. At present, the differences in signal transduction between PDGF-BB and PDGF-DD have not been elucidated at a biochemical level. Although studies in NIH-3T3 fibroblasts showed that PDGF-BB had a lower $EC_{50}$ for induction of cell proliferation than PDGF-DD *(3)*, recent data from Hudkins et al. *(11)* found little difference on the ability of PDGF-BB and PDGF-DD to stimulate mesangial cell proliferation in vitro. However, when PDGF-BB and PDGF-DD were expressed in C57BL/6 mice by administration of adenoviral (Ad) constructs, the Ad-PDGF-D mice showed a more severe nephritic phenotype than the Ad-PDGF-B mice. The authors suggested that the resulting differences in nephritis severity were the result of biological effects of the PDGF chains rather than the differences in protein expression from the Ad constructs. Further comparative analysis of the signal transduction cascade and subsequent transcriptional activation mediated by each PDGF in vivo is merited to fully explain these data.

Finally, the presence of a protease activation domain on PDGF-D chain might also regulate receptor binding and activation. Control of the biological function of PDGF-D might be mediated by appropriate protease expression and activity in the vicinity of the expressed PDGF-D chain. As protease cleavage is not required for PDGF-B activity, the presence of the CUB domain on PDGF-D might play a key role in differentiating the function and target cell specificity of the two β PDGFR ligands.

## 2.5. Expression of PDGFD

Expression of *PDGFD* transcripts and PDGF-D protein has been studied in various normal and diseased tissues. Using real-time quantitative polymerase chain reaction (RTQ-PCR) analysis, the *PDGFD* gene was shown to be expressed at relatively high levels in the adrenal gland *(3)*. Lower levels were shown in the pancreas, adipose tissue, salivary gland, pituitary gland, mammary gland, ovary, testis, and pancreas. Northern blot analysis showed highest expression in the ovary, heart, and pancreas and also demonstrated expression in the placenta, liver, small intestine, and kidney but revealed little to no expression in brain or skeletal muscle *(2)*. Message was also detected in human umbilical vein endothelial cells (HUVEC) and human microvascular endothelial cells (HMVEC) cells *(6)*, as well as adult motor neurons *(1)*. Bleomycin induces a fibrotic injury to mouse and human lungs. On examination of mRNA levels by Northern analysis, lungs from mice treated with bleomycin demonstrated a decline in *PDGFD* levels upon treatment, whereas *PDGFC* was increased, and *PDGFA* and *PDGFB* chain genes did not significantly fluctuate *(12)*. The differences in the patterns of expression of the PDGF genes whose products bind equivalent receptors hint at nonredundant biological roles for the various PDGF chains.

## 3. PDGF-D IN NEOPLASIA

Platelet-derived growth factors play a major role in cell–cell communication in normal development and also during pathogenesis. Studies during the past two decades have clearly indicated the significance of PDGF in human tumors, including glioma *(13,14)*, dermatofibrosarcoma *(15,16)*, neurofibroma *(17)*, myelomonocytic leukemia *(18)*, osteoblastoma, and osteosarcoma *(19)*. The transforming ability of *PDGFA* and *PDGFB* and subsequent tumor formation in mouse xenograft models has been thoroughly characterized. PDGFs exert biological effects on cells via binding to and activation of the PDGF receptors α PDGFR and β PDGFR. Given that PDGF-D protein is a ligand for β PDGFR, some attention has been paid to the role of *PDGFD* in the transformation and tumor formation process.

### 3.1. PDGFD Chromosomal Localization and Cancer

*PDGFD* maps near to a human chromosomal locus (11q23-24) of recognized genomic instability *(9)*. This region also encodes matrix metalloproteinases *(20)* and shows gene copy-number variations in some diseases (e.g., Jacobsen's syndrome, various cancers) that are related to the expression of aberrant growth factors *(9,20,21)*. Of particular interest is the amplification about this locus in glioblastoma multiforme *(22)* and childhood medulloblastoma *(23)*. Amplifications or deletions in the region of chromosome 11q23-24 have also been implicated in lung cancer *(24)*, ovarian cancer *(25)*, and primary sarcomas *(26)*. Considering the role of *PDGFA* and *PDGFB* in malignancy *(20,27)*, it is possible that inappropriate expression of *PDGFD* might contribute to cancers associated with chromosome 11q23-24 abnormalities.

### 3.2. PDGFD, PDGFRα, and β PDGFR
### Transcript Expression in Human Cancer Cell Lines

The mRNA expression profile of *PDGFD* in cell lines derived from cancers of multiple origins using real-time quantitative RTQ-PCR has been reported *(9)*. The primer/probe set utilized was designed to be *PDGFD*-specific and, as such, did not detect other known PDGF family members. *PDGFD* was most highly expressed in lung cancer cell lines such as NCI H596, SW900, HOP62, A549, and NCI-UMC-1. Moderate levels of *PDGFD* were found in ovarian (RL95-2), renal (Caki-2), and in several central nervous system (CNS)-derived astrocytoma/glioblastoma and neuroblastoma cell lines such as U251, SNB-19, SNB-75, SK-N-AS, and SW1783. *PDGFD* was also expressed to a lesser extent in most melanoma cell lines and it was detected in only 2 of 17 colon carcinoma cell lines tested. Autocrine signaling was suggested for 6 of 11 astrocytoma/glioblastoma cell lines and 2 of 4 medulloblastoma/neuroblastoma cell lines, ovarian carcinoma cells (OVCAR-8), and lung cancer cells (HOP62) based on coexpression of *PDGFD* mRNA with *PDGFR* transcripts. A similar observation was made by Lokker et al. *(20)*, who showed that *PDGFD* was widely expressed in almost all of the human glioblastoma cell lines and primary glioblastoma multiforme tissues studied. In comparison, normal brain tissue showed little expression of *PDGFD*. Coexpression of *PDGFD* as well as α*PDGFR* and β*PDGFR* was observed in the majority of other cancer cell lines tested.

### 3.3. Immunohistochemical Analysis of PDGF-D in Cancer

The elevated level of *PDGFD* in certain cancer cell lines suggested that PDGF-D might be expressed in human tumor tissues. The expression of PDGF-D protein was examined in human cancers by immunohistochemical analysis using an anti-PDGF-D mAb that specifically recognized PDGF-D (not PDGF-A, PDGF-B, or PDGF-C) *(9)*. The PDGF-D mAb positively stained lung tumor tissues but not normal lung tissues. Staining of ovarian tumor tissue revealed increased PDGF-D staining of tumor cells and surrounding stroma. Ovary and lung tissues, both normal and tumor, were uniformly negative when stained with the control mAb. These data confirmed and extended the observations that *PDGFD* transcripts were expressed in certain tumors, strengthening the hypothesis that PDGF-D has a role in tumorigenesis.

### 3.4. Cancer Patient Serum PDGF-D

PDGF-D was quantitated in serum of patients with various types of malignancy *(9)*. The mean PDGF-D concentration was significantly elevated in sera from patients with medulloblastoma, and astrocytoma, as well as ovarian, lung, bladder, renal, and breast cancers (exceeding 10 ng/mL in most cancer patients compared to less than 4 ng/mL in most normal volunteers). In some ovarian cancer and medulloblastoma patients, serum concentrations exceeding 40 ng/mL were detected, however, PDGF-D levels were below detection (< 4 ng/mL) in sera from patients with lymphoma and myeloma. These data demonstrate that PDGF-D was elevated in the sera of patients with certain malignancies and might be a potential biomarker of certain diseases.

### 3.5. PDGFR Signaling and Tumorigenesis

Signaling through the PDGF-D : β PDGFR complex might occur in a paracrine, juxtacrine, or autocrine manner depending on the coexpression of PDGF-D and β PDGFR on cancer cells. Autocrine PDGF expression induces PDGFR autophosphorylation on tyrosine residues, which creates the sites for physical interactions, with a number of proteins activating intracellular signaling pathways that are critical for oncogenic transformation, including cell proliferation and survival. β PDGFR tyrosine phosphorylation was observed in neuroblastoma-derived cells (T98G) and to a lesser extent in SK-N-AS cells by antiphosphotyrosine immunoblots of cell lysates immunoprecipitated with a β PDGFR-specific antibody *(9)*. Autophosphorylation of human glioma cell lines (A172, U87, U251) and a rat glioma cell line (C6) was also reported *(9,20)*. Recently, Ustach et al. *(10)* reported that prostate carcinoma cells (LNCaP) autoactivated latent PDGF-D into the active PDGF domain, which can induce phosphorylation of β PDGFR and stimulate LNCaP cell proliferation in an autocrine manner. The authors also suggest that PDGF-D expressed by the tumor cells could function in a paracrine manner by enhancing the cell motility of surrounding fibroblasts. PDGF-D could therefore function as both an autocrine and a paracrine factor for tumor progression.

### 3.6. PDGFD Induces Morphological Transformation In Vitro and Tumor Formation In Vivo

Various groups have examined the tumorigenic potential of *PDGFB*. Lokker et al. *(20)* have reported that NIH-3T3 cells stably transfected with *PDGFB* readily form solid tumors when injected subcutaneously into nude mice, and the growth of the tumor could be inhibited by a small molecule piperazinyl quinazoline kinase inhibitor (CT52923) that is highly selective for PDGFR and c-kit. To determine if ectopic *PDGFD* expression induced cell transformation, NIH-3T3 transfectants were generated by various groups *(8,9)*. pMT-*PDGFD* was engineered to express the proteolytically processed and thus activated PDGF-D p35. NIH-3T3-*PDGFD* transfectants exhibited foci of morphologically transformed cells characterized by a dense, disorganized pattern of growth, comprised of individual cells found to be spindly in shape with increased refractility, whereas NIH-3T3 cells transfected with control pMT vector retained a normal morphology. Furthermore, potent β PDGFR tyrosine phosphorylation was detected in NIH-3T3-*PDGFD* transfectants. Li et al. *(8)* also reported that PDGF-D is a potent transforming growth factor for NIH-3T3 cells, causing increased cell proliferation and anchorage independent growth in soft agar. Ustach et al. *(10)* studied the potential oncogenic activity of *PDGFD* in prostate cancer. *PDGFD*-transfected human prostate carcinoma cells (LNCaP-PDGF-D) were generated and a comparative study of cell proliferation in culture with control cells (LNCaP-neo) was executed. During the first 24 h of cultures, neither LNCaP-neo nor LNCaP-PDGF-D significantly increased in cell numbers. However, dramatic differences in cell numbers between LNCaP-neo and LNCaP-PDGF-D were observed after 48 h. Whereas LNCaP-neo cells barely doubled, LNCaP-PDGF-D exhibited a threefold to fourfold increase in cell number after 48 h, demonstrating that PDGF-D expression in prostate cancer cells had growth promoting activity through autocrine stimulation.

The tumorigenicity of NIH-3T3-*PDGFD* cells was also examined by various groups with subcutaneous implantation of the cells in severe combined immunodeficient (SCID) mice *(8,9)*. All of the animals injected with *PDGFD*-transfected cells possessed rapidly growing tumors, whereas none of the animals injected with control cells had tumors. The tumorigenicity of NIH-3T3-*PDGFD* cells was evident with a mean tumor size approaching 2500 mm$^3$ on d 25. Examination of lung and other tissues detected no metastases. The ability of NIH-3T3-*PDGFD* cells to induce tumors in nude mice and upregulate vascular endothelial growth factor (VEGF) was also reported by Li et al. *(8)*.

Using LNCaP-PDGF-D cells, Ustach et al. *(10)* reported that PDGF-D accelerated the early onset of prostate tumor growth in SCID mice and stimulated prostate carcinoma cell interaction with stromal cells. Histological examination of LNCaP-neo tumors revealed a solid tumor mass that is well capsulated from mouse stromal tissue. In contrast, a LNCaP-PDGF-D tumor showed a close interaction with the mouse stromal cells, indicating that PDGF-D facilitated interaction between tumor cells and local mesenchymal cells. The authors hypothesized that PDGF-D might play a role in cancer progression and metastasis. Although no difference was observed between the sizes of LNCaP-PDGF-D and LNCaP-neo tumors in SCID mice, the role of PDGF-D in the metastasis of prostate carcinoma was implicated. These observations clearly demonstrate that PDGF-D has potent growth-stimulating potential in vitro and oncogenic and/or metastasis potential in vivo.

It was previously reported that the proliferative activity of PDGF-D depends on the proteolytic removal of its CUB domain and that the p84 uncleaved ligand did not activate PDGFRs *(3)*. Consistent with these observations, only the p35 active form of PDGF-DD has been shown to cause transformation of NIH-3T3 cells and tumor formation in mice. Thus, PDGF-D transformation and tumorigenesis also depended on the proteolytic removal of the CUB domain. Hence, PDGF-D requires activation by proteases that remain unidentified. Ustach et al. showed that LNCaP cells, in contrast to 293 cells, were able to cleave endogenously expressed PDGF-D in serum-free conditions *(10)*. This observation illustrates the potential for control of PDGF-D function by a posttranslational modification and highlights a potential mechanism whereby tumor cells express both the growth factor and its activating protease to achieve maximal transformation.

The importance of the activation of PDGF-DD was also reported by Furuhashi et al. *(28)*. They have generated PDGF-D-transfected B16 melanoma (B16/PDGF-D) cells that express a low level of β PDGFR. PDGF-DD was secreted from the B16/PDGF-D cells as a latent product and it did not induce receptor phosphorylation. Accordingly, the proliferation of B16/PDGF-D cells in culture was not different from that of the control B16 cells. Contrary to in vitro observation, in vivo in C57Bl6 mice, compared to B16 tumors, B16/PDGF-D tumors grew significantly faster and caspase-3-mediated apoptosis of B16/PDGF-D cells was significantly decreased. The very low levels of β PDGFR expression on B16 melanoma cells and the lack of growth stimulatory effect in vitro of B16/PDGF-D cells indicated the presence of a paracrine factor. The authors have reported a paracrine β PDGFR stimulation of perivascular host cells that was associated with increased tumor growth. Other groups have shown the expression of β PDGFR on tumor vessel pericytes in both experimental tumors and human cancers *(29,30)* and that paracrine PDGF stimulation enhanced tumor growth through recruitment of a vascularized stroma *(31,32)*.

### 3.7. Inhibition of PDGFR for Cancer Therapy

Numerous studies have demonstrated the expression of α PDGFRs and β PDGFRs in glioblastomas. Immunohistochemical analysis showed that approx 80% of prostate tumor tissues express PDGFRs at both primary and metastatic sites *(33)*. Interestingly, β PDGFR staining is more prominent in endothelial cells following exposure to prostate tumor cells that express PDGF *(34)*, suggesting PDGF signaling for prostate cancer progression in a paracrine manner. The PDGFR inhibitor STI 571, in combination with paclitaxel, was shown to substantially reduce prostate cancer bone metastasis in a mouse model *(34)*. PDGF effects on tumor interstitial pressure and drug delivery have also been documented. Whether STI 571 acts through the blockade of the PDGF-D : β PDGFR pathway or another PDGF : PDGFR pathway requires further investigation.

## 4. PDGF-D: KIDNEY DEVELOPMENT AND FUNCTION

A comprehensive analysis of PDGF-D protein expression throughout the body has yet to be published. However, there is a developing body of literature demonstrating the expression of PDGF-D in the developing *(2)* and mature *(35–37)* kidney. The literature has provided a rationale for the examination of PDGF-D antagonists as a therapeutic for various nephropathies.

### 4.1. PDGF-D and Kidney Development

The crucial role for the β PDGFR in kidney development was demonstrated in mice engineered to be genetically deficient for β PDGFR. The β-receptor knockout mice are hemorrhagic, thrombocytopenic, and severely anemic, exhibit a defect in kidney glomeruli because of a lack of mesangial cells, and die at or shortly before birth *(38)*. Interestingly, mice deficient for PDGF-B chain exhibit a similar phenotype, demonstrating that PDGF-B is necessary for normal kidney development. A mouse deficient for PDGF-D has yet to be published, and it would be of considerable interest to determine if PDGF-B and PDGF-

D had overlapping roles in kidney development or if the embryonic lethality of PDGF-B reflects that PDGF-D has no role.

Although there is a lack of functional evidence for role of PDGF-D in kidney development, Bergsten et al. (2) used a polyclonal antibody raised against a peptide representing amino acids 254–272 of PDGF-D to examine in situ PDGF-D protein expression. PDGF-D was shown to be most abundantly expressed in the fibrous capsule surrounding the developing mouse kidney and the adjacent adrenal gland. Staining was also observed in the metanephric mesenchyme in the cortical region of the kidney and in the branching ureter in the medullar region. The authors noted that no PDGF-D staining was observed in the developing nephron, including the ureter buds, glomeruli, and Henle's loops. Contrasting the mouse expression data, the developing human kidney was shown to express PDGF-D in epithelial cells of comma and S-shaped structures of the developing nephron and, in later differentiation, the visceral epithelial cells in the glomerulus (35). Staining was also observed in mesenchymal cells in the interstitium of developing renal pelvis and in fetal smooth muscle cells in arterial vessels. Normal adult kidney PDGF-D staining was observed in visceral epithelial cells, and there was persistent expression in various types of smooth muscle cells (35). Some of the differences in staining between the two studies might indicate a disparity in PDGF-D expression between mouse and human or could reflect potential differences in antibody specificity. The polyclonal antibody used by Chansirikulchai et al. (35) was stated to not bind to the cleaved (activated) PDGF-D protein, whereas the antibody used by Bergsten et al. (2) would be expected to bind both full-length and cleaved (activated) protein.

## 4.2. Role of PDGF-D in Various Nephropathies

### 4.2.1. MESANGIOPROLIFERATIVE DISEASES

β PDGFR has recently been implicated in the pathogenesis of various kidney diseases. Various agents that inhibit β PDGFR signaling either by interfering with ligand binding to the receptor or inhibiting downstream signaling of the receptor have shown activity in various preclinical in vivo models. Perhaps the greatest evidence for a role of β PDGFR agonists in nephritis is seen in mesangioproliferative nephropathies, which include IgA nephritis. IgA nephritis is characterized by a process whereby patients are thought to exhibit a strong response of their IgA system to an antigenic challenge to a pathogen. Recent data point to a role for IgA-hinge region hypoglycosylation in the pathogenesis. It is thought that the hypoglycosylated IgA is preferentially deposited in the glomerular mesangium (39), whereupon it activates complement and a subsequent induction of an inflammatory response and concomitant mesangial cell proliferation and matrix deposition. The mesangium plays a crucial role in glomerular function, and deposition of the extracellular matrix by the mesangial cells results in the diminution of kidney function. Mesangial cells are found in the glomerular mesangium between the capillary endothelial cells and the basal membrane of the glomeruli. They are irregularly shaped cells that might regulate the blood flow through capillary loops. Although the mesangial cells are thought to be a specialized type of pericyte (reviewed in ref. 40), one report suggested that they have a hematopoietic origin (41), a contention not borne out by staining for CD45 (11).

The anti-Thy-1.1 model is a well-characterized rat model of mesangial cell proliferation and has been used to define the potential of therapeutics targeting IgA nephritis. Various iterations of the model have been studied; the major differences are in the time-course of disease mirroring either acute events in the disease process or more chronic models that might reflect persistent human disease. The models are generally characterized by a phenotype consisting of an initial phase of mesangiolysis, followed by mesangial cell immigration, activation and proliferation, extracellular matrix deposition, and macrophage infiltration *(42)*. Like human mesangioproliferative diseases, the glomerular inflammation leads to diminution of kidney function, resulting in albuminuria and increased serum creatinine and blood urea nitrogen (BUN) *(43)*.

### 4.2.2. ANTAGONISM OF β PDGFR SIGNALING

A role for PDGF-B in anti-Thy-1.1-mediated nephritis was demonstrated by studies utilizing a neutralizing anti-PDGF-B mAb or a PDGF-B-specific DNA-aptamer, which likewise binds to and neutralizes PDGF-B *(44)*. Supporting evidence for a role of β PDGFR signaling in the pathologic process has been obtained using STI 571 (also known as imatinib mesylate or Gleevec), a relatively specific kinase inhibitor (inhibits signal transduction by PDGFR, v-Abl, and c-kit) that is able to block the activation of α PDGFR and β PDGFR. Use of STI 571 at 50 mg/kg was able to significantly reduce mesangial cell proliferation, activation of mesangial cells, and deposition of collagen from the mesangial cells *(45)*.

### 4.2.3. PDGF-D AND MESANGIOPROLIFERATIVE DISEASES

The expression of PDGF-D in the kidney has led to specific investigation of PDGF-D as a therapeutic target for nephritis. The evidence for PDGF-D playing a role in various nephritides is expanding. Mesangial cell proliferation, an early event in the pathology of IgA nephritis, is induced upon in vitro and in vivo treatment with PDGF-D *(11,36)*. In vivo treatment of PDGF-D using adenoviral infection of vectors containing the protein coding regions of *PDGFD* leads to proliferation of mesangial cells in the kidney, with the glomeruli becoming enlarged as a result of increased cellularity *(11)*. The effects of the treatment were sustained until at least wk 8, when the experiment was terminated. PDGF-B transduction elicited a similar phenotype; however, the PDGF-D-mediated glomerulopathy was more severe than that mediated by PDGF-B (although it could be argued that much higher concentrations of PDGF-D were noted in these experiments). An interesting feature of this model of glomerulopathy was that PDGF-D induction did not result in elevation of serum creatinine or BUN. The authors did not report the effects of PDGF-D transduction on the development of albuminuria.

Anti-Thy-1.1 treatment of rats increases the expression of PDGF-D determined by both RTQ-PCR analysis and by immunohistochemistry (IHC), where mesangial expression of PDGF-D is noted in kidneys from animals treated with anti-Thy-1.1 (OX-7) but not in control rats. The expression of PDGF-D by mesangial cells is evidence that the factor can act as an autocrine growth factor in the model.

### 4.2.4. ANTAGONISM OF PDGF-D AMELIORATES ANTI-THY-1.1-MEDIATED NEPHRITIS

Final proof of a role for PDGF-D in the acute anti-Thy-1.1-treated rat model was obtained in treatment studies using CR002, a neutralizing fully human monoclonal antibody specific for PDGF-D. CR002 treatment of rats significantly reduced mesangial cell proliferation, activation of mesangial cells, deposition of extracellular matrix (ECM) proteins, and monocyte/macrophage infiltration in glomeruli *(36)*.

### 4.2.5. OTHER NEPHROPATHIES

Along with a potential role in IgA nephritis, other nephropathies might also be amenable to anti-PDGF-D therapies based on the expression of protein. Taneda et al. *(37)* reported that PDGF-D was produced *de novo* in interstitial cells in areas of tubulofibrosis in mice with unilateral ureteral obstruction (UUO) as compared to staining of mesangial cells and vascular smooth muscle cells in normal mice. The staining in mice was correlated to humans with chronic obstructive nephropathy, with good agreement in the localization of PDGF-D staining. Chronic allograft rejection in rats is prevented by treatment with STI 571 *(46)*, suggesting that a PDGFR ligand has a pathogenic role in the progressive loss of kidney function. Evidence for a role of PDGF-D in this process has yet to be published, but it might provide yet another venue for therapeutic antagonism of PDGF-D.

## 5. CONCLUSIONS

PDGF-D, a recently identified agonist of β PDGFR, has the potential to be involved in the growth of both normal and cancerous cells. The expression of PDGF-D in prostate, ovarian, lung, and brain cancers has been recently documented, and interfering with the PDGF-D : β PDGFR signaling pathway might have therapeutic benefit for cancer.

In addition, inhibiting the agonist activity of PDGF-D using mAb or PDGFR receptor signal transduction inhibitors has the potential for therapeutic utility in nephritides, where PDGF-D is upregulated, or in tumor cells that show aberrant PDGF-D expression. Inhibition of PDGF-D in key nephritis animal models has demonstrated the proof of concept, but further work will be required to translate these findings into a clinical setting.

## ACKNOWLEDGMENT

The authors thank Dr. Glennda Smithson for comments on the manuscript.

## REFERENCES

1. Hamada T, Ui-Tei K, Miyata Y. A novel gene derived from developing spinal cords, SCDGF, is a unique member of the PDGF/VEGF family. FEBS Lett 2000; 475(2):97–102.·
2. Bergsten E, Uutela M, Li X, et al. PDGF-D is a specific, protease-activated ligand for the PDGF beta-receptor. Nature Cell Biol 2001; 3(5):512–516.
3. LaRochelle WJ, Jeffers M, McDonald WF, et al. PDGF-D, a new protease-activated growth factor. Nature Cell Biol 2001; 3(5):517–521.
4. Wistow G, Bernstein SL, Ray S, et al. Expressed sequence tag analysis of adult human iris for the NEIBank Project: steroid-response factors and similarities with retinal pigment epithelium. Mol Vis 2002; 8:185–195.
5. Li X, Eriksson U. Novel PDGF family members: PDGF-C and PDGF-D. Cytokine Growth Factor Rev 2003; 14(2):91–98.
6. Uutela M, Lauren J, Bergsten E, et al. Chromosomal location, exon structure, and vascular expression patterns of the human PDGFC and PDGFC genes. Circulation 2001; 103(18):2242–2247.
7. Heldin CH, Westermark B. Mechanism of action and in vivo role of platelet-derived growth factor. Physiol Rev 1999; 79(4):1283–1316.
8. Li H, Fredriksson L, Li X, Eriksson U. PDGF-D is a potent transforming and angiogenic growth factor. Oncogene 2003; 22(10):1501–1510.
9. LaRochelle WJ, Jeffers M, Corvalan JR, et al. Platelet-derived growth factor D: tumorigenicity in mice and dysregulated expression in human cancer. Cancer Res 2002; 62(9):2468–2473.
10. Ustach CV, Taube ME, Hurst NJ Jr, et al. A potential oncogenic activity of platelet-derived growth factor d in prostate cancer progression. Cancer Res 2004; 64(5):1722–1729.
11. Hudkins KL, Gilbertson DG, Carling M, et al. Exogenous PDGF-D is a potent mesangial cell mitogen and causes a severe mesangial proliferative glomerulopathy. J Am Soc Nephrol 2004; 15(2):286–298.
12. Zhuo Y, Zhang J, Laboy M, Lasky JA. Modulation of PDGF-C and PDGF-D expression during bleomycin-induced lung fibrosis. Am J Physiol Lung Cell Mol Physiol 2004; 286(1):L182–L188.

13. Hermanson M, Funa K, Koopmann J, et al. Association of loss of heterozygosity on chromosome 17p with high platelet-derived growth factor alpha receptor expression in human malignant gliomas. Cancer Res 1996; 56(1):164–171.

14. Westermark B, Heldin CH, Nister M. Platelet-derived growth factor in human glioma. Glia 1995; 15(3): 257–263.

15. Shimizu A, O'Brien KP, Sjoblom T, et al. The dermatofibrosarcoma protuberans-associated collagen type Ialpha1/platelet-derived growth factor (PDGF) B-chain fusion gene generates a transforming protein that is processed to functional PDGF-BB. Cancer Res 1999; 59(15):3719–3723.

16. Greco A, Roccato E, Miranda C, Cleris L, Formelli F, Pierotti MA. Growth-inhibitory effect of STI571 on cells transformed by the COL1A1/PDGFB rearrangement. Int J Cancer 2001; 92(3):354–360.

17. Kadono T, Kikuchi K, Nakagawa H, Tamaki K. Expressions of various growth factors and their receptors in tissues from neurofibroma. Dermatology 2000; 201(1):10–14.

18. Golub TR, Barker GF, Lovett M, Gilliland DG. Fusion of PDGF receptor beta to a novel ets-like gene, tel, in chronic myelomonocytic leukemia with t(5;12) chromosomal translocation. Cell 1994; 77(2):307–316.

19. Sulzbacher I, Traxler M, Mosberger I, Lang S, Chott A. Platelet-derived growth factor-AA and -alpha receptor expression suggests an autocrine and/or paracrine loop in osteosarcoma. Mod Pathol 2000; 13(6): 632–637.

20. Lokker NA, Sullivan CM, Hollenbach SJ, Israel MA, Giese NA. Platelet-derived growth factor (PDGF) autocrine signaling regulates survival and mitogenic pathways in glioblastoma cells: evidence that the novel PDGF-C and PDGF-D ligands may play a role in the development of brain tumors. Cancer Res 2002; 62(13):3729–3735.

21. Kurahashi H, Shaikh TH, Hu P, Roe BA, Emanuel BS, Budarf ML. Regions of genomic instability on 22q11 and 11q23 as the etiology for the recurrent constitutional t(11;22). Hum Mol Genet 2000; 9(11): 1665–1670.

22. Weber RG, Sommer C, Albert FK, Kiessling M, Cremer T. Clinically distinct subgroups of glioblastoma multiforme studied by comparative genomic hybridization. Lab Invest 1996; 74(1):108–119.

23. Reardon DA, Michalkiewicz E, Boyett JM, et al. Extensive genomic abnormalities in childhood medulloblastoma by comparative genomic hybridization. Cancer Res 1997; 57(18):4042–4047.

24. Tarkkanen M, Huuhtanen R, Virolainen M, et al. Comparison of genetic changes in primary sarcomas and their pulmonary metastases. Genes Chromosomes Cancer 1999; 25(4):323–331.

25. Foulkes WD, Campbell IG, Stamp GW, Trowsdale J. Loss of heterozygosity and amplification on chromosome 11q in human ovarian cancer. Br J Cancer 1993; 67(2):268–273.

26. Robbins KC, Devare SG, Reddy EP, Aaronson SA. In vivo identification of the transforming gene product of simian sarcoma virus. Science 1982; 218(4577):1131–1133.

27. Fleming TP, Matsui T, Heidaran MA, Molloy CJ, Artrip J, Aaronson SA. Demonstration of an activated platelet-derived growth factor autocrine pathway and its role in human tumor cell proliferation in vitro. Oncogene 1992; 7(7):1355–1359.

28. Furuhashi M, Sjoblom T, Abramsson A, et al. Platelet-derived growth factor production by B16 melanoma cells leads to increased pericyte abundance in tumors and an associated increase in tumor growth rate. Cancer Res 2004; 64(8):2725–2733.

29. Sundberg C, Ljungstrom M, Lindmark G, Gerdin B, Rubin K. Microvascular pericytes express platelet-derived growth factor-beta receptors in human healing wounds and colorectal adenocarcinoma. Am J Pathol 1993; 143(5):1377–1388.

30. Abramsson A, Berlin O, Papayan H, Paulin D, Shani M, Betsholtz C. Analysis of mural cell recruitment to tumor vessels. Circulation 2002; 105(1):112–117.

31. Forsberg K, Valyi-Nagy I, Heldin CH, Herlyn M, Westermark B. Platelet-derived growth factor (PDGF) in oncogenesis: development of a vascular connective tissue stroma in xenotransplanted human melanoma producing PDGF-BB. Proc Natl Acad Sci USA 1993; 90(2):393–397.

32. Skobe M, Fusenig NE. Tumorigenic conversion of immortal human keratinocytes through stromal cell activation. Proc Natl Acad Sci USA 1998; 95(3):1050–1055.

33. Ko YJ, Small EJ, Kabbinavar F, et al. A multi-institutional phase ii study of SU101, a platelet-derived growth factor receptor inhibitor, for patients with hormone-refractory prostate cancer. Clin Cancer Res 2001; 7(4):800–805.

34. Uehara H, Kim SJ, Karashima T, et al. Effects of blocking platelet-derived growth factor-receptor signaling in a mouse model of experimental prostate cancer bone metastases. J Natl Cancer Inst 2003; 95(6): 458–470.

35. Changsirikulchai S, Hudkins KL, Goodpaster TA, et al. Platelet-derived growth factor-D expression in developing and mature human kidneys. Kidney Int 2002; 62(6):2043–2054.

36. Ostendorf T, van Roeyen CR, Peterson JD, et al. A fully human monoclonal antibody (CR002) identifies PDGF-D as a novel mediator of mesangioproliferative glomerulonephritis. J Am Soc Nephrol 2003; 14(9):2237–2247.

37. Taneda S, Hudkins KL, Topouzis S, et al. Obstructive uropathy in mice and humans: potential role for PDGF-D in the progression of tubulointerstitial injury. J Am Soc Nephrol 2003; 14(10):2544–2555.

38. Soriano P. Abnormal kidney development and hematological disorders in PDGF beta-receptor mutant mice. Genes Dev 1994; 8(16):1888–1896.

39. Allen AC, Bailey EM, Brenchley PE, Buck KS, Barratt J, Feehally J. Mesangial IgA1 in IgA nephropathy exhibits aberrant O-glycosylation: observations in three patients. Kidney Int 2001; 60(3):969–973.

40. Lindahl P, Hellstrom M, Kalen M, et al. Paracrine PDGF-B/PDGF-Rbeta signaling controls mesangial cell development in kidney glomeruli. Development 1998; 125(17):3313–3322.

41. Masuya M, Drake CJ, Fleming PA, et al. Hematopoietic origin of glomerular mesangial cells. Blood 2003; 101(6):2215–2218.

42. Jefferson JA, Johnson RJ. Experimental mesangial proliferative glomerulonephritis (the anti-Thy-1.1 model). J Nephrol 1999; 12(5):297–307.

43. Cheng QL, Orikasa M, Morioka T, et al. Progressive renal lesions induced by administration of monoclonal antibody 1-22-3 to unilaterally nephrectomized rats. Clin Exp Immunol 1995; 102(1):181–185.

44. Floege J, Ostendorf T, Janssen U, et al. Novel approach to specific growth factor inhibition in vivo: antagonism of platelet-derived growth factor in glomerulonephritis by aptamers. Am J Pathol 1999; 154 (1):169–179.

45. Gilbert RE, Kelly DJ, McKay T, et al. PDGF signal transduction inhibition ameliorates experimental mesangial proliferative glomerulonephritis. Kidney Int 2001; 59(4):1324–1332.

46. Savikko J, Taskinen E, Von Willebrand E. Chronic allograft nephropathy is prevented by inhibition of platelet-derived growth factor receptor: tyrosine kinase inhibitors as a potential therapy. Transplantation 2003; 75(8):1147–1153.

# V   CANCER PROGNOSTICS, DIAGNOSTICS, AND BIOMARKERS

# 22 Cancer Pharmacogenomics

## Predicting Drug Response in the Genomic Era

*Brian Z. Ring, PhD*
*and Huijun Z. Ring, PhD*

### CONTENTS

### SUMMARY

Expectations are high that pharmacogenomics, the use of a patient's genetic information to predict response to treatment, will be able to intelligently guide the discovery and development of novel successful pharmaceuticals. Cancer poses a unique challenge in this regard because the multistep carcinogenesis process compounds the diversity already present in the human population. Both inherited and acquired genetic variations in the cancer host and tumor genomes contribute to treatment and clinical outcomes. The negative clinical phenotypes associated with these polymorphisms can be grouped in three broad categories: increased toxicity, poor drug response, and high tumor aggressiveness. By characterizing the molecular mechanisms underlying treatment response to existing drugs, pharmacogenomics can suggest novel targets in key pathways for future development. Achieving a better understanding of the pharmacogenomic determinants of anticancer agents will thus aid both oncologists in serving their patients and pharmaceutical scientists in developing novel therapies to target currently unmet patient needs.

**Key Words:** Pharmacogenomics; cancer; chemoresistance; drug response; toxicity; polymorphism.

From: *Cancer Drug Discovery and Development: The Oncogenomics Handbook*
Edited by: W. J. LaRochelle and R. A. Shimkets © Humana Press Inc., Totowa, NJ

# 1. INTRODUCTION

Modern pharmacology's goals are the right drug at the right dose for the right patient—goals more easily stated than achieved. To aid meeting these goals, the relatively new field of pharmacogenomics, drawing on data amassed in the Human Genome Project and clinical studies, assesses patients' genetic makeup to predict their responses to treatment. Pharmacogenomics seeks to enhance both drug discovery and drug use, particularly in the treatment of cancer. Achieving these goals is of keen interest not only to the pharmaceutical industry but also to oncologists and, ultimately, the patient.

Pharmacogenomics is usually defined as the use of a patient's genetic information to predict response to treatment. Hopes are high that our growing knowledge of the human genome will provide an intelligent and efficient guide to the development of novel and successful pharmaceuticals. Efficacy rates of 15–20% among the target population are now usually considered sufficient for Food and Drug Administration (FDA) approval of a novel drug. Pharmacogenomics' promise is that treatment plans and novel drugs might one day be designed for individuals by adapting them to each patient's genetic makeup. A better understanding of the determinants of a patient's drug processing should allow for decreased toxicity, increased success in the prescription of effective drugs, more effective dosage, and increased ability to monitor patient progress. As the physician Sir William Osler summarized the problem appropriately in 1892: "If it were not for the great variability among individuals, medicine might as well be a science and not an art."

## 1.1. Pharmacogenomics' Beginnings

Evidence that a genetic basis underlies some of the variability in drug response dates to the 1950s. Some, however, date the birth of pharmacogenomics to the 6th century BC, given speculation that Pythagoras' injunction, *kyamon apechete* (abstain from beans), was the result of his recognition of the dangers for some individuals of ingesting fava beans—a relatively common deficiency in some Eastern Mediterranean populations of glucose-6-phosphate dehydrogenase is associated with an acute anemic response upon exposure to fava beans. The modern field of pharmacogenomics began more recently with the identification of polymorphisms in a number of genes involved with drug metabolism. For example, inherited defects of the cytochrome P450 enzyme CYP2D6 are linked to the differential metabolism of a large number of commonly used drugs (1). The associations between DNA polymorphisms and drug response have been demonstrated to have significant interethnic variability, as well as large interindividual differences. The recognition of the importance of these genetic determinants in drug response and the development of tools for discovering and measuring those determinants have prompted the rapid rise of pharmacogenomics as a critical aspect of drug development.

A major effort in preclinical and clinical drug development involves characterizing a chemical entity's metabolism and disposition in studies that are often collectively referred to as absorption, distribution, metabolism, and excretion (ADME). These four fundamental pathways of drug movement and modification in the body control the onset of drug action, the magnitude of pharmacological and toxicological response, and the duration of the drug's activity. ADME genes encode for drug-metabolizing enzymes, drug transporters, and drug regulators. Polymorphisms in the ADME genes can greatly influence the efficacy and toxicity of drug response.

## 1.2. Pharmacogenomics and Cancer

Cancer poses a unique challenge to the emerging promise of pharmacogenomics. The multistep carcinogenesis process further complicates the effects of the genetic diversity already present in the human population. Amplification and deletion seem to provide a majority of the genetic differences in solid tumors (2–4), with translocations also playing significant roles in hematologic cancers. Consequently, to benefit the cancer patient, pharmacogenomics must entail not only an understanding of the patient's genetic inheritance but also the possible effects of treatment on the genotype of the tumor itself.

Tumor progression occurs in part through the accumulation of genetic abnormalities, including point mutations, deletions, translocations, and amplifications. These changes to the tumor's genotype and phenotype can result in predictable changes in drug response and must be a component of a pharmacogenomic approach to cancer treatment. Furthermore, the tumor develops and responds to treatment in manners unique from other organs or tissues, with factors such as angiogenesis, host immune response, invasion, and metastasis coming into play.

The interplay between the patient host and tumor is another level of complexity that is just beginning to be explored. What is clear is that the contributions of the tumor and host must both be accounted for in predicting the effects of prescribing a certain drug (Fig. 1). Adverse drug responses, which usually involve enzymes localized in the liver, are, by and large, a host response. Drug response can be mediated by both host and tumor; for example, drug detoxification by the host might decrease response, whereas protein present in the tumor might affect drug availability. The aggressiveness of the tumor, which greatly influences the therapeutic regimen the oncologist chooses, is largely tumor-defined.

Although many genes can perturb drug response, the negative clinical phenotypes presented by mutations in ADME genes and other pharmacologically important genes are limited to three broad categories: increased toxicity, poor drug response, and high tumor aggressiveness (Table 1). These categories broadly define the ways in which pharmacogenomics will benefit care providers and drug developers and closely match the injunction of Hippocrates, "Declare the past, diagnose the present, foretell the future; practice these acts. As to diseases, make a habit of two things—to help, or at least to do no harm" (5). These distinctions not only have a bearing on the conceptualization of cancer pharmacogenomics but also reflect how pharmacogenomics can aid oncologists serve their patients better and how this field can target novel therapies to currently unmet patient needs. Although it is difficult to provide a complete list of known mutations and relevant genes, the following discussion addresses the genes in each category.

## 2. TOXICITY

The therapeutic window for anticancer agents is often narrow, necessitating that the drug concentration required to produce a therapeutic effect be close to the concentration that results in significant toxicities. Given the toxic effects of these drugs, the potential therapeutic regimen is therefore limited to a certain cumulative dose, and patients are frequently treated at the maximum dose levels that they can tolerate. Following the medical dictum, "Primum non nocere" ("First, do no harm"), is, therefore, difficult in the field of oncology.

Because inherited genetic variations in drug-metabolism genes have been shown to lead to differential treatment outcomes and severe toxicity in various patient subsets, it is here that pharmacogenomics have first been pressed into practice. By identifying and

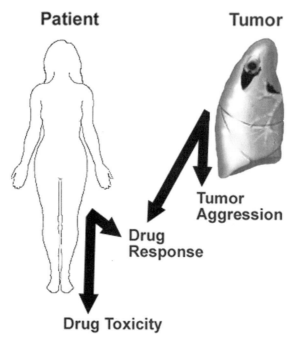

**Fig. 1.** Genetic differences in both the patient host and the tumor contribute to variable responses to therapy and to different clinical outcomes. Effective therapies must encompass prognostic and predictive elements of both the host's (the patient's) and the tumor's genomes. Toxicity is principally a host response involving liver-localized enzymes. The aggressiveness of the tumor is principally tumor-defined. Drug response can be mediated both by involving host detoxification/metabolism and tumor-governed drug availability.

understanding the relationships between genetic variations and adverse drug reactions, it is hoped that patient care with some problematic drugs can be dramatically improved.

### 2.1. 6-Mercaptopurine and Thiopurine Methyltransferase (TPMT)

6-Mercaptopurine (6-MP), is one of the most effective drugs for treating children with acute lymphoblastic leukemia (ALL). 6-MP is a prodrug that needs to be activated to 6-thioguanine nucleotides, which can then be incorporated into DNA to induce the antileukemic effect. The enzyme thiopurine methyltransferase (TPMT) converts 6-MP into inactive metabolites. Interindividual variations in TPMT enzyme activity have been observed clinically: Patients with reduced TPMT enzyme activity convert more of the drug to active thioguanine nucleotides, whereas patients with TPMT deficiency might accumulate toxic levels of metabolites and are at high risk for severe, and sometimes fatal, hematological toxicity if treated with conventional doses (reviewed in ref. 6).

The molecular mechanism for the inherited differences in human TPMT activity has been elucidated, and several inactivating mutations in the human *TPMT* gene have been identified. Specifically, three nonsynonymous single-nucleotide changes account for more than 95% of the clinically relevant *TPMT* mutations, which include *TPMT*2 (238G>C), *TPMT*3A (460G>A and 719A>G), and *TPMT*3C (719A>G). Approximately 10% of the Caucasian and African-American populations is heterozygous for *TPMT*-null mutations, which results in their being partially deficient in TPMT enzyme activity; 0.3% carries two *TPMT* mutant alleles and does not express functional TPMT (7,8).

Table 1
Polymorphic Genes Regulating Anticancer Drug Response

| Gene | Selected Polymorphisms | Drug(s) | Phenotype | Site of Action | Germline or Somatic | Selected References |
|---|---|---|---|---|---|---|
| **Drug Toxicity** | | | | | | |
| TPMT | G238C and A719G | 6-Mercaptopurine | Severe hematological toxicity when treated with conventional doses | Host (liver) | G | 7–9 |
| DPD | Splice site mutation IVS14+1G□→A | 5-Fluorouracil | Neurotoxicity and myelosuppression | Host (liver) | G | 16–18 |
| UGT1A1 | Promoter polymorphism | Irinotecan | Diarrhea and neutropenia | Host (liver) | G | 21,22 |
| **Drug Response** | | | | | | |
| MDR1 | Expression and C3435T polymorphism | Multiple | Possible involvement in the development of resistance to multiple cytotoxic drugs | Tumor, host (site of drug uptake) | G | 24,25 |
| TS | Expression and promoter polymorphism | 5-Fluorouracil | Poor response to 5-FU, although with fewer side effects | Tumor | G | 28,33–35 |
| MTHFR | C677T | Methotrexate and 5-fluorouracil | Methotrexate toxicity and 5-FU treatment response | Host | G | 38–40 |
| BCL2 | Reciprocal translocation t(14;18)(q32:q21); expression polymorphisms | Apoptosis-inducing chemotherapies | Increased resistance to some chemotherapeutics while possibly also slowing tumor growth | Tumor | S | 43–45 |
| **Tumor Aggressiveness** | | | | | | |
| BRCA1/2 | Point mutations; small deletions; small insertions | Apoptosis-inducing chemotherapies | Early-onset breast and ovarian cancer | Tumor | G/S | 54–56 |
| TP53 | Point mutations; insertions; deletions | Anthrocyclines, with possible effects on apoptosis-inducing chemotherapies | Increased susceptability to cancer; increased resistance to some chemotherapeutics | Tumor | S/G | 60,65–67 |
| RAS | Point mutations in codons 12, 13, and 61 | Ionizing radiation | Contribution to oncogenesis and radioresistance | Tumor | S | 70–72,74 |
| ERBB2 | Amplification | Tamoxifen, anthracylines, Herceptin | Resistance to tamoxifen; sensitivity to high doses of anthracylines; sensitivity to Herceptin | Tumor | S | 75–78 |

The *TPMT* genotype is an important determinant of mercaptopurine toxicity and can be used to adjust dosing. In a study of 180 childhood ALL patients treated over 2.5 yr with 6-MP, the cumulative incidence of 6-MP dose reductions resulting from toxicity was highest among patients who were homozygous for mutant *TPMT* (100%), intermediate among heterozygous patients (35%), and lowest among wild-type patients (7%) *(9)*. Clinical experience in TPMT-deficient patients suggests that they should receive 5–10% of the conventional 6-MP dose. After 6-MP dose individualization in TPMT-deficient patients, survival outcomes are similar between deficient and wild-type patients *(9)*, although TPMT deficiency has also been linked to a higher risk of second malignancies, including acute myeloid leukemia and radiation-induced brain tumors *(10–12)*.

## 2.2. 5-Fluorouracil and Dihydropyrimidine Dehydrogenase (DPD)

To treat solid tumors (e.g., breast, colorectal, head and neck cancers), 5-fluorouracil (5-FU), which is an analog of uracil, is widely used. To exert its antitumor activity, as a prodrug 5-FU needs to be converted to 5-fluoro-2-deoxyuridine monophosphate (5FdUMP), a metabolite that inhibits thymidylate synthase in the DNA synthesis pathway. More than 80% of 5-FU is inactivated by dihydropyridimide dehydrogenase (DPD) in the liver. Large interindividual variability in DPD activity has been observed. Patients with low DPD activity cannot efficiently inactivate 5-FU, and they form excessive amounts of active metabolites, which leads to hematopoietic, neurological, and gastrointestinal toxicities that can be life-threatening (reviewed in refs. *13* and *14*).

The human *DPD* gene is genetically polymorphic. About 3% of the population is heterozygous for the *DPD*-null alleles and has intermediate levels of enzyme activity. About 1 in 1000 individuals carries two mutant *DPD* alleles, which results in those individuals' being completely deficient in DPD enzyme activity (reviewed in ref. *14*). So far, at least 20 mutations in the *DPD* genes have been identified in patients suffering from severe toxicity after the administration of 5-FU *(15–18)*; those mutations include a splice site mutation, several missense mutations, and deletions. A G-to-A transition at the 5'-splice consensus sequence of exon 14 (DPD*2A) is the most common, accounting for about 50% of known nonfunctional *DPD* alleles and resulting in the production of a truncated mRNA. *DPD*\*2A has been associated with fatal outcomes in cancer patients, even in heterozygous carriers. In general, 25% of all patients suffering from grade 3–4 toxicity from 5-FU treatment prove to be heterozygous for the *DPD*\*2A allele *(17,18)*. Partial or complete DPD deficiency appears to play an important role in the etiology of 5-FU-associated toxicity.

5-Fluorouracil-related toxicities in patients with decreased levels of DPD activity are often severe. Accordingly, functional assays of DPD enzyme activity or screening for common polymorphisms in this gene in conjunction with 5-FU administration would limit the serious 5-FU-related toxicities associated with this gene. Patients at risk for 5-FU toxicity can be treated with nonfluoropyrimidine compounds. Irinotecan, oxaliplatin, and raltitrexed have been shown to be effective in colorectal cancer, and these agents have been safely used in the treatment of a patient suffering from a partial DPD deficiency *(19)*.

## 2.3. Irinotecan and UDP-Glucuronosyltransferase 1A1

Irinotecan is used to treat solid tumors, such as colon cancer and lung cancer. SN-38 (7-ethyl-10-hydroxycamptothecin), the active metabolite of irinotecan, exerts its antitumor activity by inhibiting topoisomerase I. Glucuronidation is the main detoxification pathway for SN-38, and this conjugation reaction is catalyzed by UDP-glucuronosyltransferase 1A1 (UGT1A1) in the liver.

Several common genetic polymorphisms and more than 60 rare mutations have been described in the *UGT1A1* gene (reviewed in ref. *20*). These polymorphism include a dinucleotide repeat in the atypical TATA-box region $A(TA)_nTAA$ of the *UGT1A1* promoter, with between five and eight repeats found in the general population. The increasing number of repeats is associated with a decrease in the rate of transcription initiation of the *UGT1A1* gene. The "wild-type" allele (*UGT1A1*1*) contains six TA repeats, whereas the most common variant allele (*UGT1A1*28*) contains seven repeats and is associated with Gilbert's syndrome, which is characterized by mild unconjugated hyperbilirubinemia *(21)*.

Many irinotecan-treated patients experience severe dose-limiting diarrhea and neutropenia, which can be life-threatening. Results from clinical studies with irinotecan indicate that SN-38 glucuronidation is a major determinant of irinotecan-induced diarrhea *(22)*. The *UGT1A1* promoter genotype correlates with irinotecan pharmacokinetics and toxicity, and the presence of the $(TA)_7$ repeat allele is a significant risk factor for developing severe irinotecan-induced adverse reactions. Furthermore, a missense C686A mutation in the coding region of the *UGT1A1* gene is also associated with severe toxicity. These findings suggest that individual patients' *UGT1A1* genotype could be used to tailor irinotecan dosage and to select chemotherapeutic agents.

In summary, genetic differences in drug-metabolism genes, such as *TPMT*, *DPD*, and *UGT1A1*, produce variable therapeutic outcomes in cancer chemotherapy. Prospective identification of mutations in patients is needed to avoid toxicity, choose alternative treatment, and improve dose adjustment. Tests to determine *TPMT* genotype status have been incorporated in treatment protocols for childhood ALL at some research hospitals since the early 1990s, and the case for incorporating *DPD* and *UGT1A1* phenotyping or genotyping tests in the clinical practice is also strong.

## 3. DRUG RESPONSE

As oncologists, patients, and drug developers know all too well, there is no guarantee that cancer treatment will be effective in a specific patient. Furthermore, the mutable nature of the tumor could result in changes in drug response during treatment. Genetic variations, both inherited and acquired, in a number of genes have been implicated in differential responses to a variety of cancer drugs. Although such effects are harder to study than toxicity, with clinical studies having to extend over years instead of weeks, much interest has been expressed in this application of pharmacogenomics.

### 3.1. Multidrug Resistance-1 Gene

Cancers treated with multiple anticancer drugs tend to develop or display cross-resistance to many other chemotherapy agents to which they have never been exposed. Several mechanisms contribute to the development of such multidrug resistance, including increased drug efflux from the cell by membrane transporters, activation of drug detoxification enzymes such as glutathione-*S*-transferase, decreased drug uptake into the cell, and defective apoptotic pathways (reviewed in ref. *23*).

Human multidrug resistance-1 (MDR1), also known as P-glycoprotein and ABCB1, is a membrane transporter with 12 transmembrane regions and 2 ATP-binding sites. MDR1 was originally identified as a protein abundantly expressed in multidrug-resistant cancer cells *(24)*. The principal function of the MDR1 protein is as an energy-dependent multi-drug efflux pump that exports substances from inside a cell to the outside. Because many anticancer drugs are substrates of MDR1, the expression and function of the MDR1 protein might alter the therapeutic effectiveness of such agents. Increased expression of this transporter in the presence of chemotherapy has been found to be associated with poor outcomes, and MDR1 has been implicated in the development of simultaneous resistance to multiple cytotoxic drugs in cancer cells (reviewed in ref. *23*). *MDR1* is also expressed in normal tissues, such as in intestine and at the blood–brain barrier, suggesting that MDR1 plays roles in drug uptake after ingestion and excretion of drugs and their metabolites out of the body and that it might also influence the brain's uptake of drugs.

Many genetic polymorphisms have been identified in the *MDR1* gene, and some of them can affect *MDR1* expression and function. For example, the C to T polymorphism at position 3435 of the *MDR1* gene is associated with variable gene expression and a distinct clinical phenotype *(25)*. Individuals who are homozygous for the T allele at position 3435 of the *MDR1* gene have been found to have decreased intestinal expression of P-glycoprotein and increased digoxin $C_{max}$ values, compared with homozygous *MDR1* 3435C individuals [although another study notes that the serum concentration of digoxin is lower in individuals carrying the 3445T allele *(26)*]. Recently, a comprehensive analysis of *MDR1* nucleotide diversity and haplotype structure was carried out, and 48 variant sites were identified in a collection of 247 ethnically diverse DNA samples *(27)*. However, it remains to be determined whether these genetic variations and haplotypes in *MDR1* contribute to the interindividual variability in bioavailability and tissue distribution of MDR1 substrates and whether they are correlated with the efficacy and side effects of the many anticancer drugs that are substrates of MDR1.

### 3.2. Thymidylate Synthase

Thymidylate synthase (TS) is a key enzyme in the *de novo* synthesis of thymidylate (dTMP), which is needed for the synthesis of DNA. TS is an important target for chemotherapy, and inhibition of TS by FdUMP is considered to be the main mechanism for the action of 5-FU *(28)*.

*TS* expression is a key determinant of 5-FU sensitivity. Preclinical studies in cancer cell lines have demonstrated that overexpression of *TS* is linked with 5-FU resistance *(29)*. Clinical studies have shown that lower *TS* mRNA and protein expression in tumors are associated with better response to 5-FU-based therapy *(30)*. Several genetic polymorphisms in the *TS* gene have been identified, and a tandem-repeat polymorphism in the *TS* promoter has been extensively investigated. This promoter polymorphism is associated with *TS* mRNA and protein expression; the presence of the triple tandem repeat (TSER*3) has been shown to increase *TS* expression, compared with the double repeat (TSER*2) *(31,32)*. The TSER polymorphism has been associated with 5-FU treatment outcome in several clinical studies: Individuals who were homozygous for the triple repeat had a poorer treatment outcome than those with other genotypes, although they experienced less severe side effects from the anticancer drug *(33–35)*. Genotyping of *TS* could hold the potential for identifying patients more likely to respond to 5-FU-based chemotherapy.

### *3.3. Methylenetetrahydrofolate Reductase*

Methylenetetrahydrofolate reductase (MTHFR) is a critical enzyme in folate metabolism and is involved in maintaining normal levels of reduced folates and homocysteine. The enzyme resides at a metabolic branch point, directing the folate pool either to DNA synthesis or to homocysteine remethylation. A common SNP (single-nucleotide polymorphism) in the *MTHFR* gene consists of a C to T change at nucleotide 677, which results in an alanine to valine substitution. The allele frequency of the T allele is about 35% in the general North American population. Individuals with homozygous TT or heterozygous CT genotype have reduced MTHFR activity and generally have lower folate levels than those with a CC genotype *(36)*.

The *MTHFR* C667T polymorphism could modulate the therapeutic effects of many antifolate chemotherapy agents, including 5-FU and methotrexate. In a study of colon and breast cancer cell lines, Sohn and colleagues found that the *MTHFR* 667T polymorphism leads to the decreased level of MTHFR enzyme activity and it changes the concentration and distribution of folates in cancer cells. Furthermore, the *MTHFR* 677T mutation was shown to increase the chemosensitivity of colon and breast cancer cells to 5-FU, but to decrease the chemosensitivity of breast cancer cells to methotrexate *(37)*. Several clinical studies have also suggested that patients carrying the *MTHFR* TT genotype could experience increased methotrexate toxicity *(38–40)*. Another study of 43 patients with metastatic colorectal cancer showed that the responders are more likely to carry the 677T allele *(41)*. However, most of these studies had limited sample sizes. Prospective studies in larger patient populations are needed for a better definition of the role of *MTHFR* polymorphism and the patients' response to chemotherapy.

### *3.4. BCL2*

The *BCL2* gene family consists of important regulators of programmed cell death. BCL2 is a mitochondrial membrane protein that regulates apoptosis in conjunction with p53; BCL2 also regulates caspase activation *(42)*. Because the regulation of apoptosis has well-established roles in the oncogenic process and in the activity of many chemotherapeutics, this gene has received much attention. Follicular lymphoma is associated with a reciprocal translocation, t(14;18)(q32;q21), leading to a deregulated expression of the *BCL2* gene and subsequent interference with the normal apoptosis of B-cell lymphocytes *(43,44)*. *BCL2* upregulation has been observed in many solid tumors. From BCL2's role in apoptosis, it is suspected to be a mediator of response for drugs that attack tumor cells by inducing the programmed cell death response. In vivo experiments have also shown an inverse correlation between *BCL2* expression levels and sensitivity to doxorubicin in breast cancer cell lines *(45)*. No clinical role for BCL2 in cancers besides lymphomas has yet been established. Given the large number of BCL2 family members, it might prove difficult to establish a strong relationship between an individual mutation and the efficacy of a drug. Furthermore, some evidence shows that BCL2 might promote chemoresistance while retarding tumor growth *(45)*, further confounding attempts to make associations between BCL2 and predicted outcomes.

## 4. TUMOR AGGRESSION

Because of the narrow therapeutic window proffered by most current chemotherapeutic agents, oncologists must make difficult decisions in formulating treatment plans. The expected outcome for the patient must be balanced against the potential harm associated with the proposed drug regimen. This difficulty is amplified by the inapplicability of surgery and radiation treatment for many cancers, with chemotherapy the only available therapeutic choice. In this regard, tumor or patient characteristics that can help predict outcome play an important part in therapy choice. Pathologists routinely measure a number of prognostic factors, including the presence of metastases and tumor size or histological grade. When such prognosticators are present, the oncologist might decide to treat a case more aggressively (e.g., choosing to include an adjuvant therapy). For example, a patient diagnosed with breast cancer will be assessed pathologically to determine cancer stage. Stage 1 breast cancer is usually treated with breast-conserving surgery, and whether or not adjuvant chemotherapy or more aggressive surgical options are recommended is based on a number of other prognostic factors.

However, although a number of genetic factors are known to correlate with increased cancer-related mortality, few are currently deemed clinically useful. To be of practical utility, a prognostic marker must also be a predictor of outcome with a specific therapy—an association that is more difficult to establish. Nonetheless, some mutations associated with poor outcomes have been shown to indicate specific therapeutic choices as well. Thus, the events that lead to a gene mutation presenting itself as a predictor of mortality can also often point to specific alterations in cell morphology or differentiation that impinge on tumor chemosensitivity. It is reasonable to expect that further progress will be made in defining additional prognostic polymorphisms with clinical applications.

### 4.1. BRCA1 and BRCA2

Hereditary breast cancer accounts for 5–10% of breast cancers. The majority of familial breast cancers are associated with mutations in *BRCA1* or *BRCA2*, and *BRCA1* is mutated in 80% of familial breast and ovarian cancer. These genes are rarely mutated in sporadic breast or ovarian cancers *(46)*. Carriers of mutations in these genes are also at increased risk for prostate and pancreatic cancers, although the risk is lower than for breast cancer *(47)*. BRCA1 and BRCA2 act as a tumor suppressors and negative regulators of mammary epithelial differentiation. The mechanisms through which these genes affect this role are not clear, but the proteins appear to function in the same genetic pathways, yet with distinct functions *(48,49)*. Consistent with these observations, the presentation of cancers in patients harboring mutations in *BRCA1* or *BRCA2* are similar but not identical (reviewed in ref. *50*).

BRCA1/2-related breast cancers have been shown to express a basal epithelial phenotype, a tumor subtype found in less than 15% of breast cancers *(51)*. The basal phenotype, as defined by gene expression patterns, has been associated with poor outcomes in repeated studies of breast cancer patients *(52,53)*. In addition to predicting susceptibility, recent in vivo studies have also shown that BRCA1 functions as a differential mediator of chemotherapy-induced apoptosis, indicating that diagnosis of this mutation might suggest specific appropriate therapies *(54,55)*.

For carriers of *BRCA1/2* mutations, chemoprevention (Tamoxifen, Raloxifen, aromatase inhibitors) or more aggressive surgery for early-stage tumors might be options *(56)*. This might be especially true for patients at exceptional risk for ovarian cancer, which has a much higher fatality rate than does breast cancer. Clinical trials assessing these prophylactic therapies are preliminary, but patients with *BRCA1* vs *BRCA2* mutations have responded differently to Tamoxifen, with women carrying *BRCA2* mutations showing greater benefit from the treatment *(57)*.

## 4.2. TP53

*TP53* is a critical arbitrator of the cellular response to DNA damage and thus ensures genomic stability. Its product, p53, is a DNA-binding protein that acts as a transcription factor. In conjunction with other factors, it regulates cycle senescence induced by DNA damage until repair can be effected, or apoptosis if the damage is too extensive *(58,59)*. Cell death following chemotherapy or DNA damage induced by radiation treatment are largely governed by apoptosis via the p53 pathway *(60)*. The rate of apoptosis is significantly greater in tumors with wild-type *TP53* gene than in those harboring mutations in the gene. Furthermore, mutations in *TP53* have been found in the germline of patients with Li–Fraumeni syndrome, which is characterized by early onset of a variety of tumors *(61, 62)*. *TP53* mutations also arise somatically and are often associated with aggressive tumors *(63,64)*. *TP53* and the apoptotic pathway have also been associated with sensitivity and resistance to a variety of specific agents *(60,65–67)*.

Despite the evidence that *TP53* plays a critical role in mediating response to chemotherapy, it has not yet proved to be a useful measure of outcome with specific therapeutic choices. To date, two studies have shown that *TP53* is predictive of resistance in therapies using doxorubicin, a cytotoxic antibiotic; however, attempts to associate alteration in *TP53* with response to treatment have generally been negative (reviewed in ref. *65*). The lack of evidence might reflect that the apoptosis and senescence pathways are highly regulated and that other factors play significant roles in controlling the pathways; if so, measurements of *TP53* alone might not be sufficient to predict outcome. Most studies have measured accumulation of p53 protein, given that mutations in the gene lead to a prolonged half-life for the protein. However, different mutations might exhibit different phenotypes, and studies that measure specific mutations might have differing results.

## 4.3. RAS

The members of the *RAS* gene family encode small GTPases with roles in signal transduction and regulation of cell differentiation. *RAS* was one of the first identified human oncogenes *(68)*. Further work has demonstrated that *RAS* genes are highly mutable and that these mutations can eventually give rise to tumors *(69)*. The mutations tend to consist of single-basepair changes within a few hot spots in amino acids at position 12, 13, or 61 in the protein product *(70–72)*. Mutations in *RAS* occur in 25% of human cancers, including 90% of pancreatic cancer, 50% of colon cancer, and 30% of non-small-cell lung cancer. The oncogenic mutation in RAS eliminates its GTPase activity but has little effect on its GTP-binding activity, resulting in a constitutively active protein and a cell with an impaired ability to exit the cell cycle.

Given the frequency with which these genes are mutant in human cancers, much attention has focused on the possible role of *RAS* mutations in promoting chemoresistance. However, no constant associations between *RAS* and any chemotherapeutics have been verified. The role for RAS in mediating sensitivity to ionizing radiation is better established. That role is significant, given that radiation is a primary tool in combating cancer and that response to radiation is a strong predictor of the patient's treatment prognosis. *(73)*. A number of studies have shown that the *RAS* oncogene is associated with resistance to radiation and that this resistance seems to occur through the RAS signaling pathway mediated by the phosphoinositide-3 kinase (PI3K) *(74)*. Although this association creates attractive possibilities for potential targeted therapies, it is not currently employed for treatment planning. However, detection of mutant *RAS* might aid in the early discovery of noninvasive cancer in the colon.

## 4.4. ERBB2

ERBB2 (Her2/neu) is a tyrosine kinase receptor and a member of the epidermal growth factor receptor (EGFR) family. Its roles in normal cellular physiology are not yet established, but it appears to act in the regulation of cell growth. It is genetically amplified and, thus, overexpressed at the protein level in a number of different cancers, including breast and ovarian, where it correlates with a poor outcome *(75–77)*. Numerous studies have shown that *ERBB2* amplification, in addition to indicating increased tumor proliferation, is associated with resistance to chemotherapy (reviewed in ref. *65*). This resistance can be surmounted with adjuvant therapy with doxorubicin *(78)*. The mechanism through which the protein affects the response to chemotherapy is unknown. However, because ERBB2 is involved in the activation of the Ras/Map kinase pathway, disruption of its function is likely to have pluripotent effects *(79)*.

The differential effects observed for treatment efficacy in regard to ERBB2 were among the first that demonstrated the use of a genetic marker to direct chemotherapy decisions. However, the responses measured were not dramatic, and the assessment of ERBB2 status did not become a standard part of breast cancer diagnosis until the development of Genentech's Herceptin (trastuzumab). Herceptin, a monoclonal antibody that recognizes the ERBB2 protein, has demonstrated efficacy in treating metastatic breast cancers that overexpress *ERBB2*. Its mechanism of action is uncertain, but it might have both cytostatic and cytotoxic effects *(80–82)*.

## 5. TARGET DISCOVERY AND PHARMACOGENOMICS

In addition to its initial onocologic applications in improving patient treatment design, pharmacogenomics is expected to dramatically shape future drug development as well (Fig. 2). Genetic variations that predict responses to drugs provide critical information for specifically targeting therapies to key biochemical processes and to patients whose therapeutic needs are unmet by current treatment regimens. Accordingly, this development will be a boon both to patients and to drug manufacturers.

## 5.1. Targeting Mediators of Drug Response

Proteins identified as having critical roles in the efficacy of specific drugs can become drug targets themselves, with the hope that their perturbation will increase the efficacy of the original drug. This path of drug discovery provides several benefits for the pharmaceutical industry. Because the biochemical pathways targeted by the intended therapy are clearly defined by the presence of identified polymorphisms, initial compound screens can be logically devised. Furthermore, stratifying clinical evaluations by clearly defining patients' genotypes and prescribing appropriate treatments would help increase the chance of success and limit the sizes of clinical trials. Finally, the availability of novel therapies would increase the applicability, and therefore the market, of currently employed drugs.

Because of apoptosis' central role in the mechanism of action of most chemotherapeutics, genes associated with programmed cell death have become the focus of novel drug development. The drug in this category whose development is most advanced is Genasense (Genta), an 18-mer antisense oligonucleotide targeting *BCL2*, which has passed

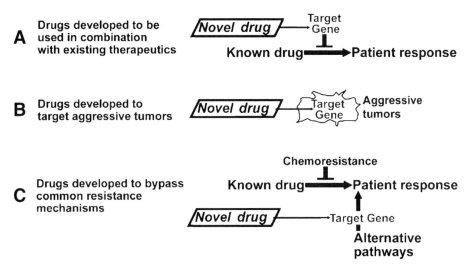

Fig. 2. Pharmacogenomics can be applied both for targeting drug discovery and for drug development. Genetic variations that have been found to predict response to existing drugs suggest novel targets in key biochemical processes that can greatly aid drug development. (**A**) Genes identified to mediate response to known drugs can become targets. Drugs developed to affect the activity of these proteins could be employed adjunctively to ensure better response to the primary therapy. (**B**) Genes identified to be targetable members of biochemical pathways critical for later stages of tumorigenesis are excellent targets because patients harboring these tumors are not being adequately served by existing therapeutics. (**C**) Pathways identified to be a significant means of resistance to existing drugs can be avoided, prompting members of other pathways to be recognized as more valuable targets.

initial trials and awaits FDA approval. Genasense is one of the first antisense therapies for cancer, with an initial proposed application in combination with dacarbazine for the treatment of patients with advanced melanoma who have not previously received chemotherapy. Other applications in combination with a variety of other chemotherapeutics in both solid and hematologic cancers are being tested. *TP53* has also received much attention, but because its mutation leads to an inactive protein, studies have largely focused on replacing *TP53* using adenovirus as a delivery mechanism. Although initial results are encouraging, the well-known problems associated with delivery in gene therapy are likely to require further advances before these drugs reach the market.

Genetic variations in drug-metabolizing genes often lead to unpredictable treatment outcomes and severe toxicity. Compounds inhibiting enzyme activity might reduce interindividual variability in drug pharmacokinetics and/or pharmacodynamics, as well as improve bioavailability for all patients. For example, the oral bioavailability of 5-FU is highly variable and unpredictable (0–80%), which limits its administration to intravenous routes *(83)*. Recently, eniluracil, a potent inactivator of DPD, became clinically available to use in combination with 5-FU. By inhibiting DPD, eniluracil permits higher and longer sustained serum levels of 5-FU while preventing the formation of 5-FU catabolites, which are toxic and have no antitumor activity. Furthermore, treatment with eniluracil removes DPD activity as a source of variability in fluorouracil pharmacokinetics *(84)*. The combination treatment of 5-FU and eniluracil allows continuous low-dose oral 5-FU to be given with predicable oral bioavailability and causes strikingly less toxicity *(85)*.

The importance of MDR1 in multidrug resistance in cancer treatment suggests that cyto-toxic drug delivery to cancer cells can be improved by modulating its function *(86,87)*. Inhibition of MDR1 might reverse existing drug resistance. Furthermore, regulating MDR1 could also provide useful intervention to improve oral uptake of drugs and reduce drug excretion, thereby reducing dosing requirements and allowing drug penetration into tar-get tissues such as the brain. Many inhibitors of MDR transporters have been identified and some are undergoing clinical trials, although clinically useful drugs have yet to make it to market.

## 5.2. Targeting Aggressive Tumors

Many genes related to the oncogenesis process could be targets in their own right, independent of current drugs. A number of genes often mutated in certain aggressive or unresponsive tumor types have been the focus of this line of attack. This method has two benefits: (1) By directing development to aggressive tumors, patients who are at most risk are targeted and (2) being able to identify these classes of patients should allow for more rapid clinical trials, given that efficacy is easier to measure when prognosis under current accepted therapies is poor.

This approach to novel drug development has made several high-profile advances in recent years. Novartis Oncology developed Gleevec (imatinib mesylate) to treat chronic myeloid leukemia (CML). CML is caused by a translocation leading to the constitutively active BCR-ABL protein. Gleevec was designed to inhibit phosphorylation of this pro-tein and thus block its activity. In breast cancer, Genentech's Herceptin (trastuzumab) has proved to be an effective therapy for patients with amplifications of the *ERBB2* gene. Although the mechanism of action of this monoclonal antibody toward this protein is uncertain, it can act both by directly inhibiting the protein and by targeting an immune response toward the expressing tumor cells *(80–82)*.

Researchers are hopeful that the RAS family or associated pathways can become pro-ductive targets for novel therapeutics, although no such drugs are currently routinely employed in cancer patients. The frequency with which *RAS* mutations occur in common cancers and their association with resistance to ionizing radiation make for a potentially powerful target. Already approved for use in treating patients with hypercholesterolemia, lovastatin is a HMG-CoA reductase inhibitor that also blocks the processing of RAS *(88)*. Application of lovastatin has been shown to increase radiosensitivity in cell lines harbor-ing mutant *RAS (89)*, and trials are under way to assess its applicability as an adjunctive therapy in a number of cancers. Also under way are attempts at inhibiting RAS processing by other farnesyltransferase inhibitors—a necessary event in ras postranslational modifi-cation. Inhibition of this step results in the radiosensitization of cells in vivo *(90)*. Cur-rently in various stages of clinical trials are the farnesyltransferase inhibitors Tipifarnib (Janssen Pharmaceutica), SCH66336 (Schering-Plough), and BAY 32-9006 (Onyx Pharma-ceuticals in partnership with Bayer), all of which have shown initially promising results.

## 5.3. Targeting Novel Pathways

On a broader note, pathways identified through pharmacogenomics to be of key impor-tance in drug response can become part of the focus of targeted drug development. Path-ways found to have few members with known clinically relevant allelic variation might be even more productive targets. Because tumorigenesis is linked to apoptosis, it is not surprising that many tumors appear to be intrinsically resistant to drugs that operate through programmed cell death. The events that lead to cell transformation disrupt the mechanisms exploited by these drugs so that the tumors are inherently resistant to their action. In addition to pointing to regulators of apoptosis as potential targets, as discussed previously, this central role of apoptosis in tumor progression and drug action suggests that drugs acting outside of this pathway might be less prone to inherent or acquired resistance. In this regard, the tyrosine kinase receptors have received much attention in this regard. Often overexpressed in proliferating cells, the constitutive activity of many receptor pathways is associated with malignant transformation. A number of new drugs directed toward members of this family have been generated; they include the therapeutic monoclonal antibody Herceptin (Genentech), which targets ERBB2, and four toward EGFR—the small molecules Iressa (AstraZeneca) and Tarceva (Genentech) and the therapeutic monoclonal antibodies Erbitux (ImClone) and ABX-EGF (Abgenix). Other pathways of interest include the Ras/Raf kinases, PI-kinases, and the cytokines.

In addition to these direct applications for targeting drug discovery, other discoveries in the pharmacogenomics field indirectly aid the drug discovery process. Acting like catalysts, advances in pharmacogenomics should allow the more rapid validation and clinical evaluation of novel drugs. Variations found to be significant in mediating adverse or poor drug responses are likely to be generalizable to broad classes of drugs. In this manner, trials of novel therapies might be able to employ established toxicity markers in trial design, helping decrease failures in early phases. Similarly, pharmacogenomics could aid in trial design by helping designate probable responder populations on the basis of find-ings for similar classes of drugs. For example, because polymorphisms of *MTHFR* are shown to modulate the therapeutic effects 5-FU and methotrexate, evaluation of the effects of variations in this gene would be prudent in the development of novel antifolate chemotherapy agents. As the predictive values of further polymorphic variations are validated in clinical trials, it is likely that bolder and more productive uses of the discipline will be realized.

## ACKNOWLEDGMENTS

The authors thank Dr. Douglas Ross for comments on the manuscript. Huijun Z. Ring is supported by grant DA016382 from the National Institute of Health and grant 12KT-0234 from the University of California Tobacco-Related Disease Research Program.

## REFERENCES

1. Gonzalez FJ, Skoda RC, Kimura S, et al. Characterization of the common genetic defect in humans deficient in debrisoquine metabolism. Nature 1988; 331:442–446.
2. Kallioniemi A, Kallioniemi OP, Sudar D, et al. Comparative genomic hybridization for molecular cytogenetic analysis of solid tumors. Science 1992; 258:818–821.
3. Pollack JR, Sorlie T, Perou CM, et al. Microarray analysis reveals a major direct role of DNA copy number alteration in the transcriptional program of human breast tumors. Proc Natl Acad Sci USA 2002; 99:12,963–12,968.
4. Pollack JR, Perou CM, Alizadeh AA, et al. Genome-wide analysis of DNA copy-number changes using cDNA microarrays. Nature Genet 1999; 23:41–46.
5. Hippocrates. Of the Epidemics Bk. I, Sect. II. (c. 400 BC), Jones WHS, transl. Loeb Classical Library No. 147: Ancient Medicine. Vol. Bk. I, Sect. II.: Cambridge, MA: Harvard University Press, 1923:432.
6. Krynetski E, Evans WE. Drug methylation in cancer therapy: lessons from the TPMT polymorphism. Oncogene 2003; 22:7403–7413.

7. Krynetski EY, Tai HL, Yates CR, et al. Genetic polymorphism of thiopurine S-methyltransferase: clinical importance and molecular mechanisms. Pharmacogenetics 1996; 6:279–290.
8. McLeod HL, Lin JS, Scott EP, Pui CH, Evans WE. Thiopurine methyltransferase activity in American white subjects and black subjects. Clin Pharmacol Ther 1994; 55:15–20.
9. Relling MV, Hancock ML, Boyett JM, Pui CH, Evans WE. Prognostic importance of 6-mercaptopurine dose intensity in acute lymphoblastic leukemia. Blood 1999; 93:2817–2823.
10. Relling MV, Rubnitz JE, Rivera GK, et al. High incidence of secondary brain tumours after radiotherapy and antimetabolites. Lancet 1999; 354:34–39.
11. Relling MV, Yanishevski Y, Nemec J, et al. Etoposide and antimetabolite pharmacology in patients who develop secondary acute myeloid leukemia. Leukemia 1998; 12:346–352.
12. Bo J, Schroder H, Kristinsson J, et al. Possible carcinogenic effect of 6-mercaptopurine on bone marrow stem cells: relation to thiopurine metabolism. Cancer 1999; 86:1080–1086.
13. Gardiner SJ, Begg EJ, Robinson BA. The effect of dihydropyrimidine dehydrogenase deficiency on outcomes with fluorouracil. Adverse Drug React Toxicol Rev 2002; 21:1–16.
14. van Kuilenburg AB, De Abreu RA, van Gennip AH. Pharmacogenetic and clinical aspects of dihydropyrimidine dehydrogenase deficiency. Ann Clin Biochem 2003; 40:41–45.
15. Van Kuilenburg AB, Vreken P, Beex LV, et al. Heterozygosity for a point mutation in an invariant splice donor site of dihydropyrimidine dehydrogenase and severe 5-fluorouracil related toxicity. Eur J Cancer 1997; 33:2258–2264.
16. Wei X, McLeod HL, McMurrough J, Gonzalez FJ, Fernandez-Salguero P. Molecular basis of the human dihydropyrimidine dehydrogenase deficiency and 5-fluorouracil toxicity. J Clin Invest 1996; 98:610–615.
17. van Kuilenburg AB, Haasjes J, Richel DJ, et al. Clinical implications of dihydropyrimidine dehydrogenase (DPD) deficiency in patients with severe 5-fluorouracil-associated toxicity: identification of new mutations in the DPD gene. Clin Cancer Res 2000; 6:4705–4712.
18. Raida M, Schwabe W, Hausler P, et al. Prevalence of a common point mutation in the dihydropyrimidine dehydrogenase (DPD) gene within the 5'-splice donor site of intron 14 in patients with severe 5-fluorouracil (5-FU)-related toxicity compared with controls. Clin Cancer Res 2001; 7:2832–2839.
19. Volk J, Reinke F, van Kuilenburg AB, et al. Safe administration of irinotecan, oxaliplatin and raltitrexed in a DPD-deficient patient with metastatic colon cancer. Ann Oncol 2001; 12:569–571.
20. Guillemette C. Pharmacogenomics of human UDP-glucuronosyltransferase enzymes. Pharmacogenomics J 2003; 3:136–158.
21. Bosma PJ, Chowdhury JR, Bakker C, et al. The genetic basis of the reduced expression of bilirubin UDP-glucuronosyltransferase 1 in Gilbert's syndrome. N Engl J Med 1995; 333:1171–1175.
22. Iyer L, Das S, Janisch L, et al. UGT1A1*28 polymorphism as a determinant of irinotecan disposition and toxicity. Pharmacogenomics J 2002; 2:43–47.
23. Gottesman MM, Fojo T, Bates SE. Multidrug resistance in cancer: role of ATP-dependent transporters. Nat Rev Cancer 2002; 2:48–58.
24. Riordan JR, Deuchars K, Kartner N, Alon N, Trent J, Ling V. Amplification of P-glycoprotein genes in multidrug-resistant mammalian cell lines. Nature 1985; 316:817–819.
25. Hoffmeyer S, Burk O, von Richter O, et al. Functional polymorphisms of the human multidrug-resistance gene: multiple sequence variations and correlation of one allele with P-glycoprotein expression and activity in vivo. Proc Natl Acad Sci USA 2000; 97:3473–3478.
26. Sakaeda T, Nakamura T, Horinouchi M, et al. MDR1 genotype-related pharmacokinetics of digoxin after single oral administration in healthy Japanese subjects. Pharm Res 2001; 18:1400–1404.
27. Kroetz DL, Pauli-Magnus C, Hodges LM, et al. Sequence diversity and haplotype structure in the human ABCB1 (MDR1, multidrug resistance transporter) gene. Pharmacogenetics 2003; 13:481–494.
28. Longley DB, Harkin DP, Johnston PG. 5-Fluorouracil: mechanisms of action and clinical strategies. Nat Rev Cancer 2003; 3:330–338.
29. Copur S, Aiba K, Drake JC, Allegra CJ, Chu E. Thymidylate synthase gene amplification in human colon cancer cell lines resistant to 5-fluorouracil. Biochem Pharmacol 1995; 49:1419–1426.
30. Johnston PG, Lenz HJ, Leichman CG, et al. Thymidylate synthase gene and protein expression correlate and are associated with response to 5-fluorouracil in human colorectal and gastric tumors. Cancer Res 1995; 55:1407–1412.
31. Horie N, Aiba H, Oguro K, Hojo H, Takeishi K. Functional analysis and DNA polymorphism of the tandemly repeated sequences in the 5'-terminal regulatory region of the human gene for thymidylate synthase. Cell Struct Funct 1995; 20:191–197.

32. Marsh S, McKay JA, Cassidy J, McLeod HL. Polymorphism in the thymidylate synthase promoter enhancer region in colorectal cancer. Int J Oncol 2001; 19:383–386.
33. Iacopetta B, Grieu F, Joseph D, Elsaleh H. A polymorphism in the enhancer region of the thymidylate synthase promoter influences the survival of colorectal cancer patients treated with 5-fluorouracil. Br J Cancer 2001; 85:827–830.
34. Pullarkat ST, Stoehlmacher J, Ghaderi V, et al. Thymidylate synthase gene polymorphism determines response and toxicity of 5-FU chemotherapy. Pharmacogenomics J 2001; 1:65–70.
35. Villafranca E, Okruzhnov Y, Dominguez MA, et al. Polymorphisms of the repeated sequences in the enhancer region of the thymidylate synthase gene promoter may predict downstaging after preoperative chemoradiation in rectal cancer. J Clin Oncol 2001; 19:1779–1786.
36. Ueland PM, Hustad S, Schneede J, Refsum H, Vollset SE. Biological and clinical implications of the MTHFR C677T polymorphism. Trends Pharmacol Sci 2001; 22:195–201.
37. Sohn KJ, Croxford R, Yates Z, Lucock M, Kim YI. Effect of the methylenetetrahydrofolate reductase C677T polymorphism on chemosensitivity of colon and breast cancer cells to 5-fluorouracil and methotrexate. J Natl Cancer Inst 2004; 96:134–144.
38. Ulrich CM, Yasui Y, Storb R, et al. Pharmacogenetics of methotrexate: toxicity among marrow transplantation patients varies with the methylenetetrahydrofolate reductase C677T polymorphism. Blood 2001; 98:231–234.
39. Toffoli G, Russo A, Innocenti F, et al. Effect of methylenetetrahydrofolate reductase 677C—>T polymorphism on toxicity and homocysteine plasma level after chronic methotrexate treatment of ovarian cancer patients. Int J Cancer 2003; 103:294–299.
40. Toffoli G, Veronesi A, Boiocchi M, Crivellari D. MTHFR gene polymorphism and severe toxicity during adjuvant treatment of early breast cancer with cyclophosphamide, methotrexate, and fluorouracil (CMF). Ann Oncol 2000; 11:373–374.
41. Cohen V, Panet-Raymond V, Sabbaghian N, Morin I, Batist G, Rozen R. Methylenetetrahydrofolate reductase polymorphism in advanced colorectal cancer: a novel genomic predictor of clinical response to fluoropyrimidine-based chemotherapy. Clin Cancer Res 2003; 9:1611–1615.
42. Cory S, Adams JM. The Bcl2 family: regulators of the cellular life-or-death switch. Nat Rev Cancer 2002; 2:647–656.
43. Tsujimoto Y, Cossman J, Jaffe E, Croce CM. Involvement of the bcl-2 gene in human follicular lymphoma. Science 1985; 228:1440–1443.
44. Reed JC. Bcl-2 family proteins: regulators of apoptosis and chemoresistance in hematologic malignancies. Semin Hematol 1997; 34:9–19.
45. Knowlton K, Mancini M, Creason S, Morales C, Hockenbery D, Anderson BO. Bcl-2 slows in vitro breast cancer growth despite its antiapoptotic effect. J Surg Res 1998; 76:22–26.
46. Futreal PA, Liu Q, Shattuck-Eidens D, et al. BRCA1 mutations in primary breast and ovarian carcinomas. Science 1994; 266:120–122.
47. Liede A, Karlan BY, Narod SA. Cancer risks for male carriers of germline mutations in BRCA1 or BRCA2: a review of the literature. J Clin Oncol 2004; 22:735–742.
48. Sharan SK, Morimatsu M, Albrecht U, et al. Embryonic lethality and radiation hypersensitivity mediated by Rad51 in mice lacking Brca2. Nature 1997; 386:804–810.
49. Gowen LC, Johnson BL, Latour AM, Sulik KK, Koller BH. Brca1 deficiency results in early embryonic lethality characterized by neuroepithelial abnormalities. Nature Genet 1996; 12:191–194.
50. Rosen EM, Fan S, Pestell RG, Goldberg ID. BRCA1 gene in breast cancer. J Cell Physiol 2003; 196: 19–41.
51. Olopade OI, Grushko T. Gene-expression profiles in hereditary breast cancer. N Engl J Med 2001; 344: 2028–2029.
52. Sorlie T, Tibshirani R, Parker J, et al. Repeated observation of breast tumor subtypes in independent gene expression data sets. Proc Natl Acad Sci USA 2003; 100:8418–8423.
53. Sorlie T, Perou CM, Tibshirani R, et al. Gene expression patterns of breast carcinomas distinguish tumor subclasses with clinical implications. Proc Natl Acad Sci USA 2001; 98:10,869–10,874.
54. Quinn JE, Kennedy RD, Mullan PB, et al. BRCA1 functions as a differential modulator of chemotherapy-induced apoptosis. Cancer Res 2003; 63:6221–6628.
55. Tassone P, Tagliaferri P, Perricelli A, et al. BRCA1 expression modulates chemosensitivity of BRCA1-defective HCC1937 human breast cancer cells. Br J Cancer 2003; 88:1285–1291.
56. Haffty BG, Harrold E, Khan AJ, et al. Outcome of conservatively managed early-onset breast cancer by BRCA1/2 status. Lancet 2002; 359:1471–1477.

57. Duffy SW, Nixon RM. Estimates of the likely prophylactic effect of tamoxifen in women with high risk BRCA1 and BRCA2 mutations. Br J Cancer 2002; 86:218–221.
58. Lane DP. Cancer. p53, guardian of the genome. Nature 1992; 358:15–16.
59. Schmitt CA, Fridman JS, Yang M, et al. A senescence program controlled by p53 and p16INK4a contributes to the outcome of cancer therapy. Cell 2002; 109:335–346.
60. Lowe SW, Ruley HE, Jacks T, Housman DE. p53-dependent apoptosis modulates the cytotoxicity of anticancer agents. Cell 1993; 74:957–967.
61. Frebourg T, Malkin D, Friend S. Cancer risks from germ line tumor suppressor gene mutations. Princess Takamatsu Symp 1991; 22:61–70.
62. Malkin D, Jolly KW, Barbier N, et al. Germline mutations of the p53 tumor-suppressor gene in children and young adults with second malignant neoplasms. N Engl J Med 1992; 326:1309–1315.
63. Kovach JS, Hartmann A, Blaszyk H, Cunningham J, Schaid D, Sommer SS. Mutation detection by highly sensitive methods indicates that p53 gene mutations in breast cancer can have important prognostic value. Proc Natl Acad Sci USA 1996; 93:1093–1096.
64. Jego N, Thomas G, Hamelin R. Short direct repeats flanking deletions, and duplicating insertions in p53 gene in human cancers. Oncogene 1993; 8:209–213.
65. Hamilton A, Piccart M. The contribution of molecular markers to the prediction of response in the treatment of breast cancer: a review of the literature on HER-2, p53 and BCL-2. Ann Oncol 2000; 11:647–663.
66. Reed JC. Dysregulation of apoptosis in cancer. J Clin Oncol 1999; 17:2941–2953.
67. Holleman A, den Boer ML, Kazemier KM, Janka-Schaub GE, Pieters R. Resistance to different classes of drugs is associated with impaired apoptosis in childhood acute lymphoblastic leukemia. Blood 2003; 102:4541–4546.
68. Parada LF, Tabin CJ, Shih C, Weinberg RA. Human EJ bladder carcinoma oncogene is homologue of Harvey sarcoma virus ras gene. Nature 1982; 297:474–478.
69. Nelson MA, Futscher BW, Kinsella T, Wymer J, Bowden GT. Detection of mutant Ha-ras genes in chemically initiated mouse skin epidermis before the development of benign tumors. Proc Natl Acad Sci USA 1992; 89:6398–6402.
70. Sweet RW, Yokoyama S, Kamata T, Feramisco JR, Rosenberg M, Gross M. The product of ras is a GTPase and the T24 oncogenic mutant is deficient in this activity. Nature 1984; 311:273–275.
71. Fasano O, Aldrich T, Tamanoi F, Taparowsky E, Furth M, Wigler M. Analysis of the transforming potential of the human H-ras gene by random mutagenesis. Proc Natl Acad Sci USA 1984; 81:4008–4012.
72. Yuasa Y, Srivastava SK, Dunn CY, Rhim JS, Reddy EP, Aaronson SA. Acquisition of transforming properties by alternative point mutations within c-bas/has human proto-oncogene. Nature 1983; 303:775–779.
73. West CM, Davidson SE, Roberts SA, Hunter RD. Intrinsic radiosensitivity and prediction of patient response to radiotherapy for carcinoma of the cervix. Br J Cancer 1993; 68:819–823.
74. Gupta AK, Bakanauskas VJ, Cerniglia GJ, et al. The Ras radiation resistance pathway. Cancer Res 2001; 61:4278–4282.
75. Yokota J, Yamamoto T, Toyoshima K, et al. Amplification of c-erbB-2 oncogene in human adenocarcinomas in vivo. Lancet 1986; 1:765–767.
76. Slamon DJ, Clark GM, Wong SG, Levin WJ, Ullrich A, McGuire WL. Human breast cancer: correlation of relapse and survival with amplification of the HER-2/neu oncogene. Science 1987; 235:177–182.
77. Slamon DJ, Godolphin W, Jones LA, et al. Studies of the HER-2/neu proto-oncogene in human breast and ovarian cancer. Science 1989; 244:707–712.
78. Thor AD, Berry DA, Budman DR, et al. erbB-2, p53, and efficacy of adjuvant therapy in lymph node-positive breast cancer. J Natl Cancer Inst 1998; 90:1346–1360.
79. von Lintig FC, Dreilinger AD, Varki NM, Wallace AM, Casteel DE, Boss GR. Ras activation in human breast cancer. Breast Cancer Res Treat 2000; 62:51–62.
80. Pietras RJ, Fendly BM, Chazin VR, Pegram MD, Howell SB, Slamon DJ. Antibody to HER-2/neu receptor blocks DNA repair after cisplatin in human breast and ovarian cancer cells. Oncogene 1994; 9:1829–1838.
81. Sliwkowski MX, Lofgren JA, Lewis GD, Hotaling TE, Fendly BM, Fox JA. Nonclinical studies addressing the mechanism of action of trastuzumab (Herceptin). Semin Oncol 1999; 26:60–70.
82. Baselga J, Norton L, Albanell J, Kim YM, Mendelsohn J. Recombinant humanized anti-HER2 antibody (Herceptin) enhances the antitumor activity of paclitaxel and doxorubicin against HER2/neu overexpressing human breast cancer xenografts. Cancer Res 1998; 58:2825–2831.
83. Diasio RB, Harris BE. Clinical pharmacology of 5-fluorouracil. Clin Pharmacokinet 1989; 16:215–237.

84. Ahmed FY, Johnston SJ, Cassidy J, et al. Eniluracil treatment completely inactivates dihydropyrimidine dehydrogenase in colorectal tumors. J Clin Oncol 1999; 17:2439–2445.

85. Smith IE, Johnston SR, O'Brien ME, et al. Low-dose oral fluorouracil with eniluracil as first-line chemotherapy against advanced breast cancer: a phase II study. J Clin Oncol 2000; 18:2378–2384.

86. Thomas H, Coley HM. Overcoming multidrug resistance in cancer: an update on the clinical strategy of inhibiting p-glycoprotein. Cancer Control 2003; 10:159–165.

87. van Zuylen L, Nooter K, Sparreboom A, Verweij J. Development of multidrug-resistance convertors: sense or nonsense? Invest New Drugs 2000; 18:205–220.

88. Jackson JH, Cochrane CG, Bourne JR, Solski PA, Buss JE, Der CJ. Farnesol modification of Kirsten-ras exon 4B protein is essential for transformation. Proc Natl Acad Sci USA 1990; 87:3042–3046.

89. Miller AC, Kariko K, Myers CE, Clark EP, Samid D. Increased radioresistance of EJras-transformed human osteosarcoma cells and its modulation by lovastatin, an inhibitor of p21ras isoprenylation. Int J Cancer 1993; 53:302–307.

90. Bernhard EJ, McKenna WG, Hamilton AD, et al. Inhibiting Ras prenylation increases the radiosensitivity of human tumor cell lines with activating mutations of ras oncogenes. Cancer Res 1998; 58:1754–1761.

# 23 Diagnosis and Treatment of Malignancies Using Gene Expression Profiling

## Jimmy C. Sung, MD, JD, Alice Y. Lee, MS, and Timothy J. Yeatman, MD

**CONTENTS**

INTRODUCTION
GENOME, TRANSCRIPTOME, AND PROTEOME
MICROARRAY TECHNOLOGY
ANALYSIS OF MICROARRAY DATA
MOLECULAR CLASSIFICATION OF CANCER
PERSONALIZED MEDICINE: "ONE PATIENT, ONE CHIP"
REFERENCES

SUMMARY

The Human Genome Project is the beginning of a new age in medicine. At the cornerstone of genomic medicine is the diagnosis and treatment of diseases using gene expression. The aim of this chapter is to provide an introduction on the microarray gene profiling technology and its application in the emerging field of molecular oncology.

**Key Words:** Molecular oncology; gene expression profiling; microarray; tumor classifier; genomics; proteomics.

## 1. INTRODUCTION

Predicting who will develop cancer and how they will respond to therapy has long been a dream of oncologists and researchers. Advancements in computer science and molecular biology have now converted this dream into a realistic expectation. The marriage of these two disciplines gave birth to the Human Genome Project, which provides the blueprint for investigating the molecular mechanism of human diseases. A genomic-based understanding of human diseases will allow us to diagnose cancer, design novel treatments, and predict therapeutic response. One of the tools widely used in genomic research is microarray technology. It is a powerful technology that enables us to profile gene expression

From: *Cancer Drug Discovery and Development: The Oncogenomics Handbook*
Edited by: W. J. LaRochelle and R. A. Shimkets © Humana Press Inc., Totowa, NJ

on the genomic scale. Using this technology, we not only can define a molecular finger-print for each type of cancer and its various stages, we can also identify molecularly distinct subgroups with different clinical outcomes that were previously categorized as a single entity. Furthermore, novel therapeutic targets can be identified in a high-throughput man-ner. The molecular classification of human malignancies will provide the basis for improv-ing prediction, diagnosis, and treatment of cancer.

## 2. GENOME, TRANSCRIPTOME, AND PROTEOME

For centuries, medicine has been grounded in the understanding of anatomy and phys-iology. Much of the medical knowledge was based on dissecting the relationship between anatomical or histological structures and pathophysiological function. With completion of the Human Genome Project, a new foundation of modern medicine has emerged. In this postgenomic era, the structure and functional paradigm has remained but the focus is on identifying the structure of the genome (genomics), interrogating critical messenger RNA transcripts expressions (transcriptome), and understanding the function of the final protein product (proteome).

The human genome is composed of 2.9 billion nucleotides. This large sequence of genetic code is made up of introns, which are the noncoding regions, and exons, which are the coding regions. However, only approx 1% of all human DNA is composed of exons. The coding region of the DNA defines nearly 55,000 genes that serve as the template for all biological functions.

The central dogma of molecular biology, although an oversimplification, summarizes the relationship among DNA, RNA, and protein. The DNA codes for the production of messenger RNA (mRNA), the recipe for protein production. By translating these unique mRNAs, distinct polypeptide chains can be made from 20 different amino acids. Once assembled, these chains of amino acids can be further modified by posttranslational pro-cesses such as glycosylation and phosphorylation and can be folded into three-dimensional structures known as proteins. It is estimated that there are 1000–5000 distinct protein structures involved in almost all biological activities. Therefore, hidden within the gene-tic code is a description of the precise mechanism of the pathophysiology of human diseases *(1)*.

Traditionally, clinicians and scientist have been focusing on single biological markers for particular diseases, especially in cancer research. This is the result of technological limitations, analytical simplicity, and the complexity of biological systems. Consequently, only a small fraction of all human diseases have clinically useful biomarkers. Not surpris-ingly, only a portion of the patients afflicted with a particular disease express the asso-ciated biological marker. This reflects that biological systems are of such complexity that a clearer understanding of their true nature can only be deciphered on a global scale. Moreover, these observations suggest that discrete subpopulations exist within each can-cer type that can be classified with informative biomarkers.

The current clinical diagnosis of cancer still largely relies upon microscopic tissue examination. Since its invention in the 17th century, microscopic examination remains a subjective operator-dependent technology. The correct diagnosis often depends on the experience of the pathologist. Furthermore, the limitation of a technology based on phe-notypical observations is illustrated by the variation in clinical outcomes of cancer patients with the same histological staging and problems such as the "unknown primary" remained;

that is, metastatic lesions arising from more than one site are often indistinguishable. The advancement in molecular biology and computer science offers attractive alternative technologies and potential solutions to these problems. The completion of the Human Genome Project provides the map necessary for a global survey of the biological activities within the human system. On the other hand, the development of microarray and computer science provides the kind of high-throughput technology needed to move biomedical research from single-gene analysis to profiling of the entire genome for any particular physiological or pathological state.

## 3. MICROARRAY TECHNOLOGY

A microarray is an ordered array of microscopic elements on a planar substrate that allows the specific binding of genes or gene products (2). Currently, gene expression profiling is accomplished by two principle microarray platforms by using either oligonucleotides or complementary DNAs (cDNAs) to interrogate RNA-derived biological samples such as normal or cancer tissues. These arrays, commonly known as "gene chips" can be homegrown or commercially produced, but all use DNA sequences from the Human Genome Project Database. Oligonucleotide arrays generally use small DNA sequences, 22- to 70-mers, to recognize and distinguish individual genes. Spotted cDNA arrays are constructed by spotting down thousands of longer portions of DNA, each representing an individual gene. The oligonucleotide arrays have the potential benefit of identifying splice products, whereas the cDNA arrays generally cannot.

The process of hybridization underlies all chip-based microarray technology. Hybridization is the chemical process by which two complementary DNA or RNA strands combine to form a double-stranded molecule. A microarray assay involves the hybridization of a copy of the mRNA (either cDNAs or cRNA) or of the DNA of a sample of interest to the DNA tethered on the microarray. The cDNA or cRNA is then labeled with fluorescent dye and hybridized to the microarray chip. Larger quantities of mRNA for any particular gene results in higher degrees of hybridization and stronger fluorescent intensity. By analyzing the digital imaging of the fluorescent intensity across the gene chip, one can determine the degree of expression of all the genes on the chip. Currently, a typical high-intensity microarray chip contains 12,000–60,000 genes, thus capable of generating large amounts of data. The huge volume of data in the backdrop of a complex biological system requires extensive computational analysis in order to uncover the intricate relationships within the entire genome.

## 4. ANALYSIS OF MICROARRAY DATA

Computational techniques for the analysis of microarray data seek to group together genes or samples (representing, for example, different experimental conditions or individual patients) that share similar patterns of gene expression. These data analysis techniques are generally divided into two groups: unsupervised methods, which can be used to discover previously unknown groupings or classes in the data, and supervised methods, which are used to learn discriminating features of already established classifications in order to classify uncategorized objects.

Hierarchical clustering is the most widely used of the unsupervised techniques. Familiar to many biologists through its use in phylogenetic analysis, hierarchical clustering is an agglomerative process that groups together closely related genes (or samples) using a distance metric that defines objects with similar patterns of gene expression as close to one another *(3)*. The process begins with each individual object as its own cluster. Subsequently, the two clusters with the smallest distance between one another are merged, with the process repeating until all clusters are joined into one. This gradual fusing of the groups results in a hierarchical tree, with branches representing the degrees of similarity among the clusters, showing relationships among genes or samples that might have previously been unknown. Although hierarchical clustering is relatively easy to understand and implement, it is known to be characterized by problems such as sensitivity to a "bad" assignment of clusters early in the process. Unsupervised methods other than hierarchical clustering include *k*-means clustering and self-organizing maps, which have been shown to be good alternatives if the number of clusters that should be contained in the data is already known.

If there is some previous knowledge about which samples should group together, such as cancer stage or length of survival, supervised methods that classify gene expression data represent a powerful alternative to unsupervised methods. The general process of classification is to train a classifier to recognize patterns from training data (a set of samples whose classification is already known) so that independent test data (new samples) can be accurately classified.

Machine learning classification techniques that have been used to analyze microarray data include artificial neural networks, the support vector machine, and the *k*-nearest-neighbor analysis. The artificial neural network (ANN) is a nonlinear machine learning paradigm modeled on how biological neural networks, such as the brain, learn and process information. An ANN is composed of large number interconnected neurons, each of which is characterized by a set of inputs, a processing element that evaluates these inputs, and a set of outputs. Each neural connection, or "synapse," has a weight assigned to it, indicating the strength of the incoming signal to the receiving neuron. A set of training data, such as the gene expression profiles of samples with known cancer types, is initially fed to a group of neurons designed to receive external information. When the neuron receives information from all its inputs, it calculates a weighted sum of these values and determines whether or not this sum meets a certain threshold value. If the threshold is met, the neuron "fires" to all other neurons to which it is connected, with each of these neurons calculating the sum of their inputs and "firing" in a similar fashion. Eventually, the information is transformed and propagated throughout the entire network until a set of neurons outputs the results, which are used to adjust the weights of the synapses in the network. In this way, the ANN is trained to recognize complex patterns and characteristic features of the classes, so that it can be used to classify new data into their appropriate categories. However, depending on the design and architecture of the ANN as well as the quality of the training data, accuracy rates for classification have been known to vary widely. In addition, with the ANN, it is difficult to determine intergene relationships.

A supervised learning technique that has been gaining popularity recently is the support vector machine (SVM), a binary linear classifier that attempts to divide genes or samples into two classes by defining a mathematical plane separating members of a class from nonmembers *(4)*. Although the SVM has been shown to be a powerful tool in classifying microarray data, it might not be able to achieve a clean separation between the classes for some datasets. Nonetheless, SVMs and other machine learning techniques that analyze microarray data could prove extremely useful in the classification and treatment of cancer.

## 5. MOLECULAR CLASSIFICATION OF CANCER

A primary challenge of cancer treatment has been to create therapies that differentiate among cancer types that are genetically distinct with unique clinical outcomes, although similar in their clinical and morphological manifestations (5). Because patients with the same type of clinically diagnosed cancer might differ in their genetic pathology, therapies that target specific cancer subtypes could minimize adverse side effects while maximizing efficacy. Molecular classification of cancer using computational analysis of microarray data is the first step toward therapy based on molecular target.

Analysis of gene expression data with respect to cancer classification is divided into two broad tasks: class discovery and class prediction. Class discovery refers to the identification of previously unknown cancer subtypes and can be achieved through the use of unsupervised machine learning, such as hierarchical clustering. Indeed, gene expression profiling with hierarchical clustering has been successfully used to discover previously undetected molecularly distinct forms of diffuse large B-cell lymphoma with significantly different survival outcomes (6).

Class prediction refers to the assignment of unknown tumor samples to previously defined classes. Classification methods such as the supervised methods discussed previously are generally used to predict the classes of unknown samples. Recently, an ANN has been trained with microarray data to classify samples tumors from 21 different sets of origin into their respective diagnostic categories with extremely high accuracy (7). Ultimately, such success with molecular classification of tumors could lead to the molecular fingerprinting of individual tumor samples, allowing practitioners to target therapies to patients with different cancer subtypes that might be similar clinically and histologically but differ in terms of gene expression. Such targeted therapies could maximize survival time while minimizing side effects, as a tumor's gene expression might play a significant, if not the deciding, role in how a tumor progresses and responds to treatment.

## 6. PERSONALIZED MEDICINE: "ONE PATIENT, ONE CHIP"

The diagnosis and treatment of malignancies using gene-expression profiling could achieve the ultimate promise of the practice of medicine—treating our patients as individuals (8). Rather than offering patients "one size fits all" therapy, where many patients are treated to benefit an unknown few, the molecular fingerprints of each patient can be used to identify cancer and guide clinicians to customize therapy based on predicted therapeutic response. This approach begins with the collection of a patient's biological specimen for gene expression profiling. This molecular fingerprint will then be used to generate an objective diagnosis that can be paired with the clinical diagnosis for accuracy. Medications will be tailored according to how the patient is predicted to respond based on his or her gene expression profile. Potential adverse reactions toward particular therapy can also be avoided using the same one patient, one gene chip approach. This concept of personalized genomic medicine will lead to a more evidence-based, outcome-driven, and cost-effective oncological care.

## REFERENCES

1. Yeatman TJ. The future of cancer management: translating the genome, transcriptome, and proteome. Ann Surg Oncol 2003; 10(1):7–14.
2. Schena M. Microarray analysis. New York: Wiley, 2003.

3. Eisen MB, Spellman PT, Brown PO, Botstein D. Cluster analysis and display of genome-wide expression patterns. PNAS 1998; 95(25):14,863–14,868.
4. Quackenbush J. Computational analysis of microarray data. Nature Rev Genet 2001; 6(2):418–427.
5. Golub TR, Slonim DK, Tamayo P, et al. Molecular classification of cancer: class discovery and class prediction by gene expression monitoring. Science 1999; 286(5439):531–537.
6. Alizadeh AA, Eisen MB, Davis RE, Ma C, Lossos IS, Rosenwald A, Boldrick JC, et al. Distinct types of diffuse large B-cell lymphoma identified by gene expression profiling. Nature 2000; 403(6769):503–511.
7. Bloom G, Yang IV, Boulware D, et al. Multi-platform, multi-site, microarray-based human tumor classification. Am J Pathol 2004; 164(1):9–16.
8. Yeatman TJ. The future of clinical cancer management: one tumor, one chip. Am Surg 2003; 69(1):41–44.

# 24

# Implications of Epigenetics for Early Cancer Diagnosis and Prevention

*Mukesh Verma, PhD and Sudhir Srivastava, PhD*

## CONTENTS

## SUMMARY

Unlike genetic regulation, the epigenetic regulation of gene expression does not involve mutations, but involves promoter methylation and histone deacetylation. It is challenging to define how promoter hypermethylation participates in gene silencing and how the loss of methylation alters chromosome structure. Nevertheless, the findings of DNA methylation abnormalities in cancer have a potential clinical impact. One of the potential targets appears to lie in the use of CpG hypermethylation events as tumor biomarkers. The promoter changes provide a positive signal for cancer cells that can be detected by conventional techniques. Based on recent research, it seems reasonable to use multiple markers for predicting one tumor type. As almost every tumor type appears to have multiple independent promoter hypermethylation events, a panel of markers might be constructed to provide indices for monitoring cancer risk assessment and early cancer detection. Because epigenetic events are reversible, chemical agents can be used to intervene epigenetic events.

**Key Words:** Acetylation; biomarkers; chromatin; early detection; epigenetics; epigenome; methylation; prevention; risk assessment.

## 1. INTRODUCTION: EPIGENETICS AND MOLECULAR MECHANISMS INVOLVED IN EPIGENETIC CHANGES

Epigenetics has been defined as the study of processes that establish metastable (i.e., somatically heritable) states of gene expression without altering the DNA sequence. We are accustomed to the idea that the coding potential of the genome lies within the arrangement

From: *Cancer Drug Discovery and Development: The Oncogenomics Handbook*
Edited by: W. J. LaRochelle and R. A. Shimkets © Humana Press Inc., Totowa, NJ

of the four bases; however, additional information that affects a phenotype is the result of the modified base 5-methylcytosine. This modification is flexible enough to be adapted for different somatic cell types and is stable enough to be retained during cell division. DNA methylation is the best studied epigenetic change that has been shown to influence gene expression. It is a postreplicative modification of DNA that occurs primarily on the 5-position of cytosine rings that are located in CpG dinucleotides (1,2). Eighty percent of CpG dinucleotides occur in repetitive sequences where they are normally dispersed. However, the dispersed CpG dinucleotides are also observed in the "bodies" of genes (coding regions, introns) (3,4). In contrast, up to 15% of CpG dinucleotides in mammals occur in clusters of CpG residues, called "CpG islands" (5,6). These CpG islands, which are about 0.5–3 kb long and occur every 100 kb in the genome, are found predominantly in the 5' region (including the promoter region, untranslated region, and exon 1) of approximately half of all human genes (2,4,7).

Epigenetics represents a leading area in biological research, which has an impact on many seemingly different areas of scientific enterprise. A partial listing includes areas of applied science, such as cancer biology (8,9), the study of viral latency (10–13), the activity of mobile elements (14), somatic gene therapy (15–20), cloning and transgenic technologies, genomic imprinting (21,22), and developmental abnormalities (21,22). Essential for normal development, epigenetic controls become misdirected in cancer cells.

Two major steps in epigenetic regulation of genes expression are changes in the chromatin structure (by deacetylation of histones) and methylation of the promoter region of the gene. It is known that methylation is needed for normal development of cells, and aberrant methylation confers a selective growth advantage to the respective cell that results in cancerous growth (23). This occurs when the promoter regions of genes, involved in the control of cell proliferation, are subjected to DNA methylation in their CpG islands, thus silencing gene expression.

## 1.1. Chromosomal Organization and Histones

The DNA of all eukaryotes is packaged into chromatin, which is composed of histone and nonhistone proteins and DNA. Covalent modifications of the tails of histone proteins play an important role in both chromosome organization and regulation of specific genes. It was demonstrated that methylation of Lys4 in the amino-terminal tail of the histone (histone H3) is specific to achromatic domains (where genes are generally active) and methylation of H3 Lys9 is specific to heterochromatic domains of chromatin (where genes are generally inactive) (24). Inverted repeats flanking the heterochromatin act as boundary elements and prevent its spread into the surrounding achromatic regions.

Histone acetylation is a dynamic process that is regulated by two classes of enzymes, the histone acetyltransferases (HATs) and histone deacetylases (HDACs). Although promoter-specific acetylation and deacetylation has received most of the recent attention, it is superimposed upon a broader-acting and dynamic acetylation mechanism that profoundly affects many nuclear processes. Kruhlak et al. (25) monitored this broader histone acetylation as cells enter and exit mitosis. In contrast to the hypothesis that HATs and HDACs remain bound to mitotic chromosomes to provide an epigenetic imprint for postmitotic activation of the genome, they observed that HATs and HDACs are spatially reorganized and displaced from condensing chromosomes when cells undergo division (mitosis). During mitosis, HATs and HDACs are unable to acetylate or deacetylate chromatin in situ despite remaining fully catalytically active when isolated from mitotic cells and assayed in vitro. Thus, HATs and HDACs do not stably bind to the genome to function as an epigenetic mechanism of selective postmitotic gene activation. Nonetheless, results do support a role for spatial organization of these enzymes within the cell nucleus. Furthermore, their relationship to euchromatin and heterochromatin postmitotically in the reactivation of the genome is also important for the active organized structure.

## 1.2. DNA Methylation

In the normal mammalian genome, methylation occurs only at the cytosines 5' to guanosines at the CpG dinucleotides. A family of enzymes, methyltransferases, are involved in methylation of the cytosine. DNMT1 maintains the methylation status of the CpG islands, whereas DNMT3A and DNMT3B are involved in *de novo* methylation of the new sites. The CpG dinucleotides have been progressively depleted from the eukaryotic genome over evolution via spontaneous deamination. The remaining CpGs have a very high frequency of methylation, facilitating chromatin arrangements to render most of the genome late replicating and repressed for the transcription of repeated regions. On the other hand, small stretches of DNA, CpG islands, contain the expected frequency of CpGs. The regions that are methylation protected are generally located in the promoter regions. It has been suggested that the lack of methylation might be a prerequisite for active transcription. Only two exceptions to this rule have been reported: fully methylated CpG islands in the silenced allele for specific imprinted autosomal genes, and multiple silenced genes on the inactivated X-chromosomes of females *(26,27)*. Deacetylation of histone is the primary step that results in the recruitment of methyltransferase to the CpG island, resulting in promoter hypermethylation. Extensive research is needed in this area, as some targets for chemoprevention could emerge from these studies. Furthermore, epigenetic regulations occur early in the development of cancer, which gives us an opportunity to develop intervention approaches to stop further development of cancer.

## 1.3. Factors Affecting Epigenetic Regulation of Genes

A variety of chemicals, base analogs, radiation, smoke, stress, hormones (such as estradiol), other agents (such as nickel, arsenic, cadmium), and reactive oxygen species can alter mammalian cells to a transformed phenotype epigenetically without changing their DNA sequence information. Within the epigenetic effects, alteration in the levels of transcription factors, such as ATF-1, p53, HIF-1, HIF-1, and NFκB, were observed by Costa's group *(28)*. The relationship between nickel and calcium metabolism and the role it plays in nickel carcinogenesis is also considered. Other considerations are reactive oxygen species and the interactions of nickel with proteins. These epigenetic events have been discussed with respect to the effects that nickel has on inducing DNA methylation in cells. It is of interest that nickel induces both a variety of signaling pathways as well as genes that seem to be important for the survival of cancer cells.

In the field of carcinogenesis research, there is growing awareness that neoplastic transformation must be viewed as an environmental process *(28)*. Breivik and Gaudernack *(29, 30)* have addressed this issue and presented a model that integrates evolution and carcinogenesis at the molecular level. This model offers new perspectives, including epigenetics, to carcinogenesis and relates the neoplastic process to the basic evolutionary concept of biology.

Nutrients can also affect epigenetic regulation of cancer-associated genes. Altered methionine metabolism has been recognized as a characteristic trait of malignant cells for two decades *(1)*. Normal cells can utilize homocysteine as a direct methionine precursor, whereas transformed cells tend to require methionine in their growth medium. As *S*-adenosylmethionine (SAM) donates its methyl group to the methyl acceptor, it is converted to *S*-adenosylhomocysteine (SAH). SAH is subsequently broken down to yield homocysteine and adenosine. Methionine is regenerated from homocysteine in a folate- and cobalamin-dependent reaction. The cycle is completed by the conversion of methionine to SAM. The methionine dependence occurs as a result of increased transmethylation and is not the result of reduced methionine biosynthesis. Finally, there is a reduced availability of free methionine in transformed cells. Reduced SAM/SAH ratios that could be reversed by SAM treatment have been observed in the early stages of liver carcinogenesis *(1)*.

## 2. EPIGENETICS AND CANCER

Genetic alterations are the hallmark of neoplastic evolution, as suggested by the analysis of chromosomal structure and determining the chromosomal number *(31)*. Based on the information available today, epigenetics is considered to play a minor role in cancer development compared to genetic events *(32)*. However, recent data suggest alternate approaches that have focused the attention on the contribution of epigenetics to tumorigenesis. Cancer appears to be a process that is developed both by mutations in DNA and by epigenetic mechanisms. These processes can complement such that one can predispose to the other in inducing cancer development.

### 2.1. Tumor Suppressor Genes Mimic Methylation Patterns in Different Tumor Types

A number of genes are regulated by epigenetic process in different tumors (Table 1), These genes are involved at different steps in cell division, differentiation, and proliferation (Table 2). Tumor suppressor genes become inactivated as a result of hypermethylation in a number of tumor types.

With the progression of the disease, a large number of cancer genes have been reported to carry high level of methylation in a normally unmethylated promoter *(33–40)*; for example, *RASSF1, RARbeta, DAPK, p16, p15, MGMT,* and *GSTP1* in lung cancer, *CDKN2A, CALCA, MGMT,* and *TIMP3p* in esophageal cancer, *14^{ARF}* in ulcerative colitis, *GSTP1* in prostate cancer, *HIC-1* and *p53* in breast cancer. It is not yet established whether methylation is an initiating event or a secondary event in gene silencing. Irrespective of the role of methylation in the initiation of tumor development, methylation both marks and plays a key role in an epigenetically mediated loss of gene function that is as critical for tumorigenesis as mutations in coding regions.

Although the functional importance of promoter hypermethylation to loss of gene expression is apparent, the actual molecular mechanisms involved remain to be established. It is possible that this will involve the integration of DNA methylation with chromatin organization and the regulation of histone acetylation and deacetylation *(32)*. The involvement of yet unidentified proteins can also not be ruled out. A critical link involved in the implication of the association of methylation with transcriptionally repressive chromatin is through proteins that bind preferentially to methylated cytosines of the DNA and participate in complexes that contain active histone deacetylases. The protein complexes so far identified include methylated DNA-binding protein MECP2 and methyl CpG-binding domain proteins MBD2 and MBD3 *(41,42)*. They contain the histone deacetylases (HDAC1

Table 1
Tumor Types and Genes Regulated by Epigenetic Mechanism

| Tumor Location | Gene |
|---|---|
| Breast | *p16, BRCA1, GSTP1, DAPK, CDH1, TIMP-3* |
| Brain | *p16, p14^{ARF}, MGMT, TIMP-3* |
| Bladder | *p16, DAPK, APC* |
| Colon | *p16, p14^{ARF}, CRBP1, MGMT, hMLH1, DAPK, TIMP-3, APC* |
| Endometrium | *hMLH1* |
| Esophagus | *p16, p14^{ARF}, GSTP1, CDH1APC* |
| Head and neck | *p16, MGMT, DAPK* |
| Kidney | *p16, p14^{ARF}, MGMT, GSTP1, TIMP-3, APC* |
| Leukemia | *p15, MGMT, DAPK1, CDH1, p73* |
| Liver | *p16, CRBP1, GSTP1, APC* |
| Lymphoma | *p16, p15, CRBP1, MGMT, DAPK, p73* |
| Lung | *p16, p14^{ARF}, CRBP1, MGMT, GSTP1, DAPK, FHIT, TIMP-3, RARbeta, RASSF1A* |
| Ovary | *p16, BRCA1, DAPK* |
| Pancreas | *p16, MGMT, APC* |
| Prostate | *GSTP1, p27(kip1)* |
| Stomach | *p14^{ARF}, P16, APC, hMLH1, MGMT* |
| Uterus | *p16, p14^{ARF}, hMLH1* |

Abbreviations: APC, adenomatous polyposis coli; CDH1, E-cathedrin; DAPK, death-associated protein kinase; FHIT, fragile histidine triad; GSTP1, glutathione-*S*-transferase P1; MGMT, $O^6$-methylguanine-DNA methyltransferase; RARbeta, retinoic acid receptor beta; RASSF1A, RAS association domain family protein 1A.

Table 2
Molecular Targets of Intervention

| Classification of Genes | Genes Regulated Epigenetically |
|---|---|
| Tumor suppressor genes | *APC, p15, p16, p73, ARF/INK4A, VHL, ER, RARbeta, AR, HIC1, Rb* |
| Invasive/metastasis suppressor genes | E-cadherin, TIMP-3, mts-1, *CD-44* |
| DNA repair genes | Methylguanine methyl transferase, *hMLH1, BRCA1, GST* |
| Angiogenesis | Thrombospondin-1 (TSP-1), *TIMP-3* |

and HDAC2) and proteins including transcriptional corepressors that are known to associate with these. The demonstration of these complexes implies that DNA methylation could target to chromatin that actively represses gene expression by undergoing remodeling and disturbing the dynamic equilibrium of histone acetylase and deacetylase *(43)*. It is possible that multiple pathways are involved in the whole process.

There are many reports of reduced levels of DNA methylation of proto-oncogenes in cancer cells *(44–46)*. For instance, reduced levels of DNA methylation of *raf, c-myc, c-fos, c-H-ras*, and *c-K-ras* associated with neoplasia have also been reported in rodent liver model system *(46,47)*. Although there have been reports documenting hypomethylation of *ras* gene in human tumors *(48–50)*, many studies do not support these findings or suggest an irrelevance of DNA methylation status to *ras* gene expression levels *(44,51)*. A good inverse correlation between methylation status and gene expression levels was seen in the *bcl-2* gene in human B-cell chronic lymphocytic leukemia *(45)*. Hypomethylation of the third exon of the *c-myc* gene has been reported in a variety of human tumors *(52)*. Sometimes, it is difficult to distinguish cause and effect, even in the few cases where associated increased levels of gene expression were documented *(1)*.

## 2.2. Colon Cancer and Epigenetics: An Example

Here, we describe genes that are deregulated by epigenetic mechanisms in colon cancer and could be used as potential biomarkers for cancer progression. The strategies to prevent these epigenetic events have also been discussed and are applicable to other tumor types also.

The study of epigenetic changes in colorectal tumors has added a new dimension to our understanding of the molecular events that underlie the disease. Colorectal cancer has provided an excellent model for studying the genetic basis of cancer and is one of the better understood malignancies in this regard. The orderly progression of the disease, with distinct genetic alterations at each step, is a useful framework for revealing the molecular basis of neoplasia. The study of DNA methylation changes in colorectal cancer has now provided additional clues into the pathogenesis of the disease. Initially, progressive methylation and silencing of a subset of genes occurs in normal tissues as a function of age or time-dependent events and predisposes these normal cells to neoplastic transformation. At a later stage of disease progression, DNA methylation plays an important role in a subset of tumors affected by the CpG island methylator phenotype (CIMP), a pathway that results in a form of epigenetic instability through the simultaneous silencing of multiple genes *(53)*. DNA methylation changes have important interactions with genetic lesions in this cancer type. CIMP+ cancers include the majority of tumors with sporadic mismatch repair deficiency through hypermethylation of the *hMLH1* promoter and also account for the majority of tumors with *Ki-ras* mutations through an unknown mechanism. On the other hand, CIMP− cases evolve along a more classic genetic instability pathway, with a high rate of *p53* mutations and chromosomal changes. Therefore, the integration of epigenetic and genetic information provides a more complete molecular understanding of colorectal cancer and might have implications for the diagnosis, prognosis, and treatment of patients affected by this disease.

Multistep carcinogenesis in the colon can now be viewed as a series of pathways that are activated (or inactivated) in populations of cells that are subsequently selected, based on growth (or survival) advantages *(53)*. In most colorectal tumors, the common pathways, which operate simultaneously, are the *APCβ*-catenin pathway, the senescence bypass pathway, and the *TGF* bypass pathway. The *APCβ*-catenin pathway provides a growth advantage via transcriptional activation of *c-myc* and other genes; the senescence bypass pathway *(54)* is required for cellular immortalization and appears to be achieved by inactivation of either the *p53* or *p16* gene; and the *TGF* bypass pathway *(55)* is required for overcoming growth inhibition by *TGF* and is activated by inactivation of *TGF RII* or activation of *Ki-ras*. The possibility of another pathway that is altered in aging cells that results in expansion of the proliferative zone and predisposition to neoplastic transformation cannot be ruled out. In this model of colon cancer, the specific pathway affected is more important than the genes altered, which partly explains the large diversity in molecular alterations described in this relatively uniform disease. Furthermore, chromosomal instability,

Table 3
A Comparison of Techniques Used to Determine Level of Methylation in Different Genes

| Technology Used | Cancer | Organ Site | Comments | Ref. |
|---|---|---|---|---|
| Methylation specific PCR | Ovarian cancer | Ovary | Highly sensitive; not quantitative; can be used on paraffin sections | 59–62 |
| COBRA | Several genes | Several sites | Not quantitative, time-consuming | 63 |
| Microarray chip technology | Acute lymphoblastic leukemia (ALL); acute myeloid leukemia (ALL); ovarian cancer | Blood, ovary | Methylation amplification DNA chip; high throughput, semiquantitative; useful for tumor class prediction | 61,62, 64,65 |
| Real-time PCR MethyLight technology | Twenty genes in esophagus cancer | Esophagus | Quantitative | 58 |
| ECIST (expressed CpG island sequence tag) | Breast cancer | Breast | Simultaneous detection of methylation and cancer-specific gene expression | 66 |

microsatellite instability, and epigenetic instability (CIMP) can now be viewed as simply the molecular mechanisms required to generate molecular diversity, which is a prerequisite to colon evolution in neoplasia.

Further clarification is needed regarding the underlying causes of chromosomal and epigenetic instability. It is now also important to determine whether the kind of instability required for tumor formation has clinical implications for disease progression and therapy. Indeed, MSI+ tumors appear to have a more favorable prognosis overall and differential responses to chemotherapy treatment. The CIMP− tumors might be expected to have a worse prognosis because of the high rate of chromosomal changes in these tumors and the high rate of *p53* mutations, which is one of the determinants of chemosensitivity in the colon *(56)*. CIMP+ tumors might be especially sensitive to therapy and prevention when targeted at methylation inhibition *(57)*. Further studies integrating patterns of molecular instability, epidemiology, and outcome are essential to answer these questions.

## 3. TECHNOLOGIES TO DETECT EPIGENETIC CHANGES

A brief description of the epigenetic technologies is presented in Table 3. Although global genomic DNA methylation content might have an important role in carcinogenesis, its measurement in cancer cells has little to offer as a molecular marker, either in sensitivity or in informational content. Conversely, methylation levels at individual CpG dinucleotides are useful for quantifying differences at important regulatory sequences. Methylation patterns have important uses in disease stratification and progression. Bisulfite genomic sequencing of cloned polymerase chain reaction (PCR) products can provide detailed information on the pattern of 5-methylcytosine distribution along a stretch of DNA, representing a single individual DNA strand. In addition, methylation-specific PCR (MSP)-based techniques can detect the presence of specific DNA patterns with very high sensitivity and specificity. Methylation profiles yield information on the methylation status across many sites in the genome, providing a unique approach to genomewide molecular diagnostics. Profiles can be constructed using measurements of individual CpG dinucleotides, as in most restriction enzyme- and microarray-based methods, or they can be compiled from multiple MSP-based analyses.

New approaches for quantitative high-throughput methylation detection, including the chip technology, and validation of different markers are needed that can be used for screening a large population for risk assessment. Laird's group utilized the MethylLight assay to analyze a panel of 20 genes *(58)*. This approach was used to analyze histologically identified clinical samples and epigenomic fingerprints for the different histological stages of esophageal carcinoma were compared. Esophageal adenocarcinoma arises through different stages (e.g., squamous mucosa, columnar epithelium Barrett's esophagus, dysplasia and malignancy). In this study, instead of analyzing a few genes, 20 genes were analyzed from more than 100 tissue specimens collected from patients with different stages of Barrett's esophagus and/or associated adenocarcinoma. The MethylLight approach differentiated distinct classes of methylation patterns in the different types of tissue. The frequency of methylation ranged from 15% to 60% for different genes. Thus, methylation patterns of specific genes at different stages of the disease progression can be used as markers and the level of methylation reflects the advancement of the disease.

## 4. FUTURE DIRECTIONS: EPIGENETIC MARKERS IN RISK ASSESSMENT AND PREVENTION OF CANCER

The fact that epigenetic changes can be reversed has great therapeutic potential. Reactivation of epigenetically silenced genes has therapeutic benefits. Indeed, 5-azacytidine and its derivatives have been used in the clinic with some beneficial therapeutic result *(67)*. However, the mechanisms underlying these effects have not been completely elucidated. Doses of 5-aza-cytidine used currently are toxic, possibly because of effects not directly related with demethylation. The recent observation that low doses of 5-azacytidine can facilitate reactivation of hypermethylated genes by inhibitors of histone deacetylase has created much interest. Trials are underway in which a clinically available drug with this activity, phenylbutyrate, will be combined with low doses of 5-azacytidine. In this approach, both hematopoietic and solid tumors will be treated and gene reactivation events monitored. It is not known whether such approaches will specifically reactivate genes for better control of the neoplastic process or whether other genes are affected that result in toxicity for normal cells. It is possible that the initial results will justify further development of this therapeutic concept and further increase the interest in clinical aspects of the epigenetics in cancer. Debinski's group has suggested immune-based therapies for X-chromosome linked malignant glioma where epigenetic and genetic regulations play a significant role *(59)*.

Knowledge of molecular events during the early stages of cancer has advanced at a rapid pace. The initiation and development of cancer involves several molecular events, including epigenetics. The promise of biomarkers to detect and diagnose cancer in its earliest stage has never been better. The field of epigenetics has seen a recent surge of interest among cancer researchers since alterations in DNA methylation has emerged as the most consistent molecular alterations in multiple neoplasms. Understanding gene regulation via epigenetics would provide biomarkers of early cancer detection and risk assessment. An important distinction between genetic and epigenetic changes in cancer is that the latter might be more easily reversed using therapeutic interventions. These facts should stimulate much additional research on the topics in years to come. For example, treatment with DNA methylation inhibitors can restore the activities of dormant genes such as *CDKN2A* and decrease the growth rate of cancer cells in a heritable manner. Similarly, DNA repair capacity can be restored by activation of *MLH1*. It should, therefore, be possible to partially reverse the cancer phenotype by the use of methylation inhibitors. In animal models, for example, experiments with *min* mice have shown that inhibition of DNA methylation can suppress tumor initiation, which suggests that this approach might be useful as a preventive strategy. Cytosine analogs are being used to treat preneoplastic syndromes in clinical trials. Antisense oligodeoxynucleotides against methyltransferase have shown a decrease in tumorigenesis. Although these trials have yielded promising preliminary clinical information, the relationship between clinical efficacy and target gene demethylation has not yet been demonstrated. The area, however, has the potential to know this relationship.

Finally, detecting cancer early has an advantage as intervention approaches can be applied for further treatment of cancer. The ubiquity of DNA methylation changes has opened the way to a host of innovative diagnostic and therapeutic strategies. Recent advances attest to the great promise of DNA methylation markers as powerful future tools in the clinic.

## REFERENCES

1. Laird PW, Jaenisch R. The role of DNA methylation in cancer genetic and epigenetics. Annu Rev Genet 1996; 30:441–464.
2. Santini V, Kantarjian HM, Issa JP. Changes in DNA methylation in neoplasia: pathophysiology and therapeutic implications. Ann Intern Med 2001; 134:573–586.
3. Esteller M, Fraga MF, Guo M, et al. DNA methylation patterns in hereditary human cancers mimic sporadic tumorigenesis. Hum Mol Genet 2001; 10:3001–3007.
4. Esteller M, Herman JG. Cancer as an epigenetic disease: DNA methylation and chromatin alterations in human tumours. J Pathol 2002; 196:1–7.
5. Robertson KD, Wolffe AP. DNA methylation in health and disease. Nat Rev Genet 2000; 1:11–19.
6. Fruhwald MC, Plass C. Global and gene-specific methylation patterns in cancer: aspects of tumor biology and clinical potential. Mol Genet Metab 2002; 75:1–16.
7. Bird AP. CpG-rich islands and the function of DNA methylation. Nature 1986; 321:209–213.
8. Baylin SB. Tying it all together: epigenetics, genetics, cell cycle, and cancer. Science 1997; 277:1948–1949.
9. Jones PA, Baylin SB. The fundamental role of epigenetic events in cancer. Nat Rev Genet 2002; 3:415–428.
10. Takacs M, Salamon D, Myohanen S, et al. Epigenetics of latent Epstein–Barr virus genomes: high resolution methylation analysis of the bidirectional promoter region of latent membrane protein 1 and 2B genes. Biol Chem 2001; 382:699–705.
11. Tierney RJ, Kirby HE, Nagra JK, Desmond J, Bell AI, Rickinson AB. Methylation of transcription factor binding sites in the Epstein-Barr virus latent cycle promoter Wp coincides with promoter down-regulation during virus-induced B-cell transformation. J Virol 2000; 74:10,468–10,479.
12. Robertson KD. The role of DNA methylation in modulating Epstein–Barr virus gene expression. Curr Topics Microbiol Immunol 2000; 249:21–34.
13. Tao Q, Swinnen LJ, Yang J, Srivastava G, Robertson KD, Ambinder RF. Methylation status of the Epstein–Barr virus major latent promoter C in iatrogenic B cell lymphoproliferative disease. Application of PCR-based analysis. Am J Pathol 1999; 155:619–625.

14. Hagan CR, Rudin CM. Mobile genetic element activation and genotoxic cancer therapy: potential clinical implications. Am J Pharmacogenomics 2002; 2:25–35.
15. Nelson WG, De Marzo AM, Deweese TL, et al. Preneoplastic prostate lesions: an opportunity for prostate cancer prevention. Ann NY Acad Sci 2001; 952:135–144.
16. Rideout WM 3rd, Eggan K, Jaenisch R. Nuclear cloning and epigenetic reprogramming of the genome. Science 2001; 293:1093–1098.
17. Nelson WG, De Marzo AM, DeWeese TL. The molecular pathogenesis of prostate cancer: Implications for prostate cancer prevention. Urology 2001; 57:39–45.
18. Howell CY, Bestor TH, Ding F, et al. Genomic imprinting disrupted by a maternal effect mutation in the Dnmt1 gene. Cell 2001; 104:829–838.
19. El-Osta A, Wolffe AP. DNA methylation and histone deacetylation in the control of gene expression: basic biochemistry to human development and disease. Gene Express 2000; 9:63–75.
20. Zuccotti M, Garagna S, Redi CA. Nuclear transfer, genome reprogramming and novel opportunities in cell therapy. J Endocrinol Invest 2000; 23:623–629.
21. Feinberg AP. Cancer epigenetics takes center stage. Proc Natl Acad Sci USA 2001; 98:392–394.
22. Feinberg AP. DNA methylation, genomic imprinting and cancer. Curr Topics Microbiol Immunol 2000; 249:87–99.
23. Hu L, Troyanovsky B, Zhang X, Trivedi P, Ernberg I, Klein G. Differences in the immunogenicity of latent membrane protein 1 (LMP1) encoded by Epstein–Barr virus genomes derived from LMP1-positive and -negative nasopharyngeal carcinoma. Cancer Res 2000; 60:5589–5593.
24. Rice JC, Allis CD. Histone methylation versus histone acetylation: new insights into epigenetic regulation. Curr Opin Cell Biol 2001; 13:263–273.
25. Kruhlak MJ, Hendzel MJ, Fischle W, et al. Regulation of global acetylation in mitosis through loss of histone acetyltransferases and deacetylases from chromatin. J Biol Chem 2001; 276:38,307–38,319.
26. Surani MA. Genetics: immaculate misconception. Nature 2002; 416:491–493.
27. Surani MA. Imprinting and the initiation of gene silencing in the germ line. Cell 1998; 93:309–312.
28. Costa M, Klein CB. Nickel carcinogenesis, mutation, epigenetics, or selection. Environ Health Perspect 1999; 107:A438–A439.
29. Breivik J, Gaudernack G. Genomic instability, DNA methylation, and natural selection in colorectal carcinogenesis. Semin Cancer Biol 1999; 9:245–254.
30. Breivik J, Gaudernack G. Carcinogenesis and natural selection: a new perspective to the genetics and epigenetics of colorectal cancer. Adv Cancer Res 1999; 76:187–212.
31. Kinzler KW, Vogelstein B. Landscaping the cancer terrain. Science 1998; 280:1036–1037.
32. Baylin SB, Herman JG. DNA hypermethylation in tumorigenesis: epigenetics joins genetics. Trends Genet 2000; 16:168–174.
33. Esteller M, Catasus L, Matias-Guiu X, et al. hMLH1 promoter hypermethylation is an early event in human endometrial tumorigenesis. Am J Pathol 1999; 155:1767–1772.
34. Esteller M, Hamilton SR, Burger PC, Baylin SB, Herman JG. Inactivation of the DNA repair gene O6-methylguanine-DNA methyltransferase by promoter hypermethylation is a common event in primary human neoplasia. Cancer Res 1999; 59:793–797.
35. Esteller M, Sanchez-Cespedes M, Rosell R, Sidransky D, Baylin SB, Herman JG. Detection of aberrant promoter hypermethylation of tumor suppressor genes in serum DNA from non-small cell lung cancer patients. Cancer Res 1999; 59:67–70.
36. Jones PA, Laird PW. Cancer epigenetics comes of age. Nat Genet 1999; 21:163–167.
37. Tycko B. Epigenetic gene silencing in cancer. J Clin Invest 2000; 105:401–407.
38. Akhtar M, Cheng Y, Magno RM, et al. Promoter methylation regulates Helicobacter pylori-stimulated cyclooxygenase-2 expression in gastric epithelial cells. Cancer Res 2001; 61:2399–2403.
39. Ahluwalia A, Yan P, Hurteau JA, et al. DNA methylation and ovarian cancer. I. Analysis of CpG island hypermethylation in human ovarian cancer using differential methylation hybridization. Gynecol Oncol 2001; 82:261–268.
40. Ahluwalia A, Hurteau JA, Bigsby RM, Nephew KP. DNA methylation in ovarian cancer. II. Expression of DNA methyltransferases in ovarian cancer cell lines and normal ovarian epithelial cells. Gynecol Oncol 2001; 82:299–304.
41. Ng HH, Zhang Y, Hendrich B, et al. MBD2 is a transcriptional repressor belonging to the MeCP1 histone deacetylase complex. Nat Genet 1999; 23:58–61.
42. Wade PA, Gegonne A, Jones PL, Ballestar E, Aubry F, Wolffe AP. Mi-2 complex couples DNA methylation to chromatin remodelling and histone deacetylation. Nat Genet 1999; 23:62–66.

43. Nan BC, Shao DM, Chen HL, et al. Alteration of N-acetylglucosaminyltransferases in pancreatic carcinoma. Glycoconj J 1998; 15:1033–1037.

44. Barbieri R, Mischiati C, Piva R, et al. DNA methylation of the Ha-ras-1 oncogene in neoplastic cells. Anticancer Res 1989; 9:1787–1791.

45. Hanada M, Delia D, Aiello A, Stadtmauer E, Reed JC. bcl-2 gene hypomethylation and high-level expression in B-cell chronic lymphocytic leukemia. Blood 1993; 82:1820–1828.

46. Ray JS, Harbison ML, McClain RM, Goodman JI. Alterations in the methylation status and expression of the raf oncogene in phenobarbital-induced and spontaneous B6C3F1 mouse live tumors. Mol Carcinog 1994; 9:155–166.

47. Rao PM, Antony A, Rajalakshmi S, Sarma DS. Studies on hypomethylation of liver DNA during early stages of chemical carcinogenesis in rat liver. Carcinogenesis 1989; 10:933–937.

48. Vachtenheim J, Horakova I, Novotna H. Hypomethylation of CCGG sites in the 3' region of H-ras protooncogene is frequent and is associated with H-ras allele loss in non-small cell lung cancer. Cancer Res 1994; 54:1145–1148.

49. Feinberg AP, Vogelstein B. Hypomethylation of ras oncogenes in primary human cancers. Biochem Biophys Res Commun 1983; 111:47–54.

50. Feinberg AP, Vogelstein B. Hypomethylation distinguishes genes of some human cancers from their normal counterparts. Nature 1983; 301:89–92.

51. Chandler LA, DeClerck YA, Bogenmann E, Jones PA. Patterns of DNA methylation and gene expression in human tumor cell lines. Cancer Res 1986; 46:2944–2949.

52. Stephenson J, Akdag R, Ozbek N, Mufti GJ. Methylation status within exon 3 of the c-myc gene as a prognostic marker in myeloma and leukaemia. Leuk Res 1993; 17:291–293.

53. Issa JP. The epigenetics of colorectal cancer. Ann NY Acad Sci 2000; 910:140–153; discussion 153–155.

54. Yeager TR, DeVries S, Jarrard DF, et al. Overcoming cellular senescence in human cancer pathogenesis. Genes Dev 1998; 12:163–174.

55. Markowitz S, Wang J, Myeroff L, et al. Inactivation of the type II TGF-beta receptor in colon cancer cells with microsatellite instability. Science 1995; 268:1336–1368.

56. Boland CR, Thibodeau SN, Hamilton SR, et al. A National Cancer Institute Workshop on Microsatellite Instability for cancer detection and familial predisposition: development of international criteria for the determination of microsatellite instability in colorectal cancer. Cancer Res 1998; 58:5248–5257.

57. Zheng M, Wang H, Zhang H, et al. The influence of the p53 gene on the in vitro chemosensitivity of colorectal cancer cells. J Cancer Res Clin Oncol 1999; 125:357–360.

58. Eads CA, Danenberg KD, Kawakami K, et al. MethyLight: a high-throughput assay to measure DNA methylation. Nucleic Acids Res 2000; 28:E32.

59. Mintz A, Debinski W. Cancer genetics/epigenetics and the X chromosome: possible new links for malignant glioma pathogenesis and immune-based therapies. Crit Rev Oncog 2000; 11:77–95.

60. Herman JG, Graff JR, Myohanen S, Nelkin BD, Baylin SB. Methylation-specific PCR: a novel PCR assay for methylation status of CpG islands. Proc Natl Acad Sci USA 1996; 93:9821–9826.

61. Wei SH, Chen CM, Strathdee G, et al. Methylation microarray analysis of late-stage ovarian carcinomas distinguishes progression-free survival in patients and identifies candidate epigenetic markers. Clin Cancer Res 2002; 8:2246–2252.

62. Chen CM, Chen HL, Hsiau TH, et al. Methylation target array for rapid analysis of CpG island hypermethylation in multiple tissue genomes. Am J Pathol 2003; 163:37–45.

63. Xiong Z, Laird PW. COBRA: a sensitive and quantitative DNA methylation assay. Nucleic Acids Res 1997; 25:2532–2534.

64. Adorjan P, Distler J, Lipscher E, et al. Tumour class prediction and discovery by microarray-based DNA methylation analysis. Nucleic Acids Res 2002; 30:e21.

65. Hatada I, Kato A, Morita S, et al. A microarray-based method for detecting methylated loci. J Hum Genet 2002; 47:448–451.

66. Shi H, Yan PS, Chen CM, et al. Expressed CpG island sequence tag microarray for dual screening of DNA hypermethylation and gene silencing in cancer cells. Cancer Res 2002; 62:3214–3220.

67. Momparler RL, Cote S, Eliopoulos N. Pharmacological approach for optimization of the dose schedule of 5-aza-2'-deoxycytidine (Decitabine) for the therapy of leukemia. Leukemia 1997; 11(Suppl 1):S1–S6.

# 25 Novel Molecular and Genetic Prognostic Biomarkers in Prostate Cancer

*Arnab Chakravarti, MD
and Gary Guotang Zhai, PhD*

### Contents

### Summary

Prostate cancer is responsible for 3% of all deaths in the Western world in men over 55 yr of age. An urgent yet challenging priority in cancer biology is to detect or identify the sequential genetic and epigenetic events early enough through characterizing cancer-associated genes and their protein products. At a specific stage, biomarkers reflect the physiologic state of a cell and might be vital for the identification of early cancer and subjects at risk of developing cancer. Biomarkers have become an important diagnostic tool in prostate cancer. With the advent and recent successes in functional genomics and proteomics, we are experiencing growing interest in discovering more molecular-based prognostic factors that could be utilized to assay the original needle biopsy specimen to tailor the primary treatment for individual prostate cancer patients. As targeted therapy in oncology becomes increasingly powerful, there is a significant interest in finding prognostic markers in prostate cancer that could be used as targets for novel biotherapies. This chapter discusses a series of existing and emerging molecular-based prognostic markers generated from the ongoing research in genomic, genetic, and proteomic approaches that identify molecular signatures such as gene expression profiles.

**Key Words:** Prostate cancer; prognosis; molecular/genetic biomarkers; cell cycle; signal transduction.

From: *Cancer Drug Discovery and Development: The Oncogenomics Handbook*
Edited by: W. J. LaRochelle and R. A. Shimkets © Humana Press Inc., Totowa, NJ

# 1. INTRODUCTION

A tumor is an unwanted organ, progressively formed through stepwise accumulation of a number of events, genetic and epigenetic, arising in a single cell over a long time interval *(1)*. An urgent yet challenging priority in cancer biology is to detect or identify these sequential events early enough through characterizing cancer-associated genes and their protein products. At a specific stage, biomarkers reflect the physiologic state of a cell and might be vital for the identification of early cancer and subjects at risk of developing cancer. Molecular profiling of cancer cell gene expression could prove to be instrumental in identifying the sensitivity of cancer cells to specific therapeutic interventions and, hence, serves as an efficient tool in discovering more molecular biomarkers for cancer control and prevention.

Prostate cancer (CaP) is responsible for 3% of all deaths in the Western world in men over 55 yr of age. Biomarkers have become an important diagnostic tool in prostate cancer. The discovery of the serum marker prostate-specific antigen (PSA) and its test have revolutionized the early detection of CaP *(2)*. Although PSA is effective in identifying men who may have CaP, it is often elevated in men with benign prostatic hyperplasia, prostatitis, and other nonmalignant disorders *(2)*. The prognostic value of the Gleason score is limited by the fact that the vast majority of prostate cancer patients presented with moderately differentiated tumors (e.g., Gleason score of 6) in the PSA era, limiting the prognostic utility of morphologic features for this subgroup of patients. Given these drawbacks, identification of additional CaP-specific molecular markers is thus needed to refine the diagnosis as well as prognosis for CaP. CaP-associated molecular genetic alterations are being uncovered through (1) analyses of genes commonly involved in human cancer, (2) positional cloning of putative genes on frequently affected chromosome loci in CaP, and (3) gene expression profiling of normal and tumor specimens of patients with CaP *(3)*.

With the advent and recent successes in functional genomics and proteomics, we are experiencing growing interest in discovering more molecular-based prognostic factors that could be utilized to assay the original needle biopsy specimen to tailor the primary treatment for individual prostate cancer patients *(4–7)*. As targeted therapy in oncology becomes increasingly powerful, there is a significant interest in finding prognostic markers in prostate cancer that could be used as targets for novel biotherapies. Many molecular- and genetic-based biomarkers have been discovered over the last two decades and are summarized in Table 1 and in ref. *8*. This chapter discusses a series of existing and emerging molecular-based prognostic markers generated from the ongoing research in genomic, genetic, and proteomic approaches that identify molecular signatures such as gene expression profiles.

# 2. CELL CYCLE AND PROLIFERATION MARKERS

It has been determined that specific cell cycle regulators are associated with adverse outcome in prostate cancer *(9)*. Through the G1- to S-phase transition of the cell cycle, cyclin D1 is a critical modulator of progression and frequently overexpressed in malignancies. *Cyclin D1* was shown to play a role in both breast and prostate tumorigenesis by mediating hormone receptor signaling *(9)* and its overexpression is linked to the subsequent development of distant metastasis in prostate cancers *(10)*. The Cip/Kip and INK4 groups of cyclin-dependent kinase inhibitors have been found to be of prognostic value in prostate cancer *(9,11,12,75–77)*. Loss of *p27* expression has been linked with adverse disease outcome in a number of studies *(9,11,12)*. Overexpression of p34$^{cdc2}$ cyclin-depen-

Table 1
List of Prognostic Markers Categorized Based on Their Biological Functions and Discussed in This Chapter

| Biomarkers | Functional Category | Prognostic Value Maturity | Method | Ref. |
|---|---|---|---|---|
| cyclin D1 | Cell cycle | Investigational | Immunoassay | 9,10 |
| p27 | Cell cycle | Investigational | Immunoassay | 9,11,12 |
| p34cdc2 | Cell cycle | Investigational | Immunoassay | 13 |
| Ki-67(MIB-1) | Cell proliferation | Investigational | Immunoassay | 14–19 |
| VEGF | Angiogenesis | Clinically employed | Immunoassay | 20–25 |
| Endothelin-1 | Angiogenesis | Investigational | Immunoassay | 23 |
| blc-2 | Apoptosis | Investigational | Immunoassay | 26–36 |
| bax | Apoptosis | Investigational | Immunoassay | 26–36 |
| bcl-x | Apoptosis | Investigational | Immunoassay | 26–36 |
| p53 | Tumor suppressor | Investigational | Immunoassay | 37–44 |
| PTEN/MMAC1 | Tumor suppressor | Investigational | Immunoassay | 45–48 |
| caveolin-1 | Signal transduction | Investigational | Immunoassay | 49–55 |
| HER-2/neu | Signal transduction | Clinically employed | Immunoassay | 14,35,56–59 |
| EGFR | Signal transduction | Clinically employed | Immunoassay | 60–66 |
| Syndecan-1 | Other type | Investigational | Immunoassay | 67 |
| TRPV6 | Other type | Investigational | mRNA expression | 68,69 |
| EBAG9/RCAS1 | Other type | Investigational | Immunoassay | 70–72 |
| Bax inhibitor-1 | Other type | Investigational | Real-time RT-PCR | 73 |
| EZH2 | Other type | Investigational | GeneChip analysis | 74 |

dent kinase in the S to $G_2M$ transition of the cell cycle has been found to have connection with aggressive high-grade disease with increased incidence of biochemical failure after primary therapy (13).

For cell proliferation markers, immunohistochemical analysis using MIB-1/Ki-67 antibody has become the standard for quantifying cell cycle progression in human tissues (14, 15), where, generally, >16–20% MIB-1 staining indicates a high proliferation rate and an adverse prognosis (14–19). Pollack et al. recently reported a study with pretreatment archival prostate biopsy tumor tissue available from stage T1–T4 prostate cancer patients treated with external beam radiotherapy (78). This investigation helped establish the significance of MIB-1/Ki-67 staining as a prognostic marker of treatment outcome for prostate cancer patients undergoing radiotherapy. The percentages of Ki-67-positive tumor cells, the Ki-67 labeling index (Ki-67 LI), were determined using immunohistochemical staining for MIB-1. Experimental analyses indicated that, for all patients, mean Ki-67 LI levels were higher with stage T3/T4 disease.

## 3. TUMOR SUPPRESSOR GENES

It has been well established that the *p53* tumor suppressor gene plays a critical role in cell cycle transition, DNA repair and apoptosis, and that *p53* or genes that affect *p53* function are mutated in most human tumors (37,38). It is also well documented that wild-type p53 is necessary to activate the signal transduction pathways involving apoptosis. The role of p53 is, therefore, important in assessing the response of tumors to ionizing radiation and chemotherapy (38). Growth arrest in wild-type *p53* is dependent on the activation of *p21* through inhibiting cyclin complexes and arresting cells in the G1- to S-phase transition (39–41). Through the activation of *bax* and downregulation of *bcl-2*, p53 plays a key role in apoptosis (42–44). However, the complex role of p53 can present opposing forces with respect to response to ionizing radiation. Xia et al. suggested that this might be the result of the fact that any decrease in apoptosis seen in *p53*-deficient cells might be offset by a defect in DNA repair (56).

Although tumor cells defective in the *p53* gene generally yield accumulation and overexpression of the p53 protein as determined by immunohistochemistry, there is often discordance between the mutation status of the *p53* gene and the evaluation of the protein levels (79–81). This experimental observation, together with the complicated role of p53 in cell cycle regulation, apoptosis, and DNA repair, has generated much confusion regarding *p53* and response to radiation. Expression of p53 has been associated with increased radiation sensitivity, decreased radiation sensitivity, or no effect (56,82–86). This confusion could be explained by the differences in techniques among studies, patient heterogeneity, relatively small patient populations, and discordance between protein expression and gene status. Further studies that determine *p53* status at both the protein and genetic levels that evaluate coexpression of p53 with other markers are needed to establish the potential clinical utility of *p53* status in assessing radiation response.

### 3.1. PTEN/MMAC1

Phosphatase and tensin homolog (PTEN) is a dual-specificity phosphatase that has activity against lipid and protein substrates. The identification of *PTEN* mutants that have defects in either lipid phosphatase activity or both lipid and protein phosphatase activities has made it possible to define the importance of each on different aspects of tumor growth. The *PTEN/MMAC1* tumor suppressor gene is deleted or mutated in a wide variety of cancers, including prostate cancer cell lines, xenografts, and clinical samples *(9,45,46)*. Biochemical and functional evidence that *PTEN/MMAC1* acted as a negative regulator of the phosphoinositide 3-kinase (PI3-kinase)/Akt pathway *(47)* was recently established. PTEN/MMAC1 was shown to exhibit the capacity of activating endogenous Akt in cells and inhibiting phosphorylation of 4E-BP1, a downstream target of the PI3-kinase/Akt pathway involved in protein translation, whereas a catalytically inactive, dominant negative PTEN/MMAC1 mutant enhances 4E-BP1 phosphorylation. More interestingly, elevated levels of Akt activation were detected in human prostate cancer cell lines and xenografts lacking PTEN/MMAC1 expression when compared with PTEN/MMAC1-positive prostate tumors or normal prostate tissue. PTEN expression loss has been associated with downregulation of the cyclin-dependent kinase inhibitor p27 and adverse outcome *(48)* and increasing grade and stage *(87)* in prostate cancer.

### *3.2. Caveolin-1*

Caveolin-1 (cav-1), the major protein component of caveolae, plays an important role in multiple signaling pathways, molecular transport, and cellular proliferation and differentiation in prostate cancer *(49–51)*. It was reported that cav-1 is secreted by androgen-insensitive prostate cancer cells and detected by Western blotting in the high-density lipoprotein fraction of serum specimens from patients with prostate cancer *(52,53)*, indicating that serum cav-1 has the power to differentiate between prostate cancer and benign prostatic hyperplasia patients and the potential to be an important biomarker for prostate cancer. It is recently established that cav-1 expression is significantly increased in primary and metastatic human prostate tumors after androgen ablation therapy *(54)*. Also, cav-1 is secreted by androgen-insensitive prostate carcinoma cells and this secretion is regulated by steroid hormones. In cases of clinically determined, localized prostate carcinoma, it was found that cav-1 expression is a novel prognostic marker with independent predictive value of biochemical recurrence. It was observed that the 5' promoter CpG islands of cav-1 were more methylated in tumor than in adjacent normal prostate cells, implying that cav-1 might serve as a tumor suppressor gene in prostate cancer *(55)*.

## 4. SIGNAL TRANSDUCTION MARKERS

### *4.1. HER-2 Oncoprotein Overexpression*

ERBB-2 or HER-2/neu, a member of the tyrosine kinase family, has been well studied in breast cancer *(88–91)*. Recent studies demonstrated poorer survival and response rates to specific chemotherapeutic agents in those patients whose primary breast tumors overexpress HER-2/neu *(91)*. It has been also shown that low *HER-2/neu* gene expression was associated with a better response to therapy *(57)*. This conclusion has led to the clinical testing of HER-2 as a useful standard of practice status for guiding treatment of breast cancer. For prostate cancer, previous studies also found that overexpression of HER-2 was associated with an adverse outcome *(9,35,56,58,59)*. For example, *HER-2* mRNA levels have been correlated with metastatic disease and androgen-independent hormone refractory progressive disease *(92)*. In a recent study, the prognostic relevance of HER-2 protein expression in patients undergoing curative radiotherapy (RT) was compared to the traditional prognostic factors such as pretreatment prostate-specific antigen (PSA) levels, biopsy Gleason score, and T category of the primary tumor *(93)*. The prognostic relevance of HER-2 expression was univariately associated with adverse outcome in terms of bio-chemical or clinical progression-free survival (B/C-PFS), clinical progression-free survival (C-PFS) and disease-specific survival (DSS). HER-2 expression, T category, and Gleason score were independently associated with clinical progression-free survival C-PFS, whereas only HER-2 expression and Gleason score were associated with DSS. Pretreatment PSA levels were associated only with B/C-PFS but not with C-PFS or DSS. This line of evidence demonstrates that expression of HER-2 is of prognostic significance in localized prostate cancer undergoing RT and alludes to that analysis for HER-2 may improve prognostic algorithms for clinically relevant end points other than biochemical relapse.

However, there are several conflicting lines of evidence showing no correlation between radiation response/local relapse and HER-2/neu expression *(94,95)*. However, most of the investigations in HER-2/neu have utilized immunohistochemical staining. Recently, fluorescent *in situ* hybridization (FISH) evaluation of gene amplification has become a more accurate and clinically meaningful measure of HER-2/neu status *(96)*. Future studies evaluating the prognostic significance of HER-2/neu and radiation sensitivity will likely employ both immunohistochemical and FISH analysis.

## 4.2. Cyclo-Oxygenase-2

It has been shown that cyclo-oxygenase-2 (COX-2) is induced by a variety of factors and is linked to carcinogenesis, tumor growth, and metastatic spread, such as upregulation in inflammatory conditions to suppress apoptosis and to promote tumor invasion and angio-genesis through metabolizing protaglandins *(97)*. Inhibitors of COX-2 can effect enhanced radiation sensitivity *(97–100)*. This, coupled with studies demonstrating that overexpres-sion of COX-2, might be related to radiation resistance, making this marker particularly appealing. Theoretically, the relatively nontoxic use of COX-2 inhibitors or nonsteroidal anti-inflammatory drugs used in combination with radiation might help to overcome the relative radioresistance of tumors overexpressing COX-2. Studies by Milas et al. *(97)* and Kishi et al. *(101)* clearly demonstrated enhancement of tumor response to gamma radiation by inhibiting the COX-2 enzyme. Pyo et al. *(98)* demonstrated that a selective COX-2 inhib-itor, NS-398, preferentially enhanced the effect of radiation on cells that overexpressed COX-2.

## 4.3. Other Growth Factor Receptors

### 4.3.1. EPIDERMAL GROWTH FACTOR RECEPTOR

The transmembrane protein epidermal growth factor receptor (EGFR) is a member of the ERBB family of tyrosine kinase receptors *(60–62)*. Significant studies have shown that molecular signaling transduction through this protein stimulates the cell cycle path-ways that control cell proliferation *(60)*. EGFR inhibitors generally produce the effects of antiproliferation, primarily inducing G1 cell cycle arrest. Moreover, EGFR inhibitors increase radiation-induced apoptosis and hinder radiation-induced DNA damage repair *(63,64)*. Recent research efforts have been focusing on utilizing antibodies to EGFR, coupling with radiation therapy so as to improve response *(64–66)*. Significantly enhanced antitumor activity in cell lines treated with a combination of radiation therapy and antibody to EGFR has been demonstrated. This kind of strategy of discovering molecular markers linked to the phenotype of radiation resistance, trying to regulate and use these markers as direct targets for therapeutic interventions, underscores the great potential of molecular markers as they relate to molecular radiation oncology.

### 4.3.2. INSULIN-LIKE GROWTH FACTOR

The type I insulin-like growth factor receptor (IGF-1R) plays a central role in mediating cell adhesion, cell growth, and protection from apoptosis (102–105). Overexpression of IGF-1R has been demonstrated in vitro to be associated with radiation resistance. For example, in mouse embryo fibroblast cell lines overexpressing IGF-1R, Tezuka et al. demonstrated clonogenic radiation resistance and resistance to the induction of apoptosis after gamma irradiation (106). Peretz and his colleagues have demonstrated a link between ATM function and IGF-1R expression, suggesting that reduced expression of IGF-1R contributes to the radiosensitivity of AT cells (105). It was also demonstrated in their experiment that interference with the IGF-1R pathway by either expression of a dominant negative IGF-1R construct or treatment of cultured cells with a neutralizing antibody to the extracellular domain can sensitize cells to ionizing radiation. High levels of IGF-1R was shown to confer radioresistance in a fibroblast cell line and the radioresistant phenotype was reversed when the cells were incubated with antisense oligonucleotides targeted to IGF-1R mRNA (107). A previous study also demonstrated that Tyrphostin AG1024, a selective inhibitor of IGF-1R, enhances radiation sensitivity and amplifies radiation-induced apoptosis in a human breast cancer cell line MCF-7.

In human glioblastoma cell lines with equivalent levels of EGFR expression, Chakravarti and his colleagues observed significantly different sensitivities to EGFR receptor tyrosine kinase inhibitor therapy (103). The resistant cell line demonstrated upregulation of IGF-1R. Cotargeting of IGF-1R and EGFR greatly promoted both spontaneous and radiation-induced apoptosis. These studies strongly support a potential role for IGF-1R as a prognostic factor for radiation resistance and as a target for therapeutic intervention to improve radiocurability.

## 5. APOPTOSIS MARKERS:
### bcl-2, bax, AND bcl-x

Suppression of overexpression of apoptosis genes or downregulation of proapoptotic genes can promote radioresistant phenotypes. For instance, the protein product of the *bcl-2* oncogene enhances cell survival by suppressing apoptosis (26). bax, a related homolog of the bcl-2 protein, can form heterodimers with bcl-2 and, therefore, antagonize its function and promote apoptosis (27,102). Therefore, the combination of overexpression of bcl-2 and low expression of bax are hypothetically associated with decreased apoptotic response to radiation and increased radiation resistance. On the contrary, increased bax and low bcl-2 should dictate increased apoptotic response and higher sensitivity to radiation. Recent studies in bcl-2 family proteins have established the connection of the overexpression of the antiapoptosis protein bcl-2 with decreased expression of the proapoptotic protein bax and adverse outcome in prostate cancer associated with resistance to cytotoxic chemotherapy in patients with hormone-refractory disease (28–30). Upregulation of bcl-2 expression upon radiation in locally recurrent tumors has been documented (31–33). Since the establishment of the experimental link of bcl-2 overexpression to clinical treatment failure, bcl-2 started to be viewed as a marker of aggressive tumor attributes and as an etiologic factor of resistance to androgen ablation and radiation (34).

bax is a proapoptotic protein and it was expected that its overexpression in tumors treated by radiation would give rise to increased cell death and improved outcome compared with tumors that had normal bax expression. For bax expression, prior studies on the usefulness of bax as a pretreatment predictor of outcome after radiotherapy in patients with prostate carcinoma were limited and the results were inconsistent *(35,36)*. In the first study, the expression levels of bax and bcl-2 were related inversely to freedom from recurrence, and a high bcl-2 : bax ratio was correlated with poor therapeutic responsiveness *(35)*.

## 6. ANGIOGENESIS MARKERS

The commonly evaluated molecular markers for angiogenesis include the microvessel density and vascular endothelial growth factor (VEGF). A number of very interesting and significant laboratory and clinical studies employing cell lines transformed to overexpress VEGF have been performed to evaluate angiogenic molecular markers as they relate to radiation sensitivity. Gupta's group demonstrated that VEGF enhanced endothelial cell survival and VEGF-positive xenografts were more resistant to the cytotoxic effects of ionizing radiation. Treatment with anti-VEGF antibody, on the other hand, enhanced radiation sensitivity *(20)*. It was demonstrated that blockade of the VEGF stress response enhanced the antitumor effects of radiation *(21)*. Geng et al. also presented evidence that inhibition of VEGF signaling can lead to reversal of radiation resistance *(22)*. Many studies have provided strong evidence that overexpression of VEGF relates to radiation resistance. Its reversal might be achieved through specific targeting of the VEGF pathway.

A different angiogenic factor, Endothelin-1, was found in high concentration in seminal fluid that appeared to be important in prostate cancer development and progression *(23)*. It stimulates prostate cancer cell proliferation in vitro and enhances the mitogenic effects of insulin-like growth factor-1 and other growth factors, and it shows increased expression in prostate cancer primary tumor specimens and metastases *(24)*. Endothelin-1 seems to play a major role in the growth and angiogenesis of prostate cancer and in the pathophysiology of its metastasis to bone *(25)*.

## 7. OTHER NEWLY IDENTIFIED MARKERS

### 7.1. EZH2 and Syndecan-1

Recent analysis by gene expression profiling shows that the polycomb group protein enhancer of zeste homolog 2 (EZH2) was overexpressed in hormone-refractory, metastatic prostate cancer. Clinically localized prostate cancers that express higher concentration of EZH2 demonstrated a poorer prognosis, suggesting that dysregulated expression of EZH2 might play a role in the progression of prostate cancer. It might be considered, given this observation, as a marker that distinguishes indolent prostate cancer from those aggressive forms *(74)*.

More recently, Zellweger et al. tested several molecular markers on a prostate tissue microarray (TMA) *(67)* that included syndecan-1 (CD-138), a proteoglycan that has been found to be of prognostic importance in various human tumors *(108–112)*. They also performed the analysis of respective expression status of Ki-67, bcl-2, p53, CD-10 (neutral endopeptidase), and syndecan-1 (CD-138) by immunohistochemistry. This tissue microarray analysis demonstrated that Gleason grade and Ki-67 Labeling Index (Ki-67 LI) were independent predictors of early recurrence and poor survival, whereas bcl-2 predicts early recurrence and p53 was associated with poor survival. It was also revealed that syndecan-1 overexpression was associated with early recurrence and with tumor-specific survival, high Gleason grade, Ki-67 LI, and bcl-2 overexpression. The results of this TMA study enforced the prognostic importance of Gleason grading and Ki-67 LI in prostate cancer, as compared to a less pronounced role of bcl-2, and p53. Most significantly, they demonstrated a very efficient approach in identifying new molecular markers such as syndecan-1, which could be developed into a new prognostic biomarker.

### 7.2. Ca²⁺-Selective Cation Channel TRPV6

The epithelial $Ca^{2+}$ cation channel TRP family members have been shown to exhibit cellular homeostatic and regulatory functions. Alterations in their expression might be associated with malignant growth. The gene of the $Ca^{2+}$-selective cation channel CaT-L or *TRPV6* is not expressed in benign prostate tissues, including benign prostate hyperplasia, but is upregulated in prostate cancer *(68)*. Fixemer et al. reported very recently on the differential expression of *TRPV6* mRNA in prostate tissue obtained from 140 patients with prostate cancer *(69)*. They showed, via *in situ* hybridization, that *TRPV6* transcripts were undetectable in benign prostate tissue, high-grade prostatic intraepithelial neoplasia, incidental adenocarcinoma, and all tumors less than 2.3 $cm^3$. Their data demonstrated that TRPV6 expression, as a plasma membrane $Ca^{2+}$ channel, has a direct relationship with prostate cancer progression, thus representing a prognostic marker and a promising target for new therapeutic intervention for prostate cancer *(69)*.

### 7.3. EBAG9/RCAS1 Expression

*EBAG9*, estrogen receptor-binding fragment-associated gene 9, has been identified as a primary estrogen-responsive gene from MCF-7 human breast cancer cells *(70)*. EBAG9 is identical to the receptor-binding cancer antigen expressed on SiSo cells (RCAS1), which has been reported as a cancer cell surface antigen implicated in immune escape *(71)*. Takahashi and his colleagues have just examined EBAG9 expression in human prostatic tissues using normal prostatic epithelial cells and PC-3, DU145, and LNCaP cancer cells by Western blot analysis and explored its prognostic value in patients with prostatic cancer *(72)*. EBAG9 was much more profusely expressed in the prostate cancer cells than the normal epithelial cells, which correlated well with advanced pathologic stages and high Gleason score. Positive EBAG9 immunoreactivity significantly correlated with poor PSA failure-free survival. Immunodetection of EBAG9/RCAS1 expression can be a negative prognostic indicator for patients with prostatic cancer.

### 7.4. bax Inhibitor-1

Grzmil et al. recently conducted some analysis work of differential gene expression of putative prostate tumor markers by comparing the expression levels of over 400 cancer-related genes using the cDNA array technique in a set of capsule-invasive prostate tumor and matched normal prostate tissue *(73)*. Using Northern blot and Western blot analyses, they confirmed the overexpression of bax inhibitor-1 (BI-1) in prostate carcinoma and prostate cancer cell lines. Using quantitative real-time reverse transcription–polymerase chain reaction (RT-PCR), they successfully detected upregulated BI-1 expression in 11 of 17 prostate tumors on intact RNAs from 17 paired laser-captured microdissected epithelial tissue samples. In addition, it was demonstrated that BI-1 expression was downregulated in stromal cells as compared to matched normal epithelial cells of the prostate. *In situ* hybridization experiments on prostate sections also revealed that BI-1 expression was mainly restricted to epithelial cells. They found no significant difference in BI-1 expression compared to normal epithelial prostate tissue via quantitative RT-PCR on RNAs derived from benign prostate hyperplasia (BPH) samples. To determine the function of BI-1 in vitro, human PC-3, LNCaP, and DU-145 prostate carcinoma cells were transfected with small interfering double-strand RNA (siRNA) oligonucleotides against the BI-1 gene, leading to a specific downregulation of BI-1 expression. Furthermore, transfection of PC-3, LNCaP, and DU-145 cells with BI-1 sequence-specific siRNAs yielded a large increase in spontaneous apoptosis in all cell lines. Their results demonstrated that the human BI-1 gene could serve as a prostate cancer expression marker and as a potential target for developing therapeutic strategies for prostate cancer.

## 8. CONCLUSIONS

The application of molecular and genetic markers in clinical oncology, including radiation oncology as prognostic factors and as potential targets for therapeutic intervention, continues to evolve rapidly, although many prognostic markers have been discovered over the last two decades. Employing molecular and genetic markers as prognostic factors has a tremendous potential because they relate to control of disease and response to therapies. There is still much to be done in evaluating molecular markers despite the rapid expansion of data and ongoing studies. It is currently lagging far behind molecular strategies in combination with chemotherapy for systemic control of disease. Discovering and using more novel molecular and genetic prognostic biomarkers in prostate cancer and beyond will prove vitally important in guiding clinical treatment, improving patient overall outcome.

## REFERENCES

1. Hanahan D, Weinberg RA. The hallmarks of cancer. Cell 2000; 100:57–70.
2. Garnick MB, Fair WR. Combating prostate cancer. Sci Am 1998; 279:74–83.
3. Augustus M, Moul JW, Srivastava S. Gene expression profiling of normal and tumor specimens of patients with prostate cancer. In: Srivastava S, Henson DE, Gazden A, eds. Molecular pathology of early cancer. Amsterdam, IOS, 1999:321–340.
4. Bubendorf L. High-throughput microarray technologies: from genomics to clinics. Eur Urol 2001; 40: 231–238.
5. Bok RA, Small EJ. Bloodborne biomolecular markers in prostate cancer development and progression. Nat Rev Cancer 2002; 2:918–926.
6. Sidransky D. Emerging molecular markers of cancer. Nat Rev Cancer 2002; 2:210–219.
7. Alers JC, Rochat J, Krijtenburg PJ, Hop WC, Kranse R, Rosenberg C, et al. Identification of genetic markers for prostatic cancer progression. Lab Invest 2000; 80:931–942.
8. Abate-Shen C, Shen MM. Molecular genetics of prostate cancer. Genes Dev 2000; 14:2410–2434.
9. Amanatullah DF, Reutens AT, Zafonte BT, Fu M, Mani S, Pestell RG. Cell-cycle dysregulation and the molecular mechanisms of prostate cancer. Front Biosci 2000; 5:D372–D390.
10. Drobnjak M, Osman I, Scher HI, Fazzari M, Cordon-Cardo C. Overexpression of cyclin D1 is associated with metastatic prostate cancer to bone. Clin Cancer Res 2000; 6:1891–1895.
11. Yang RM, Naitoh J, Murphy M, Wang HJ, Phillipson J, deKernion JB, et al. Low p27 expression predicts poor disease-free survival in patients with prostate cancer. J Urol 1998; 159:941–945.
12. Kuczyk M, Machtens S, Hradil K, Schubach J, Christian W, Knuchel R, et al. Predictive value of decreased p27Kip1 protein expression for the recurrence-free and long-term survival of prostate cancer patients. Br J Cancer 1999; 81:1052–1058.
13. Kallakury BV, Sheehan CE, Ambros RA, Fisher HA, Kaufman RP Jr, Ross JS. Prognostic significance of p34cdc2 and cyclin D1 protein expression in prostatic adenocarcinomas. Cancer 1997; 80:753–763.

14. Goel A, Abou-Ellela A, DeRose PB. The prognostic significance of proliferation in prostate cancer. J Urol Pathol 1996; 4:213–223.

15. Scalzo DA, Kallakury BV, Gaddipati RV, Sheehan CE, Keys HM, Savage D, et al. Cell proliferation rate by MIB-1immunohistochemistry predicts post-radiation recurrence of prostatic adenocarcinomas. Am J Clin Pathol 1998; 109:163–168.

16. Visakorpi T. Proliferative activity determined by DNA flow cytometry and proliferating cell nuclear anti-gen (pcna) immunohistochemistry as a prognostic factor in prostatic carcinoma. J Pathol 1992; 168: 7–13.

17. Sadasivan R, Morgan R, Jennings S, Austenfeld M, Van Veldhuizen P, Stephens R, et al. Overexpression of HER-2/neu may be an indicator of poor prognosis in prostate cancer. J Urol 1993; 150:126–131.

18. Henke RP, Kruger E, Ayhan N, Hubner D, Hammerer P. Numerical chromosomal aberrations in prostate cancer: correlation with morphology and cell kinetics. Virchows Arch Pathol Anat Histopathol 1993; 422:61–66.

19. Kaibuchi T, Furuya Y, Akakura K, Masai M, Ito H. Changes in cell proliferation and apoptosis during local progression of prostate cancer. Anticancer Res 2000; 20:1135–1139.

20. Gupta VK, Jaskowiak NT, Beckett MA, Mauceri HJ, Grunstein J, Johnson RS, et al. Vascular endothelial growth factor enhances endothelial cell survival and tumor radioresistance. Cancer J 2002b; 8: 47–54.

21. Gorski DH, Beckett MA, Jaskowiak NT, Calvin DP, Mauceri HJ, Salloum RM, et al. Blockage of the vascular endothelial growth factor stress response increases the antitumor effects of ionizing radiation. Cancer Res 1999; 59:3374–3378.

22. Geng L, Donnelly E, McMahon G, Lin PC, Sierra-Rivera E, Oshinka H, et al. Inhibition of vascular endothelial growth factor receptor signaling leads to reversal of tumor resistance to radiotherapy. Cancer Res 2001; 61:2413–2419.

23. Battistini B, D'Orleans-Juste P, Sirois P. Endothelins: circulating plasma levels and presence in other biologic fluids. Lab Invest 1993; 68:600–628.

24. Nelson JB, Hedican SP, George DJ, Reddi AH, Piantadosi S, Eisenberger MA, et al. Identification of endothelin-1 in the pathophysiology of metastatic adenocarcinoma of the prostate. Nat Med 1995; 1: 944–949.

25. Kopetz ES, Nelson JB, Carducci MA. Endothelin-1 as a target for therapeutic intervention in prostate cancer. Invest New Drugs 2002; 20:173–182.

26. Reed JC. bcl-2 family proteins. Oncogene 1998; 17:3225–3236.

27. Harima Y, Nagata K, Harima K, Oka A, Ostapenko VV, Shikata N, et al. Bax and bcl-2 protein expression following radiation therapy versus radiation plus thermoradiotherapy in stage IIIB cervical carcinoma. Cancer 2000; 88:132–138.

28. Apakama I, Robinson MC, Walter NM, Charlton RG, Royds JA, Fuller CE, et al. bcl-2 overexpression combined with p53 protein accumulation correlates with hormone-refractory prostate cancer. Br J Cancer 1996; 74:1258–1262.

29. Furuya Y, Krajewski S, Epstein JI, Reed JC, Isaacs JT. Expression of bcl-2 and the progression of human and rodent prostatic cancers. Clin Cancer Res 1996; 2:389–398.

30. Kallakury BV, Figge J, Leibovich B, Hwang J, Rifkin M, Kaufman R, et al. Increased bcl-2 protein levels in prostatic adenocarcinomas are not associated with rearrangements in the 2.8 kb major breakpoint region or with p53 protein accumulation. Mod Pathol 1996; 9:41–47.

31. Huang A, Gandour-Edwards R, Rosenthal SA, Siders DB, Deitch AD, White RW. p53 and bcl-2 immunohistochemical alterations in prostate cancer treated with radiation therapy. Urology 1998; 51:346–351.

32. Rakozy C, Grignon DJ, Sarkar FH, Sakr WA, Littrup P, Forman J. Expression of bcl-2, p53, and p21 in benign and malignant prostatic tissue before and after radiation therapy. Mod Pathol 1998; 11: 892–899.

33. Grossfeld GD, Olumi AF, Connolly JA, Chew K, Gibney J, Bhargava V, et al. Locally recurrent prostate tumors following either radiation therapy or radical prostatectomy have changes in Ki-67 labeling index, p53 and bcl-2 immunoreactivity. J Urol 1998; 159:1437–1443.

34. Gettman MT, Bergstrahl EJ, Blute M. Prediction of patient outcome in pathologic stage T2 adenocarcinoma of the prostate: lack of significance for microvessel density. Urology 1998; 51:79–85.

35. Mackey TJ, Borkowski A, Amin P, Jacobs SC, Kyprianou N. bcl-2/bax ratio as a predictive marker for therapeutic response to radiotherapy in patients with prostate cancer. Urology 1998; 52:1085–1090.

36. Szostak MJ, Kaur P, Amin P, Jacobs SC, Kyprianou N. Apoptosis and bcl-2 expression in prostate cancer: significance in clinical outcome after brachytherapy. J Urol 2001; 165(6 Pt 1):2126–2130.

37. Agarwal ML, Agarwal A, Taylor WR, Stark GR. p53 controls both the G2/M and the G1 cell cycle checkpoints and mediates reversible growth arrest in human fibroblasts. Proc Natl Acad Sci USA 1995; 92:8493–8497.
38. Agarwal ML, Taylor WR, Chernov MV, Chernova OB, Stark GR. The p53 network. J Biol Chem 1998; 273:1–4.
39. Clarke AR, Purdie CA, Harrison DJ, Morris RG, Bird CC, Hooper ML, et al. Thymocyte apoptosis induced by p53-dependent and independent pathways. Nature 1993; 362:849–852.
40. Chang EH, Jang YJ, Hao Z, Murphy G, Rait A, Fee WE Jr, et al. Restoration of the G1 checkpoint and the apoptotic pathway mediated by wild-type p53 sensitizes squamous cell carcinoma of the head and neck to radiotherapy. Arch Otolaryngol Head Neck Surg 1997; 123:507–512.
41. Bouvard V, Zaitchouk T, Vacher M, Duthu A, Canivet M, Choisy-Rossi C, et al. Tissue and cell-specific expression of the p53-target genes: bax, fas, mdm2 and waf1/p21, before and following ionising irradiation in mice. Oncogene 2000; 19:649–660.
42. Lane DP. Cancer. p53, guardian of the genome. Nature 1992; 358:15–16.
43. El-Deiry WS, Harper JW, O'Connor PM, Velculescu VE, Canman CE, Jackman J, et al. WAF1/CIP1 is induced in p53-mediated G1 arrest and apoptosis. Cancer Res 1994; 54:1169–1174.
44. Jackel MC, Sellmann L, Dorudian MA, Youssef S, Fuzesi L. Prognostic significance of p53/bcl-2 co-expression in patients with laryngeal squamous cell carcinoma. Laryngoscope 2000; 110:1339–1345.
45. Graff JR, Konicek BW, McNulty AM, Wang Z, Houck K, Allen S, et al. Increased AKT activity contributes to prostate cancer progression by dramatically accelerating prostate tumor growth and diminishing p27Kip1 expression. J Biol Chem 2000; 275:24,500–24,505.
46. McMenamin ME, Soung P, Perera S, Kaplan I, Loda M, Sellers WR. Loss of PTEN expression in paraffin embedded primary prostate cancer correlates with high Gleason score and advanced stage. Cancer Res 1999; 59:4291–4296.
47. Wu X, Senechal K, Neshat MS, Whang YE, Sawyers CL. The PTEN/MMAC1 tumor suppressor phosphatase functions as a negative regulator of the phosphoinositide 3-kinase/Akt pathway. Proc Natl Acad Sci USA 1998; 95:15,587–15,591.
48. Heidenreich B, Heidenreich A, Sesterhenn A, Srivastava S, Moul JW, Sesterhenn IA. Aneuploidy of chromosome 9 and the tumor suppressor genes p16(INK4) and p15(INK4B) detected by in situ hybridization in locally advanced prostate cancer. Eur Urol 2000; 38:475–482.
49. Brinker DA, Ross JS, Tran TA, Jones DM, Epstein JI. Can ploidy of prostate carcinoma diagnosed on needle biopsy predict radical prostatectomy and grade? J Urol 1999; 162:2036–2039.
50. Razani B, Schlegel A, Liu J, Lisanti MP. Caveolin-1, a putative tumor suppressor gene. Biochem Soc Trans 2001; 29(Pt 4):494–499.
51. Li L, Yang G, Ebara S, Satoh T, Nasu Y, Timme TL, et al. Caveolin-1 mediates testosterone-stimulated survival/clonal growth and promotes metastatic activities in prostate cancer cells. Cancer Res 2001; 61:4386–4392.
52. Mouraviev V, Li L, Tahir SA, Yang G, Timme TM, Goltsov A, et al. The role of caveolin-1 in androgen insensitive prostate cancer. J Urol 2002; 168(4 Pt 1):1589–1596.
53. Tahir SA, Ren C, Timme TL, Gdor Y, Hoogeveen R, Morrisett JD, et al. Development of an immunoassay for serum caveolin-1: a novel biomarker for prostate cancer. Clin Cancer Res 2003; 9(10 Pt 1): 3653–3659.
54. Yang G, Truong LD, Wheeler TM, Thompson TC. Caveolin-1 expression in clinically confined human prostate cancer: a novel prognostic marker. Cancer Res 1999; 59:5719–5723.
55. Cui J, Rohr LR, Swanson G, Speights VO, Maxwell T, Brothman AR. Hypermethylation of the caveolin-1 gene promoter in prostate cancer. Prostate 2001; 46:249–256.
56. Xia F, Powell SN. The molecular basis of radiosensitivity and chemosensitivity in the treatment of breast cancer. Semin Radiat Oncol 2002; 12:296–304.
57. Formenti SC, Spicer D, Skinner K, Cohen D, Groshen S, Bettini A, et al. Low HER2/neu gene expression is associated with pathological response to concurrent paclitaxel and radiation therapy in locally advanced breast cancer. Int J Radiat Oncol Biol Phys 2002; 52:397–405.
58. Ross JS, Nazeer T, Church K, Amato C, Figge H, Rifkin MD, et al. Contribution of HER-2/neu oncogene expression to tumor grade and DNA content analysis in the prediction of prostatic carcinoma metastasis. Cancer 1993; 72:3020–3028.
59. Ross JS, Fletcher JA. The HER-2/neu oncogene in breast cancer: prognostic factor, predictive factor and target of therapy. Oncologist 1998; 3:237–252.

60. Wells A. EGF receptor. Int J Biochem Cell Biol 31:637–643.
61. Nicholson RI, Gee JM, Harper ME. 2001; EGFR and cancer prognosis. Eur J Cancer 1999; 37(Suppl 4): S9–S15.
62. Nicholson RI, Hutcheson IR, Harper ME, Knowlden JM, Barrow D, McClelland RA, et al. Modulation of epidermal growth factor receptor in endocrine-resistant, estrogen-receptor-positive breast cancer. Ann NY Acad Sci 2002; 963:104–115.
63. Harari PM, Huang SM. Epidermal growth factor receptor modulation of radiation response: preclinical and clinical development. Semin Radiat Oncol 2002; 12:21–26.
64. Huang SM, Li J, Armstrong EA, Harari PM. Modulation of radiation response and tumor-induced angiogenesis after epidermal growth factor receptor inhibition by ZD1839 (Iressa). Cancer Res 2002; 62: 4300–4306.
65. Wollman R, Yahalom J, Maxy R, Pinto J, Fuks Z. Effect of epidermal growth factor on the growth and radiation sensitivity of human breast cancer cells in vitro. Int J Radiat Oncol Biol Phys 1994; 30: 91–98.
66. Ciardiello F, Tortora G. A novel approach in the treatment of cancer: targeting the epidermal growth factor receptor. Clin Cancer Res 2001; 7:2958–2970.
67. Zellweger T, Ninck C, Mirlacher M, Annefeld M, Glass AG, Gasser TC, et al. Tissue microarray analysis reveals prognostic significance of syndecan-1 expression in prostate cancer. Prostate 2003; 55: 20–29.
68. Wissenbach U, Niemeyer BA, Fixemer T, Schneidewind A, Trost C, Cavalié A, et al. Expression of cat-like, a novel calcium-selective channel, correlates with the malignancy of prostate cancer. J Biol Chem 2001; 276:19,461–19,468.
69. Fixemer T, Wissenbach U, Flockerzi V, Bonkhoff H. Expression of the $Ca^{2+}$-selective cation channel TRPV6 in human prostate cancer: a novel prognostic marker for tumor progression. Oncogene 2003; 22:7858–7861.
70. Watanabe T, Inoue S, Hiroi H, Orimo A, Kawashima H, Muramatsu M. Isolation of estrogen-responsive genes with a CpG island library. Mol Cell Biol 1998; 18:442–449.
71. Nakashima M, Sonoda K, Watanabe T. Inhibition of cell growth and induction of apoptotic cell death by the human tumor-associated antigen RCAS1. Nat Med 1999; 5:938–942.
72. Takahashi S, Urano T, Tsuchiya F, Fujimura T, Kitamura T, Ouchi Y, et al. EBAG9/RCAS1 expression and its prognostic significance in prostatic cancer. Int J Cancer 2003; 106:310–315.
73. Grzmil M, Thelen P, Hemmerlein B, Schweyer S, Voigt S, Mury D, et al. Bax inhibitor-1 is overexpressed in prostate cancer and its specific down-regulation by RNA interference leads to cell death in human prostate carcinoma cells. Am J Pathol 2003; 163:543–542.
74. Varambally S, Dhanasekaran SM, Zhou M, Barrette TR, Kumar-Sinha C, Sanda MG, et al. The polycomb group protein EZH2 is involved in progression of prostate cancer. Nature 2002; 419:624–629.
75. Cheng L, Lloyd RV, Weaver AL, Pisansky TM, Cheville JC, Ramnani DM, et al. The cell cycle inhibitors p21WAF1 and p27KIP1 are associated with survival in patients treated by salvage prostatectomy after radiation therapy. Clin Cancer Res 2000; 6:1896–1899.
76. Kuczyk MA, Bokemeyer C, Hartmann J, Schubach J, Walter C, Machtens S, et al. Predictive value of altered p27Kip1 and p21WAF/Cip1 protein expression for the clinical prognosis of patients with localized prostate cancer. Oncol Rep 2001; 8:1401–1407.
77. Omar EA, Behlouli H, Chevalier S, Aprikian AG. Relationship of p21(WAF-I) protein expression with prognosis in advanced prostate cancer treated by androgen ablation. Prostate 2001; 49:191–199.
78. Cowen D, Troncoso P, Khoo VS, Zagars GK, von Eschenbach AC, Meistrich ML, et al. Ki-67 staining is an independent correlate of biochemical failure in prostate cancer treated with radiotherapy. Clin Cancer Res 2002; 8:1148–1154.
79. Iggo R, Gatter K, Bartek J, Lane D, Harris AL. Increased expression of mutant forms of p53 oncogene in primary lung cancer. Lancet 1990; 335:675–679.
80. Wilson GD, Richman PI, Dische S, Saunders MI, Robinson B, Daley FM, et al. p53 status of head and neck cancer: relation to biological characteristics and outcome of radiotherapy. Br J Cancer 1995; 71: 1248–1252.
81. Agarwal MK, Wolfman A, Stark GR. Regulation of p53 expression by the RAS-MAP kinase pathway. Oncogene 2001; 20:2527–2536.
82. Pirollo KF, Hao Z, Rait A, Jang YJ, Fee WE Jr, Ryan P, et al. p53 mediated sensitization of squamous cell carcinoma of the head and neck to radiotherapy. Oncogene 1997; 14:1735–1746.

83. Mineta H, Borg A, Dictor M, Wahlberg P, Akervall J, Wennerberg J. p53 mutation, but not p53 over-expression, correlates with survival in head and neck squamous cell carcinoma. Br J Cancer 1998; 78: 1084–1090.

84. Wouters BG, Denko NC, Giaccia AJ, Brown JM. A p53 and apoptotic independent role for p21waf1 in tumour response to radiation therapy. Oncogene 1999; 18:6540–6545.

85. Overgaard J, Yilmaz M, Guldberg P, Hansen LL, Alsner J. TP53 mutation is an independent prognostic marker for poor outcome in both node-negative and node-positive breast cancer. Acta Oncol 2000; 39: 327–333.

86. Wang Y, Li J, Booher RN, Kraker A, Lawrence T, Leopold WR, et al. Radiosensitization of p53 mutant cells by PDD0166285, a novel G(2) checkpoint abrogator. Cancer Res 2001; 61:8211–8217.

87. Nguyen TT, Nguyen CT, Gonzales FA, Nichols PW, Yu MC, Jones PA. Analysis of cyclin-dependent kinase inhibitor expression and methylation patterns in human prostate cancers. Prostate 2000; 43:233–242.

88. Allred DC, Clark GM, Molina R, Tandon AK, Schnitt SJ, Gilchrist KW, et al. Overexpression of HER-2/neu and its relationship with other prognostic factors change during the progression of in situ to invasive breast cancer. Hum Pathol 1992; 23:974–979.

89. Slamon DJ, Leyland-Jones B, Shak S, Fuchs H, Paton V, Bajamonde A, et al. Use of chemotherapy plus a monoclonal antibody against HER2 for metastatic breast cancer that overexpresses HER2. N Engl J Med 1999; 344:783–792.

90. Agrup M, Stal O, Olsen K, Wingren S. C-erbB-2 overexpression and survival in early onset breast cancer. Breast Cancer Res Treat 2000; 63:23–29.

91. Piccart M, Lohrisch C, Di Leo A, Larsimont D. The predictive value of HER2 in breast cancer. Oncology 2001; 61(Suppl 2):73–82.

92. Signoretti S, Montironi R, Manola J, Altimari A, Tam C, Bubley G, et al. HER-2-neu expression and progression toward androgen independence in human prostate cancer. J Natl Cancer Inst 2000; 92: 1918–1925.

93. Fossa A, Lilleby W, Fossa SD, Gaudernack G, Torlakovic G, Berner A. Independent prognostic significance of HER-2 oncoprotein expression in pN0 prostate cancer undergoing curative radiotherapy. Int J Cancer 2002; 99:100–105.

94. Pierce L. Radiotherapy for breast cancer in BRCA1/BRCA2 carriers: clinical issues and management dilemmas. Semin Radiat Oncol 2002; 12:352–361.

95. Ringberg A, Anagnostaki L, Anderson H, Idvall I, Ferno M. Cell biological factors in ductal carcinoma in situ (DCIS) of the breast-relationship to ipsilateral local recurrence and histopathological characteristics. Eur J Cancer 2001; 37:1514–1522.

96. Press MF, Slamon DJ, Flom KJ, Park J, Zhou JY, Bernstein L. Evaluation of HER-2/neu gene amplification and overexpression: comparison of frequently used assay methods in a molecularly characterized cohort of breast cancer specimens. J Clin Oncol 2002; 20:3095–3105.

97. Milas L. Cyclooxygenase-2 (COX-2) enzyme inhibitors as potential enhancers of tumor radioresponse. Semin Radiat Oncol 2001; 11:290–299.

98. Pyo H, Choy H, Amorino GP, Kim JS, Cao Q, Hercules SK, et al. A selective cyclooxygenase-2 inhibitor, NS-398, enhances the effect of radiation in vitro and in vivo preferentially on the cells that express cyclooxygenase-2. Clin Cancer Res 2001; 7:2998–3005.

99. Ferrandina G, Lauriola L, Distefano MG, Zannoni GF, Gessi M, Legge F, et al. Increased cyclooxygenase-2 expression is associated with chemotherapy resistance and poor survival in cervical cancer patients. J Clin Oncol 2002a; 20:973–981.

100. Ferrandina G, Lauriola L, Zannoni GF, Distefano MG, Legge F, Salutari V, et al. Expression of cyclooxygenase-2 (COX-2) in tumour and stroma compartments in cervical cancer: clinical implications. Br J Cancer 2002b; 87:1145–1152.

101. Kishi K, Petersen S, Petersen C, Hunter N, Mason K, Masferrer JL, et al. Preferential enhancement of tumor radioresponse by a cyclooxygenase-2 inhibitor. Cancer Res 2000; 60:1326–1331.

102. Reed JC. Dysregulation of apoptosis in cancer. J Clin Oncol 1999; 17:2941–2953.

103. Chakravarti A, Loeffler JS, Dyson NJ. Insulin-like growth factor receptor I mediates resistance to antiepidermal growth factor receptor therapy in primary human glioblastoma cells through continued activation of phosphoinositide 3-kinase signaling. Cancer Res 2002; 62:200–207.

104. Hassan AB, Macaulay VM. The insulin-like growth factor system as a therapeutic target in colorectal cancer. Ann Oncol 2002; 13:349–356.

105. Peretz S, Kim C, Rockwell S, Baserga R, Glazer PM. IGF1 receptor expression protects against micro-environmental stress found in the solid tumor. Radiat Res 2002; 158:174–180.

106. Tezuka M, Watanabe H, Nakamura S, Yu D, Aung W, Sasaki T, et al. Antiapoptotic activity is dispensable for insulin-like growth factor I receptor-mediated clonogenic radioresistance after gamma-irradiation. Clin Cancer Res 2001; 7:3206–3214.

107. Turner BC, Haffty BG, Narayanan L, Yuan J, Havre PA, Gumbs AA, et al. Insulin-like growth factor-I receptor overexpression mediates cellular radioresistance and local breast cancer recurrence after lumpectomy and radiation. Cancer Res 1997; 57:3079–3083.

108. Joensuu H, Anttonen A, Eriksson M, Makitaro R, Alfthan H, Kinnula V, et al. Soluble syndecan-1 and serum basic fibroblast growth factor are new prognostic factors in lung cancer. Cancer Res 2002; 62: 5210–5217.

109. Anttonen A, Heikkila P, Kajanti M, Jalkanen M, Joensuu H. High syndecan-1 expression is associated with favorable outcome in squamous cell lung carcinoma treated with radical surgery. Lung Cancer 2001; 32:297–305.

110. Wiksten JP, Lundin J, Nordling S, Kokkola A, Haglund CA. Prognostic value of syndecan-1 in gastric cancer. Anticancer Res 2000; 20(6D):4905–4907.

111. Seidel C, Sundan A, Hjorth M, Turesson I, Dahl IM, Abildgaard N, et al. Serum syndecan-1: a new independent prognostic marker in multiple myeloma. Blood 2000; 95:388–392.

112. Anttonen A, Kajanti M, Heikkila P, Jalkanen M, Joensuu H. Syndecan-1 expression has prognostic significance in head and neck carcinoma. Br J Cancer 1999; 79:558–564.

# 26 PSA in Prostate Cancer Diagnosis

*Pradip Datta, PhD, DABCC*

## CONTENTS

## SUMMARY

Significant improvement in prostate cancer diagnosis and monitoring of therapy has been made possible by the discovery and use of prostate-specific antigen (PSA) measurement in patient serum. Widespread use of the PSA test has resulted in significant prevention of death from this major cancer disease in males. PSA measurements are used not only to stage the patient's cancer or monitor therapy but also to screen for patients who need the prostate biopsy, a costly and painful process. There are controversies present with regard to the serum PSA cutoff (4.0 µg/mL), above which level the cancer is suspected. A lower cutoff (2.5 µg/mL) improves sensitivity of cancer detection but reduces the specificity, because benign diseases of the prostate also might raise serum PSA. Measurement of serum PSA isoforms—complex or free PSA—has been reported to improve the efficiency of the PSA test. The main way serum PSA is measured is by immunoassays, of which many commercial methods, applied on automated systems, are available. It is, however, important to consider issues like hook and heterophilic interference that could affect some PSA assays. Future improvements in prostate cancer diagnosis include markers for aggressive than the slow-growth cancer and use of multiple markers to improve the efficiency of the diagnosis.

**Key Words:** Prostate cancer; prostate-specific antigen (PSA); digital rectal examination (DRE); PSA immunoassay; PSA isoforms; prostate cancer diagnosis.

## 1. INTRODUCTION

Prostate cancer (CaP) is a major cancer found in men and a leading cause of death. Like any cancer, an early detection, followed by treatment, increases the disease-free survival rate significantly. The incidence of CaP also increases with age. It is estimated from autopsy

From: *Cancer Drug Discovery and Development: The Oncogenomics Handbook*
Edited by: W. J. LaRochelle and R. A. Shimkets © Humana Press Inc., Totowa, NJ

studies that 30% of men in their eighth decade have unsuspected or latent carcinoma of the prostate. The clinical problems associated with the diagnosis and treatment of CaP are as varied as its presentation. The main screening method for the physician has so far been the digital rectal examination (DRE) and transrectal ultrasound (TRUS), both suffering from poor positive predicative value (PPV) of only 22–36% and 15–41%, respectively (1). The confirmatory test for CaP, prostate biopsy, is not suited for screening, because of the morbidity and cost associated with the process. Serum marker tests normally afford the most efficient screening for diseases. Elevated levels of serum acid phosphatase have long been taken to be indicative of the spread of prostate cancer outside of the gland, but many patients with metastatic disease have normal serum levels of acid phosphatase (2). CaP diagnosis and treatment, however, has been revolutionized by the use of prostate-specific antigen (PSA) concentration in patient serum. Several studies have shown that the measurement of serum PSA offers several advantages in the early detection of CaP (3–6). The impact of PSA on CaP incidence, mortality, and survival is evidenced by recent trends in data provided by the American Cancer Society (7,8). Estimated deaths declined from 41,800 in 1997 to 39,200 in 1998 (9). Five-year survival rates increased from 68% to 90% between 1974–1976 and 1986–1993 in Caucasian men and from 58% to 75% in African-American men (7). Using serum PSA, CaP is now detected at an earlier stage, when the malignancy is more likely to be confined to the prostate. Various treatments, including radical prostatectomy, have a high curative rate at this stage, thus reducing CaP death rate (4,5). For this reason, PSA is the only serum cancer marker approved by the Food and Drug Administration (FDA) to aid in the detection of CaP.

## 2. BIOCHEMISTRY OF PSA

First described by Wang et al. in 1979 (10), PSA is a single-chain glycoprotein neutral serine protease of 240 amino acids secreted by the prostate epithelium and CaP cells (11–13). A glycoprotein monomer with a molecular weight of 33,000–34,000, PSA contains 240 amino acids (10–14). Among the many PSA-like kallikreins that have been discovered so far, PSA is named human kallikrein 3 (hK3) (11). PSA is involved in the lysis of seminal coagulum and is one of the predominant proteins present in the prostatic fluid. PSA catalyzes the proteolytic degradation of gel-forming proteins secreted by human seminal vesicles and mediates the progressive activation of sperm motility. Even though PSA has been documented to be present in some nonprostate tissues [e.g., periurethral (15–18) and parotid glands (19) in both men and women, and in about 30% of breast tumor specimens (20)], no significant contribution of PSA from these sources to serum PSA has so far been demonstrated. The importance of PSA as a marker in prostatic diseases comes from the fact that only trace quantities of PSA are detected in the serum of all normal males. Changes in the anatomy of the prostate gland could lead to the increased diffusion of PSA in blood circulation. Thus, elevated serum PSA concentrations can suggest the existence of prostatic diseases like CaP, benign prostatic hyperplasia (BPH), prostatitis (21), and prostatic ischemia (22). Because PSA has not been found yet in any other tissue, it has so far been proved to be a highly specific prostate biochemical marker. PSA is present in the serum of normal men at concentration <4 µg/L. Women, who have no prostate, should have no PSA in their serum. However, immunoreactive PSA is detectable in about 5% of women's sera, and this is attributed to a prostate-equivalent organ called Skene's gland (17,18). No diagnostic usefulness of PSA in women has been established.

## 3. SERUM PSA CUTOFF IN DIAGNOSIS OF PROSTATE CANCER

Even though serum PSA levels increase in men with cancer of the prostate, PSA is not recommended as the only screening procedure for the diagnosis of cancer, because elevated PSA levels also are observed in patients with BPH. DeAntoni et al. showed that 90% of healthy men volunteers in the United States had serum PSA <4 µg/L (70% had <2 µg/L) (23). Of the 10% of that population with PSA >4 µg/L, about one-third would have CaP if the prostate is systematically biopsied (24). Of all CaP detected among patients tested, >75% are now impalpable, organ-confined tumors with good prospect for cure (25). Accordingly, 4 µg/L has been the most accepted cutoff in screening for CaP today. However, this cutoff does produce a low specificity (i.e., high false positive), necessitating many unnecessary biopsies, resulting in increased morbidity and cost. Various attempts have been made to improve this cutoff. For example, depending on the age and extent of the symptoms, from 21% (26) to 86% (27) of men with BPH will demonstrate elevated levels of serum PSA. These elevations are usually mild (4–10 µg/L), but as many as 25% will have elevations >10 µg/L. Because BPH progresses slowly and becomes more prevalent with advancing age, the normal range of serum PSA among men does increase with age (28). Thus, with a cutoff value of 4 µg/L, PSA has only a diagnostic sensitivity and specificity of 88% and 30%, respectively (rendering the test's PPV of 26% toward detecting CaP) (3). Instead of this fixed cutoff, this study recommends age-adjusted cutoffs: 40–49 yr, 2.5 µg/L; 50–59 yr, 3.5 µg/L; 60–69 yr, 4.5 µg/L; 70–79 yr, 6.5 µg/L. The use of age-specific PSA cutoff, however, although improving the specificity, had a lower impact on life-years gained than the 4 µg/L cutoff (29).

For this reason, serum PSA alone is not recommended by American Cancer Society to diagnose CaP. Rather, studies suggest that the measurement of PSA in conjunction with a DRE and TRUS provide a better method of detecting prostate cancer than DRE alone. Thus, the PPV of positive PSA increases from 26% to 33–52% with TRUS, to 69% with DRE, and to 62–74% when all three tests are positive (1,24). For this reason, the most common combination in screening for CaP is DRE and PSA. However, even with DRE, the PPV is still lower if the PSA is in the so-called "gray" area, 4–10 µg/L, where the specificity to detect CaP is especially low. One strategy to improve the utility of serum PSA in "screening" for CaP is to determine the PSA density, the ratio of serum PSA to the prostate volume, determined by TRUS or magnetic resonance imaging (MRI). Benson et al. (30) found that PSA density helped distinguish BPH from CaP, especially in the "gray" zone of serum PSA. Egawa et al. (31) demonstrated an improved diagnostic value of PSA for differentiating CaP from benign prostatic condition by using PSA-related parameters like PSA density for transition zone and gland volume. Another strategy to improve PPV is to use PSA velocity, or the rate of change of serum PSA over time. A retrospective study showed that PSA velocity was significantly higher among CaP patients than those with BPH and that an increase of PSA >0.75 µg/L/yr indicated CaP 90% of the time correctly (32). Another problem of the 4-µg/L cutoff for PSA is the reduced sensitivity; 25–30% men have CaP with PSA <4 µg/L. Accordingly, Catalona et al. (33) has proposed lowering the PSA cutoff to 2.5 µg/L to improve the sensitivity. Carter and Pearson developed a guideline for PSA testing for early diagnosis of CaP (34). Any such guideline must balance the conflict between two goals: Lower PSA cutoff increases sensitivity but reduces specificity and vice versa. This difficulty in the utility of PSA has produced alternate serum markers.

In addition to detecting CaP, PSA was tried in staging the cancer. Oesterling *(4)* showed poor correlation among percent patients with elevated serum PSA (>4 µg/L) and the cancer stages (from A, with prostate confined tumor, to D, with distant metastases): 67% (A), 73% (B), 80% (C), and 88% (D). However, there was <1% chance of having bone metastases for patients with PSA <10 µg/L *(35)*. PSA testing also has significant value in detecting metastatic or persistent disease in patients following surgical or medical treatment of prostate cancer *(3,36,37)*. Persistent elevation of PSA following treatment or increase in a posttreatment PSA level is indicative of recurrent or residual disease *(27, 38,39)*. The effect is most pronounced after radical prostatectomy. If the malignant tissue is successfully removed, serum PSA drops to undetectable levels. However, if the tumor is metasticized, or malignant tissue is not completely removed, serum PSA starts rising. Lange et al. *(40)* showed that with follow-up ranging from 6 to 50 mo, 16 of 16 (100%) patients who had PSA >0.4 µg/L after radical prostatectomy had recurrence of the cancer. On the other hand, a positive outcome is associated with decreasing serum PSA concentration. A longer period was required for serum PSA to come back to a normal level after successful radiation treatment; the median time to decline was 3–5 mo, with over 80% by 12 mo and 90% by 18 mo. Because the patients are monitored after the treatment, any increase in serum PSA might be indicative of relapse. This has necessitated in the development of "ultrasensitive" PSA assays, which can detect even in the range 0.002– 0.01 µg/L *(41,42)*. Diamandis has suggested that the ultrasensitive assay could detect a relapse 1 yr earlier than assays with the so-called second-generation PSA assays (detection limit = 0.1 µg/L) *(43)*.

For the correct interpretation of decreasing serum PSA levels, one must note the factors that might also decrease PSA temporarily: antiandrogen drugs, hospitalization, castration, ejaculation, prostatectomy, and radiation therapy. Hormone therapy such as with leutropin or follicle-stimulating hormone has been reported to lower serum PSA by as much as 80% *(44)*. As described earlier, therapy that reduces prostatic diseases is expected to lower the serum PSA. Other nontherapeutic, diagnostic procedures, like DRE, TRUS, or cystoscopy, which are frequently utilized in patients with suspected prostate problems, on the other hand might have a transient effect on the serum PSA *(45)*. These effects are less well defined. Whereas cystoscopy was reported to increase PSA by fourfold *(27)*, other studies showed no effect on serum PSA *(46)*. Similar conflicting effects of TRUS on serum PSA have been reported *(47)*. Based on these conflicting reports, it is probably acceptable to measure PSA anytime after these procedures; the PSA test, however, should be repeated should the earlier result be of any concern.

## 4. METHODS FOR MEASURING SERUM PSA

Serum PSA is now mostly determined by immunoassays—more specifically two-site immunometric "sandwich" assays. In these methods, commercially available from many suppliers for manual or automated assay systems, two separate antibodies to PSA are incubated with the sample. In heterogeneous assays, one antibody is conjugated to immobilized surface, including various types of particle, and the other antibody is, directly or indirectly, conjugated to a reporter molecule. The reporter molecule can provide a colorimetric, fluorescence, or chemiluminescense signal directly or through an enzyme-linked immunosorbent assay (ELISA) pathway. The bound reporter molecules with PSA sandwiched between the immobilized and the reporter antibodies) are separated, washed (if needed), and expressed into the relevant signal. Thus, the signal is directly proportional to the PSA present in the sample. Among the commercially available automated immunoassay methods to measure PSA in human serum, there are the magnetic particle chemiluminescence assay (CLIA), the microparticle enzyme assay, electrochemiluminescence assay, and radioimmunoassay. The antibody pairs used in these assays could be both monoclonal or polyclonal, or a monoclonal–polyclonal combination. Technical factors like assay design and components used do affect the assay results and, thus, the clinical utility of PSA results.

## 5. PSA FORMS IN SERUM: MEASUREMENT OF FREE OR COMPLEXED PSA

Prostate-specific antigen exists predominantly in circulation as complexes with various protease inhibitors such as $\alpha_1$-antichymotrypsin (ACT), $\alpha_2$-macroglobulin, and other acute-phase proteins *(48)*. However, complexing with the macroglobulin enfolds the PSA entity totally, resulting in the antigenic loss of PSA in those complexes *(49)*. Thus, the most prevalent form of complexed PSA (cPSA) found in CaP patient sera is the ACT complex (ACT–PSA) *(50)*. Overall in all patient samples, ACT–PSA contributes 60–95%, free PSA contributes 5–40%, and other PSA complexes contributes 1–2.5% toward the total serum PSA measured. The relative proportion of the cPSA increases in CaP and decreases in benign prostatic diseases *(50)*. Because the concentration of PSA in serum, even when elevated, is much less (100–1000 times) than the concentration of ACT, it is reasonable to conclude that the PSA isoforms in CaP or BPH could be different, the latter less able to bind ACT than the former. It has been proposed that most of the free PSA (fPSA) in serum is "nicked" or "clipped" *(51)*, lacking protease activity, and unable to bind the protease inhibitors. However, concrete data are lacking in this regard. The differential distribution of cPSA to fPSA can be used to improve the diagnosis of CaP in the "gray" serum PSA area. The percent ratio of free PSA (%fPSA) to total PSA is used for such purposes. The %fPSA increases in benign diseases *(49)*. A cutoff of 25% fPSA ratio has been in use to improve the PPV for a total PSA range of 2–12 μg/L (where total PSA alone has poor PPV) *(52)*. The use of such a ratio improves the distinction between prostate cancer and the benign prostatic diseases and helps avoid costly and painful prostate biopsies *(53)*. A new method, however, has recently been developed to measure the cPSA directly *(54)*. In this immunoassay, samples containing fPSA and cPSA are first treated with a fPSA-specific antibody, followed by a CLIA measurement for total PSA. The antibody-blocked fPSA are not available for total PSA measurement; thus, the assay results in the total cPSA that are detectable immunologically. Serum cPSA concentration has been used in monitoring prostate cancer, for determining residual disease and early recurrence after therapy when used in conjunction with other diagnostic indices. cPSA levels increase in men with cancer of the prostate, and after radical prostatectomy cPSA levels routinely falls to the undetectable range. If prostatic tissue remains after surgery or metastasis has occurred, cPSA levels can be observed. Serum cPSA has been shown to be at least as good as the %fPSA ratio in detecting prostate cancer. In a multicenter study *(55)*, the PPV of prostate cancer screening for the serum markers, PSA (cutoff = 4.0 μg/L), cPSA (cutoff = 3.75 μg/L), and %fPSA ratio (cutoff = 25%, for PSA 4–10 μg/L), were found as follows: (in this order): at site 1–31%, 40%, 37% (*n* = 75); at site 2–18%, 25%, 23% (*n* = 167); at site 3–23%, 29%, 42% (*n* = 78). The overall PPV for all three sites compared as follows (in same order): 26%, 33%,

Table 1
Commercially Available Equimolar Chemiluminescence
Immunoassay for PSA Recognizes ACT–PSA and fPSA
Equally Well Across Several Total Serum PSA Concentrations

| % Free PSA | Total PSA | | |
|---|---|---|---|
| | 4 µg/L | 10 µg/L | 30 µg/L |
| 100 | 4.25 | 10.69 | 29.77 |
| 80 | 4.13 | 10.59 | 29.49 |
| 50 | 4.23 | 10.57 | 28.94 |
| 20 | 4.44 | 10.52 | 29.15 |
| 0 | 4.39 | 10.51 | 28.64 |

and 31%. In another multicenter study *(56)* with 831 patients (of whom 37.5% had CaP), cPSA was shown to have improved specificity over total PSA. This study recommended a cPSA cutoff at 2.5 µg/L. No benefit of %fPSA or %cPSA (i.e., ratio of cPSA to total PSA) was found over cPSA alone. Such positive results with cPSA not only suggest replacement of %fPSA with cPSA, but replacement of PSA with cPSA also in CaP screening and monitoring *(55)*.

In our study, we found that the direct CLIA cPSA method correlated well with cPSA calculated from total PSA and fPSA assays *(54)*. In addition to the fact that one test (cPSA) can replace two tests (total and free PSA), use of cPSA has several analytical and preanalytical benefits as well. Use of one test over two means less error. Inherently, fPSA being 1–30% of total PSA has a higher imprecision than cPSA or total PSA. Finally, studies have shown fPSA to have much lower stability than cPSA *(57)*.

## 6. ISSUES IN PSA IMMUNOASSAYS

Because different PSA assays use different pairs of antibodies, they might recognize differently the PSA forms and isoforms that might exist in the serum. That, of course, means a possible variability among results with different assays. Foremost in this issue is the dissimilar recognition of the assays toward fPSA and ACT–PSA *(49)*. Stamey *(58)* found that some PSA assays yielded as much as twice the result than others with samples containing a higher percentage of fPSA, resulting in a false clinical diagnosis. In recognition of this problem, many of the automated PSA assays commercially available now are "equimolar"; that is, they are unaffected by the change in the relative concentrations of fPSA and cPSA. Thus, a commercially available equimolar CLIA for PSA *(59)* recognizes ACT–PSA and fPSA equally well across several total serum PSA concentrations (Table 1). A related issue in PSA assays is standardization. A large amount of variability among assays could be related to differences in their standardization. To solve this issue, an international reference material containing 90% ACT–PSA and 10% fPSA has been proposed *(60)*. Stamey *(61)* showed that with such standardization, the coefficients of variation among five monoclonal–polyclonal and four monoclonal–monoclonal assays were reduced from 28.3% to 9.5%. As more and more commercially available PSA assays standardize with respect to that reference material, the variability among assays should decrease, improving the utility of serum PSA.

Another issue that one should watch for in interpreting serum PSA immunoassay results is that of the high-dose "hook effect" observed in most one-step immunometric assays *(54)*. When serum PSA concentration is very high, instead of forming the sandwiches, PSA can form separate binary complexes with the capture and reporter antibodies separately. Under these circumstances, reduction in the ternary viable complexes could result in *false-negative* PSA concentrations. To guard against this possibility, some laboratories routinely dilute high (but within the reported assay range) PSA samples and reassay them. A third confounding issue for PSA immunoassays is the interference from heterophilic antibodies in the patient serum. For reasons of assay specificity, the use of monoclonal antibodies in PSA assays is increasing. Most such antibodies, however, are murine in nature. Existence of human anti-mouse antibody (HAMA) can either falsely bridge the immobilized and reporter antibodies, thus generating false-positive results *(62)*, or if the HAMA acts against one of the antibodies used in the PSA reagents, the complexation would result in decrease in available reagent antibody, possibly resulting in false-negative results.

## 7. FUTURE OF PSA

Most prostate cancers have very slow growth; autopsy studies show increasing occurrence of a microscopic malignant lesion in the prostate gland without any other clinical evidence of the disease among older men: 30% at >50 yr, >40% at >75 yr, and approaching 100% at >90 yr *(63)*. Because any cancer treatment has significant morbidity associated with it, a controversy in the success of PSA in detecting early CaP has been raised. If the malignancy is of slow growth, could its early detection and aggressive treatment result in "unnecessary" inconvenience of the patients and economic cost? For this reason, a search is on to detect the most dangerous of the CaP—the fast-growing, life-threatening ones. The PSA velocity has been used unsuccessfully in this regard, and newer markers are being sought. One example is the application of polymerase chain reaction (PCR) and reverse transcriptase PCR (RT-PCR) to detect micrometastatic prostate cancer cells *(64)*. Another approach is the use of neural network analysis of multiple markers, which showed better specificity (57%) with high sensitivity (90%) at PSA <4 µg/L *(65)*. Newer serum markers like the other members of the kallikrein family (e.g., hK2) *(66)*, prostate-specific membrane antigen *(67)*, insulin-like growth factor 1 *(68)*, alone or in combination of currently available markers, have been tested. The results, however, are too early to suggest any major advantage. In summary, although PSA assays have made tremendous contribution toward detecting CaP early, thus reducing CaP deaths, newer advances are needed to improve CaP diagnosis.

## REFERENCES

1. Catalona W. Prostate cancer. In: Reintgen D, Clark R, eds. Cancer Screening. St. Louis, MO: Mosby, 1996.
2. Fishman MC, Hoffman AR, Klausner RD, Thaler MS. In Medicine, 2nd ed. Philadelphia, PA: J.B. Lippincott, 1985:412–414.
3. Lange PH, Brawer MK. Serum prostate specific antigen: its use in diagnosis and management of prostate cancer. Urology 1989; 33(6 Suppl):13.
4. Oesterling JE. Prostate specific antigen: a critical assessment of the most useful tumor marker for adenocarcinoma of the prostate. J Urol 1991; 145:907–923.
5. Partin AW, Oesterling JE. The clinical usefulness of prostate specific antigen: update 1994. J Urol 1994; 152:1358.
6. Chan DW, Sokoll LJ. Prostate-specific antigen: update 1997. J Int Fed Clin Chem 1997; 9:120.

7. Parker SL, Johnston DK, Wingo PA, et al. Cancer statistics by race and ethnicity. CA Cancer J Clin 1998; 48:31.

8. Rosenthal DS. Changing trends in prostate cancer diagnosis. CA Cancer J Clin 1998; 48:49.

9. Wingo PA, Landis S, Ries LAG. An adjustment to the 1997 estimate of new prostate cancer cases. CA Cancer J Clin 1997; 47:239.

10. Wang MC, Valenzuela LA, Murphy GP, Chu TM. Purification of a human prostate specific antigen. Invest Urol 1979; 17:159–163.

11. Lilja H. A kallikrein-like serine protease in prostatic fluid cleaves the predominant seminal vesicle protein. J Clin Invest 1985; 76:1899–1903.

12. Watt KWK, Lee P-J, Timkulu T, et al. Human prostate-specific antigen: structural and functional similarity with serine proteases. Proc Natl Acad Sci USA 1986; 83:3166–3170.

13. Sokoll LJ, Chan DW. Prostate-specific antigen: its discovery and biochemical characteristics. Urol Clin North Am 1997; 24:253.

14. Ban Y, Wang MC, Watt KW, Joor R, Chu TM. The proteolytic activity of prostate specific enzyme. Biochem Biophys Res Commun 1984; 123:482.

15. Kamoshida S, Tsutsumi Y. Extraprostatic localization of prostatic acid phosphatase and prostate-specific antigen: distribution in cloacogenic glandular epithelium and sex-dependent expression in human anal gland. Hum Pathol 1990; 21:1108–1111.

16. Iwakiri J, Granbois K, Wehner N, et al. An analysis of urinary prostate specific antigen before and after radical prostatectomy: evidence for secretion of prostate specific antigen by the periurethral glands. J Urol 1993; 149:783–786.

17. Wernert N, Albrech M, Sesterhenn I, et al. The "female prostate": location, morphology, immunohistochemical characteristics and significance. Eur Urol 1992; 22:64–69.

18. Ablin RJ. Prostate-specific antigen and the female prostate. Clin Chem 1989; 35:507–508.

19. van Krieken JH. Prostate marker immunoreactivity in salivary gland neoplasms. A rare pitfall in immunohistochemistry. Am J Surg Pathol 1993; 17:410–414.

20. Yu H, Diamandis EP, Sutherland DJA. Immunoreactive prostate-specific antigen levels in female and male breast tumors and its association with steroid hormone receptors and patient age. Clin Biochem 1994; 27:75–79.

21. Robles JM, Morell AR, Redorta JP, et al. Clinical behavior of prostate specific antigen and prostatic acid phosphatase: a comparative study. Eur Urol 1988; 14:360–366.

22. Glenski WJ, Malek RS, Myrtle JF, et al. Sustained, substantially increased concentration of prostate-specific antigen in the absence of prostatic malignant disease: an unusual clinical scenario. Mayo Clin Proc 1992; 67:249–252.

23. DeAntoni EP, Crawford ED. Prostate cancer awareness week: education, service, and research in a community setting. Cancer (Suppl) 1995;75:1874–1879.

24. Catalona W, Richie J, Ahmann, et al. Comparison of digital rectal examination and serum prostate specific antigen. J Urol 1994; 151:1283–1290.

25. Stamey TA, Donaldson AN, Yemoto CE, et al. Histological and clinical findings in 896 consecutive prostates treated only by radical retropubic prostatectomy from 1988 to 1997: epidemiologic significance of annual changes. J Urol 1998; 160:2412–2417.

26. Ercole CJ, Lange PH, Mathisen M, et al. Prostate specific antigen and prostatic acid phosphatase in the monitoring and staging of patients with prostate cancer. J Urol 1987; 138:1181.

27. Stamey TA, Yang N, Hay AR, et al. Prostate-specific antigen as a serum marker for adenocarcinoma of the prostate. N Engl J Med 1987; 317:909.

28. Oesterling JE, Jacobsen SJ, Chute CG, et al. Serum prostate-specific antigen in a community-based population of healthy men: establishment of age-specific reference ranges. JAMA 1993; 270:860–864.

29. Etzioni R, Shen Y, Petteway JC, et al. Age-specific PSA: a reassessment. Prostate 1996; 7:70–77.

30. Benson MC, Whang IS, Olsson CA, et al. The use of prostate specific antigen. J Urol 1992; 147: 817–821.

31. Egawa S, Suyama K, Takashima R, et al. Prospective evaluation of prostate cancer by prostate specific antigen–related parameters. Int J Urol 1999; 6:493–501.

32. Carter HB, Morrell CH, Pearson JD, et al. Estimation of prostatic growth using serial prostate-specific antigen measurements in men with and without prostate disease. Cancer Res 1992; 52:3323–3328.

33. Catalona W, Smith DS, Ornstein DK. Prostate cancer detection in men with serum PSA concentrations of 2.6 to 4.0 ng/ml and benign prostate examination. Enhancement of specificity with free PSA measurements. JAMA 1997; 277:1452.

34. Carter HB, Pearson JD. Prostate specific antigen testing for early diagnosis of prostate cancer: formulation of guidelines. Urology 1999; 54:780–786.

35. Oesterling JE, Martin SK, Bergstralh EJ, Lowe FC. The use of prostate-specific antigen in staging patients with newly diagnosed prostate cancer. JAMA 1993; 268:57–60.

36. Killan CS, Yang N, Emrich LJ. Prognosis importance of prostate specific antigen for monitoring patients with stages B2 to D1 prostate cancer. Cancer Res 1985; 45:886.

37. Chan DW, Bruzek DJ, Oesterling JE, Rock RC, Walsh PC. Prostate specific antigen as a marker for prostatic cancer: a monoclonal and a polyclonal assay compared. Clin Chem 1987; 33:1916.

38. Brawer MK, Lange PH. Prostate specific antigen in management of prostatic carcinoma. Urology 1989; 33(5 Suppl):11.

39. Zelefsky MJ, Liebel SA, Wallner KE, et al. Significance of normal serum prostate-specific antigen in the follow-up period after definitive radiation therapy for prostate cancer. J Clin Oncol 1995; 13:459–463.

40. Lange PH, Escole CJ, Lightner DJ, et al. The value of serum prostate specific antigen determinations before and after radical prostatectomy. J Urol 1989; 141:873–879.

41. Stamey T, Graves H, Wehner N, et al. Early detection of residual prostate cancer after radical prostatectomy by an ultrasensitive assay for prostate specific antigen. J Urol 1993; 149:516–518.

42. Yu H, Diamandis EP. Ultrasensitive time-resolved immunofluorometric assay of prostatic specific antigen. Clin Chem 1993; 39:2108–2114.

43. Diamandis EP. Clinical application of ultrasensitive prostate specific antigen assays. J Natl Cancer Inst 1997; 89:1077.

44. Voges GE, Mottrie AM, Stockle M, et al. Hormone therapy prior to radical prostatectomy in patients with clinical stage C prostate cancer. Prostate 1994; 5(Suppl):4–8.

45. Yuan JJ, Coplen DE, Petros JA, et al. Effects of rectal examination, prostatic massage, ultrasonography and needle biopsy on serum prostate specific antigen levels. J Urol 1992; 147:810–814.

46. Hughes HR, Penny MD, Ryan PG, et al. Serum prostate specific antigen: in vitro stability and effect of ultrasound rectal examination in vivo. Ann Clin Biochem 1987; 24(Suppl):206.

47. Oesterling JE, Rice DC, Glenski WJ, et al. Effect of cytoscopy, prostate biopsy and transurethral resection of prostate on serum prostate-specific antigen concentration. Urology 1993; 42:276–282.

48. Lilja H, Christensson A, Dahlen U, et al. Prostate-specific antigen in serum occurs predominantly in complex with $\alpha_1$-antichymotrypsin. Clin Chem 1991; 37:1618–1625.

49. Catalona W, Partin A, Slawin K, et al. Use of percentage of free prostate specific antigen to enhance differentiation of prostate cancer from benign prostate disease. JAMA 1998; 279:1542–1547.

50. Christensson A, Bjork T, Nilsson O, et al. Serum prostate specific antigen complexed to $\alpha_1$-antichymotrypsin as an indicator of prostate cancer. J Urol 1993; 150:100–105.

51. McCormick RT, Rittenhouse HG, Finlay JA, et al. Molecular forms of prostate-specific antigen and the human kallikrein gene family: a new era. Urology 1995; 45:729.

52. Polascik TJ, Oesterling JE, Partin AW. Prostate specific antigen: a decade of discovery—what we have learned and where we are going. J Urol 1999; 162:293–306.

53. Vashi AR, Wonjo KJ, Hendricks W, et al. Determination of the "reflex-range" and appropriate cut-points for percent free prostate-specific antigen in 413 men referred for prostatic evaluation using the AxSym system. Urology 1997;49:19–27.

54. Datta P, Dasgupta A. The evaluation of an automated chemiluminescent immunoassay for complexed PSA on the Bayer ACS:180™ System. J Clin Lab Anal 2003; 17:174–178.

55. Brawer MK, Benson MC, Bostwick DG, et al. Prostate-specific antigen and other serum markers: current concepts from the World Health Organization second international consultation on prostate cancer. Semin Urol Oncol 1999; 17:206–221.

56. Partin AW, Brawer MK, Bartsch G, et al. Complexed prostate specific antigen improves specificity for prostate cancer detection: results of a prospective multicenter clinical trial. J Urol 2003; 170:1787–1791.

57. Jung K, Lein M, Brux B, et al. Different stability of free and complexed prostate-specific antigen in serum in relation to specimen handling and storage conditions. Clin Chem Lab Med 2000; 38:1271–1275.

58. Stamey TA. Second Stanford conference on international standardization of prostate specific antigen immunoassays: September 1 and 2, 1994. Urology 1995; 45:173–184.

59. Dasgupta A, Wells A, Datta P. Performance evaluation of a new chemiluminescent assay for prostate specific antigen. J Clin Lab Anal 2000; 14:164–168.

60. Stamey TA, Chen Z, Prestigiacomo AF. Reference material for PSA: the IFCC stanardization study. Clin Biochem 1998;31:475–481.

61. Stamey TA. Progress in standardization of immunoassays for prostate-specific antigen. Urol Clin North Am 1997; 24(2):269–273.
62. Camacho T, Mora J, Segura A, et al. Falsely increased prostate-specific antigen concentration attributed to heterophilic antibodies. Ann Clin Biochem 2002; 39:160.
63. Cerosimo R, Chan D. Prostate cancer: current and evolving strategies. Am J Health Syst Pharm 1996; 53:381–396.
64. Nejat R, Katz A, Olsson C. The role of RT-PCR in staging patients with clinically localized PCA. Semin Urol Oncol 1998; 16:40–45.
65. Barnhill SD, Zhang Z, Madyastha RK, et al. Artificial neural networks: a new dimension in the early diagnosis of prostate cancer. J Clin Ligand Assay 1998; 21:18–23.
66. Haese A, Becker C, Noldus J, et al. Human glandular kallikrein 2: a potential serum marker for predicting the organ confined versus non-organ confined growth of prostate cancer. J Urol 2000; 163(5):1491–1497.
67. Murphy GP, Radge H, Kenny G, et al. Comparison of prostate-specific membrane antigen and prostate-specific antigen levels in prostate cancer patients. Anticancer Res 1995; 15:1473–1480.
68. Djavan B, Bursa B, Seitz C, et al. Insulin like growth factor (IGF-1), IGF-1 density and IGF-1/PSA ratio for prostate cancer detection. Urology 1999; 54:603–606.

# 27 Tumor Targets and Biomarkers in Renal Cell Carcinoma

*Ivar Bleumer, MD*
*and Peter F. A. Mulders, MD, PhD*

## CONTENTS

## SUMMARY

Renal cell carcinoma (RCC) is the most common malignancy of the kidney. Unfortunately, 50% off all patients diagnosed with this disease will develop metastasized disease for which no adequate treatment can be offered currently. Therefore, the identification of prognostic factors and biomarkers is of the greatest importance. They might show additional prognostic value over classical prognostic factors like stage and grade. Also, these markers can be used for a better patient selection, development of specific gene immunotherapy strategies, and a better follow-up. In this chapter, we review current and future biomarkers of interest in the diagnosis, treatment, and follow-up of patients with RCC.

**Key Words:** Renal cell carcinoma; biomarkers; tumor targets; tumor markers.

## 1. INTRODUCTION

Renal cell carcinoma (RCC) is the most common renal tumor, the third malignancy within urological oncology and comprises 2–3% of all malignancies. RCC was conventionally thought to arise primarily from the proximal convoluted tubules. Indeed, this is the case for most of the clear-cell subtype of RCC (ccRCC), which accounts for 70–80% of all RCCs. However, other histological subtypes (e.g., papillary or chromophobic RCC) typically arise from more distal components of the nephron. RCC occurs twice as often in men compared to women, and the highest incidence of RCC is seen in the sixth decade *(1,2)*. The incidence of RCC is rising. A review of over 10,000 cases of RCC gathered in the Connecticut Tumor Registry indicates a sixfold increase in the incidence of RCC from 1935 to 1989, both in woman and men *(3)*. Several risk factors have been described for RCC. Tobacco smoking doubles the risk of RCC and there is a positive linear relation

From: *Cancer Drug Discovery and Development: The Oncogenomics Handbook*
Edited by: W. J. LaRochelle and R. A. Shimkets © Humana Press Inc., Totowa, NJ

between body weight and the risk for RCC, especially in women. Other factors associated with higher risk for RCC are exposure to asbestos or chemicals, thiazide drug intake, and urinary tract infections *(4)*.

At the onset of RCC, there are only few early warning signs. The classical triad of Virchow, consisting of an abdominal mass together with flank pain and macroscopic hematuria, is nowadays only seen in approx 5% of the new cases presenting with RCC. If any, the presentation of the disease is accompanied with nonspecific signs such as fatigue, weight loss, malaise, fever, and/or night sweats *(5)*. At present, more then 50% of all RCCs are found incidentally. The incidence of these so-called incidentalomas has risen from 15% to over 50% in the past decades. Typically, these incidentalomas are of smaller size, often confined within the renal capsule, and associated with a favorable clinical outcome.

Currently, the treatment of RCC is based on the anatomic extend of the disease, as addressed by the TNM staging system. Two-thirds of the patients present with localized disease, meaning that no metastatic disease is observed, and are treated by means of surgical removal of the tumor. Nevertheless, up to 30% of all patients treated with curative intent will develop distant metastasis. Together with 30% of the patient population that already has metastatic disease at onset, 50% of all patients with RCC will develop metastasized RCC (mRCC). A review of 3502 patients with mRCC treated with 1 of 72 chemotherapeutic agents revealed a cumulative objective response rate of only 2–6 % *(6)*. Combination therapy and/or radiotherapy does not significantly change these response rates or survival *(7)*. Therefore, chemotherapy and radiotherapy are considered to be of limited value for the treatment of mRCC. This treatment resistance of RCC is partly the result of overexpression of multidrug resistance 1 (*MDR1*) and/or multidrug resistance-associated protein (*MRP*) genes *(8)*. It has been shown that the intracellular accumulation of cytotoxic drug closely correlates with an alteration in the transmembrane protein P-glycoprotein (P-gp) encoded by the *MDR1* gene or *MRP (9,10)*. To what extend these genes also dictate the prognosis of the disease is less clear *(11)*.

Renal cell carcinoma is one of the few tumors for which spontaneous regression of metastatic disease after tumor nephrectomy has been documented *(12)*. Therefore, much attention has been focused on immunotherapeutic modalities for the treatment of mRCC. Indeed, nonspecific immunotherapy has convincingly shown its ability to induce long-term clinical responses in a subset of patients *(13)*. Nevertheless, the overall response rate is low and side effects are significant. Consequently, the main focus in investigating new treatment options for mRCC concerns immunotherapeutical modalities with more specificity against RCC and less side effects *(14)*. In summary, 50% of all patients with RCC will develop metastasis, and for these patients, we are not able to present an adequate treatment, hence the search for RCC-associated tumor markers for diagnostic, prognostic, and therapeutical purposes.

## 2. TUMOR MARKERS

Tumor markers can be of great value in several aspects of cancer treatment. For prostate cancer (CaP) the use of markers has become daily routine. Prostate-specific antigen (PSA) has long since been used as a serum tumor marker to detect relapse of CaP *(15)*. Moreover, PSA is used for population screening and diagnosis. Recently, DD3[PCA3] has been described as the most CaP-specific gene that is strongly overexpressed in >95% of primary CaP specimens and in CaP metastasis *(16,17)*. Evaluation of a time-resolved fluorescence-based quantitative reverse transcription–polymerase chain reaction (RT-PCR) assay for the detection of DD3[PCA3] transcripts in urinary sediments obtained after extensive prostatic massage showed a high negative predictive value for the presence of CaP *(18)*. The use of this CaP-specific marker could have a great impact for the reduction of the number of prostate-biopsies currently needed to detect CaP.

Also for RCC, numerous studies have been published that describe the potential use of tumor-associated biomarkers in the diagnosis and prognosis of RCC and as targets for (gene-immuno) therapy strategies. Tumor markers can be classified according to their origin and function:

- Apoptotic markers
- Proliferation markers
- Cell adhesion markers
- Tumor-associated antigens
- Angiogenesis
- Cytogenetics

## *2.1. Apoptotic Regulators and Cell Cycle Proteins*

As mentioned earlier, RCC shows a high degree of resistance to chemotherapy and radiation *(6,7)*. The loss of control of apoptosis might contribute to progression and resistance to treatment modalities and can be attributed to an interaction between p53 and the apoptotic regulators bcl-2 and Bax *(19)*. However, the majority of RCCs express normal function of the protein p53, and analysis of expression of p53, bcl-2, or Bax could not be significantly correlated with other parameters examined, including tumor recurrence, metastasis, or survival rate *(20)*.

Aberrations in the G1–S transition have been observed in a variety of tumors, suggesting that cell cycle defects are related to the activation of oncogenes and inactivation of suppressor genes involved in the transformation process. The frequency of G1/S aberrations in RCC has not been fully clarified. Cyclins (A and D1), pRb, p21 (waf1/cip1), and p27 (KIP1) are cellular proteins involved in the tight regulation of cell cycle events. Several groups have studied the relation between these markers and clinical and histopathological parameters, as well as clinical outcome *(21–25)*. A review of these studies suggests that cyclin-A, but mainly low expression p27, is associated with poor prognosis for patients with RCC.

## *2.2. Proliferation Markers*

Proliferation of cells is unmistakably related to cancer and, subsequently, several proliferation markers have been evaluated. AgNOR (silver-stained nucleolar-organizing regions) reflects transcription activity of ribosomal DNA and mitotic activity. PCNA (proliferating cell nuclear antigen) is a protein synthesized in the later G1- and S-phases of the cell cycle. Finally, Ki-67 (MIB1) is a monoclonal antibody that stains a proliferating-specific antigen in tumor cells. All of these markers have been correlated to histological grade and stage and even survival *(26–28)*. Comparative studies that have been performed suggest that Ki-67 is the more powerful prognostic factor of the three *(29,30)*; nevertheless, more multivariate studies are needed.

## *2.3. Cell Adhesion Markers*

Cancer metastasis is a complex multistage process. Decreased intercellular adhesion enables detachment of tumor cells and can play a role in the early steps of the metastatic process. Cell adhesion can be mediated through at least four families of adhesion molecules (integrin, immunoglobulin, selectin, and cadherin). Also, the tubular epithelium, from which the RCC originates, expresses a complex set of adhesion molecules. During carcinogenesis, the combination of cadherin expression changes in almost 50% of RCCs *(31)*. E-cadherin, a $Ca^{2+}$-dependent epithelial cadherin, is considered a critical molecule for epithelial integrity *(32)*. However, most RCCs do not express E-cadherin because renal proximal tubular epithelium from which RCCs originate does not express E-cadherin. In contrast, other studies showed that in normal kidney tubular epithelium N-cadherin and cadherin-6 are expressed *(33,34)* and that expression patterns might be related to the metastatic behavior of the tumor. The cadherin function is modulated through cytoplasmic proteins termed catenins. Immunohistochemical staining revealed that catenins were expressed in all of the segments of the nephron, including proximal tubules. The catenin family seems to be less divergent than the cadherin family. Therefore, it was reasoned that there might be a correlation between aggressiveness of RCC and a decreased expression of α-catenin, which is a member of the catenins that link cadherin to the cytoskeleton. Immunohistochemical staining on RCC using antibodies against E-cadherin and α-catenin has revealed that the ratios of abnormal staining for E-cadherin and α-catenin were 77% and 37%, respectively. The prognostic value of E-cadherin is controversial. However, a significant correlation between survival and decreased expression of α-catenin was observed. Whether α-catenin immunohistochemistry provides additional prognostic information remains to be established.

Although cell adhesion molecules are usually membrane bound, soluble forms (sICAM-1, sVCAM-1, and sELAM-1) exist and are generated by shedding of the extracellular portions from the cell surface. These molecules have been investigated along with other clinical parameters in patients with metastatic RCC *(35,36)*. The prognostic significance of sICAM-1 might indicate a role of this molecule for tumor progression, potentially in association with the abrogation of antitumor immune responses. The possibility of defining a pretreatment risk model based on sICAM-1 level, ESR and CRP also warrants further investigation, with regard to a possible linkage between acute-phase proteins and sICAM-1 levels.

CD44 is a transmembrane glycoprotein involved in cell–cell and cell–matrix interactions. *De novo* expression of CD44 and its variant isoforms have been associated with aggressive behavior in various tumors *(37,38)*. Because little data are available concerning the role of CD44 in the biological behavior of locally confined renal tumors, the expression of CD44 in a large set of conventional RCCs was analyzed to determine its prognostic value in association with other clinicopathologic variables *(38)*. The investigators concluded that CD44 expression was correlated with progression and survival of RCC patients and can be considered as a useful prognostic parameter in conventional RCC and can be used in the evaluation of the outcome of these tumors.

## *2.4. Angiogenic Markers*

Neovascularization is inextricable related to tumor growth and metastatic dissemination. Nevertheless, angiogenesis measured as intratumoral microvascular density is not an independent prognostic factor in RCC *(39,40)*. Vascular endothelial growth factor (VEGF) is definitely related to histological grade and stage; the prognostic value remains uncertain *(41)*. In addition to its association with grade and stage, VEGF might also play a role in the treatment of RCC. A recent publication described the effect of bevacizumab, a neutralizing antibody against VEGF, in the treatment of mRCC *(42)*. In this randomized, double-blind phase II trial, placebo was compared with two doses of bevacizumab. The primary end point of this study was the time to progression of disease. According to intention-to-treat analysis, progression-free survival in the group receiving the high-dose bevacizumab (10 mg/kg) was significantly longer (median: 4.8 mo) than in the placebo group (median: 2.5 mo; $p < 0.001$ by the log-rank test). The National Cancer Institute (NCI) data safety and monitoring board recommended closure of accrual on the basis of these differences in time to progression, despite an overall response rate of approx 10% and no difference in survival among the three study arms.

## 2.5. Cytogenetic Markers

Recently, it has become widely accepted that genetic alterations play an important role in the development of many cancers. The relationship of abnormal nuclear morphology to molecular genetic alterations in RCC is unknown. Nuclear morphometric analyses have been used successfully to predict the outcome of patients with cancer when classical pathologic grading systems failed. Indeed, several investigations showed a significant correlation between morphometric parameters and survival of patients with RCC (43–46). Nevertheless, in colorectal carcinoma, it was shown that nuclear morphology seemed not to be directly influenced by the individual genetic alterations but was by fractional allelic loss (i.e., a global measure of genetic changes) (47). Thus, it might be suggested that complex tumor properties such as pathologic appearance and metastatic potential cannot be understood unless most of the underlying genetic factors are taken into consideration. Therefore, several chromosomal abnormalities and subsequent overexpression of proteins have been evaluated. L-myc and C-myc, for instance, are a family of proto-oncogenes that have been studied in RCC (48); yet, so far only associations could be made with histological grade and stage, without showing independent prognostic significance (29,48,49).

## 2.6. Tumor-Associated Antigens: CA-IX^G250/MN

Markers that are in particular of interest in the optimization of gene immunotherapy are RCC-associated antigens. However, despite compelling evidence that RCC is an immunogenic tumor, until recently only a few specific tumor antigens, such as RAGE, are known. Renal antigen (RAGE), initially defined through cytotoxic T lymphocyte (CTL) technology, is expressed in a minor percentage of RCC and, therefore, a suboptimal target (50–54). In this aspect, the identification of the RCC-associated antigen CA-IX^G250/MN is of interest.

CA-IX is expressed in greater than 95% of all ccRCC tumors. Moreover, no expression can be detected in normal kidney tissue, including fetal kidney; in other normal tissues, the expression is highly restricted and limited to large bile ducts and gastric epithelium (55). Furthermore, CA-IX is also expressed in several non-RCC tumors. In RCC, the chimeric monoclonal antibody G250 (WX-G250), which recognizes the CA-IX antigen, has been identified and developed for both therapeutic and diagnostic purposes (55). Furthermore, a CA-IX-derived peptide recognized by HLA-A2.1 restricted CTL and a helper peptide recognized by HLA-DR-restricted T-helper cells have been identified (56, 57). These findings, together with the high prevalence of CA-IX in RCC make this antigen a promising tool for specific immunotherapy strategies for RCC (14,58).

The high expression of CA-IX in ccRCC implies the involvement of CA-IX in renal carcinogenesis. CA-IX is a member of the carbonic anhydrase family, which are enzymes involved in acid–base balance, $CO_2$ transport, and ion exchange, which explains their physiological expression in the gastric mucosa. Still, the involvement of CA-IX in the carcinogenesis remains to be elucidated. CA-IX cDNA transfection into CA-IX-negative cell lines did not alter the cell doubling time and did not lead to immortalization (personal communication, E. Oosterwijk, University Hospital Nijmegen, The Netherlands). Thus, CA-IX seems not to function as an oncogene. It is known that the acidic environment around tumors favor their malignant behavior, and this might explain the expression of CA-IX in a variety of tumors. However, it is also conceivable that CA-IX is upregulated only to correct the carcinogenic acidic environment, instead of creating it.

Using the clinical and data resources of the UCLA Kidney Cancer Program, Bui et al. investigated whether CA-IX is associated with progression and survival *(59)*. Immunohisto-chemical analysis using a CA-IX mAb was performed on tissue microarrays from patients treated by nephrectomy for ccRCC. CA-IX staining was correlated with response to treatment, clinical factors, pathological features, and survival. Low CA-IX staining was an independent poor prognostic factor for survival for patients with metastatic RCC, with a hazard ratio of 3.10 ($p < 0.001$). CA-IX significantly substratified patients with metastatic disease when analyzed by T stage, Fuhrman grade, nodal involvement, and performance status ($p < 0.001$, $p = 0.001$, $p = 0.009$, and $p = 0.005$, respectively). Overall expression of CA-IX decreased with development of metastasis, as demonstrated by the lower CA-IX staining levels in metastatic lesions relative to matched primary tumor specimens ($p = 0.036$). On the basis of these data, CA-IX seems to be the most significant molecular marker described in kidney cancer to date.

## 2.7. The von Hippel–Lindau Gene and RCC

The von Hippel–Lindau disease is a hereditary multisystem cancer syndrome caused by germline mutations of the VHL tumor suppressor gene on the short arm of chromosome 3 (reviewed in ref. *60*). The disease predisposes to the development of a variety of highly vascularized benign and malignant tumors of the central nervous system, adrenal glands, pancreas reproductive adnenal organs, and the kidney. VHL disease is the principal cause of inherited RCC. Furthermore, in almost 100% of the sporadic ccRCC, there is an inactivation of the VHL gene either by mutation, deletion, or methylation *(61,62)*.

VHL plays a central role in the cellular oxygen homeotasis. In normoxic conditions, the VHL protein (pVHL) binds and deactivates the hypoxia-inducible factor-1$\alpha$ (HIF-1$\alpha$). However, in the hypoxic condition, pVHL does not target HIF-1$\alpha$ for degradation leading to an increased transcription of a variety of HIF-regulated genes. Tumors (e.g., ccRCC) in which both alleles of the VHL gene are inactive mimic the hypoxic situation, leading to an overproduction of HIF-1$\alpha$ and subsequently, the HIF-1$\alpha$-targeted genes (VEGF, GLUT1, transforming growth factor [TGF]-$\alpha$, CA-IX), several of which have been discussed in this chapter *(63,64)*. In addition to carcinogenesis through the HIF-1$\alpha$ pathway, the VHL status has also been associated with effects on apoptosis (Bcl pathway) and cell cycle events (p27, cyclin-D). Many of these HIF-targeted genes are associated with aggressive tumor growth, suggesting that gene products of the VHL/HIF-1$\alpha$ pathway are important prognostic factors. Furthermore, the same VHL/HIF-1$\alpha$ pathway is of interest in developing molecular therapeutic interventions (discussed in ref. *65*).

## 3. CONCLUSION

Tumor markers are mainly used to diagnose specific malignancies. The methods commonly involve immunohistochemistry and cytogenetics, including fluorescent *in situ*

Table 1
Overview of Tumor Markers in Renal Cell Carcinoma

| Renal Cell Carcinoma | Tumor Markers | Refs. |
|---|---|---|
| Apoptotic regulators | p53 | 19,20,26 |
| | bcl-2 | |
| | Bax | |
| Cell cycle proteins | cyclin A and D1 | 21–25 |
| | p21 (waf1/cip-1) | |
| | p27 (KIP1) | |
| | pRb | |
| Proliferation markers | AgNOR | 26–30 |
| | PCNA | |
| | Ki-67 (MIB1) | |
| Cell adhesion markers | E-cadherin | 31–34 |
| | N-Cadherin | |
| | Cadherin-6 | |
| | α-catenin | |
| | sICAM1 | 35,36 |
| | sVCam-1 | |
| | sECam-1 | |
| | CD44 | 37,38 |
| Tumor-associated antigens | RAGE | 53 |
| | CA-IX$^{G250/MN}$ | 14,55 |
| Angiogenic markers | Intratumoral microvascular density | 39,40 |
| | VEGF | 41,42 |
| Cytogenic markers | Karyometry | 43–46 |
| | Myc | 48,49 |

hybridization (FISH), and reversed transcriptase (RT) and polymerase chain reaction (PCR). In RCC, several investigated tumor markers are promising (summarized in Table 1). They might show additional prognostic value over classical prognostic factors like stage and grade. Also, these markers can finally be used for a better patient selection, development of specific gene immunotherapy strategies, and a better follow-up. Ultimately, these factors should show its value in a prospective well-controlled manner and additionally, more research is needed to obtain new (better) antigens and markers in RCC. Also, the association with the carcinogenesis of RCC and the inactivation of the VHL gene with subsequent overexpression of several tumor-associated genes is intriguing and should be elucidated.

## REFERENCES

1. Motzer RJ, Bander NH, Nanus DM. Renal-cell carcinoma. N Engl J Med 1996; 335(12):865–875.
2. Mulders P, Figlin R, DeKernion JB, Wiltrout R, Linehan M, Parkinson D, et al. Renal cell carcinoma: recent progress and future directions. Cancer Res 1997; 57(22):5189–5195.
3. Katz DL, Zheng T, Holford TR, Flannery J. Time trends in the incidence of renal carcinoma: analysis of Connecticut Tumor Registry data, 1935–1989. Int J Cancer 1994; 58(1):57–63.
4. Dhote R, Pellicer-Coeuret M, Thiounn N, Debre B, Vidal-Trecan G. Risk factors for adult renal cell carcinoma: a systematic review and implications for prevention. BJU Int 2000; 86(1):20–27.

5. Mevorach RA, Segal AJ, Tersegno ME, Frank IN. Renal cell carcinoma: incidental diagnosis and natural history: review of 235 cases. Urology 1992; 39(6):519–522.

6. Yagoda A, Petrylak D, Thompson S. Cytotoxic chemotherapy for advanced renal cell carcinoma. Urol Clin North Am 1993; 20(2):303–321.

7. Harris DT. Hormonal therapy and chemotherapy of renal-cell carcinoma. Semin Oncol 1983; 10(4): 422–430.

8. Yu DS, Chang SY, Ma CP. The expression of mdr-1-related gp-170 and its correlation with anthracycline resistance in renal cell carcinoma cell lines and multidrug-resistant sublines. Br J Urol 1998; 82(4): 544–547.

9. Nooter K, Herweijer H. Multidrug resistance (mdr) genes in human cancer. Br J Cancer 1991; 63(5): 663–669.

10. Breuninger LM, Paul S, Gaughan K, Miki T, Chan A, Aaronson SA, et al. Expression of multidrug resistance-associated protein in NIH/3T3 cells confers multidrug resistance associated with increased drug efflux and altered intracellular drug distribution. Cancer Res 1995; 55(22):5342–5347.

11. Oudard S, Levalois C, Andrieu JM, Bougaran J, Validire P, Thiounn N, et al. Expression of genes involved in chemoresistance, proliferation and apoptosis in clinical samples of renal cell carcinoma and correlation with clinical outcome. Anticancer Res 2002; 22(1A):121–128.

12. Gleave ME, Elhilali M, Fradet Y, Davis I, Venner P, Saad F, et al. Interferon gamma-1b compared with placebo in metastatic renal-cell carcinoma. Canadian Urologic Oncology Group. N Engl J Med 1998; 338(18):1265–1271.

13. Fisher RI, Rosenberg SA, Fyfe G. Long-term survival update for high-dose recombinant interleukin-2 in patients with renal cell carcinoma. Cancer J Sci Am 2000; 6(Suppl 1):S55–S57.

14. Bleumer I, Oosterwijk E, de Mulder P, Mulders PF. Immunotherapy for renal cell carcinoma. Eur Urol 2003; 44(1):65–75.

15. Gregorakis AK, Holmes EH, Murphy GP. Prostate-specific membrane antigen: current and future utility. Semin Urol Oncol 1998; 16(1):2–12.

16. Bussemakers MJ, Van Bokhoven A, Verhaegh GW, Smit FP, Karthaus HF, Schalken JA, et al. DD3: a new prostate-specific gene, highly overexpressed in prostate cancer. Cancer Res 1999; 59(23):5975–5979.

17. de Kok JB, Verhaegh GW, Roelofs RW, Hessels D, Kiemeney LA, Aalders TW, et al. DD3(PCA3), a very sensitive and specific marker to detect prostate tumors. Cancer Res 2002; 62(9):2695–2698.

18. Hessels D, Klein Gunnewiek JM, van Oort I, Karthaus HF, van Leenders GJ, van Balken B, et al. DD3 (PCA3)-based molecular urine analysis for the diagnosis of prostate cancer. Eur Urol 2003; 44(1):8–15.

19. Tomasino RM, Morello V, Tralongo V, Nagar C, Nuara R, Daniele E, et al. p53 expression in human renal cell carcinoma: an immunohistochemical study and a literature outline of the cytogenetic characterization. Pathologica 1994; 86(3):227–233.

20. Vasavada SP, Novick AC, Williams BR. P53, bcl-2, and Bax expression in renal cell carcinoma. Urology 1998; 51(6):1057–1061.

21. Aaltomaa S, Lipponen P, Ala-Opas M, Eskelinen M, Syrjanen K, Kosma VM. Expression of cyclins A and D and p21(waf1/cip1) proteins in renal cell cancer and their relation to clinicopathological variables and patient survival. Br J Cancer 1999; 80(12):2001–2007.

22. Hedberg Y, Davoodi E, Ljungberg B, Roos G, Landberg G. Cyclin E and p27 protein content in human renal cell carcinoma: clinical outcome and associations with cyclin D. Int J Cancer 2002; 102(6):601–607.

23. Haitel A, Wiener HG, Neudert B, Marberger M, Susani M. Expression of the cell cycle proteins p21, p27, and pRb in clear cell renal cell carcinoma and their prognostic significance. Urology 2001; 58(3): 477–481.

24. Anastasiadis AG, Calvo-Sanchez D, Franke KH, Ebert T, Heydthausen M, Schulz WA, et al. p27KIP1-expression in human renal cell cancers: implications for clinical outcome. Anticancer Res 2003; 23(1A): 217–221.

25. Migita T, Oda Y, Naito S, Tsuneyoshi M. Low expression of p27(Kip1) is associated with tumor size and poor prognosis in patients with renal cell carcinoma. Cancer 2002; 94(4):973–979.

26. Rioux-Leclercq N, Turlin B, Bansard J, Patard J, Manunta A, Moulinoux JP, et al. Value of immunohistochemical Ki-67 and p53 determinations as predictive factors of outcome in renal cell carcinoma. Urology 2000; 55(4):501–505.

27. Morell-Quadreny L, Clar-Blanch F, Fenollosa-Enterna B, Perez-Bacete M, Martinez-Lorente A, Llombart-Bosch A. Proliferating cell nuclear antigen (PCNA) as a prognostic factor in renal cell carcinoma. Anticancer Res 1998; 18(1B):677–682.

28. Yasunaga Y, Shin M, Miki T, Okuyama A, Aozasa K. Prognostic factors of renal cell carcinoma: a multivariate analysis. J Surg Oncol 1998; 68(1):11–18.

29. Rini BI, Vogelzang NJ. Prognostic factors in renal carcinoma. Semin Oncol 2000; 27(2):213–220.

30. Hofmockel G, Tsatalpas P, Muller H, Dammrich J, Poot M, Maurer-Schultze B, et al. Significance of conventional and new prognostic factors for locally confined renal cell carcinoma. Cancer 1995; 76(2): 296–306.

31. Shimazui T, Oosterwijk-Wakka J, Akaza H, Bringuier PP, Ruijter E, Debruyne FM, et al. Alterations in expression of cadherin-6 and E-cadherin during kidney development and in renal cell carcinoma. Eur Urol 2000; 38(3):331–338.

32. Nose A, Nagafuchi A, Takeichi M. Expressed recombinant cadherins mediate cell sorting in model systems. Cell 1988; 54(7):993–1001.

33. Nouwen EJ, Dauwe S, van der Biest I, De Broe ME. Stage- and segment-specific expression of cell-adhesion molecules N-CAM, A-CAM, and L-CAM in the kidney. Kidney Int 1993; 44(1):147–158.

34. Shimazui T, Schalken JA, Giroldi LA, Jansen CF, Akaza H, Koiso K, et al. Prognostic value of cadherin-associated molecules (alpha-, beta-, and gamma-catenins and p120cas) in bladder tumors. Cancer Res 1996; 56(18):4154–4158.

35. Tanabe K, Campbell SC, Alexander JP, Steinbach F, Edinger MG, Tubbs RR, et al. Molecular regulation of intercellular adhesion molecule 1 (ICAM-1) expression in renal cell carcinoma. Urol Res 1997; 25(4): 231–238.

36. Hoffmann R, Franzke A, Buer J, Sel S, Oevermann K, Duensing A, et al. Prognostic impact of in vivo soluble cell adhesion molecules in metastatic renal cell carcinoma. Br J Cancer 1999; 79(11–12):1742–1745.

37. Gilcrease MZ, Guzman-Paz M, Niehans G, Cherwitz D, McCarthy JB, Albores-Saavedra J. Correlation of CD44S expression in renal clear cell carcinomas with subsequent tumor progression or recurrence. Cancer 1999; 86(11):2320–2326.

38. Heider KH, Ratschek M, Zatloukal K, Adolf GR. Expression of CD44 isoforms in human renal cell carcinomas. Virchows Arch 1996; 428(4–5):267–273.

39. Gelb AB, Sudilovsky D, Wu CD, Weiss LM, Medeiros LJ. Appraisal of intratumoral microvessel density, MIB-1 score, DNA content, and p53 protein expression as prognostic indicators in patients with locally confined renal cell carcinoma. Cancer 1997; 80(9):1768–1775.

40. MacLennan GT, Bostwick DG. Microvessel density in renal cell carcinoma: lack of prognostic significance. Urology 1995; 46(1):27–30.

41. Jacobsen J, Rasmuson T, Grankvist K, Ljungberg B. Vascular endothelial growth factor as prognostic factor in renal cell carcinoma. J Urol 2000; 163(1):343–347.

42. Yang JC, Haworth L, Sherry RM, Hwu P, Schwartzentruber DJ, Topalian SL, et al. A randomized trial of bevacizumab, an anti-vascular endothelial growth factor antibody, for metastatic renal cancer. N Engl J Med 2003; 349(5):427–434.

43. Murphy GF, Partin AW, Maygarden SJ, Mohler JL. Nuclear shape analysis for assessment of prognosis in renal cell carcinoma. J Urol 1990; 143(6):1103–1107.

44. Bibbo M, Galera-Davidson H, Dytch HE, Gonzalez DC, Lopez-Garrido J, Bartels PH, et al. Karyometry and histometry of renal-cell carcinoma. Anal Quant Cytol Histol 1987; 9(2):182–187.

45. Gilchrist KW, Hogan TF, Harberg J, Sonneland PR. Prognostic significance of nuclear sizing in renal cell carcinoma. Urology 1984; 24(2):122–124.

46. van der Poel HG, Mulders PF, Oosterhof GO, Schaafsma HE, Hendriks JC, Schalken JA, et al. Tumor heterogeneity as prognostic factor in patients with low-stage (T1-3N0M0) renal-cell carcinoma. Investig Urol (Berl) 1994; 5:60–65.

47. Mulder JW, Offerhaus GJ, de Feyter EP, Floyd JJ, Kern SE, Vogelstein B, et al. The relationship of quantitative nuclear morphology to molecular genetic alterations in the adenoma–carcinoma sequence of the large bowel. Am J Pathol 1992; 141(4):797–804.

48. Lipponen P, Eskelinen M, Syrjanen K. Expression of tumour-suppressor gene Rb, apoptosis-suppressing protein Bcl-2 and c-Myc have no independent prognostic value in renal adenocarcinoma. Br J Cancer 1995; 71(4):863–867.

49. Mejean A, Oudard S, Thiounn N. Prognostic factors of renal cell carcinoma. J Urol 2003; 169(3):821–827.

50. Koo AS, Tso CL, Shimabukuro T, Peyret C, DeKernion JB, Belldegrun A. Autologous tumor-specific cytotoxicity of tumor-infiltrating lymphocytes derived from human renal cell carcinoma. J Immunother 1991; 10(5):347–354.

51. Finke JH, Rayman P, Edinger M, Tubbs RR, Stanley J, Klein E, et al. Characterization of a human renal cell carcinoma specific cytotoxic CD8+ T cell line. J Immunother 1992; 11(1):1–11.
52. Schendel DJ, Gansbacher B, Oberneder R, Kriegmair M, Hofstetter A, Riethmuller G, et al. Tumor-specific lysis of human renal cell carcinomas by tumor-infiltrating lymphocytes. I. HLA-A2-restricted recognition of autologous and allogeneic tumor lines. J Immunol 1993; 151(8):4209–4220.
53. Gaugler B, Brouwenstijn N, Vantomme V, Szikora JP, Van der Spek CW, Patard JJ, et al. A new gene coding for an antigen recognized by autologous cytolytic T lymphocytes on a human renal carcinoma. Immunogenetics 1996; 44(5):323–330.
54. Brandle D, Brasseur F, Weynants P, Boon T, Van den EB. A mutated HLA-A2 molecule recognized by autologous cytotoxic T lymphocytes on a human renal cell carcinoma. J Exp Med 1996; 183(6):2501–2508.
55. Oosterwijk E, Ruiter DJ, Hoedemaeker PJ, Pauwels EK, Jonas U, Zwartendijk J, et al. Monoclonal antibody G 250 recognizes a determinant present in renal-cell carcinoma and absent from normal kidney. Int J Cancer 1986; 38(4):489–494.
56. Vissers JL, De Vries IJ, Schreurs MW, Engelen LP, Oosterwijk E, Figdor CG, et al. The renal cell carcinoma-associated antigen G250 encodes a human leukocyte antigen (HLA)-A2.1-restricted epitope recognized by cytotoxic T lymphocytes. Cancer Res 1999; 59(21):5554–5559.
57. Vissers JL, De Vries IJ, Engelen LP, Scharenborg NM, Molkenboer J, Figdor CG, et al. Renal cell carcinoma-associated antigen G250 encodes a naturally processed epitope presented by human leukocyte antigen-DR molecules to CD4(+) T lymphocytes. Int J Cancer 2002; 100(4):441–444.
58. Bleumer I, Knuth A, Oosterwijk E, Hoffmann R, Varga Z, Lamers CH, et al. A phase II trial of chimeric monoclonal antibody G250 for advanced renal cell carcinoma patients. Br J Cancer 2004; 90(5):985–990.
59. Bui MH, Seligson D, Han KR, Pantuck AJ, Dorey FJ, Huang Y, et al. Carbonic anhydrase IX is an independent predictor of survival in advanced renal clear cell carcinoma: implications for prognosis and therapy. Clin Cancer Res 2003; 9(2):802–811.
60. Lonser RR, Glenn GM, Walther M, Chew EY, Libutti SK, Linehan WM, et al. von Hippel–Lindau disease. Lancet 2003; 361(9374):2059–2067.
61. Gnarra JR, Tory K, Weng Y, Schmidt L, Wei MH, Li H, et al. Mutations of the VHL tumour suppressor gene in renal carcinoma. Nat Genet 1994; 7(1):85–90.
62. Pavlovich CP, Schmidt LS, Phillips JL. The genetic basis of renal cell carcinoma. Urol Clin North Am 2003; 30(3):437–454.
63. Pugh CW, Ratcliffe PJ. The von Hippel–Lindau tumor suppressor, hypoxia-inducible factor-1 (HIF-1) degradation, and cancer pathogenesis. Semin Cancer Biol 2003; 13(1):83–89.
64. Wykoff CC, Beasley NJ, Watson PH, Turner KJ, Pastorek J, Sibtain A, et al. Hypoxia-inducible expression of tumor-associated carbonic anhydrases. Cancer Res 2000; 60(24):7075–7083.
65. Pantuck AJ, Zeng G, Belldegrun AS, Figlin RA. Pathobiology, prognosis, and targeted therapy for renal cell carcinoma: exploiting the hypoxia-induced pathway. Clin Cancer Res 2003; 9(13):4641–4652.

# VI   EMERGING APPROACHES TO CANCER THERAPY

# VI-A   TARGETING THE VASCULATURE

# 28

# Tumor Vasculature as a Target for Cancer Therapy

*Grzegorz Korpanty, MD,*
*Xianming Huang, PhD,*
*and Rolf A. Brekken, PhD*

## Contents

## Summary

The delivery of nutrients to and the removal of waste products from cells are required for the development, growth, and maintenance of all tissues, including ones that have undergone malignant transformation. Therefore, both normal and tumor tissues are dependent on a functional circulatory system. Blood vessels, which consist of endothelial cells, support cells (smooth muscle cells or pericytes), and a basement membrane, are responsible for the efficient transport of nutrients and wastes to and from tissues. In the context of a solid tumor, blood vessels are the supply lines that are required for the persistence, expansion, and metastasis of the tumor. Vascular targeting aims at developing strategies to selectively block the flow of blood in tumors, resulting in damage (e.g., coagulation) of the tumor's blood supply while not perturbing blood flow in normal tissue. Thus, there has been an increased interest in finding tumor vasculature-specific markers that can be exploited as vascular targeting agents. Although a marker that is absolutely specific for tumor vasculature has not yet been found, there are a variety of candidates under investigation that warrant our attention. These include markers of endothelial cell activation and proliferation, markers of stress and hypoxia, ligand : receptor pairs, undefined endothelial cell antigens, and proteins that are expressed in newly formed or remodeled basement membrane. In this chapter, we will discuss some of the strategies that are being investigated to utilize these markers to selectively attack the vasculature of tumors.

**Key Words:** Tumor vasculature; vascular targeting; angiogenesis; VEGF; drug delivery; cancer therapeutics.

From: *Cancer Drug Discovery and Development: The Oncogenomics Handbook*
Edited by: W. J. LaRochelle and R. A. Shimkets © Humana Press Inc., Totowa, NJ

# 1. INTRODUCTION

An adequate blood supply is crucial for the growth and metastasis of solid tumors. Angiogenesis, or the development of new blood vessels, is therefore a requirement for tumor progression *(1,2)*. Angiogenesis occurs through endothelial cell sprouting, bridging, and intussusception from pre-existing vessels *(3–5)*, as well as contributions from circulating endothelial precursor (stem) cells *(6)*. The angiogenic process is initiated more frequently in neoplastic tissue than normal tissue because of a shift in the balance of angiogenic regulators in the tumor microenvironment that favors blood vessel growth and remodeling *(7)*. The proangiogenic environment promotes endothelial cell expression of markers that are consistent with proliferation, migration, growth factor activation, and basement membrane remodeling. Further, blood vessels that are formed or activated in the tumor microenvironment differ morphologically and functionally from vasculature in normal tissue. Tumor blood vessels are characterized typically as tortuous, leaky, and inefficient, with irregular diameters and thinner walls that are supported by fewer pericytes than blood vessels in normal tissue *(8,10)*. The functional, morphological, and protein expression differences between blood vessels in tumor and normal tissue present the opportunity for the selective attack of the supply lines of tumors. There are two types of vascular targeting agents (VTAs) under investigation for the treatment of cancer. Ligand-directed VTAs are targeted to tumor vasculature through the use antibodies, peptides, or proteins that bind specific targets on tumor endothelial cells. In contrast, there are a few examples of small molecules (e.g., combretastatin and DMXAA) that do not localize specifically to tumor endothelium but, nonetheless, exploit the pathophysiological differences between tumor and normal tissue vasculature to induce vascular damage specifically in solid tumors. For more information on small-molecule VTAs, see recent reviews by Tozer et al. *(11)* and Zhou et al. *(12)*.

# 2. VASCULAR TARGETING

The concept of vascular targeting as originally proposed by Denekamp in 1984 *(13,14)* has many advantages over targeting tumor cells themselves *(15,16)*. First, the target cell is accessible. Tumor endothelial cells are freely accessible to targeting moieties that are delivered intravenously. This allows the efficient delivery and the rapid accumulation of a VTA at the target site. Second, unlike traditional chemotherapy, directed against tumor cells, not all target cells in a tumor vessel need to be bound by the VTA or express the target antigen to generate an occlusive thrombus that shuts down blood flow throughout the entire tumor vessel *(17,18)*. Third, antigen-negative mutant tumor endothelial cells are unlikely to emerge as a result of vascular targeting because the endothelium in tumors is nonmalignant with stable genomes *(19,20)*. Fourth, vascular targeting is potent. Coagulation of the vasculature of a tumor has a built-in amplification mechanism because, as Tannock *(21,22)* has shown, tumor proliferation is limited by vascular density, demonstrating that there is little vascular redundancy in solid tumors. Finally, this approach has the potential to be applicable to a broad spectrum of human tumors, because tumor vessels in histologically distinct tumors express common markers *(14)*, such as those listed in Table 1.

Vascular targeting has been validated experimentally by a number of groups as an effective way to treat solid tumors in mice. The first of these studies used a VTA directed against

Table 1
Potential Markers of Tumor Blood Vessels

| Targeting Moiety | Antigen | Location of Marker | Refs. |
|---|---|---|---|
| Multiple | VEGF : VEGFR | Angiogenic BV | 3–26 |
| MKID2 | $a_3b_{11}$ | Angiogenic BV | 27 |
| GoH3 | $a_6b_1$ | Angiogenic BV | 27 |
| EN7/44 | p30.5 | Proliferating EC | 28 |
| Multiple | CD105 (endoglin) | Proliferating EC | 29–34 |
| FB5 | Endosialin | Proliferating EC | 35 |
| MK 2.7 | VCAM-1 | Activated EC | 36 |
|  | E-selectin, CD62E | Activated EC | 36 |
| 4A11 | H-5-2, Lewis$^y$-6 | Activated EC | 37 |
|  | CD44 | Activated EC | 38 |
| Metastatin | Hyaluronan | Activated EC | 39 |
| Vitaxin; RGD cyclic peptide | $\alpha_V\beta_3$; $\alpha_V\beta_5$ | Activated EC | 40–42 |
| Multiple | $\alpha_1\beta_1$; $\alpha_2\beta_1$ | Activated EC | 43,44 |
| Multiple | $\alpha_5\beta_1$ | Activated EC | 45 |
| 3SB, 3G4 | Phosphatidylserine | Activated EC | 36 |
| TV-1 | FN | Basement membrane | 46 |
| L19 | ED-B isoform of FN | Basement membrane | 47–50 |
| HUIV26, HUI77 | Denatured collagens | Proteolyzed basement membrane | 51,52 |
| Multiple | NG2 proteoglycan | Pericytes | 53 |
| NGR peptide | CD13/APN | Tumor EC | 54 |

Abbreviations: APN, aminopeptidase N; BV, blood vessels; EC, endothelial cells; FN, fibronectin; MMP, matrix metalloproteinases; PSMA, prostate specific membrane antigen; SMC, smooth muscle cell; TEM, tumor endothelial marker; VEGF : VEGFR, complex of VEGF and its receptor.

a genetically engineered tumor endothelial cell marker (18,55). These studies demonstrated that large solid tumors could be dramatically and safely debulked by either toxin-linked or tissue factor (TF)-linked VTAs. More recent studies have utilized VTAs directed against VCAM-1 (56) and the ED-B domain of fibronectin (47), both naturally occurring markers of tumor blood vessels. One of the key points to come out of the study of Ran et al. (56) was the demonstration that initiation of coagulation with a TF-linked VTA is dependent on the luminal expression of phosphatidylserine (PS) in the outer leaflet of the endothelial cell plasma membrane. PS is found exclusively in the inner leaflet of the plasma membrane in healthy normal cells and, therefore, is not available to participate in TF-mediated coagulation under normal circumstances. However, tumor endothelial cells flip PS to the outer leaflet of the plasma membrane, which enables TF to activate the coagulation cascade in tumor blood vessels. The study by Nilsson et al. (47) demonstrated that it is possible to initiate tumor blood vessel coagulation with TF that is targeted to a basement membrane component, namely a unique domain of fibronectin. This is an important and exciting finding, as it should expand the potential target molecules that are evaluated for vascular targeting to include those expressed in the basement membrane of tumor blood vessels.

## *2.1. Endothelial Cell Markers*

### 2.1.1. VEGF : VEGFR Complex

A class of tumor endothelial cells markers that hold particular promise are ligand-induced targets. The best characterized ligand-induced target is the VEGF : VEGFR complex *(58)*. Vascular endothelial growth factor (VEGF) is a prominent proangiogenic growth factor that is expressed abundantly in most tumors *(59,60)*. Tumor cells express and secrete VEGF as a result of hypoxic conditions in the tumor mass and also as a result of genetic mutations. The increased expression of VEGF by tumor cells and the hypoxic conditions in the tumor result in an increase in the expression of the receptors VEGFR1 (Flt-1) and VEGFR2 (KDR/Flk-1) on endothelial cells lining the vasculature of the tumor. Upregulation of both the ligand and its receptor(s) specifically in the tumor leads to a high concentration of the VEGF : VEGFR complex on tumor endothelium as compared with endothelium in normal tissue. Initial studies using rabbit polyclonal antibodies against the $NH_2$-terminus of VEGF demonstrated that the VEGF : VEGFR complex could be localized to tumor vasculature *(23)*. Monoclonal antibodies, Gv39M, 11B5, and 3E7 *(24)*, and recently described scFv *(25)*, which are selective for the VEGF : VEGFR complex, also localize to tumor vasculature while not binding to endothelium in most normal tissues.

These antibodies been utilized to demonstrate VEGF-activated blood vessels in human and mouse tumors. Bergers et al. *(61)* using a transgenic mouse model (RIP1-Tag2) of multistage carcinogenesis *(62)* demonstrated that Gv39M reactivity with tumor blood vessels correlated with the induction of angiogenesis in the progression of islet tumor cell carcinogenesis. Furthermore, Koukourakis et al. *(63)* used 11B5 reactivity as a measure of activated microvessel density (aMVD) and compared it to standard MVD (sMVD) evaluated by anti-CD31 reactivity. The study showed that VEGF activation of VEGFR is a tumor-specific feature in more than 50% of non-small-cell lung cancer (NSCLC) cases and is associated with poor outcome. Both Bergers et al. *(61)* and Koukourakis et al. *(64)* showed distinct staining of blood vessels in tumor tissue with monoclonal antibodies (mAbs) specific for the VEGF : VEGFR complex. In both studies, blood vessel selective reactivity occurred in spite of a significant amount of VEGF being present in and around the extracellular matrix (ECM) and tumor cells (demonstrated by non-$NH_2$-terminal anti-VEGF antibodies). It is conceivable that antibodies specific for other ligand : receptor pairs could also be specific markers of "activated" endothelium. Other members of the VEGF family of proteins and their respective receptors, including VEGF-B bound to VEGFR1, and VEGF-C and VEGF-D bound to VEGFR3, as well as the angiopoietin : Tie-receptor system might be especially useful to target in this manner.

### 2.1.2. Markers of Endothelial Cell Activation

Integrins are heterodimeric transmembrane receptors made up of $\alpha$- and $\beta$-subunits that bind to ligands located in the ECM or to their counterreceptors on adjacent cells *(65)*. Endothelial cells express several integrins, which function as receptors for ECM proteins such as fibronectin, collagen, and laminins *(66)*. The expression of some integrins (e.g., $\alpha_v\beta_3$, $\alpha_4\beta$, $\alpha_v\beta_5$, $\alpha_5\beta_1$) is linked both functionally and spatially with growth factor activation of endothelial cells. These integrins are expressed abundantly on the surface of endothelial cells in tumor vessels during vascular remodeling *(67)*. For example, activation of endothelial cells with either VEGF or platelet-derived growth factor (PDGF) induces association of VEGFR2 or PDGFR, respectively with integrin $\alpha_v\beta_3$. The association of the growth factor receptor with the integrin results in increased $\alpha_v\beta_3$ expression and promigratory function, whereas $\alpha_v\beta_3$, in turn, facilitates the mitogenic action of VEGF and PDGF *(68,69)*. Similar interactions have also been reported for fibroblast growth factor (FGF)-2 and $\alpha_5\beta_1$ integrin *(70)*. Outside-in signals mediated by integrins not only cooperate with growth factor receptors to promote cell proliferation and motility but integrins by themselves are able to activate growth factor receptors in a ligand-independent way *(71)*. Because there is evidence of spatial and functional crosstalk among integrins, growth factors and their receptors, targeting integrins involved in angiogenesis might be very beneficial and of great importance in inhibiting tumor growth and angiogenesis.

The most promising and most studied integrin linked to tumor angiogenesis is $\alpha_v\beta_3$, which is instrumental in guiding endothelial cells through the angiogenic process *(72,73)*. Antibodies against or peptide ligands specific for $\alpha_v\beta_3$ integrin localize to angiogenic blood vessels in solid tumors and have been used for imaging the vasculature of solid tumors in experimental animals *(40)*. This integrin coordinates an activated endothelial cell's interaction with the ECM and serves as a docking site for matrix metalloproteinase-2 (MMP-2), which allows the endothelial cells to degrade the immediate surroundings and migrate toward the angiogenic stimuli *(74)*. Blocking $\alpha_v\beta_3$ function through the use of antibodies, peptides, or organic small molecules results in apoptosis of endothelial cells *(75)*. This in itself is an appropriate way to block the process of angiogenesis in tumors.

Activated and proliferating endothelial cells lining tumor vessels express endoglin (CD105), a 180-kDa transmembrane protein, which serves as an accessory receptor for transforming growth factor $\beta1$ and 3 (TGF-$\beta1$, TGF-3) *(76)*. The density of endoglin-positive microvessels was determined to be an independent prognostic factor in breast carcinoma, whereas sMVD based on CD3-1 positive vessels was not predictive *(77)*. These results mirror those of the VEGF : VEGFR complex *(64)* and strongly suggest that the use of a marker of angiogenic endothelium might be more predictive than vascular density determined by a pan-endothelial marker. Furthermore, a number of studies have demonstrated that CD105 is an attractive candidate for targeting tumor vasculature. Delivery of deglycosylated ricin A chain (dgA), a protein synthesis inhibitor, to endoglin/CD105 on endothelial cells was effective at killing cells that were proliferating but did not damage endoglin/CD105-positive cells that were quiescent *(29)*. Anti-endoglin/CD105-based immunoconjugates under in vivo conditions were able to prevent the growth of human MCF-7 tumors in nude mice without any apparent toxicity to normal tissues *(29,77,78)*. Additionally, [125]I-labeled mAb anti-endoglin/CD105 conjugates have been used to effectively image spontaneous canine mammary adenocarcinomas with tumor : background ratios of greater than 8 : 1 *(79)*.

E-selectin (CD62E), a cell adhesion molecule that facilitates and enables adhesion and rolling of leukocytes along the surface of endothelial cells, is also a promising marker of activated endothelium. CD62E is expressed on endothelial cells under inflammatory conditions while being absent in normal, noninflammatory tissue. Inflammatory cytokines such as tumor necrosis factor-$\alpha$ (TNF-$\alpha$), interleukin-1 (IL-1), or interferon-$\gamma$ (IFN-$\gamma$) stimulate endothelial cells to express CD62E. A variety of human tumors, including breast, colorectal, NSCLC, and hemangiomas have been shown to have CD62E-positive blood vessels *(80)*. Expression of CD62E on the luminal side of activated endothelium makes it a leading candidate for vascular targeting. Because CD62E is similar to VCAM-1 in its regulation and expression, and VCAM-1 has already proven to be a suitable target for vascular targeting, it is expected that targeting CD62E will also be effective *(81)*. CD62E might have a role in facilitating transendothelial migration of tumor cells during metastatic invasion *(82)*; therefore, targeting CD62E might be an effective method of interfering with tumor cell metastasis as well initiating tumor infarction. Another very promising marker for targeting proliferating endothelial cells is the 30.5-kDa antigen that is recognized by the EN7/44 antibody. This antigen is present in vessels of both tumors and inflammatory tissues. Its presence is associated with budding and proliferating endothelial cells within the tumors and it is often coexpressed with E-selectin *(83)*.

### 2.1.3. PROSTATE-SPECIFIC MEMBRANE ANTIGEN

Prostate-specific membrane antigen (PSMA) is a 750-amino-acid type II transmembrane glycoprotein of approximately 100 kDa. It has at least two enzymatic activities: (1) *N*-acetylated α-linked L-amino dipeptidase (NAALADase), an enzyme involved in regulation of excitatory signaling in the brain, and (2) γ-glutamyl carboxypeptidase (folate hydrolase). PSMA was defined originally by mAb 7E11, which binds to an intracellular epitope of human PSMA *(84,85)*. A number of other anti-PSMA mAbs have since been developed that bind to the extracellular domain of human PSMA, such as mAbs J591, J415, J533, and E99 *(86)*. Expression of PSMA is restricted to prostatic tissue, including normal prostatic epithelium, benign prostatic secretory-acinar epithelium, prostatic intraepithelial neoplasia, and prostatic adenocarcinoma cells *(87,88)*. Interestingly, PSMA is also expressed consistently and abundantly on vascular endothelium in a wide variety of primary and metastatic solid tumors in humans, such as cancers of the breast, lung, ovary, kidney, bladder, and intestinal tract but not on blood vessels in normal tissues *(86,89)*. In addition, in vivo localization with $^{111}$In-labeled 7E11 mAb to a conventional (clear cell) renal cell carcinoma demonstrated that anti-PSMA mAbs have utility for targeting and imaging tumor vasculature in nonprostatic cancers *(90)*. Based on these exciting observations, PSMA is an attractive candidate for targeting tumor vasculature for both therapy and imaging of cancer.

Studies on the expression of PSMA in normal and tumor tissue in the mouse have proven difficult. We have recently generated a rat mAb, which recognizes both mouse and human PSMA. Surprisingly, PSMA was not detected immunohistochemically on the vessels of any tumors grown in mice, regardless the type of tumor, site of implantation, or tissue of origin *(91)*. It is unclear why vascular endothelium in murine tumors does not express detectable levels of PSMA. A potential difference is the growth rate of most mouse tumor systems compared to the growth rate of typical carcinomas in man. However, blood vessels in slow-growing spontaneous mammary tumors that arise in Apc$^{min}$ mice (doubling time is approx 4 wk) were also negative for PSMA. Another possible explanation might be species differences between human and mouse with regard to PSMA expression on tumor vessels, as is true of prostatic epithelium *(92)*. Thus, because of the lack of appropriate animal models, PSMA as a target for vascular targeting has not been explored fully.

### 2.1.4. PHOSPHATIDYLSERINE

The phospholipids of the plasma membrane are distributed asymmetrically. Choline-containing lipids are located on the outer leaflet, whereas the amino phospholipids are restricted largely to the inner leaflet. Under normal conditions, phosphatidylserine (PS) is restricted exclusively to the inner leaflet of the plasma membrane in most cell types, including vascular endothelial cells *(93)*. PS asymmetry is maintained by an ATP-dependent aminophospholipid translocase that is responsible for inward movement of aminophospholipids *(94)*. Loss of PS asymmetry is caused by either decreased aminophospho-lipid translocase activity *(95)* and/or activation of scramblase, a $Ca^{2+}$-dependent enzyme that transports lipids bidirectionally *(96)*.

Exposure of PS on the outer leaflet of the cell membrane has been found under certain pathologic and physiologic conditions, such cell apoptosis *(97)*, cell migration *(98)*, and activation of platelets *(99)*. PS exposure has also been observed in some malignant cells in the absence of exogenous activators or cell injury *(100)*. A series of studies have shown that PS exposure is a general feature of tumor vascular endothelium *(36,56,101)*. A recent study *(36)* examined PS exposure in six tumor models through the use of in vivo local-ization studies in which anti-PS antibodies were found to localize specifically to tumor endothelium after intravenous injection into mice bearing various types of solid tumors. The percentage of PS-positive vessels was found to be 4–40% depending on tumor type and tumor size, in contrast, none of the blood vessels in normal tissues had detectable externalized PS. It is worth noting that PS exposure on tumor vessels is not a result of endothelial cell apoptosis. It is hypothesized that PS is exposed on tumor vasculature as a result of stress conditions in the tumor microenvironment, such as tumor-associated cytokines, leukocytes, metabolites, and hypoxia, and subsequent reoxygenation. These factors might act individually or collectively in tumors to induce PS exposure on tumor endothelial cells. Using cultured endothelial cells, it was found that subtoxic levels of inflammatory cytokines (IL-1, TNF-$\alpha$, and interferon), hypoxia, acidity, thrombin, and hydrogen peroxide induce PS exposure without inducing apoptosis. Hydrogen peroxide was the most potent inducer of PS exposure *(36)*. Because PS exposed on endothelial cells is involved in and can promote coagulation *(102)*, PS might be particularly well suited for vascular targeting strategies that employ soluble tissue factor as the effector. Various coaguligands, VTAs that employ tissue factor as the effector, have shown impressive anti-tumor effects by a number of laboratories *(47,55,56,103,104)*. PS exposure on tumor vascular endothelium not only potentiates VTA-induced coagulation but also limits the extent of thrombosis to tumor vessels, therefore increasing the specificity of the VTA. This was demonstrated by Ran et al. *(56)*, who showed that a coaguligand targeted to VCAM-1 (which is present on tumor vessels as well as on vessels in heart and lung) selec-tively induced coagulation in tumor vessels only; no thromboses were seen in the heart or lung in spite of coaguligand localization to vessels in the heart and lung.

In summary, PS is specifically and abundantly expressed on tumor vascular endothe-lium; it is present on a high percentage of tumor endothelial cells in various solid tumors; it is absent from normal vessels; and it is on the luminal side of tumor endothelium, readily accessible for targeting agents. Naked antibodies and antibody conjugates directed against PS could potentially be used for cancer therapy and imaging.

## 2.2. Basement Membrane Targets

Markers present on the surface of cells that support vessels together with the compo-nents of remodeled basement membrane (BM) within the tumor blood vessels can also serve as vascular targets. One of the most promising and extensively studied examples is the ED-B domain of fibronectin, bound by the human antibody fragment L19 *(105)*. Intravenous administration of soluble tissue factor fused with L19 into tumor-bearing mice mediated the complete and selective infarction of tumor blood vessels, which resulted in significant tumor regression *(47)*.

Another candidate is collagen type IV (Col IV), which is a major component of the blood vessel's basement membrane. Col IV is proteolytically digested in the process of vascular remodeling during angiogenesis. Through the use of subtractive immunization, Xu et al. *(51,52)* raised monoclonal antibodies that bind selectively to denatured or proteolyzed collagen type I and type IV. The mAbs bind to the basement of tumor blood vessels and could be used as targeting agents for selective delivery of TF or other effectors that might cause infarction of tumor vasculature. Interestingly, these mAbs possess antiangiogenic activity by themselves and are being investigated for use as therapeutic "naked" mAbs, as well as VTAs.

Vascular BM components are required for the initiation and resolution of angiogenesis. Most of these components under physiological conditions sustain the growth, survival, and health of vascular endothelium. The primary signals originating from capillary BM inhibit proliferation and promote an environment that facilitates appropriate cell–cell adhesion. Proteolytic cleavage of basement membrane and the ECM by MMPs during the process of remodeling releases endogenous inhibitors of angiogenesis that consist of fragments of constituents of the ECM. These "cryptic domains" are hidden in folded or assembled protein structures, especially of collagen types: IV [arrestin, canstatin, tumstatin and $\alpha6(IV)NC1$ domain], XV (endostatinlike protein), and XVIII (endostatin). They are biologically inactive until released during basement membrane and ECM remodeling *(106–108)*. These molecules not only have antiangiogenic properties but their presence can serve as an exclusive marker for sites with ongoing angiogenesis. This fact makes them attractive VTAs that can help to attack the exterior part of the forming tumor vasculature and modulate tumor cell–ECM–vessel wall interaction.

## 3. OVERVIEW AND FUTURE DIRECTIONS

To move vascular targeting into the clinic, current candidate targets must be validated and new targets must be identified. The technique of phage display is currently being used to identify new specific markers of tumor vasculature. Phage display libraries contain bacteriophages, which display as many as $10^9$ specific peptides. Peptides that bind specifically to a target cell can be found by panning. Panning can be performed both in vitro and in vivo. In vivo panning is especially intriguing for identifying tumor vascular targets, because pure tumor vascular endothelial cells are technically difficult to obtain and in vitro cultivation changes the characteristics of isolated endothelial cells. To perform panning in vivo, phage display libraries are injected intravenously into tumor-bearing mice, and the tumor is harvested and phage are extracted. Peptides specific for tumor vasculature can be enriched and selected by several rounds of biopanning. Using in vivo panning, a number of potentially tumor vasculature specific markers have been identified *(109,110)*. For example, recently Joyce et al. *(111)* identified several peptides specific for angiogenic stages in mouse pancreatic islet carcinogenesis. In vivo biopanning has also been done in human patients *(112)*. Given the potential specificity of peptides identified by biopanning, there is great hope that this technology will identify tumor stage-specific and organ-specific vascular targets. Identification of these targets will facilitate vascular targeting and antiangiogenic therapeutic approaches for the treatment of cancer.

Tumor vessels are formed by the process of angiogenesis and vasculogenesis *(113)*. During vasculogenesis, hematopoietic and vascular stem cells are mobilized from the bone marrow and incorporated into tumor vessel structures *(114,115)*. Circulating endothelial progenitor cells (CEPs) and hematopoietic stem cells (HSCs) localize to sites of neovascularization and, therefore, could be potentially useful for identifying or targeting tumor blood vessels *(116)*. After being modified genetically, CEPs can be exploited in the future as "molecular shuttles" that deliver therapeutic genes or therapeutic agents to tumor endothelial cells *(117)*.

New effectors for VTAs are also under investigation. Microbubbles, which are ultrasound contrast agents that are used widely in echocardiographic examination, are an exciting new potential effector. Microbubbles provide a very promising, tissue-specific, noninvasive new tool for vascular-based tumor imaging and therapy *(118)*. By targeting microbubbles to markers expressed on activated endothelial cells, it is possible to image noninvasively and specifically sites of tumor angiogenesis *(119,120)*. It is conceivable that therapeutic agents (e.g., drugs, genes) could be attached to microbubbles and released within the target tissue during ultrasound-triggered destruction of the microbubbles *(121,122)*.

Solid tumors, which make up over 90% of all human cancers, have proven resistant thus far to antitumor antibody-based therapies. This is largely the result of the inaccessibility of tumor cells in solid masses to macromolecular agents *(123–125)*. A potential solution to this problem is to attack the endothelium lining the vasculature of solid tumors instead of the tumor cells themselves (reviewed in ref. *126*). This is consistent with the hypothesis put forth by Folkman in 1971 *(1)*, in which he proposed that if neovascularization of solid tumors could be prevented, then the tumors would not be able to expand their volume beyond that allowed by the existing host vasculature. He argued that small tumors and metastases would be able to grow only to a size of approx 2–3 mm$^3$ before inhibition of neovascularization would limit further tumor growth. These predictions have proven to be substantially correct: Inhibitors of angiogenesis that act by diverse mechanisms retard or prevent the growth of angiogenic tumors in experimental animals and in man *(127)*. That blood vessels in tumors are a viable therapeutic target is no longer questioned; however, the optimum method of attacking those blood vessels is still under investigation. Vascular targeting will likely evolve to be an adjuvant therapy used after surgical resection and/or radiation therapy in most cases, while in some nonoperable tumors, VTAs might be considered as a first line of therapy, provided specific markers combined with effective and safe effectors are utilized.

## REFERENCES

1. Folkman J. Tumor angiogenesis: therapeutic implications. N Engl J Med 1971; 285:1182–1186.
2. Hanahan D, Weinberg RA. The hallmarks of cancer. Cell 2000; 100:57–70.
3. Folkman J. Fundamental concepts of the angiogenic process. Curr Mol Med 2003; 3:643–651.
4. Tonini T, Rossi F, Claudio PP. Molecular basis of angiogenesis and cancer. Oncogene 2003; 22:6549–6556.
5. Carmeliet P. Angiogenesis in health and disease. Nat Med 2003; 9:653–660.
6. Drake CJ. Embryonic and adult vasculogenesis. Birth Defects Res Part C Embryo Today 2003; 69: 73–82.
7. Bergers G, Benjamin LE. Tumorigenesis and the angiogenic switch. Nat Rev Cancer 2003; 3:401–410.
8. Pasqualini R, Arap W, McDonald DM. Probing the structural and molecular diversity of tumor vasculature. Trends Mol Med 2002; 8:563–571.
9. Baluk P, Morikawa S, Haskell A, Mancuso M, McDonald DM. Abnormalities of basement membrane on blood vessels and endothelial sprouts in tumors. Am J Pathol 2003; 163:1801–1815.
10. McDonald DM, Choyke PL. Imaging of angiogenesis: from microscope to clinic. Nat Med 2003; 9: 713–725.
11. Tozer GM, Kanthou C, Parkins CS, Hill SA. The biology of the combretastatins as tumour vascular targeting agents. Int J Exp Pathol 2002; 83:21–38.

12. Zhou S, Kestell P, Baguley BC, Paxton JW. 5,6-Dimethylxanthenone-4-acetic acid (DMXAA): a new biological response modifier for cancer therapy. Invest New Drugs 2002; 20:281–295.
13. Denekamp J. Vasculature as a target for tumour therapy. Prog Appl Microcirc 1984; 4:28–38.
14. Denekamp J. Vascular attack as a therapeutic strategy for cancer. Cancer Metastasis Rev 1990; 9:267–282.
15. Brekken RA, Li C, Kumar S. Strategies for vascular targeting in tumors. Int J Cancer 2002; 100:123–130.
16. Thorpe PE, Chaplin DJ, Blakey DC. The first international conference on vascular targeting: meeting overview. Cancer Res 2003; 63:1144–1147.
17. Denekamp J. Endothelial cell attack as a novel approach to cancer therapy. Cancer Topics 1986; 6:6–8.
18. Burrows FJ, Thorpe PE. Eradication of large solid tumors in mice with an immunotoxin directed against tumor vasculature. Proc Natl Acad Sci USA 1993; 90:8996–9600.
19. Denekamp J, Hobson B. Endothelial-cell proliferation in experimental tumours. Br J Cancer 1982; 46: 711–720.
20. Folkman J. Tumor angiogenesis. Adv Cancer Res 1985; 43:175–230.
21. Tannock IF. The relation between cell proliferation and the vascular system in a transplanted mouse mammary tumor. Br J Cancer 1968; 22:258–273.
22. Tannock IF. Population kinetics of carcinoma cells, capillary endothelial cells, and fibroblasts in a transplanted mouse mammary tumor. Cancer Res 1970; 30:2470–2476.
23. Ke L, Qu H, Nagy JA, et al. Vascular targeting of solid and ascites tumours with antibodies to vascular endothelial growth factor. Eur J Cancer 1996; 32A:2467–2473.
24. Brekken RA, Huang X, King SW, Thorpe PE. Vascular endothelial growth factor as a marker of tumor endothelium. Cancer Res 1998; 58:1952–1959.
25. Cooke SP, Boxer GM, Lawrence L, et al. A strategy for antitumor vascular therapy by targeting the vascular endothelial growth factor: receptor complex. Cancer Res 2001; 61:3653–3659.
26. Molema G, Meijer DK, de Leij LF. Tumor vasculature targeted therapies: getting the players organized. Biochem Pharmacol 1998; 55:1939–1945.
27. Gonzalez AM, Gonzales M, Herron GS, et al. Complex interactions between the laminin alpha 4 subunit and integrins regulate endothelial cell behavior in vitro and angiogenesis in vivo. Proc Natl Acad Sci USA 2002; 99:16,075–16,080.
28. Hagemeier H-H, Vollmer E, Goerdt S, Schulze-Osthoff K, Sorg C. A monoclonal antibody reacting with endothelial cells of budding vessels in tumors and inflammatory tissues, and non-reactive with normal adult tissues. Int J Cancer 1986; 38:481–488.
29. Burrows FJ, Derbyshire EJ, Tazzari PL, et al. Up-regulation of endoglin on vascular endothelial cells in human solid tumors: implications for diagnosis and therapy. Clin Cancer Res 1995; 1:1623–3164.
30. Seon BK, Matsuno F, Haruta Y, Kondo M, Barcos M. Long-lasting complete inhibition of human solid tumors in SCID mice by targeting endothelial cells of tumor vasculature with antihuman endoglin immunotoxin. Clin Cancer Res 1997; 3:1031–1044.
31. Thorpe PE, Burrows FJ. Antibody-directed targeting of the vasculature of solid tumors. Breast Cancer Res.Treat . 1995; 36:237–251.
32. Westphal JR, Willems HW, Schalkwijk CJ, Ruiter DJ, deWaal RM. A new 180-kDa dermal endothelial cell activation antigen: in vitro and in situ characteristics. J Invest Dermatol 1993; 100:27–34.
33. Wang JM, Kumar S, Pye D, Vanagthoven AJ, Krupinski J, Hunter RD. A monoclonal antibody detects heterogeneity in vascular endothelium of tumours and normal tissues. Int J Cancer 1993; 54:363–370.
34. Wang JM, Kumar S, van Agthoven A, Kumar P, Pye D, Hunter RD. Irradiation induces up-regulation of E9 protein (CD105) in human vascular endothelial cells. Int J Cancer 1995; 62:791–796.
35. Rettig WJ, Garinchesa P, Healey JH, Su SL, Jaffe EA, Old LJ. Identification of endosialin, a cell surface glycoprotein of vascular endothelial cells in human cancer. Proc Natl Acad Sci USA 1992; 89: 10,832–10,836.
36. Ran S, Thorpe PE. Phosphatidylserine is a marker of tumor vasculature and a potential target for cancer imaging and therapy. Int J Radiat Oncol Biol Phys 2002; 54:1479–1484.
37. Koch AE, Nickoloff BJ, Holgersson J, et al. 4A11, a monoclonal antibody recognizing a novel antigen expressed on aberrant vascular endothelium. Upregulation in an in vivo model of contact dermatitis. Am J Pathol 1994; 144:244–259.
38. Griffioen AW, Coenen MJ, Damen CA, et al. CD44 is involved in tumor angiogenesis; an activation antigen on human endothelial cells. Blood 1997; 90:1150–1159.
39. Liu N, Lapcevich RK, Underhill CB, et al. Metastatin: a hyaluronan-binding complex from cartilage that inhibits tumor growth. Cancer Res 2001; 61:1022–1028.

40. Sipkins DA, Cheresh DA, Kazemi MR, Nevin LM, Bednarski MD, Li KC. Detection of tumor angiogenesis in vivo by alphaVbeta3-targeted magnetic resonance imaging. Nat Med 1998; 4:623–626.

41. Gasparini G, Brooks PC, Biganzoli E, et al. Vascular integrin alpha(v)beta3: a new prognostic indicator in breast cancer. Clin Cancer Res 1998; 4:2625–2634.

42. Pasqualini R, Koivunen E, Ruoslahti E. Alpha v integrins as receptors for tumor targeting by circulating ligands. Nat Biotechnol 1997; 15:542–546.

43. Senger DR, Claffey KP, Benes JE, Perruzzi CA, Sergiou AP, Detmar M. Angiogenesis promoted by vascular endothelial growth factor: regulation through alpha1beta1 and alpha2beta1 integrins. Proc Natl Acad Sci USA 1997; 94:13,612–13,617.

44. Senger DR, Perruzzi CA, Streit M, Koteliansky VE, de Fougerolles AR, Detmar M. The alpha(1)beta(1) and alpha(2)beta(1) integrins provide critical support for vascular endothelial growth factor signaling, endothelial cell migration, and tumor angiogenesis. Am J Pathol 2002; 160:195–204.

45. Kim S, Bell K, Mousa SA, Varner JA. Regulation of angiogenesis in vivo by ligation of integrin alpha5 beta1 with the central cell-binding domain of fibronectin. Am J Pathol 2000; 156:1345–1362.

46. Epstein AL, Khawli LA, Hornick JL, Taylor CR. Identification of a monoclonal antibody, TV-1 directed against the basement membrane of tumor vessels, and its use to enhance the delivery of macromolecules to tumors after conjugation with interleukin 2. Cancer Res 1995; 55:2673–2680.

47. Nilsson F, Kosmehl H, Zardi L, Neri D. Targeted delivery of tissue factor to the ED-B domain of fibronectin, a marker of angiogenesis, mediates the infarction of solid tumors in mice. Cancer Res 2001; 61:711–716.

48. Carnemolla B, Neri D, Castellani P, et al. Phage antibodies with pan-species recognition of the oncofoetal angiogenesis marker fibronectin ED-B domain. Int J Cancer 1996; 68:397–405.

49. Marty C, Odermatt B, Schott H, et al. Cytotoxic targeting of F9 teratocarcinoma tumours with anti-ED-B fibronectin scFv antibody modified liposomes. Br J Cancer 2002; 87:106–112.

50. Borsi L, Balza E, Bestagno M, et al. Selective targeting of tumoral vasculature: comparison of different formats of an antibody (L19) to the ED-B domain of fibronectin. Int J Cancer 2002; 102:75–85.

51. Xu J, Rodriguez D, Kim JJ, Brooks PC. Generation of monoclonal antibodies to cryptic collagen sites by using subtractive immunization. Hybridoma 2000; 19:375–385.

52. Xu J, Rodriguez D, Petitclerc E, et al. Proteolytic exposure of a cryptic site within collagen type IV is required for angiogenesis and tumor growth in vivo. J Cell Biol 2001; 154:1069–1079.

53. Burg MA, Pasqualini R, Arap W, Ruoslahti E, Stallcup WB. NG2 proteoglycan-binding peptides target tumor neovasculature. Cancer Res 1999; 59:2869–2874.

54. Pasqualini R, Koivunen E, Kain R, et al. Aminopeptidase N is a receptor for tumor-homing peptides and a target for inhibiting angiogenesis. Cancer Res 2000; 60:722–727.

55. Huang X, Molema G, King S, Watkins L, Edgington TS, Thorpe PE. Tumor infarction in mice by antibody-directed targeting of tissue factor to tumor vasculature. Science 1997; 275:547–550.

56. Ran S, Gao B, Duffy S, Watkins L, Rote N, Thorpe PE. Infarction of solid Hodgkin's tumors in mice by antibody-directed targeting of tissue factor to tumor vasculature. Cancer Res 1998; 58:4646–4653.

57. Abramovitch R, Frenkiel D, Neeman M. Analysis of subcutaneous angiogenesis by gradient echo magnetic resonance imaging. Magn Reson Med 1998; 39:813–824.

58. Brekken RA, Thorpe PE. VEGF–VEGF receptor complexes as markers of tumor vascular endothelium. J Control Release 2001; 74:173–181.

59. Dvorak HF. Vascular permeability factor/vascular endothelial growth factor: a critical cytokine in tumor angiogenesis and a potential target for diagnosis and therapy. J Clin Oncol 2002; 20:4368–4380.

60. Dvorak HF. Rous-Whipple Award Lecture. How tumors make bad blood vessels and stroma. Am J Pathol 2003; 162:1747–1757.

61. Bergers G, Brekken R, McMahon G, et al. Matrix metalloproteinase-9 triggers the angiogenic switch during carcinogenesis. Nat Cell Biol 2000; 2:737–744.

62. Hanahan D. Heritable formation of pancreatic beta-cell tumours in transgenic mice expressing recombinant insulin/simian virus 40 oncogenes. Nature 1985; 315:115–122.

63. Giatromanolaki A, Koukourakis MI, Sivridis E, et al. Tumor specific activation of the VEGF/KDR angiogenic pathway in a subset of locally advanced squamous cell head and neck carcinomas. Clin Exp Metastasis 2000; 18:313–319.

64. Koukourakis MI, Giatromanolaki A, Thorpe PE, et al. Vascular endothelial growth factor/KDR activated microvessel density versus CD31 standard microvessel density in non-small cell lung cancer. Cancer Res 2000; 60:3088–3095.

65. Stupack DG, Cheresh DA. Get a ligand, get a life: integrins, signaling and cell survival. J Cell Sci 2002; 115:3729–3738.

66. Hynes RO. Integrins: bidirectional, allosteric signaling machines. Cell 2002; 110:673–687.

67. Ruegg C, Mariotti A. Vascular integrins: pleiotropic adhesion and signaling molecules in vascular homeostasis and angiogenesis. Cell Mol Life Sci 2003; 60:1135–1157.

68. Soldi R, Mitola S, Strasly M, Defilippi P, Tarone G, Bussolino F. Role of alphavbeta3 integrin in the activation of vascular endothelial growth factor receptor-2. EMBO J 1999; 18:882–892.

69. Woodard AS, Garcia-Cardena G, Leong M, Madri JA, Sessa WC, Languino LR. The synergistic activity of alphavbeta3 integrin and PDGF receptor increases cell migration. J Cell Sci 1998; 111(Pt 4): 469–478.

70. Klein S, Bikfalvi A, Birkenmeier TM, Giancotti FG, Rifkin DB. Integrin regulation by endogenous expression of 18-kDa fibroblast growth factor-2. J Biol Chem 1996; 271:22,583–22,590.

71. Moro L, Dolce L, Cabodi S, et al. Integrin-induced epidermal growth factor (EGF) receptor activation requires c-Src and p130Cas and leads to phosphorylation of specific EGF receptor tyrosines. J Biol Chem 2002; 277:9405–9414.

72. Eliceiri BP, Cheresh DA. Role of alpha v integrins during angiogenesis. Cancer J 2000; 6(Suppl 3): S245–S249.

73. Kumar CC. Integrin alpha v beta 3 as a therapeutic target for blocking tumor-induced angiogenesis. Curr Drug Targets 2003; 4:123–131.

74. Brooks PC, Silletti S, von Schalscha TL, Friedlander M, Cheresh DA. Disruption of angiogenesis by PEX, a noncatalytic metalloproteinase fragment with integrin binding activity. Cell 1998; 92:391–400.

75. Silletti S, Kessler T, Goldberg J, Boger DL, Cheresh DA. Disruption of matrix metalloproteinase 2 binding to integrin alpha vbeta 3 by an organic molecule inhibits angiogenesis and tumor growth in vivo. Proc Natl Acad Sci USA 2001; 98:119–124.

76. Li C, Hampson IN, Hampson L, Kumar P, Bernabeu C, Kumar S. CD105 antagonizes the inhibitory signaling of transforming growth factor beta1 on human vascular endothelial cells. FASEB J 2000; 14: 55–64.

77. Kumar S, Ghellal A, Li C, et al. Breast carcinoma: vascular density determined using CD105 antibody correlates with tumor prognosis. Cancer Res 1999; 59:856–861.

78. Matsuno F, Haruta Y, Kondo M, Tsai H, Barcos M, Seon BK. Induction of lasting complete regression of preformed distinct solid tumors by targeting the tumor vasculature using two new anti-endoglin monoclonal antibodies. Clin Cancer Res 1999; 5:371–382.

79. Fonsatti E, Jekunen AP, Kairemo KJ, et al. Endoglin is a suitable target for efficient imaging of solid tumors: in vivo evidence in a canine mammary carcinoma model. Clin Cancer Res 2000; 6:2037–2043.

80. Langley RR, Russell J, Eppihimer MJ, et al. Quantification of murine endothelial cell adhesion molecules in solid tumors. Am J Physiol 1999; 277:H1156–H1166.

81. Chiu GN, Bally MB, Mayer LD. Targeting of antibody conjugated, phosphatidylserine-containing liposomes to vascular cell adhesion molecule 1 for controlled thrombogenesis. Biochim Biophys Acta 2003; 1613:115–121.

82. Laferriere J, Houle F, Huot J. Regulation of the metastatic process by E-selectin and stress-activated protein kinase-2/p38. Ann NY Acad Sci 2002; 973:562–572.

83. Mayer B, Spatz H, Funke I, Johnson JP, Schildberg FW. De novo expression of the cell adhesion molecule E-selectin on gastric cancer endothelium. Langenbecks Arch Surg 1998; 383:81–86.

84. Horoszewicz JS, Kawinski E, Murphy GP. Monoclonal antibodies to a new antigenic marker in epithelial prostatic cells and serum of prostatic cancer patients. Anticancer Res 1987; 7:927–935.

85. Israeli RS, Powell CT, Fair WR, Heston WD. Molecular cloning of a complementary DNA encoding a prostate-specific membrane antigen. Cancer Res 1993; 53:227–230.

86. Liu H, Moy P, Kim S, et al. Monoclonal antibodies to the extracellular domain of prostate-specific membrane antigen also react with tumor vascular endothelium. Cancer Res 1997; 57:3629–3634.

87. Silver DA, Pellicer I, Fair WR, Heston WD, Cordon-Cardo C. Prostate-specific membrane antigen expression in normal and malignant human tissues. Clin Cancer Res 1997; 3:81–85.

88. Israeli RS, Powell CT, Corr JG, Fair WR, Heston WD. Expression of the prostate-specific membrane antigen. Cancer Res 1994; 54:1807–1811.

89. Chang SS, Reuter VE, Heston WD, Bander NH, Grauer LS, Gaudin PB. Five different anti-prostate-specific membrane antigen (PSMA) antibodies confirm PSMA expression in tumor-associated neovasculature. Cancer Res 1999; 59:3192–3198.

90. Michaels EK, Blend M, Quintana JC. [111]Indium-capromab pendetide unexpectedly localizes to renal cell carcinoma. J Urol 1999; 161:597–598.

91. Huang X, Bennet M, Thorpe PE. Antitumor effects and lack of side effects in mice of an immunotoxin directed against human and mouse prostate specific membrane antigen. Prostate 2004; 61:1–11.

92. Bacich DJ, Pinto JT, Tong WP, Heston WD. Cloning, expression, genomic localization, and enzymatic activities of the mouse homolog of prostate-specific membrane antigen/NAALADase/folate hydrolase. Mamm Genome 2001; 12:117–123.

93. Williamson P, Schlegel RA. Back and forth: the regulation and function of transbilayer phospholipid movement in eukaryotic cells. Mol Membr Biol 1994; 11:199–216.

94. Devaux PF. Protein involvement in transmembrane lipid asymmetry. Annu Rev Biophys Biomol Struct 1992; 21:417–439.

95. Comfurius P, Senden JMG, Tilly RHJ, Schroit AJ, Bevers EM, Zwaal RFA. Loss of membrane phospholipid asymmetry in platelets and red cells may be associated with calcium-induced shedding of plasma membrane and inhibition of aminophospholipid translocase. Biochim Biophys Acta: Biomembranes 1990; 1026:153–160.

96. Zhou Q, Zhao J, Stout JG, Luhm RA, Wiedmer T, Sims PJ. Molecular cloning of human plasma membrane phospholipid scramblase. A protein mediating transbilayer movement of plasma membrane phospholipids. J Biol Chem 1997; 272:18,240–18,244.

97. Blankenberg FG, Katsikis PD, Tait JF, et al. In vivo detection and imaging of phosphatidylserine expression during programmed cell death. Proc Natl Acad Sci USA 1998; 95:6349–6354.

98. Vogt E, Ng AK, Rote NS. A model for the antiphospholipid antibody syndrome: monoclonal antiphosphatidylserine antibody induces intrauterine growth restriction in mice. Am J Obstet Gynecol 1996; 174: 700–707.

99. Rote NS, Ng A-K, Dostal-Johnson DA, Nicholson SL, Siekman R. Immunologic detection of phosphatidylserine externalization during thrombin-induced platelet activation. Clin Immunol Immunopathol 1993; 66:193–200.

100. Utsugi T, Schroit AJ, Connor J, Bucana CD, Fidler IJ. Elevated expression of phosphatidylserine in the outer membrane leaflet of human tumor cells and recognition by activated human blood monocytes. Cancer Res 1991; 51:3062–3066.

101. Ran S, Downes A, Thorpe PE. Increased exposure of anionic phospholipids on the surface of tumor blood vessels. Cancer Res 2002; 62:6132–6140.

102. Bombeli T, Karsan A, Tait JF, Harlan JM. Apoptotic vascular endothelial cells become procoagulant. Blood 1997; 89:2429–2442.

103. Thorpe PE, Ran S. Tumor infarction by targeting tissue factor to tumor vasculature. Cancer J 2000; 6(Suppl 3):S237–S244.

104. Liu C, Huang H, Donate F, et al. Prostate-specific membrane antigen directed selective thrombotic infarction of tumors. Cancer Res 2002; 62:5470–5475.

105. Tarli L, Balza E, Viti F, et al. A high-affinity human antibody that targets tumoral blood vessels. Blood 1999; 94:192–198.

106. Schenk S, Quaranta V. Tales from the crypt[ic] sites of the extracellular matrix. Trends Cell Biol 2003; 13:366–375.

107. Kalluri R. Basement membranes: structure, assembly and role in tumour angiogenesis. Nat Rev Cancer 2003; 3:422–433.

108. Kerbel R, Folkman J. Clinical translation of angiogenesis inhibitors. Nat Rev Cancer 2002; 2:727–739.

109. Zurita AJ, Arap W, Pasqualini R. Mapping tumor vascular diversity by screening phage display libraries. J Control Release 2003; 91:183–186.

110. Hoffman JA, Giraudo E, Singh M, et al. Progressive vascular changes in a transgenic mouse model of squamous cell carcinoma. Cancer Cell 2003; 4:383–391.

111. Joyce JA, Laakkonen P, Bernasconi M, Bergers G, Ruoslahti E, Hanahan D. Stage-specific vascular markers revealed by phage display in a mouse model of pancreatic islet tumorigenesis. Cancer Cell 2003; 4:393–403.

112. Arap W, Kolonin MG, Trepel M, et al. Steps toward mapping the human vasculature by phage display. Nat Med 2002; 8:121–127.

113. Carmeliet P, Jain RK. Angiogenesis in cancer and other diseases. Nature 2000; 407:249–257.

114. Lyden D, Hattori K, Dias S, et al. Impaired recruitment of bone-marrow-derived endothelial and hematopoietic precursor cells blocks tumor angiogenesis and growth. Nat Med 2001; 7:1194–1201.

115. Marchetti S, Gimond C, Iljin K, et al. Endothelial cells genetically selected from differentiating mouse embryonic stem cells incorporate at sites of neovascularization in vivo. J Cell Sci 2002; 115:2075–2085.

116. Rafii S, Lyden D, Benezra R, Hattori K, Heissig B. Vascular and haematopoietic stem cells: novel targets for anti-angiogenesis therapy? Nat Rev Cancer 2002; 2:826–835.

117. Ferrari N, Glod J, Lee J, Kobiler D, Fine HA. Bone marrow-derived, endothelial progenitor-like cells as angiogenesis-selective gene-targeting vectors. Gene Ther 2003; 10:647–656.

118. Stewart MJ. Contrast echocardiography. Heart 2003; 89:342–348.

119. Ellegala DB, Leong-Poi H, Carpenter JE, et al. Imaging tumor angiogenesis with contrast ultrasound and microbubbles targeted to alpha(v)beta3. Circulation 2003; 108:336–341.

120. Leong-Poi H, Christiansen J, Klibanov AL, Kaul S, Lindner JR. Noninvasive assessment of angiogenesis by ultrasound and microbubbles targeted to alpha(v)-integrins. Circulation 2003; 107:455–460.

121. Unger EC, Matsunaga TO, McCreery T, Schumann P, Sweitzer R, Quigley R. Therapeutic applications of microbubbles. Eur J Radiol 2002; 42:160–168.

122. Unger EC, Hersh E, Vannan M, Matsunaga TO, McCreery T. Local drug and gene delivery through microbubbles. Prog Cardiovasc Dis 2001; 44:45–54.

123. Burrows FJ, Watanabe Y, Thorpe PE. A murine model for antibody-directed targeting of vascular endothelial cells in solid tumors. Cancer Res. 1992; 52:5954–5962.

124. Dvorak HF, Nagy JA, Dvorak AM. Structure of solid tumors and their vasculature: implications for therapy with monoclonal antibodies. Cancer Cells 1991; 3:77–85.

125. Baxter LT, Jain RK. Transport of fluid and macromolecules in tumors. Microvasc Res 1991; 41:5–23.

126. Burrows FJ, Thorpe PE. Targeting the vasculature of solid tumors. J Control Release Soc 1994; 28: 195–202.

127. St Croix B, Man S, Kerbel RS. Reversal of intrinsic and acquired forms of drug resistance by hyaluronidase treatment of solid tumors. Cancer Lett 1998; 131:35–44.

# 29

## Targeting the VEGF/VEGFR Axis for Cancer Therapy

*Frank A. Scappaticci, MD, PhD*

### SUMMARY

Promising new antiangiogenic strategies are emerging for the treatment of cancer. Numerous candidate drugs that target vascular endothelial growth factor (VEGF), VEGF receptors (VEGFR), integrins, matrix metalloproteinases, and other blood vessel targets are being developed and tested in clinical trials. Many approaches have been taken to interfere or completely block angiogenesis. These include antibodies, small molecules, gene therapy, vaccine strategies, and antiangiogenic radioligands. New insight has been gained from completed phase III trials with antiangiogenic drugs, including trial design, dosing, toxicities, and resistance. This chapter will focus on the VEGF/VEGFR axis and the clinical trial results of interfering with this axis by the VEGF-targeting agent Avastin™ (bevacizumab, rhuMAb VEGF).

**Key Words:** Angiogenesis; antiangiogenic agents; VEGF; VEGF/VEGFR axis; chemotherapy; cancer therapy.

## 1. VEGF AS A TARGET FOR CANCER THERAPY

Folkman and colleagues have provided strong evidence linking tumor growth and metastases with new blood vessel growth or "angiogenesis" *(1)*. Several investigators have shown a statistically significant correlation between the density of microvessels in

From: *Cancer Drug Discovery and Development: The Oncogenomics Handbook*
Edited by: W. J. LaRochelle and R. A. Shimkets © Humana Press Inc., Totowa, NJ

tumor specimens of human breast cancer and clinical outcome, including the incidence of metastases as well as overall and relapse-free survival (2,3).

Of the multitude of angiogenic factors that have been identified, vascular endothelial growth factor (VEGF; also known as vascular permeability factor) is the most potent and specific and has been identified as critical to both normal and pathologic angiogenesis (4). VEGF has been shown to be upregulated in most human tumors examined to date. These include cancers of the lung, breast, thyroid, gastrointestinal tract, kidney, bladder, ovary, cervix, angiosarcomas, glioblastomas, and others (4).

Vascular endothelial growth factor has pleiotrophic effects, including endothelial cell growth/migration, induction of proteinases leading to remodeling of the extracellular matrix, and increased vascular permeability. It is also a survival factor for newly formed blood vessels (4). The biologic effects of VEGF are mediated through binding and engagement of two tyrosine kinase receptors on the surface of endothelial cells: Flt-1 (fms-like tyrosine kinase) and KDR (kinase domain region) (4).

Inhibition of VEGF using an anti-VEGF monoclonal antibody has been shown to block the growth of numerous human cancer cell lines in mouse models (4). Human cancer cell lines that are inhibited by anti-VEGF antibody include non-small-cell lung cancer (Calu-6), colorectal cancer (LS174T, HM-7, LSLiM6), breast cancer (MCF-7), prostate cancer (D-145), head and neck cancer (KB), ovarian cancer (SK-OV-3), and others (4). Furthermore, treatment of nude mice harboring human cancer xenografts with anti-VEGF antibody and chemotherapy resulted in an increased antitumor effect compared with antibody or chemotherapy treatment alone (5).

To assess VEGF as a target for cancer therapy, a recombinant humanized version of a murine anti-human VEGF monoclonal antibody, named Avastin™ (bevacizumab, rhuMAb VEGF), was created at Genentech (6). Preclinical toxicology studies had shown that this antibody was relatively safe and it subsequently entered clinical trials.

## 2. CLINICAL TRIAL RESULTS WITH AVASTIN

### 2.1. Efficacy

Avastin, a humanized monoclonal antibody directed against VEGF A, has emerged as the lead antiangiogenic agent to become part of the armamentarium against metastastic colorectal cancer. The results of a recently completed large, randomized, multicenter, double-blinded clinical trial for untreated metastatic colorectal cancer was presented at the May 2003 American Society of Clinical Oncology meeting (7). Over a 2-yr period, 925 patients were randomized into 3 arms: bolus irinotecan/5-fluorouracil (5-FU)/leucovorin (IFL), IFL + Avastin (5 mg/kg q 2 wk), and 5-FU/leucovorin (LV) + Avastin (5 mg/kg q 2 wk). The addition of Avastin to IFL resulted in a 34% reduction in the daily hazard of death compared with IFL alone ($p < 0.01$; median survival increased from 15.6 to 20.3 mo) (7). The addition of Avastin to IFL not only resulted in increased survival, but also increased progression-free survival, response rate, and duration of response as compared with bolus-IFL chemotherapy alone (Table 1).

Results of the addition of Avastin to 5-FU/LV in the above trial have also been reported. This arm was discontinued after the Data Safety Monitoring Committee determined that combination of Avastin with IFL was safe. Approximately 100 patients per arm had been enrolled at the time of discontinuation. Compared with patients who received bolus IFL alone, those that had received Avastin + 5-FU/LV had an improvement in objective

Table 1
Efficacy Summary of Phase III Trial of Avastin in Metastatic Colorectal Cancer

| | IFL + Placebo (n = 412) | IFL + Avastin (n = 403) | p-value |
|---|---|---|---|
| Median survival (mo) | 15.6 | 20.3 | 0.00003 |
| PFS (mo) | 6.24 | 10.6 | <0.00001 |
| ORR (%) | 35 | 45 | 0.0029 |
| CR | 2.2 | 3.7 | |
| PR | 32.5 | 41.2 | |
| Duration of response (mo) | 7.1 | 10.4 | 0.0014 |

*Abbreviations:* ORR, overall response; CR, complete response; PR, partial response.

response rate, duration of response, and survival without significant toxicity. Avastin added to 5-FU/LV appeared to have significant activity as first-line therapy for metastatic colorectal cancer. These results, along with a completed phase II study of combining Avastin with 5-FU/LV *(8)* and a second phase II trial of Avastin in combination with 5-FU/LV for patients that are not optimal candidates for irinotecan (data unpublished), demonstrate that combining Avastin with either 5-FU- or irinotecan-containing chemotherapy regimens provides substantial survival benefit for first line treatment of metastatic colorectal cancer.

A phase II trial of Avastin in combination with carboplatin/taxol chemotherapy for treatment of metastatic non-small-cell lung carcinoma (NSCLC) has shown promising results. This was a randomized, three-arm study that compared chemotherapy alone versus chemotherapy with low-dose Avastin (7.5 mg/kg every 3 wk) versus chemotherapy with high-dose Avastin (15 mg/kg every 3 wk). The data, as assessed by the investigator, revealed an advantage for the high-dose Avastin arm compared with the low-dose Avastin arm or chemotherapy alone (31.5%, 28.1%, and 18.8% response rate, 7.4, 4.3, and 4.2 mo time to progression, and 17.7, 11.6, and 14.9 mo overall survival, respectively). Although this was an underpowered phase II trial with approx 32–35 patients per arm, the trends for each of these end points in favor of high-dose Avastin, was encouraging *(9)*.

Avastin has also been studied in refractory metastatic breast cancer. In this phase III trial, Avastin + capecitabine was evaluated against capecitabine alone and a doubling of the response rate in the combination arm (19% vs 9%) was observed *(10)*. However, statistically significant improvement in progression-free survival and overall survival were not seen. Possibilities for this are as follows. First, the patients in this trial had advanced disease and their tumors might have been expressing multiple angiogenic factors. The therapy might have selected for tumor cells that were not dependent or not expressing VEGF, thus allowing for return of rapid tumor growth and subsequent short-lived responses. Second, the chemotherapy agent itself was not antiangiogenic and, thus, a potential synergistic interaction would not have occurred. Taxol and taxotere might have been better choices in this regard. Administration of these agents using weekly or metronomic dosing to optimize endothelial cell killing might also be ideal. A randomized ECOG phase III trial is currently evaluating weekly Taxol versus Taxol + Avastin in metastatic breast cancer patients. Similarly, there are also two phase II trials evaluating docetaxel in combination with Avastin in inflammatory and locally advanced breast cancer *(10)*.

Avastin as a single agent has shown encouraging results in renal cancer as a second-line therapy. A recently published report comparing two doses of Avastin (3 mg/kg and 10 mg/kg q 2 wk) with placebo for second-line therapy of renal cancer patients that had failed IL-2 therapy showed clinical benefit of the higher dose *(11)*. This trial was stopped early when the 10-mg dose revealed a statistically significant prolongation of time to progression from 2.5 mo in the placebo arm to 4.8 mo ($p < 0.5$). This high-dose arm also showed a 10% response rate versus 0% in the other arms. Although there was no increase in survival, this trial allowed crossover to Avastin in patients who progressed on placebo. Other phase II trials evaluating Avastin with chemotherapy (pancreas, prostate) have been undertaken with very early promising results *(12)*. Results of Avastin in trials of other tumor types are too early to report.

## 2.2. Safety

A previous phase II trial of Avastin in metastatic colorectal cancer revealed that the drug was well tolerated but with safety signals of hypertension, thrombosis, hemorrhage, proteinuria, and minor epistaxis *(8)*. However, a completed large phase III trial in colorectal cancer with more than 400 patients per arm showed that compared with chemotherapy alone, the addition of Avastin to chemotherapy increased the incidence of grade 3 hypertension (this was managed with oral antihypertensive medication), but there was no statistically significant increase in the rates of grade 3/4 thrombosis, hemorrhage, or proteinuria. These data indicated the limited usefulness of phase II trials with regard to determination of drug-related safety signals.

With regard to hemorrhage, this was not observed to be a safety concern in a large phase III trial in metastatic colorectal cancer; however, there were six cases of pulmonary hemorrhage (four of which were fatal) observed in a completed phase II trial of Avastin combined with carboplatin/taxol in NSCLC *(8,13)*. Two-thirds of patients with pulmonary hemorrhage had squamous cell histology. Other risk factors appeared to include cavitation, centrally located tumors invading major vessels, and hemoptysis. Based on these results, a current phase III trial of Avastin combined with carboplatin/Taxol has excluded patients with squamous cell histology. Interim safety results have not been formally reported as to whether the bleeding risk has been reduced by the exclusion of squamous cell histology in this trial, but after review of the safety data by the data safety monitoring board, a recommendation has been made to continue the trial.

In the phase III colorectal cancer trial, gastrointestinal perforations were seen in 6 patients out of approx 400 patients in the Avastin + IFL arm compared with none in the IFL-alone arm *(7)*. These events were rare, and predisposing factors for this infrequent condition have not been identified because of the small numbers. The cases were heterogeneous in nature, ranging from a perforated stomach ulcer, to hemorrhage in the setting of carcinomatosis, to abscess. There was only one fatality out of these six patients and efforts are underway in other metastatic colorectal cancer trials to learn more about this rare condition.

Based on the efficacy and safety of phase II trials, four phase III clinical trials are currently underway (Table 2). These trials are testing Avastin in metastatic colorectal, non-small-cell lung (nonsquamous), breast, and renal cancers. In all studies, Avastin has been added to chemotherapy or cytokine therapy in order to enhance the effects of standard therapies. Furthermore, the potentially greater benefit of antiangiogenic therapy in early

**Table 2**
**Ongoing Avastin Phase III Trials**

| Trial | Tumor Type | Disease Setting | Treatment Setting | Chemotherapy | Design | Primary End Point | No. of Patients |
|---|---|---|---|---|---|---|---|
| ECOG 3200 | Colorectal | Metastatic | Second line | Yes | FOLFOX ± Avastin | Overall survival | 840 |
| ECOG 4599 | NSCLC (nonsquamous) | Metastatic | First line | Yes | Carbo/Taxol ± Avastin | Overall survival | 840 |
| ECOG 2100 | Breast | Metastatic | First line | Yes | Taxol ± Avastin | Disease-free survival | 685 |
| CALGB 90206 | Renal | Metastatic | First line | No | Interferon ± Avastin | Overall survival | 700 |

433

disease settings where there is minimal residual disease has spurred activity in using this agent in the adjuvant setting. Avastin will be tested in the adjuvant setting for colorectal cancer in combination with chemotherapy (infusional 5-FU with oxaliplatin otherwise known as FOLFOX) in large cooperative group trials that are being planned to start this year. It would not be a leap to speculate that this approach might also be undertaken for the adjuvant setting after resection of advanced NSCLC.

### 3. WHAT IS THE MECHANISM FOR ENHANCED ACTIVITY OF CHEMOTHERAPY IN COMBINATION WITH AVASTIN?

The mechanism for the enhanced activity of chemotherapy with the addition of Avastin is not completely understood. There are several potential mechanisms by which an anti-angiogenic agent might enhance antitumor activity in combination with a standard chemotherapy for colorectal cancer. First, the activity of Avastin in killing endothelial cells could potentially impede the angiogenic repair of tumors after initial cytoreduction of tumor cells by chemotherapy and might kill poorly oxygenated tumor cells that are highly dependent on the vasculature. Second, antiangiogenic agents might mediate a "pruning" effect on tumor blood vessels that might allow for better penetration of chemotherapy (14). As a result, a decreased interstitial fluid pressure could enable better penetration of chemotherapy and allow higher intratumoral drug levels. Third, antiangiogenic therapy might synergize with chemotherapy in killing endothelial cells. Perhaps the choice of a cytotoxic agent that has antiangiogenic activity as well as the appropriate scheduling of the drug might synergize with antiangiogenic agents (15,16). Fourth, inhibition of VEGF could lead to enhanced maturation of dendritic cells and allow for more robust immune responses against the tumor (17). Finally, the expression of VEGF/VEGFR (VEGF receptor) in cancer cells cannot be excluded with the possibility of direct antitumor effects. A large effort is currently underway to further understand the mechanism of Avastin in vivo. Various imaging modalities are currently being employed including dynamic contrast magnetic resonance imaging. Techniques such as these are being used to measure blood flow through tumors and to correlate changes in blood flow with antiangiogenic treatment as with the VEGFR inhibitor PTK787 (18,19).

### 4. COMBINING TARGETED THERAPIES

It is known that as breast tumors develop after the angiogenic switch, they secrete multiple angiogenic growth factors that allow for continued growth and expansion of tumor cells (20). Smaller tumors secrete fewer of these factors and might, thus, be amenable to treatment with one or fewer agents targeting angiogenesis. It is likely, then, that successful treatment of larger tumors would entail the use of multiple antiangiogenic agents in combination (21).

For optimal synergistic effects on tumor kill, it might be advantageous to target intracellular signaling pathways that are distinct but critical to growth, differentiation, and apoptosis of tumor cells. Examples might include the combination of an antiangiogenic agent, EGFR inhibitor, an agent that targets the PI3K–AkT pathway, and an agent that targets the TRAIL/TNF (tumor necrosis factor) receptor pathway (10). Such combinations might work best in settings of small tumor burden when there might be limited growth factors and escape mechanisms that are driving the tumor. Efforts to combine Avastin with anti-EGFR (epidermal growth factor) therapies are currently being explored in NSCLC, renal cancer, breast cancer, and other solid tumor types.

Targeted therapies might be used in combination with chemotherapy for optimal reduction of tumor bulk *(13)*. Similarly, in clinical settings of recurrent or metastatic disease, the use of combinations of biological agents alone or with chemotherapy might be useful in palliation, especially when response might be critical for better quality of life as, for example, in treatment of bony metastases. Combinations of biological agents might also be used after cytoreductive therapy with standard chemotherapeutic agents such as adriamycin, cytoxan, paclitaxel, and docetaxel. In this scenario, they might be considered in maintenance programs that could stabilize disease and prevent tumor progression or allow tumor progression at a very slow pace. Targeted therapies might also function as radiation sensitizers and be incorporated for treatment of local disease *(22,23)*. Safety of these agents must be considered, especially when combining these agents with chemotherapy or with each other *(24)*. Overall, combining targeted therapies represents a rational approach in controlling cancer with potentially less toxicity.

## 5. NOVEL ANTIANGIOGENIC STRATEGIES

Table 3 shows the multitude of other agents being developed to target VEGF and its receptors. These agents are in all phases of clinical trials as single agents or in combination with chemotherapy. In addition to the VEGF/VEGFR axis, other targets are also being explored, including angiopoietin/Tie receptors, EGF/EGFR, ephrins/Eph receptors, PlGF, bFGF, TNF, and others. Many of these strategies have undertaken antibodies as drugs with the advantage of specificity and stability of these large molecules. However, small-molecule drugs and peptides are also being widely explored. Finally, novel experimental approaches using gene therapy, vaccines, and antiangiogenic radioligands are being evaluated in the preclinical setting for potential use in future clinical trials *(13)*.

## 6. SUMMARY

The promise of antiangiogenic therapy is now being realized in the cancer clinic some 30 yrs after the theory of angiogenesis was postulated. The potential advantages of drugs that target this process include easy access to targets because of intravascular receptor–ligand interactions, broad applicability to many tumor types, and avoidance of tumor-resistance mechanisms *(25)*. Because angiogenesis is infrequent in the adult, there is the potential to develop very specific anticancer drugs that could avoid toxicities to bone marrow and gastrointestinal organs.

The vasculature throughout the body is very heterogeneous with differences that exist between normal versus quiescent vasculature, one organ versus another, and proliferating endothelium of physiologic versus pathophysiologic states *(26)*. The blood vessels of one type of tumor differ compared with another tumor type. Even within a single tumor, there are regions of the vasculature that have quiescent versus proliferating endothelial cells. To develop such specific agents, new endothelial cell markers need to be identified. Ideally, these would be markers that target tumor-specific endothelial cells *(27)*.

Identifying new endothelial cell markers is the goal of many biotechnology companies and laboratories. Screening methods include microarray and serial analysis of gene expression (SAGE) methods for analyses of gene expression in normal versus quiescent endothe-

Table 3
Inhibitors of the VEGF/VEGFR Axis

| Agent | Mechanism | Clinical Trials | Company |
|---|---|---|---|
| **Phase III** | | | |
| Avastin (bevacizumab) | Blocks VEGF | Phase III trials in colorectal cancer, NSCLC (nonsquamous), breast, and renal; phase II trials for advanced solid malignancies, hematopoietic malignancies, and MDS | Genentech, Inc. |
| PTK787 | VEGFR inhibitor | Phase III colorectal cancer | Novartis AG |
| Interferon α-2a | Decrease bFGF, VEGF | Phase II/III advanced tumors | Roche |
| Thalidomide | Decrease TNF-α, bFGF, VEGF | Phase III NSCLC, nonmetastatic prostate, refractory multiple myeloma, renal cancer phase I and II in advanced solid tumors | Celgene Corp. |
| Fenretinide | FGF and VEGF antagonism | Phase III chemoprevention of breast cancer, phase I prostate cancer | McNeil Pharmaceuticals Inc. |
| **Phase II** | | | |
| SU11248 | Inhibitor of PDGF/ VEGF/ Kit/ Flt-3 receptor tyrosine kinases | Phase II in advanced solid tumors | Pfizer |
| RPI-4610 (angiozyme) | VEGF R1 mRNA cleavage | Phase II breast, colorectal, and advanced solid tumors | Ribozyme Pharmaceuticals Inc. |
| Vatalanib | VEGF receptor tyrosine kinase inhibitor | Phase II advanced solid malignancies, phase I myeloid leukemia | Novartis AG |
| Flavopiridol | Decrease VEGF | Phase II esophageal, leukemia, lung, lymphoma, stomach, Phase I advanced solid tumors | NCI |
| Bay 43-9006 | Inhibitor of VEGFR, PDGFR-β, and multiple tyrosine kinase receptors | Phase II renal, hepatomas, other advanced solid malignancies | Bayer Pharmaceuticals Inc./Onyx |

| Phase I | | | |
|---|---|---|---|
| VEGF Trap | Binds VEGF | Phase I advanced cancer and NHL | Regeneron Pharmaceuticals, Inc. |
| IMC-1C11 | Inhibition of VEGF-R2 | Phase I metastatic colorectal cancer | ImClone Systems Inc. |
| Midostaurin | VEGF inhibition | Phase I leukemia, NHL, advanced cancers | Novartis AG |
| CP-547632 | VEGF receptor tyrosine kinase inhibitor | Phase I advanced solid malignancies | OSI Pharmaceuticals and Pfizer Inc. |
| AZD-2171 | VEGF receptor tyrosine kinase inhibitor | Phase I refractory solid tumors | AstraZeneca plc |
| ZD6474 | VEGFR inhibitor | Phase I advanced solid tumors | AstraZeneca |
| CEP-7055 | VEGF antagonist | Phase I refractory solid tumors | Cephalon Inc. |
| NM-3 | VEGF antagonist | Phase I in advanced solid tumors | ILEX Oncology Inc. |

*Abbreviations:* VEGF, vascular endothelial growth factor; NSCLC, non-small-cell lung cancer; FGF, fibroblast growth factor; TNF, tumor necrosis factor; PDGF, platelet-derived growth factor; NHL, non-Hodgkin's lymphoma; MDS, myelodysplastic syndromes.

lial cells, phage display to identify new endothelial cell receptors, and proteomic technologies to discover peptides and proteins that regulate endothelial cell growth (27–29). Functional genomic methods using retroviral cDNA and peptide library systems will allow perturbation of endothelial cells for discovery of novel genes and peptides that could counteract or promote physiologic changes.

As new markers on endothelial cells are discovered, so too will be development of novel therapies directed against them for cancer therapy. Experimental therapies include gene therapies with viral and nonviral methods that can downregulate growth and proliferation of endothelial cells or induce apoptosis (30,31). Liposomal delivery methods of genes has shown promise in preclinical studies and are being considered in clinical trials (32,33). The use of new endothelial cell antigens to stimulate immune responses in the host may be a novel way of creating anticancer vaccines that target proliferating endothelial cells (34–36). These novel vaccines can be useful for primary and secondary prevention strategies in cancer treatment. Finally, the delivery of radiation to proliferating endothelial cells with antiangiogenic radioligands offers the possibility of systemic radiotherapy directed toward and selective for sites of tumor growth (35). Such an approach might be useful in eradicating both endothelial cells and tumors cells and could, in some instances, provide imaging data for detection of metastatic tumor growth at very early stages during the angiogenic switch.

Numerous clinical trials with antiangiogenic drugs are ongoing. Various obstacles have impaired early trials with antiangiogenic agents. These include the selection of appropriate dose/schedule, choosing appropriate biological correlates and clinical trial end points, and incorporating these agents in optimal clinical settings with chemotherapy, radiation, and other antiangiogenic compounds (13).

Most of these clinical trials have focused on single-agent administration. Moving forward, newer trials need to be designed to test multiple antiangiogenic compounds in combination akin to how combination chemotherapy developed. Thus, combination antiangiogenic therapy could be effective in late-stage disease, when endothelial cell heterogeneity, abundant angiogenic growth factors, and epigenetic resistance mechanisms are present.

Finally, toxicities of antiangiogenic therapies must be closely monitored with regard to both acute and chronic effects. Effects on hemostasis such as thrombosis and bleeding must be monitored as well as effects on fertility/reproduction and wound healing (11). These types of therapy could potentially exacerbate ischemic states and must be scrutinized for long-term side effects (37).

Overall, antiangiogenic therapy remains an exciting and potentially effective new arm in cancer therapy. The success of Avastin in prolonging survival in combination with chemotherapy for metastatic colorectal cancer is a clear example of the benefit that can be achieved by targeting angiogenesis. VEGF and its receptors on endothelial cells have been shown to be a part of a critical pathway for tumor growth. Multiple agents are currently in development to target this pathway, and a combination of these agents with each other and with chemotherapy will make up some of the newer generation of clinical trials in oncology. Efficacy of Avastin in metastatic colorectal cancer will herald in new clinical trials for evaluating this agent in the adjuvant setting for this disease, perhaps yielding enhanced clinical benefit in a setting of minimal residual disease. From these and other trials, new information will be obtained that will provide insight on antiangiogenic agents not only in the treatment of established disease but also in preventing cancer growth.

# REFERENCES

1. Folkman J. Angiogenesis in cancer, vascular, rheumatoid and other disease. Nat Med 1995; 1:27–31.
2. Weidner N SJ, Welch WR, Folkman J. Tumor angiogenesis and metastasis—correlation in invasive breast carcinoma. N Engl J Med 1991; 324:1–8.
3. Weidner N FJ, Pozza F, Bevilacqua P, Allred EN, Moore DH, Meli S, et al. Tumor angiogenesis: a new significant and independent prognostic indicator in early-stage breast carcinoma. J Natl Cancer Inst 1992; 84:1875–1887.
4. Ferrara N, Davis-Smyth T. The biology of vascular endothelial growth factor. Endocr Rev 1997; 18: 4–25.
5. Borgstrom P GD, Hillan KJ, Ferrara N. Importance of VEGF for breast cancer angiogenesis in vivo: implications from intravital microscopy of combination treatments with an anti-VEGF neutralizing monoclonal antibody and doxorubicin. Anticancer Res 1999; 19:4203–4214.
6. Presta LG, Chen H, O'Connor SJ, et al. Humanization of an anti-vascular endothelial growth factor monoclonal antibody for the therapy of solid tumors and other disorders. Cancer Res 1997; 57:4593–4599.
7. Hurwitz H, Fehrenbacher L, Novotny W, et al. Bevacizumab plus irinotecan, fluorouracil, and leucovorin for metastatic colorectal cancer. N Engl J Med 2004; 350:2335–2342.
8. Kabbinavar F, Hurwitz HI, Fehrenbacher L, et al. Phase II, randomized trial comparing bevacizumab plus fluorouracil (FU)/leucovorin (LV) with FU/LV alone in patients with metastatic colorectal cancer. J Clin Oncol 2003; 21:60–65.
9. Johnson DH, Fehrenbacher L, Novotny W, et al. Randomized Phase II trial comparing bevacizumab plus carboplatin and paclitaxel with carboplatin and paclitaxel alone in previously untreated locally advanced or metastatic non-small-cell lung cancer. J Clin Oncology 2004; 22:2184–2191.
10. Scappaticci FA, Mass RD. The Syed/Rowinsky article reviewed. Oncology 2003; 17:1352–1355.
11. Yang JC, Naworth L, Sherry RM, et al. A randomized trial of bevacizumab, an anti-vascular endothelial growth factor antibody, for metastatic renal cancer. N Engl J Med 2003; 349:427–434.
12. Scappaticci FA. The therapeutic potential of novel antiangiogenic therapies. Expert Opin Invest Drugs 2003; 12:923–932.
13. Scappaticci F. Mechanisms and future directions for angiogenesis-based cancer therapies. J Clin Oncol 2002; 20:3906–3927.
14. Jain RK. Normalizing tumor vasculature with anti-angiogenic therapy: a new paradigm for combination therapy. Nat Med 2001; 7:987–989.
15. Hanahan D, Bergers G, Bergsland E. Less is more, regularly: metronomic dosing of cytotoxic drugs can target tumor angiogenesis in mice. J Clin Invest 2000; 105:1045–1047.
16. Kerbel RS, Klement G, Pritchard KI, Kamen B. Continuous low-dose anti-angiogenic/metronomic chemotherapy: from the research laboratory into the oncology clinic. Ann Oncol 2002; 13:12–15.
17. Gabrilovich DI, Chen HL, Girgis KR, et al. Production of vascular endothelial growth factor by human tumors inhibits the functional maturation of dendritic cells. Nat Med 1996; 2:1096–1103.
18. Li WW. Tumor angiogenesis: molecular pathology, therapeutic targeting, and imaging. Acad Radiol 2000; 7:800–811.
19. Morgan BTA, Drevs J, Hennig J, Buchert M, Jivan A, Horsfield MA, et al. Dynamic contrast-enhanced magnetic resonance imaging as a biomarker for the pharmacological response of PTK787/ZK 222584, an inhibitor of the vascular endothelial growth factor receptor tyrosine kinases, in patients with advanced colorectal cancer and liver metastases: results from two phase I studies. J Clin Oncol 2003; 21:3955–3964.
20. Relf M, LeJeune S, Scott PA, et al. Expression of the angiogenic factors vascular endothelial cell growth factor, acidic and basic fibroblast growth factor, tumor growth factor beta-1, platelet-derived endothelial cell growth factor, placenta growth factor, and pleiotrophin in human primary breast cancer and its relation to angiogenesis. Cancer Res 1997; 57:963–969.
21. Folkman J. Antiangiogenic gene therapy. Proc Natl Acad Sci USA 1998; 95:9064–9066.
22. Gorski DH, Beckett MA, Jaskowiak NT, et al. Blockage of the vascular endothelial growth factor stress response increases the antitumor effects of ionizing radiation. Cancer Res 1999; 59:3374–3378.
23. Paris F, Fuks Z, Kang A, et al. Endothelial apoptosis as the primary lesion initiating intestinal radiation damage in mice. Science 2001; 293:293–297.
24. Kuenen BC, Rosen L, Smit EF, et al. Dose-finding and pharmacokinetic study of cisplatin, gemcitabine, and SU5416 in patients with solid tumors. J Clin Oncol 2002; 20:1657–1667.

25. Folkman J. Antiangiogenic therapy. In: Devita VT, Rosenberg SA, eds. Principles and practice of oncology. Philadelphia: Lippincott–Raven, 1997:3075–3085.

26. McDonald DM, Foss AJ. Endothelial cells of tumor vessels: abnormal but not absent. Cancer Metastasis Rev 2000; 19:109–120.

27. St Croix B, Rago C, Velculescu V, et al. Genes expressed in human tumor endothelium. Science 2000; 289:1197–1202.

28. Pasqualini R, Ruoslahti E. Organ targeting in vivo using phage display peptide libraries. Nature 1996; 380:364–366.

29. Liotta LA, Kohn EC. The microenvironment of the tumour-host interface. Nature 2001; 411:375–379.

30. Scappaticci FA, Smith R, Pathak A, et al. Combination angiostatin and endostatin gene transfer induces synergistic antiangiogenic activity in vitro and antitumor efficacy in leukemia and solid tumors in mice. Mol Ther 2001; 3:186–196.

31. Kuo CJ, Farnebo F, Yu EY, et al. Comparative evaluation of the antitumor activity of antiangiogenic proteins delivered by gene transfer. Proc Natl Acad Sci USA 2001; 98:4605–4610.

32. Chen QR, Kumar D, Stass SA, Mixson AJ. Liposomes complexed to plasmids encoding angiostatin and endostatin inhibit breast cancer in nude mice. Cancer Res 1999; 59:3308–3312.

33. Sacco MG, Caniatti M, Cato EM, et al. Liposome-delivered angiostatin strongly inhibits tumor growth and metastatization in a transgenic model of spontaneous breast cancer. Cancer Res 2000; 60:2660–2665.

34. Wei Y, Wang Q, Zhao X, et al. Immunotherapy of tumors with xenogeneic endothelial cells as a vaccine. Nat Med 2000; 6:1160–1166.

35. Scappaticci FA, Contreras A, Boswell CA, Lewis JS, Nolan GP. Polyclonal antibodies to xenogeneic endothelial cells induce apoptosis and block support of tumor growth in mice. Vaccine 2003; 21: 2667–2677.

36. Scappaticci FA, Nolan GP. Induction of anti-tumor immunity using a syngeneic endothelial cell vaccine. Anticancer Res 2003; 23:1165–1172.

37. Kong HL, Crystal RG. Gene therapy strategies for tumor antiangiogenesis. J Natl Cancer Inst 1998; 90: 273–286.

# 30

## Inhibiting Cancer Angiogenesis With Molecular Therapy

*Qixin Leng, PhD and A. James Mixson, MD*

**CONTENTS**

INTRODUCTION
PROANGIOGENIC FACTORS
"ENDOGENOUS" ANGIOGENIC INHIBITORS
TUMOR ANGIOGENESIS VACCINES
CONCLUSION AND SUMMARY
ACKNOWLEDGMENT
REFERENCES

**SUMMARY**

An exciting approach in cancer molecular therapy is the ability to target the developing blood supply of the tumor. In contrast to several other molecular therapy approaches, antiangiogenic molecular therapy can readily access its target—the tumor vasculature. Numerous viral and nonviral vectors that target tumor angiogenesis have demonstrated antitumor efficacy in preclinical models in vivo. Molecular therapy strategies that inhibit proangiogenic growth factors such as vascular endothelial growth factor (VEGF) or its receptors include antisense methods, RNAzymes, DNAzymes, RNAi, or a dominant-negative protein encoded from a gene. These therapeutic molecules could be incorporated within mammalian expression vectors (plasmids or viruses) and/or delivered as small therapeutic polynucleotide molecules. Alternatively, tumor angiogenesis could be inhibited by in vivo expression of "endogenous" antiangiogenic proteins or peptides such as thrombospondin 1 or 2. In this chapter, we discuss the current status and strategies of antiangiogenic molecular therapy.

**Key Words:** Molecular therapy; antiangiogenic; tumor; angiogenic; vaccine; endothelial; p53; cytokines; VEGF; Raf-1.

## 1. INTRODUCTION

Angiogenesis is a tightly controlled dynamic process through which new blood vessels develop from pre-existing vessels. Angiogenesis is critical not only for several physiological processes, including wound repair and ovulation, but also for tumor growth. The

From: *Cancer Drug Discovery and Development: The Oncogenomics Handbook*
Edited by: W. J. LaRochelle and R. A. Shimkets © Humana Press Inc., Totowa, NJ

realization that tumor growth was dependent on angiogenesis significantly advanced our understanding of tumor biology. Activation of growth factors that stimulate angiogenesis together with suppression of angiogenic inhibitors thus contribute to tumor growth. As a result, antiangiogenic molecular therapy attempts to inhibit tumor growth either by reducing angiogenic growth factors (and their signal pathways) or by augmenting angiogenic inhibitors within a tumor.

Several reports have described the efficacy of antiangiogenic molecular therapy in tumor-bearing mouse models. Investigators have successfully inhibited tumor growth by molecular therapy approaches designed to inhibit angiogenic inducers (vascular endothelial growth factor [VEGF], angiopoietin 2) and/or their receptors (1–4). To inhibit these proangiogenic factors, a wide variety of molecular nucleotide-based tools have been used, including dominant-negative strategies, antisense, ribozymes, DNAzymes, and RNAi methods. Alternatively, molecular therapy with "endogenous" angiogenic inhibitors has shown promise for antitumor action in animal models; examples of these "endogenous" inhibitors include angiostatin, endostatin, p53, thrombospondin 1 and 2, and tissue inhibitory metalloproteinases (TIMPs) (5–7). Most recently, DNA vaccines targeting tumor endothelial cells are being developed (8–17). Because angiogenesis occurs in both normal tissue and tumors, it will be essential to identify those factors that are preferentially or solely expressed in the tumor vessels to develop successful vaccines.

With these experiments demonstrating efficacy in tumor-bearing animal models, there has been increased interest in antiangiogenic molecular therapy by utilizing DNA- or RNA-based methods. Most studies with antiangiogenic therapy have thus far shown their efficacy in preclinical models, and no antiangiogenic agents have yet been approved by the Food and Drug Administration (FDA) for cancer treatment. Currently, genes encoding three proteins (p53, interferon [INF]-γ, and interleukin [IL]-12) with multiple tumor-inhibitory mechanisms in addition to antiangiogenesis are currently being evaluated in clinical trials (18). In subsequent sections, we review the following antiangiogenic therapeutic strategies for reducing tumor growth: first, inhibition of proangiogenic factors, then expression of "endogenous" antiangiogenic inhibitors, and, finally, tumor vaccines targeting tumor angiogenesis.

## 2. PROANGIOGENIC FACTORS

### 2.1. VEGF

Tumor angiogenesis is dependent on VEGF and its cognate receptors (*flt-1* or VEGFR1, *flk-1* or VEGFR2). Not unexpectedly, these have frequently been targeted to limit tumor growth (Table 1). VEGF was first targeted by antisense strategies and later by siRNA strategies. Stable transfection of tumor cells with plasmids expressing antisense VEGF did not affect the growth of tumor cells in vitro but reduced tumor growth in vivo (2). Targeting VEGF with a retrovirus-producing antisense RNA also prolonged survival in a glioma-bearing rat model (19). Injection of tumors with adenoviral constructs expressing VEGF in the antisense orientation has resulted in marked decreases in tumor size (20,21). Similar to antisense strategies, ribozymes targeting VEGF have resulted in tumor inhibition (22). VEGF levels could also be decreased indirectly through inhibition of the adenosine 2B receptor by use of an antisense oligonucleotide (23). The major obstacle of targeting VEGF in vivo with antisense approaches either directly or indirectly is that if most of the VEGF is expressed in tumor cells and not in the tumor endothelial cells, it might

Table 1

Strategies for Inhibiting Proangiogenic Factors

| Name | Dominant-negative | Antisense | RNAzymes, DNAzymes | siRNA | Decoy | DNA Vaccine |
|---|---|---|---|---|---|---|
| VEGF | | Riedel, 2003[a-c] | | Yin, 2003; Filleur, 2003[a-c]; Reich, 2003[a,b] | Holash, 2002[a,b] | Niethammer, 2002[a-c]; Liu, 2003[a-c]; Wei, 2001[a-c] |
| VEGF receptors | Millauer, 1993[a-c] Machein, et al., 1999[a-c] | | Weng, 2001[a-c] Zhang, 2002[a-c] | | | |
| HIF-α | | Sun, 2003[b,c] | | | | |
| FGF and receptors | Auguste, 2001[a-c] | Wang, 1997[a-c] | | | | He, 2003[a-c] |
| Raf-1 | Hood et al., 2002[a-c] Pourtier-Manzanedo, 2003[b,c] | Zavaglia, 2003[a-c] Lincoln, 2003[a]; Tomita, 2003[a,b]; Lavenburg, 2003[a-c] | | Cioca, 2003[d] | | |
| ETS-1 | | Kobayashi, 2003[a-c]; Zhu, 2003[a] | | | | |
| PI3K | Kawasaki, 2003[a,b] | | | Barbieri, 2003[a] | | |
| ERK-1 STAT3D | Chandrasekar, 2003[a] Wei, 2003[b,c]; Niu, 2002[a,b] | | | | | |
| SPK FAK Sp1 | Dormond, 2002[a] Qi, 2002[a] | | | | Novak, 2003[b,c] | |

[a] Inhibition of angiogenesis demonstrated with in vitro assays.
[b] Inhibition of angiogenesis demonstrated with in vivo assays (dependent or independent of tumors).
[c] Antitumor activity of solid tumors demonstrated with xenograft models.
[d] In vitro antitumor activity.

443

be difficult to attain adequate expression of the antisense construct in the tumor. The latest method to reduce VEGF levels is with small interfering (si)RNA and this approach might ameliorate inadequate expression of the therapeutic molecule. In some cases, a single siRNA molecule within the cell can markedly inhibit its target mRNA. To date, VEGF siRNA has been shown to reduce significantly hypoxia-driven stimulation of VEGF levels in vitro, and when administered intravenously, it inhibits growth of fibrosarcomas in vivo *(24)*.

In addition to VEGF, its receptors VEGFR1 and VEGFR2 have been targeted. Unlike VEGF, its receptors are located and upregulated primarily on mitogenic endothelial cells. Therefore, these receptors might be more accessible targets than their ligand VEGF. An early study showed that injection of a retrovirus-truncated VEGFR2 construct together with tumor cells inhibited tumor growth *(1)*. It has been suggested that this retrovirus-transduced receptor acts through a dominant-negative mechanism to inhibit the wild-type VEGF receptor. More recently, antiangiogenic therapy with a dominant-negative truncated VEGF receptor has been shown to suppress angiogenesis and growth of an intracerebral glioma in a rat model *(25)*. Although therapy with dominant-negative receptors might have limited clinical utility owing to the low transfection efficiencies of the vector delivery systems injected directly into a tumor, one approach to circumvent the low transfection efficiency is to engineer a secreted therapeutic protein. This was demonstrated in a mouse model in which tumor cells transduced with a secreted soluble VEGF receptor (sVEGFR1) inhibited implantation of a primary tumor *(4)*. Furthermore, the mice had fewer lung metastases when tumor cells expressing elevated levels of sVEGFR1 were injected intravenously. To prevent the potential unwanted antiangiogenic side effects of systemic therapy, peritumoral injection of an adenovirus expressing a secreted form of VEGFR1 markedly inhibited tumor growth *(26)*.

An alternative to gene therapy is the use of catalytic oligonucleotides to inhibit VEGF receptors. A ribozyme targeting VEGFR1, upregulated in mitogenic endothelial cells, has been reported to have significant antitumor activity in animal models *(27)*. Similar to ribozymes, VEGFR2 DNAzymes have demonstrated marked antitumor efficacy in vivo with a 75% reduction in tumor size compared to controls; the potential advantages of DNAzymes compared to RNAzymes include greater resistance to nucleases and the ability to digest mRNA at the start site, a region with little secondary structure *(28)*. (In Section 4, antitumor vaccines directed toward VEGFR2 and FGFR2 are discussed.)

## 2.2. Angiopoietin 2

In addition to VEGF, antiangiogenic molecular therapy has targeted other ligands with receptors that are located specifically on endothelial cells. Elevated levels of angiopoietin 2, the ligand to the Tie2 receptor, have been associated with increased tumor angiogenesis. Consequently, angiopoietin 2 is a logical therapeutic target. When injected intravenously, an adenovirus expressing a soluble Tie 2 receptor was recently shown to inhibit tumor growth by binding to angiopoietin 2 *(3)*. In this study, established tumors that were treated with plasma concentrations of the soluble recombinant Tie2 receptor exceeding 1 mg/mL for an 8-d period were significantly reduced in size. In addition, coadministration of the adenovirus–Tie2 vector with tumor cells greatly reduced the number of lung metastases. A possible drawback to this approach is that the adenovirus–Tie2 construct might decrease levels of angiopoietin 1, a protein known to stabilize blood vessels.

## 2.3. Basic Fibroblast Growth Factor

In contrast to VEGF and the angiopoietins, fibroblast growth factor 1 (FGF-1, acidic) and fibroblast growth factor 2 (FGF-2, basic) exhibit a variety of biological functions in many tissues and organs *(29)*. Although FGF2 most certainly is involved in tumor angiogenesis, its direct role is inconclusive. Many investigators have extrapolated from in vitro and in vivo angiogenic assays that utilized FGF-2 to explain the promotion of tumor angiogenesis and growth in vivo. The lack of measurable fibroblast growth factor receptors (FGFRs) on the tumor endothelium is in marked contrast to the expression of VEGF receptors. Although there is little direct evidence to show that FGFRs are present in microvessels of a tumor *(30)*, there is at least one effective antitumor therapeutic strategy that is based on activation of both FGFR- and VEGFR-induced pathways within the tumor endothelium *(31,32)*.

It has also been suggested that FGF-2 might increase angiogenesis in vivo by inducing other angiogenic factors such as VEGF *(33)*. A number of molecular therapy studies targeting FGF or its receptor by antisense and dominant-negative methods have shown marked tumor inhibition *(34–36)*. For instance, with a liposomal delivery system, antisense targeting FGF or FGFR-2 inhibited tumor growth and angiogenesis *(36)*. In a second study in which glioma cells expressed a dominant-negative form of FGFR, tumor growth and tumor microvessel density were substantially reduced and angiogenesis was inhibited in an in vivo assay *(35)*. Thus, molecular therapy strategies targeting FGF or FGFR-2 could be particularly effective for antitumor efficacy *(35)*.

## 2.4. Cytosolic Mediators

Raf-1 is a central regulator of endothelial cell survival during angiogenesis. Both basic FGF (bFGF) and VEGF differentially activate Raf-1 by phosphorylating different domains of the molecule, providing protection from apoptosis by these distinct pathways *(32)*. Recently, systemic injection of a plasmid encoding a dominant-negative Raf induced massive apoptosis of the tumor endothelium and tumor after just one injection in a mouse model *(31)*. To deliver the dominant-negative Raf-1 plasmid to the tumor vessels, the investigators used a cationic liposome in which an integrin $\alpha v \beta 3$-targeted ligand was attached. Although the tumor biology in humans is far more complex, the results of this molecular therapy study hold promise.

In addition to Raf-1, signal transduction proteins such as phosphatidylinositol (PI)-3 kinase or regulators of these pathways including PTEN might be associated with either endothelial growth or inhibition of apoptosis and these might be suitable antiangiogenic targets *(37)*; because these factors can be upregulated in a number of different cells and tissues not related to the tumor, specific carriers will need to be designed to target the tumor endothelial cells. Although small therapeutic molecules (LY294002) targeting PI-3 kinase have resulted in tumor regression and are antiangiogenic, to date no in vivo gene therapy experiments have been done. A complete list of signal transduction factors that have been downregulated by various strategies with in vitro angiogenic assays is given in Table 1.

## 2.5. Transcriptional Factors

The Ets-1 proto-oncoprotein is a member of the Ets family of transcription factors that is involved in the control of the endothelium-specific expression of genes that are important for the formation of new blood vessels. For example, Ets-1 regulates several metalloproteinases (MMP1, MMP3, MMP9, and uPA), and VEGF and its receptors. It has also been well documented that Ets-1 is required for endothelial cells to adopt an angiogenic, blood-vessel-forming phenotype *(38–42)*. Only one in vivo experiment with an antisense oligodeoxynucleotide (ODN) directed against Ets-1 in endothelial cells has been done. In an ischemic hind-leg mouse model, an antisense ODN toward *Ets* inhibited angiogenesis, probably by downregulating VEGF and hepatocyte growth factors in endothelial cells *(43)*. Because Ets-1 is important in cellular differentiation in several cell lines and tissues, specific carriers to tumor endothelial cells will likely be necessary to prevent unwanted side effects. Inhibition of the transcriptional factor Sp1 with a decoy oligonucleotide strategy has also been shown to inhibit VEGF and tumor necrosis factor (TNF)-$\alpha$ levels, inhibit angiogenesis, and reduce tumor growth *(44)* (Table 1).

## 3. "ENDOGENOUS" ANGIOGENIC INHIBITORS

### *3.1. Extracellular Inhibitors*

#### 3.1.1. ANGIOSTATIN AND ENDOSTATIN

Angiostatin and endostatin are proteolytically cleaved from plasminogen and collagen XVIII, respectively, to become angiogenic inhibitors. The specific molecular targets for these inhibitors have not been clearly identified. It has recently, however, been found that angiostatin binds tightly to an ATP synthase on the endothelial cell surface *(45)*. For endostatin, one study suggests that tropomyosin binds to endostatin and plays a role in its tumor-inhibitory function *(46)*, whereas another study shows that interaction between $\alpha5$ and $\alpha3$ integrins on endothelial cell membranes occurs and might be critical for its antitumor mechanism *(47)*. Both angiostatin and endostatin polypeptides clearly inhibited a variety of tumors in animal models *(48,49)*. Moreover, there has been no evidence of resistance developing to endostatin in these tumor-bearing mice. Identification of the receptors for endostatin and angiostatin might lead to more potent antiangiogenic analogs.

Several molecular therapy studies with angiostatin or endostatin have shown antitumor efficacy in animal models (Table 2) *(6,7,50–59)*. Proteins encoded by genes have mainly been delivered intratumorally or intravenously by adenoviruses to inhibit tumor growth. Nevertheless, nonviral delivery via polyvinylpyrrolidione (PVP), liposomes, or "naked" DNA injection has also demonstrated efficacy. With "naked" DNA intratumoral injections of endostatin, not only were the tumors decreased as expected, but, interestingly, VEGF levels increased intratumorally. Thus, there appeared to be a compensatory increase in VEGF levels when endostatin was administered in this manner. A second nonviral study with cationic liposomes as a carrier of endostatin showed moderate reduction in the tumor size of mice bearing MDA-MB-435 cells after the third injection *(6)*. Cationic liposomes as carriers of their DNA cargo administered intravenously could achieve higher selectivity and lower toxicity than their viral counterparts. Thurston et al. demonstrated that liposome : DNA complexes selectively target the mitogenic tumor endothelial cells rather than quiescent endothelial cells *(60)*. Adding ligands that specifically target the tumor endothelial cells might further increase the specificity and efficacy of cationic liposomes *(61,62)*. In addition to nonviral carriers, two recent particularly interesting viral studies show the potential of adeno-associated virus (AAV) as carriers of angiostatin. Injection of the AAV–angiostatin construct intratumorally or intramuscularly prolonged the survival of mice with orthotopically implanted glioblastoma in a mouse model *(58,59)*.

Table 2
"Endogenous" Inhibitors

| | |
|---|---|
| Angiostatin/endostatin | Ma et al., 2002; |
| | Dell'Eva et al., 2002; |
| | Kuo et al., 2001; |
| | Scappaticci et al., 2001 |
| Angiostatic cytokines | Ruehlmann et al., 2001; |
| | Chada et al., 2003; |
| | Wigginton and Wiltrout, 2002 |
| Thrombospondin 1 and 2 | Streit et al., 2002; |
| | Jin et al., 2000; |
| | Kyriakides et al., 2002 |
| TIMPS | Fernandez et al., 2003; |
| | Tran et al., 2003; |
| | Valente et al., 1998 |
| p53 | Dameron et al., 1994; |
| | Roth et al., 1996; |
| | Lesoon-Wood et al., 1995; |
| | Daniel et al., 2003 |

Cell-based therapy is an alternative molecular therapeutic strategy for increasing angiostatin levels in tumors. Investigators have recently demonstrated that by administering the gene encoding pancreatic elastase I, angiostatin levels were increased *(63)*. Increased levels of the antiangiogenic angiostatin, a breakdown product of plasminogen, is the putative mechanism of elastase molecular therapy. In this study, endothelial cells transduced with elastase I showed marked growth inhibition in vitro, but the growth of transduced Lewis lung carcinoma in vitro was not inhibited. In addition, Lewis lung cells transduced with elastase I and then implanted into mice showed reduced growth compared to controls. In a second study, cells encapsulated with alginate-poly-L-lysine showed prolonged secretion of endostatin compared to nonencapsulated cells *(64)*. A particularly attractive feature of the alginate-poly-L-lysine material is that it has low immunogenicity. A single intratumoral injection of these encapsulated endostatin-secreting cells inhibited U87 glioma xenografts by 72.3% compared to untreated controls.

### 3.1.2. ANGIOSTATIC CYTOKINES

Inhibitory cytokines that lack the N-terminal glutamic acid-leucine-arginine (ELR) motif are angiostatic and could carry out their antiangiogenic activity through the CXCR3 receptor on endothelial cells *(65)*. These antiangiogenic cytokines include platelet factor-4 (PF-4), interferon-inducible protein 10 (IP-10), monokine induced by interferon-γ (MIG), and IFN-γ-inducible T-cell α chemoattractant (I-TAC) *(66)*. Whereas earlier in vivo molecular therapy experiments targeting angiogenesis had demonstrated antitumor efficacy, molecular therapy with the angiogenic inhibitor platelet factor 4 (PF-4) was probably the first to show efficacy in a clinically relevant model. In this study, an adenovirus expressing PF-4 *(67)* was injected into established glioma tumors and found to inhibit tumor growth and prolong animal survival. PF-4 belongs to a family of C-X-C chemokines; in addition to its antiangiogenic effect mediated through the CXCR3, PF-4 might inhibit angiogenesis by altering the affinity of VEGF for its receptors (68). A second CXC cytokine used in molecular therapy has also demonstrated its antitumor efficacy in an immunocompetent model. Compared to endostatin, adenoviral delivery of IP-10 was significantly more effective; however, both intratumoral and intravenous injection of IP-10 were required to regress tumors completely (54).

Molecular therapy of non-CXC cytokines such as interleukin-12 (IL-12) has been shown to inhibit tumor angiogenesis (69) and growth (70,71). The antiangiogenic activity of IL-12 is mediated by interferon-γ and the CXC chemokine IP-10 (72,73). Mice receiving IL-12 molecular therapy were found to survive significantly longer (median survival = 43 d) than mice treated with control plasmid/lipid complexes (median survival = 35 d). These data demonstrated that nonviral IL-12 molecular therapy with a cationic liposome carrier could inhibit the development of lung metastases (74). IL-12 might mediate its antiangiogenic effect through immune effector cells (75). In addition to its angiostatic mechanism of action, IL-12 probably inhibits tumor growth by several other mechanisms, and it is difficult to distinguish the relative roles of these mechanisms in reducing tumor growth. Although the antitumor activity of IL-12 could, in part, be mediated by IP-10 and MIG, combined molecular therapy with IL-12 and IP-10, and/or MIG delivered by adenoviral vectors resulted in significantly more tumor regression and prolonged survival time than did either IL-12 or IP-10 alone (76).

### 3.1.3. THROMBOSPONDIN

Thrombospondins (TSP1 and TSP2) are secreted angiostatic proteins and are potent inhibitors of various cancers (77–79). Both TSPs are large multifunctional proteins that share significant homology and have been found to be important prognostic indicators. In breast tumors, decreased secretion of TSP-1 in a variety of cell lines correlates with a more malignant phenotype (80). In another study, the microvessel density and histological grade of gliomas from patients correlated inversely with TSP-2 levels (81). In vitro experiments in which TSP-1 was used to reduce endothelial cell growth gave conflicting results. Nonetheless, peptides have been isolated from TSP-1 that clearly have antiangiogenic effects in vitro (82), and synthetic antiangiogenic thrombospondin peptides in the D-conformation have exhibited antitumor activity in vivo (83).

Several studies have indicated that antiangiogenic molecular therapy with TSP-1 or peptides derived from TSP-1 has antitumor activity (51,79,84,85). Initially, an ex vivo study demonstrated that a tumor clone expressing high levels of TSP-1 peptide reduced tumor growth (84). Recently, an ex vivo study showed that tumor cell clones expressing TSP-2 had significantly more antitumor efficacy than clones expressing TSP-1. More impressively, tumor clones expressing TSP-1 and TSP-2 were synergistic in their antitumor efficacy as demonstrated by the complete inhibition of tumor growth (79). In addition, p53 and an antiangiogenic peptide of TSP-1 in complex with liposomes, delivered intravenously at a site distant from the tumor, were found to be synergistic in their inhibition of tumors (85).

### 3.1.4. TISSUE INHIBITORY METALLOPROTEINASES

Turnover of the extracellular matrix (ECM) mediated by the matrix metalloproteinases (MMPs) is an important event in cancer growth and progression. Tissue inhibitors of matrix metalloproteinases (TIMPs) limit the activity of MMPs, suggesting their use in cancer molecular therapy (86,87). In one in vitro study, adenovirus-mediated overexpression of TIMP-1, TIMP-2, and TIMP-3 inhibited invasion of several different tumor cells through an artificial basement membrane *(86,87)*, but of these, only TIMP-3 promoted apoptosis. An in vivo study showed that nonviral delivery of a plasmid expressing TIMP-2 reduced microvessel density and tumor growth after intratumoral administration. In this study, tumor reduction by TIMP-2 and angiostatin was 84% and 71%, respectively, and when both genes were administered together intratumorally by nonviral gene delivery, tumor reduction was 96%. Conflicting results have been observed for molecular therapy with TIMP-4. In one study, nonviral delivery of TIMP-4 in a mouse model significantly inhibited Wilms' tumor growth in nude mice. In this mouse model, sustained systemic levels of TIMP-4 were accomplished by intramuscular electroporation of TIMP-4 expression plasmid *(88)*. Nevertheless, systemic delivery of a TIMP-4 after its naked plasmid was electroporated intramuscularly augmented the growth of implanted breast tumors by its antiapoptotic mechanism.

## *3.2. Transcriptional Factors: p53*

In contrast to the preceding angiogenic inhibitors, which are secreted or proteolytically activated extracellularly, p53 is a nuclear transcriptional protein. Nevertheless, p53 might induce secreted antiangiogenic protein, including thrombospondin I *(51,89)*, and p53 might inhibit angiogenesis by several additional mechanisms: (1) decrease endothelial cell growth by affecting p21 and the cell cycle or by downregulation of VEGF *(90)* or bFGF *(91,92)*; (2) promote endothelial cell apoptosis *(93,94)*; (3) inhibit endothelial cell differentiation *(95)*; (4) inhibit breakdown of the extracellular matrix *(96)*.

Therapy with p53 is one of the few molecular approaches that has shown efficacy in humans *(97)* and it is likely that this antitumor activity is mediated in part by its antiangiogenic mechanism. In one clinical study in which the transfection efficiency with p53-containing retrovirus was at most 20%, some of the injected tumors regressed completely. As a result, the authors concluded that apoptosis or cell cycle inhibition of the transfected tumor cell could not account for the amount of tumor inhibition observed and that a bystander effect was responsible. It appears that the bystander antitumor effect of p53 in this and many other studies was partially the result of its antiangiogenic mechanism *(51,90,94, 95)*. With both viral *(90,95)* and nonviral carriers *(51,94,98–100)*, p53 has demonstrated an antiangiogenic and antitumor effect on an array of different tumors.

## 4. TUMOR ANGIOGENESIS VACCINES

In addition to discovering more potent angiogenic inhibitors, new approaches are on the horizon for antiangiogenic molecular therapy. Vaccines toward tumor angiogenesis are now being developed with purified proteins *(8,10)* or with whole-cell endothelial extracts from tumors *(15)*. In one study, fixed xenogeneic whole endothelial cells were effective as a vaccine in protecting against tumor growth, inducing regression of established tumors, and prolonging survival of tumor-bearing mice. In three other studies, purified angiogenic receptors were used as antigens to develop a tumor neovascularization vaccine. Vaccination with FGFR-1 *(8)* and VEGR-2 *(10,101)* effectively induced antitumor immunity and activity in vivo. There was marked tumor reduction and prolonged survival with few side effects in the vaccinated animals in all three studies. Although these results in preclinical models have been encouraging, the success of active immunization will depend on specificity toward tumor angiogenesis *(15)*. In the aforementioned studies, none of the targets chosen thus far for vaccination is likely to be sufficiently specific to avoid untoward side effects in humans. To achieve this specificity, profiles of gene and protein expression between the tumor and other tissue endothelial cells are necessary. A recent study that used serial analysis of gene expression (SAGE) showed that nearly 80 genes were increased in tumor endothelial cells compared to quiescent endothelial cells *(102)*. Nevertheless, all of these genes (with the possible exception of tissue endothelial marker 8) were also found to be expressed in endothelial cells involved in wound healing or the corpus luteum *(102)*. Many such studies are essential to identify attractive targets for tumor endothelial vaccines. Nevertheless, antiangiogenic vaccines offer new therapeutic opportunities to target tumor angiogenesis.

## 5. CONCLUSION AND SUMMARY

In this chapter, we have discussed several angiogenic targets and approaches that investigators have used to inhibit tumor angiogenesis and growth. To reduce proangiogenic factors, one must select from an array of molecular nucleotide-based tools, including antisense, ribozymes, DNAzymes, and RNAi methods or genes encoding dominant-negative proteins. Alternatively, the investigator might choose a molecular therapy strategy that inhibits tumor growth with an "endogenous" angiogenic inhibitor. Selection of a particular angiogenic inhibitor and the method by which to deliver this inhibitor (e.g., exogenously sythesized siRNA versus plasmid promoter expression of the siRNA within tissues) are clearly critical issues to maximize antitumor activity. Nevertheless, the most important obstacle for an effective molecular therapy angiogenic inhibitor is the development of a specific carrier that targets tumor angiogenesis. Efficient transfection is a problem that antiangiogenic molecular therapy shares with the rest of molecular therapy, notwithstanding that the tumor vasculature is accessible to systemic therapy.

There have been several recent advances for nonviral and viral carriers of antiangiogenic genes to inhibit tumor growth. For instance, liposomes modified by αvβ3-ligands augmented delivery of a luciferase expression plasmid by eightfold to the tumor compared to the unmodified carriers *(31)*. Furthermore, there was increased specificity of the αvβ3-ligand nanoparticle in that no luciferase activity was detected in extratumoral tissues. Perhaps most important, one injection of the αvβ3-ligand nanoparticle in complex with a dominant-negative Raf-1 plasmid resulted in complete tumor regression of the tumor for several weeks. In another study that utilized the intramuscular platform, AAVs provided high systemic levels of antiangiogenic gene products *(58)*. In contrast to other viral vectors, AAVs appear to be safer to administer, in that chromosomal integration is minimal and immunogenicity to the virus is low. This was exemplified by 40% of mice with glioblastomas surviving for the duration of the experiment (greater than 10 mo) after a single administration of an AAV construct expressing angiostatin; in contrast, in the control mice tumors progressed rapidly and all died by 6 wk *(58)*. In mice administered the AAV–angiostatin construct, angiostatin levels remained elevated for more than 250 d. If systemic proteins do not affect to a significant degree normal physiological processes and obligatory compensatory angiogenesis in certain disease states (e.g., coronary disease, peripheral vascular disease), then this therapy will be beneficial. Although these studies are promising, the safety and efficacy of these different molecular therapy treatments will become clearer as these studies progress toward and through clinical trials.

In addition to selection of the optimal carrier and angiogenic inhibitor, the investigator must consider the likely emergence of drug resistance to antiangiogenic molecular therapy for human cancers. Until quite recently, acquired anticancer drug resistance was thought to occur rarely, if at all, with antiangiogenic therapy because of the relative genomic stability of endothelial cells *(103,104)*. However, current studies suggest that tumors and/or their vessels can adapt to become more resistant to angiogenic chemotherapy (for a review, see ref. *105*). For example, p53-deficient tumors are more resistant to antiangiogenic therapy than are wild-type p53 tumors *(106,107)*. To circumvent antiangiogenic resistance, multiple strategies are currently being tried, including combined standard chemotherapy regimens with the antiangiogenic agents *(108)*. Although antiangiogenic therapy is commonly effective in animal models, further knowledge of the tumor and its microenvironmental biology will be required for antiangiogenic (molecular) therapy to be effective in clinical studies. Despite these challenges, marked advances in antiangiogenic molecular therapy have occurred in the last few years.

## ACKNOWLEDGMENT

This work was supported by the National Institutes of Health (CA70394).

## REFERENCES

1. Millauer B, Shawver LK, Plate KH, Risau W, Ullrich A. Glioblastoma growth inhibited *in vivo* by a dominant-negative Flk-1 mutant. Nature 1994; 367:576–579.
2. Saleh M, Stacker SA, Wilks AF. Inhibition of growth of C6 glioma cells *in vivo* by expression of antisense vascular endothelial growth factor sequence. Cancer Res 1996; 56:383–401.
3. Lin P, Buxton JA, Acheson A, et al. Antiangiogenic gene therapy targeting the endothelium-specific receptor tyrosine kinase Tie2. Proc Natl Acad Sci USA 1998; 95:8829–8834.
4. Goldman CK, Kendall FL, Cabrera G, et al. Paracrine expression of a native soluble vascular endothelial growth factor receptor inhibits tumor growth, metastasis, and mortality rate. Proc Natl Acad Sci USA 1998; 95:8795–8800.
5. Griscelli F, Li H, Griscelli AB, et al. Angiostatin gene transfer: inhibition of tumor growth *in vivo* by blockage of endothelial cell proliferation associated with a mitosis arrest. Proc Natl Acad Sci USA 1998; 95:6367–6372.
6. Chen QR, Kumar D, Stass SA, Mixson AJ. Liposomes complexed to plasmids encoding angiostatin and endostatin inhibit breast cancer in nude mice. Cancer Res 1999; 59:3308–3312.
7. Blezinger P, Wang J, Gondo M, Quezada A, Mehrens D, French M, et al. Systemic inhibition of tumor growth and tumor metastases by intramuscular administration of the endostatin gene. Nat Biotechnol 1999; 17:623–632.
8. He QM, Wei YQ, Tian L, et al. Inhibition of tumor growth with a vaccine based on xenogeneic homologous fibroblast growth factor receptor-1 in mice. J Biol Chem 2003; 278:21,831–21,836.
9. Mengiardi B, Berger R, Just M, Gluck R. Virosomes as carriers for combined vaccines. Vaccine 1995; 13:1306–1315.
10. Niethammer AG, Xiang R, Becker JC, et al. A DNA vaccine against VEGF receptor 2 prevents effective angiogenesis and inhibits tumor growth. Nat Med 2002; 8:1369–1375.
11. O'Reilly MS. Vessel maneuvers: vaccine targets tumor vasculature. Nat Med 2002; 8:1352–1353.
12. Poltl-Frank F, Zurbriggen R, Helg A, et al. Use of reconstituted influenza virus virosomes as an immunopotentiating delivery system for a peptide-based vaccine. Clin Exp Immunol 1999; 117:496–503.
13. Rafii S. Vaccination against tumor neovascularization: promise and reality. Cancer Cell 2002; 2:429–431.
14. Scappaticci FA. The therapeutic potential of novel antiangiogenic therapies. Expert Opin Investig Drugs 2003; 12:923–932.
15. Wei YQ, Wang QR, Zhao X, et al. Immunotherapy of tumors with xenogeneic endothelial cells as a vaccine. Nat Med 2000; 6:1160–1166.
16. Wloch MK, Pasquini S, Ertl HC, Pisetsky DS. The influence of DNA sequence on the immunostimulatory properties of plasmid DNA vectors. Hum Gene Ther 1998; 9:1439–1447.
17. Zhang ZL, Wang JH, Liu XY. Current strategies and future directions of antiangiogenic tumor therapy. Acta Biophys Sin 2003; 35:873–880.

18. Gene therapy clinical trials. New York: Wiley (accessed 12/15/03, 2003, at http://www.wiley.co.uk/genetherapy/clinical/index.html).

19. Sasaki M, Wizigmann-Voos S, Risau W, Plate KH. Retrovirus producer cells encoding antisense VEGF prolong survival of rats with intracranial GS9L gliomas. Int J Dev Neurosci 1999; 17:579–591.

20. Im SA, Gomez-Manzano C, Fueyo J, et al. Antiangiogenesis treatment for gliomas: transfer of anti-sense-vascular endothelial growth factor inhibits tumor growth in vivo. Cancer Res 1999; 59:895–900.

21. Im SA, Kim JS, Gomez-Manzano C, et al. Inhibition of breast cancer growth in vivo by antiangiogenesis gene therapy with adenovirus-mediated antisense-VEGF. Br J Cancer 2001; 84:1252–1257.

22. Yan RL, Qian XH, Xin XY, et al. Experimental study of anti-VEGF hairpin ribozyme gene inhibiting expression of VEGF and proliferation of ovarian cancer cells. Ai Zheng 2002; 21:39–44.

23. Grant MB, Tarnuzzer RW, Caballero S, et al. Adenosine receptor activation induces vascular endothe-lial growth factor in human retinal endothelial cells. Circ Res 1999; 85:699–706.

24. Filleur S, Courtin A, Ait-Si-Ali S, et al. SiRNA-mediated inhibition of vascular endothelial growth factor severely limits tumor resistance to antiangiogenic thrombospondin-1 and slows tumor vascular-ization and growth. Cancer Res 2003; 63:3919–3922.

25. Machein MR, Risau W, Plate KH. Antiangiogenic gene therapy in a rat glioma model using a dominant-negative vascular endothelial growth factor receptor 2. Hum Gene Ther 1999; 10:1117–1128.

26. Kong HL, Hecht D, Song W, et al. Regional suppression of tumor growth by in vivo transfer of a cDNA encoding a secreted form of the extracellular domain of the flt-1 vascular endothelial growth factor receptor. Hum Gene Ther 1998; 9:823–833.

27. Weng DE, Usman N. Angiozyme: a novel angiogenesis inhibitor. Curr Oncol Rep 2001; 3:141–146.

28. Zhang L, Gasper WJ, Stass SA, Ioffe OB, Davis MA, Mixson AJ. Angiogenic inhibition mediated by a DNAzyme that targets vascular endothelial growth factor receptor 2. Cancer Res 2002; 62:5463–5469.

29. Colville-Nash PR, Willoughby DA. Growth factors in angiogenesis: current interest and therapeutic potential. Mol Med 1997; 3:14–23.

30. Risau W. What, if anything, is an angiogenic factor? Cancer Metastasis Rev 1996; 15:149–151.

31. Hood JD, Bednarski M, Frausto R, et al. Tumor regression by targeted gene delivery to the neovascu-lature. Science 2002; 296:2404–2407.

32. Alavi A, Hood JD, Frausto R, Stupack DG, Cheresh DA. Role of Raf in vascular protection from dis-tinct apoptotic stimuli. Science 2003; 301:94–96.

33. Dedhar S, Hannigan GE, Rak J, Kerbel RS. The extracellular environment and cancer. In: Tannock IF, Hill RP, eds. The basic science of oncology, 3rd ed. New York: McGraw-Hill, 1998:197–218.

34. Aoki T, Kato S, Fox JC, et al. Inhibition of autocrine fibroblast growth factor signaling by the adeno-virus-mediated expression of an antisense transgene or a dominant negative receptor in human glioma cells in vitro. Int J Oncol 2002; 21:629–636.

35. Auguste P, Gursel DB, Lemiere S, et al. Inhibition of fibroblast growth factor/fibroblast growth factor receptor activity in glioma cells impedes tumor growth by both angiogenesis-dependent and -indepen-dent mechanisms. Cancer Res 2001; 61:1717–1726.

36. Wang Y, Becker D. Antisense targeting of basic fibroblast growth factor and fibroblast growth factor receptor-1 in human melanomas blocks intratumoral angiogenesis and tumor growth. Nat Med 1997; 3:887–893.

37. Su JD, Mayo LD, Donner DB, Durden DL. PTEN and phosphatidylinositol 3'-kinase inhibitors up-regulate p53 and block tumor-induced angiogenesis: evidence for an effect on the tumor and endo-thelial compartment. Cancer Res 2003; 63:3585–3592.

38. Naito S, Shimizu S, Matsuu M, et al. Ets-1 upregulates matrix metalloproteinase-1 expression through extracellular matrix adhesion in vascular endothelial cells. Biochem Biophys Res Commun 2002; 291: 130–138.

39. Ishikawa H, Nakao K, Matsumoto K, et al. Antiangiogenic gene therapy for hepatocellular carcinoma using angiostatin gene. Hepatology 2003; 37:696–704.

40. Chen Z, Fisher RJ, Riggs CW, Rhim JS, Lautenberger JA. Inhibition of vascular endothelial growth factor-induced endothelial cell migration by ETS1 antisense oligonucleotides. Cancer Res 1997; 57: 2013–2019.

41. Oda N, Abe M, Sato Y. ETS-1 converts endothelial cells to the angiogenic phenotype by inducing the expression of matrix metalloproteinases and integrin beta3. J Cell Physiol 1999; 178:121–132.

42. Lincoln DW 2nd, Phillips PG, Bove K. Estrogen-induced Ets-1 promotes capillary formation in an in vitro tumor angiogenesis model. Breast Cancer Res Treat 2003; 78:167–178.

43. Tomita N, Morishita R, Taniyama Y, et al. Angiogenic property of hepatocyte growth factor is dependent on upregulation of essential transcription factor for angiogenesis, ets-1. Circulation 2003; 107: 1411–1417.

44. Novak EM, Metzger M, Chammas R, et al. Downregulation of TNF-alpha and VEGF expression by Sp1 decoy oligodeoxynucleotides in mouse melanoma tumor. Gene Ther 2003; 10:1992–1997.

45. Moser TL, Stack MS, Asplin I, et al. Angiostatin binds ATP synthase on the surface of human endothelial cells. Proc Natl Acad Sci USA 1999; 96:2811–2816.

46. MacDonald NJ, Shivers WY, Plum SM, Sim BKL. Endostatin proteins binds tropomyosin: potential for modulation of the anti-angiogenic activity of endostatin protein. In: Presentation at the American Association of Cancer Research Conference on Molecular Targets and Cancer Therapeutics 1999.

47. Rehn M, Veikkola T, Kukk-Valdre E, et al. Interaction of endostatin with integrins implicated in angiogenesis. Proc Natl Acad Sci USA 2001; 98:1024–1029.

48. O'Reilly MS, Holmgren L, Chen C, Folkman J. Angiostatin induces and sustains dormancy of human primary tumors in mice. Nat Med 1996; 2:689–692.

49. O'Reilly MS, Boehm T, Shing Y, et al. Endostatin: an endogenous inhibitor of angiogenesis and tumor growth. Cell 1997; 88:277–285.

50. Cao Y, O'Reilly MS, Marshall B, Flynn E, Ji RW, Folkman J. Expression of angiostatin cDNA in a murine fibrosarcoma suppresses primary tumor growth and produces long-term dormancy of metastases. J Clin Invest 1998; 101:1055–1063.

51. Liu Y, Thor A, Shtivelman E, et al. Systemic gene delivery expands the repertoire of effective antiangiogenic agents. J Biol Chem 1999; 274:13,338–13,344.

52. Ding I, Sun JZ, Fenton B, et al. Intratumoral administration of endostatin plasmid inhibits vascular growth and perfusion in MCa-4 murine mammary carcinomas. Cancer Res 2001; 61:526–531.

53. Feldman AL, Restifo NP, Alexander HR, et al. Antiangiogenic gene therapy of cancer utilizing a recombinant adenovirus to elevate systemic endostatin levels in mice. Cancer Res 2000; 60:1503–1506.

54. Regulier E, Paul S, Marigliano M, et al. Adenovirus-mediated delivery of antiangiogenic genes as an antitumor approach. Cancer Gene Ther 2001; 8:45–54.

55. Sauter BV, Martinet O, Zhang WJ, Mandeli J, Woo SL. Adenovirus-mediated gene transfer of endostatin *in vivo* results in high level of transgene expression and inhibition of tumor growth and metastases. Proc Natl Acad Sci USA 2000; 97:4802–4807.

56. Wen XY, Bai Y, Stewart AK. Adenovirus-mediated human endostatin gene delivery demonstrates strain-specific antitumor activity and acute dose-dependent toxicity in mice. Hum Gene Ther 2001; 12:347–358.

57. Szary J, Szala S. Intra-tumoral administration of naked plasmid DNA encoding mouse endostatin inhibits renal carcinoma growth. Int J Cancer 2001; 91:835–839.

58. Ma HI, Guo P, Li J, et al. Suppression of intracranial human glioma growth after intramuscular administration of an adeno-associated viral vector expressing angiostatin. Cancer Res 2002; 62:756–763.

59. Ma HI, Lin SZ, Chiang YH, et al. Intratumoral gene therapy of malignant brain tumor in a rat model with angiostatin delivered by adeno-associated viral (AAV) vector. Gene Ther 2002; 9:2–11.

60. Thurston G, McLean JW, Rizen B, et al. Cationic liposomes target angiogenic endothelial cells in tumors and chronic inflammation in mice. J Clin Invest 1998; 101:1410–1413.

61. Arap W, Pasqualini R, Ruoslahti E. Cancer treatment by targeted drug delivery to tumor vasculature in a mouse model. Science 1998; 279:377–380.

62. Pasqualini R, Koivunen E, Ruoslahti E. Alpha v integrins as receptors for tumor targeting by circulating ligands. Nat Biotechnol 1997; 15:542–546.

63. Matsuda KM, Madoiwa S, Hasumi Y, et al. A novel strategy for the tumor angiogenesis-targeted gene therapy: generation of angiostatin from endogenous plasminogen by protease gene transfer. Cancer Gene Ther 2000; 7:589–596.

64. Joki T, Machluf M, Atala A, et al. Continuous release of endostatin from microencapsulated engineered cells for tumor therapy. Nat Biotechnol 2001; 19:35–39.

65. Lasagni L, Francalanci M, Annunziato F, et al. An alternatively spliced variant of CXCR3 mediates the inhibition of endothelial cell growth induced by IP-10, Mig, and I-TAC, and acts as functional receptor for platelet factor 4. J Exp Med 2003; 197:1537–1549.

66. Romagnani P, Annunziato F, Lasagni L, et al. Cell cycle-dependent expression of CXC chemokine receptor 3 by endothelial cells mediates angiostatic activity. J Clin Invest 2001; 107:53–63.

67. Tanaka T, Manome Y, Wen P, Kufe DW, Fine HA. Viral vector-mediated transduction of a modified platelet factor 4 cDNA inhibits angiogenesis and tumor growth. Nat Med 1997; 3:437–442.

68. Gengrinovitch S, Greenberg SM, Cohen T, et al. Platelet factor-4 inhibits the mitogenic activity of VEGF121 and VEGF165 using several concurrent mechanisms. J Biol Chem 1995; 270:15,059–15,065.

69. Voest EE, Kenyon BM, O'Reilly MS, Truitt G, D'Amato RJ, Folkman J. Inhibition of angiogenesis *in vivo* by interleukin 12. J Natl Cancer Inst 1995; 87:581–586.

70. Boggio K, Di Carlo E, Rovero S, et al. Ability of systemic interleukin-12 to hamper progressive stages of mammary carcinogenesis in HER2/neu transgenic mice. Cancer Res 2000; 60:359–364.

71. Sharpe RJ, Byers HR, Scott CF, Bauer SI, Maione TE. Growth inhibition of murine melanoma and human colon carcinoma by recombinant human platelet factor 4. J Natl Cancer Inst 1990; 82:848–853.

72. Sgadari C, Angiolillo AL, Tosato G. Inhibition of angiogenesis by interleukin-12 is mediated by the interferon-inducible protein 10. Blood 1996; 87:3877–3882.

73. Angiolillo AL, Sgadari C, Tosato G. A role for the interferon-inducible protein 10 in inhibition of angiogenesis by interleukin-12. Ann NY Acad Sci 1996; 795:158–167.

74. Blezinger P, Freimark BD, Matar M, et al. Intratracheal administration of interleukin 12 plasmid-cationic lipid complexes inhibits murine lung metastases. Hum Gene Ther 1999; 10:723–731.

75. Yao L, Sgadari C, Furuke K, Bloom ET, Teruya-Feldstein J, Tosato G. Contribution of natural killer cells to inhibition of angiogenesis by interleukin-12. Blood 1999; 93:1612–1621.

76. Palmer K, Hitt M, Emtage PC, Gyorffy S, Gauldie J. Combined CXC chemokine and interleukin-12 gene transfer enhances antitumor immunity. Gene Ther 2001; 8:282–290.

77. Hawighorst T, Oura H, Streit M, et al. Thrombospondin-1 selectively inhibits early-stage carcinogenesis and angiogenesis but not tumor lymphangiogenesis and lymphatic metastasis in transgenic mice. Oncogene 2002; 21:7945–7956.

78. Hawighorst T, Velasco P, Streit M, et al. Thrombospondin-2 plays a protective role in multistep carcinogenesis: a novel host anti-tumor defense mechanism. EMBO J 2001; 20:2631–2640.

79. Streit M, Riccardi L, Velasco P, et al. Thrombospondin-2: a potent endogenous inhibitor of tumor growth and angiogenesis. Proc Natl Acad Sci USA 1999; 96:14,888–14,893.

80. Zabrenetzky V, Harris CC, Steeg PS, Roberts DD. Expression of the extracellular matrix molecule Thrombospondin inversely correlates with malignant progression in melanoma, lung, and breast carcinoma. Int J Cancer 1994; 59:191–195.

81. Kazuno M, Tokunaga T, Oshika Y, et al. Thrombospondin-2 (TSP2) expression is inversely correlated with vascularity in glioma. Eur J Cancer 1999; 35:502–506.

82. Tolsma VS, Volpert OV, Good DJ, Frazier WA, Polverini PJ, Bouck N. Peptides derived from two separate domains of the matrix protein thrombospondin I have anti-angiogenic activity. J Cell Biol 1993; 122:497–511.

83. Guo NH, Krutzsch HC, Inman JK, Shannon CS, Roberts DD. Antiproliferative and antitumor activities of D-reverse peptides derived from the second type-1 repeat of thrombospondin-1. J Pept Res 1997; 50:210–221.

84. Weinstat-Saslow D, Zabrenetzky VS, VanHoutte K, Frazier WA, Roberts DD, Steeg PS. Transfection of thrombospondin I complementary DNA into a human breast carcinoma cell line reduces primary tumor growth, metastatic potential, and angiogenesis. Cancer Res 1994; 54:6504–6511.

85. Xu M, Kumar D, Stass SA, Mixson AJ. Gene therapy with p53 and a fragment of thrombospondin I inhibits human breast cancer *in vivo*. Mol Genet Metab 1998; 63:103–109.

86. Baker AH, George SJ, Zaltsman AB, Murphy G, Newby AC. Inhibition of invasion and induction of apoptotic cell death of cancer cell lines by overexpression of TIMP-3. Br J Cancer 1999; 79:1347–1355.

87. Valente P, Fassina G, Melchiori A, et al. TIMP-2 over-expression reduces invasion and angiogenesis and protects B16F10 melanoma cells from apoptosis. Int J Cancer 1998; 75:246–253.

88. Celiker MY, Wang M, Atsidaftos E, et al. Inhibition of Wilms' tumor growth by intramuscular administration of tissue inhibitor of metalloproteinases-4 plasmid DNA. Oncogene 2001; 20:4337–4343.

89. Folkman J. Antiangiogenic therapy. In: DeVita VT, Hellman S, Rosenberg SA, eds. Principles and practice of oncology. Philadelphia: Lippincott–Raven, 1997:3075–3085.

90. Bouvet M, Ellis LM, Nishizaki M, Fujiwara T, Liu W, Bucana CD, et al. Adenovirus-mediated wild-type p53 gene transfer down-regulates vascular endothelial growth factor expression and inhibits angiogenesis in human colon cancer. Cancer Res 1998; 58:2288–2292.

91. Galy B, Creancier L, Prado-Lourenco L, Prats AC, Prats H. p53 directs conformational change and translation initiation blockade of human fibroblast growth factor 2 mRNA. Oncogene 2001; 20:4613–4620.

92. Sherif ZA, Nakai S, Pirollo KF, Rait A, Chang EH. Downmodulation of bFGF-binding protein expression following restoration of p53 function. Cancer Gene Ther 2001; 8:771–782.

93. Yonish-Rouach E, Resnitzky D, Lotem J, Sachs L, Kimch A, Oren M. Wild-type p53 induces apoptosis of myeloid cells that is inhibited by interleukin-6. Nature 1991; 352:345–347.

94. Xu M, Kumar D, Srinivas S, et al. Parenteral gene therapy with p53 inhibits human breast tumors *in vivo* through a bystander mechanism without evidence of toxicity. Hum Gene Ther 1996; 8:177–185.

95. Riccioni T, Cirielli C, Wang X, Passaniti A, Capogrossi MC. Adenovirus-mediated wild-type p53 over-expression inhibits endothelial cell differentiation *in vitro* and angiogenesis *in vivo*. Gene Ther 1998; 5:747–754.

96. Toschi E, Rota R, Antonini A, Melillo G, Capogrossi MC. Wild-type p53 gene transfer inhibits invasion and reduces matrix metalloproteinase-2 levels in p53-mutated human melanoma cells. J Invest Dermatol 2000; 114:1188–1194.

97. Roth JA, Nguyen D, Lawrence DD, et al. Retrovirus-mediated wild-type p53 gene transfer to tumors of patients with lung cancer. Nat Med 1996; 2:985–991.

98. Lesoon-Wood LA, Kim WH, Kleinman HK, Weintraub BD, Mixson AJ. Systemic gene therapy with p53 reduces growth and metastases of a malignant human breast cancer in nude mice. Hum Gene Ther 1995; 6:395–405.

99. Hsiao M, Tse V, Carmel J, et al. Intracavitary liposome-mediated p53 gene transfer into glioblastoma with endogenous wild-type p53 *in vivo* results in tumor suppression and long-term survival. Biochem Biophys Res Commun 1997; 233:359–364.

100. Xu L, Pirollo KF, Tang WH, Rait A, Chang EH. Transferrin-liposome-mediated systemic p53 gene therapy in combination with radiation results in regression of human head and neck cancer xenografts. Hum Gene Ther 1999; 10:2941–2952.

101. Wei YQ, Huang MJ, Yang L, et al. Immunogene therapy of tumors with vaccine based on *Xenopus* homologous vascular endothelial growth factor as a model antigen. Proc Natl Acad Sci USA 2001; 98: 11,545–15,550.

102. St Croix B, Rago C, Velculescu V, et al. Genes expressed in human tumor endothelium. Science 2000; 289:1197–1202.

103. Kerbel RS. Inhibition of tumor angiogenesis as a strategy to circumvent acquired resistance to anti-cancer therapeutic agents. Bioessays 1991; 13:31–36.

104. Boehm T, Folkman J, Browder T, O'Reilly MS. Antiangiogenic therapy of experimental cancer does not induce acquired drug resistance. Nature 1997; 390:404–407.

105. Sweeney CJ, Miller KD, Sledge GW Jr. Resistance in the anti-angiogenic era: nay-saying or a word of caution? Trends Mol Med 2003; 9:24–29.

106. Yu JL, Coomber BL, Kerbel RS. A paradigm for therapy-induced microenvironmental changes in solid tumors leading to drug resistance. Differentiation 2002; 70:599–609.

107. Yu JL, Rak JW, Coomber BL, Hicklin DJ, Kerbel RS. Effect of p53 status on tumor response to anti-angiogenic therapy. Science 2002; 295:1526–1528.

108. Sweeney CJ, Miller KD, Sissons SE, et al. The antiangiogenic property of docetaxel is synergistic with a recombinant humanized monoclonal antibody against vascular endothelial growth factor or 2-methoxyestradiol but antagonized by endothelial growth factors. Cancer Res 2001; 61:3369–3372.

# VI-B SUPPORTIVE AND ADJUVANT THERAPIES

# 31

# Development of Palifermin (rHuKGF) for Mucositis

*Ping Wei, PhD and Catherine L. Farrell, PhD*

## Contents

## Summary

Mucositis is a painful adverse event caused by chemo- and/or radiation therapy in cancer patients. It occurs in about 40% of patients receiving chemoradiotherapy and can have profound effects on their quality of life and treatment protocol. Mucositis patients are more susceptible to infections and frequently require longer hospital stays, which lead to significant increases in medical costs. At present, effective treatment against mucositis is lacking. Palifermin, a recombinant form of the human keratinocyte growth factor (KGF) developed by Amgen Inc., has been shown to reduce the incidence and duration of oral mucositis in patients with hematologic malignancies who have undergone myelo-ablative chemoradiotherapy and peripheral blood progenitor cell transplantation. Our chapter reviews the current knowledge on KGF, including its molecular biology, its role in epithelial repair and regeneration of the alimentary tract, and its effect on wound healing, lung repair, bladder injury, and graft-vs-host disease. In addition, we discuss preclinical data on the effects of KGF on different tumors and review the palifermin clinical development.

**Key Words:** Keratinocyte growth factor; KGF; palifermin; oral mucositis; chemotherapy; radiotherapy; hematologic malignancies; peripheral blood progenitor cell transplantation; clinical development; Amgen Inc.

From: *Cancer Drug Discovery and Development: The Oncogenomics Handbook*
Edited by: W. J. LaRochelle and R. A. Shimkets © Humana Press Inc., Totowa, NJ

# 1. MUCOSITIS

Mucositis is a common, debilitating, and often dose-limiting complication of cancer therapy *(1–4)*. The condition results from the inhibitory effects of chemotherapy and/or radiotherapy on rapidly dividing cells, leading to reduction in the renewal capabilities of the basal epithelium. The disease is characterized by sequential mucosal changes, including erythema resulting from inflammation, atrophy, collagen breakdown, and, ultimately, painful ulcerative lesions affecting the alimentary tract, including the mouth (oral mucositis) and the gastrointestine (GI mucositis). In the United States alone, approx 400,000 patients per year develop acute or chronic oral complications during chemoradiotherapy, with about 40% developing oral mucositis *(2,3)*. More than 75% of patients who receive conditioning regimens in preparation for bone marrow transplantation (BMT) or peripheral blood progenitor cell transplantation (PBPCT) and more than 90% of patients receiving head and neck irradiation develop oral mucositis *(2,3)*.

Patients receiving high-dose cytotoxic therapy with hematopoietic stem cell support cite mucositis as the most painful and debilitating side effect of myeloablative regimens *(5)*. Mucositis significantly affects the quality of life of cancer patients, often leading to pain so severe that it interferes with basic functions such as eating, swallowing, talking, and sleeping. Systemic analgesics, adjunctive medications such as antibiotics, and physical and/or psychological therapy might be required. Patients are also more susceptible to serious infections (e.g., sepsis) because of the disruption of the natural mucosal barrier, and septicemia is associated with 6–30% mortality *(4)*.

Currently, available mucositis treatments are purely symptomatic and include analgesics (for pain control), parenteral nutrition (to support patients alimentation and hydration), and/or modification of the chemoradiotherapy regimens (dose delay/reduction). Such measures result in longer hospitalization and increased health care costs and could affect disease outcome. In one study, total hospital charges were almost $43,000 higher in patients with ulcerative oral mucositis than in patients with milder, nonulcerative disease *(6)*.

There is a clear unmet need for effective mucositis therapies. About a dozen mucositis treatments are in development, but few have been tested in phase III trials. Among the most promising agents is keratinocyte growth factor (KGF), which has been evaluated in several murine models of chemo/radio-induced mucositis. A recombinant form of human KGF (rHuKGF, palifermin) is being clinically evaluated and results of a pivotal phase III trial indicate that it is effective in reducing the incidence and duration of severe oral mucositis in patients receiving high-dose chemoradiotherapy prior to PBPCT for hematologic malignancies (see Section 4).

# 2. MOLECULAR BIOLOGY OF KGF

## 2.1. Expression and Regulation

Human KGF is a 194-amino-acid polypeptide and a member of the fibroblast growth factor (FGF) family. It was originally isolated from the conditioned medium of a human embryonic lung fibroblast cell line *(7)*. It was then found to be produced by a variety of mesenchymal cells, including fibroblasts *(8)*, microvascular endothelial cells *(9)*, and smooth muscle cells *(10)*. Activated γδT-cells from skin and intestine also express KGF, whereas other types of lymphocyte, monocytes/macrophages, umbilical vein endothelial cells, and most epithelial cells do not *(8,11)*.

Keratinocyte growth factor expression is significantly upregulated in several epithelial injury conditions, including incisional and excisional skin wounds *(12,13)*, surgical bladder injury *(14)*, lung and kidney chemical injury *(15,16)*, inflammatory diseases such as inflammatory bowel disease (IBD) *(17–19)*, and psoriasis *(20)*. Although KGF does not appear to be important for organogenesis because the KGF knockout mice develop normally *(21)*, this pattern of expression strongly suggests that KGF plays an important role in epithelial homeostasis in adult organs, particularly during epithelial regeneration and repair.

The mechanism of induction of KGF could be via cytokines known to regulate KGF expression: Interleukin-1 (IL-1) has been shown to strongly induce the expression of KGF mRNA and protein in fibroblasts from multiple sources, whereas platelet-derived growth factor-BB (PDGF-BB), IL-6, and transforming growth factor-$\alpha$ (TGF-$\alpha$) have also been shown to produce moderate induction *(22,23)*. Glucocorticoids such as dexamethasone have been demonstrated to inhibit KGF expression *(24–26)*, whereas nonsteroidal anti-inflammatory agents had no effect on KGF production. KGF has been proposed as a primary mediator of steroid hormone action in organs in the male and female reproductive tracts, including the prostate, seminal vesicle, and endometrium *(27–31)*. This is because testosterone stimulates KGF expression in prostate stromal cells *(27,28)*. Similarly, estrogen induces KGF expression in mammary stromal cells *(29)*, endometrial epithelial cells *(30)*, and isolated thecal cells from bovine ovarian follicles *(31)*.

Unlike other members of the FGF family that bind to a variety of FGF receptors, KGF targets exclusively the KGF receptor, KGFR, which is a splicing variant of FGFR2 and belongs to the FGF receptor family of tyrosine kinase receptors *(32,33)*. Patterns of expression of KGF and KGFR in mouse embryo indicate that organs within the integumentary, respiratory, gastrointestinal, and urogenital systems, which depend on mesenchymal–epithelial interactions to develop, show KGF mRNA in mesenchymal cells, whereas epithelial cells express transcripts for the KGFR *(34)*. Similar patterns of expression of KGF and KGFR mRNA are also seen throughout the adult tissues, such as lung *(35)*, skin *(36)*, breast *(29)*, GI tract *(37)*, and the reproductive organs *(38,39)*.

## 2.2. Action of KGF

The earliest in vitro studies showed that KGF promoted proliferation of a variety of cultured epithelial cells but had no effect on fibroblasts, saphenous vein endothelial cells, melanocytes, or myoblasts *(8)*, suggesting that KGF was an epithelial-specific mitogen. It was also shown to induce epithelial migration *(40,41)* and differentiation *(42,43)* but inhibit terminal differentiation and apoptosis *(44,45)*. Together, these data suggested that KGF could function as a paracrine survival factor for epithelial cells.

Keratinocyte growth factor is also active on lung cells, pancreatic cells, and hepatocytes. In the lung, alveolar type II cells differentiate into type I cells in vitro. KGF prolonged the type II phenotype and increased the synthesis of surfactant proteins *(46,47)*. KGF also stimulated lipogenesis and the conversion of fatty acids into phospholipids in these cells *(48)*. In the adult rat, systemic daily KGF resulted in proliferation of pancreatic exocrine cells and differentiation into ductal epithelial cells *(49,50)* while repressing the development of endocrine cells *(51)*. KGF decreased apoptosis in hepatocytes treated with actinomycin D and tumor necrosis factor (TNF) *(52)*. The mechanism by which KGF exerts these effects has been partially elucidated. KGF increased expression of antiapoptotic protein Bcl-2 in intestinal epithelial cells *(53)* and inhibited the expression of proapoptotic protein p53, p21, Bax, and Bcl-x in alveolar epithelial cells (54,55). KGF was also shown to induce the Akt pathway, and inhibition of this pathway abolished the protection that KGF gave to the epithelium (56). KGF was further shown to have cytoprotective effect on epithelial cells through its ability to reduce radiation- or chemical-induced DNA strand breaks (57,58) and its induction of antioxidant enzymes (59,60).

# 3. PRECLINICAL STUDIES OF KGF
# IN EPITHELIAL REPAIR AND REGENERATION

## 3.1. KGF in Mucositis

Epithelia have a hierarchical proliferative organization, with cell loss through differentiation and mechanical stress at the surface, replenished by continuous cell production in the basal epithelial layers. Chemotherapy and radiation directly affect cell proliferation, reducing regeneration of the epithelial lining. The high rate of cellular turnover in the alimentary tract, including the oral mucosa, makes these areas particularly susceptible to damage from cytotoxic therapies.

There is substantial evidence demonstrating that KGF is a muco-protective agent in both normal animals and radiation and/or chemotherapy animal models. Consistent with the finding that KGF and KGFR mRNAs are expressed throughout the entire alimentary tract (38,61), KGF has been shown to promote cell proliferation, differentiation, and survival of alimentary epithelial cells (61–64). In healthy animals, KGF causes epithelial thickening of nonkeratinized layers of oral epithelium, including the tongue, esophagus, and buccal mucosa (61), and it also increases the total cellularity in mouse ventral tongue (64). In adult rats, KGF causes a marked increase in the proliferation of epithelial cells from the foregut to the colon and the selective induction of mucin-producing goblet cells throughout the GI tract (38). This enhanced epithelial thickness and increased cell number might play a role in epithelial survival and regeneration.

In a mouse model of oral mucositis, the ventral tongue epithelium was irradiated with X-rays to induce ulcer formation. Recombinant human KGF (rHuKGF) given before, after, or during the radiation exposure significantly reduced the incidence of oral mucosal ulceration (65). The maximum protection was observed when KGF was given either from d –3 to +1 or from d 0 to +2 with radiation given on d 0. In a similar model, mouse tongue ulceration was induced by five daily doses of fractionated irradiation followed with graded test doses of X-ray to approximate the fractionated irradiation in a clinical setting. rHuKGF given before radiotherapy, during fractionated radiotherapy, over the weekend break, or in a combination of these schedules, significantly enhanced oral mucosal radiation tolerance (66). Interestingly, KGF appeared to be ineffective when given at the time of ulcer manifestation (67), suggesting that appropriate scheduling might be needed for optimal clinical management of radiotherapy-induced mucositis.

Further rodent studies showed that short-term administration of rHuKGF (5 mg/kg/ d ×3 d) prior to chemotherapy and/or radiotherapy was beneficial in reducing GI injury and improving survival (62). In models using multiple-dose 5-fluorouracil (5-FU) (Fig. 1), methotrexate, and radiation in combination, or total-body irradiation followed by BMT, rHuKGF increased survival by 55% or greater and significantly reduced weight loss (62). At the cellular level, pretreatment with rHuKGF promoted an increase in mucosal thickness that was sustained during a 5-FU course and resulted in a 3.5-fold improvement in crypt survival in the small intestine (Fig. 2 and Color Plate 11 following p. 302). The

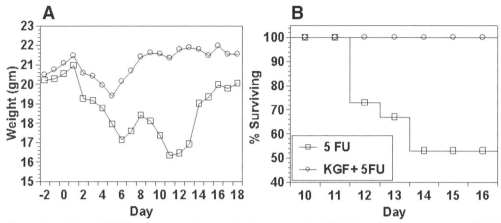

**Fig. 1.** The effect of KGF on mouse body weight (**A**) and survival (**B**) following chemotherapy. BDF1 mice were pretreated with KGF (5 mg/kg/d, subcutaneous) or vehicle for 3 d (d −2 to 0) before treatment with 5-FU (50 mg/kg/d, intraperitoneal) for 4 d (d 1 to 4, $n$ = 15/group).

increased survival was attributed to regeneration of the GI mucosa by rHuKGF (Fig. 3), enabling normal feeding, better nutrient and water absorption in the gut, and better protection against invasion by micro-organisms through a more intact epithelial barrier *(62,68)*. rHuKGF had a similar, muco-protective effect in reversing oral epithelial atrophy caused by irradiation of the oral epithelia and esophagus in mice *(61)*.

As a key mediator controlling the viability of the GI colonic mucosa, KGF might be beneficial in diseases of the GI tract other than mucositis. Consistent with this notion, it was discovered that KGF expression was markedly increased in surgical specimens from patients with ulcerative colitis or Crohn's disease *(17–19)*. Subsequent studies demonstrated that rHuKGF ameliorated mucosal damage in several colitis models *(69–71)*. A specific role of KGF in colon mucosal protection and repair was demonstrated by a study using KGF-null mice, which were more susceptible to dextran sulfate-mediated colonic injury than their wild-type counterparts *(72)*. In rats that had undergone large bowel surgery, rHuKGF promoted healing of colonic anastomoses, possibly by accelerating reparative processes and enhancing protection of the anastomotic wound bed by increasing epithelial proliferation and mucus production *(73,74)*. KGF also reduced the extent of intestinal atrophy in animals maintained on total parenteral nutrition *(75)*.

The proliferative, differentiation-promoting, and protective/survival effects of KGF on epithelial cells contribute to the overall defense of the alimentary tract and heightened reparative functions. By conferring a higher resistance to cytotoxic injury, KGF might be useful in preventing or ameliorating the side effects of cancer therapy.

### 3.2. KGF in Skin Wound Healing and Hair Loss

The role of KGF in skin wound repair was first suggested by the fact that whereas KGFR is localized to the epithelium, KGF is expressed in the dermis of skin and dramatically upregulated upon injury *(12)*. Its putative role as a paracrine skin survival factor is substantiated by a number of studies showing its protective function in wound repair and epithelial regeneration *(76)*. KGF significantly increased the rate of re-epithelialization in partial

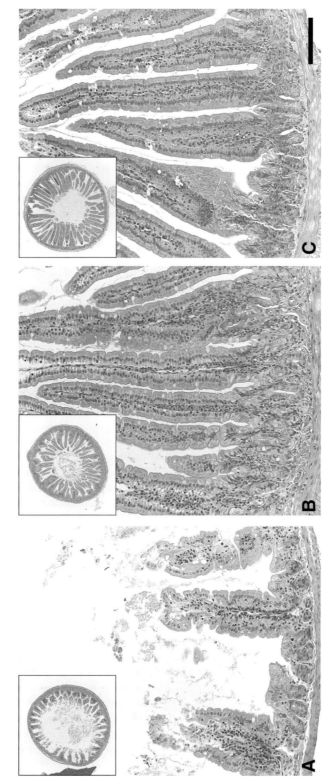

**Fig. 2.** Effect of KGF on the small intestine of 5-FU-treated mice (50 mg/kg/d for 4 d). (**A**) Intestinal mucosa of a 5-FU-treated mouse showing the thinned mucosa and the shortened villa; (**B**) KGF pretreatment restored thickness of the mucosa and the length of the villa; (**C**) mucosa of a control normal mouse. (*See* Color Plate 11 following p. 302.)

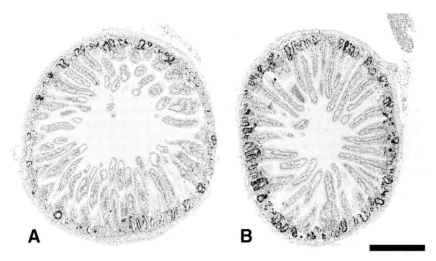

**Fig. 3.** Effect of KGF on BrdU labeling in intestinal mucosa. BDF1 mice irradiated with 12 Gy before BMT have few numbers of BrdU-labeled crypts (**A**) compared with mice pretreated with three doses of KGF at 5 mg/kg (**B**).

thickness excisional wounds of the porcine epidermis *(77)*. It also accelerated re-epithelialization and increased the thickness of the epithelium in a rabbit ear wound model *(78)*. In partial and full thickness burns in porcine models, daily rHuKGF induced an increase in new epithelial tissue area and doubled the number of fully re-epithelialized burns at 13 d after injury *(79)*. KGF also induced granulation tissue in ischemic dermal wounds in the rabbit ear *(80)*. Thus, KGF might have a role in skin wound repair.

A number of growth factors and cytokines control the growth and development of hair follicles. Although of little clinical significance, hair loss is a distressing side effect of cancer therapy. KGF was found to stimulate proliferation and differentiation of early progenitor cells within hair follicles and sebaceous glands in the wound site *(78)*. The potential therapeutic effect of KGF on hair follicles was investigated in distinct murine models of alopecia *(81)*. Intraperitoneal or subcutaneous rHuKGF given for 17–18 d to athymic nude mice dose-dependently induced hair growth over most of the body. The most extensive growth was at subcutaneous injection sites. At the cellular level, rHuKGF induced significant follicular and sebaceous gland hypertrophy, restoring the nude mouse keratinocyte defect and increasing follicular keratinocyte proliferation. In a neonatal rat model of cytarabine-induced alopecia, rHuKGF had a dose-dependent cytoprotective effect on alopecia, with up to 50% attenuation when given 1 d before chemotherapy *(81)*. In another mouse model of induced cytotoxic injury, KGF increased hair follicle survival and regeneration after irradiation *(82)*.

### 3.3. KGF in Lung Injuries

Alveolar epithelial cell damage is common in respiratory illnesses, as well as a consequence of chemotherapy or radiotherapy. Both KGF and KGFR are expressed in fetal and adult lung, suggesting their involvement in lung development and homeostasis *(35)*. KGF stimulates human bronchial cell proliferation in vitro and in vivo *(83)* and specifically induces proliferation and differentiation of alveolar type II cells and the synthesis of surfactant proteins *(35,83–85)*. A series of in vivo studies have established that KGF is an important cytoprotective factor in acute lung injury.

In an acid instillation model of lung damage in rats, treatment with intratracheal KGF 72 h before insult improved survival and ameliorated histological changes in the lung *(86)*. In a rat model of radiation- and bleomycin-induced lung injury, rHuKGF ameliorated respiratory death and enhanced lung function *(87)*. Pretreatment with KGF increased survival from 40% to 100% in mice receiving bleomycin. It also prolonged survival after a lethal challenge with a combination of bleomycin and radiation. At the cellular level, 72 h pretreatment with KGF in murine models of bleomycin insult preserved the number of type II alveolar cells and decreased pulmonary edema, expression of cytokines, TGF-$\beta$, and PDGF-BB compared with controls *(88)*. In rats with hyperoxic lung injury, both intratracheal *(89)* and intravenous (IV) *(90)* rHuKGF stimulated alveolar/bronchial cell proliferation and reduced tissue damage. KGF protects both alveolar epithelium and endothelium from hyperoxia-induced injury in this model *(55)*. Clinically, it was found that a high concentration of KGF in the airways correlated with the lack of bronchopulmonary dysplasia in premature infants *(91)*.

The mechanisms that govern these processes have still to be elucidated. Studies have shown that KGF attenuates oxidant-mediated injury and enhances the DNA repair capacity in cultured lung epithelial cells exposed to radiation *(57)*. It also upregulates active sodium transport in rat alveolar epithelial cells in vitro and prevents hyperoxia-induced reduction of active sodium ion transport *(46,92)*. In human airway epithelial cells, pretreatment with rHuKGF can completely abolish the increase in permeability induced in a hydrogen peroxide damage model *(93)*.

### 3.4. KGF in Bladder Injury

Hemorrhagic cystitis is a complication often associated with chemotherapy using cyclophosphamide (CP) or its derivatives, but less frequently with radiotherapy. Remarkably, KGF was shown to almost completely ameliorate CP-induced ulcerative hemorrhagic cystitis in a rat model. This effect was achieved with a single iv injection of KGF 24 h before CP administration and maintained until at least 48 h later *(94)*. Consistent with this observation, KGF has been shown previously in rats and rhesus monkeys to promote rapid proliferation of urothelial transitional epithelial cells *(95)*. These studies support the clinical testing of Palifermin (rHuKGF) for the treatment of CP-induced bladder cystitis.

### 3.5. Graft-vs-Host Disease, KGF, and the Thymus

Graft-vs-host disease (GVHD) is a common side effect of allogeneic BMT or PBPCT induced by donor alloreactive T-cells targeting the host organs, including the lung, GI tract, liver, spleen, and thymus. It represents a major cause of morbidity and mortality after allogeneic transplantation. Interestingly, KGF was shown to ameliorate GVHD and to protect thymic functions in murine models. When recipient mice were conditioned with total-body irradiation (TBI) with or without chemotherapy before allogeneic BMT with spleen cells as a source of GVHD-inducing T-cells, pretreatment with KGF (5 mg/kg/d × 3 d) significantly increased survival and reduced body weight loss *(96)*. KGF also ameliorated GVHD-related pathologic changes in the liver, lung, and skin. Similar results were seen in a severe combined immunodeficient (SCID) model without cytotoxic conditioning *(97)*. Longer treatment of KGF (from day −3 to +7) in a GVHD model enhanced leukemia-free survival and reduced the severity of GVHD in the GI tract *(98)*.

The protective effect of KGF appears to be associated with a reduction of inflammatory cytokines, such as TNF and interferon-γ (IFN-γ), and an increase of type II cytokines (interleukin [IL]-4, -IL-6, and IL-13) *(97,98)*. In GVHD models, KGF also exerted a cytoprotective effect on thymic epithelial cells in the cortex and medulla and resulted in better T-cell alloengraftment *(97)*.

### *3.6. KGF and Tumors*

A theoretical concern regarding clinical use of KGF in oncology relates to its stimulatory activity of epithelial cell growth. In this context, a number of growth factors and their receptors are known to be important in tumorigenesis. However, not all growth factors act as positive regulators of tumor growth; there are instances in which they have been shown to act in a negative manner, and the loss of their receptors or alteration of signaling pathways is associated with poor prognosis. KGF and KGFR expression has been examined in tumors of various biological origins (*see* following paragraphs), but the role of this pathway in tumorigenesis remains unclear.

In patients with advanced stage squamous cell carcinoma of the head and neck, levels of KGF mRNA were significantly lower than in normal mucosa *(99)*. KGF expression was also lower in endometrial adenocarcinoma tissue than in normal cycling endometrium, without any corresponding reduction in KGFR expression *(100)*. In normal human bladder, KGFR is expressed throughout most of the urothelium; however, in transitional cell bladder carcinomas, receptor expression was markedly reduced *(101)*. Moreover, the extent of this reduction correlated with prognosis, and reintroducing KGFR was later found to inhibit the growth of bladder tumors *(102)*. In human and rat prostate cancer cells, loss of KGFR resulting from splicing events was thought to be a trigger for androgen independence and tumor progression *(103,104)*. Similar to human bladder tumor cells, introducing KGFR in rat prostatic cancer cells inhibited tumor cell growth *(105)*. Furthermore, KGFR was shown to be absent in salivary gland adenocarcinomas and its reintroduction induced differentiation and apoptosis instead of growth *(106)*. These data suggest that loss of KGF or KGFR expression might favor tumor development, and KGF signaling is associated with tumor suppression.

Although some tumors do express KGFR, most of them when tested do not respond to KGF in either in vitro proliferation assays or in xenograft tumor models *(62,107,108)*. One out of seven human tumor lines showed a 45% increase in tumor growth in vivo only after prolonged exposure (three times weekly for 6 wk) to KGF at 1500–4000 µg/kg/dose *(108)*. Transient exposure to KGF at low doses (three to six times 60 µg/kg), albeit protected epithelial cells in preclinical models, did not appear to enhance tumor growth or interfere with the cytoablative effects of cancer treatment on tumor cells in xenograft models. Farrell et al. demonstrated that KGF as a pretreatment in mouse models of chemotherapy- and/or radiation-induced GI injury significantly improved mouse survival, with no detectable stimulation of tumor growth or protection of tumor cells from cytoablative therapy *(62)*. In human squamous cell carcinoma cell lines in vitro, and in corresponding xenografts in mice, rHuKGF exposure resulted in little or no stimulation of cell proliferation and did not compromise radiosensitivity *(107)*. Furthermore, Palifermin was found to have a short half-life of 2–4 h in human and mouse *(108)*, and histological analysis showed that the effect of Palifermin on epithelia is transient and reversible. Nonetheless, the real effect and clinical significance of exogenous KGF administration on tumor can only be determined in appropriately designed clinical studies. So far, no significant differences in long-term survival have been observed between patients who received placebo or Palifermin in clinical trials, although the total number of patients evaluated is relatively limited (about 700) with short follow-up time (about 24 mo). Nonetheless, the real effect and clinical significance of KGF on tumor can only be determined in clinical studies.

## 4. CLINICAL DEVELOPMENT OF PALIFERMIN (rHuKGF)

Extensive preclinical animal studies have identified KGF as an important cytoprotective factor for the regeneration and repair of a variety of epithelial organs, including the upper and lower alimentary track, lung, skin, bladder, and others. Based on this preclinical evidence, Amgen, Inc. carried out clinical investigations into Palifermin as a cytoprotective agent in chemotherapy- and/or radiation-induced oral mucositis in humans.

Palifermin clinical development program focused on the evaluation of the safety and efficacy of Palifermin in reducing the severity and duration of oral mucositis in three clinical settings in which oral mucositis is an important clinical complication of anticancer therapy:

1. Patients receiving high-dose cytotoxic therapy with hematopoietic stem cell support
2. Patients receiving fractionated radiotherapy with/without concomitant chemotherapy (e.g. advanced head and neck cancer)
3. Patients receiving certain regimen of cyclic chemotherapy (e.g., 5-FU/leucovorin for colorectal cancer)

A phase III trial is complete in the first clinical setting, and phase II trials are complete in the second and third settings.

The phase III study investigated the efficacy of iv Palifermin in reducing the severity and duration of oral mucositis and related sequelae in patients with hematologic malignancies receiving TBI and high-dose chemotherapy with autologous peripheral blood stem cells. The trail was a two-arm, randomized, double-blind, placebo-controlled study in which patients received Palifermin at the dose of 60 µg/kg/d for three consecutive days before TBI and three consecutive days after PBPCT. The results from this study demonstrate that Palifermin, at this dose and schedule, reduced the incidence and duration of severe oral mucositis. These reductions were associated with a clinically meaningful improvement in patients' reported mouth and throat soreness and consequent reduction in mucositis-related sequelae such as the need for parental nutrition and opiod analgesia *(109)*. In this study palifermin was well tolerated with the most common treatment-related adverse events being mild-to-moderate skin rash and flushing, and transient asymptomatic elevation of serum amylase and lipase. Current trials are designed to determine the appropriate dose and schedule in patients receiving fractionated radiotherapy with concomitant chemotherapy or cyclic chemotherapy.

## 5. FUTURE STUDIES

Palifermin is a promising agent for of cancer-therapy-induced oral mucositis. However, despite recent advances in understanding the function of KGF, much remains to be learned: relatively little is known about the downstream mechanisms it uses for signal transduction in epithelial cells, and its wide-ranging and diverse activities in a number of epithelial systems throughout the body hold promise in a number of areas. Further preclinical studies and carefully designed and executed clinical studies would help to fully exploit the potential benefit of this exciting new molecule.

## ACKNOWLEDGMENTS

We thank Dr. Glenn Begley, Dr. Alessandra Cesano, and Dr. Andy Partridge for reviewing the manuscript and helpful comments. The authors also thank James Bready, Karen Rex, and Sheila Scully for preparation of the figures.

## REFERENCES

1. Pico J-L, Avila-Garavito A, Nacchache P. Mucositis: its occurrence, consequences, and treatment in the oncology setting. Oncologist 1998; 3:446–451.
2. Duncan M, Grant G. Oral and intestinal mucositis—causes and possible treatments. Aliment Pharmacol Ther 2003; 18:853–874.
3. Epstein JB, Schubert MM. Oropharangeal mucositis in cancer therapy: review of pathogenesis, diagnosis and management. Oncology 2003; 17:1767–1779.
4. Woo SB, Teister N. Chemotherapy-induced oral mucositis. Available online at http://www.emedicine. com/derm/topic682.htm.
5. Bellm LA, Epstein JB, Rose-Ped A, Martin P, Fuchs HJ. Patients' reports of complications of bone marrow transplantation. Support Care Cancer 2000; 8:33–39.
6. Sonis ST, Oster G, Fuchs H, Bellm L, Bradford WZ, Edelsberg J, et al. Oral mucositis and the clinical and economic outcomes of hematopoietic stem-cell transplantation. J Clin Oncol 2001; 19:2201–2205.
7. Rubin JS, Osada H, Finch PW, Taylor WG, Rudikoff S, Aaronson SA. Purification and characterization of a newly identified growth factor specific for epithelial cells. Proc Natl Acad Sci USA 1989; 86: 802–806.
8. Rubin JS, Bottaro DP, Chedid M, Miki T, Ron D, Cheon G, et al. Keratinocyte growth factor. Cell Biol Int 1995; 19:399–411.
9. Smola H, Thiekotter G, Fusenig NE. Mutual induction of growth factor gene expression by epidermal–dermal cell interaction. J Cell Biol 1993; 122:417–429.
10. Winkles JA, Alberts GF, Chedid M, Taylor WG, DeMartino S, Rubin JS. Differential expression of the keratinocyte growth factor (KGF) and KGF receptor genes in human vascular smooth muscle cells and arteries. J Cell Physiol 1997; 173:380–386.
11. Boismenu R, Havran WL. Modulation of epithelial cell growth by intraepithelial gamma delta T cells. Science 1994; 266:1253–1255.
12. Werner S, Peters KG, Longaker MT, Fuller-Pace F, Banda MJ, Williams LT. Large induction of keratinocyte growth factor in the dermis during wound healing. Proc Natl Acad Sci USA 1992; 89:6896–6900.
13. Marchese C, Chedid M, Dirsch OR, Csaky KG, Santanelli F, Latini C, et al. Modulation of keratinocyte growth factor and its receptor in reepithelializing human skin. J Exp Med 1995; 182:1369–1376.
14. Baskin LS, Sutherland RS, Thomson AA, Nguyen HT, Morgan DM, Hayward SW, et al. Growth factors in bladder wound healing. J Urol 1997; 157:2388–2395.
15. Ichimura T, Finch PW, Zhang G, Kan M, Stevens JL. Induction of FGF-7 after kidney damage: a possible paracrine mechanism for tubule repair. Am J Physiol 1996; 271:F967–F976.
16. Adamson IY, Bakowska J. Relationship of keratinocyte growth factor and hepatocyte growth factor levels in rat lung lavage fluid to epithelial cell regeneration after bleomycin. Am J Pathol 1999; 155: 949–954.
17. Brauchle M, Madlener M, Wagner AD, Agnermeyer K, Ulich L, Hofschneider PH, et al. Keratinocyte growth factor is highly overexpressed in inflammatory bowel disease. Am J Pathol 1996; 149:521–529.
18. Finch PW, Pricolo V, Wu A, Finkelstein SD. Increased expression of keratinocyte growth factor messenger RNA associated with inflammatory bowel disease. Gastroenterology 1996; 110:441–451.
19. Bajaj-Elliott M, Breese E, Poulsom R, Fairclough PD, MacDonald TT. Keratinocyte growth factor in inflammatory bowel disease. Increased mRNA transcripts in ulcerative colitis compared with Crohn's disease in biopsies and isolated mucosal myofibroblasts. Am J Pathol 1997; 151:1469–1476.
20. Finch PW, Murphy F, Cardinale I, Krueger JG. Altered expression of keratinocyte growth factor and its receptor in psoriasis. Am J Pathol 1997; 151:1619–1628.

21. Guo L, Degenstein L, Fuchs E. Keratinocyte growth factor is required for hair development not for wound healing. Genes Dev 1996; 10:165–175.
22. Chedid M, Rubin JS, Csaky KG, Aaronson SA. Regulation of keratinocyte growth factor gene expression by interleukin 1. J Biol Chem 1994; 269:10,753–10,757.
23. Brauchle M, Angermeyer K, Hubner G, Werner S. Large induction of keratinocyte growth factor expression by serum growth factors and pro-inflammatory cytokines in cultured fibroblasts. Oncogene 1994; 9:3199–31204.
24. Brauchle M, Fassler R, Werner S. Suppression of keratinocyte growth factor expression by glucocorticoids in vitro and during wound healing. J Invest Dermatol 1995; 105:579–584.
25. Chedid M, Hoyle JR, Csaky KG, Rubin JS. Glucocorticoids inhibit keratinocyte growth factor production primary dermal fibroblasts. Endocrinology 1996; 137:2232–2237.
26. Tang A, Gilchrest BA. Regulation of keratinocyte growth factor gene expression in human skin fibroblasts. J Dermatol Sci 1996; 11:41–50.
27. Yan G, Fukabori Y, Nikolaropoulos S, Wang F, McKeehan WL. Heparin-binding keratinocyte growth factor is a candidate for stromal-to-epithelial-cell andromedin. Mol Endocrinol 1992; 6:2123–2128.
28. Levine AC, Liu XH, Greenberg PD, Eliashvili M, Schiff JD, Aaronso SA, et al. Androgens induce the expression of vascular endothelial growth factor in human fetal prostatic fibroblasts. Endocrinology 1998; 139:4672–4678.
29. Pedchenko VK, Imagawa W. Estrogen treatment in vivo increases keratinocyte growth factor expression in the mammary gland. J Endocrinol 2000; 165:39–49.
30. Ka H, Spencer TE, Johnson GA, Bazer FW. Keratinocyte growth factor: expression by endometrial epithelia of the porcine uterus. Biol Reprod 2000; 62:1772–1778.
31. Parrott JA, Skinner MK. Thecal cell-granulosa cell interactions involve a positive feedback loop among keratinocyte growth factor, hepatocyte growth factor, and Kit ligand during ovarian follicular development. Endocrinology 1998; 139:2240–2245.
32. Miki T, Fleming TP, Bottaro DP, Rubin JS, Ron D, Aaronson SA. Expression cDNA cloning of the KGF receptor by creation of a transforming autocrine loop. Science 1991; 251(4989):72–75.
33. Ornitz DM, Xu J, Colvin JS, McEwen DG, MacArthur CA, Coulier F, et al. Receptor specificity of the fibroblast growth factor family. J Biol Chem 1996; 271:15,292–15,297.
34. Finch PW, Cunha GR, Rubin JS, Wong J, Ron D. Pattern of keratinocyte growth factor and keratinocyte growth factor receptor expression during mouse fetal development suggests a role in mediating morphogenetic mesenchymal-epithelial interactions. Dev Dyn 1995; 203:223–240.
35. Ulich TR, Yi ES, Longmuir K, Yin S, Biltz R, Morris CF, et al. Keratinocyte growth factor is a growth factor for type II pneumocytes in vivo. J Clin Invest 1994; 93:1298–1306.
36. Werner S. Keratinocyte growth factor: a unique player in epithelial repair processes. Cytokine Growth Factor Rev 1998; 9:153–165.
37. Housely RM, Morris CF, Boyle W, Ring B, Blitz R, Tarpley JE, et al. Keratinocyte growth factor induces proliferation of hepatoctyes and epithelial cells throughout the rat gastrointestinal tract. J Clin Invest 1994; 94:1764–1777.
38. Koji T, Chedid M, Rubin JS, Slayden OD, Csaky KG, Aaronson SA, et al. Progesterone-dependent expression of keratinocyte growth factor mRNA stromal cells of the primate endometrium: keratinocyte growth factor as a progestomedin. J Cell Biol 1994; 125:393–401.
39. Thomson AA, Foster BA, Cunha GR. Analysis of growth factor and receptor mRNA levels during development of the rat seminal vesicle and prostate. Development 1997; 124:2431–2439.
40. Tsuboi R, Sato C, Kurita Y, Ron D, Rubin JS, Ogawa H. Keratinocyte growth factor (FGF-7) stimulates migration and plasminogen activator activity of normal human keratinocytes. J Invest Dermatol 1993; 101:49–53.
41. Atabai K, Ishigaki M, Geiser T, Ueki I, Matthay MA, Ware LB. Keratinocyte growth factor can enhance alveolar epithelial repair by nonmitogenic mechanisms. Am J Physiol Lung Cell Mol Physiol 2002; 283: L163–L169.
42. Marchese C, Rubin J, Ron D, Faggioni A, Torrisi MR, Messina A, et al. Human keratinocyte growth factor activity on proliferation and differentiation of human keratinocytes: differentiation response distinguishes KGF from EGF family. J Cell Physiol 1990; 144:326–332.
43. Marchese C, Sorice M, De Stefano C, Frati L, Torrisi MR. Modulation of keratinocyte growth factor receptor expression in human cultured keratinocytes. Cell Growth Differ 1997; 8:989–997.
44. Hines MD, Allen-Hoffman BL. Keratinocyte growth factor inhibits cross-linked envelope formation and nucleosomal fragmentation in cultured human keratinocytes. J Biol Chem 1996; 271:6254–6251.

45. Andreadis ST, Hamoen KE, Yarmush ML, Morgan JR. Keratinocyte growth factor induces hyperproliferation and delays differentiation in a skin equivalent model system. FASEB J 2001; 15:898–906.

46. Borok Z, Danto SI, Dimen LL, Zhang X-L, Lubman RL. $Na^+$-$K^+$-ATPase expression in alveolar epithelial cells: upregulation of active transport by KGF. Am J Physiol 1998; 274:L149–L158.

47. Isakson BE, Lubman RL, Seedorf GJ, Boitano S. Modulation of pulmonary alveolar type II cell phenotype and communication by extracellular matrix and KGF. Am J Physiol Cell Physiol 2001; 281: C1291–C1299.

48. Mason M, Johnson P, Rudd R. MRC Gastrointestinal and Gynaecological Cancer Trials Steering Committee. Combination chemotherapy for advanced colorectal cancer. Br J Cancer 2003; 88:1152–1153.

49. Yi ES, Yin S, Harclerode DL, Bedoya A, Bikhazi NB, Housley RM, et al. Keratinocyte growth factor induces pancreatic ductal epithelial proliferation. Am J Pathol 1994; 145:80–85.

50. Miralles F, Czernichow P, Ozaki K, Itoh N, Scharfman R. Signaling through fibroblast growth factor receptor 2b plays key role in the development of the exocrine pancreas. Proc Natl Acad Sci USA 1999; 96:6267–6272.

51. Elghazi L, Cras-Meneur C, Czernichow P, Scharfmann R. Role for FGFR2IIIb-mediated signals in controlling pancreatic endocrine progenitor cell proliferation. Proc Natl Acad Sci USA 2002; 99:3884–3889.

52. Senaldi G, Shaklee CL, Simon B, Rowan CG, Lacey DL, Hartung T. Keratinocyte growth factor protects murine hepatocytes from tumor necrosis factor-induced apoptosis in vivo and in vitro. Hepatology 1998; 27:1584–1591.

53. Wildhaber BE, Yang H, Teitelbaum DH. Keratinocyte growth factor decreases total parenteral nutrition-induced apoptosis in mouse intestinal epithelium via Bcl-2. J Pediatr Surg 2003; 38:92–96.

54. Buckley S, Barsky L, Driscoll B, Weinberg K, Anderson KD, Warburton D. Apoptosis and DNA damage in type 2 alveolar epithelial cells cultured from hyperoxic rats. Am J Physiol 1998; 274:L714–L720.

55. Barrazone C, Donati YR, Rochat AF, Vesin C, Kan C-D, Pache JC, et al. Keratinocyte growth factor protects alveolar epithelium and endothelium from oxygen-induced injury in mice. Am J Path 1999; 154: 1479–1487.

56. Ray R, Cabal-Manzano R, Moser AR, Waldman T, Zipper LM, Aigner A, et al. Up-regulation of fibroblast growth factor-binding protein, by beta-catenin during colon carcinogenesis. Cancer Res 2003; 63:8085–8089.

57. Takeoka M, Ward WF, Polack H, Kamp DW, Panos RJ. KGF facilitates repair of radiation-induced DNA damage in alveolar epithelial cells. Am J Physiol 1997; 272:L1174–L1180.

58. Wu KI, Pollack N, Panos RJ, Sporn PH, Kamp DW. Keratinocyte growth factor promotes alveolar epithelial cell DNA repair after $H2O2$ exposure. Am J Physiol 1998; 275:L780–L787.

59. Frank S, Munz B, Werner S. The human homologue of a bovine non-selenium glutathione peroxidase is a novel keratinocyte growth factor-regulated gene. Oncogene 1997; 14:915–921.

60. Jonas CR, Farrell CL, Scully S, Eli A, Estivariz CF, Gu LH, et al. Enteral nutrition and keratinocyte growth factor regulate expression of glutathione-related enzyme messenger RNAs in rat intestine. JPEN J Parenter Enteral Nutr 2000; 24:67–75.

61. Farrell CL, Rex KI, Kaufman SA, DiPalma CR, Chen JN, et al. Effects of keratinocyte growth factor in the squamous epithelium of the upper aerodigestive tract of normal and irradiated mice. Int J Radiat Biol 1999; 75:609–620.

62. Farrell CL, Bready JV, Rex KL, Chen JN, DiPalma CR, Lane Whitcomb K, et al. Keratinocyte growth factor protects mice from chemotherapy and radiation-induced gastro-intestinal injury and mortality. Cancer Res 1998; 58:933–939.

63. Farrell CL, Rex KL, Chen JN, Bready JV, DiPalma CR, Kaufman SA, et al. The effects of keratinocyte growth factor in preclinical models of mucositis. Cell Prolif 2002; 35(Suppl 1):78–85.

64. Potten CS, Booth D, Cragg NJ, O'Shea JA, Tudor GL, Booth C. Cell kinetic studies in the murine ventral tongue epithelium: the effects of repeated exposure to keratinocyte growth factor. Cell Prolif 2002; 35(Suppl 1):22–31.

65. Dörr W, Noack R, Spekl K, Farrell CL. Modification of oral mucositis by keratinocyte growth factor: single radiation exposure. Int J Radiat Biol 2001; 77:342–347.

66. Dörr W, Spekl K, Farrell CL. The effect of keratinocyte growth factor on healing of manifest radiation ulcers in mouse tongue epithelium. Cell Prolif 2002; 35:86–92.

67. Dörr W, Spekl K, Farrell CL. Ameriolation of acute oral mucositis by keratinocyte growth factor: fractionated irradiation. Int J Radiat Oncol Biol Phys 2002; 54:245–251.

68. Khan WB, Shui C, Ning S, Knox SJ. Enhancement of murine intestinal stem cell survival after irradiation by keratinocyte growth factor. Radiat Res 1997; 148:248–253.

69. Zeesh JM, Procaccino F, Hoffman P, Aukerman SL, McRoberts JA, Soltani S, et al. Keratinocyte growth factor ameliorates mucosa injury in an experimental model of colitis in rats. Gastroenterology 1996; 110:1077–1083.

70. Egger B, Procaccino F, Sarosi I, Tolmos J, Buchler MW, Eysselein VE. Keratinocyte growth factor ameliorates dextran sodium sulfate colitis in mice. Dig Dis Sci 1999; 44:836–844.

71. Byrne FR, Farrell CL, Aranda R, Rex KL, Scully S, Brown HL, et al. rHuKGF ameliorates symptoms in DSS and CD4(+)CD45RB(Hi) T cell transfer mouse models of inflammatory bowel disease. Am J Physiol Gastrointest Liver Physiol 2002; 282:G690–G701.

72. Chen Y, Chou K, Fuchs E, Havran WL, Boismenu R. Protection of the intestinal mucosa by intraepithelial gamma delta T cells. Proc Natl Acad Sci USA 2002; 99:14,338–14,343.

73. Egger B, Tolmos J, Procaccino F, Sarosi I, Friess H, Büchler MW, et al. Keratinocyte growth factor promotes healing of left-sided colon anastomoses. Am J Surg 1998; 176:18–24.

74. Egger B, Inglin R, Zeeh J, Dirsch O, Huang Y, Buchler MW. Insulin-like growth factor I and truncated keratinocyte growth factor accelerate healing of left-sided colonic anastomoses. Br J Surg 2001; 88: 90–98.

75. Yang H, Wildhaber B, Tazuke Y, Teitelbaum DH. 2002 Harry M. Vars Research Award. Keratinocyte growth factor stimulates the recovery of epithelial structure and function in a mouse model of total parenteral nutrition. J Parenter Enteral Nutr 2002; 26:333–340.

76. Werner S. Keratinocyte growth factor: a unique player in epithelial repair processes. Cytokine Growth Factor Rev 1998; 9:153–165.

77. Taino-Coico L, Krueger JG, Rubin JS, D'Iimi S, Vallat VP, Valentino L, et al. Human keratinocyte growth factor effects in a porcine model of epidermal wound healing. J Exp Med 1993; 178:865–878.

78. Pierce GF, Yanagihara D, Klopchin K, Danilenko DM, Hsu E, Kenney WC, et al. Stimulation of all epithelial elements during skin regeneration by keratinocyte growth factor. J Exp Med 1994; 179(3): 831–840.

79. Danilenko DM, Ring BD, Tarpley JE, Morris B, Van GY, Morawiecki A, et al. Growth factor in porcine full and partial thickness burn repair. Differing targets and effects of keratinocyte growth factor, platelet-derived growth factor-BB, epidermal growth factor, and neu differentiation factor. Am J Pathol 1995; 147:1261–1277.

80. Wu L, Pierce GF, Galiano RD, Mustoe TA. Keratinocyte growth factor induces granulation in ischemic dermal wounds. Importance of epithelial–mesenchymal cell interactions. Arch Surg 1996; 131:660–666.

81. Danilenko DM, Ring BD, Yanagihara D, Benson W, Wiemann B, Starnes CO, et al. Keratinocyte growth factor is an important endogenous mediator of hair follicle growth, development, and differentiation. Am J Pathol 1995; 147:145–154.

82. Booth C, Potten CS. Keratinocyte growth factor increases hair follicle survival following cytotoxic insult. J Invest Dermatol 2000; 114:667–673.

83. Michelson PH, Tigue M, Panos RJ, Sporn PH. Keratinocyte growth factor stimulates bronchial epithelial cell proliferation in vitro and in vivo. Am J Physiol 1999; 277:L737–L742.

84. Sughara K, Rubin JS, Mason RJ, Aronsen EL, Shankon JM. Keratinocyte growth factor increases mRNAs for SP-A and SP-B in adult rat alveolar type II cells in culture. Am J Physiol 1995; 269:L344–L350.

85. Xu X, McCormick-Shannon, Voelker DR, Mason RJ. KGF increases SP-A and SP-D mRNA levels and secretion in cultured rat alveolar type II cells. Am J Respir Cell Mol Biol 1998; 18:168–178.

86. Yano T, Deterding RR, Simonet WS, Shannon JM, Mason RJ. Keratinocyte growth factor reduces lung damage due to acid installation in rats. Am J Respir Cell Mol Biol 1996; 15:433–442.

87. Yi ES, Williams ST, Lee H, Malicke DM, Chin EM, Yin S, et al. Keratinocyte growth factor ameliorates radiation- and bleomycin-induced lung injury and mortality. Am J Pathol 1996; 149:1963–1970.

88. Yi ES, Salgado M, Williams S, Kim SJ, Masliah E, Yin S, et al. Keratinocyte growth factor decreases pulmonary edema, transforming growth factor-beta and platelet-derived growth factor-BB expression, and alveolar type II cell loss in bleomycin-induced lung injury. Inflammation 1998; 22:315–325.

89. Panos RJ, Bak PM, Simonet WS, Rubin JS, Smith LJ. Intratracheal instillation of keratinocyte growth factor decreases hyperoxia-induced mortality in rats. J Clin Invest 1995; 96:2026–2033.

90. Guo J, Yi ES, Havill AM, Sarosi I, Whitcomb L, Yin S, et al. Intravenous keratinocyte growth factor protects against experimental pulmonary injury. Am J Physiol 1998; 275:L800–L805.

91. Danan C, Franco ML, Jarreau PH, Dassieu G, Chailley-Heu B, Bourbon J, et al. High concentrations of keratinocyte growth factor in airways of premature infants predicted absence of bronchopulmonary dysplasia. Am J Respir Crit Care Med 2002; 165:1384–1387.

92. Borok Z, Mihyu S, Fernandes VFJ, Zhang X-L, Kim KJ, Lubman RL. KGF prevents hyperoxia-induced reduction of active ion transport in alveolar epithelial cells. Am J Physiol 1999; 274:C1352–C1360.
93. Waters CM, Savla U, Panos RJ. KGF prevents hydrogen peroxide-induced increases in airway epithelial cell permeability. Am J Physiol 1997; 272:L681–L689.
94. Ulich TR, Whitcomb L, Tang W, Tressel PO, Tarpley J, Yi ES, et al. Keratinocyte growth factor ameliorates cyclophosphamide-induced ulcerative hemorrhagic cystitis. Cancer Res 1997; 57:472–475.
95. Yi ES, Shabaik AS, Lacey DL, Bedoya AA, Yin S, Housely RM, et al. Keratinocyte growth factor causes proliferation of urothelium in vivo. J Urol 1995; 154:1566–1570.
96. Panoskaltsis-Mortari A, Lacey DL, Vallera DA, Blazar BR. Keratinocyte growth factor administered before conditioning ameliorates graft-versus-host disease after allogeneic bone marrow transplantation in mice. Blood 1998; 92:3960–3967.
97. Panoskaltsis-Mortari A, Ingbar DH, Jung P, Haddad IY, Bitterman PB, Wangensteen OD, et al. KGF pre-treatment decreases B7 and granzyme B expression and hastens repair in lungs of mice after allogeneic BMT. Am J Physiol Lung Cell Mol Physiol 2000; 278:L988–L999.
98. Krijanovski OI, Hill GR, Cooke KR, Teshima T, Crawford JM, Brinson YS, et al. Keratinocyte growth factor separates graft-versus-leukemia effects from graft-versus-host disease. Blood 1999; 94:825–831.
99. Knerer B, Formanek M, Temmel A, Martinek H, Schickinger B, Kornfehl J. The role of fibroblasts from oropharyngeal mucosa in producing proinflammatory and mitogenic cytokines without prior stimulation. Eur Arch Otorhinolaryngol 1999; 256:266–270.
100. Siegfried S, Pekonen F, Nyman T, Ämmälä M, Rutanen E-M. Distinct patterns of keratinocyte growth factor and its receptor in endometrial carcinoma. Cancer 1997; 79:1166–1171.
101. Diez de Medina SG, Chopin D, El Marjou A, Delouvee A, LaRochelle WJ, et al. Decreased expression of keratinocyte growth factor receptor in a subset of human transitional cell bladder carcinomas. Oncogene 1997; 14:323–330.
102. Ricol D, Cappellen D, El Marjou A, Gil-Diez-de-Medina S, Girault JM, Yoshida T, et al. Tumour suppressive properties of fibroblast growth factor receptor 2-IIIb in human bladder cancer. Oncogene 1999; 18:7234–7243.
103. Yan G, Fukabori Y, McBride G, Nikolaropolous S, McKeehan WL. Exon switching and activation of stromal and embryonic fibroblast growth factor (FGF)-FGF receptor genes in prosta epithelial cells accom-pany stromal independence and malignancy. Mol Cell Biol 1993; 13:4513–4522.
104. Carstens Diaz de Medina SG, Chopin D, El Marjou A, Delouvee A, LaRochelle WJ, Hoznek A, et al. Decreased expression of keratinocyte growth factor receptor in a subset of human transitional cell bladder carcinomas. Oncogene 1997; 14:323–330.
105. Matsubara A, Kan M, Feng S, Mckeehan WL. Inhibition of growth of malignant rat prostate tumor cells by restoration of fibroblast growth factor receptor 2. Cancer Res. 1998; 58:1509-1514.
106. Zhang Y, Wang H, Toratani S, Sato JD, Kan M, McKeehan WL, et al. Growth inhibition by keratinocyte growth factor receptor of human salivary adenocarcinoma cells through induction of differentiation and apoptosis. Proc Natl Acad Sci USA 2001; 98:11,336–11,340.
107. Ning S, Shui C, Khan WB, Benson W, Lacey DL, Knox SJ. Effects of keratinocyte growth factor on the proliferation and radiation survival of human squamous cell carcinoma cell lines in vitro and in vivo. Int J Radiat Oncol Biol Phys 1998; 40:177–187.
108. Amgen data on file.
109. Spielberger R, Emmananouilides C, Stiff P, Bensinger W, Gentile T, Weisdorf D, et al. Use of recombinant human keratinocyte growth factor (rHuKGF) can reduce severe oral mucositis in patients (pts) with hematologic malignancies undergoing autologous peripheral blood progenitor cell transplantation (auto-PBPCT) after radiation-based conditioning—results of a phase 3 trial. American Society of Clinical Oncology Thirty-Ninth Annual Meeting. Meeting May 31–June 3 2003. Proc ASCO 2003; 22:3642.

# 32 Immune Modulation

## The B7 Family Cosignaling Molecules as Emerging Targets for Enhancing Cancer Therapy

*Sheng Yao, PhD and Lieping Chen, MD, PhD*

## Contents

## Summary

To breach host immune defense, cancer cells deploy elaborate tactics to reduce its immunogenicity and to induce immune tolerance. To counter these evasion mechanisms, manipulation of the T-cell cosignaling pathway has become an attractive approach. The B7 family costimulatory molecules deliver crucial signals through receptors on the T-cell surface for effective T-cell priming, differentiation, survival, and function. New B7 and B7-receptor family homologs that control distinct T-cell costimulatory and/or coinhibitory pathways continue to be discovered. Modulation of the B7 family molecules could enhance tumor immunogenicity and reverse tumor-induced tolerance, providing us promising immune-modulating arsenals against tumor.

**Key Words:** B7 family; costimulation; immune evasion; immunotherapy.

## 1. INTRODUCTION

Ample evidence indicates the presence of cellular and humoral immune response against tumor antigens in cancer patients *(1)*. These observations indicate that adoptive immune responses could be mounted against cancer cells, although these immune responses are often incapable of controlling cancer growth. What is still unclear is whether or not immune responses could be elicited against newly transformed cancer cells. It is widely believed that tumors often develop a unique microenvironment to suppress immune responses.

From: *Cancer Drug Discovery and Development: The Oncogenomics Handbook*
Edited by: W. J. LaRochelle and R. A. Shimkets © Humana Press Inc., Totowa, NJ

According to the "Cancer Immunoediting" theory *(2)*, the immune response eliminates the majority of neoplastic cells at early stages of tumorigenesis and creates a selection pressure for the development of poorly immunogenic tumors capable of evading immune attack. This chapter will first overview possible tumor evasion mechanisms. Subsequently, we will discuss tumor immunotherapy strategies through manipulating T-cell cosignaling pathways, focusing on the fast-expanding B7 family costimulatory molecules.

## 2. TUMOR EVASION OF IMMUNE SYSTEM

It is well accepted that the qualitative and quantitative nature of T-cell activation is determined by at least two signals upon engagement of T-cells and antigen-presenting cells (APCs) *(3)*. The primary signal is provided by the ligation of T-cell receptor with major histocompatibility complex (MHC) molecules loaded with antigenic peptides; the second signal is generated by the interactions of cosignaling receptors and ligands on T-cells and APCs, respectively. Without the primary signal, no immune response will be launched. In light of the coexistence of both positive (costimulator) and negative (coinhibitor) cosignaling molecules, the absence or imbalance of the second signal will lead to T-cell anergy or inappropriate T-cell activation *(4)*. The significance of the two-signal mechanism for T-cell activation also makes it a breach point for the tumor to overcome the host immunity. In persistent confrontation with host immune surveillance, tumor acquires and utilizes two major defense arsenals: One is to tone down its intrinsic immunogenicity and the second one is to induce apoptosis or unresponsiveness of tumor-specific effector cells.

### 2.1. Reduced Antigen Presentation by Tumor Cells

Because tumor-specific cytotoxic T lymphocytes (CTL) recognize tumor antigen associated with MHC class I molecules expressed on the tumor surface, any alteration in the tumor antigen processing and presentation will greatly affect CTL immunity. In fact, downregulation or complete loss of MHC I molecules have been demonstrated in a wide array of tumors, particularly prostate, colon, lung, and breast cancers *(5–12)*. Disruption or downregulation of antigen processing components, such as TAP (transporters associated with antigen processing) and LMP (components of the proteasome complex) genes have also been observed in several tumor types, including breast, prostate, and renal cancers *(13–15)*. Another tactic tumors exploit is downregulation or alteration of tumor antigens. Several independent research groups described the loss of melanoma-associated antigen either during treatment by adoptive transfer of ex vivo expanded antigen-specific CTL *(16)* or during immune therapy by tumor vaccinations *(12,17,18)*.

### 2.2. Deletion or Unresponsiveness of Antitumor Effector Cells

In addition to passive defense against the host immune system by minimizing its immunogenicity, the tumor also mounts active immune resistance by surface expression or secreting inhibitory/proapoptotic molecules against tumor-specific effector cells.

Secretion of immunosuppressive cytokine transforming growth factor (TGF)-β by numerous tumor types could limit local inflammatory responses and profoundly suppress APC functions, which, in turn, inhibit T-cell activation *(19,20)*.

Overexpression of indoleamine 2,3-dioxygenase (IDO) by a large number of human tumor types has been recently described as a new resistance mechanism *(21)*. T-Cell proliferation is heavily dependent on tryptophan metabolism, and IDO is an enzyme that catalyzes tryptophan degradation. In a mouse model, systematic administration of IDO inhibitors partially reversed the progression of an IDO-positive tumor, indicating a therapeutic value *(21)*.

The T regulatory cell (T-reg), vital for maintaining peripheral tolerance against auto-immunity, has been shown to play a negative role in antitumor immunity *(22)*. Recent evidence suggests that the tumor might utilize the host T-reg cell to suppress immune response. Wang and colleagues identified a tumor antigen-specific CD4+ CD25+ T-reg cell clone generated from human tumor-infiltrating lymphocytes (TILs) and demonstrated that the T-reg clone could strongly suppress T-cell response *(23)*. Depletion of CD25+ T-reg cells with antibodies abrogated the unresponsiveness of CTL to syngeneic tumors in vivo and in vitro and led to regression of various tumors in animal models *(24–27)*. These studies support the T-reg cell as an emerging target for cancer immunotherapy.

### 2.3. Aberrant Expression of T-Cell Cosignaling Molecules

Given the importance of cosignaling for T-cell activation, it is conceivable that the poor immunogenicity of many tumors could be caused by the lack of positive costimulatory ligands. Indeed, most human solid tumors do not express appropriate costimulatory molecules such as B7s *(28)*; thus, they are unable to directly prime a T-cell. Therefore, presentation of tumor antigens will employ a relatively inefficient cross-priming mechanism. In animal models, vaccinations of modified tumors that ectopically expressed various co-stimulators had been shown to promote tumor regression and even generate long-lasting immunity against the challenge of parental tumor cells *(29)*. An immunotherapy targeting costimulatory pathway will be discussed in detail later in this chapter.

The recent studies on coinhibitors have shed light on another novel tumor evasion mechanism. B7-H1, a B7 family member *(30)*, has been demonstrated to have an unusually high expression on the cell membrane and cytoplasm in a majority of freshly isolated human carcinomas of the lung, ovary, colon, breast, and head and neck and melanomas *(31,32)*. Expression of B7-H1 stimulated apoptosis of tumor antigen-specific T-cells and promoted tumor growth. Inclusion of B7-H1 monoclonal antibody (mAb) could partially neutralize the apoptotic effect in vitro. From the perspective of cancer immunotherapy, these findings suggest that in addition to magnifying immune-activating signals through costimulators, it is equally important to block coinhibitors presented by tumors from reaching activated T-cells.

## 3. THE B7-CD28: RAPIDLY EXPANDING FAMILY OF PROMISING IMMUNOTHERAPY TARGETS

The first pair of costimulatory ligand-receptor B7-CD28 was described by Linsley and his colleagues in 1990 *(33,34)*. In the last 5 yr, the costimulation field has witnessed a spurt of expansion *(35)*. The concept of costimulation has also evolved over the years, from simply promoting T-cell activation, to a complex coordinated regulation of priming, differentiation, survival, and effector function of T-cells through interaction of a network of ligands and receptors *(4)*. The dynamic interaction of both positive and negative cosignals ultimately determines the outcome of a T-cell response.

### 3.1. Immunoglobulin Superfamily

The majority of cosignaling molecules fall into two main groups: the immunoglobulin (Ig) superfamily (mainly the B7-CD28 family) and the tumor necrosis factor family of

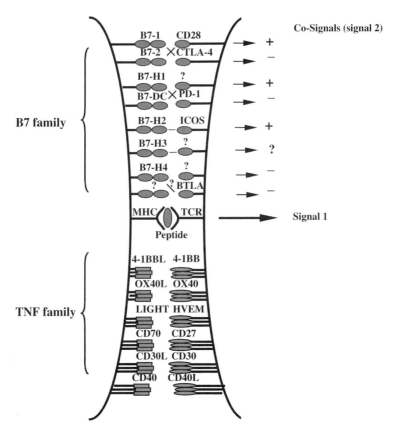

**Fig. 1.** The B7 and TNF families of cosignaling receptors/ligands.

ligands and receptors (TNF-TNFR) (Fig. 1). Chapter 34 in this book covers the application of TNF ligands and receptors in cancer therapy. Here, we will focus on the B7-CD28 family.

The B7 receptor family molecules universally contain a single Ig variable regionlike (IgV) motif in their extracellular domains, including CD28, cytotoxic T-lymphocyte antigen-4 (CTLA-4), inducible costimulator (ICOS), program death 1 (PD-1), and B- and T-lymphocyte attenuator (BTLA) *(36)*. Their known ligands all belong to the B7 family, with a structural feature of two Ig-like extracellular domains, Ig variable regionlike (IgV) and Ig constant regionlike (IgC) domains (Fig. 1).

### 3.2. The Classical B7-1, B7-2, and CD28 CTLA-4 Pathways

Constitutively expressed on naïve peripheral T-cell, CD28 plays an essential role for effective T-cell activation. It delivers a primary costimulatory signal upon the engagement of its ligands B7-1 (CD80) or B7-2 (CD86) expressed on APCs *(37)*. CD28 signaling promotes antigen-specific T-cell proliferation, produces of an array of cytokines, and leads to the differentiation of effector T-cells *(37–40)*. To the contrary, ligation of the homologous CTLA-4 receptor on activated T-cells with the same B7-1 or B7-2 ligands will attenuate T-cell response *(41–43)*. Unlike CD28, surface expression of CTLA-4 is only induced on activated T-cells. CTLA-4 also has a much higher binding affinity with B7 ligands than CD28 *(44)* and, thus, could effectively compete for ligand binding. The critical negative regulatory role of CTLA-4 for T-cell activation was best demonstrated in CTLA-4-deficient mice, which had massive enlargement of lymphoid organs resulting from uncontrolled T-cell proliferation, and fatal multiorgan destruction caused by lymphocyte infiltration *(45,46)*.

More than a decade ago, introduction of the costimulatory molecule B7-1 into tumor cells was shown to enhance antitumor immunity *(47)*. An immunogenic melanoma (K1735) expressing E7 viral gene product could grow progressively in immunocompetent murine hosts. Transfection of E7+ K1735 with B7-1 resulted in tumor regression by a B7-1-dependent response mediated by CD8+ T-cells. The induced host antitumor response also led to the regression of a parental B7-1-negative tumor at distal site, indicating a therapeutic potential for even metastatic tumors. Mechanistic studies demonstrated that enhanced priming of tumor-specific CTLs, through both direct priming (antigen presented by tumor) *(47)* and cross-priming (antigen presented by tumor site APCs) *(48)*, played major roles in B7+ tumor-induced immunity. Subsequent studies, however, revealed that the effectiveness of T-cell immunity enhanced by B7-1 transfection correlates directly to tumor immunogenicity. Poorly immunogenic tumors, such as sarcomas MCA101 and melanoma B16, remained progressive despite expression of the B7-1 *(49)*.

To treat less immunogenic tumors and achieve a better response against large established tumors, several independent groups have reported synergistic antitumor effects with combined strategies of B7 overexpression with either systemic treatment or overexpression of immune response stimulatory cytokines, including interferon (IFN)-γ *(50)*, interleukin (IL)-2 *(51,52)*, IL-7 *(53)*, IL-10 *(54)*, IL-12 *(55)*, IL-15 *(56)*, and granulocyte-macrophage colony-stimulating factor (GM-CSF) *(57)*. In all of these models, the combined strategies led to effective tumor rejection and establishment of immunity against the parental unmodified tumor. An even greater antitumor effect was observed when both MHC class II and B7-1 were cotransfected into mouse sarcoma I tumor, indicating that the induction of both CD4+ and CD8+ tumor-specific T-cell response will boost the antitumor effects *(58)*.

In addition to enhancement of positive signals, suppression of coinhibitory pathways has also been explored and successfully implemented to induce strong T-cell-mediated antitumor response in animal models. The ability of CTLA-4 to prevent continuous T-cell activation makes it an ideal target. First shown by Leach and colleagues in 1995, then further investigated by other groups, systemic administration of CTLA-4 blocking antibody could enhance the potency of tumor vaccine and generate a stronger antitumor immunity *(59–62)*. Another potential mechanism behind the CTLA-4 mAb antitumor effect is that CD4+ CD25+ T-reg cells constitutively express a high level of cell surface CTLA-4, which is essential for T-reg cell function in some models *(63,64)*. Application of CTLA-4 mAb will directly inhibit T-reg cell or cause T-reg cell depletion in vivo. Similar to the combined strategy with B7 transfection, systematic administration of GM-CSF also has a synergistic effect when applied with CTLA-4 blockade *(60,65)*. This reveals a promising approach that is undergoing clinical trials: enhancement of host APC function together with modulation of costimulatory pathway to maximize antitumor immunity. Soluble antibodies hold practical advantages clinically because they bypass the requirement of complicated in vitro tumor manipulation. In theory, agonistic CD28 antibody should also have antitumor effects because it could significantly costimulate T-cell proliferation and cytokine production in vitro. Ironically, there is no in vivo antitumor activity reported for CD28 mAb to date. One possible explanation is that CD28 antibody could not fully mimic the binding of B7 ligands, which might depend on cell–cell contact and coordination of other costimulatory molecules.

Two recent reports showed that significant autoimmune responses could be induced by infusion of anti-CTLA-4 mAb in cancer patients with metastatic melanoma (66,67), although autoreactivity was relatively mild in mouse tumor models (60). Six out of fourteen patients manifested severe autoimmune responses, which were mediated by massive infiltration of lymphoid cells into various organs with the symptoms of dermatitis, colitis, and hepatitis. The antitumor effect of the anti-CTLA-4 mAb was moderate: Out of fourteen total patients, two experienced complete tumor regression and one had partial response (67). These studies thus highlighted the critical role of CTLA-4 in the control of autoimmune responses and demand further studies on mechanistic aspects of CTLA-4-mediated suppression before further extensive clinical trials.

### 3.3. The B7-H1 (PD-L1), B7-DC (PD-L2), and PD-1 Pathway

Database searching for molecules with similar extracellular domain organization and overall homology with B7-1 and B7-2 has revealed a novel group of B7 family ligands with immune modulation activities (Table 1). For a more comprehensive review, refer to ref. 68.

Human B7-H1 (B7 Homologue-1), the third member of B7 family, was identified in 1999 (30). Its extracellular domain shares 22% amino acid sequence identity with both B7-1 and B7-2. The hB7-H1 messenger RNA has a broad tissue distribution, including the heart, skeletal muscle, placenta, lung, thymus, spleen, kidney, and liver (30). In contrast, hB7-H1 protein was undetectable in most normal tissues, except on limited macrophage-like cells, such as Kupffer cells in liver and macrophages in the lung. Surface expression of hB7-H1 could be induced in response to immune stimulatory IFN-γ on skeleton muscle and endothelial cells, indicating the existence of a post-transcriptional regulatory mechanism of B7-H1 in peripheral tissues (69,70). Freshly isolated T- and B-cells from peripheral blood mononuclear cell (PBMC) have a negligible amount of surface B7-H1, whereas 16% of CD14+ macrophage cells are B7-H1-positive. Upon activation, B7-H1 was upregulated on T-cells and macrophages, but to a lesser extent on B-cells (30,71). Human monocyte-derived dendritic cells constitutively express high levels of B7-H1, which could be further induced by lipopolysaccharide (LPS) or IFN-γ treatment (30).

Mouse B7-H1 shares 69% overall identity with its human counterpart. Likewise, mB7-H1 mRNA has wide tissue distribution with no cell surface expression (72). Mouse B7-H1 protein was detected on activated T-lymphocytes and antigen-presenting cells (B-cell, macrophage, and dendritic cell [DC]) (72,73). In general, constitutive surface expression of B7-H1 is limited to a small fraction of hematopoietic cells, but it is highly inducible in various tissues and cells.

The immunological function(s) of B7-H1 is controversial, as both positive and negative roles have been implicated. Using an immobilized suboptimal amount of anti-CD3 on plastic plates as antigen mimicry, both human and mouse B7-H1Ig fusion proteins promoted proliferation of resting T-cells and preferentially enhanced T-cell IL-10 production (30,72). In a different setting using beads as the immobilization matrix, inclusion of B7-H1Ig with an optimal amount of anti-CD3 inhibited T-cell proliferation and cytokine production (71). This discrepancy is still not fully understood, but several lines of evidence suggest the presence of at least two B7-H1 receptors on T-cells with opposing effects

Table 1
Protein Sequence[a] Identities (%) Among Human and Mouse B7 Family Members

| Human | B7-1 | B7-2 | B7-H1 | B7-DC | B7-H2 | B7-H3 | B7-H4 |
|---|---|---|---|---|---|---|---|
| B7-1 | 100 | 25 | 22 | 23 | 23 | 25 | 22 |
| B7-2 | | 100 | 22 | 20 | 22 | 23 | 23 |
| B7-H1 | | | 100 | 39 | 21 | 29 | 23 |
| B7-DC | | | | 100 | 20 | 24 | 25 |
| B7-H2 | | | | | 100 | 29 | 21 |
| B7-H3 | | | | | | 100 | 27 |
| B7-H4 | | | | | | | 100 |

| Mouse | B7-1 | B7-2 | B7-H1 | B7-DC | B7-H2 | B7-H3 | B7-H4 |
|---|---|---|---|---|---|---|---|
| B7-1 | 100 | 27 | 22 | 22 | 22 | 26 | 24 |
| B7-2 | | 100 | 23 | 20 | 24 | 26 | 26 |
| B7-H1 | | | 100 | 35 | 22 | 28 | 28 |
| B7-DC | | | | 100 | 19 | 26 | 20 |
| B7-H2 | | | | | 100 | 28 | 21 |
| B7-H3 | | | | | | 100 | 30 |
| B7-H4 | | | | | | | 100 |

| Mouse/Human | hB7-1 | hB7-2 | hB7-H1 | hB7-DC | hB7-H2 | hB7-H3 | hB7-H4 |
|---|---|---|---|---|---|---|---|
| mB7-1 | **50**[b] | 27 | 24 | 23 | 23 | 27 | 24 |
| mB7-2 | 21 | **56** | 21 | 19 | 21 | 24 | 25 |
| mB7-H1 | 24 | 20 | **73** | 40 | 21 | 28 | 26 |
| mB7-DC | 22 | 19 | 36 | **71** | 20 | 24 | 22 |
| mB7-H2 | 25 | 25 | 21 | 17 | **49** | 29 | 21 |
| mB7-H3 | 27 | 22 | 30 | 25 | 28 | **92** | 28 |
| mB7-H4 | 24 | 23 | 24 | 22 | 23 | 31 | **89** |

[a]Extracellular domain only, without signal peptide, transmembrane, and intracellular regions.
[b]Boldface indicates sequence identities shared by mouse and human B7 family member orthologs, such as mB7-1 and hB7-1.

*(31,74)*. An emerging model casts B7-H1 in spatially and functionally divergent roles in vivo. During T-cell priming on lymphoid organs, B7-H1 expressed on APCs costimulates naïve T-cells, whereas on peripheral tissues, B7-H1 is upregulated by proinflammatory cytokines to suppress activated or memory T-cells to maintain self-tolerance *(69,70,75,76)*.

The function of B7-H1 to sustain peripheral tolerance is employed by various tumors to evade host immune attack *(31)*. Immunohistochemistry studies demonstrated that B7-H1 was expressed on several tumor cell lines and various types of freshly isolated human cancer tissue *(31,32)*. The B7-H1-transfected human melanoma cell line 624mel increased apoptosis of the antigen-specific CTL clone M15 in vitro. The addition of B7-H1 mAb can partially inhibit the apoptotic effect *(31)*. In the mouse P815 tumor model, inoculation of B7-1-transfected P815 in syngeneic mice could cause complete tumor regression and generate immunity against rechallenge of unmodified P815. Expression of B7-H1 in B7-1+ P815, however, led to progressive tumor growth, indicating that B7-H1 could oppose the curative effect of B7-1 *(31)*. Injection of mB7-H1 blocking mAb had no effect on the P815 or B7-1+ P815 tumor, but induced a regression of the B7-H1+ B7-1+ P815 tumor and further confirmed that the protective effect for tumor was provided through surface B7-H1 *(77)*. These findings had a profound impact on the design of T-cell-based immunotherapy. Conceivably, when adoptive transferred preactivated T-cells encounter a B7-H1-positive tumor in vivo, the majority of tumor-specific CTLs would be deleted at the tumor site. A combination of B7-H1 mAb treatment with either cancer vaccine or T-cell adoptive transfer would be essential to protect CTL and enhance the killing of tumor cells.

B7-DC, a new B7 family member discovered in 2001 *(78,79)*, shares a high sequence identity with B7-H1 in their extracellular domains (39% in human, 35% in mouse). Surface expression of B7-DC is restricted to dendritic cells and activated macrophages *(73, 78)*. Similar to B7-H1, both costimulatory *(78)* and inhibitory *(79)* functions of B7-DC were also reported. In contrast, B7-DC had an overall costimulatory role in antitumor immunity. Ectopic expression of B7-DC on the J558 mouse tumor cells promoted CD8$^+$ T-cell-mediated tumor rejection *(80)*. Interestingly, crosslinking of B7-DC by a human IgM antibody augmented the immune function of DC to induce potent T-cell response *(81,82)*. Therefore, the B7-DC crosslinking antibody could be utilized in tumor immunotherapy.

PD-1, an inducible molecule on activated T- and B-cells *(83)*, is a receptor for both B7-H1 and B7-DC *(71,78)*. The cytoplasmic domain of PD-1 contains an immunoreceptor tyrosine-based inhibitory motif (ITIM) and an immunoreceptor tyrosine-based switch motif (ITSM) *(84)*. The ITIM domain has been implicated in transmitting negative signals to suppress T- and B-cell responses by recruiting SHP family phosphatases *(85)*. Cumulative evidence indicates that PD-1 is important for the maintenance of peripheral tolerance. PD-1-deficient mice in BALB/c background had dilated cardiomyopathy, congestive heart failure, and frequent sudden death *(86)*. The cardiomyopathy was caused by the generation of high-titer autoantibodies against a heart-specific protein cardiac troponin I *(87)*. In C57BL/6 background, PD-1-deficient mice had enlarged lymphoid organs and spontaneously developed lupuslike arthritis and glomerulonephritis with predominant IgG3 deposition at advanced age (14 mo) *(88)*. The negative role of PD-1 in immune response was further supported in various animal models. PD-1 pathway blockade by systematic administration of mPD-1-blocking mAb accelerated experimental autoimmune encephalitis (EAE) *(89)*, autoimmune diabetes *(90)*, hapten-induced allergic inflammatory response *(91)*, and graft-vs-host disease (GVHD) *(92)*. Furthermore, in the mouse P815 tumor model, injection of mPD-1-blocking mAb instead of mB7-H1 mAb could also lead to partial regression of B7-H1$^+$ B7-1$^+$ tumor, indicating the resistance mechanism for B7-H1$^+$ B7-1$^+$ tumor was at least partly provided through the B7-H1-PD-1 pathway. The current hypothesis is that after ligation with tumor surface B7-H1, T-cell PD-1 delivered a negative or proapoptotic signal to inhibit activated T-cell response *(77)*.

A large amount of evidence indicated PD-1 as a coinhibitory receptor and the negative functions of B7-H1 and B7-DC appeared to be mediated through PD-1. Meanwhile, several lines of evidence strongly supported the presence of a secondary costimulatory receptor for B7-H1 and B7-DC. First, the B7-DC and B7-H1 fusion protein could costimulate the proliferation and cytokine production of T-cells purified from PD-1-deficient mice *(74)*. Second, B7-DC$^+$ tumor-vaccine-induced immunity was mediated through a PD-1-independent mechanism *(80)*. Third, B7-H1 blockade suppressed the development of T-cell-mediated inflammatory bowel disease *(93)*. Finally, B7-H1 tissue-specific transgenic expression on islet β-cells increased the incidence of insulitis and diabetes in mouse models *(94)*. Cloning the potential secondary receptor is an important goal in future experiments that will yield important insights into the complicated costimulatory and coinhibitory functions of B7-H1.

In summary, the B7-H1/B7-DC and PD-1/unknown receptor pathway closely resembles the classical B7-1/B7-2 and CD28/CTLA-4 pathway, both of which bidirectionally regulate immune response and could be exploited to enhance the antitumor immunity. Blocking mAbs against B7-H1 and PD-1 are especially promising immunotherapy bioreagents.

### 3.4. The ICOSL (B7-H2) and ICOS Pathway

The inducible costimulator (ICOS) was identified by expression cloning using mAb-recognizing activated T-cell surface antigens (95). In human, ICOS, CD28 and CTLA-4 are closely clustered within a 300-kb region on chromosome 2q33, suggesting that they were originated by gene duplications (95). Absent on resting T-cells, both human and mouse ICOS were quickly induced upon T-cell activation (95,96). The crucial role of ICOS in regulating activated T-cells was demonstrated by defective T-cell activation and cytokine production in ICOS-deficient mice (97). Interestingly, ICOS-deficient mice also had defects in immunoglobulin isotype class switching with impaired germinal center formation (98), suggesting an involvement in T-cell-dependent B-cell response.

The ICOS ligand (ICOSL), also known as B7-H2, B7RP-1, B7h, or GL50, was identified by several independent groups (96,99–101). The ICOSL expression is mainly restricted to APCs and could be further induced by IFN-γ and TNF-α (101). Immobilized with a suboptimal amount of CD3 mAbs, the mouse ICOSL–Ig fusion protein promoted T-cell proliferation, whereas with optimal CD3 mAbs, ICOSL-Ig preferentially stimulated IL-10 production (99).

Similar to the classical B7, ectopic expression of ICOSL on multiple tumor types could induce tumor rejection mediated by CD8+ T-cells (102,103). ICOSL costimulated clonal expansion of tumor-specific CTL and facilitated tumor destruction in vivo (103). It is worth noting that systematic administration of the ICOSL fusion protein caused complete or partial regression of immunogenic Meth A, SA-1, and EMT6 tumors in syngeneic mice, but it was less effective on poorly immunogenic tumor, such as P815 and EL4 (104). When combined with pretreatment with an antineoplastic agent cyclophosphamide, soluble ICOSL-Ig had a synergistic effect against EL-4 tumor (104).

### 3.5. The B7-H3 Pathway

B7-H3, discovered in 2001 as a B7 homolog, remains an orphan B7 family ligand without known receptor (105). Human B7-H3 extracellular domain shares 25% identity with B7-1, 23% with B7-2, and 29% with both B7-H1 and B7-H2. Although B7-H3 mRNA was found in various normal tissues of human and mouse (105), characterization of B7-H3 protein expression remains elusive. It was weakly detected on activated dendritic cells treated by IFN-γ or a combination of phorbol myristate acetate (PMA) and ionomycin (105). In addition to a typical two domain (IgV-IgC) molecule, a long transcript of B7-H3 encoding an unusual IgV-IgC-IgV-IgC (4Ig-B7-H3) extracellular domain was detected in human and monkey but not in mouse and hamster (106,107). A recent report further confirmed the presence of 4Ig-B7-H3 protein product in human monocyte-derived DC (108). No mouse transcript corresponding to the human 4Ig-B7-H3 is yet found in either reverse transcription–polymerase chain reaction (RT-PCR) experiment or current NCBI database. The biological significance of these 4Ig-B7-H3 isoforms remains to be investigated.

The expression of human B7-H3 receptor was detected on PHA-activated T-cells while none of the known B7 receptor family member interacts with B7-H3. The receptor for B7-H3 still waits to be discovered.

The in vivo function of B7-H3 is currently under debate. In the presence of CD3 mAb, immobilized or surface expressed B7-H3 was found to be either costimulatory *(105,109)* or inhibitory *(110)* or no effect *(108)* for T-cell proliferation and cytokine production in vitro. B7-H3-deficient mice developed more severe Th1-mediated hypersensitivity in an airway inflammation model *(110)*, supporting an inhibitory role of B7-H3 in vivo. In contrast, expression of B7-H3 showed costimulatory antitumor activity in mouse tumor models. Intratumoral injection of mouse B7-H3 expression plasmid into EL-4 led to complete regression of 50% tumors mediated by CD8+ T-cells and natural killer (NK) cells *(111)*. Expression of B7-H3 in P815 tumor costimulated expansion of antigen-specific CD8+ CTL clone and led to enhanced recognition and destruction of tumor cell by CTL in vivo *(109)*. Therefore, B7-H3 is a potential candidate for cancer therapy.

### 3.6. The B7-H4 and BTLA Pathway(s)

B7-H4 (B7S1, B7x) is the most recent addition to the B7 family *(112–114)*. Human B7-H4 shares 22% and 23% sequence identities with B7-1 and B7-2, respectively. As a common scene for B7 family members, mRNA of B7-H4 also show a wide tissue distribution, whereas surface B7-H4 protein is undetectable in normal tissues *(113)*. Absent from freshly isolated human hematopoietic cells, B7-H4 surface expression can be induced after in vitro activation on T-cell, B-cell, monocyte, and DC *(113)*. Putative receptor for B7-H4 is detected on activated T-cells *(112,113)*.

Three groups reported the negative function of B7-H4 on T-cell immunity *(112–114)*. Coimmobilized with CD3 mAb, B7-H4Ig inhibited T-cell proliferation and cytokine production by inducing cell cycle arrest at the G0/G1-phase *(113)*. In a parent-to-F1 GVHD model, blockade of B7-H4 by mAb promoted alloreactive CTL activity *(113)*. In addition, B7-H4-blocking mAb aggravated the disease progression in the EAE model *(112)*, further supporting the inhibitory role of B7-H4 in vivo. Interestingly, immunohistochemistry analysis demonstrated that B7-H4 was expressed on a high percentage of freshly isolated ovarian and lung carcinomas *(115)*. The correlation between B7-H4 expression and the progression of ovarian and lung cancers is yet to be established. However, a possible role for B7-H4 in tumor escape could be envisioned based on the suppressive function of B7-H4 in T-cell immunity.

BTLA (B- and T-lymphocyte attenuator) is a recently identified Ig superfamily molecule with similar domain organization but limited sequence homology to CTLA-4 (14%) and PD-1 (13%) *(36)*. BTLA mRNA expression was detected in T- and B-cells. Cytoplasmic region of BTLA contains two immunosuppressive ITIM domains. Crosslinking BTLA with TCR led to tyrosine phosphorylation within ITIM and subsequent recruitment of SHP-1 and SHP-2. Furthermore, BTLA-deficient mice showed increased T-cell activation and enhanced disease susceptibility in the EAE model *(36)*, indicating a negative role of BTLA upon T-cell activation.

BTLA had been suggested to be a receptor for B7-H4, based on the fact that the B7-H4 fusion protein could bind wild-type but not BTLA-deficient T-cells *(36,114)*. However, no direct interaction between B7-H4 and BTLA has been detected in vitro. It is possible that the real receptor for B7-H4 is downregulated in BTLA-deficient mice. It remains to be verified whether B7-H4 and BTLA are involved in the same pathway. Nevertheless, because of their strong inhibitory functions in T-cell response, BTLA and B7-H4 are interesting new targets to be suppressed in cancer immunotherapy.

## 4. PERSPECTIVES

Studies on both costimulatory and coinhibitory molecules in recent years have provided us with a better understanding of the interactions between tumor and host immune system and thus afforded us novel windows of opportunities to battle cancer. Multiple human clinical trials have been carried out to treat cancer by modulating cosignaling pathways.

Nonreplicating canarypoxvirus (ALVAC) vector expressing both human carcinoembryonic antigen (CEA) and the B7-1 costimulatory molecule was used as cancer vaccine to treat patients with advanced CEA-positive adenocarcinomas in two phase I trials *(116, 117)*. Cancer progressions in three out of six patients were stabilized with increased CEA-specific precursor T-cells in vivo. As discussed earlier, in two other recent phase I trials, combination of CTLA-blocking mAb with GM-CSF treatment or tumor antigen vaccines were tested. Administration of CTLA-4 antibody (MDX-CTLA4) induced moderate antitumor response and led to tumor stabilization in several metastatic melanoma and ovarian carcinoma patients while unfavorably inducing significant autoimmunity *(66,67)*. More complicated combined strategies such as using tumor vaccine transfected with recombinant viral vector expressing multiple costimulatory molecules, given along with immune stimulatory cytokines, are currently under clinical trial.

Future successful cancer treatment would likely be dependent on multidisciplinary strategies with logical design and modulation of various cosignaling pathways, including both ectopic expression of costimulatory molecules on tumor cells and blockade of coinhibitory molecules. A combination of chemotherapy, radiation therapy or surgery with immunotherapy would have a promising therapeutic value.

## ACKNOWLEDGMENTS

We thank Kathy Jensen for editing the manuscript. This work has been supported by the National Institutes of Health grants CA79915, CA85721, CA97085, CA98731, and AI55028, the American Cancer Society, the United States Army, the National Natural Science Foundation in China, and the Mayo Foundation.

## REFERENCES

1. Pardoll D. Does the immune system see tumors as foreign or self? Annu Rev Immunol 2003; 21: 807–839.
2. Dunn GP, Bruce AT, Ikeda H, Old LJ, Schreiber RD. Cancer immunoediting: from immunosurveillance to tumor escape. Nat Immunol 2002; 3:991–998.
3. Mueller DL, Jenkins MK, Schwartz RH. Clonal expansion versus functional clonal inactivation: a costimulatory signalling pathway determines the outcome of T cell antigen receptor occupancy. Annu Rev Immunol 1989; 7:445–480.
4. Chen L. Co-inhibitory molecules of the B7-CD28 family in the control of T cell immunity. Nat Rev Immunol 2004; 4:336–347.
5. Doyle A, Martin WJ, Funa K, et al. Markedly decreased expression of class I histocompatibility antigens, protein, and mRNA in human small-cell lung cancer. J Exp Med 1985; 161:1135–1151.
6. Esteban F, Concha A, Delgado M, Perez-Ayala M, Ruiz-Cabello F, Garrido F. Lack of MHC class I antigens and tumour aggressiveness of the squamous cell carcinoma of the larynx. Br J Cancer 1990; 62:1047–1051.

7. Ferrone S, Marincola FM. Loss of HLA class I antigens by melanoma cells: molecular mechanisms, functional significance and clinical relevance. Immunol Today 1995; 16:487–494.

8. Lopez-Nevot MA, Esteban F, Ferron A, et al. HLA class I gene expression on human primary tumours and autologous metastases: demonstration of selective losses of HLA antigens on colorectal, gastric and laryngeal carcinomas. Br J Cancer 1989; 59:221–226.

9. Ruiz-Cabello F, Perez-Ayala M, Gomez O, et al. Molecular analysis of MHC-class-I alterations in human tumor cell lines. Int J Cancer 1991; 6(Suppl):123–130.

10. van den Ingh HF, Ruiter DJ, Griffioen G, van Muijen GN, Ferrone S. HLA antigens in colorectal tumours —low expression of HLA class I antigens in mucinous colorectal carcinomas. Br J Cancer 1987; 55: 125–130.

11. Whitwell HL, Hughes HP, Moore M, Ahmed A. Expression of major histocompatibility antigens and leucocyte infiltration in benign and malignant human breast disease. Br J Cancer 1984; 49:161–172.

12. Jager E, Ringhoffer M, Altmannsberger M, et al. Immunoselection in vivo: independent loss of MHC class I and melanocyte differentiation antigen expression in metastatic melanoma. Int J Cancer 1997; 71:142–147.

13. Alpan RS, Zhang M, Pardee AB. Cell cycle-dependent expression of TAP1, TAP2, and HLA-B27 messenger RNAs in a human breast cancer cell line. Cancer Res 1996; 56:4358–4361.

14. Sanda MG, Restifo NP, Walsh JC, et al. Molecular characterization of defective antigen processing in human prostate cancer. J Natl Cancer Inst 1995; 87:280–285.

15. Seliger B, Hohne A, Knuth A, et al. Reduced membrane major histocompatibility complex class I density and stability in a subset of human renal cell carcinomas with low TAP and LMP expression. Clin Cancer Res 1996; 2:1427–1433.

16. Yee C, Thompson JA, Byrd D, et al. Adoptive T cell therapy using antigen-specific CD8+ T cell clones for the treatment of patients with metastatic melanoma: in vivo persistence, migration, and antitumor effect of transferred T cells. Proc Natl Acad Sci USA 2002; 99:16,168–16,173.

17. Jager E, Ringhoffer M, Karbach J, Arand M, Oesch F, Knuth A. Inverse relationship of melanocyte differentiation antigen expression in melanoma tissues and CD8+ cytotoxic-T-cell responses: evidence for immunoselection of antigen-loss variants in vivo. Int J Cancer 1996; 66:470–476.

18. Ohnmacht GA, Wang E, Mocellin S, et al. Short-term kinetics of tumor antigen expression in response to vaccination. J Immunol 2001; 167:1809–1820.

19. Wojtowicz-Praga S, Verma UN, Wakefield L, et al. Modulation of B16 melanoma growth and metastasis by anti-transforming growth factor beta antibody and interleukin-2. J Immunother Emphasis Tumor Immunol 1996; 19:169–175.

20. Moretti S, Pinzi C, Berti E, et al. In situ expression of transforming growth factor beta is associated with melanoma progression and correlates with Ki67, HLA-DR and beta 3 integrin expression. Melanoma Res 1997; 7:313–321.

21. Uyttenhove C, Pilotte L, Theate I, et al. Evidence for a tumoral immune resistance mechanism based on tryptophan degradation by indoleamine 2,3-dioxygenase. Nat Med 2003; 9:1269–1274.

22. Wei WZ, Morris GP, Kong YC. Anti-tumor immunity and autoimmunity: a balancing act of regulatory T cells. Cancer Immunol Immunother 2004; 53:73–78.

23. Wang HY, Lee DA, Peng G, et al. Tumor-specific human CD4+ regulatory T cells and their ligands: implications for immunotherapy. Immunity 2004; 20:107–118.

24. Shimizu J, Yamazaki S, Sakaguchi S. Induction of tumor immunity by removing CD25+CD4+ T cells: a common basis between tumor immunity and autoimmunity. J Immunol 1999; 163:5211–5218.

25. Jones E, Dahm-Vicker M, Simon AK, et al. Depletion of CD25+ regulatory cells results in suppression of melanoma growth and induction of autoreactivity in mice. Cancer Immun 2002; 2:1.

26. Golgher D, Jones E, Powrie F, Elliott T, Gallimore A. Depletion of CD25+ regulatory cells uncovers immune responses to shared murine tumor rejection antigens. Eur J Immunol 2002; 32:3267–3275.

27. Tanaka H, Tanaka J, Kjaergaard J, Shu S. Depletion of CD4+ CD25+ regulatory cells augments the generation of specific immune T cells in tumor-draining lymph nodes. J Immunother 2002; 25:207–217.

28. Denfeld RW, Dietrich A, Wuttig C, et al. In situ expression of B7 and CD28 receptor families in human malignant melanoma: relevance for T-cell-mediated anti-tumor immunity. Int J Cancer 1995; 62:259–265.

29. Vesosky B, Hurwitz AA. Modulation of costimulation to enhance tumor immunity. Cancer Immunol Immunother 2003; 52:663–669.

30. Dong H, Zhu G, Tamada K, Chen L. B7-H1, a third member of the B7 family, co-stimulates T-cell proliferation and interleukin-10 secretion. Nat Med 1999; 5:1365–1369.

31. Dong H, Strome SE, Salomao DR, et al. Tumor-associated B7-H1 promotes T-cell apoptosis: a potential mechanism of immune evasion. Nat Med 2002; 8:793–800.

32. Iwai Y, Ishida M, Tanaka Y, Okazaki T, Honjo T, Minato N. Involvement of PD-L1 on tumor cells in the escape from host immune system and tumor immunotherapy by PD-L1 blockade. Proc Natl Acad Sci USA 2002; 99:12,293–12,297.

33. Linsley PS, Clark EA, Ledbetter JA. T-cell antigen CD28 mediates adhesion with B cells by interacting with activation antigen B7/BB-1. Proc Natl Acad Sci USA 1990; 87:5031–5035.

34. Linsley PS, Brady W, Urnes M, Grosmaire LS, Damle NK, Ledbetter JA. CTLA-4 is a second receptor for the B cell activation antigen B7. J Exp Med 1991; 174:561–569.

35. Chen L. The B7-CD28 family molecules. In: Chen L, ed. Molecular biology intelligence unit. New York: Kluwer/Plenum, 2003.

36. Watanabe N, Gavrieli M, Sedy JR, et al. BTLA is a lymphocyte inhibitory receptor with similarities to CTLA-4 and PD-1. Nat Immunol 2003; 4:670–679.

37. Lenschow DJ, Walunas TL, Bluestone JA. CD28/B7 system of T cell costimulation. Annu Rev Immunol 1996; 14:233–258.

38. Linsley PS, Brady W, Grosmaire L, Aruffo A, Damle NK, Ledbetter JA. Binding of the B cell activation antigen B7 to CD28 costimulates T cell proliferation and interleukin 2 mRNA accumulation. J Exp Med 1991; 173:721–730.

39. Damle NK, Linsley PS, Ledbetter JA. Direct helper T cell-induced B cell differentiation involves interaction between T cell antigen CD28 and B cell activation antigen B7. Eur J Immunol 1991; 21: 1277–1282.

40. Carreno BM, Collins M. The B7 family of ligands and its receptors: new pathways for costimulation and inhibition of immune responses. Annu Rev Immunol 2002; 20:29–53.

41. Chambers CA, Kuhns MS, Egen JG, Allison JP. CTLA-4-mediated inhibition in regulation of T cell responses: mechanisms and manipulation in tumor immunotherapy. Annu Rev Immunol 2001; 19: 565–594.

42. Krummel MF, Allison JP. CD28 and CTLA-4 have opposing effects on the response of T cells to stimulation. J Exp Med 1995; 182:459–465.

43. Cross AH, Girard TJ, Giacoletto KS, et al. Long-term inhibition of murine experimental autoimmune encephalomyelitis using CTLA-4-Fc supports a key role for CD28 costimulation. J Clin Invest 1995; 95:2783–2789.

44. Linsley PS, Greene JL, Brady W, Bajorath J, Ledbetter JA, Peach R. Human B7-1 (CD80) and B7-2 (CD86) bind with similar avidities but distinct kinetics to CD28 and CTLA-4 receptors. Immunity 1994; 1:793–801.

45. Tivol EA, Borriello F, Schweitzer AN, Lynch WP, Bluestone JA, Sharpe AH. Loss of CTLA-4 leads to massive lymphoproliferation and fatal multiorgan tissue destruction, revealing a critical negative regulatory role of CTLA-4. Immunity 1995; 3:541–547.

46. Waterhouse P, Penninger JM, Timms E, et al. Lymphoproliferative disorders with early lethality in mice deficient in Ctla-4. Science 1995; 270:985–988.

47. Chen L, Ashe S, Brady WA, et al. Costimulation of antitumor immunity by the B7 counterreceptor for the T lymphocyte molecules CD28 and CTLA-4. Cell 1992; 71:1093–1102.

48. Huang AY, Bruce AT, Pardoll DM, Levitsky HI. Does B7-1 expression confer antigen-presenting cell capacity to tumors in vivo? J Exp Med 1996; 183:769–776.

49. Chen L, McGowan P, Ashe S, et al. Tumor immunogenicity determines the effect of B7 costimulation on T cell-mediated tumor immunity. J Exp Med 1994; 179:523–532.

50. Hurwitz AA, Townsend SE, Yu TF, Wallin JA, Allison JP. Enhancement of the anti-tumor immune response using a combination of interferon-gamma and B7 expression in an experimental mammary carcinoma. Int J Cancer 1998; 77:107–113.

51. Emtage PC, Wan Y, Muller W, Graham FL, Gauldie J. Enhanced interleukin-2 gene transfer immunotherapy of breast cancer by coexpression of B7-1 and B7-2. J Interferon Cytokine Res 1998; 18:927–937.

52. Emtage PC, Wan Y, Bramson JL, Graham FL, Gauldie J. A double recombinant adenovirus expressing the costimulatory molecule B7-1 (murine) and human IL-2 induces complete tumor regression in a murine breast adenocarcinoma model. J Immunol 1998; 160:2531–2538.

53. Cayeux S, Beck C, Aicher A, Dorken B, Blankenstein T. Tumor cells cotransfected with interleukin-7 and B7.1 genes induce CD25 and CD28 on tumor-infiltrating T lymphocytes and are strong vaccines. Eur J Immunol 1995; 25:2325–2331.

54. Yang G, Hellstrom KE, Mizuno MT, Chen L. In vitro priming of tumor-reactive cytolytic T lympho-cytes by combining IL-10 with B7-CD28 costimulation. J Immunol 1995; 155:3897–3903.
55. Coughlin CM, Wysocka M, Kurzawa HL, Lee WM, Trinchieri G, Eck SL. B7-1 and interleukin 12 synergistically induce effective antitumor immunity. Cancer Res 1995; 55:4980–4987.
56. Brentjens RJ, Latouche JB, Santos E, et al. Eradication of systemic B-cell tumors by genetically targeted human T lymphocytes co-stimulated by CD80 and interleukin-15. Nat Med 2003; 9:279–286.
57. Sumimoto H, Tani K, Nakazaki Y, et al. GM-CSF and B7-1 (CD80) co-stimulatory signals co-operate in the induction of effective anti-tumor immunity in syngeneic mice. Int J Cancer 1997; 73:556–561.
58. Baskar S, Glimcher L, Nabavi N, Jones RT, Ostrand-Rosenberg S. Major histocompatibility complex class II+B7-1+ tumor cells are potent vaccines for stimulating tumor rejection in tumor-bearing mice. J Exp Med 1995; 181:619–629.
59. Kwon ED, Foster BA, Hurwitz AA, et al. Elimination of residual metastatic prostate cancer after sur-gery and adjunctive cytotoxic T lymphocyte-associated antigen 4 (CTLA-4) blockade immunotherapy. Proc Natl Acad Sci USA 1999; 96:15,074–15,079.
60. van Elsas A, Hurwitz AA, Allison JP. Combination immunotherapy of B16 melanoma using anti-cyto-toxic T lymphocyte-associated antigen 4 (CTLA-4) and granulocyte/macrophage colony-stimulating factor (GM-CSF)-producing vaccines induces rejection of subcutaneous and metastatic tumors accom-panied by autoimmune depigmentation. J Exp Med 1999; 190:355–366.
61. Leach DR, Krummel MF, Allison JP. Enhancement of antitumor immunity by CTLA-4 blockade. Science 1996; 271:1734–1736.
62. Hernandez J, Ko A, Sherman LA. CTLA-4 blockade enhances the CTL responses to the p53 self-tumor antigen. J Immunol 2001; 166:3908–3914.
63. Read S, Malmstrom V, Powrie F. Cytotoxic T lymphocyte-associated antigen 4 plays an essential role in the function of CD25(+)CD4(+) regulatory cells that control intestinal inflammation. J Exp Med 2000; 192:295–302.
64. Takahashi T, Tagami T, Yamazaki S, et al. Immunologic self-tolerance maintained by CD25(+)CD4(+) regulatory T cells constitutively expressing cytotoxic T lymphocyte-associated antigen 4. J Exp Med 2000; 192:303–310.
65. Hurwitz AA, Yu TF, Leach DR, Allison JP. CTLA-4 blockade synergizes with tumor-derived granu-locyte-macrophage colony-stimulating factor for treatment of an experimental mammary carcinoma. Proc Natl Acad Sci USA 1998; 95:10,067–10,071.
66. Hodi FS, Mihm MC, Soiffer RJ, et al. Biologic activity of cytotoxic T lymphocyte-associated antigen 4 antibody blockade in previously vaccinated metastatic melanoma and ovarian carcinoma patients. Proc Natl Acad Sci USA 2003; 100:4712–4717.
67. Phan GQ, Yang JC, Sherry RM, et al. Cancer regression and autoimmunity induced by cytotoxic T lymphocyte-associated antigen 4 blockade in patients with metastatic melanoma. Proc Natl Acad Sci USA 2003; 100:8372–8377.
68. Chen L. The B7-CD28 family molecules. Georgetown, TX. New York, NY: Landes Bioscience/Eurekah. com; Kluwer Academic/Plenum, 2003:141.
69. Mazanet MM, Hughes CC. B7-H1 is expressed by human endothelial cells and suppresses T cell cyto-kine synthesis. J Immunol 2002; 169:3581–3588.
70. Wiendl H, Mitsdoerffer M, Schneider D, et al. Human muscle cells express a B7-related molecule, B7-H1, with strong negative immune regulatory potential: a novel mechanism of counterbalancing the immune attack in idiopathic inflammatory myopathies. FASEB J 2003; 17:1892–1894.
71. Freeman GJ, Long AJ, Iwai Y, et al. Engagement of the PD-1 immunoinhibitory receptor by a novel B7 family member leads to negative regulation of lymphocyte activation. J Exp Med 2000; 192:1027–1034.
72. Tamura H, Dong H, Zhu G, et al. B7-H1 costimulation preferentially enhances CD28-independent T-helper cell function. Blood 2001; 97:1809–1816.
73. Yamazaki T, Akiba H, Iwai H, et al. Expression of programmed death 1 ligands by murine T cells and APC. J Immunol 2002; 169:5538–5545.
74. Wang S, Bajorath J, Flies DB, Dong H, Honjo T, Chen L. Molecular modeling and functional mapping of B7-H1 and B7-DC uncouple costimulatory function from PD-1 interaction. J Exp Med 2003; 197:1083–1091.
75. Rodig N, Ryan T, Allen JA, et al. Endothelial expression of PD-L1 and PD-L2 down-regulates CD8+ T cell activation and cytolysis. Eur J Immunol 2003; 33:3117–3126.

76. Cao Y, Zhou H, Tao J, et al. Keratinocytes induce local tolerance to skin graft by activating interleukin-10-secreting T cells in the context of costimulation molecule B7-H1. Transplantation 2003; 75:1390–1396.

77. Hirano F, Kaneko K, Tamura H, et al. Molecular shield: a new mechanism for cancer resistance to immunotherapy. Cancer Res 2004; in press.

78. Tseng SY, Otsuji M, Gorski K, et al. B7-DC, a new dendritic cell molecule with potent costimulatory properties for T cells. J Exp Med 2001; 193:839–846.

79. Latchman Y, Wood CR, Chernova T, et al. PD-L2 is a second ligand for PD-1 and inhibits T cell activation. Nat Immunol 2001; 2:261–268.

80. Liu X, Gao JX, Wen J, et al. B7DC/PDL2 promotes tumor immunity by a PD-1-independent mechanism. J Exp Med 2003; 197:1721–1730.

81. Radhakrishnan S, Nguyen LT, Ciric B, et al. Naturally occurring human IgM antibody that binds B7-DC and potentiates T cell stimulation by dendritic cells. J Immunol 2003; 170:1830–1838.

82. Nguyen LT, Radhakrishnan S, Ciric B, et al. Cross-linking the B7 family molecule B7-DC directly activates immune functions of dendritic cells. J Exp Med 2002; 196:1393–1398.

83. Agata Y, Kawasaki A, Nishimura H, et al. Expression of the PD-1 antigen on the surface of stimulated mouse T and B lymphocytes. Int Immunol 1996; 8:765–772.

84. Ishida Y, Agata Y, Shibahara K, Honjo T. Induced expression of PD-1, a novel member of the immunoglobulin gene superfamily, upon programmed cell death. Embo J 1992; 11:3887–3895.

85. Okazaki T, Maeda A, Nishimura H, Kurosaki T, Honjo T. PD-1 immunoreceptor inhibits B cell receptor-mediated signaling by recruiting src homology 2-domain-containing tyrosine phosphatase 2 to phosphotyrosine. Proc Natl Acad Sci USA 2001; 98:13,866–13,871.

86. Nishimura H, Okazaki T, Tanaka Y, et al. Autoimmune dilated cardiomyopathy in PD-1 receptor-deficient mice. Science 2001; 291:319–322.

87. Okazaki T, Tanaka Y, Nishio R, et al. Autoantibodies against cardiac troponin I are responsible for dilated cardiomyopathy in PD-1-deficient mice. Nat Med 2003; 9:1477–1483.

88. Nishimura H, Nose M, Hiai H, Minato N, Honjo T. Development of lupus-like autoimmune diseases by disruption of the PD-1 gene encoding an ITIM motif-carrying immunoreceptor. Immunity 1999; 11:141–151.

89. Salama AD, Chitnis T, Imitola J, et al. Critical role of the programmed death-1 (PD-1) pathway in regulation of experimental autoimmune encephalomyelitis. J Exp Med 2003; 198:71–78.

90. Ansari MJ, Salama AD, Chitnis T, et al. The programmed death-1 (PD-1) pathway regulates autoimmune diabetes in nonobese diabetic (NOD) mice. J Exp Med 2003; 198:63–69.

91. Tsushima F, Iwai H, Otsuki N, et al. Preferential contribution of B7-H1 to programmed death-1-mediated regulation of hapten-specific allergic inflammatory responses. Eur J Immunol 2003; 33:2773–2782.

92. Blazar BR, Carreno BM, Panoskaltsis-Mortari A, et al. Blockade of programmed death-1 engagement accelerates graft-versus-host disease lethality by an IFN-gamma-dependent mechanism. J Immunol 2003; 171:1272–1277.

93. Kanai T, Totsuka T, Uraushihara K, et al. Blockade of B7-H1 suppresses the development of chronic intestinal inflammation. J Immunol 2003; 171:4156–4163.

94. Subudhi SK, Zhou P, Yerian LM, et al. Local expression of B7-H1 promotes organ-specific autoimmunity and transplant rejection. J Clin Invest 2004; 113:694–700.

95. Hutloff A, Dittrich AM, Beier KC, et al. ICOS is an inducible T-cell co-stimulator structurally and functionally related to CD28. Nature 1999; 397:263–266.

96. Yoshinaga SK, Whoriskey JS, Khare SD, et al. T-cell co-stimulation through B7RP-1 and ICOS. Nature 1999; 402:827–832.

97. Dong C, Juedes AE, Temann UA, et al. ICOS co-stimulatory receptor is essential for T-cell activation and function. Nature 2001; 409:97–101.

98. McAdam AJ, Greenwald RJ, Levin MA, et al. ICOS is critical for CD40-mediated antibody class switching. Nature 2001; 409:102–105.

99. Wang S, Zhu G, Chapoval AI, et al. Costimulation of T cells by B7-H2, a B7-like molecule that binds ICOS. Blood 2000; 96:2808–2813.

100. Ling V, Wu PW, Finnerty HF, et al. Cutting edge: identification of GL50, a novel B7-like protein that functionally binds to ICOS receptor. J Immunol 2000; 164:1653–1657.

101. Swallow MM, Wallin JJ, Sha WC. B7h, a novel costimulatory homolog of B7.1 and B7.2, is induced by TNFalpha. Immunity 1999; 11:423–432.

102. Wallin JJ, Liang L, Bakardjiev A, Sha WC. Enhancement of CD8+ T cell responses by ICOS/B7h costimulation. J Immunol 2001; 167:132–139.

103. Liu X, Bai XF, Wen J, et al. B7H costimulates clonal expansion of, and cognate destruction of tumor cells by, CD8(+) T lymphocytes in vivo. J Exp Med 2001; 194:1339–1348.

104. Ara G, Baher A, Storm N, et al. Potent activity of soluble B7RP-1-Fc in therapy of murine tumors in syngeneic hosts. Int J Cancer 2003; 103:501–507.

105. Chapoval AI, Ni J, Lau JS, et al. B7-H3: a costimulatory molecule for T cell activation and IFN-gamma production. Nat Immunol 2001; 2:269–274.

106. Sun M, Richards S, Prasad DV, Mai XM, Rudensky A, Dong C. Characterization of mouse and human B7-H3 genes. J Immunol 2002; 168:6294–6297.

107. Ling V, Wu PW, Spaulding V, et al. Duplication of primate and rodent B7-H3 immunoglobulin V- and C-like domains: divergent history of functional redundancy and exon loss. Genomics 2003; 82:365–377.

108. Steinberger P, Majdic O, Derdak SV, et al. Molecular characterization of human 4Ig-B7-H3, a member of the B7 family with four Ig-like domains. J Immunol 2004; 172:2352–2359.

109. Luo L, Chapoval AI, Flies DB, et al. B7-H3 enhances tumor immunity in vivo by costimulating rapid clonal expansion of antigen-specific CD8+ cytolytic T cells. J Immunol 2004; 173:5445–5450.

110. Suh WK, Gajewska BU, Okada H, et al. The B7 family member B7-H3 preferentially down-regulates T helper type 1-mediated immune responses. Nat Immunol 2003; 4:899–906.

111. Sun X, Vale M, Leung E, Kanwar JR, Gupta R, Krissansen GW. Mouse B7-H3 induces antitumor immunity. Gene Ther 2003; 10:1728–1734.

112. Prasad DV, Richards S, Mai XM, Dong C. B7S1, a novel B7 family member that negatively regulates T cell activation. Immunity 2003; 18:863–873.

113. Sica GL, Choi IH, Zhu G, et al. B7-H4, a molecule of the B7 family, negatively regulates T cell immunity. Immunity 2003; 18:849–861.

114. Zang X, Loke P, Kim J, Murphy K, Waitz R, Allison JP. B7x: a widely expressed B7 family member that inhibits T cell activation. Proc Natl Acad Sci USA 2003; 100:10,388–10,392.

115. Choi IH, Zhu G, Sica GL, et al. Genomic organization and expression analysis of B7-H4, an immune inhibitory molecule of the B7 family. J Immunol 2003; 171:4650–4654.

116. von Mehren M, Arlen P, Tsang KY, et al. Pilot study of a dual gene recombinant avipox vaccine containing both carcinoembryonic antigen (CEA) and B7.1 transgenes in patients with recurrent CEA-expressing adenocarcinomas. Clin Cancer Res 2000; 6:2219–2228.

117. Horig H, Lee DS, Conkright W, et al. Phase I clinical trial of a recombinant canarypoxvirus (ALVAC) vaccine expressing human carcinoembryonic antigen and the B7.1 co-stimulatory molecule. Cancer Immunol Immunother 2000; 49:504–514.

# VI-C TUMOR-TARGETED THERAPIES

# 33 Proteasome Inhibition and Its Clinical Application in Solid Tumors

*David J. Park, MD and Heinz-Josef Lenz, MD, FACP*

## CONTENTS

## SUMMARY

The proteasome is a multicatalytic protein complex whose principal function is the degradation of vital proteins many of which are involved in cell cycle regulation, tumor suppression, apoptosis, transcription, and angiogenesis. The inhibition of the proteasome is a promising novel therapeutic approach to cancer treatment. Bortezomib (Velcade) is the first proteasome inhibitor to have shown anticancer activity and reach clinical trials. Preclinical and early clinical trials in both solid tumors and hematological malignancies demonstrate that bortezomib is a relatively well-tolerated and active agent, either alone or in combination with traditional chemotherapeutic drugs. Most recently, its efficacy has been shown in multiple myeloma. Currently, clinical trials are ongoing in order to determine the efficacy as well as safety of bortezomib in the management of solid tumors, especially in combination with traditional cytotoxic agents.

**Key Words:** Bortezomib; proteasome inhibition; PS-341; NF-κB; novel target.

## 1. INTRODUCTION

The degradation of intracellular proteins into their component amino acids is a highly complex and closely regulated process that leads to downstream effects on a wide array of essential cellular activities. This degradative process fulfills two main functions: (1) It eliminates defective proteins that could potentially harm the cell and (2) it ensures proper

From: *Cancer Drug Discovery and Development: The Oncogenomics Handbook*
Edited by: W. J. LaRochelle and R. A. Shimkets © Humana Press Inc., Totowa, NJ

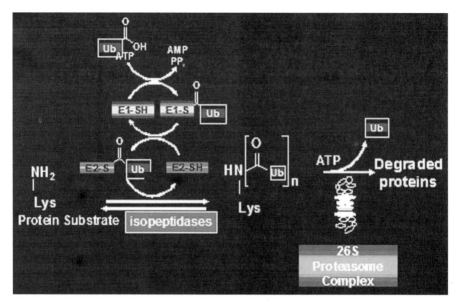

**Fig. 1.** Ubiquitin–proteasome pathway. Ubiquination of a proteins substrate starts with the linkage of ubiquitin with E1 through a thiolester bond (ATP-dependent process). This "activated" ubiquitin is transferred to E2. With the aid of ubiquitin ligase (E3), ubiquitin is covalently linked to the lysine residue of the protein substrate. This now "marked" protein substrate is recognized by the proteasome, deubiquination occurs, and the protein enters the proteolytic core for degradation. (Courtesy of Millenium Pharmaceuticals, Inc., Cambridge, MA. Used with permission.)

regulation of cellular metabolism by maintaining adequate levels of enzymes and regulatory proteins. Interestingly, prior to the discovery of the "ubitiquitin–proteasome pathway," intracellular protein degradation was believed to be an unregulated process conducted principally through nonselective lysosomal protein degradation.

A substrate protein begins its degradative pathway by being "marked" through covalent linkage with ubiquitin. Ubiquitin is a highly conserved 76-amino-acid protein that attaches to a target protein through a three-step process involving several enzymes. First, ubiquitin is activated by ubiquitin-activating enzyme (E1) in an ATP-requiring reaction. Activated ubiquitin is then transferred to ubiquitin-conjugating enzyme (E2), which, in turn, presents it to ubiquitin protein ligase (E3). Finally, E3 facilitates covalent linkage of the activated ubiquitin to a target protein. Multiple ubitiquin molecules could tandemly bind to a target protein, resulting in polyubiquination. This ubiquitin-marked protein is then recognized by the proteasome and it is degraded within its proteolytically active 20S chamber, thus the term "ubiquitin–proteasome pathway" (UPP) *(1–4)* (see Fig. 1).

The 26S proteasome is a 2.5-kDa multiprotein complex that consists of a 20S core particle, flanked by one or two 19S regulatory proteins. It is expressed in all eukaryotic cells, both in the nucleus and cytoplasm, and its main function is the degradation of a large number of intracellular proteins. These include proteins involved in cell cycle regulation *(5)*, apoptosis *(6)*, angiogenesis, transcription factors *(7,8)*, growth factor receptors *(9)*, and signal transduction molecules. Interfering with the normal cycling of these proteins through proteasome inhibition could lead to derangement of key processes, such as cell mitosis,

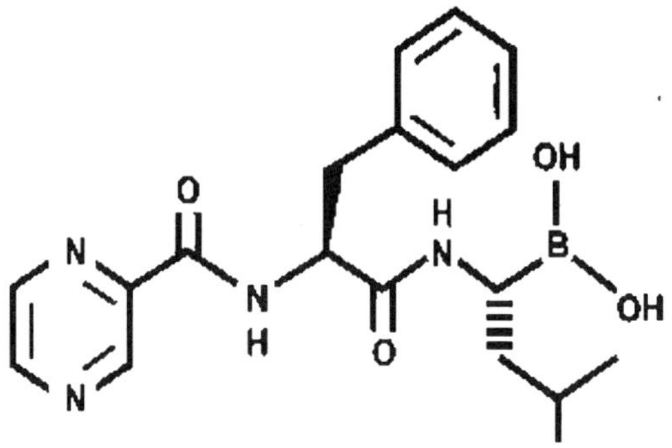

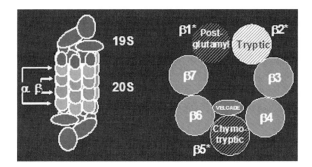

**Fig. 2.** Chemical structure of bortezomib. (Courtesy of Millenium Pharmaceuticals, Inc., Cambridge, MA. Used with permission.)

**Fig. 3.** Structure of the proteasome. (**Left**) The 26S proteasome has a proteolytically active 20S core, usually flanked by one or two 19S regulatory subunits, which act as "gate-keepers," recognizing and controlling access of ubiquinated proteins into the core; (**right**) cross-sectional view of the proteolytic core. Bortezomib binds to the proteolytically active β-subunit, thus inhibiting its chymotrypsin-like activity. (Courtesy of Millenium Pharmaceuticals, Inc., Cambridge, MA. Used with permission.)

cell adhesion, neoplastic growth, and metastasis, and cause cell apoptosis. Consequently, proteasome inhibition has drawn considerable attention as a potential novel approach for anticancer therapy.

A large number of molecules that interfere with proteasome function, both naturally occurring and synthetic, have been described. Many bind either irreversibly or reversibly to the proteolytically active sites within the 20S core particle, thus inhibiting its function. Among them, boronic acid peptides have shown great promise from the clinical standpoint because of their high potency, selectivity for the proteasome, and stability under physiologic conditions.

Bortezomib (VELCADE; formerly PS-341) is a boronic acid dipeptide derivative and is the first proteasome inhibitor to have progressed to clinical trials (see Fig. 2). It inhibits the proteasome in a highly selective manner through the stability of the boron–Thr'Ogdative bond that forms at the active site of the proteosome, inhibiting its chymotrypsinlike activity (see Fig. 3). Its highly selective property allows other common proteases to be unaffected by this molecule. Bortezomib has shown activity in both preclinical and clinical studies

in both solid tumors and hematological malignancies. Its clinical activity in multiple myeloma was found to be especially impressive in phase II trials, leading to its accelerated
approval by the Federal Drug Administration (FDA) for the treatment of multiple myeloma in heavily pretreated patients *(10)*. Most recently, a phase III trial in multiple myeloma
comparing bortezomib to high-dose dexamethasone in refractory patients was terminated
early because of significant advantage of the bortezomib arm.

This chapter will present the molecular rationale, key preclinical data, as well as current
clinical trials data evaluating proteasome inhibitors, namely bortezomib, in the management of solid tumors.

## 2. TARGETS OF THE PROTEASOME

The list of substrate proteins degraded by the UPP reported in the literature is rather
extensive and continues to expand with differing levels of impact in cell cycle regulation,
apoptosis, and angiogenesis.

Proteins involved in cell cycle progression and regulation are among the key substrates
for UPP degradation. Included among them are the cyclins (A, B, D, E) *(5,11)*. Cyclins are
expressed in a cell-cycle-dependent manner (e.g., cyclins D and E during progression from
the G1- to S-phase) and mediate progression through the cell cycle. After activation via
its association with cyclin-dependent protein kinases (cdk) and phosphorylation of cdk, the
cyclin–cdk complex causes a disruption of the *Rb–E2F1* repressor complex, through phosphorylation of tumor suppressor *Rb*. Transcription factor *E2F1*, which is also degraded
by via the UPP *(12)*, is then allowed to activate the expression of various genes involved
in DNA synthesis, thus progressing the cell into the S-phase. Activated cyclin–cdk complexes are also involved in the G2 to M transition.

Cyclin-dependent protein kinase inhibitors (CKIs) $p21^{WAF1/CIP1}$ and $p27^{KIP1}$ are also
degraded through the UPP *(13,14)*. CKIs form a complex with cyclin–cdk, inhibiting its
activity and thus inducing G1/S cell cycle arrest *(15)*. In fact, low expression of $p27^{KIP1}$ has
been shown to be associated with tumor aggressiveness and poor prognosis in various neoplasms, including breast *(16)*, colon *(17)*, prostate *(18)*, and non-small-cell lung cancer *(19)*.

Consequently, the dysregulation of "activator" and "inhibitor" proteins involved in the
cell cycle via their stabilization by proteasome inhibition might cause conflicting growth
and arrest signals and eventually lead to cell apoptosis *(20)*.

Another substrate degraded via the UPP is tumor suppressor *p53*, the most highly
mutated gene in human malignancies *(21)*. Tumor suppressor *p53* plays an important role
in cell cycle regulation as well as cell apoptosis. It acts as a negative regulator of cell
growth causing G1 arrest, and there is evidence that the S-phase and G2/M arrest might
partly be influenced by *p53* as well *(22,23)*. G1 arrest is mainly mediated through induction
of the CKI $p21^{WAF1/CIP1}$ by *p53*, although initial rapid induction of G1 arrest occurs via
*p53*-independent phosphatase activity of *Cdc25A* *(24)*. Moreover, it is a well established
fact that the *p53* gene plays a key role in damage-induced cell apoptosis *(25)*. Interestingly,
studies exploring the role of *p53* in inducing cell cycle arrest and apoptosis after bortezomib
treatment have yielded inconsistent results across different cell lines *(26–29)*.

A key transcription factor affected by the ubiquitin–proteasome pathway is nuclear factor-κB (*NF-κB*) *(7)*. *NF-κB* activates the expression of a number of genes involved in the
cell survival, proliferation, and chemoresistance, especially under conditions of physiologic stress. Specifically, *NF-κB* downregulates the apoptotic action of tumor necrosis

factor (*TNF-α*) *(30–32)* and oncogenic *Ras (33)*, whereas activating antiapoptotic factors such as inhibitors of apoptosis (IAPs) and the *Bcl-2* family *(34)*. It also causes upregulation of cell adhesion molecules such as *E-selectin*, intracellular adhesion molecule (*ICAM-1*), and vascular cell adhesion molecule (*VCAM-1*) *(35)*, which might be involved in tumor metastasis and angiogenesis. Various studies have demonstrated *NF-κB*'s role in chemoresistance and cell survival *(36–38)*. In addition, *NF-κB* has been shown to be constitutively activated in several neoplasms, including multiple myeloma *(39)*, lymphoma *(40)*, leukemia *(41,42)*, breast *(43,44)*, colon, pancreatic *(45)*, and lung cancer cells *(46)*, thus underscoring its importance as a potential therapeutic target.

This UPP-mediated process takes place indirectly through degradation of *NF-κB*'s inhibitor protein, *IκB*, by the proteasome *(47)*. *IκB* is bound to *NF-κB*, and the inactive *IκB/NF-κB* complex remains in the cytoplasm under normal conditions. However, when the cell is "stressed" by any number of factors (chemotherapy, ionizing radiation, *TNF-α*, lipopolysaccharides, etc.), *IκB* is phosphorylated, ubiquinated, and, subsequently, degraded by the proteasome *(48)*. *NF-κB* is then released for its translocation into the nucleus where it activate multiple target genes, including cytokines, cell adhesion molecules, and antiapoptotic factors that can lead to cell proliferation, survival, and potential tumor metastasis. Therefore, stabilization of *IκB* via proteasome inhibition can aid in overcoming chemoresistance and promote cell apoptosis, even in chemorefractory tumors.

## 3. PRECLINICAL ACTIVITY OF PROTEASOME INHIBITORS

Various in vitro and in vivo studies have demonstrated the cytotoxic property of proteasome inhibitors—in particular, bortezomib. A few salient studies testing the cytotoxic properties of bortezomib either as a single agent of in combination with more conventional chemotherapeutic drugs are reviewed herein.

Bortezomib's cytotoxic activity was first demonstrated in a broad range of human tumor cells in a 60 tumor cell line panel from the National Cancer Institute (NCI), used for preclinical assays. This panel includes cell lines from nine different cancer types (colon, brain, melanoma, prostate, lung, breast, renal, and ovarian). In the study, bortezomib was able to achieve growth inhibition of 50% ($GI_{50}$) at low concentrations (average $GI_{50} = 7$ n$M$). Moreover, bortezomib was shown to penetrate into cells and inhibit proteolysis of long-lived proteins by the proteasome with concentrations of 0.1 μ$M$, achieving 50% inhibition. The study investigators were also able to show a unique cytotoxic mechanism by bortezomib, not exhibited by other compounds, by comparing its "fingerprint" with NCI's historical database of 60,000 investigational agents via the NCI COMPARE algorithm *(28)*.

Further examination of bortezomib's antitumor activity in *p53*-null PC-3 prostate tumor xenografts was performed in the same study. Interestingly, application of bortezomib was able to induce an increase in CKI *p21*[WAF1/CIP1] levels and lead to accumulation of PC-3 cells at the G2/M-phase. Weekly intravenous administration of bortezomib for 4 wk in nude mice caused significant decrease in tumor growth of approx 60%. Moreover, injecting bortezomib directly into the tumor also caused a significant (70%) decrease in tumor volume. It is worth mentioning that at the end of the study, two of five mice (40%) treated with bortezomib had no detectable tumors. Finally, pharmacodynamics studies showed a significant dose-dependent effect on 20S proteasome activity by bortezomib *(28)*.

In MCF-7 human breast carcinoma cells, bortezomib was also found to be a potent cytotoxic agent, with an $IC_{90}$ of 0.05 μ$M$ on 24 h of exposure of the drug. After 48 h of exposure, the drug achieved a 99% kill of MCF-7 cells. In vivo evaluation of bortezomib's cytotoxicity was performed in mice bearing the EMT-6/Parent murine mammary carcinoma xenografts. In the parent cell lines, bortezomib was shown to increase the cytotoxicity of cyclophosphamide, radiation therapy, and cisplatin. However, the addition of bortezomib in the treatment regiment of resistant EMT-6 cell lines did not lead to chemosensitivity (49).

Antitumor activity by bortezomib was shown in the same study in Lewis lung carcinoma implants. Animals receiving bortezomib per os (po) showed significant decreased tumor burden from Lewis lung carcinoma implants, both primary and metastatic disease, and bortezomib combination regimens with 5-fluorouracil [5-FU], cisplatin, taxol, adriamycin, and fractionated radiation therapy demonstrated its additive cytotoxic property (49).

Antitumor activity of bortezomib has been shown in squamous cell cancer (SCC) as well. One study examined the effects of bortezomib on activation of *NF-κB* and cell survival, growth, and angiogenesis in murine and human SCC cell lines. In this study, bortezomib was able to inhibit activation of *NF-κB* DNA-binding and functional reporter activity at concentrations between $10^{-8}$ *M* and $10^{-7}$ *M*. Moreover, bortezomib was shown to inhibit growth of murine and human SCC xenografts in mice at doses of 1–2 mg/kg given three times weekly for 25 d. Dose-limiting toxicity (DLT) occurred at 2 mg/kg. Tumor growth inhibition was associated with decreased blood vessel density. In fact, bortezomib was able to inhibit expression of the proangiogenic cytokines' growth-regulated *oncogene-α* and vascular endothelial growth factor (*VEGF*) in the range at which it inhibited *NF-κB*. This study showed that bortezomib was able to neutralize *NF-κB* pathway components related to cell survival, tumor growth, and angiogenesis in SCC (50).

An important chemotherapeutic agent in the treatment of a variety of neoplasms is the camptothecin analog irinotecan (CPT-11). In fact, CPT-11 has been approved as first-line therapy for metastatic colorectal cancer in combination with 5-FU/leucovorin (LV). This topoisomerase I inhibitor forms a tertiary complex with the enzyme and DNA, preventing resealing of single-strand breaks mediated by *topoisomerase I*, eventually leading to double-stranded breaks in the DNA. Although the exact mechanism of cell death is unclear, CPT-11 causes inhibition of DNA synthesis, G2 arrest, and, consequently, cell apoptosis. Activation of *NF-κB* by CPT-11 has been shown to increase transcription of antiapoptotic factors and is seen as an important mechanism of chemoresistance (38).

The addition of bortezomib to CPT-11 has been shown to potentiate its cytotoxic effectiveness in LoVo colon cancer cell lines. In this study, pretreatment of LoVo colon cancer cells with bortezomib prior to exposure to SN-38 (the active metabolite of CPT-11) resulted in a significantly higher level of growth inhibition (64–75%) compared to either bortezomib (20–30%) or SN-38 alone (24–47%). The same study showed that combination therapy with bortezomib and CPT-11 led to a significant tumoricidal effect compared to either single agent alone, and to a 94% decrease in tumor size compared to the control group. The level of apoptosis was 80–90% in the treatment group that received combination treatment compared with single-agent therapy (10%). The effect of bortezomib on *NF-κB* inhibition and consequent stabilization of *p21*, *p27*, and *p53* was also evaluated. Again, the combination of bortezomib and CPT-11 led to a much higher stabilization of the aforementioned cell cycle inhibitory factors (51).

A study utilizing BxPC3 human pancreatic cells also demonstrated bortezomib's effectiveness in combination with CPT-11. In vitro, bortezomib was able to block mitogen fetal calf serum (FCS)-induced proliferation of BxPC3 human pancreatic cancer cells, stop cell cycle progression, and induce apoptosis by 24 h. Also, bortezomib-induced CKI *p21* stability was correlated with cell cycle arrest. When bortezomib's tumoricidal property was evaluated in tumor xenograft models, weekly administration of bortezomib led to significant reduction in tumor growth. However, inhibition of tumor xenograft growth was greatest (89%) when bortezomib was combined with CPT-11 versus either agent alone *(52)*.

The synergistic property of bortezomib with other chemotherapeutic agents in a variety of tumor models have been demonstrated both in vitro and in vivo. These agents include gemcitabine, cisplatin, docetaxel, and 5-FU, among others *(49,53,54)*.

An interesting clinical challenge in the use of combination chemotherapy is that of the optimal sequence of drug administration, especially when the two agents work on very different targets. At times, the given sequence can lead to synergistic or antagonistic effects even with the same regimen. Recently, a study examining this very question in the use of bortezomib was published. In this experiment human pancreatic cancer cells were treated either before, simultaneously, or after gemcitabine treatment. Then, surrogate markers for bortezomib's activity ($p21^{WAF1/CIP1}$, $p27^{KIP1}$, and *bcl-2*) and differential cell growth were evaluated. The administration of gemcitabine followed by bortezomib led to the greatest induction of apoptosis and long-term cell growth inhibition. It seems that this observation might be true in other tumor types and agents *(55)*. Whether these findings translate in actual clinical efficacy differences remain to be demonstrated.

In essence, preclinical studies have shown promising in vitro and in vivo evidence on the cytotoxic properties of bortezomib either as a single agent or in combination in a variety of neoplasms. Molecular effects of proteasome inhibition on major cell cycle regulators, antiapoptotic proteins, and growth and angiogenic factors have been documented. Among the remaining questions, optimal sequencing in bortezomib administration during combined therapy might be an important issue in future clinical trials.

## 4. PHASE I CLINICAL TRIALS IN SOLID TUMORS

Currently, a large number of phase I trials for bortezomib either as a single agent or in combination with conventional chemotherapy are underway (see Table 1). In this section, we expound on the details of some of these trials. Most results are available only in abstract form at the present.

Recently, results of a phase I trial by Aghajanian et al. have been published. In this study, 43 patients in a variety of neoplasms were treated with single-agent bortezomib in doses ranging from 0.13 to 1.56 mg/m²/dose. The tumor types included were non-small-cell lung cancer (NSCLC), colon, head and neck, melanoma, ovary, renal, prostate, bladder, cervix, endometrial, esophagus, gastric, and unknown primary. A total of 89 doses were administered, with an average of 2 cycles per patient. The median number of previous chemotherapeutic regimens was four. Reported DLTs were diarrhea and sensory neurotoxicity. Other side effects seen were fatigue, fever, anorexia, nausea, vomiting, rash, pruritus, and headache. There was no dose-limiting hematological toxicity. One partial response was seen in a patient with NSCLC. The maximum tolerated dose (MTD) was established at 1.56 mg/m². Pharmacodynamics studies showed a dose-related inhibition of 20S proteasome activity with increasing dose of bortezomib *(56)*.

Other phase I trials for single-agent bortezomib have preliminary results that have been presented in abstract form *(62,63)*. In one study, bortezomib was given twice a week for 4 out 6 wk cycles in 22 patients with advanced cancer in doses ranging from 0.5 to 1.7 mg/m². Common reported toxicities were fatigue, anorexia, diarrhea, nausea, vomiting, fever,

Table 1
Bortezomib Phase I Solid Tumor Trials

| Solid Tumor | Treatment | MTD ($mg/m^2$) | DLTs | Site/Status |
|---|---|---|---|---|
| Advanced solid tumors | Bortezomib, paclitaxel, carboplatin | Pending | | Mayo Clinic |
| Breast (57) | Bortezomib, docetaxel | Pending | Neutropenic fever, neurotoxicity, lover, GI, mucositis | |
| Advanced solid tumors (56) | Bortezomib | 1.56 | GI, neurotoxicity | |
| Ovarian (58) | Bortezomib, carboplatin | Pending | | Memorial Sloan–Kettering Cancer Center (open) |
| Glioma | Bortezomib | | | Johns Hopkins (open) |
| Advanced solid tumors (59) | Bortezomib, gemzar | 1.00 1000 | Hematologic, GI, cardiac, liver | |
| Advanced solid tumors | Bortezomib, docetaxel | Pending | | Johns Hopkins |
| Lung (NSCLC) | Bortezomib, gemcitabine, carboplatin | Pending | | City of Hope Cancer Center (open) |
| Advanced solid tumors | Bortezomib, carboplatin, etoposide | Pending | | University of Colorado (open) |
| Advanced malignancies | Bortezomib, oxaliplatin | Pending | | NYU (open) |
| Advanced solid tumors (60) | Bortezomib, fluorouracil, leucovorin | 0.7 500 20 | GI | University of Southern California (closed) |
| Advanced solid tumors or lymphomas | Bortezomib | Pending | | NYU |
| Advanced malignancies and renal insufficiency | Bortezomib | Pending | | University of Wisconsin (open) |
| Metastatic or unresectable malignancy | Bortezomib, topotecan | Pending | | Yale (open) |
| Advanced solid tumors (61) | Bortezomib, irinotecan | 1.3 125 | Hematologic, GI, partial small bowel obstruction | |
| Locally advanced or metastatic solid tumors | Bortezomib, paclitaxel | Pending | | Ohio State (open) |
| Advanced solid tumors | Bortezomib, doxorubicin | Pending | | University of Wisconsin |
| Head and neck | Bortezomib, radiotherapy | Pending | | NIH (open) |

Source: www.cancer.gov unless otherwise specified.

and thrombocytopenia. Dose-dependent decreases in 20S proteasome activity in peripheral blood mononuclear cells (PBMNCs) were observed as well as increases in levels of *p53*. The MTD was not reported at the time; and in 18 evaluable patients, no objective responses were observed.

Bortezomib was administered in escalating doses ranging from 0.5 to 1.3 mg/m$^2$ twice weekly, followed by 500 mg/m$^2$ 5-FU and 20 mg/m$^2$ LV for 4 wk with 2 wk of rest, in a combination study with 5-FU/LV. Twenty-one patients were enrolled (15 colorectal, 1 esophageal, 1 breast, 1 anal, and 2 unknown). With 19 patients evaluable for response, 8 patients had stable disease, 10 had disease progression, and 1 (esophageal) had a partial response to the treatment. The MTD was determined to be 0.7 mg/m$^2$ and the major DLT was gastrointestinal toxicity *(60)* (updated via personal communication with Dr. Iqbal and Dr. Lenz).

In another combination study, bortezomib and docetaxel were administered in patients with anthracycline-pretreated metastatic breast cancer. Bortezomib was given on d 1, 4, 8, and 11, and docetaxel was given 1 h before bortezomib on d 1. Dose levels evaluated were (mg/m$^2$ bortezomib/mg/m$^2$ docetaxel):1.0/60, 1.0/75, 1.3/75, and 1.0/100. The MTD was not reached at the time of abstract publication, and the DLTs reported were febrile neutropenia, neuropathy, transaminitis, mucositis, vomiting, and diarrhea *(64)*.

Fifty-one patients with advanced solid tumors were enrolled in a phase I bortezomib/irinotecan dose escalation study. Bortezomib dosing levels were 1.0, 1.3, and 1.5 mg/m$^2$, and the dose of irinotecan ranged from 50 to 125 mg/m$^2$. Secondary end-points included tumor response, 20S proteosome inhibition, and pharmacokinetics. Major DLTs reported were neutropenia, partial small bowel obstruction, diarrhea, rash, vomiting, and thrombocytopenia. Most frequent complaints were fatigue, diarrhea, and nausea. The combination therapy did not appear to result in additive toxicities, and pharmacokinetic interactions were not seen. The MTD was established at the1.3/125 (bortezomib/irinotecan) level, and two patients (gastroesophageal [GE] junction adenocarcinoma and ovarian cancer) had a response to the treatment *(61)*.

The toxicity and efficacy of bortezomib/gemcitabine combination therapy was recently evaluated. Thirty-one patients with various advanced malignancies were enrolled. The MTD was determined to be 1.0/1000 (bortezomib/gemcitabine) mg/m$^2$. DLTs reported included thrombocytopenia, leucopenia, neutropenia, nausea, vomiting, myocardial infarction, and hyperaminotransferasemia. Out of five patients with refractory NSCLC, one achieved a partial response under the combination regimen. The pharmacokinetics of bortezomib and its effect on proteasome inhibition in peripheral blood cells was similar to that when used as a single agent. Furthermore, combination therapy did not affect significantly the pharmacokinetics of each individual agent *(62)*.

Recently, preliminary results of a dose-escalation trial of bortezomib with concurrent radiation therapy in patients with recurrent or metastatic head and neck were presented. Bortezomib was given twice weekly starting at 0.6 mg/m$^2$/dose with radiation at 1.8 Gy and daily fractions to 60–72 Gy. At the time of abstract presentation, seven patients had been treated at two dose levels (0.6 and 0.9 mg/m$^2$), with four patients showing marked reduction in tumor size. However, three of these patients subsequently progressed after 3 mo. No DLTs were observed at 0.6 mg/m$^2$. At 0.9 mg/m$^2$, G3 orthostatic hypotension and hyponatremia were seen *(65)*.

To summarize, numerous phase I trials have shown the relative tolerability of bortezomib either as a single agent or in combination with chemotherapy or radiation. Major toxicities were hematological, gastrointestinal, and neuropathic. It is especially encouraging to see that combination therapy did not seem to cause a marked increase in toxicity.

## 5. PHASE II TRIALS OF BORTEZOMIB IN SOLID TUMORS

Various phase II studies are currently underway in order to evaluate the efficacy and toxicity of bortezomib in an array of neoplasms either as a single agent or in combination with conventional chemotherapy (see Table 2). Many of these trials also include pharmacodynamic and biologic correlative data.

Most recently, results from a multicenter phase II study of single-agent bortezomib in patients with metastatic renal cell cancer have been published. Twenty-three patients were enrolled and 21 were evaluable for response. Bortezomib was administered at a dose of 1.5 mg/m$^2$ twice weekly for 2 wk in a 3 wk cycle. The median number of cycles received was 3, and 18 patients (86%) completed at least 3 cycles of therapy. If there were no grade 3 or 4 toxicities, the dose was escalated to 1.7 mg/m$^2$. Only one objective response (5%) was seen, and six patients (28%) had stable disease. Grade 3/4 toxicities were arthralgia, diarrhea, vomiting, thrombocytopenia, anemia, febrile neutropenia, gastrointestinal toxicity, pain, fatigue, neuropathy (one sensory, one mixed sensorimotor), and electrolyte disturbances. The trial was terminated after planned analysis revealed only one response to treatment. Because to insufficient biopsy and whole-blood sample numbers, no meaningful information regarding proteasome inhibition within the tumor was obtained. The authors concluded that although bortezomib was a relatively well-tolerated regimen, it did not offer clinically significant activity in metastatic renal cell cancer as a single agent *(66)*. Preliminary results of another recently presented phase II trial showed are more modest response. In that trial, 3 out 31 patients (9%) with metastatic renal cell cancer had a response to single-agent bortezomib. Interestingly, all the patients who responded were of clear cell histology with a 13% (3/24) response rate. The starting bortezomib dose for that trial was 1.5 mg/m$^2$, which was later reduced to 1.3 mg/m$^2$ because of toxicities *(67)*. Although bortezomib alone did not show significant clinical efficacy in metastatic renal cell carcinoma, combination with other active agents might lead to greater clinical effectiveness through synergism.

Preliminary results from a still ongoing phase II study of bortezomib as a single agent in patients with metastatic or recurrent sarcoma were presented in abstract form. Arm A comprised patients with Ewing's, osteogenic, or rhabdomyosarcoma; and arm B included other soft tissue sarcomas. The primary end point was response rate evaluation. Secondary end points included analysis of 20S proteasome inhibition in patients' lymphocytes, urine *VEGF* and *fibroblast growth factor* (*FGF*) levels, tumor *p53*, *murine double minute 2* (*MDM2*), and *cyclin D* and *E* expression. Bortezomib was given 1.5 mg/m$^2$ twice weekly for 2 wk, then 1-wk rest. At the time of abstract presentation, 13 patients were enrolled in arm B and no patients in arm A. The median number of cycles administered was 2. Out of 11 evaluable patients, 7 had progressive disease and 2 had stable disease. For two patients, it was too early for evaluation. Major reported toxicities were constipation, abdominal pain, myalgias, and persistent neuropathy. Urine *VEGF* and *FGF* levels were within normal limits in the nine patients evaluated so far *(68)*.

Single-agent bortezomib was evaluated in 14 patients with metastatic, well-differentiated neuroendocrine carcinomas. Primary sites included the small bowel, pancreas, stomach, lung, and unknown. Bortezomib was given for 6 mo at a dose of 1.5 mg/m$^2$ twice a week

Table 2
Bortezomib Phase II Solid Tumor Trials

| Solid tumor | Treatment | Projected Accrual | Status | Response Rate | Site |
|---|---|---|---|---|---|
| Ovarian | Bortezomib | 22–60 | Closed | | Gynecologic Oncology Group |
| Pancreas | Bortezomib ± gemcitabine | 88 | Closed | | North Central Cancer Treatment Group |
| Breast | Bortezomib | 12–35 | Closed | | MD Anderson |
| Lung (NSCLC) | Gemcitabine, carboplatin, bortezomib | 99 | Open | | Southwest Oncology Group (open) |
| Renal cell (67) | Bortezomib | 32 (actual) | Closed | 9% | Memorial Sloan–Kettering Cancer Center |
| Lung (NSCLC) | Bortezomib ± docetaxel | 155 | Open | | Johnson Cancer Center, UCLA |
| Breast | Bortezomib | 12–35 | Closed | | Northwestern University |
| Lung (SCLC) | Bortezomib | 40–80 | Open | | Southwest Oncology Group |
| Sarcoma (68) | Bortezomib | 20–41 | Open | | Memorial Sloan–Kettering Cancer Center |
| Melanoma | Bortezomib | 22–50 | Closed | | Mayo Clinic |
| Colorectal | Bortezomib | 21–41 | Open | | Princess Margaret Hospital, Toronto |
| Advanced TCC | Bortezomib | 15–40 | Open | | |
| Neuroendocrine (69) | Bortezomib | 16–25 | Closed | | Ohio State University |
| Stomach, GE junction | Bortezomib | 15–33 | Open | | Memorial Sloan–Kettering Cancer Center |
| Renal cell (66) | Bortezomib | 23 (actual) | Closed | 5% | University of Chicago |
| Lung (NSCLC) (70) | Bortezomib | 23–56 | Open | 8% | University of Pennsylvania |
| Stomach, GE junction | Bortezomib ± irinotecan | 33–58 | Open | | Cornell University |
| Bladder, renal pelvis, ureter (TCC) | Bortezomib | 20–35 | Open | | Princess Margaret Hospital, Toronto |

Source: www.cancer.gov unless otherwise specified.
GE, gastroesophageal; TCC, transitional cell carcinoma.

for 2 wk, then 1-wk rest. Six patients with carcinoid syndrome were allowed to be on a stable dose of long-acting octreotide. Preliminary results of this ongoing study are available. Eight patients were evaluable for response. Sixty-two percent (5/8) of patients had stable disease and 38% (3/8) had progressive disease, with no responders. Major toxicities included ileus, peripheral neuropathy, transient thrombocytopenia, neutropenia, fatigue, conjunctivitis, and hypertension/atrial flutter. Ileus was not an expected toxicity by the investigators but was resolved in all three patients after conservative management. Patients should be evaluated for ileus if clinically indicated. Bortezomib was found to be a relatively well-tolerated regimen in this cohort and might increase progression-free survival in metastatic neuroendocrine tumors (69).

Most recently, a phase II trial intended to test bortezomib alone or in combination with irinotecan in patients with metastatic colorectal cancer who progressed under irinotecan-based therapy was terminated early. It was a multicentered clinical trial where the primary objective was to determine tumor response to either bortezomib alone or bortezomib plus irinotecan in refractory colorectal cancer. Secondary objectives were to determine time to progression and survival and to assess tolerability and safety of the treatments. The dose of bortezomib was 1.5 mg/m$^2$ in the single-agent arm (given intravenously twice a week for 2 wk, followed by a 10-d rest period), whereas in the combination arm, it was 1.3 mg/m$^2$ (given intravenously twice a week for 2 wk, followed by a 10-d rest period). Bortezomib was administered immediately after a 90-min infusion of irinotecan at 125 mg/m$^2$ (d 1 and 8) when given on the same day. The decision for early termination was based after an interim analysis where both treatment arms failed meet preset efficacy criteria required to continue the study. Unfortunately, no further details regarding this trial are available at this time.

## 6. CONCLUSION

Proteosome inhibition might be a viable and potentially useful adjunct in solid tumor management. This novel approach achieves antitumor activity via multiple levels and pathways, interfering with tumor growth, angiogenesis, and metastasis, and it might allow overcoming of intrinsic chemoresistance. Numerous preclinical studies have demonstrated the potential usefulness of bortezomib alone or in combination in a variety of neoplasms. Furthermore, results from numerous phase I and early phase II trials show that bortezomib is a relatively well-tolerated agent, even in combination regimens. Currently, phase II studies are under way in order to better understand its efficacy and toxicity, as well as synergistic possibilities of this novel agent with the chemotherapeutic drugs already in use in major tumor types. Clinical data on the efficacy of bortezomib in solid tumors are limited at this time, although early results with bortezomib as a single agent are not as encouraging as with trials in multiple myeloma. In fact, a recent phase II trial of bortezomib alone or in combination with irinotecan in refractory colorectal patients was stopped early because of the lack of efficacy of either treatment arm. Further studies are needed to determine bortezomib's efficacy, ideal sequence regimen, as well as insights into clinical resistance and systemic toxicity in the treatment of solid tumors.

## ACKNOWLEDGMENT

This work was supported by National Institutes of Health–National Cancer Institute grants K24 CA 82754, 5 P30 CA14089, and U01CA62505 grants.

## REFERENCES

1. Coux O, Tanaka K, Goldberg AL. Structure and functions of the 20S and 26S proteasomes. Annu Rev Bio-chem 1996; 65:801–847.
2. Ciechanover A. The ubiquitin-proteasome pathway: on protein death and cell life. EMBO J 1998; 17(24): 7151–7160.
3. Spataro V, Norbury C, Harris AL. The ubiquitin-proteasome pathway in cancer. Br J Cancer 1998; 77(3): 448–455.
4. Pickart CM. Mechanisms underlying ubiquitination. Annu Rev Biochem 2001; 70:503–533.
5. King RW, Deshaies RJ, Peters JM, Kirschner MW. How proteolysis drives the cell cycle. Science 1996; 274(5293):1652–1659.
6. Chadebech P, Brichese L, Baldin V, Vidal S, Valette A. Phosphorylation and proteasome-dependent degradation of Bcl-2 in mitotic-arrested cells after microtubule damage. Biochem Biophys Res Commun 1999; 262(3):823–827.

7. Palombella VJ, Rando OJ, Goldberg AL, Maniatis T. The ubiquitin–proteasome pathway is required for processing the NF-kappa B1 precursor protein and the activation of NF-kappa B. Cell 1994; 78(5):773–785.

8. Conaway RC, Brower CS, Conaway JW. Emerging roles of ubiquitin in transcription regulation. Science 2002; 296(5571):1254–1258.

9. Lipkowitz S. The role of the ubiquitination–proteasome pathway in breast cancer: ubiquitin mediated degradation of growth factor receptors in the pathogenesis and treatment of cancer. Breast Cancer Res 2003; 5(1):8–15.

10. Kane RC, Bross PF, Farrell AT, Pazdur R. Velcade: U.S. FDA approval for the treatment of multiple myeloma progressing on prior therapy. Oncologist 2003; 8(6):508–513.

11. Glotzer M, Murray AW, Kirschner MW. Cyclin is degraded by the ubiquitin pathway. Nature 1991; 349 (6305):132–138.

12. Hateboer G, Kerkhoven RM, Shvarts A, Bernards R, Beijersbergen RL. Degradation of E2F by the ubiquitin–proteasome pathway: regulation by retinoblastoma family proteins and adenovirus transforming proteins. Genes Dev 1996; 10(23):2960–2970.

13. Blagosklonny MV, Wu GS, Omura S, El-Deiry WS. Proteosome-dependent regulation of p21$^{WAF/CIP1}$ expression. Biochem Biophys Res Commun 1996; 227:564–569.

14. Pagano M, Tam SW, Theodoras AM, Beer-Romero P, Del Sal G, Chau V, et al. Role of the ubiquitin–proteasome pathway in regulating abundance of the cyclin-dependent kinase inhibitor p27. Science 1995; 269(5224):682–685.

15. Machiels BM, Henfling ME, Gerards WL, Broers JL, Bloemendal H, Ramaekers FC, et al. Detailed analysis of cell cycle kinetics upon proteasome inhibition. Cytometry 1997; 28(3):243–252.

16. Catzavelos C, Bhattacharya N, Ung YC, Wilson JA, Roncari L, Sandhu C, et al. Decreased levels of the cell-cycle inhibitor p27Kip1 protein: prognostic implications in primary breast cancer. Nat Med 1997; 3(2):227–230.

17. Loda M, Cukor B, Tam SW, Lavin P, Fiorentino M, Draetta GF, et al. Increased proteasome-dependent degradation of the cyclin-dependent kinase inhibitor p27 in aggressive colorectal carcinomas. Nat Med 1997; 3(2):231–234.

18. Tsihlias J, Kapusta LR, DeBoer G, Morava-Protzner I, Zbieranowski I, Bhattacharya N, et al. Loss of cyclin-dependent kinase inhibitor p27Kip1 is a novel prognostic factor in localized human prostate adenocarcinoma. Cancer Res 1998; 58(3):542–548.

19. Catzavelos C, Tsao MS, DeBoer G, Bhattacharya N, Shepherd FA, Slingerland JM. Reduced expression of the cell cycle inhibitor p27Kip1 in non-small cell lung carcinoma: a prognostic factor independent of Ras. Cancer Res 1999; 59(3):684–688.

20. Mack PC, Davies AM, Lara PN, Gumerlock PH, Gandara DR. Integration of the proteasome inhibitor PS-341 (Velcade) into the therapeutic approach to lung cancer. Lung Cancer 2003; 41(Suppl 1):S89–S96.

21. Maki CG, Huibregtse JM, Howley PM. In vivo ubiquitination and proteasome-mediated degradation of p53(1). Cancer Res 1996; 56(11):2649–2654.

22. Cox LS, Lane DP. Tumour suppressors, kinases and clamps: how p53 regulates the cell cycle in response to DNA damage. Bioessays 1995; 17(6):501–508.

23. Ling YH, Liebes L, Jiang JD, Holland JF, Elliott PJ, Adams J, et al. Mechanisms of proteasome inhibitor PS-341-induced G(2)-M-phase arrest and apoptosis in human non-small cell lung cancer cell lines. Clin Cancer Res 2003; 9(3):1145–1154.

24. Bartek J, Lukas J. Mammalian G1- and S-phase checkpoints in response to DNA damage. Curr Opin Cell Biol 2001; 13(6):738–747.

25. Wu X, Levine AJ. p53 and E2F-1 cooperate to mediate apoptosis. Proc Natl Acad Sci USA 1994; 91(9): 3602–3606.

26. Herrmann JL, Briones F Jr, Brisbay S, Logothetis CJ, McDonnell TJ. Prostate carcinoma cell death resulting from inhibition of proteasome activity is independent of functional Bcl-2 and p53. Oncogene 1998; 17(22):2889–2899.

27. An WG, Hwang SG, Trepel JB, Blagosklonny MV. Protease inhibitor-induced apoptosis: accumulation of wt p53, p21WAF1/CIP1, and induction of apoptosis are independent markers of proteasome inhibition. Leukemia 2000; 14(7):1276–1283.

28. Adams J, Palombella VJ, Sausville EA, Johnson J, Destree A, Lazarus DD, et al. Proteasome inhibitors: a novel class of potent and effective antitumor agents. Cancer Res 1999; 59(11):2615–2622.

29. Dietrich C, Bartsch T, Schanz F, Oesch F, Wieser RJ. p53-dependent cell cycle arrest induced by N-acetyl-L-leucinyl-L-leucinyl-L-norleucinal in platelet-derived growth factor-stimulated human fibroblasts. Proc Natl Acad Sci USA 1996; 93(20):10,815–10,819.

30. Beg AA, Baltimore D. An essential role for NF-kappaB in preventing TNF-alpha-induced cell death. Science 1996; 274(5288):782–784.

31. Van Antwerp DJ, Martin SJ, Kafri T, Green DR, Verma IM. Suppression of TNF-alpha-induced apoptosis by NF-kappaB. Science 1996; 274(5288):787–789.

32. Wang CY, Mayo MW, Baldwin AS Jr. TNF- and cancer therapy-induced apoptosis: potentiation by inhibition of NF-kappaB. Science 1996; 274(5288):784–787.

33. Mayo MW, Wang CY, Cogswell PC, Rogers-Graham KS, Lowe SW, Der CJ, et al. Requirement of NF-kappaB activation to suppress p53-independent apoptosis induced by oncogenic Ras. Science 1997; 278(5344):1812–1815.

34. Zong WX, Edelstein LC, Chen C, Bash J, Gelinas C. The prosurvival Bcl-2 homolog Bfl-1/A1 is a direct transcriptional target of NF-kappaB that blocks TNFalpha-induced apoptosis. Genes Dev 1999; 13(4): 382–387.

35. Baldwin AS Jr. The NF-kappa B and I kappa B proteins: new discoveries and insights. Annu Rev Immunol 1996; 14:649–683.

36. Mayo MW, Madrid LV, Westerheide SD, Jones DR, Yuan XJ, Baldwin AS Jr, et al. PTEN blocks tumor necrosis factor-induced NF-kappa B-dependent transcription by inhibiting the transactivation potential of the p65 subunit. J Biol Chem 2002; 277(13):11,116–11,125.

37. Jones DR, Broad RM, Madrid LV, Baldwin AS Jr, Mayo MW. Inhibition of NF-kappaB sensitizes non-small cell lung cancer cells to chemotherapy-induced apoptosis. Ann Thorac Surg 2000; 70(3):930–936; discussion 936–937.

38. Wang CY, Cusack JC Jr, Liu R, Baldwin AS Jr. Control of inducible chemoresistance: enhanced antitumor therapy through increased apoptosis by inhibition of NF-kappaB. Nat Med 1999; 5(4):412–417.

39. Ni H, Ergin M, Huang Q, Qin JZ, Amin HM, Martinez RL, et al. Analysis of expression of nuclear factor kappa B (NF-kappa B) in multiple myeloma: downregulation of NF-kappa B induces apoptosis. Br J Haematol 2001; 115(2):279–286.

40. Izban KF, Ergin M, Huang Q, Qin JZ, Martinez RL, Schnitzer B, et al. Characterization of NF-kappaB expression in Hodgkin's disease: inhibition of constitutively expressed NF-kappaB results in spontaneous caspase-independent apoptosis in Hodgkin and Reed–Sternberg cells. Mod Pathol 2001; 14(4): 297–310.

41. Kordes U, Krappmann D, Heissmeyer V, Ludwig WD, Scheidereit C. Transcription factor NF-KB is constitutively activated in acute lymphoblastic leukemia cells. Leukemia 2000; 14(3):399–402.

42. Tricot G. New insights into the role of microenvironment in multiple myeloma. Lancet 2000; 355(9200): 248–250.

43. Nakshatri H, Bhat-Nakshatri P, Martin DA, Goulet RJ Jr, Sledge GW Jr. Constitutive activation of NF-kappaB during progression of breast cancer to hormone-independent growth. Mol Cell Biol 1997; 17(7): 3629–3639.

44. Patel NM, Nozaki S, Shortle NH, Bhat-Nakshatri P, Newton TR, Rice S, et al. Paclitaxel sensitivity of breast cancer cells with constitutively active NF-kappaB is enhanced by IkappaBalpha super-repressor and parthenolide. Oncogene 2000; 19(36):4159–4169.

45. Wang W, Abbruzzese JL, Evans DB, Larry L, Cleary KR, Chiao PJ. The nuclear factor-kappa B RelA transcription factor is constitutively activated in human pancreatic adenocarcinoma cells. Clin Cancer Res 1999; 5(1):119–127.

46. Mukhopadhyay T, Roth JA, Maxwell SA. Altered expression of the p50 subunit of the NF-kappa B transcription factor complex in non-small cell lung carcinoma. Oncogene 1995; 11(5):999–1003.

47. Henkel T, Machleidt T, Alkalay I, Kronke M, Ben-Neriah Y, Baeuerle PA. Rapid proteolysis of I kappa B-alpha is necessary for activation of transcription factor NF-kappa B. Nature 1993; 365(6442):182–185.

48. Alkalay I, Yaron A, Hatzubai A, Orian A, Ciechanover A, Ben-Neriah Y. Stimulation-dependent I kappa B alpha phosphorylation marks the NF-kappa B inhibitor for degradation via the ubiquitin-proteasome pathway. Proc Natl Acad Sci USA 1995; 92(23):10,599–10,603.

49. Teicher BA, Ara G, Herbst R, Palombella VJ, Adams J. The proteasome inhibitor PS-341 in cancer therapy. Clin Cancer Res 1999; 5(9):2638–2645.

50. Sunwoo JB, Chen Z, Dong G, Yeh N, Crowl Bancroft C, Sausville E, et al. Novel proteasome inhibitor PS-341 inhibits activation of nuclear factor-kappa B, cell survival, tumor growth, and angiogenesis in squamous cell carcinoma. Clin Cancer Res 2001; 7(5):1419–1428.

51. Cusack JC Jr, Liu R, Houston M, Abendroth K, Elliott PJ, Adams J, et al. Enhanced chemosensitivity to CPT-11 with proteasome inhibitor PS-341: implications for systemic nuclear factor-kappaB inhibition. Cancer Res 2001; 61(9):3535–3540.

52. Shah SA, Potter MW, McDade TP, Ricciardi R, Perugini RA, Elliott PJ, et al. 26S proteasome inhibition induces apoptosis and limits growth of human pancreatic cancer. J Cell Biochem 2001; 82(1):110–122.

53. Bold RJ, Virudachalam S, McConkey DJ. Chemosensitization of pancreatic cancer by inhibition of the 26S proteasome. J Surg Res 2001; 100(1):11–17.

54. Nawrocki ST, Sweeney-Gotsch B, Takamori R, McConkey DJ. The proteasome inhibitor bortezomib enhances the activity of docetaxel in orthotopic human pancreatic tumor xenografts. Mol Cancer Ther 2004; 3(1):59–70.

55. Fahy BN, Schlieman MG, Virudachalam S, Bold RJ. Schedule-dependent molecular effects of the proteasome inhibitor bortezomib and gemcitabine in pancreatic cancer. J Surg Res 2003; 113(1):88–95.

56. Aghajanian C, Soignet S, Dizon DS, Pien CS, Adams J, Elliott PJ, et al. A phase I trial of the novel proteasome inhibitor PS341 in advanced solid tumor malignancies. Clin Cancer Res 2002; 8(8):2505–2511.

57. Albanell J, Baselga J, Guix M, Twelves CJ, Glasspool R, Awada A, et al. Phase I study of bortezomib in combination with docetaxel in anthracycline-pretreated advanced breast cancer. In: American Society of Clinical Oncology; Chicago, IL, 2003 (abstract).

58. Aghajanian C, Dizon D, Yan XJ, Raizer J, Sabbatini P, Pezzulli S, et al. Phase I trial of PS-341 and carboplatin in recurrent ovarian cancer. In: American Society of Clinical Oncology; Chicago, IL, 2003 (abstract).

59. Appleman LJ, Ryan DP, Clark JW, Eder JP, Fishman M, Cusack JC, et al. Phase I dose escalation study of bortezomib and gemcitabine safety and tolerability in patients with advanced solid tumors. In: American Society of Clinical Oncology, Chicago, IL; 2003 (abstract).

60. Iqbal S, Lenz H-J, Groshen S, Wei Y, Gandara DR, Lara PN, et al. Phase I study of PS-341 in combination with 5-FU/LV in solid tumors. In: American Society of Clinical Oncology, Orlando, FL; 2002 (abstract).

61. Ryan DP, O'Neil B, Lima CR, Eder JP, Lynch TL, Cusack JC, et al. Phase I dose-escalation study of the proteasome inhibitor, bortezomib, plus irinotecan in patients with advanced solid tumors. In: American Society of Clinical Oncology, Chicago, IL; 2003 (abstract).

62. Papandreou C, Daliani D, Millikan RE, Tu S, Pagliaro L, Adams J, et al. Phase I study of intravenous (I.V.) Proteasome inhibitor PS-341 in patients (pts) with advanced malignancies. In: American Society of Clinical Oncology, 2001 (abstract).

63. Erlichman C, Adjei AA, Thomas JP, Wilding G, Reid JM, Sloan JA, et al. A phase I trial of the proteasome inhibitor PS-341 in patients with advanced cancer. In: American Society of Clinical Oncology, San Francisco, CA; 2001 (abstract).

64. Albanell J, Baselga J, Guix M, Twelves CT, Glasspool R, Awada A, et al. Phase I study of bortezomib in combination with docetaxel in anthracycline-pretreated advanced breast cancer. In: American Society of Clinical Oncology, Chicago, IL; 2003 (abstract).

65. Lebowitz PF, Harkins C, Conley B, Headlee D, Camphausen K, Guis D, et al. Concomitant therapy with proteasome inhibitor, bortezomib, and radiation in patients with recurrent or metastatic head and neck squamous cell carcinoma (HNSCC). In: American Society of Clinical Oncology, Chicago, IL; 2003 (abstract).

66. Davis NB, Taber DA, Ansari RH, Ryan CW, George C, Vokes EE, et al. Phase II trial of PS-341 in patients with renal cell cancer: a University of Chicago phase II consortium study. J Clin Oncol 2004; 22(1):115–119.

67. Drucker BJ, Schwartz L, Bacik J, Mazumdar M, Marion S, Motzer RJ. Phase II trial of PS-341 shows response in patients with advanced renal cell carcinoma. In: American Society of Clinical Oncology; Chicago, IL, 2003 (abstract).

68. Maki R, Kraft A, Demetri GD, Siegel E, Hirst C, Connors S, et al. A phase II multicenter study of proteasome inhibitor PS-341 (LDP-341, bortezomib) for untreated recurrent or metastatic soft tissue sarcoma (STS); CTEP study 1757. In: American Society of Clinical Oncology, Chicago, IL; 2003 (abstract).

69. Shah MH, Martin E, Ellison C, Kraut E, Kindler H, Young D, et al. A phase II study of proteasome inhibitor PS-341 in metastatic neuroendocrine tumors. In: American Society of Clinical Oncology, Orlando, FL; 2002 (abstract).

70. Stevenson J, Nho CW, Schick J, Johnson SW, Algazy K, Miller D, et al. Phase II clinical/pharmacodynamic trial of the proteasome inhibitor PS-341 in advanced non-small cell lung cancer. In: American Society of Oncology; Chicago, IL, 2003 (abstract).

# 34 Tumor Necrosis Factor Family of Ligands and Receptors in Cancer Therapy

*Anas Younes, MD and Andrea Cerutti, MD*

**SUMMARY**

The tumor necrosis factor (TNF) family members are membrane-bound and soluble proteins that play an important physiological role in lymphocyte homeostasis, immunity, inflammation, and calcium metabolism. Abnormalities in the expression or function of these ligands and their receptors have been linked to several human diseases, including autoimmunity and cancer. These observations provided the background for exploring this system to design novel treatment strategies for autoimmune diseases, bone disorders, and cancer. Because the systemic administration of some TNF family members is toxic to normal cells, only a few have a potential therapeutic value. In this concise review, we focus on the potential role of six TNF family members in cancer therapy: CD30 ligand, CD40 ligand, receptor activator of nuclear factor-κB (RANK)/ RANK ligand, TNF-related apoptosis-inducing ligand (TRAIL) Apo-2L/TRAIL, BAFF, and APRIL and their receptors.

**Key Words:** Hodgkin; TRAIL; apoptosis; CD30; CD40; RANK; BAFF; TACI; IL-13; BlyS.

## 1. INTRODUCTION

The current membership of the tumor necrosis factor (TNF) family include 26 receptors and 18 ligands. The complexity of this family is illustrated by the fact that some ligands have more than one receptor, and some receptors are shared between more than one ligand

From: *Cancer Drug Discovery and Development: The Oncogenomics Handbook*
Edited by: W. J. LaRochelle and R. A. Shimkets © Humana Press Inc., Totowa, NJ

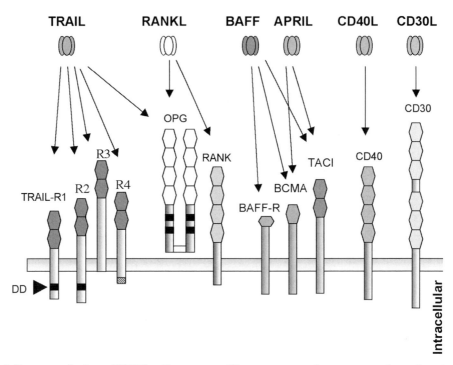

**Fig. 1.** Structure of selected TNF family receptors. These receptors share sequence homology in their extracellular domains that contain a variable number of cysteine-rich pseudorepeats (hexagons). Some of these ligands bind to more than one receptor, and some receptors are shared with more than one ligand. Both TRAIL-R1 and TRAIL-R2 cytoplasmic tails contain a death domain (DD) sequence, which is important for their ability to induce cell death. TRAIL-R3 and TRAIL-R4 do not induce cell death, as TRAIL-R3 lacks a cytoplasmic tail and TRAIL-R4 has an incomplete DD.

(Fig. 1). The majority of these ligands exist as membrane-bound type II proteins (N-terminal inside the cell and C-terminal outside the cell) or as secreted soluble proteins *(1,2)*. The biologically active forms of the ligands and their receptors are self-assembled protein trimers that share 25–30% sequence homology at their trimerization sites, but not at the binding sites. The receptors also exist in either membrane-bound (type I proteins, or type III) or soluble forms. These receptors are characterized by the presence of 40-amino-acid cysteine-rich repeats in the extracellular domains (Fig. 1) *(1,3)*. Each cysteine-rich domain typically contains two motifs with three disulfide bonds. The intracellular tails of these receptors share minimal or no sequence homology, accounting for their diverse biologic functions. The cytoplasmic tails signal by interacting with two major groups of intracellular proteins: TNF receptor-associated factors (TRAFs) *(4,5)* and death domain (DD)-containing proteins (Fig. 2) *(6–8)*. There are at least six human TRAFs that can interact with TRAF-binding sites on the cytoplasmic tail of some of these receptors to initiate several signaling pathways, including mitogen-activated protein kinases (MAPK), AKT, and nuclear factor-κB (NF-κB). TNF family receptors that have a DD sequence in their cytoplasmic tail are called death receptors. The DD binds to adaptor proteins called FADD (Fas-associated death domain) or TRADD (TNF-receptor-associated death domain (Fig. 2).

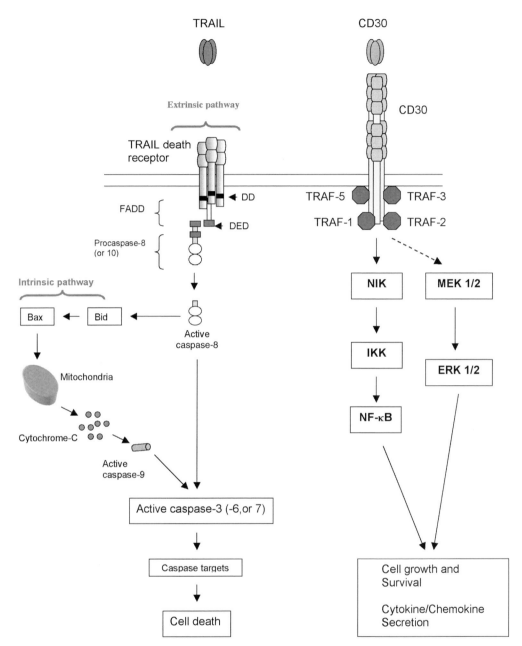

**Fig. 2.** Examples of signaling pathways of a death receptor (TRAIL-R1 or TRAIL-R2) and a survival receptor (CD30). DED, death effector domain.

## 2. STRUCTURE AND EXPRESSION

### 2.1. CD30 and CD30 Ligand

CD30 is a 120-kDa type I transmembrane protein that contains six extracellular cysteine-rich domains (Fig. 1) *(9)*. CD30 is shed in a soluble form (sCD30), which can be detected in sera of patients with CD30+ tumors, autoimmune disease, and viral infection

Table 1
Characteristics of Selected TNF and TNF Receptor Family Members

| Member | Other Names | Human Gene | Phenotype Associated With Loss of Function |
|--------|-------------|------------|--------------------------------------------|
| CD30 | — | 1p36 | Unknown |
| CD30L | CD153 | 9q33 | Conflicting data on possible role in T-cell selection |
| CD40 | — | 20q12-q13.2 | Defect in germinal center formation and immunoglobulin class switch |
| CD40L | CD154 | Xq26 | Hyper IgM syndrome, defective cellular and humoral immunity |
| BAFF | BlyS, TALL-1, THANK, zTNF-4 | 13q34 | Loss of mature follicular and marginal zone B-cells |
| APRIL | TALL-2, TRDL-1 | 17p13 | Normal phenotype |
| BAFFR | BR3 | 22q13 | Similar phenotype to BAFF −/− |
| BCMA | — | 16p13 | Normal phenotype |
| TACI | — | 17p11 | B-Cell proliferation and autoimmunity |
| RANK | TRANCE receptor | 18q22.1 | Osteopetrosis, absence of lymph nodes, defective B-cell development, defective mammary gland development |
| RANKL | TRANCE, OPGL, ODF | 13q14 | Osteoporosis, absence of lymph nodes, defective lymphocyte development, defective mammary gland development |
| OPG | Osteoprotegerin, OCIF, TR1 | 8q24 | Osteopetrosis |
| TRAIL | Apo2L | 3q26 | Decreases antitumor immune surveillance |
| TRAIL-R1 | DR4, Apo2 | 8p21 | Unknown |
| TRAIL-R2 | DR5, KILLER, TRICK2A, TRICKB | 8p22-p21 | Unknown |
| TRAIL-R3 | DcR1, LIT, TRID | 8p22-p21 | Unknown |
| TRAIL-R4 | DcR2, TRUND | 8p21 | Unknown |
| TRAIL-R4 | DcR2, TRUND | 8p21 | Unknown |

(10). Elevated levels of serum-soluble CD30 correlates with poor prognosis in patients with anaplastic large cell lymphoma or Hodgkin's disease (11–13). The expression of CD30 in healthy individuals is restricted to a small number of activated B- and T-lymphocytes. CD30 is also expressed in several types of malignancy, including Hodgkin's disease, anaplastic large cell lymphoma, immunoblastic lymphoma, multiple myeloma, adult T-cell lymphoma leukemia, mycosis fungoides, germ cell malignancies, and thyroid carcinoma, in addition to several nonmalignant disorders (10,14).

CD30L (CD153) was identified in 1993 as a member of the TNF family, and its gene is mapped to human chromosome 9q33 (Table 1) (15). Although CD30 receptor is rarely expressed in healthy individuals, CD30L is expressed by a wide variety of hematopoietic cells, epithelial cells, and Hassall's corpuscles in the thymus medulla. CD30L is also expressed by several types of lymphoid tumor, including by chronic lymphocytic leukemia (CLL), follicular B-cell lymphoma, Hairy cell leukemia, T-cell lymphoblastic lymphoma, and adult T-cell leukemia lymphoma *(2,16–19)*.

## 2.2. CD40 and CD40L

CD40 receptor was identified in the mid-1980s by two independent groups, and almost a decade later, its ligand (CD40L) was identified *(20,21)*. The extracellular domain of CD40 contains four cysteine-rich repeats and shares sequence homology with receptor activator of nuclear factor-κB (RANK) and CD30 (Fig. 1) *(22)*. CD40 and CD40L genes are mapped to human chromosomes 20 and X, respectively (Table 1).

CD40 is more widely expressed than CD30; it is expressed by normal B-lymphocytes, monocytes, and dendritic cells, a subset of T-cells, in addition to epithelial (urinary bladder, ovary, breast, and endobronchial cells) and endothelial cells *(10,22)*. CD40 is also expressed in several types of malignant cell, including B- and T-cell lymphomas, Reed–Sternberg cells of Hodgkin's disease, and several carcinomas *(10,23,24)*.

CD40 ligand (CD40L, CD154) is predominantly expressed by activated T-lymphocytes (more frequently in CD4+ than in CD8+ lymphocytes), but can also be expressed by activated B-lymphocytes, natural killer (NK) cells, monocytes, basophils, eosinophils, dendritic cells, and platelets, in addition to nonhematopoietic cells, including endothelial and smooth muscle cells *(10)*. Solube CD40L (sCD40L) is detected in sera of patients with lymphoma, chronic lymphocytic leukemia, autoimmune disease, and essential thrombocythemia *(25–27)*. Recently, a new gene called AKNA was reported to regulate the expression of both CD40 and CD40L *(28)*.

CD40L has diverse physiologic functions, including priming dendritic cells to activate CD8+ cytotoxic T-cells, B-cell selection and survival, and immunoglobulin isotype switching. CD40 plays a role in enhancing antigen presentation by upregulating CD80 (B7.1) and CD86 (B7.2) costimulatory molecules and in regulating cytokine and chemokine secretion *(22)*. An inherited deficiency of CD40L causes the X-linked hyper IgM syndrome and severe immune impairment, whereas sustained expression of CD40L in transgenic mice causes both benign and malignant T-cell lymphoproliferative diseases *(27,29–32)*.

The function of CD40 in B-cell lymphoma and leukemia has extensively been examined by several groups *(14)*. In some studies, conflicting results were reported perhaps as a result of the different methods that were used (activating CD40 with CD40L vs agonistic antibodies, cell lines vs primary tumor cells, and mouse vs human cells). CD40 is also expressed by the malignant H/RS cells of Hodgkin's disease *(24,33–35)*. Activation of CD40 on Reed–Sternberg cells induces NF-κB, cytokine and chemokine secretion, and, perhaps, survival *(33)*. Although H/RS cells do not express CD40L or CD30L, they could receive these cytokines from the surrounding benign infiltrating cells in the microenvironment, including B-cells, T-cells, and eosinophils *(36–39)*.

## 2.3. BAFF, APRIL, and Their Receptors

BAFF (also known as BLyS, TALL-1, ZANK, zTNF4, and TNFS 13B) was identified in 1999 by several independent groups as a type II transmembrane protein that belongs to the TNF family *(40–42)*. BAFF is expressed by macrophages, monocytes, and dendritic cells but not by benign B- or T-lymphocytes. BAFF is also secreted in a soluble form. BAFF binds to three receptors (Fig. 1); the BAFF-R (also known as BR-3) is the shortest one and is specific for BAF. The other two receptors are called TACI (transmembrane activator and calcium modulator and cyclophylin ligand interactor) and BCMA·(B-cell maturation antigen). TACI and BCMA are shared with a related TNF family member called APRIL (a proliferation-inducing ligand; also called TRDL-1 or TALL-2) *(43–45)*. These three receptors are almost exclusively expressed by B-lymphocytes, although TACI transcripts have been observed in T-lymphocytes. BAFF-R has one partial extracellular cystein-rich domain, BCMA has one complete cystein-rich domain, and TACI has two of them (Fig. 1). The genes for BAFF-R, TACI, and BCMA are located on human chromosomes 22, 16, and 17, respectively (Table 1). BAFF is an important survival factor for B-lymphocytes. Mice lacking BAFF or having mutant BAFF-R display almost a total loss of B-lymphocytes (marginal zone B-cells and follicular B-cells) (Table 1) *(46–50)*. Overproduction of BAFF in transgenic mice has been associated with autoimmune diseases *(51,52)*, and elevated levels of soluble BAFF has been detected in sera from patients with several autoimmune diseases, including rheumatoid arthritis, systemic lupus erythematosus (SLE), and Sjogren's syndrome *(53,54)*.

APRIL (TRDL-1 or TALL-2) is a secreted soluble protein that shares the highest sequence homology with BAFF. APRIL is expressed in monocytes, macrophages, dendritic cells, and T-lymphocytes. APRIL protein is cleaved inside the cell before it is secreted as a soluble protein. APRIL can form homotrimers and heterotrimers with BAFF. APRIL binds to TACI and BCMA receptors that are also shared with BAFF. Although no APRIL-specific receptor has been identified yet, it is believed that such a receptor is likely to exist.

## 2.4. RANK Ligand and Its Receptors

The RANK ligand binds to two distinctive receptors: RANK and osteoprotegerin (OPG) *(55–57)*. RANK exhibits the highest similarity to CD40 and TNF receptor-2. RANK protein expression is restricted to dendritic cells, CD4+ and CD8+ T-cells, and osteoclast hematopoietic precursor cells. OPG is a secreted receptor dimer that binds to both RANKL and TRAIL. It has four cysteine-rich pseudorepeats followed by two functional DDs and a dimerization motif. RANK ligand (RANKL; also known as OPG ligand, or TRANCE, or osteoclast differentiation factor [ODF]) exists in a 40-kDa to 45-kDa transmembrane form and in a smaller 31-kDa soluble form. RANKL is expressed primarily by activated T-cells and osteoblasts. In cancer patients, the malignant cells could secrete several cytokines and hormones that can upregulate RANKL expression in osteoblasts (Fig. 3). However, some cancer cells might express RANKL, which can directly activate osteoclasts.

## 2.5. TRAIL and Its Receptors

TRAIL (Apo2 ligand) is a death protein that shares the highest sequence homology with Fas ligand (28%) and TNF-α (23%). TRAIL has four exclusive receptors: TRAIL-R1 (DR4), TRAIL-R2 (DR5, KILLER, TRICK2), TRAIL-R3 (DcR1, TRID, LIT), and TRAIL-R4 (DcR2, TRAIL-R4, TRUNDD) *(2,6,8)*. TRAIL also shares OPG receptor with RANKL, but it binds to it with a lower affinity *(58)*. TRAIL-R1 and TRAIL-R2 are death receptors that contain a death domain (DD) sequence in their intracellular tail, whereas TRAIL-R3 and TRAIL-R4 are decoy receptors (Fig. 1) *(59)*. TRAIL-R3 lacks an intracellular tail, whereas TRAIL-R4 has an incomplete DD in its intracellular tail. The genes for all four TRAIL receptors are clustered on the short arm of chromosome 8 (Table 1). Normal tissues usually do not express TRAIL-R1 and TRAIL-R2; therefore, they are protected from TRAIL-induced apoptosis. In contrast, most tumors express TRAIL-R1 and TRAIL-R2, making them more sensitive to TRAIL-induced cell death. TRAIL-R3 and TRAIL-R4

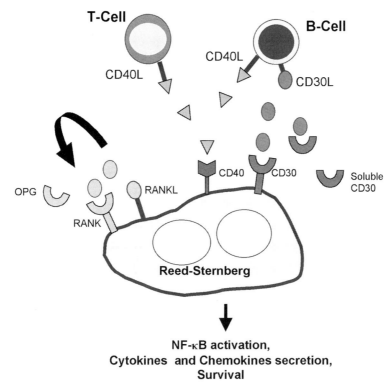

**Fig. 3.** The complexity of Reed–Sternberg of Hodgkin's disease. These cells express several TNF-receptor family members, including CD30, CD40, RANK, and TRAIL receptors. The ligands for these receptors are either expressed by the cancer cells (RANKL) or by the surrounding cells in the microenvironment (CD30L and CD40L).

can be expressed by both normal and malignant tissues. Although TRAIL mRNA is constitutively expressed in most normal tissues, the protein expression is restricted to activated T-cells and NK cells. However, several tumor cells can aberrantly express functional TRAIL.

## 3. BIOLOGIC FUNCTIONS AND SIGNALING PATHWAYS

### 3.1. CD30L

CD30 cytoplasmic tail contains several TRAF-binding motifs that can bind TRAF-1, TRAF-2, TRAF-3, and TRAF-5 and activate NF-κB and ERK (Fig. 2) (60–65). The exact function of CD30 and CD30L in healthy individuals remains poorly understood, as no human diseases have been linked to defects in the CD30 and CD30L genes (Table 1). The involvement of this ligand/receptor pair in T-cell-negative selection and removal of autoreactive thymocytes remains somewhat controversial. Proposed physiologic functions of CD30L include a role in T-cell costimulation, cytokine and chemokine secretion, regulation of class-switch DNA recombination, and antibody production in subsets of human B-cells (66,67). CD30L might induce cell cycle arrest and cell death in some CD30+ tumors, perhaps because of its differential effect on NF-κB activation (18,68–72).

## 3.2. CD40L

CD40 binds TRAF-2, TRAF-3, TRAF-5, and TRAF-6, leading to the activation of diverse signaling pathways, including ERK, c-jun amino terminal kinase (JNK), p38 MAPK, and NF-κB. CD40L has several biologic functions, including priming dendritic cells to activate CD8+ cytotoxic T-cells, in addition to promoting B-cell survival, proliferation, differentiation, and immunoglobulin isotype switching (73–80). Furthermore, CD40L enhances antigen presentation by upregulating CD80 (B7.1) and CD86 (B7.2) costimulatory molecules. The CD40L gene is located on chromosome X, and an inherited deficiency of CD40L causes the X-linked hyper IgM syndrome.

## 3.3. BAF and APRIL

As discussed earlier, BAFF binds with high affinity to three different receptors: BAFF-R, TACI, and BCMA. These three receptors activate B-cells mainly through the NF-κB–Rel family of transcription factors (53,81). By recruiting TRAF adaptor proteins, TACI and BCMA activate the IκB kinase (IKK) complex, which includes two catalytic α- and β-subunits and a regulatory γ-subunit (82,83). Phosphorylation of IκB, an NF-κB inhibitor that retains p50, p65, and c-Rel NF-κB–Rel proteins in an inactive cytoplasmic state, by the IKK complex is followed by IκB ubiquitination, proteasome-mediated IκB degradation and p50, p65, and c-Rel translocation from the cytoplasm to the nucleus. Unlike TACI and BCMA, BAFF-R binds TRAF-3 and activates an alternative NF-κB pathway, in which p100 phosphorylation by TRAF-induced NIK-activated IKKκ is followed by p100 ubiquitination and processing to p52, which then translocates to the nucleus in association with RelB (44,84–86). Once in the nucleus, NF-κB–Rel proteins activate survival genes, such as Bcl-2, as well as genes involved in B-cell activation, proliferation, and differentiation, including Ig class switching (81,87–89).

BAFF is expressed by monocytes, macrophages, dendritic cells, and neutrophils (40–43, 45,90–92). The membrane-bound trimer can also be cleaved by a furinlike convertase to yield a soluble BAFF (93). BAFF expression can be further increased by cytokines, including interferon (IFN)-α, IFN-γ, ligand (CD40L), and lymphotoxin-α/β (LT) (94–96). BAFF binds to three receptors called BAFF-R, TACI, and BCM (Table 1) (47,49,50,83,89,97). BAFF-R is essential for peripheral survival and would collaborate with TACI and BCMA to initiate/amplify B-cell antibody production in response to T-cell-independent and T-cell-dependent antigens (53,81).

Several lines of evidence show that BAFF is critical for the conservation of the peripheral B-cell repertoire. BAFF-deficient mice show severe depletion of marginal zone (MZ) and follicular B-cells, including naïve, germinal center (GC), memory, and antibody-secreting plasma cells (98,99). This results in hypogammaglobulinemia and impaired IgM, IgG, and IgA production in response to T-cell-dependent and T-cell-independent antigens. A similar phenotype is observed in mice injected with soluble TACI–Ig, BCMA–Ig and BAFF-R–Ig decoy receptors, which sequester BAFF from B-cell-bound receptors (100). Conversely, BAFF transgenic mice display B-cell hyperplasia, hypergammaglobulinemia, autoimmune manifestations, and enhanced T-cell-dependent and T-cell-independent antibody responses (47,51,52).

BAFF transmits B-cell survival signals through BAFF-R, because BAFF-R-deficient mice and A/WySnJ mice, which express a functionally inactive BAFF-R, show a phenotype similar to that of BAFF-deficient mice (88,89,98). The role of TACI appears to be more complex. TACI deficiency is associated with B-cell hyperplasia, enhanced T-cell-dependent antibody production, autoimmune disorders, and B-cell tumors *(44,101)*. In addition, TACI engagement triggers B-cell apoptosis and impairs B-cell responses to BAFF and the CD40 ligand *(44)*. This latter is a TNF family member mainly expressed by antigen-activated CD4[+] T-cells and induces CD40-expressing B-cells to undergo antibody production, including IgG and IgA class switching, in response to T-cell-dependent antigens *(102)*. Thus, TACI might regulate the homeostasis of the B-cell compartment by inhibiting BAFF-R and CD40 signaling. Interestingly, TACI-deficient mice show impaired IgG and IgA production in response to T-cell-independent antigens *(101)*. This indicates that TACI might account for the ability of BAFF to trigger CD40-independent IgG and IgA class switching *(96,103)*. The role of BCMA remains unclear. Although BCMA-deficient mice lack an overt phenotype, recent findings suggest that BCMA is important for the survival of Ig-secreting plasma cells *(81,104)*.

APRIL is expressed and secreted by myeloid cells and binds to TACI and BCMA receptors on B-cells with lower and higher affinity than BAFF, respectively *(96,97,105)*. Unlike BAFF-deficient mice, APRIL-deficient mice show conserved peripheral B-cell numbers and normal antibody responses (Table 1) *(106)*. This is in line with the inability of APRIL to bind and activate BAFF-R. Nevertheless, APRIL collaborates with BAFF to enhance plasma cell survival through BCMA *(81,104)*. In addition, APRIL triggers T-cell-independent IgG and IgA class switching *(96)*, possibly through TACI *(101)*. Finally, APRIL stimulates the growth and survival of nonimmune cell types *(107)*. Because these cells lack TACI, BCMA, and BAFF-R, it is believed that these biologic functions are mediated through an APRIL-specific receptor that is yet to be identified.

### *3.4. RANK*

RANK signals through TRAF-1, TRAF-2, TRAF-3, TRAF-5, and TRAF-6 to activate several signaling pathways, including NF-κB, AKT, JNK, ERK, p38, and STAT3 *(73, 108–112)* RANK$^{-/-}$ or RANKL$^{-/-}$ mice have profound defects in bone resorption (osteopetrosis), lymph node formation, and B-cell development *(113–115)*. In contrast, OPG$^{-/-}$ mice developed osteoporosis and hypercalcemia, and homozygous deletion of the OPG gene has been recently linked to Paget's disease *(116,117)*. In addition to the critical role of RANKL/RANK in bone metabolism, RANKL also enhances survival and function of dendritic cells and plays a role in mammary gland development and angiogenesis *(118–121)*. The functional balance between RANKL and its two receptors is critical for bone and calcium homeostasis. This balance is shifted toward bone destruction and calcium resorption in several human cancers, including multiple myeloma *(122,123)* (Fig. 4). In fact, the cancer cells can secrete several cytokines and hormones that induce RANKL expression on osteoblasts, with subsequent activation of osteoclasts. Alternatively, some cancer cells might express and secrete RANKL and directly activate osteoclasts (Fig. 4). OPG inhibits the effects of RANKL on osteoclasts both in vitro and in vivo. It is, therefore, not surprising that serum OPG levels are decreased in patients with lytic bone lesions such as multiple myeloma and Paget's disease *(117,124,125)*. In contrast, patients with blastic bone lesions, such as advanced prostate carcinoma, have elevated serum OPG levels *(126,127)*. Interestingly, the malignant cells of Hodgkin's disease and non-Hodgkin's lymphoma have been reported to express OPG, and serum OPG is also elevated in these patients, but the significance of this observation remains unknown *(112,125)*.

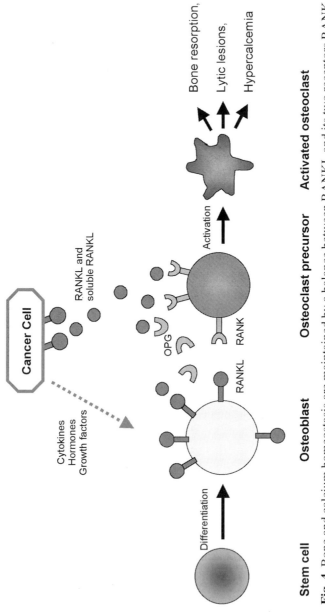

**Fig. 4.** Bone and calcium homeostasis are maintained by a balance between RANK and its two receptors RANK and OPG. This balance is frequently disturbed in patients with cancer favoring hypercalcemia and lytic bone lesions. Cancer cells can secrete cytokines and hormones to upregulate RANKL on osteoblasts or they can express RANKL bypassing the need for osteoblasts.

### 3.5. TRAIL

The primary physiologic function of TRAIL is immune surveillance *(128,129)*. This is predominantly achieved by NK cells that express TRAIL, which will kill target cells that express TRAIL death receptors TRAIL-R1 and TRAIL-R2. Both TRAIL-deficient (TRAIL$^{-/-}$) mice and mice that receive treatment using an anti-TRAIL blocking antibody are more susceptible to tumor initiation and metastasis *(128,129)*. TRAIL could also play a role in regulating cytokine and chemokine expression and inflammation, perhaps by activating NF-κB *(130–134)*. TRAIL induces cell death by recruiting and activating caspase-8 and caspase-10 to R1 and R2 receptors, followed by a cascade of caspases (extrinsic receptor-mediated pathway) *(6,8,14,135)*. In some cell types, TRAIL might also activate the mitochondria and caspase-9 intrinsic pathway (Fig. 2). In the extrinsic receptor-mediated pathway, R1 and R2 recruit a Fas-associated DD adapter protein (FADD), which, in turn, recruits caspase-8 and caspase-10, leading to activation of the execution caspase-3, caspase-6, and caspase-7 and subsequent cell death (Fig. 2). TRAIL activates the intrinsic pathway by cleaving Bid, which promotes Bax and Bak activation and oligomerization, leading to mitochondrial membrane damage and cytochrome-*c* release *(136,137)*. Subsequently, caspase-9 is activated, which then activates the execution caspase-3, caspase-6, and caspase-7 (Fig. 2), in addition to activating death pathways. It remains unclear how cells resist TRAIL-induced cell death. However, several mechanisms of resistance to TRAIL have been proposed in different cell lines, including TRAIL R1 and R2 receptor mutations, cFLIP overexpression, caspase-8 deficiency, Bax deficiency, Bcl-2 overexpression, inhibitor of apoptosis (IAP) family of proteins overexpression, NF-κB activation, protein kinase C activation, caspase-8 hypermethylation, and constitutive ERK 1/2 and AKT expression *(137–147)*. Aberrant but functional expression of TRAIL has been reported in tumor cells, including myeloid, lymphoid, breast, and brain tumor cells *(148–150)*. However, whether this expression can make tumor cells escape immune surveillance or enable tumor cells to invade tissues remains undetermined.

## 4. POTENTIAL ROLES IN CANCER THERAPY

### 4.1. CD30/CD30L

Because CD30 expression is restricted to a small number of normal cells, its expression in malignant cells makes it a good target for antibody therapy (Table 2). However, because CD30 triggering might produce paradoxical effects in different CD30+ cells, choosing a therapeutic anti-CD30 antibody should be performed carefully. Recently, a chimeric anti-CD30 antibody was reported to induce cell cycle arrest and apoptosis in Hodgkin's-derived cell lines and is currently being evaluated in a phase I study in patients with relapsed Hodgkin's disease and other CD30+ hematologic malignancies *(151)*. Unconjugated anti-CD30 antibodies have been effective in prolonging survival of mice bearing chemotherapy-resistant human CD30+ anaplastic large cell lymphomas. In addition to the use of unconjugated anti-CD30 antibodies, both bispecific antibodies and immune-toxin conjugates have been evaluated with promising results.

### 4.2. CD40/CD40L

The optimal use of the CD40L/CD40 pathway in cancer therapy remains controversial because of conflicting reports of CD40L activity against cultured and primary cancer cells in vivo and in vitro *(2,80)*. CD40 is expressed in B-cell lymphoid malignancies and

Table 2
Planned or Ongoing Clinical Trials
of Selected TNF Ligand and Receptor Family Members in Patients With Cancer

| Pathway | Clinical Development | Potential Disease Target |
|---------|---------------------|--------------------------|
| CD30 | Anti-CD30 antibody | Hodgkin's lymphoma, anaplastic large cell lymphoma, multiple myeloma |
| CD40 | Anti-CD40 antibody Anti-CD40L antibody | Non-Hodgkin's lymphoma, Hodgkin's disease, multiple myeloma, epithelial tumors |
| BAFF | Anti-BAFF, soluble BAFFR or BR3 | B-Cell lymphoma, chronic lymphocytic leukemia, multiple myeloma, autoimmune disease |
| RANK | Anti-RANKL, soluble OPG | Multiple myeloma, malignancy-associated hypercalcemia and osteoporosis |
| TRAIL | Soluble TRAIL, agonistic anti-TRAIL-R1 and TRAIL-R2 | Non-Hodgkin's lymphoma, multiple myeloma, solid tumors |

in several types of solid tumor. Depending on the tumor type, CD40 activation can lead to cell survival or growth arrest and apoptosis in vitro. However, in vivo activation of CD40 is complicated by the added immunologic functions of the CD40/CD40L system. CD40L is a survival factor for normal germinal center B cells, and this prosurvival function is maintained in the primary B-cell lymphoma and leukemia (2,80). Furthermore, when freshly isolated primary malignant B-cell lymphoma or leukemia cells were stimulated with CD40L or activating anti-CD40 antibodies, they became resistant to chemotherapy and Fas ligand, presumably because of upregulation of antiapoptotic molecules, including Bcl-xL, Mcl-1, NF-κB, survivin, and cFLIP (152–156). However, in a few cell lines, CD40 activation might promote survival or induce apoptosis. Finally, because CD40L and CD40 can be coexpressed by several types of B-cell malignancies, an autocrine/paracrine CD40L/CD40 survival loop has been proposed to play a role in the pathogenesis and survival of some B-cell neoplasms (157). Because of the complexity of CD40/CD40L functions, the optimal use of the CD40/CD40L system in the treatment of lymphoid malignancies and in cancer has not been determined. One proposed strategy is to therapeutically interrupt the CD40/CD40L survival loop by using blocking antibodies to either CD40L or CD40 (157). An opposing but intriguing strategy is to activate CD40 to generate therapeutically effective T-cell-mediated antitumor responses. This observation generated some enthusiasm about the potential use of CD40L in cancer immunotherapy and vaccines (158–160). Some of these strategies were recently evaluated in phase I clinical trials. In one study, the safety and efficacy of recombinant human CD40L (rhuCD40L) trimer was examined in patients with relapsed solid tumors or aggressive lymphoma (161, 162). One patient with T-cell lymphoma achieved a partial response, whereas none of the eight patients with B-cell lymphoma responded. A second phase I study used a CD40L gene transfer approach in patients with relapsed chronic lymphocytic leukemia (CLL) (163). Patients were treated with a single infusion of autologous CLL cells transfected with adenovirus CD40L. An increase in plasma levels of interleukin (IL)-12 and INF-γ and in total peripheral blood and CLL-specific T-cell counts were observed in some patients.

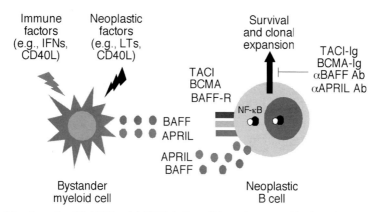

**Fig. 5.** Model for the role of BAFF and APRIL in B-cell lymphoma and leukemia. Neoplastic B-cells evade apoptosis upon engagement of TACI, BCMA, and BAFF-R by paracrine (provided by bystander myeloid cells, including dendritic cells and macrophages ) and autocrine BAFF and APRIL.

## 4.3. BAFF and APRIL

As discussed earlier, several mouse studies, such as *BAFF*-transgenic mice and TACI-deficient mice, develop lymphoproliferative disorders, including marginal zone (MZ) B-cell lymphoma *(44,53)*. This tendency increases in the absence of TNF-α *(164)*. Recently, dysregulated BAFF and APRIL have also been observed in patients with lymphomas. Soluble BAFF is increased in patients with certain types of non-Hodgkin's lymphoma (NHL), including germinal center B cell-derived follicular lymphoma. Soluble BAFF and APRIL are also increased in patients with CLL and multiple myeloma (MM) *(165, 166)*. Interestingly, soluble BAFF is also increased in patients with autoimmune diseases such as Sjoegren's syndrome, which is often associated with low-grade B-cell lymphoma *(53)*. Moreover, the chromosomal 13q32-34 region, which encompasses the *BAFF* gene, is often amplified in non-Hodgkin's lymphomas (NHLs).

The importance of BAFF and APRIL in B-cell tumors is further confirmed by recent studies showing that malignant B-cells from CLL, MM, and different types of NHLs aberrantly express BAFF and APRIL *(167–169)*. These tumor cells also express TACI, BCMA and BAFF-R, suggesting that the autonomous accumulation of B-cell tumors might be supported at least in part by an autocrine BAFF- and APRIL-mediated loop (Fig. 5). Consistent with this observation, neutralization of BAFF and APRIL by soluble TACI or BCMA decoy receptors have been shown to decrease the survival of neoplastic B-cells *(167–169)*. This effect is associated with reduced activation of NF-κB–Rel and downregulation of intracellular prosurvival proteins, including Bcl-2 *(164,165)*. Conversely, external BAFF or APRIL, which are likely provided in vivo by bystander myeloid and stromal cells, rescues neoplastic B-cells from spontaneous apoptosis or from apoptosis induced by antineoplastic drugs *(169–171)*. This effect is associated with activation of NF-κB–Rel and upregulation of intracellular antiapoptotic proteins, including Bcl-2 *(167–169)*. Collectively, these findings suggest that malignant cells from different types of B-cell neoplasia evade apoptosis through autocrine and paracrine BAFF and APRIL.

The mechanism by which neoplastic B-cells dysregulate BAFF and APRIL expression remains unclear. In most NHLs, somatic hypermutation of Ig V(D)J genes is actively ongoing and might alter *BAFF* and *APRIL* gene transcription by aberrantly targeting their

5' promoters. Abnormal BAFF expression might also stem from 13q32-34 amplification or aberrant activation of NF-κB–Rel *(172)*, a key inducer of *BAFF* gene transcription *(173)*. Genetic alterations of genes encoding endogenous IKK-activating proteins, such as Bcl-10 and Malt *(172)*, or IKK activation by proteins produced by B-cell lymphotropic viruses, including Epstein–Barr virus *(173)*, might also play an important role in the upregulation of BAFF and APRIL. It is also possible that bystander "nurselike" cells might aberrantly increase BAFF and APRIL upon exposure to products released by or expressed on the pro-gressively expanding malignant B-cell clone, including lymphotoxin and CD40L (Fig. 5) *(10,95,170)*.

Finally, high levels of APRIL expression have been observed in tumor cell lines. In one study, APRIL overexpression increased the growth of neoplastic NIH-3T3 epithelial cells in vivo *(107)*. Furthermore, APRIL has been reported to protect glioma cells against apoptosis induced by FasL or TRAIL *(174)*.

## 4.4. RANKL and Its Receptors

Therapeutic inhibition of the RANKL pathway by soluble OPG receptor or by blocking antibodies to RANKL or RANK was recently examined in murine models of human multiple myeloma and prostate carcinoma *(123,175)*. In both examples, soluble RANK or OPG prevented bone destruction and metastasis. Collectively, these data suggest that OPG, soluble RANK, or an anti-RANKL/RANK blocking antibodies might be of therapeutic value for patients with multiple myeloma and metastatic bony tumors. Tumor cells that express RANK might also be targeted anti-RANK antibody, similar to anti-CD20 antibody therapy of NHL. This approach could be tested in Hodgkin's disease, whereas RANK expression is restricted to the malignant Reed–Sternberg cells *(112)*.

## 4.5. TRAIL and Its Receptors

The preferential activity of TRAIL against cancer cells has generated hopes for its potential use in cancer therapy *(2,176,177)*. In fact, TRAIL has some antitumor activity against the majority of human cancer cell lines,including those derived from colon, lung, breast, kidney, prostate, brain, pancreas, skin, lymphoma, myeloma, and leukemia *(2)*. TRAIL activity is independent of p53 status, which makes it potentially effective against tumors that are resistant to chemotherapy *(178)*. Recently, the use of an anti-TRAIL-R1 or TRAIL-R2 monoclonal antibody was found to be as effective as TRAIL in killing tumor cells, and it was not toxic to normal human hepatocytes *(179,180)*. Furthermore, the activity of TRAIL and anti-TRAIL-R1 or anti-TRAIL-R2 was enhanced by chemotherapy or radiation therapy in vitro and in vivo *(181)*. Clinical trials using anti-TRAIL-R1 and anti-TRAIL-R2 are ongoing in patients with multiple myeloma and solid tumors. These important trials will provide valuable information on the safety and efficacy of these novel antibodies in cancer patients.

## REFERENCES

1. Locksley RM, Killeen N, Lenardo MJ. The TNF and TNF receptor superfamilies: integrating mammalian biology. Cell 2001; 104:487–501.
2. Younes A, Kadin ME. Emerging applications of the tumor necrosis factor family of ligands and receptors in cancer therapy. J Clin Oncol 2003; 21:3526–3534.
3. Kwon B, Youn BS, Kwon BS. Functions of newly identified members of the tumor necrosis factor receptor/ligand superfamilies in lymphocytes. Curr Opin Immunol 1999; 11:340–345.

4. Inoue J, Ishida T, Tsukamoto N, et al. Tumor necrosis factor receptor-associated factor (TRAF) family: adapter proteins that mediate cytokine signaling. Exp Cell Res 2000; 254:14–24.
5. McWhirter SM, Pullen SS, Werneburg BG, et al. Structural and biochemical analysis of signal transduction by the TRAF family of adapter proteins. Cold Spring Harb Symp Quant Biol 1999; 64:551–562.
6. Bhardwaj A, Aggarwal BB. Receptor-mediated choreography of life and death. J Clin Immunol 2003; 23:317–332.
7. Aggarwal BB. Signalling pathways of the TNF superfamily: a double-edged sword. Nat Rev Immunol 2003; 3:745–756.
8. Ashkenazi A. Targeting death and decoy receptors of the tumour-necrosis factor superfamily. Nat Rev Cancer 2002; 2:420–430.
9. Durkop H, Latza U, Hummel M, Eitelbach F, Seed B, Stein H. Molecular cloning and expression of a new member of the nerve growth factor receptor family that is characteristic for Hodgkin's disease. Cell 1992; 68:421–427.
10. Younes A, Carbone A. CD30/CD30 ligand and CD40/CD40 ligand in malignant lymphoid disorders. Int J Biol Markers 1999; 14:135–143.
11. Gause A, Pohl C, Tschiersch A, et al. Clinical significance of soluble CD30 antigen in the sera of patients with untreated Hodgkin's disease. Blood 1991; 77:1983–1988.
12. Zinzani PL, Pileri S, Bendandi M, et al. Clinical implications of serum levels of soluble CD30 in 70 adult anaplastic large-cell lymphoma patients. J Clin Oncol 1998; 16:1532–1537.
13. Nadali G, Vinante F, Ambrosetti A, et al. Serum levels of soluble CD30 are elevated in the majority of untreated patients with Hodgkin's disease and correlate with clinical features and prognosis. J Clin Oncol 1994; 12:793–797.
14. Younes A, Aggarwall BB. Clinical implications of the tumor necrosis factor family in benign and malignant hematologic disorders. Cancer 2003; 98:458–467.
15. Smith CA, Gruss HJ, Davis T, et al. CD30 antigen, a marker for Hodgkin's lymphoma, is a receptor whose ligand defines an emerging family of cytokines with homology to TNF. Cell 1993; 73:1349–1360.
16. Pera MF, Bennett W, Cerretti DP. Expression of CD30 and CD30 ligand in cultured cell lines from human germ-cell tumors. Lab Invest 1997; 76:497–504.
17. Gattei V, Degan M, Gloghini A, et al. CD30 ligand is frequently expressed in human hematopoietic malignancies of myeloid and lymphoid origin. Blood 1997; 89:2048–2059.
18. Younes A, Consoli U, Snell V, et al. CD30 ligand in lymphoma patients with CD30+ tumors. J Clin Oncol 1997; 15:3355–3362.
19. Younes A, Consoli U, Zhao S, et al. CD30 ligand is expressed on resting normal and malignant human B lymphocytes. Br J Haematol 1996; 93:569–571.
20. Clark EA. CD40: a cytokine receptor in search of a ligand. Tissue Antigens 1990; 36:33–36.
21. Armitage RJ, Maliszewski CR, Alderson MR, Grabstein KH, Spriggs MK, Fanslow WC. CD40L: a multi-functional ligand. Semin Immunol 1993; 5:401–412.
22. van Kooten C, Banchereau J. CD40-CD40 ligand. J Leukocyte Biol 2000; 67:2–17.
23. Carbone A, Gloghini A. Diagnostic significance of CD40, CD40L, and CD26 expression in Hodgkin's disease and other lymphomas. Am J Clin Pathol 1996; 105:522–523.
24. Carbone A, Gloghini A, Gruss HJ, Pinto A. CD40 antigen expression on Reed–Sternberg cells. A reliable diagnostic tool for Hodgkin's disease [letter; comment]. Am J Pathol 1995; 146:780–781.
25. Kato K, Santana-Sahagan E, Rassenti LZ, et al. The soluble CD40 ligand sCD154 in systemic lupus erythematosus. J Clin Invest 1999; 104:947–955.
26. Viallard JF, Solanilla A, Gauthier B, et al. Increased soluble and platelet-associated CD40 ligand in essential thrombocythemia and reactive thrombocytosis. Blood 2002; 99:2612–2614.
27. Younes A, Snell V, Consoli U, et al. Elevated levels of biologically active soluble CD40 ligand in the serum of patients with chronic lymphocytic leukaemia. Br J Haematol 1998; 100:135–141.
28. Siddiqa A, Sims-Mourtada JC, Guzman-Rojas L, et al. Regulation of CD40 and CD40 ligand by the AT-hook transcription factor AKNA. Nature 2001; 410:383–387.
29. Trentin L, Zambello R, Sancetta R, et al. B lymphocytes from patients with chronic lymphoproliferative disorders are equipped with different costimulatory molecules. Cancer Res 1997; 57:4940–4947.
30. Storz M, Zepter K, Kamarashev J, Dummer R, Burg G, Haffner AC. Coexpression of CD40 and CD40 ligand in cutaneous T-cell lymphoma (mycosis fungoides). Cancer Res 2001; 61:452–454.
31. Koshy M, Berger D, Crow MK. Increased expression of CD40 ligand on systemic lupus erythematosus lymphocytes. J Clin Invest 1996; 98:826–837.

32. Berner B, Wolf G, Hummel KM, Muller GA, Reuss-Borst MA. Increased expression of CD40 ligand (CD154) on CD4+ T cells as a marker of disease activity in rheumatoid arthritis. Ann Rheum Dis 2000; 59:190–195.
33. Gruss HJ, Ulrich D, Braddy S, Armitage RJ, Dower SK. Recombinant CD30 ligand and CD40 ligand share common biological activities on Hodgkin and Reed–Sternberg cells. Eur J Immunol 1995; 25: 2083–2089.
34. Carbone A, Gloghini A, Zagonel V, et al. The expression of CD26 and CD40 ligand is mutually exclusive in human T-cell non-Hodgkin's lymphomas/leukemias. Blood 1995; 86:4617–4626.
35. Carbone A, Gloghini A, Gattei V, et al. Expression of functional CD40 antigen on Reed-Sternberg cells and Hodgkin's disease cell lines. Blood 1995; 85:780–789.
36. Clodi K, Asgari Z, Younes M, et al. Expression of CD40 ligand (CD154) in B and T lymphocytes of Hodgkin disease: potential therapeutic significance. Cancer 2002; 94:1–5.
37. Carbone A, Gloghini A, Gruss HJ, Pinto A. CD40 ligand is constitutively expressed in a subset of T cell lymphomas and on the microenvironmental reactive T cells of follicular lymphomas and Hodgkin's disease. Am J Pathol 1995; 147:912–922.
38. Molin D, Fischer M, Xiang Z, et al. Mast cells express functional CD30 ligand and are the predominant CD30L-positive cells in Hodgkin's disease. Br J Haematol 2001; 114:616–623.
39. Pinto A, Aldinucci D, Gloghini A, et al. Human eosinophils express functional CD30 ligand and stimulate proliferation of a Hodgkin's disease cell line. Blood 1996; 88:3299–3305.
40. Harless Smith S, Cancro MP. BLyS: the pivotal determinant of peripheral B cell selection and lifespan. Curr Pharm Des 2003; 9:1833–1847.
41. Laabi Y, Egle A, Strasser A. TNF cytokine family: more BAFF-ling complexities. Curr Biol 2001; 11: R1013–R1016.
42. Schneider P, Tschopp J. BAFF and the regulation of B cell survival. Immunol Lett 2003; 88:57–62.
43. Mackay F, Ambrose C. The TNF family members BAFF and APRIL: the growing complexity. Cytokine Growth Factor Rev 2003; 14:311–324.
44. Gordon NC, Pan B, Hymowitz SG, et al. BAFF/BLyS receptor 3 comprises a minimal TNF receptor-like module that encodes a highly focused ligand-binding site. Biochemistry 2003; 42:5977–5983.
45. Medema JP, Planelles-Carazo L, Hardenberg G, Hahne M. The uncertain glory of APRIL. Cell Death Differ 2003; 10:1121–1125.
46. Gross JA, Dillon SR, Mudri S, et al. TACI-Ig neutralizes molecules critical for B cell development and autoimmune disease: impaired B cell maturation in mice lacking BLyS. Immunity 2001; 15:289–302.
47. Gross JA, Johnston J, Mudri S, et al. TACI and BCMA are receptors for a TNF homologue implicated in B-cell autoimmune disease. Nature 2000; 404:995–999.
48. Schneider K, Kothlow S, Schneider P, et al. Chicken BAFF—a highly conserved cytokine that mediates B cell survival. Int Immunol 2004; 16:139–148.
49. Thompson JS, Schneider P, Kalled SL, et al. BAFF binds to the tumor necrosis factor receptor-like molecule B cell maturation antigen and is important for maintaining the peripheral B cell population. J Exp Med 2000; 192:129–135.
50. Yan M, Marsters SA, Grewal IS, Wang H, Ashkenazi A, Dixit VM. Identification of a receptor for BLyS demonstrates a crucial role in humoral immunity. Nat Immunol 2000; 1:37–41.
51. Mackay F, Woodcock SA, Lawton P, et al. Mice transgenic for BAFF develop lymphocytic disorders along with autoimmune manifestations. J Exp Med 1999; 190:1697–1710.
52. Khare SD, Sarosi I, Xia XZ, et al. Severe B cell hyperplasia and autoimmune disease in TALL-1 transgenic mice. Proc Natl Acad Sci USA 2000; 97:3370–3375.
53. Groom J, Kalled SL, Cutler AH, et al. Association of BAFF/BLyS overexpression and altered B cell differentiation with Sjogren's syndrome. J Clin Invest 2002; 109:59–68.
54. Zhou T, Zhang J, Carter R, Kimberly R. BLyS and B cell autoimmunity. Curr Dir Autoimmun 2003; 6:21–37.
55. Khosla S. Minireview: the OPG/RANKL/RANK system. Endocrinology 2001; 142:5050–5055.
56. Takahashi N, Udagawa N, Suda T. A new member of tumor necrosis factor ligand family, ODF/OPGL/TRANCE/RANKL, regulates osteoclast differentiation and function. Biochem Biophys Res Commun 1999; 256:449–455.
57. Yasuda H, Shima N, Nakagawa N, et al. Osteoclast differentiation factor is a ligand for osteoprotegerin/osteoclastogenesis-inhibitory factor and is identical to TRANCE/RANKL. Proc Natl Acad Sci USA 1998; 95:3597–3602.

58. Emery JG, McDonnell P, Burke MB, et al. Osteoprotegerin is a receptor for the cytotoxic ligand TRAIL. J Biol Chem 1998; 273:14,363–14,367.

59. Degli-Esposti M. To die or not to die—the quest of the TRAIL receptors. J Leukocyte Biol 1999; 65: 535–542.

60. Horie R, Watanabe T, Ito K, et al. Cytoplasmic aggregation of TRAF2 and TRAF5 proteins in the Hodgkin–Reed–Sternberg cells. Am J Pathol 2002; 160:1647–1654.

61. Boucher LM, Marengere LE, Lu Y, Thukral S, Mak TW. Binding sites of cytoplasmic effectors TRAF1, 2, and 3 on CD30 and other members of the TNF receptor superfamily. Biochem Biophys Res Commun 1997; 233:592–600.

62. Duckett CS, Gedrich RW, Gilfillan MC, Thompson CB. Induction of nuclear factor kappaB by the CD30 receptor is mediated by TRAF1 and TRAF2. Mol Cell Biol 1997; 17:1535–1542.

63. Kieff E. Tumor necrosis factor receptor-associated factor (TRAF)-1, TRAF-2, and TRAF-3 interact in vivo with the CD30 cytoplasmic domain; TRAF-2 mediates CD30-induced nuclear factor kappa B activation. Proc Natl Acad Sci USA 1997; 94:12732.

64. Aizawa S, Nakano H, Ishida T, et al. Tumor necrosis factor receptor-associated factor (TRAF) 5 and TRAF2 are involved in CD30-mediated NFkappaB activation. J Biol Chem 1997; 272:2042–2045.

65. Ansieau S, Scheffrahn I, Mosialos G, et al. Tumor necrosis factor receptor-associated factor (TRAF)-1, TRAF-2, and TRAF-3 interact in vivo with the CD30 cytoplasmic domain; TRAF-2 mediates CD30-induced nuclear factor kappa B activation. Proc Natl Acad Sci USA 1996; 93:14,053–14,058.

66. Cerutti A, Kim EC, Shah S, et al. Dysregulation of CD30+ T cells by leukemia impairs isotype switching in normal B cells. Nat Immunol 2001; 2:150–156.

67. Cerutti A, Schaffer A, Goodwin RG, et al. Engagement of CD153 (CD30 ligand) by CD30+ T cells inhibits class switch DNA recombination and antibody production in human IgD+ IgM+ B cells. J Immunol 2000; 165:786–794.

68. Hubinger G, Muller E, Scheffrahn I, et al. CD30-mediated cell cycle arrest associated with induced expression of p21(CIP1/WAF1) in the anaplastic large cell lymphoma cell line Karpas 299. Oncogene 2001; 20:590–598.

69. Hsu PL, Hsu SM. Autocrine growth regulation of CD30 ligand in CD30-expressing Reed–Sternberg cells: distinction between Hodgkin's disease and anaplastic large cell lymphoma. Lab Invest 2000; 80: 1111–1119.

70. Mori M, Manuelli C, Pimpinelli N, et al. CD30–CD30 ligand interaction in primary cutaneous CD30(+) T-cell lymphomas: a clue to the pathophysiology of clinical regression. Blood 1999; 94:3077–3083.

71. Gruss HJ, Ulrich D, Dower SK, Herrmann F, Brach MA. Activation of Hodgkin cells via the CD30 receptor induces autocrine secretion of interleukin-6 engaging the NF-kappabeta transcription factor. Blood 1996; 87:2443–2449.

72. Gruss HJ, Boiani N, Williams DE, Armitage RJ, Smith CA, Goodwin RG. Pleiotropic effects of the CD30 ligand on CD30-expressing cells and lymphoma cell lines. Blood 1994; 83:2045–2056.

73. Zheng B, Fiumara P, Li YV, et al. MEK/ERK pathway is aberrantly active in Hodgkin disease: a signaling pathway shared by CD30, CD40, and RANK that regulates cell proliferation and survival. Blood 2003; 102:1019–1027.

74. Dadgostar H, Zarnegar B, Hoffmann A, et al. Cooperation of multiple signaling pathways in CD40-regulated gene expression in B lymphocytes. Proc Natl Acad Sci USA 2002; 99:1497–1502.

75. Werneburg BG, Zoog SJ, Dang TT, Kehry MR, Crute JJ. Molecular characterization of CD40 signaling intermediates. J Biol Chem 2001; 276:43,334–43,342.

76. Pullen SS, Dang TT, Crute JJ, Kehry MR. CD40 signaling through tumor necrosis factor receptor-associated factors (TRAFs). Binding site specificity and activation of downstream pathways by distinct TRAFs. J Biol Chem 1999; 274:14,246–14,254.

77. Lomaga MA, Yeh WC, Sarosi I, et al. TRAF6 deficiency results in osteopetrosis and defective interleukin-1, CD40, and LPS signaling. Genes Dev 1999; 13:1015–1024.

78. Lee HH, Dempsey PW, Parks TP, Zhu X, Baltimore D, Cheng G. Specificities of CD40 signaling: involvement of TRAF2 in CD40-induced NF-kappaB activation and intercellular adhesion molecule-1 up-regulation. Proc Natl Acad Sci USA 1999; 96:1421–1426.

79. Kosaka Y, Calderhead DM, Manning EM, et al. Activation and regulation of the IkappaB kinase in human B cells by CD40 signaling. Eur J Immunol 1999; 29:1353–1362.

80. Fiumara P, Younes A. CD40 ligand (CD154) and tumour necrosis factor-related apoptosis inducing ligand (Apo-2L) in haematological malignancies. Br J Haematol 2001; 113:265–274.

81. Avery DT, Kalled SL, Ellyard JI, et al. BAFF selectively enhances the survival of plasmablasts generated from human memory B cells. J Clin Invest 2003; 112:286–297.

82. von Bulow GU, Bram RJ. NF-AT activation induced by a CAML-interacting member of the tumor necrosis factor receptor superfamily. Science 1997; 278:138–141.

83. Xia XZ, Treanor J, Senaldi G, et al. TACI is a TRAF-interacting receptor for TALL-1, a tumor necrosis factor family member involved in B cell regulation. J Exp Med 2000; 192:137–143.

84. Cancer vaccine—antigenics. BioDrugs 2002; 16:72–74.

85. Hatada EN, Do RK, Orlofsky A, et al. NF-kappa B1 p50 is required for BLyS attenuation of apoptosis but dispensable for processing of NF-kappa B2 p100 to p52 in quiescent mature B cells. J Immunol 2003; 171:761–768.

86. Claudio E, Brown K, Park S, Wang H, Siebenlist U. BAFF-induced NEMO-independent processing of NF-kappa B2 in maturing B cells. Nat Immunol 2002; 3:958–965.

87. Batten M, Groom J, Cachero TG, et al. BAFF mediates survival of peripheral immature B lymphocytes. J Exp Med 2000; 192:1453–1466.

88. Kayagaki N, Yan M, Seshasayee D, et al. BAFF/BLyS receptor 3 binds the B cell survival factor BAFF ligand through a discrete surface loop and promotes processing of NF-kappaB2. Immunity 2002; 17:515–524.

89. Thompson JS, Bixler SA, Qian F, et al. BAFF-R, a newly identified TNF receptor that specifically interacts with BAFF. Science 2001; 293:2108–2111.

90. Steed PM, Hubert RS. The TNF superfamily is on the TRAIL to BlyS. Drug Discov Today 2003; 8:114–117.

91. Schneider P, MacKay F, Steiner V, et al. BAFF, a novel ligand of the tumor necrosis factor family, stimulates B cell growth. J Exp Med 1999; 189:1747–1756.

92. Harless Smith S, Cancro MP. Integrating B cell homeostasis and selection with BLyS. Arch Immunol Ther Exp (Warsz). 2003; 51:209–218.

93. Scaffidi C, Schmitz I, Krammer PH, Peter ME. The role of c-FLIP in modulation of CD95-induced apoptosis. J Biol Chem 1999; 274:1541–1548.

94. Nardelli B, Belvedere O, Roschke V, et al. Synthesis and release of B-lymphocyte stimulator from myeloid cells. Blood 2001; 97:198–204.

95. Dejardin E, Droin NM, Delhase M, et al. The lymphotoxin-beta receptor induces different patterns of gene expression via two NF-kappaB pathways. Immunity 2002; 17:525–535.

96. Litinskiy MB, Nardelli B, Hilbert DM, et al. DCs induce CD40-independent immunoglobulin class switching through BLyS and APRIL. Nat Immunol 2002; 3:822–829.

97. Wu Y, Bressette D, Carrell JA, et al. Tumor necrosis factor (TNF) receptor superfamily member TACI is a high affinity receptor for TNF family members APRIL and BLyS. J Biol Chem 2000; 275:35,478–35,485.

98. Schiemann B, Gommerman JL, Vora K, et al. An essential role for BAFF in the normal development of B cells through a BCMA-independent pathway. Science 2001; 293:2111–2114.

99. Huard B, Schneider P, Mauri D, Tschopp J, French LE. T cell costimulation by the TNF ligand BAFF. J Immunol 2001; 167:6225–6231.

100. Alizadeh AA, Eisen MB, Davis RE, et al. Distinct types of diffuse large B-cell lymphoma identified by gene expression profiling [see comments]. Nature 2000; 403:503–511.

101. von Bulow GU, van Deursen JM, Bram RJ. Regulation of the T-independent humoral response by TACI. Immunity 2001; 14:573–582.

102. Van Kooten C, Banchereau J. CD40-CD40 ligand: a multifunctional receptor–ligand pair. Adv Immunol 1996; 61:1–77.

103. Hanada T, Yoshida H, Kato S, et al. Suppressor of cytokine signaling-1 is essential for suppressing dendritic cell activation and systemic autoimmunity. Immunity 2003; 19:437–450.

104. O'Connor BP, Raman VS, Erickson LD, et al. BCMA Is essential for the survival of long-lived bone marrow plasma cells. J Exp Med 2004; 199:91–98.

105. Yu G, Boone T, Delaney J, et al. APRIL and TALL-I and receptors BCMA and TACI: system for regulating humoral immunity. Nat Immunol 2000; 1:252–256.

106. Varfolomeev E, Kischkel F, Martin F, et al. APRIL-deficient mice have normal immune system development. Mol Cell Biol 2004; 24:997–1006.

107. Kataoka T, Schroter M, Hahne M, et al. FLIP prevents apoptosis induced by death receptors but not by perforin/granzyme B, chemotherapeutic drugs, and gamma irradiation. J Immunol 1998; 161:3936–3942.

108. Darnay BG, Ni J, Moore PA, Aggarwal BB. Activation of NF-kappaB by RANK requires tumor necrosis factor receptor-associated factor (TRAF) 6 and NF-kappaB-inducing kinase. Identification of a novel TRAF6 interaction motif. J Biol Chem 1999; 274:7724–7731.
109. Wong BR, Josien R, Lee SY, Vologodskaia M, Steinman RM, Choi Y. The TRAF family of signal transducers mediates NF-kappaB activation by the TRANCE receptor. J Biol Chem 1998; 273:28,355–28,359.
110. Darnay BG, Haridas V, Ni J, Moore PA, Aggarwal BB. Characterization of the intracellular domain of receptor activator of NF-kappaB (RANK). Interaction with tumor necrosis factor receptor-associated factors and activation of NF-kappab and c-Jun N-terminal kinase. J Biol Chem 1998; 273:20,551–20,555.
111. Mukhopadhyay A, Fiumara P, Li Y, Darnay BG, Aggarwal B, Younes A. Receptor activator of nuclear factor-kB (RANK) ligand activates mitogen-activated protein kinases signaling pathways in Hodgkin/Reed–Sternberg cells. Blood 2002; 99:3485–3486.
112. Fiumara P, Snell V, Li Y, et al. Functional expression of receptor activator of nuclear factor kappaB in Hodgkin disease cell lines. Blood 2001; 98:2784–2790.
113. Kong YY, Yoshida H, Sarosi I, et al. OPGL is a key regulator of osteoclastogenesis, lymphocyte development and lymph-node organogenesis. Nature 1999; 397:315–323.
114. Dougall WC, Glaccum M, Charrier K, et al. RANK is essential for osteoclast and lymph node development. Genes Dev 1999; 13:2412–2424.
115. Li J, Sarosi I, Yan XQ, et al. RANK is the intrinsic hematopoietic cell surface receptor that controls osteoclastogenesis and regulation of bone mass and calcium metabolism. Proc Natl Acad Sci USA 2000; 97:1566–1571.
116. Mizuno A, Amizuka N, Irie K, et al. Severe osteoporosis in mice lacking osteoclastogenesis inhibitory factor/osteoprotegerin. Biochem Biophys Res Commun 1998; 247:610–615.
117. Whyte MP, Obrecht SE, Finnegan PM, et al. Osteoprotegerin deficiency and juvenile Paget's disease. N Engl J Med 2002; 347:175–184.
118. Josien R, Wong BR, Li HL, Steinman RM, Choi Y. TRANCE, a TNF family member, is differentially expressed on T cell subsets and induces cytokine production in dendritic cells. J Immunol 1999; 162:2562–2568.
119. Josien R, Li HL, Ingulli E, et al. TRANCE, a tumor necrosis factor family member, enhances the longevity and adjuvant properties of dendritic cells in vivo. J Exp Med 2000; 191:495–502.
120. Kim YM, Lee YM, Kim HS, et al. TNF-related activation-induced cytokine (TRANCE) induces angiogenesis through the activation of Src and phospholipase C (PLC) in human endothelial cells. J Biol Chem 2002; 277:6799–6805.
121. Fata JE, Kong YY, Li J, et al. The osteoclast differentiation factor osteoprotegerin-ligand is essential for mammary gland development. Cell 2000; 103:41–50.
122. Roux S, Meignin V, Quillard J, et al. RANK (receptor activator of nuclear factor-kappaB) and RANKL expression in multiple myeloma. Br J Haematol 2002; 117:86–92.
123. Pearse RN, Sordillo EM, Yaccoby S, et al. Multiple myeloma disrupts the TRANCE/osteoprotegerin cytokine axis to trigger bone destruction and promote tumor progression. Proc Natl Acad Sci USA 2001; 98:11,581–11,586.
124. Seidel C, Hjertner O, Abildgaard N, et al. Serum osteoprotegerin levels are reduced in patients with multiple myeloma with lytic bone disease. Blood 2001; 98:2269–2271.
125. Lipton A, Ali SM, Leitzel K, et al. Serum osteoprotegerin levels in healthy controls and cancer patients. Clin Cancer Res 2002; 8:2306–2310.
126. Brown JM, Vessella RL, Kostenuik PJ, Dunstan CR, Lange PH, Corey E. Serum osteoprotegerin levels are increased in patients with advanced prostate cancer. Clin Cancer Res 2001; 7:2977–2983.
127. Brown JM, Corey E, Lee ZD, et al. Osteoprotegerin and rank ligand expression in prostate cancer. Urology 2001; 57:611–616.
128. Cretney E, Takeda K, Yagita H, Glaccum M, Peschon JJ, Smyth MJ. Increased susceptibility to tumor initiation and metastasis in TNF-related apoptosis-inducing ligand-deficient mice. J Immunol 2002; 168:1356–1361.
129. Takeda K, Smyth MJ, Cretney E, et al. Critical role for tumor necrosis factor-related apoptosis-inducing ligand in immune surveillance against tumor development. J Exp Med 2002; 195:161–169.
130. Chou AH, Tsai HF, Lin LL, Hsieh SL, Hsu PI, Hsu PN. Enhanced proliferation and increased IFN-gamma production in T cells by signal transduced through TNF-related apoptosis-inducing ligand. J Immunol 2001; 167:1347–1352.

131. Choi C, Kutsch O, Park J, Zhou T, Seol DW, Benveniste EN. Tumor necrosis factor-related apoptosis-inducing ligand induces caspase- dependent interleukin-8 expression and apoptosis in human astroglioma cells. Mol Cell Biol 2002; 22:724–736.

132. Li JH, Kirkiles-Smith NC, McNiff JM, Pober JS. TRAIL induces apoptosis and inflammatory gene expression in human endothelial cells. J Immunol 2003; 171:1526–1533.

133. Schneider P, Thome M, Burns K, et al. TRAIL receptors 1 (DR4) and 2 (DR5) signal FADD-dependent apoptosis and activate NF-kappaB. Immunity 1997; 7:831–836.

134. Lin Y, Devin A, Cook A, et al. The death domain kinase RIP is essential for TRAIL (Apo2L)-induced activation of IkappaB kinase and c-Jun N-terminal kinase. Mol Cell Biol 2000; 20:6638–6645.

135. Green DR, Evan GI. A matter of life and death. Cancer Cell 2002; 1:19–30.

136. Deng Y, Lin Y, Wu X. TRAIL-induced apoptosis requires Bax-dependent mitochondrial release of Smac/DIABLO. Genes Dev 2002; 16:33–45.

137. LeBlanc H, Lawrence D, Varfolomeev E, et al. Tumor-cell resistance to death receptor—induced apoptosis through mutational inactivation of the proapoptotic Bcl-2 homolog Bax. Nat Med 2002; 8:274–281.

138. Griffith TS, Chin WA, Jackson GC, Lynch DH, Kubin MZ. Intracellular regulation of TRAIL-induced apoptosis in human melanoma cells. J Immunol 1998; 161:2833–2840.

139. Jeremias I, Kupatt C, Baumann B, Herr I, Wirth T, Debatin KM. Inhibition of nuclear factor kappaB activation attenuates apoptosis resistance in lymphoid cells. Blood 1998; 91:4624–4631.

140. Zhang XD, Franco A, Myers K, Gray C, Nguyen T, Hersey P. Relation of TNF-related apoptosis-inducing ligand (TRAIL) receptor and FLICE-inhibitory protein expression to TRAIL-induced apoptosis of melanoma. Cancer Res 1999; 59:2747–2753.

141. Mitsiades N, Mitsiades CS, Poulaki V, Anderson KC, Treon SP. Intracellular regulation of tumor necrosis factor-related apoptosis-inducing ligand-induced apoptosis in human multiple myeloma cells. Blood 2002; 99:2162–2171.

142. Chen X, Thakkar H, Tyan F, et al. Constitutively active Akt is an important regulator of TRAIL sensitivity in prostate cancer. Oncogene 2001; 20:6073–6083.

143. Shiiki K, Yoshikawa H, Kinoshita H, et al. Potential mechanisms of resistance to TRAIL/Apo2L-induced apoptosis in human promyelocytic leukemia HL-60 cells during granulocytic differentiation. Cell Death Differ 2000; 7:939–946.

144. Fulda S, Meyer E, Debatin KM. Inhibition of TRAIL-induced apoptosis by Bcl-2 overexpression. Oncogene 2002; 21:2283–2294.

145. Bin L, Li X, Xu LG, Shu HB. The short splice form of Casper/c-FLIP is a major cellular inhibitor of TRAIL-induced apoptosis. FEBS Lett 2002; 510:37–40.

146. Lincz LF, Yeh TX, Spencer A. TRAIL-induced eradication of primary tumour cells from multiple myeloma patient bone marrows is not related to TRAIL receptor expression or prior chemotherapy. Leukemia 2001; 15:1650–1657.

147. Teitz T, Wei T, Valentine MB, et al. Caspase 8 is deleted or silenced preferentially in childhood neuroblastomas with amplification of MYCN [see comments]. Nat Med 2000; 6:529–535.

148. Herrnring C, Reimer T, Jeschke U, et al. Expression of the apoptosis-inducing ligands FasL and TRAIL in malignant and benign human breast tumors. Histochem Cell Biol 2000; 113:189–194.

149. Nakamura M, Rieger J, Weller M, Kim J, Kleihues P, Ohgaki H. APO2L/TRAIL expression in human brain tumors. Acta Neuropathol (Berl) 2000; 99:1–6.

150. Zhao S, Asgary Z, Wang Y, Goodwin R, Andreeff M, Younes A. Functional expression of TRAIL by lymphoid and myeloid tumour cells. Br J Haematol 1999; 106:827–832.

151. Wahl AF, Cerveny CH, Klussman K, et al. SGN-30, a chimeric antibody to CD30, for the treatment of Hodgkin's disease. Proc Am Assoc Cancer Res 2002; 43:4979a.

152. Kitada S, Zapata JM, Andreeff M, Reed JC. Bryostatin and CD40-ligand enhance apoptosis resistance and induce expression of cell survival genes in B-cell chronic lymphocytic leukaemia. Br J Haematol 1999; 106:995–1004.

153. Romano MF, Lamberti A, Tassone P, et al. Triggering of CD40 antigen inhibits fludarabine-induced apoptosis in B chronic lymphocytic leukemia cells. Blood 1998; 92:990–995.

154. Ghia P, Boussiotis VA, Schultze JL, et al. Unbalanced expression of bcl-2 family proteins in follicular lymphoma: contribution of CD40 signaling in promoting survival. Blood 1998; 91:244–251.

155. Lomo J, Blomhoff HK, Jacobsen SE, Krajewski S, Reed JC, Smeland EB. Interleukin-13 in combination with CD40 ligand potently inhibits apoptosis in human B lymphocytes: upregulation of Bcl-xL and Mcl-1. Blood 1997; 89:4415–4424.

156. Clodi K, Asgary Z, Zhao S, et al. Coexpression of CD40 and CD40 ligand in B-cell lymphoma cells. Br J Haematol 1998; 103:270–275.

157. Younes A. The dynamics of life and death of malignant lymphocytes. Curr Opin Oncol 1999; 11: 364–369.

158. French RR, Chan HT, Tutt AL, Glennie MJ. CD40 antibody evokes a cytotoxic T-cell response that eradicates lymphoma and bypasses T-cell help. Nat Med 1999; 5:548–553.

159. Kato K, Cantwell MJ, Sharma S, Kipps TJ. Gene transfer of CD40-ligand induces autologous immune recognition of chronic lymphocytic leukemia B cells. J Clin Invest 1998; 101:1133–1141.

160. Tutt AL, O'Brien L, Hussain A, Crowther GR, French RR, Glennie MJ. T cell immunity to lymphoma following treatment with anti-CD40 monoclonal antibody. J Immunol 2002; 168:2720–2728.

161. Vonderheide RH, Dutcher JP, Anderson JE, et al. Phase I study of recombinant human CD40 ligand in cancer patients. J Clin Oncol 2001; 19:3280–3287.

162. Younes A. CD40 ligand therapy of lymphoma patients. J Clin Oncol 2001; 19:4351–4353.

163. Wierda WG, Cantwell MJ, Woods SJ, Rassenti LZ, Prussak CE, Kipps TJ. CD40-ligand (CD154) gene therapy for chronic lymphocytic leukemia. Blood 2000; 96:2917–2924.

164. Batten M, Fletcher C, Ng LG, et al. TNF deficiency fails to protect BAFF transgenic mice against auto-immunity and reveals a predisposition to B cell lymphoma. J Immunol 2004; 172:812–822.

165. Klein B, Tarte K, Jourdan M, et al. Survival and proliferation factors of normal and malignant plasma cells. Int J Hematol 2003; 78:106–113.

166. Kolb JP, Kern C, Quiney C, Roman V, Billard C. Re-establishment of a normal apoptotic process as a therapeutic approach in B-CLL. Curr Drug Targets Cardiovasc Haematol Disord 2003; 3:261–286.

167. Novak AJ, Bram RJ, Kay NE, Jelinek DF. Aberrant expression of B-lymphocyte stimulator by B chronic lymphocytic leukemia cells: a mechanism for survival. Blood 2002; 100:2973–2979.

168. Moreaux J, Legouffe E, Jourdan E, et al. BAFF and APRIL protect myeloma cells from apoptosis induced by IL-6 deprivation and dexamethasone. Blood 2003; 103:3148–3157.

169. Novak AJ, Darce JR, Arendt BK, et al. Expression of BCMA, TACI, and BAFF-R in multiple myeloma: a mechanism for growth and survival. Blood 2004; 103:689–694.

170. He B, Raab-Traub N, Casali P, Cerutti A. EBV-encoded latent membrane protein 1 cooperates with BAFF/BLyS and APRIL to induce T cell-independent Ig heavy chain class switching. J Immunol 2003; 171:5215–5224.

171. Kern C, Cornuel JF, Billard C, et al. Involvement of BAFF and APRIL in the resistance to apoptosis of B-CLL through an autocrine pathway. Blood 2004; 103:679–688.

172. Staudt LM. Gene expression profiling of lymphoid malignancies. Annu Rev Med 2002; 53:303–318.

173. Abbasi. Phase I trial of fludarabine and paclitaxel in non-Hodgkin's lymphoma. Med Oncol 2003; 20: 53–58.

174. Benimetskaya L, Miller P, Benimetsky S, et al. Inhibition of potentially anti-apoptotic proteins by antisense protein kinase C-alpha (Isis 3521) and antisense bcl-2 (G3139) phosphorothioate oligodeoxy-nucleotides: relationship to the decreased viability of T24 bladder and PC3 prostate cancer cells. Mol Pharmacol 2001; 60:1296–1307.

175. Croucher PI, Shipman CM, Lippitt J, et al. Osteoprotegerin inhibits the development of osteolytic bone disease in multiple myeloma. Blood 2001; 98:3534–3540.

176. Nagane M, Huang HJ, Cavenee WK. The potential of TRAIL for cancer chemotherapy. Apoptosis 2001; 6:191–197.

177. French LE, Tschopp J. The TRAIL to selective tumor death. Nat Med 1999; 5:146–147.

178. El-Deiry WS. Insights into cancer therapeutic design based on p53 and TRAIL receptor signaling. Cell Death Differ 2001; 8:1066–1075.

179. Dobson C, Edwards BF, Main S, et al. Generation of human therapeutic anti-TRAIL-R1 agonistic anti-bodies by phage display. Proc Am Assoc Cancer Res 2002; 43:2869a.

180. Ichikawa K, Liu W, Zhao L, et al. Tumoricidal activity of a novel anti-human DR5 monoclonal anti-body without hepatocyte cytotoxicity. Nat Med 2001; 7:954–960.

181. Ohtsuka T, Buchsbaum D, Oliver P, Makhija S, Kimberly R, Zhou T. Synergistic induction of tumor cell apoptosis by death receptor antibody and chemotherapy agent through JNK/p38 and mitochon-drial death pathway. Oncogene 2003; 22:2034–2044.

# 35 Small-Molecule Receptor Tyrosine Kinase Inhibitors in Targeted Cancer Therapy

*Carlos García-Echeverría, PhD*

## CONTENTS

## SUMMARY

ATP site-directed competitive and irreversible inhibitors of receptor tyrosine kinases have been extensively investigated in the search for new targeted antitumor agents. This chapter provides a comprehensive overview of key results and achievements for three receptor tyrosine kinases, EGFR, c-Kit, and FLT3, in which drug discovery and development activities have advanced with some success. Three additional receptor tyrosine kinases (IGF-IR, c-Met, and RET) have been selected to illustrate new opportunities and challenges in the identification of drugs for tailored cancer treatment.

**Key Words:** Signal transduction inhibitors; cancer therapy; signaling pathways; drugs; leukemia; tumors; receptor; kinase; antitumor; ATP; EGFR; c-Kit; FLT3; IGF-IR; IGF-1; IGF-II; c-Met; RET.

## 1. INTRODUCTION

In the past few years, molecular biology has produced important advances in the identification of dysregulated signal transduction pathways that affect cell transformation and tumor growth. This knowledge, together with the data obtained from epidemiological studies, can be exploited to create rational, mechanism-based inhibitors of specific biochemical processes that are essential for the malignant phenotype of tumor cells.

From: *Cancer Drug Discovery and Development: The Oncogenomics Handbook*
Edited by: W. J. LaRochelle and R. A. Shimkets © Humana Press Inc., Totowa, NJ

Many of the critical elements identified in signal transduction cascades that affect tumor growth and survival are kinases and, among the members of this large family of enzymes, a set of receptor tyrosine kinases (RTKs) has emerged as suitable targets for oncology drug discovery.

The complexity and number of RTKs being targeted in oncology drug discovery has greatly increased in the past few years, and it is impossible to capture all of the available information herein. Among the different approaches used to target these enzymes (e.g., monoclonal antibodies and kinase inhibitors), this chapter focuses on contributions in the inhibition of receptor tyrosine kinase activity by ATP-site directed competitive and irreversible compounds. The intent is to provide a comprehensive, rather than an exhaustive overview of the pertinent literature in this fascinating and challenging area of research. To start, we briefly describe key results and achievements for three RTKs (EGFR, c-Kit and FLT3) in which drug discovery and development activities have advanced with some success. After this, we have selected representative examples of a new wave of therapeutic targets (IGF-IR, c-MET, and RET) to illustrate new opportunities and challenges in the identification of drugs for tailored cancer treatment.

## 2. FROM THE BENCH TO THE CLINIC: RECEPTOR TYROSINE KINASE INHIBITORS IN CLINICAL TRIALS

### 2.1. Inhibitors of the Epidermal Growth Factor Receptor System

The epidermal growth factor (EGF) family of type I receptor tyrosine kinases is composed of four structurally related proteins: EGFR (erbB-1, HER1); erbB-2 (Her2, Neu), erbB-3 (HER3), and erbB-4 (HER4) (1). The functions of these receptors are intimately interrelated, and their activation by a broad spectrum of ligands[*,†] triggers a network of signaling pathways that are involved in cellular proliferation, apoptosis, differentiation, angiogenesis, motility, and invasion. The EGF receptor (EGFR) system was first implicated in cancer when the avian erythroblastosis tumor virus was found to encode an aberrant form of the human EGFR. Additional studies have supported an important role for this family of RTKs in the development and progression of numerous human tumors (2–6). Overexpression of EGFR or coexpression of both receptor and ligand(s) is a frequent event in a large variety of epithelial cancers (7) and is associated with advanced disease and poor prognosis (3). In a significant proportion of these tumors, gene amplification is accompanied by rearrangements that result in constitutively active receptors. This effect has also been observed in mutated forms of the EGFR. The most common mutation (EGFRvIII), which is found in gliomas, non-small-cell lung cancer, and breast cancer, lacks domains I and II of the extracellular domain and, despite being unable to bind to the ligands, displays constitutive kinase activity (8).

Targeting EGFR as a potential anticancer strategy was first proposed by Mendelsohn in the early 1980s (9), and since then, the identification and development of monoclonal antibodies and ATP-competitive/irreversible inhibitors of EGFR has been a major area

---

[*]erbB-3 lacks tyrosine kinase activity and so far there are no known ligands for erbB-2. This protein can be transactivated by heterodimerisation with other EGF family members.

[†]There are currently six known endogenous ligands for EGFRs: EGF, transforming growth factor-α, amphiregulin, betacellulin, heparin-binding EGF, and epiregulin.

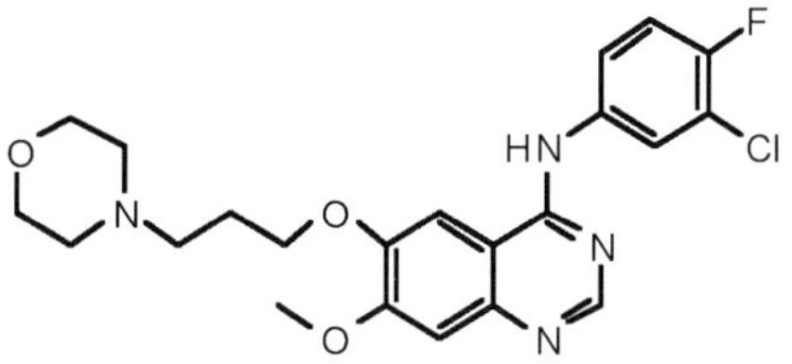

Gefitinib
**1**

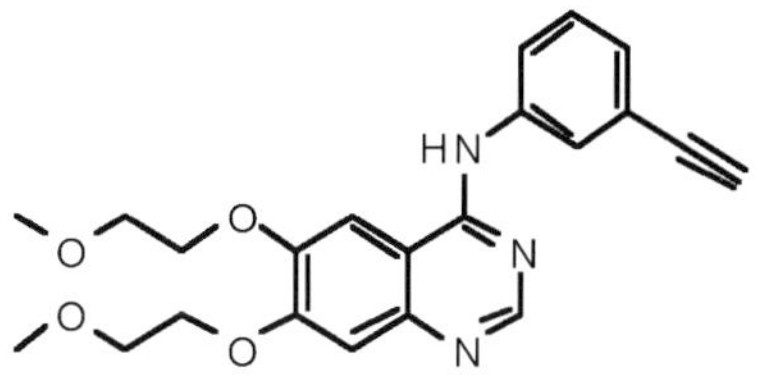

Erlotinib
**2**

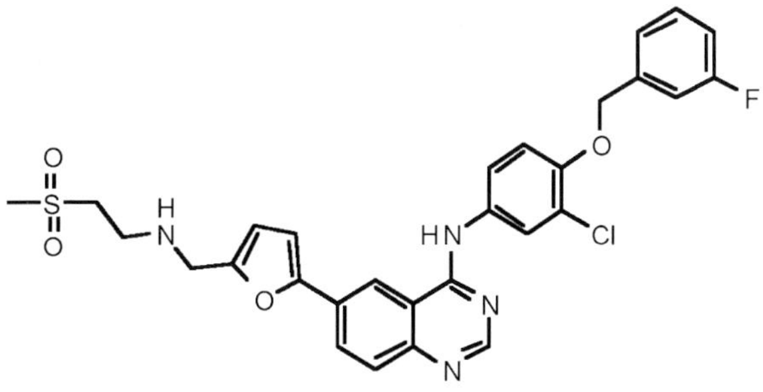

Lapatinib
**3**

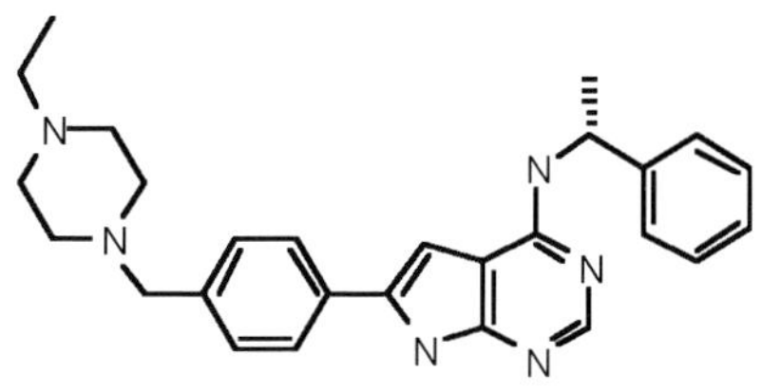

NVP-AEE788
**4**

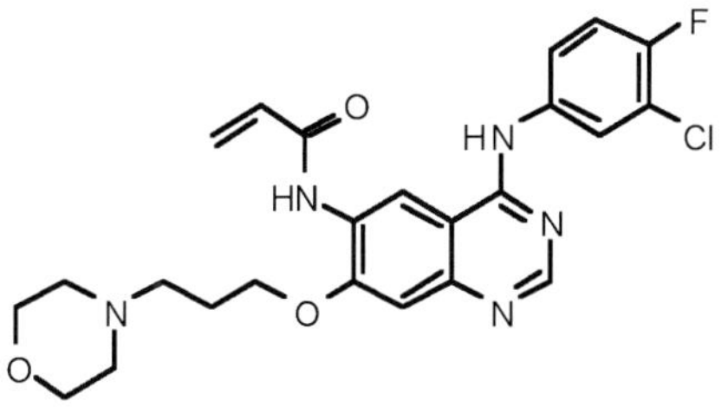

Canertinib
**5**

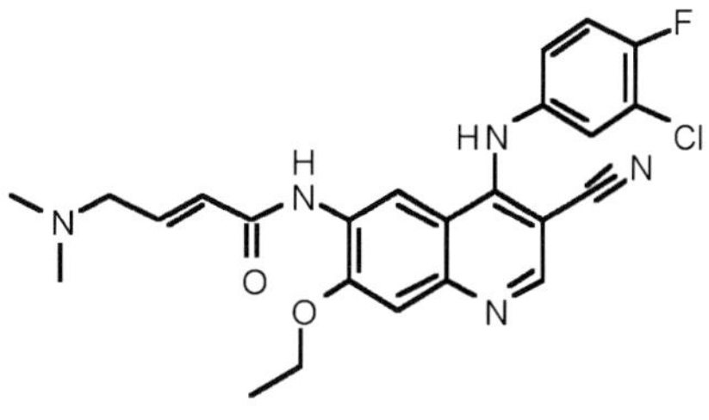

EKB-569
**6**

**Fig. 1.** Kinase inhibitors of members of the EGFR family.

of research *(10–16)*‡. The EGFR kinase inhibitors undergoing clinical trials or known to be in late-stage preclinical development are discussed in this section.

Gefitinib (Iressa™, ZD-1839; AstraZeneca plc; **1** in Fig. 1) has been the first EGFR kinase inhibitor to be approved for marketing in any country. This 4-phenylamino-quinazoline derivative *(17)* selectively inhibits the kinase activity of EGFR in biochemical assays ($K_i$ = 2.1 n*M* on a purified receptor) *(18)*. In cellular settings, the compound blocks

‡Trastuzumab (Herceptin™; Genentech Inc.), which is a recombinant monoclonal antibody against erbB-2, has been the first growth factor receptor-targeted agent approved for the treatment of metastatic breast tumor that overexpresses erbB-2 *(13)*.

receptor autophosphorylation in a range of tumor cell lines *(19)* and potently inhibits the proliferation of cancer cells that overexpressed the EGFR ($IC_{50}$ = 7–90 n*M*) *(20)*.

In preclinical in vivo studies, gefitinib demonstrated antitumor activity against a panel of human xenografts derived from cell lines that expressed high levels of EGFR *(21,22)*, and complete regression of large tumors (e.g., A431 xenografts) was obtained when the compound was administered orally at high doses (200 mg/kg/d for 2 wk). Tumor growth was suppressed for as long as 4 mo, but regrowth occurred when treatment was suspended. Interestingly, the antitumor activity of gefitinib seems to be partly mediated by its anti-angiogenic effects on EGFR-expressing endothelial cells *(23)* and is accompanied by a decreased production of autocrine and paracrine proangiogenic factors *(24)*. Additional in vitro and in vivo preclinical studies showed additive to synergistic effects when gefitinib was used in combination with cytotoxic agents (e.g., doxorubicin, etoposide, or cisplatin) *(25,26)*, radiotherapy *(27)*, or trastuzumab[‡] *(28)*.

The Japanese Ministry of Health, Labor and Welfare was the first institution to approve gefitinib in July 2002 for the treatment of inoperable or recurrent non-small-cell lung cancer (NSCLC). The approval was based on data from two pivotal phase II studies (Iressa Dose Evaluation in Advanced Lung Cancer, IDEAL 1 and 2). The results of these clinical trials showed that gefitinib provides clinical significant symptom relief for patients with extensively pretreated advanced NSCLC. This improvement in disease-related symptoms correlated with improved survival and tumor response *(29)*. Doubts about its approval in other countries arise when the results of the INTACT (Iressa NSCLC Trials Assessing Combination Therapy) trials were reported in 2002. In these phase III trials, gefitinib showed no added benefit in survival or any other efficacy end points in NSCLC patients when combined with gemcitabine/cisplatin or paclitaxel/carboplatin. In spite of these disappointing results, gefitinib was approved by the US Food and Drug Administration (FDA) in May 2003 as a single-agent treatment for advanced NSCLC after failure with two standard of care treatments and, the same month, by the Australian Therapeutic Goods Administration for the treatment of NSCLC in patients who have previously received treatment with chemotherapy. The compound is currently under review by the European Agency for the Evaluation of Medical Products.

Erlotinib (Tarceva[TM], CP-358774, OSI-774; OSI Pharmaceuticals Inc./Genentech Inc./ Roche Holdings AG; **2** in Fig. 1) is another EGFR kinase inhibitor of the 4-phenlyamino-quinazoline class being developed as a stand-alone treatment for solid tumors and for use in combination with existing chemotherapy. The compound inhibits EGFR kinase activity in biochemical assays with an $IC_{50}$ value of 1–2 n*M*, shows high selectivity against other kinases, and effectively reduces cellular EGFR autophosphorylation ($IC_{50}$ = 20 n*M*) *(30, 31)*. In preclinical studies, the compound showed substantial in vivo antitumor activity against various human EGFR-expressing tumor xenografts alone or in combination with chemotherapeutic agents *(32–35)*. Ex vivo analyses of some of these tumors showed that the compound produced a long-lasting inhibition of EGFR autophosphorylation (70% reduction over a period of 24 h) after a single dose of 100 mg/kg/per os (po) *(35)*. The inhibition of the PKB/Akt and MAPK pathways by erlotinib seems to be required for optimal antitumor effect *(32,35)*.

Partial responses (14–16%) were reported in a phase II clinical trials with NSCLC patients treated orally with erlotinib (150 mg/d). The median survival duration was 257 d and the 1-yr survival rate was estimated to be 48%. Recently, the companies involved in the development of this compound announced that two first-line phase III studies of erlotinib in combination with standard chemotherapy in metastatic NSCLC patients did not meet their primary end point of improving overall survival. In another phase II study, oral administration of erlotinib to patients with advanced head and neck cancer showed three confirmed and two unconfirmed partial responses. Encouraging responses have also been observed in a phase I glioblastoma study: 8 patients (16%) had a partial response, 3 patients (6%) had a minor response, and 11 patients (22%) had stable disease. Based on these results, the US FDA has granted orphan drug status for erlotinib in patients with glioblastoma.

Diarrhea and acneiform rashes are the main adverse events observed in the clinical studies with erlotinib, and fatigue, headache, nausea, and transient increases in serum bilirubin and transaminases have been reported as minor side effects *(36,37)*.

An alternative strategy to block EGFR signaling has been the dual inhibition of EGFR and erbB-2 receptor kinase activities. ErbB-2 participates in type I receptor signaling by heterodimerization with members of the EGFR family *(38)*. Dimerization leads to receptor transautophosphorylation and initiation of signal transduction pathways linked to cell survival and division *(39)*. The epidemiological evidence implicating these two receptors in cancer patients (e.g., overexpression of erbB-2 occurs in around 30% of breast cancers and coexpression of elevated levels of these two receptors has been observed in ovarian cancer patients) *(40,41)* suggested that a dual EGFR/erbB-2 inhibitor could provide a therapeutic opportunity in patients with tumors expressing either or both of these receptors. EGFR and erbB2 have homologous kinase domains and optimization of quinazoline and pyrido-[3,4-*d*]-pyrimidine derivatives *(42)* lead to lapatinib (GW2016, GW572016, GlaxoSmithKline plc; **3** in Fig. 1), which is a potent dual inhibitor of the EGFR and erbB-2 receptor tyrosine kinases ($IC_{50} = 11$ n*M* and 9.2 n*M*, respectively) *(43)*. The antiproliferative effects of lapatinib on EGFR/erbB-2 overexpressing tumor cell lines are in the 100-n*M* range and selectivity against normal cell lines is retained ($IC_{50} = 10$ μ*M*). In preclinical studies, lapatinib (100 mg/kg po bid) showed potent in vivo antitumor activity in several xenograft models [e.g., head and neck cancer *(44)* and BT-474 model *(45)* with no adverse effects]. In a phase II multicenter study with patients with tumors that overexpress EGFR and/or erbB-2, among the 30 women with advanced breast cancer, 26 received lapatinib for at least 8 wk. Within this group, 4 patients experienced a partial response (treatment duration ranging from 15 to 27+ wk), and 10 had disease stabilization (treatment duration from 10 to 41+ weeks). Last year, lapatinib received fast-track status from the US FDA for the treatment of patients with refractory advanced or metastatic breast cancer who have failed previous therapies. Phase III studies are underway in advanced/metastatic breast cancer patients and early-phase studies are ongoing for other solid tumors.

Another dual inhibitor of EGFR and erbB-2 is NVP-AEE788 (Novartis Pharma AG; **4** in Fig. 1), a pyrrolo[2,3-*d*]pyrimidine derivative that has recently entered phase I clinical trials. This compound is a potent inhibitor of EGFRs in biochemical assays ($IC_{50} = 2$ n*M* and 6 n*M* for EGFR and erbB-2, respectively) as well as in cellular settings *(46)*. An important feature of NVP-AEE788 is that it also blocks the kinase activity of VEGFR2 ($IC_{50} = 77$ n*M*) and Flt-1 ($IC_{50} = 59$ n*M*) and inhibits the proliferation of EGF- and vascular endothelial growth factor (VEGF)-stimulated human umbilical vein endothelial cells (HUVECs). Combining activity against EGF and VEGF receptor kinases in a single molecule could lead to improved antitumor activity by targeting both tumor cell proliferation and vascularization. These properties, combined with a favorable physicochemical profile, most likely contribute to the in vivo antitumor and antiangiogenic activities observed for NVP-AEE788 in several animal models *(47–49)*.

As an alternative strategy to target EGFR and EGFR/erbB-2, selective erbB-2 kinase inhibition has also been pursued. TAK-165 (structure not disclosed; Takeda Chemical Industries Ltd.) is a potent erbB-2 inhibitor ($IC_{50} = 6$ n$M$) that has a remarkable selectivity over the homologous EGFR ($IC_{50} > 25$ µ$M$). Preclinical data showed significant in vivo efficacy in hormone refractory prostate cancer and bladder xenografts when the compound was administered orally (10 or 20 mg/kg/d) for 14 d *(50)*. This new kinase inhibitor is currently undergoing phase I clinical trials in patients with tumors known to express erbB-2. CP 724714 (structure not disclosed; Pfizer Inc.) is another example of a potent and selective oral inhibitor of erbB-2 receptor undergoing clinical studies.

The potential utility of compounds that effectively block the function of the EGFR family but do not inhibit more structurally diverse kinases has also being explored with pan-EGFR inhibitors *(51,52)*. The goal of this approach is to achieve greater efficacy and a broader spectrum of activity by blocking the kinase activity of all the members of the EGFR family and the crosstalk between them *(38)*. One way to accomplish this is by using site-directed irreversible inhibitors *(52)*. This medicinal chemistry strategy has been extensively used to target proteolytic enzymes, and its use in the kinase field came as a surprise. The pan-EGFR inhibitors described today contain a Michael acceptor-type substituent and exploit the presence of a cysteine residue at the "sugar pocket" of the ATP-binding site *(53,54)*. Cysteine-773, which is located on the extended coil stretch of the EGFR, is unique for the EGFR family and forms an adduct with the inhibitor when bound to the enzyme. The covalent interaction provides selectivity (ratio of nearly $10^5$–fold) against other receptor or intracellular kinases, but it is unclear if the prolonged suppression of kinase activity caused by these agents might be limited by the rate of receptor regeneration.

The preclinical performance of this type of derivative has improved to the point where several of these compounds have entered clinical trials. Canertinib (CI-1033, PD-183805; Pfizer Inc; **5** in Fig. 1) *(55)* is an irreversible inhibitor of the kinase activity of EGFR ($IC_{50}$ = 1.5 n$M$, in vitro enzyme assay) as well as that of erbB-2, erbB-4 *(56)*, and EGFRvIII *(57)*. This compound potently inhibits EGFR autophosphorylation ($IC_{50}$ = 7.4 n$M$) in tumor cells that are EGF dependent *(58)*. Several studies have shown that canertinib can synergize with a variety of cytotoxic agents (e.g., gemcitabine, cisplatin, 7-ethyl-10-hydroxy-camptothecin) and radiation *(59–62)*. The compound enhances the cytotoxicity of gemcitabine through inhibition of PKB/Akt and mitogen-activated protein kinase (MAPK) *(59)*. In combination with 7-ethyl-10-hydroxy-camptothecin, it increases the steady-state accumulation of the topoisomerase I inhibitor by blocking drug efflux in breast cancer resistance protein transporter-expressing cells *(62)*. Preclinical data have shown that canertinib is efficacious against a variety of human tumors in mouse xenograft models (e.g., A431, H125, BCA-1, SF767, or MCF-7), and, for example, it demonstrated optimal efficacy (T/C of 4%) at 5 mg/kg/d in A431 xenografts with a minimal weight loss (< 10%) *(58)*.

Canertinib has progressed through phase I clinical studies using oral dosing, and acneiform rash, emesis, hematological, and diarrhea have been reported as the most common adverse events. In a phase I study, the compound was administered daily for 7 d every 21 d *(63)*. Of the 37 treated patients, there was a partial response in 1 patient with squamous cell carcinoma of the head and neck and disease stabilization in 10 patients. A second phase I study administered the compound on d 1, 8, and 15 every 28 d, and 1 disease stabilization in a patient with osteosarcoma was documented out of 34 patients *(64)*. Ongoing clinical trials include a randomized phase II study of canertinib in patients with advanced ovarian cancer.

EKB-569 (Howard Hughes Medical Institute/Wyeth Research; **6** in Fig. 1) is a cyano-quinoline derivative that also binds covalently and irreversibly to the EGFR. It potently inhibits the autophosphorylation of EGFR ($IC_{50}$ = 0.08 $\mu M$; solid-phase enzyme-linked immunosorbent assay [ELISA]) but shows lower activity against erbB-2 ($IC_{50}$ = 1.23 $\mu M$) *(65)*. In spite of this in vitro profile, EKB-569 is equipotent in inhibiting the proliferation of cells expressing EGFR or erbB-2, and a 50-fold higher concentration is needed to inhibit cells that do not overexpress either receptor.

In a nude mouse xenograft model and at the highest dose investigated (80 mg/kg), EKB-569 inhibits the growth of the human A431 cell line by over 90% even 20 d after terminating dosing *(65)*. EKB-569 either alone or in combination with the nonsteroidal anti-inflammatory sulindac reduces the incidence of intestinal polyps in a murine model of human familial adenomatous polyposis *(66)*. Sulindac (5 mg/kg/d) had no effect on polyp formation, whereas EKB-559 (20 mg/kg/d) reduced polyp formation by 87% compared with controls. The combination therapy produced a 95% reduction in polyp numbers, and 47% of the treated mice had no evidence of tumors at all. This synergistic effect might be the result of the convergence of EGFR and cyclo-oxygenase-2 (COX-2) signaling and point to the potential clinical use of EGFR plus COX-2 inhibitors. Following this preclinical finding, EKB-569 in combination with sulindac is currently in phase I/IIa clinical trials as a chemopreventative agent against colon cancer. Other phase I studies are also underway in patients with a variety of cancers known to overexpress EGFR. Toxicity patterns in the clinical trials appear to be similar to other agents in this class and include diarrhea and skin rash.

### 2.2. Inhibitors of c-Kit

c-Kit is a transmembrane glycoprotein that is expressed by hematopoietic progenitor cells, mast cells, germs cells, and the interstitial cells of Cajal. A member of the type III split-kinase domain family of RTKs, this enzyme has been implicated in the pathophysiology of a number of tumors, including, among others, gastrointestinal stromal tumors (GISTs), seminoma, acute myelogenous leukemia, small-cell lung cancer, and ovarian cancer *(67)*. Activation of c-Kit in tumor cells occurs primarily by two general mechanisms: (1) autocrine and/or paracrine stimulation by its cognate ligand, the stem cell factor *(68)*, and (2) somatic mutations *(69)*. The transforming mechanism of these mutations (single or multiple amino acid changes) results in constitutive ligand-independent kinase activation and stimulation of downstream signaling pathway. The finding that somatic mutations are common in several tumors made c-Kit kinase activity a logical therapeutic target for these malignancies. Proof-of-concept of this approach has been obtained with imatinib mesylate (Gleevec™/Glivec™, STI-571, CGP57148, Novartis Pharma AG; **7** in Fig. 2) in the treatment of patients with advanced GISTs.

Gastrointestinal stromal tumors are the most common mesenchymal tumors of the gastrointestinal tract *(70)*, and gain-of-function mutations of c-Kit occur in over half of these tumors *(71)*. The constitutive c-Kit kinase activity observed in GISTs was hypothesized to provide growth and survival signal to GISTs cells and to be crucial to the pathogenesis of this malignancy *(68,72,73)*. Preclinical studies showed that imatinib mesylate, which was originally developed as a bcr-abl kinase inhibitor *(74–77)*,[§] inhibited c-Kit

---

[§]Imatinib mesylate received US FDA approval in May 2001 for the treatment of patients with chronic myelogenous leukemia after failure of interferon-α therapy.

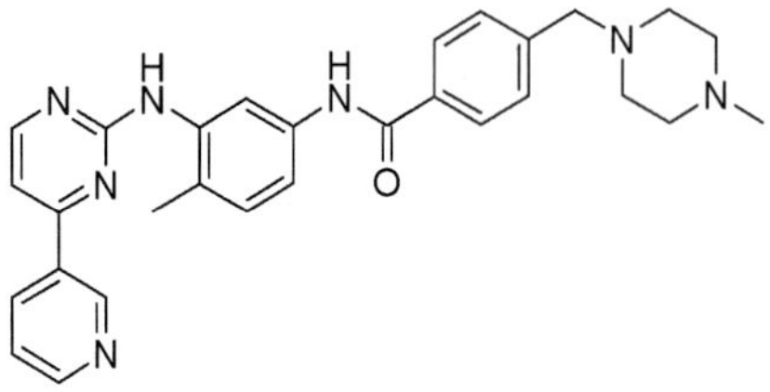

Imatinib
**7**

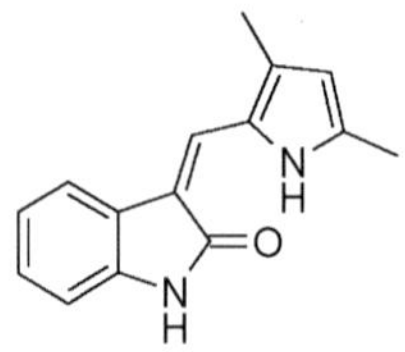

SU5416
**8**

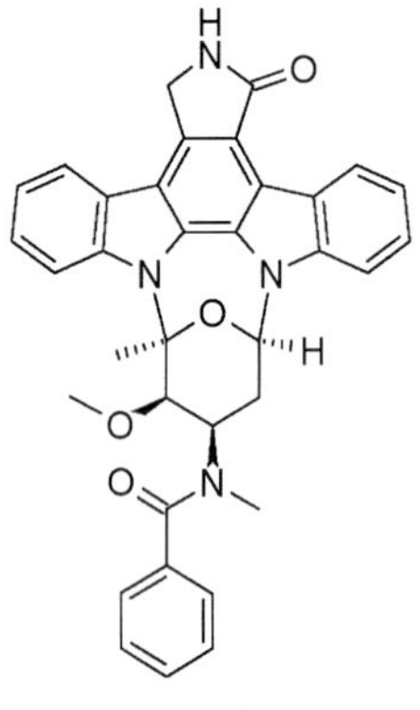

Midostaurin
**9**

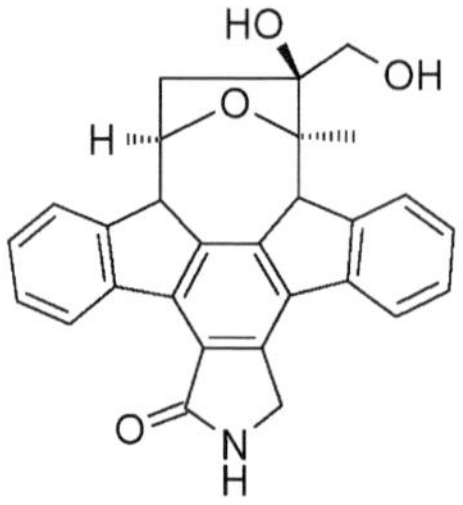

CEP-701
**10**

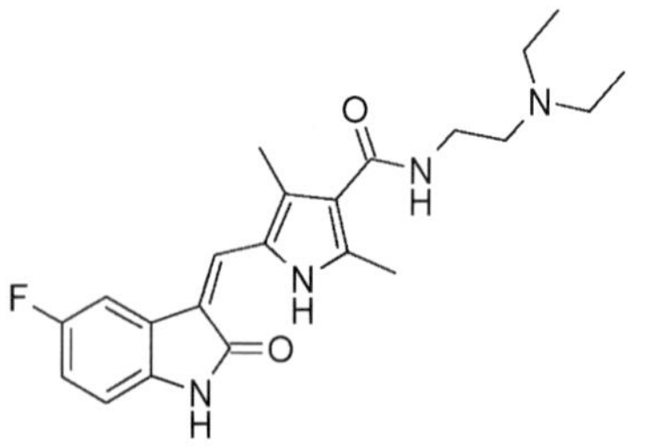

SU11248
**11**

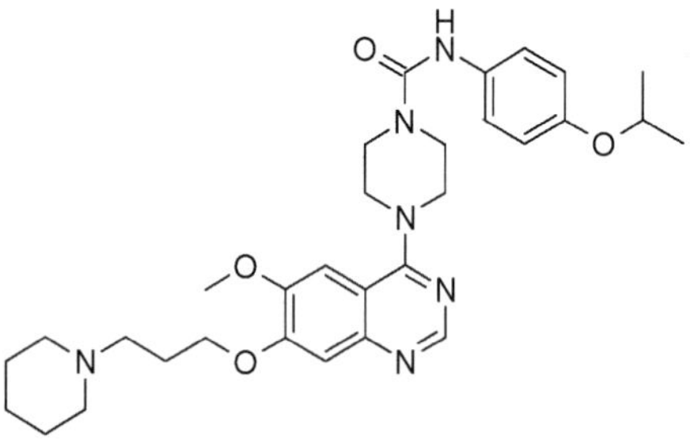

MLN-518
**12**

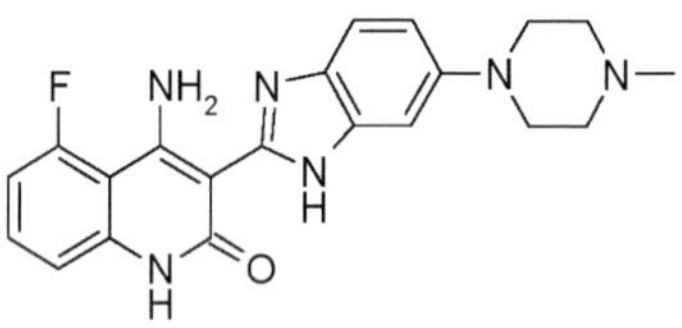

CHIR258
**13**

**Fig. 2.** Kinase inhibitors of c-Kit receptor of stem-cell growth factor and fms-like tyrosine kinase 3 (FLT3).

kinase activity also in a biochemical assay ($IC_{50} = 0.1\ \mu M$), blocked autophosphorylation of wild-type and activated mutant forms of c-Kit in different tumor cell lines, and decreased cellular proliferation of GIST cells *(78–80)*. These results provided the rationale to move forward with clinical testing of imatinib mesylate as an anticancer therapy for GISTs. In an open-label, randomized, multicenter trial, 147 c-Kit-positive GIST patients received imatinib mesylate at oral daily doses of 400 or 600 mg/d. Overall, 59 patients (40.1%) had a partial response, 61 patients (41.5%) had stable disease, and, for technical reasons, response could not be evaluated in 7 patients (4.8%). Early resistance to imatinib mesylate was noted in 20 patients (13.6%) *(81)*. In another study, tolerable doses were found to be up to 800 mg/d. There was a partial remission rate of 36%, a minor remission rate of 33%, and a stable disease rate of 19% *(82,83)*. Clinical responses in GIST patients following treatment with imatinib mesylate appear to be associated with the presence of activating mutations of c-Kit, as patients whose tumor had no detectable c-Kit mutations were more likely to have primary progression in response to the drug *(84)*. The most common adverse events observed with imatinib mesylate in patients with GISTs were edema, fatigue, nausea, and diarrhea. Most of these events were mild or moderate in intensity. Gastrointestinal or abdominal hemorrhages occurred in some patients with large tumors *(81)*.

The objective responses observed in the GISTs clinical trails lead to approval of imatinib mesylate in February 2002 by the US FDA for the treatment of patients with c-Kit (CD117)-positive unresectable (inoperable) and/or metastatic malignant GISTs *(84–86)*. The compound has now been launched for this indication in numerous countries worldwide.

Other compounds in clinical development inhibit c-Kit kinase activity in biochemical and cellular assays (see Section 2.3). The kinase domain of the members of the type III split-kinase domain family of RTKs is strongly conserved and, so far, specific c-Kit kinase inhibitors have not been reported. For example, SU5416 (SUGEN Inc./Pfizer Inc.; **8** in Fig. 2) is a potent kinase inhibitor of VEGFR-1 and -2 ($K_i = 0.16\,\mu M$, c-Kit ($IC_{50} = 0.1\,\mu M$), and wild-type and mutated FLT3 ($IC_{50} = 0.1$–$0.25\,\mu M$, cellular data) *(87)*. On the basis of this inhibitory profile, a phase II clinical study was performed with SU5416 to evaluate the combined effect of inhibiting c-Kit and FLT3 and impeding bone marrow neoangiogenesis (inhibition of VEGFRs) in patients with advanced acute myeloid leukemia (AML, see section 2.3). The overall observed response rate with SU5416 (145 mg/m$^2$, 1-h (intravenous [iv] infusion twice weekly) was low and responses consisted mainly of partial remissions of short duration *(87)*.

## 2.3. Inhibitors of FLT3

FLT3 (fms-related tyrosine kinases) is a member of the type III split-kinase domain family of RTKs that is expressed by normal bone marrow stem and early progenitor cells *(88,89)*. This receptor, which regulates survival and proliferation of hematopoietic cells, has been recently implicated in acute myeloid leukemia (AML), the most common type of leukemia in adults *(90–94)*. Internal tandem duplications (ITDs) of amino acids within the juxtamembrane domain or point mutations in the activation loop of the FLT3 receptor (e.g., missense mutation of aspartic acid-835) have been found in about 30% of patients with AML and in a small number of patients with acute lymphocytic leukemia or myelodysplastic syndrome *(93,95,96)*. These mutations, which result in constitutive FLT3 tyrosine kinase activity, confer a poor clinical prognosis and lower response rate in retrospective clinical studies *(97–99)*, suggesting that FLT3 could play a causative role in the progression of tumors with activating mutations in this RTK. Collectively, the epidemiological data *(90)* and the experimental results obtained with inhibitors that abrogate FLT3 kinase activity *(100–105)* indicate that this receptor might be a viable therapeutic target for the treatment of AML.

Currently, five kinase inhibitors are in phase I/II clinical trials in patients with AML harboring FLT3-activating mutations *(106)*: (1) midostaurin (PKC-412, CGP41251; Novartis AG; **9** in Fig. 2), a staurosporine derivative with broad inhibitory activity against PKC, VEGFR2, PDGFR, c-Kit, syk, and FLT3 *(100,107)*; (2) CEP-701 (KT-5555, Cephalon Inc./ Kyowa Hakko Kogyo Co Ltd; **10** in Fig. 2), another indolocarbazole derivative reported to inhibit Trk and FLT3 *(101,108)*; (3) SU11248 (SUGEN Inc./Pfizer Inc.; **11** in Fig. 2), an indolin-2-one derivative that inhibits PDGFR, VEGFR-2, FGFR-1, c-kit, and FLT3 *(102–104)*; (4) SU5416 (SUGEN Inc./Pfizer Inc.; **8** in Fig. 2), another 3-substituted indolin-2-one that was originally developed to target VEGFR-1 and 2 and was found later to inhibit also FLT3; and (5) MLN-518 (CT-53518, Millennium Pharmaceuticals Inc; **12** in Fig. 2), a quinazoline-piperazine derivative with activity against PDGFR, c-kit, and FLT3 *(105)*. In human FLT3–ITD-positive AML cell lines, these compounds induced apoptosis and inhibited ligand-independent FLT3-ITD phosphorylation, cellular proliferation, and signaling through the phosphatidylinositol-3 kinase (PI3K) and MAPK pathways. In some cases, the cytotoxic effects are observed at concentrations that are lower than those required for FLT3 inhibition. This discrepancy is likely to be caused by the simultaneous inhibition of the other kinases targeted by these compounds. It remains to be seen in clinical settings whether this lack of selectivity has a therapeutic benefit or can lead to increased side effects. Oral administration of FLT3 kinase inhibitors to athymic mice previously injected with cells carrying FLT3 mutations caused tumor regression and enhanced survival *(100–102, 105,109)*. Other compounds (e.g., tyrphostins, indolinones, bis($^1$H-indolyl)-1-methanones, and amino-benzimidozol-equinolines) are able to inhibit the kinase activity of wild-type and mutant FLT3 in vitro and in cellular settings *(110–112)*, and some of the new inhibitors also show potent in vivo activity in AML xenograft tumors (e.g., CHIR258, Chiron Corp.; **13** in Fig. 2) *(112)*.

Overall, the FLT3 inhibitors in clinical trials with AML patients are well tolerated and preliminary results have provided evidence of antitumor activity. The most advanced compounds seem to be CEP-701 and PKC412. In a phase II trial, 4 of 10 patients treated with 60 mg/d po bid of CEP-701 had their peripheral blood leukemia blasts decreased to less than 5%, and one patient had a decrease in bone marrow blasts from >25% to <5% after 1 mo *(113)*. A phase II trial with PKC412 involved 14 patients with advanced AML harboring mutations in the FLT3 gene. Twelve of 14 patients treated with PKC412 (75 mg/d po tid) had the number of blasts in their blood decreased by more that 50% compared with baseline, and in 2 of them, blasts completely disappeared. Five of the 14 patients also experienced a reduction of more than 50% of the number of blasts in their bone marrow *(114)*. The responses in these trials seem so far to be transient. Because of the similarities between AML and blast crisis in chronic myeloid leukemia (CML), hematological response rates in AML patients treated with FLT3 kinase inhibitors should be similar to those found with imatinib in blast crisis CML *(115,116)*, and resistance in relapsed AML patients is likely to occur following single therapy with the FLT3 inhibitors.

## 3. EMERGING THERAPEUTIC TARGETS:
## NEW OPPORTUNITIES AND CHALLENGES IN DRUG DISCOVERY

### 3.1. Insulin-Like Growth Factor I Receptor

The insulin-like growth factor I receptor (IGF-IR) is a member of the insulin receptor (InsR) subclass of RTKs that is activated by insulin-like growth factor I (IGF-I) and II

(IGF-II; 2- to 15-fold lower affinity). Signaling mediated by the IGF-IR has been reported to result in neoplastic transformation, tumor cell growth, survival, angiogenesis, and metastasis *(117–119)*. Parallel to the findings obtained in cellular settings and in vivo animal models *(120)*, a substantial number of clinical studies also support an important role for this receptor in human cancer. Increased expression of IGF-IR, IGF-I, or both has been documented in carcinomas of the lung, breast, thyroid, colon, and prostate *(121)*, and although contradictory among some studies, it is generally accepted that increased risk of solid tumors is associated with high levels of IGF-1 in plasma *(122–124)*.

It is probably the antiapoptotic activity of the IGF-I/IGF-II/IGF-IR axis *(125,126)* that makes IGF-IR an attractive therapeutic target in anticancer drug discovery. Activation of IGF-IR signaling has been shown to protect cancer cells from apoptosis induced by DNA damaging agents, targeted anticancer drugs, and radiation *(127–129)*. Conversely, inhibition of IGF-IR signaling by various means was reported to enhance the in vitro or in vivo sensitivity of selected cancer cells to radiation and antitumor agents *(130–132)*. Thus, the use of an IGF-IR signaling antagonist could be envisioned as a single agent in IGF-I/IGF-II/IGF-IR-dependent malignancies or in combination with established therapeutic modalities.

Blocking the expression and/or activation of IGF-IR has led to the reversal of the transformed phenotype in different types of cancer cell line and suppressed tumor growth in vivo. These studies have been performed using dominant negative mutants, kinase domain mutagenesis, antisense oligonucleotides, plasmids expressing IGF-IR antisense cDNA, IGF-I peptide antagonists, soluble IGF-IRS, or anti-IGR-IR antibodies *(133–137)*. Although these approaches have been able to provide biological tools for studying this receptor, the identification of specific low-molecular-mass kinase inhibitors of this receptor has proven to be a major challenge for medicinal chemistry. The sequence identify at the kinase domain of IGF-IR and InsR is around 84%, and the residues that line the ATP-binding cleft are strictly conserved between these two receptors *(138,139)*. Initial attempts to inhibit IGF-IR kinase activity resulted in the identification of tyrphostin derivatives that showed weak activity in blocking IGF-IR autophosphorylation but some selectivity over InsR (fourfold to eightfold) *(140)*. Improved IGF-IR inhibitory activity and cellular selectivity has been reported recently for a new class of pyrrolo[2,3-*d*]pyrimidine derivatives. For example, NVP-ADW742 (Novartis Pharma AG; **14** in Fig. 3) inhibits IGF-1-dependent IGF-IR autophosphorylation with an $IC_{50}$ value of 170 n*M*, and, under similar experimental conditions, it shows 16-fold selectivity over the native InsR and weak activity ($IC_{50}$ >5 µ*M*) against other RTKs *(141)*. The compound shows antiangiogenic activity in an IGF-I-driven porous chamber model *(141)*, and when used alone or in combination with cytotoxic agents, it suppresses tumor growth and prolongs survival of mice with diffuse bone lesions of multiple myeloma *(142)*. These preclinical findings and additional studies *(143)* support the potential application of targeted therapeutic strategies directed at IGF-IR in the treatment of multiple myeloma *(144,145)* or other IGFs-responsive neoplasias *(146–149)*.

### 3.2. c-Met

The c-Met proto-oncogene encodes a receptor tyrosine kinase that is activated by the hepatocyte growth factor/scatter factor (HGF/SF) *(150)*. Although the c-Met/HGF signaling mediates a variety of normal cellular events, its induction in inappropriate contexts has been clearly implicated in cancer *(151,152)*. Activation of this receptor in target cells can lead to proliferation, scattering, branching, angiogenesis, enhanced cell motility, invasion of extracellular matrices, and metastasis *(153–155)*. Constitutive activation of and

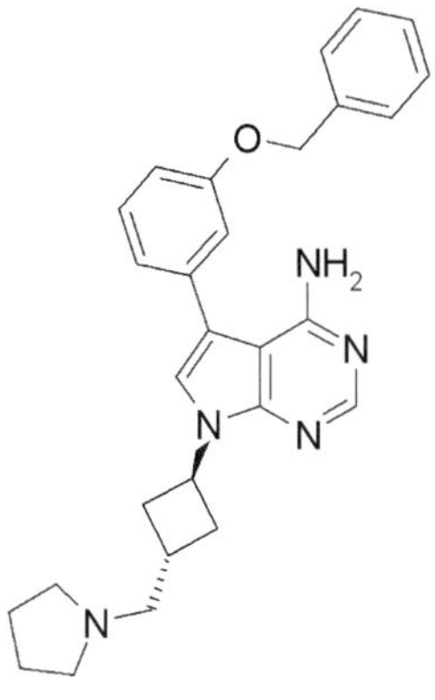

NVP-ADW742
**14**

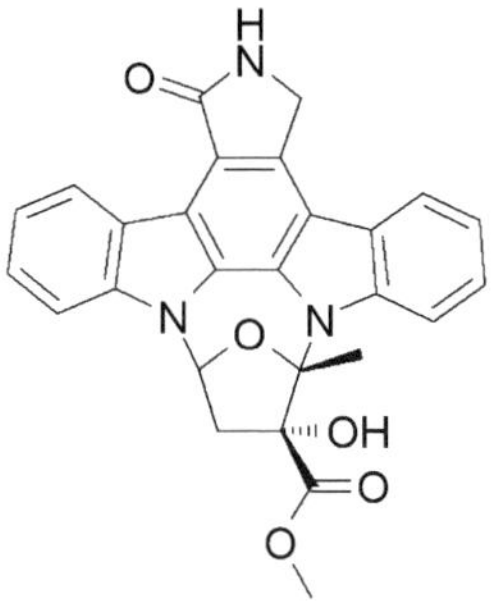

K-252a
**15**

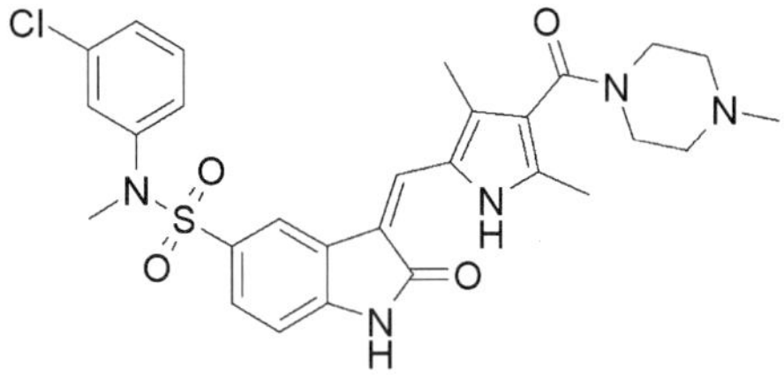

SU11274
**16**

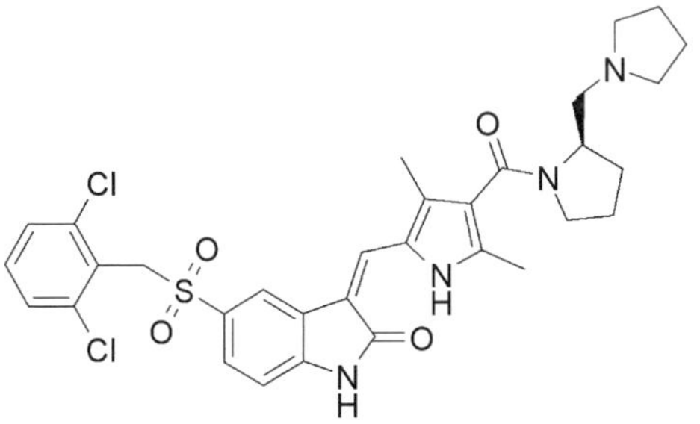

PHA-665752
**17**

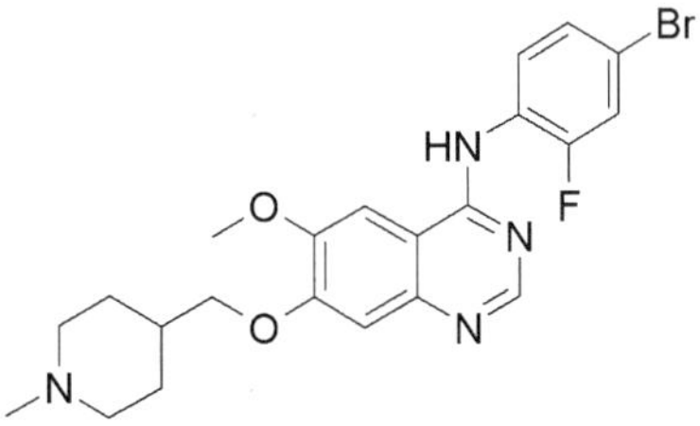

AZD-6474
**18**

**Fig. 3.** Kinase inhibitors of insulin-like growth factor-1 receptor (IGF-IR), c-Met (hepatocyte growth factor receptor) and RET (rearranged during transfection).

transformation by the c-Met tyrosine kinase domain in the form of the Tpr-Met oncoprotein was the first indication that inappropriate c-Met activation could mediate oncogenesis *(156,157)*. Although this form of activation is rarely found in human cancers (e.g., gastric carcinomas) *(158)*, the c-Met receptor is frequently activated in tumors by overexpression or by the presence of an ectopic HGF loop *(159)*. Epidemiological studies have shown that c-Met is overexpressed in tumors of specific histotypes, including thyroid, pancreatic, lung, and liver metastases of colorectal carcinomas *(152,160)*. In addition, germline and somatic missense mutations in the tyrosine kinase domain of this receptor have been identified in papillary renal and childhood hepatocellular carcinomas, as well as in ovarian cancer and lymph node metastases of head and neck squamous cell carcinomas *(151,161–163)*. These activating mutations point to the potential acquisition of a metastatic phenotype by c-Met-transformed cancer cells *(164,165)*.

Different approaches have been explored to target c-Met function in tumor cells (e.g., antagonists of HGF *(166–169)*, substrate kinase inhibitors *(170)*, or Hsp90 inhibitors *(171, 172)*, but, as for the other therapeutic targets in this section, the number of c-Met kinase inhibitors in public domain is low in comparison with other RTKs. K-252a (**15** in Fig. 3), which is a microbial alkaloid active against serine/threonine and tyrosine kinases, has been shown to inhibit the activating Met/Thr-1268 mutation in cultured cells ($IC_{50} < 0.5$ $\mu M$) and completely block HGF-induced scattering of MLP-20 cells at 33 n$M$ (173). More compelling data about the feasibility of blocking c-Met catalytic site with ATP-competitive inhibitors have been reported in two recent publications. SU11274 (SUGEN Inc./Pfizer Inc.; **16** in Fig. 3), which inhibits c-Met receptor kinase activity in a biochemical assay ($IC_{50}$ = 20 n$M$) and shows greater than 50-fold selectivity over other tyrosine kinases (e.g., EGFR, PDGFR$\beta$, Tie-2), blocks receptor autophosphorylation and induces apoptosis and cell cycle arrest in Tpr-Met-transformed BaF3 at concentration in the low micromolar range (174). PHA-665752 (SUGEN Inc./Pfizer Inc.; **17** in Fig. 3), which is another indolin-2-one derivative, inhibits c-Met kinase activity in vitro with a $K_i$ value of 4 n$M$ ($IC_{50}$ = 9 n$M$) and has an excellent selectivity profile over other kinases, with the exceptions of Ron ($IC_{50}$ = 68 n$M$) and VEGFR-2 ($IC_{50}$ = 200 n$M$) (175). This compound modulates c-Met-dependent phenotypes in cellular settings, and exhibits in vivo antitumor activity in c-Met-dependent tumor models upon intravenous administration. As mentioned by the authors of this work (175), the diverse roles of c-Met in the biology of primary and metastatic tumors could represent major challenges in the characterization of c-Met inhibitors in a clinical setting. To date, no c-Met inhibitors are known to be in clinical trials.

### 3.3. RET

The RET (rearranged during transfection) proto-oncogene encodes an evolutionary conserved RTK that is activated by growth factors of the glial cell-line-derived neurotrophic factor family. This receptor plays an important role in kidney development and promotes neural cell survival and differentiation, but the chronic activation of RET can specifically cause certain type of human cancers (176,177). Thus, germline point mutations of RET are responsible for multiple endocrine neoplasia type 2 (MEN2), an inherited cancer syndrome characterized by medullary thyroid carcinoma (MTC) (178,179). The clinical syndromes associated with MTC are caused by three types of RET mutations (180). The subtype RET/MEN2A is characterized by mutations in the extracellular domain (e.g., Cys634Arg) that result in constitutive receptor dimerization and gain of function (179). The mutations in the familial medullary thyroid carcinoma subtype are more homogenously distributed on three cysteines of the extracellular domain or occur in the intracellular tyrosine kinase domain. The less prevalent subtype RET/MEN2B carries a mutation in the activation loop (Met918Thr, 95%; Ala883Phe, 3%) (181) that causes constitutive activation of the RET transformation potential and eventually modifies its kinase substrate specificity (e.g., autophosphorylation sites and intracellular substrates) (179). RET/MEN2B remains also responsive to its ligands, and temporal and spatial expression of neurotrophic factors could further enhanced RET kinase activity in patients harboring MEN2B mutations.

In addition to the MEN2 syndromes, papillary thyroid carcinoma (PTC), which is the most common type of thyroid tumor (182), is associated with specific alterations of the RET proto-oncogene (183,184). The rearranged PTC oncogene (RET/PTC), which is found with variable frequency (from 2.5% to 40%) in papillary carcinomas (185), is the product of the fusion of the tyrosine kinase domain of the proto-RET to other genes (e.g., H4, R1$\alpha$ and RFG/ELE1) (186). These rearrangements (e.g., PCT1, PCT2, and PCT3) (184) allow the expression of RET in thyroid cells, generate constitutively active chimeric oncoproteins, and alter the cellular localization of this kinase from the plasma membrane to the cytosol.

Inhibition of RET kinase activity has been reported so far with compounds designed to target other RTKs. For example, AZD6474 (AstraZeneca plc; **18** in Fig. 3), which is a potent VEGFR-2 tyrosine kinase inhibitor, blocks the enzymatic ($IC_{50} = 100$ n$M$ against RET/PTC3, biochemical assay) and the transforming effects (morphological transformation, proliferation, and anchorage-independent growth) of RET-derived oncoproteins *(187)*. This compound completely arrests the growth of NIH-RET/PTC3 xenografts *(188)* in nude mice when administered intraperitoneally (1 mg/mouse/d, 10 d). Ex vivo analyses of tumor tissue showed that tumor growth inhibition in the treated animals was associated with a remarkable reduction of RET/PTC3 phosphotyrosine content. Similar cellular effects have been observed with other ATP-competitive inhibitors active against constitutive activated RET/PTC and RET/MEN2 oncoproteins *(189–191)*. Overall, these experimental findings support the idea that targeting the kinase activity of RET oncoproteins might offer a potential tailored therapeutic strategy for carcinomas sustaining chronic activation of this RTK.

# 4. CONCLUSIONS

In spite of the enormous efforts devoted to the identification and development of receptor tyrosine kinase inhibitors as new antitumor agents, only two compounds have so far been approved for the treatment of malignancies in which the importance of the targeted kinase is well established. Although it is impossible to predict if new receptor tyrosine kinase inhibitors are going to reach the marketplace in the near future, some of the disappointing clinical results obtained with early kinase inhibitors call for improvements in the selection of clinical candidates and in the clinical development of these targeted antitumor agents. We can only hope that attention to the problems and issues already identified in this challenging area of drug discovery *(192)* could increase the odds of these agents to alter the natural course of the disease they are targeting and positively impact the lives of cancer patients.

# REFERENCES

1. Yarden Y, Slimkowski MX. Untangling the erbB signalling network. Nat Rev 2001; 2:127–137.
2. Yarden Y. The EGFR family and its lignad in human cancer signalling mechanisms and therapeutic opportunities. Eur J Cancer 2001; 37:S3–S8.
3. Mendelsohn J, Baselga J. The EGF receptor family as targets for cancer therapy. Oncogene 2000; 19: 6550–6565.
4. Voldborg BR, Damstrup L, Spang-Thomsen M, Poulsen HS. Epidermal growth factor receptor (EGFR) and EGFR mutations, function and possible role in clinical trials. Ann Oncol 1997; 12:1197–1206.
5. Moscatello DK, Holgado-Madruga M, Godwin AK, Ramirez G, Gunn G, Zoltick PW, et al. Frequent expression of a mutant epidermal growth factor receptor in multiple human tumours. Cancer Res 1995; 55:5536–5539.
6. Salomon DS, Brandt R, Ciardiello F, Normanno N. Epidermal growth facctor-related peptides and their receptors in human malignancies. Crit Rev Oncol Hematol 1995; 19:183–232.
7. Scambia G, Benedetti-Panici P, Ferrandine G, Distefano M, Salerno G, Romanini ME, et al. Epidermal growth factor, estrogen and progesterone receptor expression in primary ovarian cancer: correlation with clinical outcome and response to chemotherapy. Br J Cancer 1995; 72:361–366.
8. Tang CK, Gong XQ, Moscatello DK, Wong AJ, Lippman ME. Epidermal growth factor receptor vIII enhances tumorogenicity in human breast cancer. Cancer Res 2000; 60:3081–3087.
9. Sato JD, Kawamoto T, Le AD, Mendelsohn J. Biological effects of monoclonal antibodies to human epidermal growth factor receptors. Mol Biol Med 1983; 1:511–529.
10. Ciardiello F, Tortora G. Anti-epidermal growth factor receptor drugs in cancer therapy. Expert Opin Invest Drugs 2002; 11:755–768.

11. Adjei AA. Epidermal growth factor receptor tyorsine kinase inhibitors in cancer therapy. Drugs Future 2001; 21:1087–1092.

12. Baselga J, Albanell J, Molina MA, Arribas J. Mechanism of action of trastuzumab and scientific update. Semin Oncol 2001; 28:4–11.

13. Slamon D, Pegram M. Rationale for trastuzumab (Herceptin) in adjuvant breast cancer trials. Semin Oncol 2001; 28:13–19.

14. Noonberg SB, Benz CC. Tyrosine kinase inhibitors targeted to the epidermal growth factor receptor subfamily: role as anticancer agents. Drugs 2000; 59:753–767.

15. Gibbs JB. Anticancer drug targets: growth factors and growth factor signaling. J Clin Invest 2000; 105 :9–13.

16. Woodburn JR. The epidermal growth factor receptor and its inhibition in cancer therapy. Pharmacol Ther 1999; 82:241–250.

17. Herbst RS. ZD1839: targeting the epidermal growth factor receptor in cancer therapy. Expert Opin Invest Drugs 2002; 11(6):837–849.

18. Woodburn JR, Kendrew J, Fennell M, Wakeling AE. ZD1839 (Iressa) a selective epidermal growth factor receptor tyrosine kinase inhibitor (EGFR-TKI): inhibition of c-fos mRNA, an intermediate marker of EGFR activation, correlates with tumour growth inhibition. Proc Am Assoc Cancer Res 2000; 41: 2552 (abstract).

19. Woodburn JR, Barker AJ, Wakeling A, Valcaccia BE. 6-Amino-4-(3-methylphenylamino)-quinazoline: an EGF receptor tyrosine kinase inhibitor with activity in a range of human tumour xenografts. Proc Am Assoc Cancer Res 1996; 37:2665 (abstract).

20. Anderson NG, Ahmad T, Chan KC, Bundred NJ. Effects of ZD1839 (Iressa), a novel EGF receptor tyrosine kinase inhibitor, on breast cancer cell proliferation and invasiveness. Breast Cancer Res Treat 2000; 64:32.

21. Lavelle F. American Association for Cancer Research 1997: progress and new hope in the fight against cancer, April 12–16, 1997, San Diego, California. Expert Opin Invest Drugs 1997; 6:771–775.

22. Woodburn JR, Barker AJ, Gibson KH, Ashton SE, Wakeling AE, Curry BJ, et al. ZD 1839, an epidermal growth factor tyrosine kinase inhibitors selected for clinical development. Proc Am Assoc Cancer Res 1997; 38:633 (abstract).

23. Hirata A, Ogawa S, Kometani T, Kuwano T, Naito S, Kuwano M, et al. ZD1839 (Iressa) induces antiangiogenic effects through inhibiiton of epidermal growth factor receptor tyrosine kinase. Cancer Res 2002; 62:2554–2560.

24. Ciardiello F, Caputo R, Bianco R, Damiano V, Fontanini G, Cuccato S, et al. Inhibitionn of growth factor production and angiogenesis in human cancer cells by ZD1839 (Iressa), a selective epidermal growth factor receptor tyrosine kinase inhibitor. Clin Cancer Res 2001; 7:1459–1465.

25. Ciardiello F, Caputo R, Bianco R, et al. Antitumor effect and potentiation of cytotoxic drugs activity in human cancer cells by ZD1839 (Iressa), a selective epidermal growth factor receptor tyrosine kinase inhibitor. Clin Cancer Res 2000; 6:2053–2063.

26. Sirotnak FM, Zakowski MF, Miller VA, Scher HI, Kris MG. Efficacy of cytotoxic agents against human tumor xenografts markedly enhanced by coadministration of ZD1839 (Iressa), an inhibitor of EGFR tyrosine kinase. Clin Cancer Res 2000; 6:4885–4892.

27. Williams KJ, Telfer BA, Stratford IJ, Wedge SR. ZD1839 (Iressa), a specific oral epidermal growth factor recepto-tyrosine kinase inhibitors, potentitates radiotherapy in a human colorectal cancer xenograft model. Br J Cancer 2002; 86:1157–1161.

28. Normanno N, Campiglio M, De L, Somenzi G, Maiello M, Ciardiello F, et al. Cooperative inhibitory effect of ZD1839 (Iressa) in combination with trastuzumab (Herceptin) on human breast cancer cell growth. Ann Oncol 2002; 13:65–72.

29. Natale RB, Zaretsky SL. ZD1839 (Iressa): what's in it for the patient? Oncologist 2002; 7:25–30.

30. Moyer JD, Barbacci EG, Iwata KK, Arnold L, Boman B, Cunningham A, et al. Induction of apoptosis and cell cycle arrest by CP-358,774, an inhibitor of epidermal growth factor receptor tyrosine kinase. Cancer Res 1997; 57:4838–4848.

31. Iwata K, Miller PE, Barbacci EG, Arnold L, Doty J, DiOrio CI, et al. CP-358,774: a selective EGFR kinase inhibitor with potent antiproliferative activity against HN5 head and neck tumor cells. Proc Am Assoc Cancer Res 1997; 38:633 (abstract).

32. Hidalgo M. Erlotinib: preclinical investigations. Oncology 2003; 17:11–16.

33. Akita RW, Sliwkowski MX. Preclinical studies with erlotinib (Tarceva). Semin Oncol 2003; 30:15–24.

34. Herbst RS. Erlotinib (Tarceva): an update on the clinical program. Semin Oncol 2004; 30:34–46.

35. Pollack VA, Savage DM, Baker DA, Tsaparikos KE, Sloan DE, Moyer JD, et al. Inhibition of epidermal growth factor receptor-associated tyrosine phosphorylation in humna carcinomas wiht CP-358,774: dynamics of receptor inhibition in situ and antitumor effects in athymic mice. J Pharmacol Exp Ther 1999; 291:739–748.

36. Siu LL, Hidalgo M, Heumanaitis J, et al. Dose and schedule-duration escalation of the epidermal growth factor receptor tyrosine kinase inhibitors CP-358,774: a phase I and pharmacokinetic study. Proc Am Soc Clin Oncol 1999; 18:388 (abstract).

37. Karp DD, Silberman SL, Csudae R, et al. Phase I dose escalation study of epidermal growth factor receptor tyrosine kinase inhibitor CP-358,774 in patients with advanced solid tumors. Proc Am Soc Clin Oncol 1999; 18:1499 (abstract).

38. Tzahar E, Waterman H, Chen X, Levkowitz G, Karunagaran D, Lav S, et al. A hierarchical network of interreceptor interactions determines signal transduction by Neu differentiation factor/neuregulin and epidermal growth factor. Mol Cell Biol 1996; 16:5276–5287.

39. Riese DJ, Stern DF. Specificity within the EGF family/ErbB receptor family signaling network. BioEssays 1998; 20:41–48.

40. Simpson BJ, Phillips HA, Lessels AM, Langdon SP, Miller WR. c-erB growth-factor-receptor proteins in ovarian tumours. Int J Cancer 1995; 64:202–206.

41. Slamon DJ, Clark GM, Wong SG, Levin WJ, Ullrich A, McGuire WL. Human breast cancer: correlation of relapse and survival with amplification of the HER-2/new oncogene. Science 1987; 235:177–182.

42. Rusnak DW, Affeck K, Cockerill SG, Stubberfield C, Harris R, Page M, et al. The characterization of novel, dual ErbB-2/EGFR, tyrosine kinase inhibitors: potential therapy for cancer. Cancer Res 2001; 61:7196–7203.

43. Rusnak DW, Lackey K, Affleck K, Wood ER, Alligood KJ, Rhodes N, et al. The effects of the novel, reversible EGFR/ErbB-2 tyrosine kinase inhibitor, GW2016, on the growth of human normal and tumor-derived cell lines in vitro and in vivo. Mol Cancer Ther 2001; 1:85–94.

44. Mullin RJ, Alligood KJ, Allen PP, Crosby RM, Keith BR, et al. Antitunmor activity of GW2016 in the EGFR positive human head and neck cancer xenograft, HN5. Proc Am Assoc Cancer Res 2001; 42:854 (abstract).

45. Keith BR, Allen PP, Alligood KJ, Crosby RM, Lackey K, et al. Antitumor activity of GW2016 in the ErbB-2 positive human breast cancer xenograft, BT474. Proc Am Assoc Cancer Res 2001; 42:803 (abstract).

46. Caravatti G, Guido B, Brueggen J, Furet P, Lane H, Mestan J, et al. Preclinical activity of AEE788, a potent inhibitor of the erbB and VEGF receptor tyrosine kinases. Discovery and in vitro profile of AEE788. Proceedings of the AACR-NCI-EORTC International Conference 2003:118 (abstract).

47. Traxler P, Allegrini PR, Brandt R, Brueggen J, Cozens R, Grosios K, et al. Preclinical activity of AEE788, a potent new inhibitor of the erbB and VEGF receptor tyrosine kinases. In vivo profile of AEE788. Proceedings of the AACR-NCI-EORTC International Conference 2003:87 (abstract).

48. Kim S, Schiff BA, Younes MA, Jasser SA, Doan D, Yigitbasi OG, et al. Treatment with NVP-AEE788 —a dual inhibitor of EGFR and VEGFR tyrosine kinase—inhibits anaplastic thyroid carcinioma growth. Proceedings of the AACR–NCI–EORTC International Conference 2003:128 (abstract).

49. Yigitbasi OG, Younes MN, Schiff BA, Doan D, Jasser SA, Al-Muhtaseb Z, et al. Dual inhibition of EGFR and VEGFR in squamous cell carcinoma of the head and neck: the role of the new EGFR/VEGFR inhibitor NVP-AEE788. Proceedings of the AACR–NCI–EORTC International Conference 2003:102 (abstract).

50. Nagasawa J, Mizokami A, Asahi H, Iwasa Y, Kosida K, Yoshida S, et al. TAK-165, a selective inhibitor of HER2 tyrosine kinase: antitumor effect of TAK-165 on hormone refractory prostate cancer and bladder cancer in vitro and in vivo. Proc Am Assoc Cancer Res 2003; 44:4690 (abstract).

51. Denny WA. Irreversible inhibitors of the erbB family of protein tyrosine kinases. Pharmacol Ther 2002; 93:253–261.

52. Fry DW. Site-directed irreverersible inhibitors of the erbB family of receptor tyrosine kinases as novel chemotherapeutic agents for cancer. Anti-Cancer Drug Des 2000; 15:3–16.

53. Smaill JB, Palmer BD, Rewcastle GF, Denny WA, McNamara DJ, Dobrusin EM, et al. Tyrosine kinase inhibitors. 15. 4-(Phenylamino)quinazoline and 4-(phenylamino)pyrido[d]pyrimidine acrylamides as irreversible inhibitors of the ATP binding site of the epidermal growth factor receptor. J Med Chem 1999; 42:1803–1815.

54. Fry DW, Bridges AJ, Denny WA, Doherty AM, Greis KD, Hicks JL, et al. Specific, irreversible inactivation of the epidermal growth factor receptor and erbB2, by a new class of tyrosine kinase inhibitor. Proc Natl Acad Sci USA 1998; 95:12,022–12,027.

55. Allen LF, Eiseman IA, Fry DW, Lenehan PF. CI-1033, an irreversible pan-erbB receptor inhibitor and its potential application for the treatment of breast cancer. Semin Oncol 2003; 5:65–78.

56. Slichenmyer WJ, Elliott WL, Fry DW. CI-1033, a pan-erbB tyrosine kinase inhibitor. Semin Oncol 2001; 28:80–85.

57. Allen LF, Lenehan PF, Eiseman IA, Elliott WL, Fry DW. Potential benefits of the irreversible pan-erbB inhibitor, CI-1033, in the treatment of breast cancer. Semin Oncol 2002; 30:11–21.

58. Smaill JB, Rewcastle GW, Loo JA, Greis KD, Chan OH, Reyner EL, et al. Tyrosine kinase inhibitors. 17. Irreversible inhibitors of the epidermal growth factor recetpor: 4.(phenylamino)quinazoline- and 4-(phenylamino)pyrido[3,2-d]pyrimidine-6-acrylamides bearing additional solubilizing functions. J Med Chem 2000; 43:1380–1397.

59. Nelson JM, Fry DW. Akt, MAPK (Erk1/2), and p38 act in concert to promote apoptosis in response to ErbB receptor family inhibition. J Biol Chem 2001; 276:14,842–14,847.

60. Rao GS, Murray S, Ethier SP. Radiosensitization of human breast cancer cells by a novel ErbB family receptor tyrosine kinase inhibitor. Int J Radiat Oncol Biol Phys 2000; 48:1519–1528.

61. Gieseg MA, De Block C, Ferguson LR, Denny WA. Evidence for receptor enhanced chemosensitivity in combinations of cisplatin and the new irreversible tyrosine kinase inhibitor CI-1033. Anti-Cancer Drugs 2001; 12:681–690.

62. Erlichman C, Boerner SA, Hallgren CG, Spieker R, Wang XY, James CD, et al. The HER tyrosine kinase inhibitor CI1033 enhances cytoxicity of 7-ethyl-10-hydroxycamtothecin and topotecan by inhibiting breast cancer resistance protein-mediated drug efflux. Cancer Res 2001; 61:739–748.

63. Shin DM, Nemunaitis J, Zinner RG, et al. A phase I clinical and biomarker study of CI-1033, a novel pan-ErbB tyrosine kinase inhibitor in patients with solid tumors. Proc Am Soc Clin Oncol 2001; 20:324 (abstract).

64. Garrison MA, Tolcher A, McCreery H, et al. A phase I and pharmacokinetic study of CI-1033, a pan-ErbB tyrosine kinase inhibitor, given orally on days 1, 8, and 15 every 28 days to patients with solid tumors. Proc Am Soc Clin Oncol 2001; 20:283 (abstract).

65. Wissner A, Overbeek E, Reich MF, Floyd B, Johnson BD, Namuya N, et al. Synthesis and structure–activity relationships of 6,7-disubstituted 4-anilinoquinoline-3-carbonitriles. The design of an orally activa, irreversible inhibitor of the tyrosine kinase activity of the epidermal growth factor receptor (EGFR) and the human epidermal growth factor receptor-2 (HER-2). J Med Chem 2003; 46:49–63.

66. Torrance CJ, Jackson PE, Montgomery E, Kinzler KW, Vogelstein B, Wissner A, et al. Combinatorial chemoprevention of intestinal neoplasia. Nat Med 2000; 6:1024–1028.

67. Heinrich MC, Blanke CD, Druker BJ, Corless CL. Inhibition of KIT tyrosine kinase activity: a novel molecular approach to the treatment of KIT-positive malignancies. J Clin Oncol 2002; 20:1692–1703.

68. Heinrich MC, Blanke CD, Druker BJ, Corless CL. Inhibition of KIT tyrosine kinase activity: a novel molecular approach to the treatment of KIT-positive malignancies. J Clin Oncol 2002; 20:1692–1703.

69. Blume-Jensen P, Hunter T. Oncogenic kinase signalling. Nature 2001; 411:355–365.

70. Blanke CD, Eisenberg BL, Heinrich MC. Gastrointestinal stromal tumors. Curr Treat Options Oncol 2001; 2:485–491.

71. Chandu de Silva MV, Reid R. Gastrointestinal stromal tumours (GIST): c-Kit mutations, CD117 expression, differential diagnosis and targeted cancer therapy with imatinib. Pathol Oncol Res 2003; 9:13–19.

72. Joensuu H, Fletcher C, Dimitrijevic S, Silberman S, Roberts P, Demetri G. Management of malignant gastrointestinal stromal tumours. Lancet Oncol 2002; 3:655–664.

73. Demetri GD. Targeting c-kit mutations in solid tumors: scientific rationale and novel therapeutic options. Semin Oncol 2002; 28:19–26.

74. Savage DG, Antman KH. Imatinib mesylate; a new oral targeted therapy. N Engl J Med 2002; 346: 683–693.

75. Druker BJ. STI571 (Gleevec™) as a paradigm for cancer therapy. Trends Mol Med 2002; 8:S14–S18.

76. de Bree F, Sorbera LA, Fernandez R, Castaner J. Imatinib mesylate. Drugs 2001; 26:545–552.

77. Zimmermann J, Buchdunger E, Mett H, Meyer T, Lydon NB. Potent and selective inhibitors of the ABL-kinase: phenylaminopyridine (PAP) derivatives. Bioorg Med Chem Lett 1997; 7:187–192.

78. Frost MJ, Ferrao PT, Hughes TP, Ashman LK. Juxtamebrane mutant V560GKit is more sensitive to imatinib (STI571) compared with wild.type c-kit whereas the kinase domain mutant D816VKit is resistant. Mol Cancer Ther 2002; 1:1115–1124.

79. Buchdunger E, Cioffi CL, Law N, Stover D, Ohno-Jones S, Druker BJ, et al. Abl protein–tyrosine kinase inhibitor STI571 inhibits in vitro signal transduction mediated by c-Kit and platelet-derived growth factor receptors. J Pharmacol Exp Ther 2000; 295:139–145.

80. Heinrich MC, Griffith DJ, Druker BJ, Wait CL, Ott KA, Zigler AJ. Inhibition of c-kit receptor tyrosine kinase activity by STI 571, a selective tyrosine kinase inhibitor. Blood 2000; 96: 925–932.

81. Demetri GD, von Mehren M, Blanke CD, Van den Abbeele AD, Eisenberg B, Roberts PJ, et al. Efficacy and safety of imatinib mesylate in advanced gastrointestinal stromal tumors. N Engl J Med 2002; 347:472–480.

82. Drevs J, Medinger M, Schmidt-Gersbach C, Weber R, Unger C. Receptor tyrosine kinases: the main targets for new anticancer therapy. Curr Drug Targets 2003; 4:113–121.

83. Joensuu H. Treatment of inoperable gastrointestinal stromal tumor (GIST) with imatinib (Glivec, Gleevec). Med Klin 2002; 97:28–30.

84. Blanke CD, von Mehren M, Joensuu H, Roberts PJ, Eisenberg B. Evaluation of the safety and efficacy of an oral molecularly-targeted therapy, STI571, in patients with unresectable or metastatic gastrointestinal stromal tumors (GISTS) expressing c-Kit. Proc Am Soc Clin Oncol 2001; 20:1a (abstract).

85. Kantarjian H, Sawyers C, Hochhaus A, Guilhot F, Schiffer C, Gambacorti-Passerini C, et al. Hematologic and cytogenetic responses to imatinib mesylate in chronic myelogenous leukemia. N Engl J Med 2002; 346:645–652.

86. van Oosterom AT, Judson I, Verweij J, Stroobants S, Donato di Paola E, Dimitrijevic S, et al. Safety and efficacy of imatinib (STI571) in metastatic gastrointestinal stromal tumours: a phase I study. Lancet 2001; 358:1421–1423.

87. Fiedler W, Mesters R, Tinnefeld H, Loges S, Staib P, Dührsen U, et al. A phase 2 clinical study of SU5416 in patients with refractory acute myeloid leukemia. Blood 2003; 102:2763–2767.

88. Rosnet O, Buhring HJ, deLapeyriere O, Beslu N, Lavagana C, Marchetto S, et al. Expression and signal transduction of the FLT3 tyrosine kinase receptor. Acta Haematol 1996; 95:218–223.

89. Rosnet O, Marchetto S, de Lapyriere O, Birnbaum D. Murine Flt3, a gene encoding a novel tyrosine kinase receptor of the PDGFR/CS1R family. Oncogene 1991; 6:1641–1650.

90. Redaelli A, Lee JM, Stephens JM, Pashos CL. Epidemiology and clinical burden of acute myeloid leukemia. Expert Rev Anticancer Ther 2003; 3:695–710.

91. Sawyers CL. Finding the next Gleevec: FLT3 targeted kinase inhibitor therapy for acute myeloid leukemia. Cancer Cell 2002; 1:413–415.

92. Levis M, Allebach J, Tse KF, Zheng R, Baldwin BR, Smith BD, et al. A FLT3-targeted tyrosine kinase inhibitor is cytotoxic to leukemia cells in vitro and in vivo. Blood 2002; 99:3885–3891.

93. Gilliland DG, Griffin JD. Role of FLT3 in leukemia. Curr Opin Hematol 2002; 9:274–281.

94. Kiyoi H, Naoe T. FLT3 in human hematologic malignancies. Leuk Lymphoma 2002; 43:1541–1547.

95. Yamamoto Y, Kiyoi H, Nakano Y, et al. Activating mutation of D835 within the activation loop of FLT3 in human hematologic malignancies. Blood 2001; 97:2434–2439.

96. Iwai T, Yokota S, Nakao M, et al. Internal tandem duplication of the FLT3 gene and clinical evaluation in childhood acute myeloid leukemia. The Childen's Cancer and Leukemia Study Group, Japan. Leukemia 1999; 13:38–43.

97. Kottaridis PD, Gale RE, Frew ME, Harrison G, Langabeer SE, Belton AA, et al. The presence of a FLT3 internal tandem duplication in patients with acute myeloid leukemia (AML) adds important prognostic information to cytogenetic risk group and response to the first cycle of chemotherapy: analysis of 854 patients from the United Kingdom Medical Research Council AML 10 and 12 trials. Blood 2001; 98:1752–1759.

98. Meshinchi S, Woods WG, Stirewalt DL, Sweetser DA, Buckley JD, Tjoa TK, et al. Prevalence and prognostic significance of Flt3 internal tandem duplication in pediatric acute myeloid leukemia. Blood 2001; 97:89–94.

99. Abu-Duhier FM, Goodeve AC, Wilson GA, Gari MA, Peake IR, Rees DC, et al. FLT3 internal tandem duplication mutations in adult acute myeloid leukaemia define a high-risk group. Br J Haematol 2000; 111:190–195.

100. Weisberg E, Boulton C, Kelly LM, Manley P, Fabbro D, Meyer T, et al. Inhibition of mutant FLT3 receptors in leukemia cells by the small molecule tyrosine kinase inhibitors PKC412. Cancer Cell 2002; 1:433–443.

101. Levis M, Allebach J, Tse KF, Zheng R, Baldwin BR, Smith BD, et al. A FLT3-targeted tyrosine kinase inhibitor is cytotoxic to leukemia cells in vitro and in vivo. Blood 2002; 99:3885–3891.

102. O'Farrell AM, Abrams TJ, Yuen HA, Ngai TJ, Louie SG, Yee KW, et al. SU11248 is a novel FLT3 tyrosine kinase inhibitors with potent activity in vitro and in vivo. Blood 2003; 101:3597–3605.

103. Mendel DB, Laird AD, Xin X, Louie SG, Christensen JG, Li G, et al. In vivo antitumor activityof SU11248, a novel tyrosine kianse inhibitor targeting vascular endothelial growth factor and platelet-derived growth factor receptors: determination of a pharmacokinetic/pharmacodynamic relationship. Clin Cancer Res 2003; 9:327–337.

104. Abrams TJ, Lee LB, Murray LJ, Mendel DB, Cherrington JM. Inhibition of Kit-positive SCLC growth by SU11248, a novel tyrosine kinase inhibitors. Proceedings of the AACR–NCI–EORTC International Conference 2002:1669 (abstract).

105. Kelly LM, Yu J-C, Boulton CL, Apatira M, Li J, Sullivan CM, et al. CT53518, a novel selective FLT3 antagonist for the treatment of acute myelogenous leukemia (AML). Cancer Cell 2002; 1:421–432.

106. Levis M, Small D. Novel FLT3 tyrosine kinase inhibitors. Expert Opin Invest Drugs 2003; 12:1951–1962.

107. Fabbro D, Ruetz S, Bodis S, Pruschy M, Csermak K, Man A, et al. PKC412-a protein kinase inhibitor with a broad therapeutic potential. Anti-Cancer Drug Des 2000; 15:17–28.

108. Pinski J, Weeraratna A, Uzgare AR, Arnold JT, Denmeade SR, Isaacs JT. Trk receptor inhibition induces apoptosis of proliferating but not quiescent human osteoblasts. Cancer Res 2002; 62:986–989.

109. Sawyers CL. Finding the next Gleevec: FLT3 targeted kinase inhibitor therapy for acute myeloid leukemia. Cancer Cell 2002; 1:413–415.

110. Yee KWH, O'Farrell AM, Smolich BD, Cherrington JM, McMahon G, et al. SU5416 nad SU5614 inhibit kinase activity of wild-type and mutant FLT3 receptor tyrosine. Blood 2002; 100:2941–2949.

111. Teller S, Kraemer D, Boehmer S-A, Tse KF, Small D, Mahboobi S, et al. Bis($^1$H-2-indolyl)-1-methanones as inhibitors of the hematopoietic tyrosine kinase Flt3. Leukemia 2002; 16:1528–1534.

112. Menezes D, Lee SH, Wiesmann M, Vora J, Peng J, Shephard L, et al. CHIR258: a potent inhibitor of FLT-3 kinase in experimental tumor xenografts models of human acute myelogenous leukemia. Proceedings of the AACR–NCI–EORTC International Conference 2003:C127 (abstract).

113. Smith BD, Levis M, Beran M, Giles F, Brown P, Russell L, et al. Single agent CEP-701, a novel FLT3 inhibitor, shows initial response in patients with refractory acutre myeloid leukemia. Proc Am Assoc Cancer Res 2003; 39:779 (abstract).

114. Stone RM, Klimek V, Deangelo I, Galinsky I, Fox E, Nimer S, et al. Oral PKC412 has activitiy in patients with mutant FLT3 in acute myeloid leukemia (AML): a phase II trial. Proc Am Assoc Cancer Res 2003; 39:2265 (abstract).

115. Druker BJ, Sawyers CL, Kantarjian H, Resta DJ, Reese SF, Ford JM, et al. Activity of a specific inhibitor of the BCR-ABL tyrosine kinase in the blast crisis of chronic myeloid leukemia and acute lymphoblastic leukemia with the Philadelphia chromosome. N Engl J Med 2002; 344:1038–1042.

116. Sawyers CL, Hochhaus A, Feldman E, Goldman JM, Miller CB, Ottmann OG, et al. Imatinib induces hematologic and cytogenetic responses in patients with chronic myeloid leukemia in myeloid blast crisis: results of a phase II study. Blood 2002; 99:3530–3539.

117. Mauro L, Salerno M, Morelli C, Boterberg T, Bracke ME, Surmacz E. Role of the IGF-I receptor in the regulation of cell-cell adhesion: implications in cancer development and progression. J Cell Physiol 2003; 194:108–116.

118. Valentinis B, Baserga R. IGF-I receptor signalling in transformation and differentiation. Mol Pathol 2001; 54:133–137.

119. Baserga R. The contradictions of the insulin-like growth factor 1 receptor Oncogene 2000; 19:5574–5581.

120. Brodt P, Samani A, Navab R. Inhibition of the type I insulin-like growth factor receptor expression and signaling: novel strategies for antimetastatic therapy. Biochem Pharmacol 2000; 60:1101–1107.

121. Macaulay VM. Insulin-like growth factors and cancer. Br J Cancer 1992; 65:311–320.

122. Ma J, Pollak MN, Giovannucci E, Chan JM, Tao Y, Hennekens CH, et al. Prospective study of colorectal cancer risk in men and plasma levels of insulin-like growth factor (IGF)-I and IGF-binding protein-3. J Natl Cancer Inst 1999; 91:620–625.

123. Yu H, Spitz MR, Mistry J, Gu J, Hong WK, Wu X. Plasma levels of insulin-like growth factor-I and lung cancer risk: a case-control analysis. J Natl Cancer Inst 1999; 91:151–156.

124. Hankinson SE, Willette WC, Colditz GA, Hunter DJ, Michaud DS, Deroo B, et al. Circulating concentrations of insulin-like growth factor-I and risk of breast cancer. Lancet 1998; 351:1373–1375.

125. O'Connor R. Survival factors and apoptosis. Adv Biochem Eng Biotechnol 1998; 62:137–166.

126. Werner H, Le Roith D. The insulin-like growth factor-I receptor signaling pathways are important for tumorigenesis and inhibition of apoptosis. Crit Rev Oncog 1997; 8:71–92.

127. Yu D, Watanabe H, Shibuya H, Miura M. Redundancy of radioresistant signaling pathways originating from insulin-like growth factor I receptor. J Biol Chem 2003; 278:6702–6709.

128. Lu Y, Zi X, Mascarenhas D, Pollak M. Insulin-like growth factor-I receptor signaling and resistance to trastuzumab (Herceptin). J Natl Cancer Inst 2001; 93:1852–1857.

129. Grothey A, Voigt W, Schober C, Muller T, Dempke W, Schmoll HJ. The role of insulin-like growth factor I and its receptor in cell growth, transformation, apoptosis, and chemoresistance in solid tumors. J Cancer Res Clin Oncol 1999; 125:166–173.

130. Wen B, Deutsch E, Marangoni E, Frascona V, Maggiorella L, Abdulkarim B, et al. Tyrphostin AG1024 modulates radiosensitivity in human breast cancer cells. Br J Cancer 2001; 85:2017–2021.

131. Scotlandi K, Avnet S, Benini S, Manara MC, Serra M, Cerisano V, et al. Expression of an IGF-I receptor dominant negative mutant induces apoptosis, inhibits tumorogenesis and enhances chemosensitivity in Ewing's sarcoma cells. Int J Cancer 2002; 101:11–16.

132. Beech DJ, Parekh N, Pang Y. Insulin-like growth factor receptor antagonism results in increased cytotoxicity of breast cancer cells to doxorubicin and taxol. Oncol Rep 2001; 8:325–329.

133. Sachdev D, Li SL, Hartell JS, Fujita-Yamaguchi Y, Miller JS, Yee D. A chimeric humanized single-chain antibody against the type I insulin-like growth factor (IGF) receptor renders breast cancer cells refractory to the mitogenic effects of IGF-I. Cancer Res 2003; 63:627–635.

134. Scotlandi K, Maini C, Manara MC, Benini S, Serra M, Cerisano V, et al. Effectiveness of insulin-like growth factor I receptor antisense strategy against Ewing's sarcoma cells. Cancer Gene Ther 2002; 9: 296–307.

135. Wang Y, Sun Y. Insulin-like growth factor receptor-1 as an anti-cancer target: blocking transformation and inducing apoptosis. Curr Cancer Drug Targets 2002; 2:191–207.

136. Nakamura K, Hongo A, Kodama J, Miyagi Y, Yoshinouchi M, Kudo T. Down-regulation of the insulin-like growth factor I receptor by antisense RNA can reverse the transformed phenotype of human cervical cancer cell lines. Cancer Res 2000; 60:760–765.

137. Wang H, Liu Y, Wei L, Guo Y. Antisense IGF and antisense IGF-IR therapy of malignancy. Adv Exp Med Biol 2000; 465:265–272.

138. Adams TE, Epa VC, Garrett TP, Ward CW. Structure and function of the type 1 insulin-like growth factor receptor.Cell Mol Life Sci 2000; 57:1050–1093.

139. Dupont J, LeRoith D. Insulin and insulin-like growth factor I receptors: similarities and differences in signal transduction. Horm Res 2001; 55(Suppl 2):22–26.

140. Parrizas M, Gazit A, Levitzki A, Wertheimer E, LeRotih D. Specific inhibition of insulin-like growth factor-1 and insulin receptor tyrosine kinase activity and biologicyl function by tyrphostins. Endocrinology 1997; 138:1427–1433.

141. Garcia-Echeverria C, Brueggen J, Capraro H-G, Evans DB, Ferrari S, Fabbro D, et al. Characterization of potent and selective kinase inhibitors of IGF-IR. Proc Am Assoc Cancer Res 2003; 44:1008 (abstract).

142. Mitsiades C, Kung A, Garcia-Echeverria C, Pearson MA, Hofmann F, Anderson KC. The IGF-I/IGF-IR system is a major therapeutic target for multiple myeloma, other malignancies and solid tumours. Proc Am Assoc Cancer Res 2003; 44:4005 (abstract).

143. Surmacz E. Growth factor receptors as therapeutic targets: strategies to inhibit the insulin-like growth factor I receptor. Oncogene 2003; 22:6589–6597.

144. Mitsiades C, Catley LP, Podar K, Akiyama M, Burger R, Shringarpure R, et al. Insulin-like growth factor-1 induces adhesion and migration in multiple myeloma cells via activation of β1-integrin and phosphatidylinositol 3-kinase/Akt signaling. Proc Am Assoc Cancer Res 2003; 44:3967 (abstract).

145. Qiang Y-W, Yao L, Tosato G, Rudikoff S. Insulin-like growth factor I induces migration and invasion of human multiple myeloma cells. Blood 2004; 103:301–308.

146. Furstenberger G, Morant R, Senn HJ. Insulin-like growth factors and breast cancer. Onkologie 2003; 26:290–294.

147. Byron SA, Yee D. Potential therapeutic strategies to interrupt insulin-like growth factor signaling in breast cancer. Semin Oncol 2003; 30(5 Suppl 16):125–132.

148. Khalili K, Del Valle L, Wang JY, Darbinian N, Lassak A, Safak M, et al. T-antigen of human polyomavirus JC cooperates withIGF-IR signaling system in cerebellar tumors of the childhood-medulloblastomas. Anticancer Res 2003; 23:2035–2041.

149. Min Y, Adachi Y, Yamamoto H, Ito H, Itoh F, Lee CT, et al. Genetic blockade of the insulin-like growth factor-I receptor: promising strategy for human pancreatic cancer. Cancer Res 2003; 1:6432–6441.

150. Bottaro DP, Rubin JS, Faletto DL, Chan AM, Kmiecik TE, Vande Woude GF, et al. Science 1991; 251: 802–804.

151. Ma P, Maulik G, Christensen J, Salgia R. c-Met: structure, functions and potential for therapeutic inhibition. Cancer Metastasis Rev 2003; 22:309–325.

152. Longati P, Comoglio PM, Bardelli A. Receptor tyrosine kinases as therapeutic targets: the model of the MET oncogene. Curr Drug Targets 2001; 2:41–55.

153. Fan S, Wang JA, Yuan RQ, Rockwell S, Andres J, Zlatapolskiy A, et al. Oncogene 1998; 17:131–141.

154. Bardelli A, Longati P, Gramaglia D, Stella MC, Comoglio PM. Oncogene 1997; 15:3103–3111.

155. Jeffers M, Rong S, Vande Woude GF. Hepatocyte growth factor/scatter factor–Met signaling in tumorigenicity and invasion/metastasis. J Mol Med 1996; 74:505–513.

156. Park M, Dean M, Cooper CS, Schmidt M, O'Brien SJ, Blair DG, et al. Mechanism of met oncogene activation. Cell 1986; 45:895–904.

157. Cooper CS, Park M, Blair DG, Tainsky MA, Huebner K, Croce CM, et al. Molecular cloning of a new transforming gene from a chemically transformed human cell line. Nature 1984; 311:29–33.

158. Yu J, Miehlke S, Ebert MP, Hoffmann J, Breidert M, Alpen B, et al. Frequency of TPR–MET rearrangements in patients with gastric carcinomas and in first-degree relatives. Cancer 2000; 88:1801–1806.

159. Jeffers M, Rong S, Anver M, Vande Woude GF. Autocrine hepatocyte growth factor/scatter factor signaling induces transformation and the invasive/metastatic phenotype in C127 cells. Oncogene 1996; 13:853–861.

160. Rong S, Jeffers M, Resau JH, Tsarfaty I, Oskarsson M, Vande Woude GF. Met expression and sarcoma tumorigenicity. Cancer Res 1993; 53:5355–5360.

161. Park WS, Dong SM, Kim SY, et al. Somatic mutations in the kinase domain of the Met/hepatocyte growth factor receptor gene in childhood hepatocellular carcinomas. Cancer Res 1999; 59:307–310.

162. Schmidt L, Junker K, Nakaigawa N, Kinjerski T, Wierich G, Miller M, et al. Novel mutations of the MET proto-oncogene in papillary renal carcinomas. Oncogene 1999; 18:2343–2350.

163. Schmidt L. Germline and somatic mutations in the tyrosine kinase domain of the Met proto-oncogene in papillary renal carcinomas. Nat Genet 1997; 16:68–73.

164. Maulik G, Shrikhande A, Kijima T, Ma PC, Morrison PT, Salgai R. Role of the hepatocyte growth factor receptor, c-Met, in oncogenesis and potential for therapeutic inhibition. Cytokine Growth Factor Rev 2002; 13:41–59.

165. Jiang W, Hiscox S, Matsumoto K, Nakamura T. Hepatocyte growth factor/scatter factor, its molecular, cellular and clinical implications in cancer. Crit Rev Oncol Hematol 1999; 29:209–248.

166. Tomioka D, Maehara N, Kuba K, Mizumoto K, Tanaka M, Matsumoto K, et al. Inhibition of growth, invasion, and metastasis of human pancreatic carcinoma cells by NK4 in an orthotopic mouse model. Cancer Res 2001; 61:7518–7524.

167. Parr C, Davies G, Nakamura T, Matsumoto K, Mason MD, Jiang WG. The HGF/SF-induced phosphorylation of paxillin, matrix adhesion, and invasion of prostate cancer cells were suppressed by NK4, an HGF/SF variant. Biochem Biophys Res Commun 2001; 285:1330–1337.

168. Maehara N, Matsumoto K, Kuba K, Mizumoto K, Tanaka M, Nakamura T. NK4, a four-kringle antagonist of HGF, inhibits spreading and invasion of human pancreatic cancer cells. Br J Cancer 2001; 84: 864–873.

169. Matsumoto K, Nakamura T. Suppression of tumor malignancy by NK4/malignostatin: a new cancer therapy by inhibition of tumor invasion-metastasis and angiogenesis. Saishin Igaku 2000; 55:1960–1968.

170. Bardelli A, Longati P, Williams TA, Benvenuti S, Comoglio PM. A peptide representing the carboxyl-terminal tail of the met receptor inhibits kinase activity and invasive growth. J Biol Chem 1999; 274: 29,274–29,281.

171. Maulik G, Kijima T, Ma PC, Ghosh SK, Lin J, Shapiro GI, et al. Modulation of the c-Met/hepatocyte growth factor pathway in small cell lung cancer. Clin Cancer Res 2002; 8:620–627.

172. Webb CP, Hose CD, Koochekpour S, Jeffers M, Oskarsson M, Sausville E, et al. The geldanamycins are potent inhibitors of the hepatocyte growth factor/scatter factor-met-urokinase plasminogen activator–plasmin proteolytic network. Cancer Res 2000; 60:342–349.

173. Morotti A, Mila S, Accornero P, Tagliabue E, Ponzetto C. K252a inhibits the oncogenic properties of Met, the HGF receptor. Oncogene 2002; 21:4885–4893.

174. Sattler M, Pride YB, Ma P, Gramlich JL, Chu SC, Quinnan LA, et al. A novel small molecule Met inhibitor induces apoptosis in cells transformed by the oncogenic Tpr-Met tyrosine kinase. Cancer Res 2003; 63:5462–5469.

175. Christensen JG, Schreck R, Burrows J, Kuruganti P, Chan E, Le P, et al. A selective small molecular inhibitors of c-Met kinase inhibits c-Met-dependent phenotypes in vitro and exhibits cytoreductive antitumor activity in vivo. Cancer Res 2003; 63:7345–7355.

176. Santoro M., Melillo RM, Carlomagno F., Fusco A, Vecchio G. Molecular mechanisms of RET activation in human cancer. Ann NY Acad Sci 2002; 963:116–121.

177. Pasini B, Ceccherini I, Romeo G. RET mutations in human disease. Trends Genet 1996; 12:138–144.

178. Santoro M, Carlomagno F, Romano A, Bottaro DP, Datha NA, Grieco M, et al. Activation of RET as a dominant transforming gene by germline mutations of MEN2A and MEN2B. Science 1995; 267: 381–383.

179. Takahashi M. Oncogenic activation of the ret protooncogene in thyroid cancer. Crit Rev Oncog 1995; 6:35–46.

180. Takahashi M, Asai N, Iwashita T, Murakami H, Ito S. Molecular mechanisms of development of multiple endocrine neoplasia 2 by RET mutations. J Intern Med 1998; 243:509–513.

181. Ponder BA. The phenotypes associated with ret mutations in the multiple endocrine neoplasia type 2. Cancer Res 1999; 59:1736–1741.

182. Tallini G. Molecular pathobiology of thyroid neoplasms. Endocr Pathol 2002; 13(4):271–288.

183. Santoro M, Papotti M, Chiappetta G, Garcia-Rostan G, Volante M, Johnson C, et al. RET activation and clinicopathologic features in poorly differentiated thyroid tumors. J Clin Endocrinol Metab 2002; 87:370–379.

184. Tallini G, Asa SL. RET oncogene activation in papollary thyroid carcinoma. Adv Anat Pathol 2001; 8:345–354.

185. Tallini G, Santoro M, Helie M, Carlomagno F, Salvatore G, Chiappetta G, et al. RET/PTC oncogene activation defines a subset of papillary thyroid carcinomas lacking evidence of progession to poorly differentiated or undifferentiated tumor phenotypes. Clin Cancer Res 1998; 4:287–294.

186. Grieco M, Santoro M, Berlingieri MT, Melillo RM, Donghi R, Bongarzone I, et al. PTC is a novel rearranged form of the ret proto-oncogene and is frequently detected in vivo in human thyroid papillary carcinomas. Cell 1990; 60:557–563.

187. Carlomagno F, Vitagliano D, Guida T, Ciardiello F, Tortora G, Vecchio G, et al. ZD6474, an orally available inhibitor of KDR tyrosine kinase activity, efficiently blocks oncogenic RET kinases. Cancer Res 2002; 62:7284–7290.

188. Xing S, Smanik PA, Oglesbee MJ, Trosko JE, Mazzaferri EL, Jhiang SM. Characterization of ret oncogenic activation in MEN2 inherited cancer syndromes. Endocrinology 1996; 137:1512–1519.

189. Carniti C, Perego C, Mondellini P, Pierotti MA, Bongarzone I. PP1 inhibitor induces degradation of RETMEN2A and RETMEN2B oncoproteins through proteosomal targeting. Cancer Res 2003; 63: 2234–2243.

190. Lanzi C, Cassinelli G, Cuccuru G, Zaffaroni N, Supino R, Vignati S, et al. Inactivation of Ret/PTC oncoprotein and inhibition of papillary thyroid carcinoma cell proliferation by indolinone RP1-1. Cell Mol Life Sci 2003; 60:1449–1459.

191. Carlomagno F, Vitagliano D, Guida T, Napolitano M, Vecchio G, Fusco A, et al. The kinase inhibitor PP1 blocks tumorigenesis induced by RET oncogenes. Cancer Res 2002; 62:1077–1082.

192. Dancey J, Sausville EA. Issues and progress with protein kinase inhibitors for cancer treatment. Nature Rev 2003; 2:296–313.

# 36 The mTOR Pathway and Its Inhibitors

*John B. Easton, PhD and Peter J. Houghton, PhD*

## Contents

## Summary

The mammalian target of rapamycin (mTOR) plays a central role in the regulation of cell growth and proliferation by controlling translation in response to nutrients, energy levels, and growth factors. A number of proteins both upstream and downstream in the mTOR signaling pathway have been found to be modified in multiple cancers. As a result, significant interest has been generated in developing small-molecule inhibitors directed against mTOR. Over 30 yr ago a naturally occurring macrolide antibiotic, rapamycin, was isolated that subsequently was identified as a specific inhibitor of mTOR. Rapamycin has played a critical role as a chemical probe for defining the role of mTOR and served as a template for developing compounds with improved therapeutic properties. This chapter will describe our current understanding of the cellular functions of mTOR, modifications of the mTOR pathway currently identified in various types of cancer, the status of clinical trials using rapamycin analogs targeting mTOR, and future possibilities for novel small-molecule inhibitors of mTOR.

**Key Words:** TOR; signaling; inhibitors; rapamycin; cancer; chemotherapy; clinical trials.

## 1. IDENTIFICATION OF mTOR

The identification of the mammalian target of rapamycin (mTOR) was the end result of a series of studies that began with the screen of a soil sample from Easter Island *(1)*. Rapamycin, a macrocyclic lactone produced by *Streptomyces hygroscopicus*, a bacterium

From: *Cancer Drug Discovery and Development: The Oncogenomics Handbook*
Edited by: W. J. LaRochelle and R. A. Shimkets © Humana Press Inc., Totowa, NJ

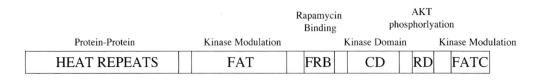

| | Protein-Protein | | Kinase Modulation | | Rapamycin Binding | | Kinase Domain | | AKT phosphorlyation Kinase Modulation |
|---|---|---|---|---|---|---|---|---|---|
| | HEAT REPEATS | | FAT | | FRB | | CD | RD | FATC |

1                                                                                              2549

**Fig. 1.** Functional regions of the PIKK family member mTOR: mTOR contains a number of motifs that are found in other proteins. In additions, mTOR also contains a domain that is required for rapamycin binding (*see* text for details). PIKK, PI-3K related protein kinase; HEAT, Huntington, EF3, A subunit of PP2A, TOR1; FAT, FRAP, ATM, TRAPP; FRB, FKBP12 rapamycin binding domain; CD, catalytic domain; RD, regulatory domain; FATC, FRAP ATM TRAPP carboxy terminus.

present in the soil sample, was demonstrated to have potent antifungal properties *(1–3)*. Subsequent screens in the budding yeast *Saccharomyces cereviseae*, using rapamycin as a selection agent, ultimately led to the identification of both TOR (the yeast ortholog of mTOR) and FPR1 (the yeast ortholog of FKBP12), a protein that also binds rapamycin and is required for its suppressive effects on TOR function *(4,5)*. In yeast, there are two forms of TOR: TOR1 and TOR2 *(6)*. Deletion of TOR1 was shown to have to a profound effect on cell cycle with a G1 delay phenotype, reduced protein synthesis, and decreased amino acid transport *(7)*. The G1 delay and reduction of protein synthesis observed with TOR1 deletion closely correlates with the observed effects of inhibiting the function of the single form of TOR present in higher organisms *(8)*. Deletion of TOR2 generated a lethal phenotype that did not a have a specific cell cycle component *(7,9)*. In addition, TOR2 has a rapamycin-independent function that affects cytoskeletal structure *(10,11)*. Currently, there is little evidence as to whether any the functions of TOR2 are present in the metazoan form of TOR.

## 2. mTOR STRUCTURE

A number laboratories identified mTOR (FRAP, RAFT1, SEP) around the same time *(8,12–14)*. Cloning and sequence analysis revealed that mTOR was a 289-kDa serine threonine kinase with approx 44% homology to the yeast TORs. The homology in the C-terminus of mTOR with the catalytic kinase domain (CD) of the lipid kinase phospho-insitide-3 kinase (PI3K) led to its characterization as a phosphotidylinositol-3 kinase related protein kinase (PIKK) *(15)*. Members of the PIKK family include TEL1, ATM, ATR, and TRRAP. There are a number of HEAT repeats (Huntington, EF3, A subunit of PP2A, TOR1) present in the amino terminus half of the protein that are thought to mediate protein–protein interactions (Fig. 1) *(16)*. There is also a FAT (FRAP, ATM, TRRAP) and FATC domain that are thought to modulate kinase activity, possibly by interaction with each other *(17)*. The FRB (FKBP12 rapamycin-binding domain) is required for binding of the rapamycin FKBP12 complex to mTOR *(18,19)*. Point mutations within this domain generate rapamycin-resistant forms of mTOR *(18)*. The RD (regulatory domain) region of mTOR contains sites that are phosphorylated in response to growth factors, although it is not clear exactly how this phosphorylation affects mTOR function *(20–22)*.

## 3. mTOR SIGNALING PATHWAY

In yeast, TOR, through interaction with various proteins, regulates the rate of protein translation, protein turnover, and transcription in response to the availability of nutrients

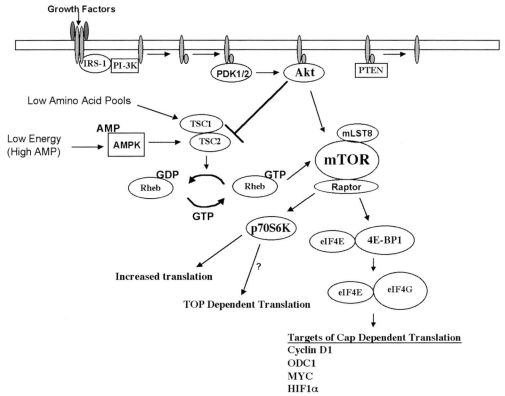

**Fig. 2.** Conditions regulating mTOR and the proteins involved in the mTOR pathway: Low amino acid pools, low energy levels, and growth factor deprivation all downregulate mTOR through a series of kinase cascades (*see* text for details). IRS1, insulin receptor substrate; PI-3K, phosphoinositide 3 kinase; PDK1/2, phosphoinositide 3 phosphate dependent kinase 1/2; AKT, oncogene from AKR mouse thymoma; PTEN, phosphatase and tension homolog; TSC, tuberous sclerosis complex; Gbl, G protein beta subunit-like; AMP, adenosine monophosphate; AMPK, AMP-activated protein kinase; ATP, adenosine triphosphate; mLST8, mammalian homolog of lethal with sec-thirteen gene 8; mTOR, mammalian target of rapamycin; Rheb, RAS-homolog enriched in brain; RAPTOR, regulatory associated protein of mTOR; GDP, guanosine diphosphate; GTP, guanosine triphosphate; p70S6K, P70 ribosomal protein S6 kinase; eIF4E, elongation initiation factor 4E; 4EBP1, EIF4E binding protein 1; eIF4G, elongation initiation factor 4G; TOP, tract of pyrimidine; Myc, myelocytomatosis oncogene; ODC, ornithine decarboxylase; HIF1α, hypoxia inducible factor 1 alpha.

such as amino acids and glucose *(23)*. Although our knowledge of TOR signaling and the proteins involved might not be quite as extensive for metazoans as it is for yeast, a significant amount of knowledge has been gained about the function of mTOR and its regulation over the last several years. For mammalian cells, it has been determined that TOR is regulated by growth factors, cellular energy levels, hypoxia, and nutrients *(24)*.

### 3.1. Growth Factors Activate mTOR Signaling

A number of growth factors have been shown to activate mTOR signaling, including platelet-derived growth factor (PDGF), epidermal growth factor (EGF), insulin, and the insulin-like growth factors (Fig. 2) *(25)*. These growth factors bind to their respective growth factor receptors, which results in the activation of the receptor by autophosphory-lation *(26)*. A number of downstream signals are then transduced as result of proteins binding to the phosphorylated receptor. One of the principal proteins recruited to these activated receptors via its regulatory domain is PI3K *(27)*. As a result of being recruited to the cell membrane, PI3K phosphorylates the membrane lipid phosphatidyl inositol 4-5 bisphosphate at the D3 position to generate phosphatidyl inositol 3,4,5, trisphosphate (PIP3) *(28)*. PIP3, in turn, recruits the phosphoinositide-dependent kinase 1 (PDK1) to the cell membrane. AKT, a substrate of PDK1, is also recruited to the cell membrane by PIP3 via binding to the protein's plexin homology (PH) domain. AKT is activated as a result of phosphorylation by PDK1 plus phosphorylation by another unidentified kinase termed PDK2 *(29)*. AKT then phosphorylates mTOR in the RD domain (serine 2448) and also phosphorylates and inhibits the activity of the GTPase-activating protein (GAP) TSC2 (tuberin) *(30–33)*. As a result, the small G-protein target of the TSC2 GAP activity, Ras homology enriched in brain (RHEB), remains in its active GTP-bound form *(34)*. GTP-bound RHEB then activates mTOR signaling *(34–38)*. The exact details by which GTP : RHEB accomplishes this activation are not currently understood. The function of mLST8 (GbetaL) is not clearly understood either, but its binding to mTOR significantly enhances mTOR signaling *(39)*. mTOR phosphorylates downstream targets, including eukariotic initiation factor-binding protein 4 (4E-BP1) and p70 S6 kinase (S6K1) *(40,41)*. These phos-phorylation events are mediated by sequences present on both 4EBP1 and S6K termed TOS (target of rapamycin signaling) sequences *(42)*. RAPTOR is thought to act as an adaptor protein that binds to both the TOS sequence and mTOR *(43–46)*. Phosphoryla-tion of 4E-BP1 results in the release of eIF4E from 4EBP1 *(47)*. Free eIF4E is then able to bind eIF4G and, in association with other initiation factors, translate RNAs containing a m7GTP Cap *(48)*. This includes the transcripts for c-MYC, cyclin D1, ODC1, and HIF1α *(49–54)*. Phosphorylation of S6K leads to its activation; this, in turn, leads to phosphoryl-ation of the 40S ribosomal protein S6. Phosphorylation of S6 has been linked to an increase in translation of RNA transcripts with the 5 tract of pyrimidine (TOP) sequence *(55)*. TOP sequences are present in a number of transcripts that code for components of translation such as elongation factors 1A (EF1A) and (EF2) and the polyA-binding protein (PABP) *(56,57)*. Increasing the level of proteins responsible for translation has previously been thought to lead to an increase in the rate of translation *(58)*. However, conflicting data have been generated recently with respect to the role of S6K in this pathway *(59)*. Currently, it is not clear to what extent mTOR-dependent phosphorylation of S6K regulates TOP-dependent translation. The exact mechanisms by which mTOR mediates changes in the level of translation is not understood, but it might involve the rate of elongation during pro-tein synthesis and the regulation of transcription of proteins required for translation *(60)*.

### 3.2. Energy Levels Regulate mTOR

Recently, it was demonstrated that in mammalian cells, the levels of AMP (which reflect cellular energy levels) regulate mTOR function *(61)*. This function is a result of the acti-vation of the AMP-dependent protein kinase (AMPK) *(61)*. Activated AMPK directly phosphorylates TSC2 and activates its GAP function, leading to an increase in the inac-tive GDP-bound form of RHEB and consequent downregulation of mTOR signaling *(61)*. This is in contrast to the phosphorylation of TSC2 by AKT that inhibits TSC2 and, hence, activates mTOR signaling.

### 3.3. Amino Acid Availability Regulates mTOR

Amino acid deprivation is known to rapidly inactivate mTOR. Tor deletion in *Drosophila* results in a phenotype that resembles amino-acid-starved flies *(62,63)* Although the exact mechanism is not understood, experimental evidence indicates that this function is also mediated through the TSC1/TSC2 complex *(36,64)*. Loss of TSC1/TSC2 results in an mTOR-dependent increase in S6K activity and blocks the inactivation of S6K in response to the removal of amino acids from the growth media *(65)*. *Drosophila* starved for amino acids during development normally have reduced cell size in the fat bodies. In *Drosophila* that overexpress RHEB, cells in the fat body reach normal size despite the starvation conditions *(66)*. Thus, modulation of RHEB GTPase activity appears to be a common mechanism by which mTOR signaling is regulated in response to nutritional and energy status.

## 4. CELL PROLIFERATION AND mTOR

There is considerable evidence that signaling components of the mTOR pathway control both cell size and proliferation. *Drosophila* that lack S6K are developmentally delayed and approximately half the size of wild-type flies *(67)*. Deletion of proteins upstream of S6, such as mTOR and AKT, leads to flies with both decreased size and cell number *(67)*. Mice homozygous for a mutant form of mTOR exhibit an embryonic lethal phenotype, with effects on both pattern development and cell proliferation *(68,69)*. The deletion of S6K in mice results in reduced embryo size because of reduction in the size of individual cells *(70)*.

## 5. CELL CYCLE PROGRESSION IS REGULATED BY mTOR

Deletion of TOR1 in yeast leads to a G1 arrest phenotype *(6)*. In mammalian cells, a similar effect is observed in cells treated with rapamycin *(7)*. However, the extent of the arrest varies among different cell lines. This is likely to be a function of both cell type and the genetic modifications present in the cell line because modification of downstream targets of mTOR are likely to reduce the effectiveness of inhibiting mTOR function. For instance, cells that overexpress eIF4E are able to partially overcome the effects of the G1 delay induced by rapamycin *(71)*. This is not a surprise given eIF4E's regulation of translation of a number of cell cycle proteins. Less easily explained is the observation that U2OS cells overexpressing S6K are able to partially overcome the G1 delay of cells treated with rapamycin *(71)*. In cell lines selected for resistance to rapamycin, 4EBP1 levels are downregulated, thereby relieving inhibition of eIF4E *(72)*. Cells that have reverted back to rapamycin sensitivity have levels of 4EBP similar to those observed in wild-type cells *(72)*. However, the effects of inhibiting mTOR function on cell cycle progression and proliferation are complicated, and the mechanism by which mTOR regulates some cell cycle regulatory components is not well understood. For instance, in a number of cell lines, the levels of p27[kip1], an inhibitor of the cell division control kinase 2 (CDK2), increase in response to inhibition of mTOR by treatment with rapamycin *(73–75)*. In support of a role for p27[kip1] in mTOR-mediated cell cycle control is the observation that splenic thymocytes derived from p27[kip1] –/– mice are partially resistant the antiproliferative effects of rapamycin treatment *(73)*. If a constitutively active form of 4EBP1 is expressed in MCF7 breast cancer cells, the level of p27[kip1] increases and proliferation is inhibited, indicating that this effect is directly or indirectly related to cap-dependent translation *(76)*.

## 6. INHIBITION OF mTOR CAN CAUSE APOPTOSIS

Although the principal effect of rapamycin in most normal cells and many cell lines is cytostatic, treatment with rapamycin for some cell types leads to apoptosis. These cell types include B-cells, dendritic cells, and renal tubular cells (77–81). Under serum-free conditions, rapamycin treatment causes apoptosis in tumor cell lines with mutated p53 (77,79). Overexpression of wild-type p53 or $p21^{Cip1}$ protects against these cells from rapamycin-dependent apoptosis (82). This effect is a result of the activation the stress response pathway in cells treated with rapamycin and dependent on the expression of 4EBP1 and concomitant inhibition of eIF4E. MEF cells from PTEN –/– mice have increased levels of phosphorylated 4EBP1 and active S6K, which is consistent with increased mTOR signaling (83,84). In some instances, PTEN –/– cells are extremely sensitive to rapamycin (83–85). It is believed that as a result of the increased PI3K activity in PTEN –/– cells during development, the cells become more dependent on mTOR function. In contrast to wild-type cells, the mRNAs for cyclin D1 and c-Myc becomes associated with the monosomal fraction in rapamycin-treated cells lacking PTEN.

## 7. mTOR AND ANGIOGENESIS

Activation of the mTOR pathway is also involved in angiogenesis via regulation of the levels of the transcription factor HIF1α (86–92). HIF1-α is a primary activator of vascular endothelial growth factor (VEGF) (92). The expression level of HIF1α is regulated in response to the activation of mTOR, presumably through eIF4E because HIF1α is a $m^7$GTP Cap-containing transcript (90,92). Treatment of endothelial cells with rapamycin significantly reduces the production of VEGF (93). These results are complicated by the fact that hypoxia also appears to downregulate mTOR function (94). It is likely that there are cell-type-specific and perhaps temporal responses to hypoxic conditions with regard to mTOR regulation, the details of which remain to be determined.

## 8. CANCER AND THE mTOR PATHWAY

Pathways upstream of mTOR are activated in many human cancers. The dual-function phosphatase that negatively regulates PI3K, PTEN, is mutated, silenced, or deleted in a number of tumor types, including glioblastoma, hepatocellular carcinoma, lung carcinoma, melanoma, endometrial carcinomas, and prostate cancer (95–97). The net effect of loss of function is an upregulation or constitutive activation of AKT and, consequently, mTOR signaling. Mutation and activation of AKT2 or gene amplification occurs frequently. Similarly, mutations in TSC proteins, associated with the tuberous sclerosis syndrome, are associated not only with well-vascularized hamartomas (benign lesions) but also with an increased risk of renal cell carcinoma. Mutations in the LKB1 kinase gene are associated with the Peutz–Jehgers cancer prone syndrome. LKB1 kinase positively regulates AMPK, an activator of TSC2 function. Cancer-related changes in pathways downstream of mTOR are also reported. S6K is overexpressed or constitutively active in tumor cell lines and in early stages of transformation in ovarian surface epithelium associated with BRCA1 mutations. The S6K1 gene is also amplified in some breast carcinomas, although this is not necessarily associated with overexpression. eIF4E is altered in a number in a number of tumors. Progressive amplification of the eIF4E gene is associated with late-stage head and neck carcinoma, ductal cell breast carcinoma, and thyroid carcinoma

*(98–100).* Levels of eI4E are elevated in some colon carcinomas in comparison to normal colon cells *(101,102).* The levels of eIF4E are also increased in some bladder and breast cancers that have a poor outcome *(103,104).* In these cancers, a corresponding increase in VEGF was also observed *(104,105).* The levels of 4EBP1 or the presence of inactivating mutations have not been rigorously investigated in tumors samples. However, based on its inhibitory effect on eIF4E, one might predict that such alterations in 4EBP1 might also be observed in some cancers. It is likely that the ratio 4EBP1 to eIF4E is not only an important determinant in tumor progression but also might predict the extent to which inhibition of mTOR will prove to be an effective treatment. In support of this, cell lines in which 4EBP1 is overexpressed become more sensitive to rapamycin, whereas cells over-expressing eIF4E are less sensitive to rapamycin *(71,72).* Currently, the strongest clinical data to support this hypothesis have been observed in colon carcinoma. In these tumors, both EIF4e and 4EBP1 are overexpressed, but the 4EBP1 levels are higher in patients without significant metastatic disease *(106).* Although a daunting task, ultimately the molecular fingerprints of individual tumors are likely to prove at least as important in the successful application of inhibitors of mTOR as treatment based on the tumor's origin.

## 9. INHIBITORS OF mTOR

Rapamycin, has proven to be extremely valuable in elucidating the functions of mTOR and the components of its signaling pathway. Currently, rapamycin and its analogs are the only specific small-molecule inhibitors of mTOR. The screen that identified rapamycin led to its initial development as an antifungal compound. However, in animal studies, it became apparent that it had potent immunosuppressive properties. In addition, as a compound tested in the NCI screening program, it was shown to have significant inhibitory effects against a number of solid tumors *(107–109).* Problematic was its instability and extreme lack of solubility because of its hydrophobic nature, which has slowed its development and translation to the clinic. Initially, the proteins that interact with rapamycin, TOR (mTOR) and FPR1 (FKBP12), were identified in yeast *(4,5).* Genetic experiments demonstrated that both FKBP12 and rapamycin were required for inhibition of mTOR. From structural analysis using crystals containing the FRB domain of mTOR, FKBP12, and rapamycin, it was determined that one hydrophobic face of rapamycin binds to FKBP12 and another hydrophobic face binds to the FRB domain of mTOR (see Fig. 3) *(19).* There are relatively few contacts between FKBP12 and mTOR. FKB12 might bind rapamycin and stabilize it in a conformation that is favorable for interaction with mTOR. Thus, the hydrophobic nature of rapamycin accounts for its unique properties and extreme specificity as an inhibitor of mTOR. To date, no other targets of rapamycin other than mTOR have been identified. Because of its potent immunosuppressive properties, rapamycin has been developed as an immunosuppressive agent by Wyeth (Rapamune) for use in organ transplantation and received Food and Drug Administration (FDA) approval for that application in 1999. Two analogs of rapamycin, RAD001 (Novartis) and CCI-779 (Wyeth), have been developed to improve the solubility and stability of the drug (see Fig. 3). RAD001 has been developed as an oral formulation, whereas CCI-779 is available as an intravenous (iv) and oral formulation. Two additional rapamycin analogs have recently been developed by Ariad: AP23573 and AP23841. AP23481 has a modification that facilitates accumulation in bone and is being developed with intent to treat bone metastases. The structures for AP23573 and AP23481 are not currently available.

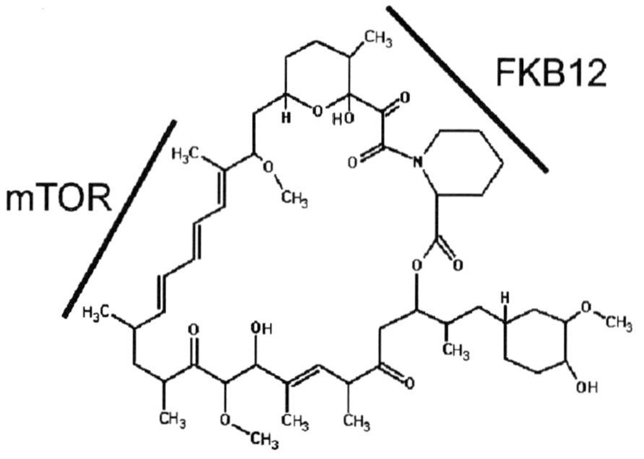


Rapamycin

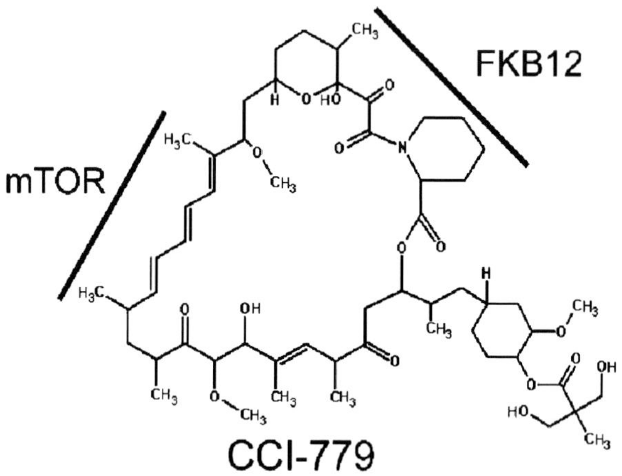


CCI-779

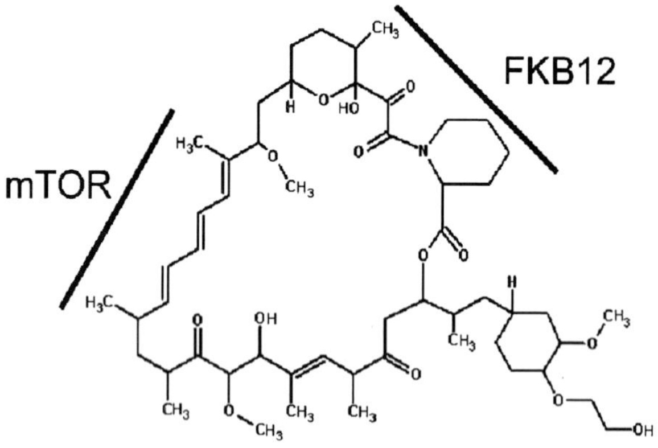


RAD001

**Fig. 3.** Chemical structure of rapamycin and related ester analogs. Shown is the structure of rapamycin in the conformation known to bind FKBP12 and the FRB domain of mTOR. The conformation and interactions with the FKBP12 and the FRB domain for the ester analogs RAD001 and CCI-779 are predicted based on the data from rapamycin. FKB12, FK506 binding protein 12 kiloDalton; mTOR, mammalian target of rapamycin.

## 9.1. Inhibitors of mTOR: Results from Preclinical Models

Since the original identification of the tumor suppressing properties of rapamycin in the NCI cancer screen, rapamycin, and, later, the analogs CCI-779 and RAD001 have been tested for their effects on a number of tumor-derived cell lines and mouse xenograft tumor models *(107–109)*. Treatment of rapamycin or its analogs inhibits proliferation in a large number of cell lines, and in some instances treatment leads to apoptosis. These cell lines are derived from a number of tumor types, including rhabdomyosarcoma, neuroblastoma, glioblastoma, small-cell lung carcinoma, osteosarcoma, pancreatic carcinoma, renal cell carcinoma, Ewing's sarcoma, prostate cancer, and breast cancer *(110–125)*. The breadth of tumor types that are affected is impressive but not surprising given the role of mTOR as a nutrient sensor, cell cycle regulator, and growth regulator, all of which are important for tumor progression. However, the results also provide a cautionary note, because for most of the tumor types, only a proportion of the cell lines respond to rapamycin, and for some of these tumor types, it is a very small proportion. This illustrates the critical importance of understanding the molecular characteristics of individual tumors and if any of the proteins in the mTOR signaling pathways are modified.

## 9.2. Inhibitors of mTOR: Clinical Trials

Based on the preclinical data, a phase I trial evaluating the safety of CCI-779 was implemented *(126)*. The results indicate that with daily intravenous treatment, there are significant grade 3 toxicities, including hypocalcemia, vomiting, thrombocytopenia, and increase in the level of hepatic transaminase. One patient had an objective response (non-small-cell carcinoma), and a number of patients had minor responses or stable disease (cervical carcinoma, uterine carcinoma, renal cell carcinoma, and soft tissue sarcoma). On a weekly treatment schedule, patients experienced no grade 3 toxicities regardless of dosage. Three patients had a partial tumor regression (renal cell, neuroendocrine, and breast carcinomas). Subsequently, based on the phase I results, phase II trials were initiated to study the effects treating advanced-stage refractory renal cell carcinoma with CCI-779 *(127,128)*. The results of the two completed trials were positive, with an objective response rate of 5–7%, a minor response rate of 26–29%, and stable disease in approx 40% of the patients. Currently, phase III trials are in progress to test the efficacy of CCI-779 either alone or in combination with interferon-α as a first-line treatment of renal cell carcinoma. Results from the initial dose-finding and safety trials have prompted the development of a number of additional phase I and phase II trials for various forms of cancer. These include trials for breast cancer, prostate cancer, pancreatic cancer, malignant glioma, glioblastoma multiforme, endometrial cancer, renal cell carcinoma, and endometrial cancer. For a few of these studies, such as a prostate cancer study in which CCI-779 is used as a neoadjuvant to shrink tumors prior to prostatectomy, a comprehensive examination of the phosphorylation status and expression levels of the various components of the mTOR signaling pathway will be performed, including examination of the PTEN status in these tumors. This study will also monitor the S6K activity in peripheral blood mononuclear cells (PBMCs) because data from animal models indicate that this activity might serve as an indirect biomarker of the drug activity within the tumors *(129)*. However, few of the other studies will collect comprehensive data about the mTOR pathway. This is unfortunate, because it is likely that such information would prove valuable in the future for targeting patient populations more likely to respond to CCI-779 treatment. This would, however, require a change in the design of clinical trials from a tumor-classification approach to a biomarker-based approach.

Table 1
Summary of Current Clinical Trials Using Rapamycin or Its Analogs

| Drug | Title | Disease | Phase |
|------|-------|---------|-------|
| CCI-779 | Phase II Randomized Study of Neoadjuvant CCI-779 Followed by Radical Prostatectomy in Patients With Newly Diagnosed Prostate Cancer Who Have a High Risk of Relapse | Adenocarcinoma of the prostate Stage II prostate cancer Stage I prostate cancer | II |
| CCI-779 | Phase II Randomized Study of Letrozole With or Without CCI-779 in Postmenopausal Women With Locally Advanced or Metastatic Breast Cancer | Stage IIIB breast cancer Stage IIIC breast cancer Stage IV breast cancer Recurrent breast cancer | II |
| CCI-779 | Phase II Study of CCI-779 in Patients With Locally Advanced or Metastatic Pancreatic Cancer | Stage II pancreatic cancer Stage III pancreatic cancer Stage IVA pancreatic cancer Stage IVB pancreatic cancer Recurrent pancreatic cancer Adenocarcinoma of the pancreas | II |
| CCI-779 | Phase II Study of CCI-779 in Patients With Metastatic or Locally Advanced Recurrent Endometrial Cancer | Endometrial cancer | II (not yet open) |
| CCI-779 | Phase II Study of CCI-779 in Patients With Recurrent Glioblastoma Multiforme | Recurrent adult brain tumor Glioblastoma multiforme | II |
| CCI-779 | Phase I/II Study of CCI-779 in Patients With Malignant Glioma | Recurrent adult brain tumor Adult glioblastoma multiforme Adult anaplastic astrocytoma Adult anaplastic Oligodendroglioma Mixed gliomas | I–II |

As a result of the development of CCI-779, there are few clinical cancer trials testing rapamycin. However, there is currently an ongoing phase II trial examining the effect of rapamycin treatment on refractory renal cell carcinoma. There is also a phase I trial establishing safety in treatment of pediatric patients with refractory acute leukemias or lymphomas.

The initial results of the RAD001 phase I MTD trial using a fixed dosing schedule indicated mild toxicity with tumor responses observed in several patients (130).

Clinical data are lacking for the more recently developed inhibitors from Ariad. An initial phase I trial is currently underway for AP23573, and AP23841 is still in preclinical development. The current clinical trials that are open and recruiting for the various analogs of rapamycin are summarized in Table 1.

### Table 1 (Continued)

| Drug | Title | Disease | Phase |
|------|-------|---------|-------|
| CCI-779 | A Phase 3, Three-Arm, Randomized, Open-Label Study of Interferon Alfa Alone, CCI-779 Alone, and the Combination of Interferon Alfa and CCI-779 in First-Line Poor-Prognosis Subjects With Advanced Renal Cell Carcinoma | Carcinoma Renal cell Kidney Neoplasms | III |
| CCI-779 | Phase III Randomized Study of Interferon Alfa Versus CCI-779 Versus Interferon Alfa and CCI-779 in Patients With Poor Prognosis Stage IV or Recurrent Renal Cell Carcinoma | Recurrent renal cell cancer Stage IV renal cell cancer | III |
| CCI-779 | Phase II Study of CCI-779 in Patients With Previously Treated Mantle Cell Non-Hodgkin's Lymphoma | Recurrent mantle cell lymphoma | II (suspended) |
| CCI-779 | Phase II Randomized Study of CCI-779 in Patients With Extensive-Stage Small Cell Lung Cancer | Extensive stage small-cell lung cancer | II |
| CCI-779 | Phase II Study of CCI-779 in Patients With Metastatic Melanoma | Stage IV melanoma Recurrent melanoma | II |
| Rapamycin | Phase I/II Study of Sirolimus in Patients With Glioblastoma Multiforme | Recurrent adult brain tumor Adult glioblastoma multiforme | I–II |
| Rapamycin | Phase I Study of Sirolimus in Pediatric Patients With Relapsed or Refractory Acute Leukemia or Non-Hodgkin's Lymphoma | Recurrent childhood Lymphoblastic lymphoma Recurrent childhood small noncleaved cell lymphoma Recurrent childhood large-cell lymphoma Recurrent childhood acute myeloid leukemia Recurrent childhood acute lymphoblastic leukemia | I |
| AP23573 | A Phase I, Sequential Cohort, Dose Escalation Trial to Determine the Safety, Tolerability, and Maximum Tolerated Dose of Daily × 5 Administration of AP23573, an mTOR Inhibitor, in Patients with Refractory or Advanced Malignancies | Advanced, refractory or recurrent solid tumors Lymphoma Multiple myeloma | I |

## 10. THE FUTURE OF mTOR AS A TARGET FOR CHEMOTHERAPY

Because the development of rapamycin as a chemotherapeutic agent is still at an early stage, there are a many possibilities that can be explored in identifying areas where rapamycin might be an effective treatment for cancer.

### 10.1. Combination Therapy

Most of the studies examining the analogs of rapamycin have focused on establishing the safety of these compounds and it use as a single agent usually in patients previously treated with other drugs. However, like many past regimens developed to treat cancer, it is quite likely that compounds that target mTOR will prove more effective in combination with other chemotherapeutic agents directed against other molecular targets. There is already some preliminary data indicating that this might be the case in mouse models of prostate cancer. A number of possible approaches with combination therapy could be imagined. Treatment with rapamycin followed by the timed addition of drugs targeting S-phase, such as irinotecan, might have an additive effect in tumors. For tumors where treatment with mTOR inhibitors might cause a general slowing of growth without a significant accumulation of G1-phase cells, concomitant therapy with compounds such as interferon-α or other compounds inducing general apoptosis might prove more appropriate. This combination is currently a component of the phase III trials in the treatment of renal cell carcinoma. Targeting multiple proteins in the same pathway might also prove effective. This is especially true where mutations have generated drug resistance. For chronic myelogenous leukemia (CML) patients who have developed resistance to imatinib, in the vast majority of cases it is the result of a point mutation in BCR-ABL (131). Because activation of the tyrosine kinase fusion product BCR–ABL is absolutely required and defines the disease, and since the effects of BCR-ABL are dependent on upregulation of PI3K activity and its downstream effectors, it is predicted that mTOR might have a significant effect in either stabilizing or regressing the disease. Also, targeting both proteins simultaneously might prevent the development of resistant tumor cells by slowing proliferation.

Regardless of which therapies are considered, careful preclinical studies in tumor models such as the mouse xenograft or transgenic model should be conducted to study various dosing and timing considerations as well as the effects on the various molecular components of mTOR signaling before the use of these new combination therapies are applied in the clinic.

### 10.2. Novel Inhibitors of mTOR

The success of the ATP mimetic imanitib in targeting the BCR-ABL tyrosine kinase proves that the use of ATP mimetics can be a successful strategy in diseases where a clearly defined kinase function is required for tumor viability. An interesting discovery as a result of the development of imanitib is that the ATP mimetic does not have to be absolutely specific. Imanitib also targets activated c-KIT and the PDGF receptor (132). Perhaps not surprisingly, in tumors in which expression of these genes is altered, imanitib has been demonstrated to have potential as a treatment (133,134). For mTOR, the situation might be more complicated. As described earlier, the rapamycin–FKBP12 complex, although a specific inhibitor of mTOR function, probably does not inhibit kinase activity per se but, rather, is thought to function, by interfering with the association of mTOR with other proteins that bind in this region, or perhaps proteins binding allosterically. For example, mTOR substrates or adaptor proteins that recruit substrates to mTOR. Therefore, the activity of ATP mimetics directed against mTOR are less certain and might result in unexpected biological effects because the loss of TOR function in lower organisms is developmentally lethal. Thus, potent inhibitors of the kinase activity might result in apoptosis rather than the cytostatic effect most frequently observed with rapamycins. Currently, there are no reported ATP mimetic inhibitors of mTOR; however, if the rapamycin analogs prove to be clinically successful in defined tumor types, this is likely to change because there are a limited number of patentable alterations that can be made to rapamycin. Another approach to disrupt mTOR signaling could be to attempt to disrupt the mTOR complex by using small inhibitors designed against the TOS motif, which would disrupt both S6K and 4EBP1 interactions. Other novel approaches include the use of RNA interference to downregulate components of the mTOR pathway that are overexpressed or amplified. Because of delivery considerations however, this therapy might be restricted to certain types of cancer. In the final analysis, whether or not these types of compounds will be developed depends in large part on the success of currently ongoing clinical trials of the rapamycin analogs.

## ACKNOWLEDGMENTS

This work was supported by USPHS Awards CA23099, CA77776, CA96966, and CA21765 (Cancer Center Support Grant) and by American, Lebanese, Syrian, Associated Charities (ALSAC).

## REFERENCES

1. Vezina C, Kudelski A, Sehgal SN. Rapamycin (AY-22,989), a new antifungal antibiotic. I. Taxonomy of the producing streptomycete and isolation of the active principle. J Antibiot (Tokyo) 1975; 28:721–726.
2. Sehgal SN, Baker H, Vezina C. Rapamycin (AY-22,989), a new antifungal antibiotic. II. Fermentation, isolation and characterization. J Antibiot (Tokyo) 1975; 28:727–732.
3. Sehgal SN. Rapamune (RAPA, rapamycin, sirolimus): mechanism of action immunosuppressive effect results from blockade of signal transduction and inhibition of cell cycle progression. Clin Biochem 1998; 31:335–340.
4. Heitman J, Movva NR, Hall MN. Targets for cell cycle arrest by the immunosuppressant rapamycin in yeast. Science 1991; 253:905–909.
5. Koltin Y, et al. Rapamycin sensitivity in *Saccharomyces cerevisiae* is mediated by a peptidyl-prolyl cis-trans isomerase related to human FK506-binding protein. Mol Cell Biol 1991; 11:1718–1723.
6. Cafferkey R, McLaughlin MM, Young PR, Johnson RK, Livi GP. Yeast TOR (DRR) proteins: amino-acid sequence alignment and identification of structural motifs. Gene 1994; 141:133–136.
7. Helliwell SB, Wagner P, Kunz J, Deuter-Reinhard M, Henriquez R, Hall MN. TOR1 and TOR2 are structurally and functionally similar but not identical phosphatidylinositol kinase homologues in yeast. Mol Biol Cell 1994; 5:105–118.
8. Brown EJ, Albers MW, Shin TB, Ichikawa K, Keith CT, Lane WS, et al. A mammalian protein targeted by G1-arresting rapamycin-receptor complex. Nature 1994; 369:756–758.
9. Kunz J, Henriquez R, Schneider U, Deuter-Reinhard M, Movva NR, Hall MN. Target of rapamycin in yeast, TOR2, is an essential phosphatidylinositol kinase homolog required for G$_1$ progression. Cell 1993; 73:585–596.
10. Zheng XF, Florentino D, Chen J, Crabtree GR, Schreiber SL. TOR kinase domains are required for two distinct functions, only one of which is inhibited by rapamycin. Cell 1995; 82:121–130.
11. Schmidt A, Kunz J, Hall MN. TOR2 is required for organization of the actin cytoskeleton in yeast. Proc Natl Acad Sci USA 1996; 93:13,780–13,785.
12. Sabatini DM, Erdjument-Bromage H, Lui M, Tempst P, Snyder SH. Raft1: a mammalian protein that binds to FKBP12 in a rapamycin-dependent fashion and is homologous to yeast TORs. Cell 1994; 78: 35–43.
13. Sabers CJ, Martin MM, Brunn GJ, Williams JM, Dumont FJ, Wiederrecht G, et al. Isolation of a protein target of the FKBP12-rapamycin complex in mammalian cells. J Biol Chem 1995; 270:815–822.

14. Chen Y, et al. A putative sirolimus (rapamycin) effector protein. Biochem Biophys Res Commun 1994; 203:1–7.
15. Abraham RT. Cell cycle checkpoint signaling through the ATM and ATR kinases. Genes Dev 2001; 15: 2177–2196.
16. Andrade MA, Bork P. HEAT repeats in the Huntington's disease protein. Nat Genet 1995; 11:115–116.
17. Bosotti R, Isacchi A, Sonnhammer EL. FAT: a novel domain in PIK-related kinases. Trends Biochem Sci 2000; 25:225–227.
18. Chen J, Zheng XF, Brown EJ, Schreiber SL. Identification of an 11-kDa FKBP12–rapamycin-binding domain within the 289-kDa FKBP12-rapamycin-associated protein and characterization of a critical serine residue. Proc Natl Acad Sci USA 1995; 92:4947–4951.
19. Choi J, Chen J, Schreiber SL, Clardy J. Structure of the FKBP12–rapamycin complex interacting with the binding domain of human FRAP. Science 1996; 273:239–242.
20. Scott PH, Brunn GJ, Kohn AD, Roth RA, Lawrence JC. Evidence of insulin-stimulated phosphorylation and activation of the mammalian target of rapamycin mediated by a protein kinase B signaling pathway. Proc Natl Acad Sci USA 1998; 95:7772–7777.
21. Nave B, Ouwens M, Withers DJ, Alessi DR, Shepherd PR. Mammalian target of rapamycin is a direct target for protein kinase B: identification of a convergence point for opposing effects of insulin and amino acid deficiency on protein translation. Biochem J 1999; 344:427–431.
22. Sekulic A, Hudson CC, Homme JL, Yin P, Otterness DM, Karnitz LM, et al. A direct linkage between the phosphoinositide 3-kinase-AKT signaling pathway and the mammalian target of rapamycin (mTOR) in mitogen-stimulated and transformed cells. Cancer Res 2000; 60:3504–3513.
23. Thomas G, Sabatini DM, Hall MN. Tor (target of rapamycin). In: Thomas G, Sabatini DM, Hall MN, eds. Current Topics in Microbiology and Immunology, Vol. 279. Berlin: Springer-Verlag, 2004.
24. Huang S, Bjornsti MA, Houghton PJ. Rapamycins: mechanisms of action and cellular resistance. Cancer Biol Ther 2003; 2:222–232.
25. Chung J, Grammer TC, Lemon KP, Kazlauskas A, Blenis J. PDGF- and insulin-dependent pp70[S6k] activation mediated by phosphatidylinositol-3-OH kinase. Nature 1994; 370:71–75.
26. Ullrich A, Schlessinger J. Signal transduction by receptors with tyrosine kinase activity. Cell 1990; 61: 203–212.
27. Ueki K, Algenstaedt P, Mauvais-Jarvis F, Kahn CR. Positive and negative regulation of phosphoinositide 3-kinase-dependent signaling pathways by three different gene products of the p85 regulatory subunit. Mol Cell Biol 2000; 20:8035–8046.
28. Whitman M, Downes CP, Keeler M, Keller T, Cantley L. Type I phosphatidylinositol kinase makes a novel inositol phospholipid, phosphatidylinositol-3-phosphate. Nature 1988; 332:644–646.
29. Chan T, Rittenhouse S, Tsichlis P. AKT/PKB and other D3 phosphoinostide regulated kinases: kinase acitivation by phosphoimositide-dependent phosporylation. Annu Rev Biochem 1998; 68:965–1014.
30. Jacinto E, Hall MN. Tor signalling in bugs, brain and brawn. Nat Rev Mol Cell Biol 2003; 4:117–126.
31. Inoki K, Li Y, Zhu T, Wu J, Guan KL. TSC2 is phosphorylated and inhibited by Akt and suppresses mTOR signalling. Nat Cell Biol 2002; 4:648–657.
32. Potter CJ, Pedraza LG, Xu T. Akt regulates growth by directly phosphorylating Tsc2. Nat Cell Biol 2002; 4:658–665.
33. Manning BD, Tee AR, Logsdon MN, Blenis J, Cantley LC. Identification of the tuberous sclerosis complex-2 tumor suppressor gene product tuberin as a target of the phoshpoinositide-3-kinase/akt pathway. Mol Cell 2002; 10:151–162.
34. Tee AR, et al. Tuberous sclerosis complex-1 and -2 gene products function together to inhibit mammalian target of rapamycin (mTOR)-mediated downstream signaling. Proc Natl Acad Sci USA 2002; 99: 13,571–13,576.
35. Zhang Y, et al. Rheb is a direct target of the tuberous sclerosis tumour suppressor proteins. Nat Cell Biol 2003; 5:578–581.
36. Saucedo LJ, et al. Rheb promotes cell growth as a component of the insulin/TOR signalling network. Nat Cell Biol 2003; 5:566–571.
37. Stocker H, et al. Rheb is an essential regulator of S6K in controlling cell growth in *Drosophila*. Nat Cell Biol 2003; 5:559–565.
38. Inoki K, Li Y, Xu T, Guan KL. Rheb GTPase is a direct target of TSC2 GAP activity and regulates mTOR signaling. Genes Dev 2003; 15:1829–1834.

39. Kim DH, Sarbassov dos D, Ali SM, Latek RR, Guntur KV, Erdjument-Bromage H, et al. GbetaL, a positive regulator of the rapamycin-sensitive pathway required for the nutrient-sensitive interaction between raptor and mTOR. Mol Cell 2003; 4:895–904.
40. Brunn SJ, Hudson CC, Sekulic A, Williams JM, Hosoi H, Houghton PJ, et al. Phosphorylation of the translational repressor PHAS-I by the mammalian target of rapamycin. Science 1997; 277:99–101.
41. Burnett PE, Barrow RK, Cohen NA, Snyder SH, Sabatini DM. RAFT1 phosphorylation of the translational regulators p70 S6 kinase and 4E-BP1. Proc Natl Acad Sci USA 1998; 95:1432–1437.
42. Schalm SS, Blenis J. Identification of a conserved motif required for mTOR signaling. Curr Biol 2002; 12:632–639.
43. Hara K, Maruki Y, Long X, Yoshino K, Oshiro N, Hidayat S, et al. Raptor, a binding partner of target of rapamycin (TOR), mediates TOR action. Cell 2002; 110:177–189.
44. Kim DH, Sarbassov DD, Ali SM, King JE, Latek RR, Erdjument-Bromage H, et al. mTOR interacts with raptor to form a nutrient-sensitive complex that signals to the cell growth machinery. Cell 2002; 110:163–175.
45. Schalm SS, Fingar DC, Sabatini DM, Blenis J. TOS motif-mediated raptor binding regulates 4E-BP1 multisite phosphorylation and function. Curr Biol 2003; 13:797–806.
46. Nojima H, Tokunaga C, Eguchi S, Oshiro N, Hidayat S, Yoshino K, et al. The mammalian target of rapamycin (mTOR) partner, raptor, binds the mTOR substrates p70 S6 kinase and 4E-BP1 through their TOR signaling (TOS) motif. J Biol Chem 2003; 278:15,461–15,464.
47. Mader S, Lee H, Pause A, Sonenberg N. The translation initiation factor eIF-4E binds to a common motif shared by the translation factor eIF-4G and the translational repressor 4E-binding proteins. Mol Cell Biol 1995; 15:4990–4997.
48. Pause A, Belsham GJ, Gingras AC, Donze O, Lin TA, Lawrence JC, et al. Insulin-dependent stimulation of protein synthesis by phosphorylation of a regulator of 5'-cap function. Nature 1994; 371:762–767.
49. Rosenwald IB, Kaspar R, Rousseau D, Gehrke L, Lebouch P, Chen JJ, et al. Eukaryotic translation initiation factor 4E regulates expression of cyclin D1 at transcriptional and post-transcriptional levels. J Biol Chem 1995; 270:21,176–21,180.
50. Hashemolhosseini S, Nagamine Y, Morley SJ, Desrivieres S, Mercep L, Ferrari S. Rapamycin inhibition of the G1 to S transition is mediated by effects on cyclin D1 mRNA and protein stability. J Biol Chem 1998; 273:14,424–14,429.
51. Shantz LM, Pegg AE. Overproduction of ornithine decarboxylase caused by relief of translational repression is associated with neoplastic transformation. Cancer Res 1994; 54:2313–2316.
52. DeBenedetti A, Joshi B, Graff JR, Zimmer SG. CHO cells transformed by the translation factor eIF4E display increased c-myc expression but require overexpression of Max for tumorigenicity. Mol Cell Differ 1994; 2:347–371.
53. Zhong H, Chiles K, Feldser D, Laughner E, Hanrahan C, Georgescu MM, et al. Modulation of hypoxia-inducible factor 1alpha expression by the epidermal growth factor/phosphatidylinositol3-kinase/PTEN/AKT/FRAP pathway in human prostate cancer cells: implications for tumor angiogenesis and therapeutics. Cancer Res 2000; 60:1541–1545.
54. Mayerhofer M, Valent P, Sperr WR, Griffin JD, Sillaber C. BCR/ABL induces expression of vascular endothelial growth factor and its transcriptional activator, hypoxia inducible factor-1alpha, through a pathway involving phosphoinositide 3-kinase and the mammalian target of rapamycin. Blood 2002; 100:3767–3775.
55. Jefferies HB, Reinhard C, Kozma SC, Thomas G. Rapamycin selectively represses translation of the "polypyrimidine tract" mRNA family. Proc Natl Acad Sci USA 1994; 91:4441–4445.
56. Terada N, et al. Rapamycin selectively inhibits translation of mRNAs encoding elongation factors and ribosomal proteins. Proc Natl Acad Sci USA 1994; 91:11,477–11,481.
57. Jefferies HB, et al. Rapamycin suppresses 5'TOP mRNA translation through inhibition of p70s6k. EMBO J 1997; 16:3693–3704.
58. Gingras AC, Raught B, Sonenberg N. mTOR signaling to translation. Curr Topics Microbiol Immunol 2004; 279:169–197.
59. Tang H, et al. Amino acid-induced translation of TOP mRNAs is fully dependent on phosphatidylinositol 3-kinase-mediated signaling, is partially inhibited by rapamycin, and is independent of S6K1 and rpS6 phosphorylation. Mol Cell Biol 2001; 21:8671–8683.
60. Wang X, et al. Regulation of elongation factor 2 kinase by p90(RSK1) and p70 S6 kinase. EMBO J 2001; 20:4370–4379.

61. Inoki K, Zhu T, Guan KL. TSC2 mediates cellular energy response to control cell growth and survival. Cell 2003; 115:577–590.
62. Zhang H, Stallock JP, Ng JC, Reinhard C, Neufeld TP. Regulation of cellular growth by the *Drosophila* target of rapamycin dTOR. Genes Dev 2000; 14:2712–2724.
63. Oldham S, Montagne J, Radimerski T, Thomas G, Hafen E. Genetic and biochemical characterization of dTOR, the *Drosophila* homolog of the target of rapamycin. Genes Dev 2000; 14:2689–2694.
64. Tee AR, Manning BD, Roux PP, Cantley LC, Blenis J. Tuberous sclerosis complex gene products, Tuberin and Hamartin, control mTOR signaling by acting as a GTPase-activating protein complex toward Rheb. Curr Biol 2003; 13:1259–1268.
65. Gao X, et al. Tsc tumour suppressor proteins antagonize amino-acid-TOR signalling. Nat Cell Biol 2002; 4:699–704.
66. Stocker H, et al. Rheb is an essential regulator of S6K in controlling cell growth in Drosophila. Nat Cell Biol 2003; 5:559–565.
67. Montagne J, et al. *Drosophila* S6 kinase: a regulator of cell size. Science 1999; 285:2126–2129.
68. Hentges KE, et al. FRAP/mTOR is required for proliferation and patterning during embryonic development in the mouse. Proc Natl Acad Sci USA 2001; 98:13,796–13,801.
69. Hentges K, Thompson K, Peterson A. The flat-top gene is required for the expansion and regionalization of the telencephalic primordium. Development 1999; 126:1601–1609.
70. Shima H, et al. Disruption of the p70(s6k)/p85(s6k) gene reveals a small mouse phenotype and a new functional S6 kinase. EMBO J 1998; 17:6649–6659.
71. Fingar DC, Richardson CJ, Tee AR, Cheatham L, Tsou C, Blenis J. mTOR controls cell cycle progression through its cell growth effectors S6K1 and 4E-BP1/eukaryotic translation initiation factor 4E. Mol Cell Biol 2004; 24:200–216.
72. Dilling MB, et al. 4E-binding proteins, the suppressors of eukaryotic initiation factor 4E, are down-regulated in cells with acquired or intrinsic resistance to rapamycin. J Biol Chem 2002; 277:13,907–13,917.
73. Law BK, et al. Rapamycin potentiates transforming growth factor beta-induced growth arrest in nontransformed, oncogene-transformed, and human cancer cells. Mol Cell Biol 2002; 22:8184–8198.
74. Nourse J, et al. Interleukin-2-mediated elimination of the p27Kip1 cyclin-dependent kinase inhibitor prevented by rapamycin. Nature 1994; 372:570–573.
75. Barata JT, Cardoso AA, Nadler LM, Boussiotis VA. Interleukin-7 promotes survival and cell cycle progression of T-cell acute lymphoblastic leukemia cells by down-regulating the cyclin-dependent kinase inhibitor p27(kip1). Blood 2001; 98:1524–1531.
76. Jiang H, Coleman J, Miskimins R, Miskimins WK. Expression of constitutively active 4EBP-1 enhances p27Kip1 expression and inhibits proliferation of MCF7 breast cancer cells. Cancer Cell Int 2003; 3:2.
77. Huang S, et al. p53/p21(CIP1) cooperate in enforcing rapamycin-induced G(1) arrest and determine the cellular response to rapamycin. Cancer Res 2001; 61:3373–3381.
78. Lieberthal W, et al. Rapamycin impairs recovery from acute renal failure: role of cell-cycle arrest and apoptosis of tubular cells. Am J Physiol Renal Physiol 2001; 281:693–706.
79. Thimmaiah KN, et al. Insulin-like growth factor I-mediated protection from rapamycin-induced apoptosis is independent of Ras-Erk1-Erk2 and phosphatidylinositol 3'-kinase-Akt signaling pathways. Cancer Res 2003; 63:364–374.
80. Woltman AM, et al. Rapamycin specifically interferes with GM-CSF signaling in human dendritic cells, leading to apoptosis via increased p27KIP1 expression. Blood 2003; 101:1439–1445.
81. Kenerson HL, Aicher LD, True LD, Yeung RS. Activated mammalian target of rapamycin pathway in the pathogenesis of tuberous sclerosis complex renal tumors. Cancer Res 2002; 62:5645–5650.
82. Huang S, et al. Sustained activation of the JNK cascade and rapamycin-induced apoptosis are suppressed by p53/p21(Cip1). Mol Cell 2003; 11:1491–1501.
83. Neshat MS, et al. Enhanced sensitivity of PTEN-deficient tumors to inhibition of FRAP/mTOR. Proc Natl Acad Sci USA 2001; 98:10,314–10,319.
84. Podsypanina K, et al. An inhibitor of mTOR reduces neoplasia and normalizes p70/S6 kinase activity in Pten+/– mice. Proc Natl Acad Sci USA 2001; 98:10,320–10,325.
85. Shi Y, et al. Enhanced sensitivity of multiple myeloma cells containing PTEN mutations to CCI-779. Cancer Res 2002; 62:5027–5034.
86. Treins C, Giorgetti-Peraldi S, Murdaca J, Semenza GL, Van Obberghen E. Insulin stimulates hypoxia-inducible factor 1 through a phosphatidylinositol 3-kinase/target of rapamycin-dependent signaling pathway. J Biol Chem 2002; 277:27,975–27,981.

87. Zhong H, et al. Modulation of hypoxia-inducible factor 1alpha expression by the epidermal growth factor/phosphatidylinositol 3-kinase/PTEN/AKT/FRAP pathway in human prostate cancer cells: implications for tumor angiogenesis and therapeutics. Cancer Res 2000; 60:1541–1545.

88. Zundel W, et al. Loss of PTEN facilitates HIF-1-mediated gene expression. Genes Dev 2000; 14:391–396.

89. Jiang BH, et al. Phosphatidylinositol 3-kinase signaling controls levels of hypoxia-inducible factor 1. Cell Growth Differ 2001; 12:363–369.

90. Laughner E, Taghavi P, Chiles K, Mahon PC, Semenza GL. HER2 (neu) signaling increases the rate of hypoxia-inducible factor 1alpha (HIF-1alpha) synthesis: novel mechanism for HIF-1-mediated vascular endothelial growth factor expression. Mol Cell Biol 2001; 21:3995–4004.

91. Mayerhofer M, Valent P, Sperr WR, Griffin JD, Sillaber C. BCR/ABL induces expression of vascular endothelial growth factor and its transcriptional activator, hypoxia inducible factor-1alpha, through a pathway involving phosphoinositide 3-kinase and the mammalian target of rapamycin. Blood 2002; 100:3767–3775.

92. Brugarolas JB, Vazquez F, Reddy A, Sellers WR, Kaelin WG. TSC2 regulates VEGF through mTOR-dependent and -independent pathways. Cancer Cell 2003; 4:147–158.

93. Guba M, et al. Rapamycin inhibits primary and metastatic tumor growth by antiangiogenesis: involvement of vascular endothelial growth factor. Nat Med 2002; 8:128–135.

94. Arsham AM, Howell JJ, Simon MC. A novel hypoxia-inducible factor-independent hypoxic response regulating mammalian target of rapamycin and its targets. J Biol Chem 2003; 278:29,655–29,660.

95. Li J, et al. PTEN, a putative protein tyrosine phosphatase gene mutated in human, brain, breast, and prostate cancer. Science 1997; 275:1943–1947.

96. Steck PA, et al. Identification of a candidate tumour suppressor gene, MMAC1, at chromosome 10q23.3 that is mutated in multiple advanced cancers. Nat Genet 1997; 15:356–362.

97. Risinger JI, Hayes AK, Berchuck A, Barrett JC. PTEN/MMAC1 mutations in endometrial cancers. Cancer Res 1997; 57:4736–4738.

98. Haydon MS, Googe JD, Sorrells DS, Ghali GE, Li BD. Progression of eIF4e gene amplification and overexpression in benign and malignant tumors of the head and neck. Cancer 2000; 88:2803–2810.

99. Sorrells DL, Meschonat C, Black D, Li BD. Pattern of amplification and overexpression of the eukaryotic initiation factor 4E gene in solid tumor. J Surg Res 1999; 85:37–42.

100. Wang S, et al. Expression of eukaryotic translation initiation factors 4E and 2alpha correlates with the progression of thyroid carcinoma. Thyroid 2001; 11:1101–1107.

101. Berkel HJ, Turbat-Herrera EA, Shi R, de Benedetti A. Expression of the translation initiation factor eIF4E in the polyp-cancer sequence in the colon. Cancer Epidemiol Biomarkers Prev 2001; 10:663–666.

102. Rosenwald IB, et al. Upregulation of protein synthesis initiation factor eIF-4E is an early event during colon carcinogenesis. Oncogene 1999; 18:2507–2517.

103. Li BD, et al. Prospective study of eukaryotic initiation factor 4E protein elevation and breast cancer outcome. Ann Surg 2002; 235:732–738.

104. Crew JP, et al. Eukaryotic initiation factor-4E in superficial and muscle invasive bladder cancer and its correlation with vascular endothelial growth factor expression and tumour progression. Br J Cancer 2000; 82:161–166.

105. Scott PA, et al. Differential expression of vascular endothelial growth factor mRNA vs protein isoform expression in human breast cancer and relationship to eIF-4E. Br J Cancer 1998; 77:2120–2128.

106. Martin ME, et al. 4E binding protein 1 expression is inversely correlated to the progression of gastrointestinal cancers. Int J Biochem Cell Biol 2000; 32:633–642.

107. Douros J, Suffness M. New antitumor substances of natural origin. Cancer Treat Rev 1981; 8:63–87.

108. Houchens DP, Ovejera AA, Riblet SM, Slagel DE. Human brain tumor xenografts in nude mice as a chemotherapy model. Eur J Cancer Clin Oncol 1983; 19:799–805.

109. Eng CP, Sehgal SN, Vezina C. Activity of rapamycin (AY-22,989) against transplanted tumors. J Antibiot (Tokyo) 1984; 37:1231–1237.

110. Dilling MB, Dias P, Shapiro DN, Germain GS, Johnson RK, Houghton PJ. Rapamycin selectively inhibits the growth of childhood rhabdomyosarcoma cells through inhibition of signaling via the type I insulin-like growth factor receptor. Cancer Res 1994; 54:903–907.

111. Shi Y, Frankel A, Radvanyi LG, Penn LZ, Miller RG, Mills GB. Rapamycin enhances apoptosis and increases sensitivity to cisplatin in vitro. Cancer Res 1995; 55:1982–1988.

112. Seufferlein T, Rozengurt E. Rapamycin inhibits constitutive p70[s6k] phosphorylation, cell proliferation, and colony formation in small cell lung cancer cells. Cancer Res 1996; 56:3895–3897.

113. Hosoi H, Dilling MB, Liu LN, Danks MK, Shikata T, Sekulic A, et al. Studies on the mechanism of resistance to rapamycin in human cancer cells. Mol Pharmacol 1998; 54:815–824.

114. Hosoi H, Dilling MB, Shikata T, Liu LN, Shu L, Ashmun RA, et al. Rapamycin causes poorly reversible inhibition of mTOR and induces p53-independent apoptosis in human rhabdomyosarcoma cells. Cancer Res 1999; 59:886–894.

115. Geoerger B, Kerr K, Tang CB, Fung KM, Powell B, Sutton LN, et al. Antitumor activity of the rapamycin analog CCI-779 in human primitive neuroectodermal tumor/medulloblastoma models as single agent and in combination chemotherapy. Cancer Res 2001; 61:1527–1532.

116. Ogawa T, Tokuda M, Tomizawa K, Matsui H, Itano T, Konishi R, et al. Osteoblastic differentiation is enhanced by rapamycin in rat osteoblast-like osteosarcoma (ROS 17/2.8) cells. Biochem Biophys Res Commun 1998; 249:226–230.

117. Grewe M, Gansauge F, Schmid RM, Adler G, Seufferlein T. Regulation of cell growth and cyclin D1 expression by the constitutively active FRAP-S6K1 pathway in human pancreatic cancer cells. Cancer Res 1999; 59:3581–3587.

118. Shah SA, Potter MW, Ricciardi R, Perugini RA, Callery MP. Frap-S6K1 signaling is required for pancreatic cancer cell proliferation. J Surg Res 2001; 97:123–130.

119. Gibbons JJ, Discafani C, Peterson R, Hernandez R, Skotnicki J, Frost P. The effect of CCI-779, a novel macrolide anti-tumor agent, on the growth of human tumor cells in vitro and in nude mouse xenografts in vivo. Proc Am Assoc Cancer Res 1999; 40:301.

120. Yu K, Zhang W, Lucas J, Toral-Barza L, Peterson R, Skotnicki J, et al. Deregulated PI3K/AKT/TOR pathway in PTEN-deficient tumor cells correlates with an increased growth inhibition sensitivity to a TOR kinase inhibitor CCI-779. Proc Am Assoc Cancer Res 2001; 42:802.

121. Yu K, Toral-Barza L, Discafani C, Zhang WG, Skotnicki J, Frost P, et al. mTOR, a novel target in breast cancer: the effect of CCI-779, an mTOR inhibitor, in preclinical models of breast cancer. Endocr Relat Cancer 2001; 8:249–258.

122. Hultsch T, Martin R, Hohman RJ. The effect of the immunophilin ligands rapamycin and FK506 on proliferation of mast cells and other hematopoietic cell lines. Mol Biol Cell 1992; 3:981–987.

123. Gottschalk AR, Boise LH, Thompson CB, Quintans J. Identification of immunosuppressant-induced apoptosis in a murine B-cell line and its prevention by bcl-x but not bcl-2. Proc Natl Acad Sci USA 1994; 91:7350–7354.

124. Muthukkumar S, Ramesh TM, Bondada S. Rapamycin, a potent immunosuppressive drug, causes programmed cell death in B lymphoma cells. Transplantation 1995; 60:264–270.

125. Mateo-Lozano S, Tirado OM, Notario V. Rapamycin induces the fusion-type independent downregulation of the EWS/FLI-1 proteins and inhibits Ewing's sarcoma cell proliferation. Oncogene 2003; 22:9282–9287.

126. Dancey JE. Clinical development of mammalian target of rapamycin inhibitors. Hematol Oncol Clin North Am 2002; 16:1101–1114.

127. Atkin MB, et al. A randomized double-blind phase 2 study of intraveneous CCI-779 administered weekly to patients with advanced renal cell carcinoma. Proc Am Soc Clin Oncol 2002; 21:36A

128. Atkins MB, et al. Randomized phase II study of multiple dose levels of CCI-779, a novel mTOR kinase inhibitor, in patients with advanced refractory renal cell carcinoma. Clin Cancer Res 2004; J Clin Oncol 22:909–918.

129. Boulay A, et al. Antitumor efficacy of intermittent treatment schedules with the rapamycin derivative RAD001 correlates with prolonged inactivation of ribosomal protein S6 kinase 1 in peripheral blood mononuclear cells. Cancer Res 2004; 64:252–261.

130. O'Donnell A, et al. A phase I study of the oral mTOR inhibitor RAD001 as monotherapy to identify the optimal biologically effective dose using toxicity, pharmacokinetic (PK) and pharmacodynamic (PD) endpoints in patients with solid tumours. Proc Am Soc Clin Oncol 2003; 22:200.

131. Gorre ME, Mohammed M, Ellwood K, Hsu N, Paquette R, Rao PN, et al. Clinical resistance to STI-571 cancer therapy caused by BCR-ABL gene mutation or amplification. Science 2001; 293:876–880.

132. Sawyers CL. Finding the next Gleevec: FLT3 targeted kinase inhibitor therapy for acute myeloid leukemia. Cancer Cell 2002; 5:413–415.

133. Verweij J, et al. Imatinib mesylate (STI-571 Glivec, Gleevec) is an active agent for gastrointestinal stromal tumours, but does not yield responses in other soft-tissue sarcomas that are unselected for a molecular target. Results from an EORTC Soft Tissue and Bone Sarcoma Group phase II study. Eur J Cancer 2003; 39:2006–2011.

134. Schittenhelm M, Aichele O, Krober SM, Brummendorf T, Kanz L, Denzlinger C. Complete remission of third recurrence of acute myeloid leukemia after treatment with imatinib (STI-571). Leuk Lymphoma 2003; 44:1251–1253.

# 37

# Cyclo-Oxygenase-2 Enzyme and Its Inhibition in Tumor Growth and Therapy

*Zhongxing Liao, MD, Uma Raju, PhD,*
*Kathryn A. Mason, MSc,*
*and Luka Milas, MD, PhD*

**CONTENTS**

**SUMMARY**

Cyclo-oxygenase-2 (COX-2) is an enzyme induced in pathologic states such as inflammatory disorders and cancer, where it mediates production of prostanoids. The enzyme is commonly expressed in both premalignant lesions and overt cancer of different types. A growing body of evidence links COX-2 with tumor development, aggressive biological tumor behavior, resistance to standard cancer treatment, and adverse patient outcome. Preclinical investigations have demonstrated that inhibition of this enzyme with selective COX-2 inhibitors enhances tumor response to radiation and chemotherapeutic agents. These preclinical findings have been rapidly advanced to clinical oncology. Clinical trials of the combination of selective COX-2 inhibitors with radiotherapy, chemotherapy, or both in patients with a number of cancers have been initiated, and preliminary results are encouraging. This chapter discusses the role of COX-2, its products (prostaglandins), and inhibitors of the enzyme in tumor growth and treatment.

**Key Words:** COX-2; COX-2 inhibitors; tumor biology; radiotherapy; chemotherapy.

From: *Cancer Drug Discovery and Development: The Oncogenomics Handbook*
Edited by: W. J. LaRochelle and R. A. Shimkets © Humana Press Inc., Totowa, NJ

# 1. INTRODUCTION

Over the past decade, significant advances have been made in our understanding of the fundamental biology of cancer. Many molecular processes and signaling pathways that normally regulate survival, proliferation, and function of normal cells have been found to be dysregulated and dysfunctional in cancer cells. Many of these have been shown to be involved in the development and growth of malignant tumors and in rendering tumors resistant to standard cancer treatments. Because of these properties, the abnormal molecular processes and pathways in cancer cells have increasingly been used as potential targets for cancer therapy. Molecular targeting is particularly appealing as a therapeutic approach in combination with radiotherapy, chemotherapy, or their combination. Radiotherapy has traditionally been the treatment of choice for locally or regionally advanced, surgically unresectable cancers. More recently, radiotherapy has been increasingly combined with chemotherapy delivered during the course of radiotherapy (concurrent chemoradiotherapy) and, compared to radiotherapy alone, has resulted in increased local tumor control and improved survival rate of patients *(1–4)*. Unfortunately, these improvements have been achieved at the expense of increased rate and severity of normal tissue toxicity. Incorporating molecular targeting into chemoradiotherapy strategies could further improve local tumor control and reduce metastases. Theoretically, because most normal tissues lack such dysregulated molecular targets, these improvements might be achieved without increasing treatment-induced normal tissue toxicity. Novel agents that specifically target molecular pathways linked to tumor resistance to cytotoxic agents are being developed at an increasing rate and are rapidly moving from preclinical investigations to the clinical arena. Among these are agents that inhibit cyclo-oxygenase-2 (COX-2), an enzyme linked to tumor development, stimulation of tumor growth, and metastatic spread, and tumor resistance to cytotoxic agents. This enzyme mediates production of prostaglandins (PGs) in pathologic states, principally in inflammatory diseases and cancer. Selective COX-2 inhibitors have recently been used extensively to treat patients with arthritis and have been found to have excellent safety profiles. These agents have shown antitumor activity and a potential to enhance tumor response to cytotoxic agents in a variety of preclinical tumor models and have already entered clinical testing. This chapter discusses the rationale and preclinical findings for targeting COX-2 as a cancer treatment strategy, focusing mainly on the combination with radiotherapy, and describes initial observations obtained in clinical trials.

# 2. COX ENZYMES AND PROSTANOID SYNTHESIS

Cyclo-oxygenase is the key enzyme involved in synthesis of prostanoids, a collective term for PGs and thromboxanes (TXs). There are two major isoforms of COX enzyme: COX-1 and COX-2 *(5)*. Whereas COX-1 is ubiquitous, constitutively expressed in virtually all normal tissues, COX-2 is an inducible enzyme that appears rapidly in pathological states, such as in inflamed tissues and tumors *(6,7)*. COX-2 is induced by a variety of substances including pro-inflammatory cytokines (i.e., tumor necrosis factor [TNF]-$\alpha$, interleukin [IL]-1$\beta$, platelet activity factors), growth factors (i.e., epidermal growth factor [EGF], platelet-derived growth factor [PDGF], basic fibroblastic growth factor [bFGF], transforming growth factor [TGF]-1$\beta$), mitogenic substances, oncogenes, and hypoxia.

Both COX-1 and COX-2 are genetically independent proteins with different properties, encoded by genes located on different chromosomes. The COX-1 gene is located on chro-

Table 1
Major Characteristics of COX-1 and COX-2

|  | *COX-1* | *COX-2* |
|---|---|---|
| Regulation | Constitutive | Inducible |
| Molecular weight | 67 kDa | 72 kDa |
| Gene size | 22 kb | 8.3 kb |
| Human chromosome | Chromosome 9 | Chromosome 1 |
| mRNA size | 2.7 kb | 4.3 kb |
| Localization | Endoplasmic reticulum | Endoplasmic reticulum, perinuclear envelope |
| Tissue expression | Ubiquitous | Mainly pathological states |
| TATA motif (5' end) | No | Yes |
| Promoter | Unknown | NF-κB, NF-IL-6, CRE, TCF |

*Source:* Ref. *12*, with permission, copyright 2003 Springer-Verlag New York.

mosome 9 (9q32-q33.3) and has a size of 22 kb which is composed of 11 exons producing a 2.7-kb mRNA message. The COX-2 gene is located on chromosome 1 (1q25.2-q25.3), has a size of 8.3 kb, which is much smaller than that of COX-1, and includes 10 exons generating a 4.3- to 4.5-kb message. Although the intron/exon structures of these genes are nearly identical and the encoded proteins are 75% homologous, the regulatory elements within the genes are quite different. The greater size of the COX-2 mRNA is the result of a larger 3'-untranslated region *(8,9)*. Unlike COX-1, COX-2 is an immediate, early-response gene whose expression is regulated by transcriptional activation sites as well as motifs controlling message stability. The COX-2 promoter contains a TATA box absent from COX-1 and cis-acting elements responsive to factors upregulated during inflammation, specifically nuclear factor (NF)-κB, NF-IL-6, and adenosine 3', 5'-cyclic monophosphate. In addition, the first exon of COX-2 contains a TPA-response element. The 3'-untranslated region contains 17 copies of the Shaw–Kamen motif (AUUUnA) that controls message stability and three polyadenylation signals.

Both COX-1 and COX-2 are membrane bound, localized in the endoplasmic reticulum. Additionally, COX-2 is present in the perinuclear envelope. The molecular weight of COX-1 protein is 67 kDa and that of COX-2 is 72 kDa *(10)*. COX-2 has a variable molecular weight, depending on its glycosylation *(11)*. Each protein has three structural domains: an EGF domain, a membrane-binding domain, and a large catalytic domain that is structurally similar to mammalian peroxidase. Both the cyclo-oxygenase and peroxidase regions are conserved between the two enzyme isoforms, but the amino acid sequence of COX-2 is truncated at its amino-terminus and contains an additional block of 18 amino acids at the carboxy-terminus. Table 1 *(12)* lists major characteristics of COX-1 and COX-2; for additional details, see recent reviews *(7,13–15)*.

Figure 1 shows schematic diagram of prostanoid synthesis by COX-1 and COX-2. Upon physiological signals, stress, or injury, cells produce prostanoids via enzymatic metabolism of arachidonic acid, a polyunsaturated fatty acid bound as an ester to cell membrane phospholipids. Arachidonic acid is first liberated from the membrane phospholipids by phospholipase $A_2$ and then catalyzed by COX enzymes to prostaglandin (PG) $G_2$. Being

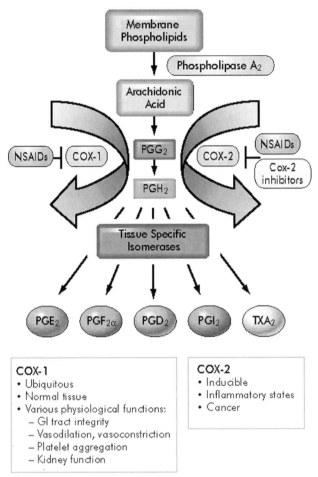

**Fig. 1.** A flow diagram of prostanoid synthesis from arachidonic acid and the involvement of COX-1 and COX-2. Phospholipase A2 generates free arachidonic acid from membrane phospholipids. COX-1 or COX-2 convert arachidonic acid to prostaglandin (PG) G$_2$ via a cyclo-oxygenase activity followed by conversion to PGH$_2$ into other prostaglandin isoforms or thromboxane (TX) A$_2$. Nonsteroidal anti-inflammatory drugs (NSAIDs) inhibit both COX-1 and COX-2, whereas specific COX-2 inhibitors inhibit COX-2 only. (From ref. *16* with permission.)

unstable, this prostaglandin is rapidly converted to PGH$_2$ by the peroxidase activity of COX. The cyclo-oxygenase and peroxidase sites are located on opposite sides of the catalytic domain of COX. Because COX catalyzes two sequential enzymatic reactions, it is also called prostaglandin peroxide synthase, PGH synthase, or PGG/H synthase. Once generated, PGH$_2$ undergoes further metabolism to PGs and TXA$_2$ through the action of specific isomerases that exert a wide range of biological actions specific to an individual prostanoid. There are several PGs, including PGE$_2$, PGF$_{2\alpha}$, PGD$_2$, and PGI$_2$ (prostacyclin).

In normal tissues, prostanoids regulate numerous homeostatic physiological functions, including vasomotility (constriction and dilation), platelet aggregation, gastrointestinal mucosal integrity, immunomodulation, and regulation of cell growth and differentiation. Different PGs might have agonistic or antagonistic effects, and the final biological effect on tissues depends on the balance of similar and opposing actions of the prostanoids involved. Prostanoids are short-lived locally acting substances (autocoids) released from cells immediately after being synthesized. They bind to membrane receptors and might exert both autocrine and paracrine activities. Each prostanoid has a single receptor, with the exception of $PGE_2$, which has four separate receptors. The receptors couple to G (guanine nucleotide)-binding proteins and generate second messengers, primarily cAMP, $Ca^{2+}$, and inositol triphosphate [17,18]. A number of protein kinases are activated, including protein kinases C and A and likely protein tyrosine kinase. Each receptor primarily binds to its own ligand, but most prostanoids can crossbind to receptors other than their own. Prostanoids can also initiate signaling not only via binding to membrane receptors but also through nuclear hormone receptors, notably the peroxisome proliferator-activated receptors (PPARs) [19–23].

## 3. COX-2 IN TUMOR DEVELOPMENT

Prostaglandins have long been suspected to play a role in tumor development, leading to the use of aspirin and other nonsteroidal anti-inflammatory drugs (NSAIDs) as possible cancer-preventive agents. Retrospective and epidemiologic studies have demonstrated that prolonged regular intake (more than 2 yr) of NSAIDs can decrease the relative risk of developing certain types of cancer. This decrease has most consistently been observed for colon cancer, where reduction in tumor development up to 50% was achieved [24–26]. Protection has also been reported against development of other cancers, including esophageal, stomach, breast, and bladder [27]. These studies indirectly implicated the involvement of COX enzymes and their products in tumor development; however, more recent investigations provided solid evidence directly linking COX-2 to pathogenesis in tumor development.

Cyclo-oxygenase-2 is expressed in a high percentage of both premalignant lesions and established tumors. For example, it was detected in about 40–50% of malignant adenomas and in more than 80% of adenocarcinomas [28,29]. Genetic studies in Apc$^{\Delta716}$ knockout mice that have mutations in the APC (adenopolyposis coli) gene [30] provided the most compelling evidence of a causal relationship between COX-2 and colon carcinogenesis [30]. The Apc$^{\Delta716}$ knockout mouse is an experimental animal model for human familial adenomatous polyposis (FAP), a heritable condition characterized by the formation of multiple colonic polyps in young adults and a near 100% probability of developing colon cancer. Apc$^{\Delta716}$ knockout mice engineered homozygous for *COX-2* gene, having both copies of the gene, spontaneously developed an average of 652 polyps. The number of polyps was 66% lower in mice having a single copy of the *COX-2* gene (heterozygous) and was 86% lower in mice lacking both copies of the *COX-2* gene. Another preclinical genetic study provided solid evidence for the role of COX-2 in mammary cancer development [31]. Transgenic mice were engineered to express human COX-2 in their mammary glands. Low levels of human COX-2 were expressed in the mammary glands of virgin mice, but these levels increased substantially during pregnancy and lactation. In these virgin transgenic mice and in nontransgenic multiparous mice, mammary tumors were rarely observed. In contrast, however, an exaggerated incidence of focal hyperplasia and dysplasia and at least one tumor were observed in mammary tissue from 85% of the multiparous transgenic

Table 2
COX-2 is Overexpressed in a Variety of Malignant Conditions

| Organ | Malignancy | COX-2 Expression Rate | Ref. |
|---|---|---|---|
| Head an neck | Squamous cell carcinoma | 100% | 83 |
| Esophagus | Adenocarcinoma, squamous cell carcinoma | 76–100% | 51,53 |
| Stomach | Adenocarcinoma | 51–58% | 48,87 |
| Colon | Adenocarcinoma | 83–100% | 46,88,89 |
| Liver | Hepatocellular carcinoma | 83–97% | 59 |
| Pancreas | Adenocarcinoma | 67–90% | 54,56 |
| Breast | Adenocarcinoma | 37.4% | 86 |
| Lung | Adenocarcinoma, squamous cell carcinoma | 72–100% | 61,63 |
| Bladder | Transitional cell carcinoma, squamous cell carcinoma | 66% | 70 |
| Cervix | Squamous cell carcinoma or adenocarcinoma of cervix, endometrial carcinoma | 98–100% | 75,78 |
| Ovarian | Ovarian carcinoma | 42% | 81 |
| Prostate | Adenocarcinoma | 83% | 65 |
| Skin | Melanoma | 93% | 84 |

animals. Further evidence in support of a crucial role of COX-2 in tumor development comes from a large number of preclinical studies showing that selective COX-2 inhibiting agents are highly potent in preventing tumor development (32–37). An illustrative example is a study by Jacoby et al. (32) showing that treatment of Min mice with the selective COX-2 inhibitor celecoxib reduced total tumor load (a reflection of both tumor number and volume) by more than 83%.

Selective COX-2 inhibitors have already entered clinical trials of chemoprevention, but, at present, only limited information is available on their efficacy. A study by Steinbach et al. (38) showed celecoxib was effective in reducing both the number and size of polyps in FAP patients. Celecoxib, given twice daily for 6 mo at a dose of 400 mg, reduced the number of polyps by 28% and the size of polyps by 31% at the end of this 6-mo treatment.

## 4. COX-2 IN CANCER PROGRESSION

There is ample information, both preclinical and clinical, that COX-2 and its products might play a stimulatory role in tumor growth and metastases (39,40). Both experimental and human cancers have long been known to often produce excessive amounts of PGs (39, 41,42), most commonly $PGE_2$. Since the discovery of COX-2 enzyme more than a decade ago, there has been an increase of clinical studies assessing the expression of COX-2 in tumors and its relevance to tumor growth behavior, patient prognosis, and response to conventional treatments. Elevated COX-2 has been reported in a broad range of human cancers, including at least 80% of cancers of the colon, esophagus, lung, pancreas, and head and neck (Table 2) (28,43–86). Although there is often broad variation in tumors that overexpress COX-2, overexpression generally correlates with a more malignant phenotype. In several cancers, COX-2 overexpression correlates with aggressive behavior, worse prognosis *(46,52,53,61–63,90,97)* and the development of metastatic disease *(46,92)*. The following results of a few studies illustrate these relationships. Colorectal carcinomas usually display high levels of COX-2 expression *(46,88,93)* that positively relates to more aggressive tumor behavior, such as advanced bowel wall invasion, lymph node metastasis, and poorer patient survival *(46)*. A positive relationship between COX-2 overexpression and poor survival of patients with lung carcinoma was reported *(63,90)*. Khuri et al. *(90)* analyzed COX-2 positivity in 185 patients with stage I non-small-cell lung carcinoma (NSCLC) treated with surgical resection and found an inverse correlation between the level of COX-2 positivity and 5-yr survival. The level of COX-2 expression was an independent prognostic factor for survival in the multivariate analysis. Ang et al. *(94)* reported that more than 85% of head and neck carcinomas were positive for COX-2 and that the percentage of tumor cells positive and the intensity of staining broadly varied from tumors with no tumor cells positive to tumors in which all tumor cells were positive. COX-2 positivity significantly correlated with local tumor failure to radiotherapy and poor patient survival.

Both COX-2 and PGs are involved in multiple sequential processes of cancer metastasis. There are reports of (1) positive correlation between COX-2 expression and in vitro cancer cell motility and invasion as well as in vivo metastasis *(95)*, (2) a direct link between COX-2 and enhanced adhesion of carcinoma cells to endothelial cells, and enhanced liver metastasis potential has been reported *(96)*, (3) frequent coexpression of COX-2 and Laminin-5, an extracellular matrix protein that plays a key role in cell migration and tumor invasion at the invasive front of early-stage adenocarcinoma of the lung *(97)*, and (4) a positive correlation between COX-2 expression and lymphatic invasion and metastasis in human gastrointestinal tract cancers *(92)*. On the other hand, treatment with selective COX-2 inhibitors have been reported to inhibit COX-2 activity and the proliferation of malignant cells in vitro *(62,98)*, and to retard tumor growth and to reduce metastasis in vivo *(28,45, 99)*. Treatment with celecoxib, a selective COX-2 inhibitor, showed a dose-dependent inhibitory effect on both tumor growth and the number of lung metastases that developed in tumor-bearing mice. Celecoxib treatment retarded growth of HT-29 human colon tumor xenografts by up to 67% and reduced the development of lung metastases by as much as 91% *(45)*. Selective COX-2 inhibitors have also demonstrated antitumor activity against murine mammary cancer *(36)*, canine bladder cancer *(100)*, and human head and neck cancer xenografts in mice *(101)*.

## 5. MECHANISMS OF ACTION OF COX-2 AND ITS INHIBITORS

Multiple mechanisms operate in COX-2 involvement in tumor development, growth, and metastasis. Through its peroxidase activity, COX enzymes can generate mutagens and carcinogens, this activity being important in xenobiotic metabolism and particularly relevant to the gastrointestinal and upper aerodigestive tracts where cells are constantly exposed to a variety of xenobiotics *(102–104)*. For example, peroxidase reaction converts chemicals present in tabacco smoke into carcinogens that bind to DNA *(105)*. COX-2 and prostanoids can deregulate ordinary cell growth and death in tissues, particularly the apoptotic mode of cell death. Most PGs stimulate cell growth and proliferation by autocrine or paracrine signaling involving the G protein family of receptors. They might act on their own or cooperate with other cell growth stimulatory molecules, such as the epidermal growth factor receptor (EGFR).

There exists solid evidence that COX-2 is involved in resistance of cells to undergo apoptotic cell death, and via this mechanism, COX-2 can exert its procarcinogenic effect as well as its stimulatory actions on tumor growth *(106,107)*. Transfection-type experiments showed that COX-2 rendered intestinal epithelial cells resistant to butyrate-induced apoptosis *(108)*. The transfected cells acquired an increased ability to attach to extracellular matrix and showed an augmented expression of the apoptosis inhibitory protein Bcl-2. The effects of COX-2 transfection were abrogated by treatment of cells with the NSAID sulindac sulfide. Both NSAIDs and selective COX-2 inhibitors have been reported to induce apoptosis in a variety of tumor cell types *(29,109)*. Thus, COX-2 and PGs promote cell survival either by increasing their proliferation or by inhibiting apoptosis. This would increase the chance for accumulated sequential genetic changes to result in malignant transformation and, in the case of already established tumors, to stimulate tumor growth.

Stimulation of angiogenesis is perhaps the most important mechanism by which COX-2 and PGs support the growth of tumors. As early as the 1980s it was established that PGs possess angiogenic properties *(110,111)*. COX-2 can regulate not only the production of PGs but also of other angiogenic factors such as vascular endothelial growth factor (VEGF) and fibroblast growth factor (FGF). The expression of VEGF was reported to be weak in tumor cells lacking COX-2 *(112)*, COX-2-generated PGs can enhance bFGF-induced angiogenesis through induction of VEGF *(113)*, or PGs can stimulate IL-6 production, which, in turn, stimulates VEGF production *(114)*. These examples illustrate complex interplay in production of angiogenic factors, but they definitely implicate COX-2 as a regulator of tumor angiogenesis.

Standard NSAIDs and selective COX-2 inhibitors are potent inhibitors of tumor angiogenesis. Milas et al. *(115)* were first to report on this aspect, demonstrating that indomethacin reduces formation of new blood vessels at the site of tumor cell injection. More recently, this observation was extended to the selective COX-2 inhibitor SC-236 *(116)* (Fig. 3). Inhibition of angiogenesis by either indomethacin or SC-236 was associated with tumor growth retardation. Subsequent studies revealed that other selective COX-2 inhibitors, including celecoxib *(117)* and rofecoxib *(118)*, exert potent antiangiogenic activity. Studies by Masferrer et al. *(45)* show that in contrast to COX-2 inhibitors, COX-1 inhibitors are not capable of inhibiting angiogenesis. Although selective COX-2 inhibitors, SC-236 and celecoxib, profoundly reduced corneal neovascularization induced in rats or mice by bFGF, a selective COX-1 inhibitor, a regioisomer of celecoxib, had no effect.

Immunosupression, a condition long recognized to be conducive to tumor development and growth, is another mechanism of COX-2 and PGs actions on tumors. Most PGs—in particular, $PGE_2$—are potent immunosuppressants. $PGE_2$ can block the antitumor activity of lymphocytes, natural killer cells, and macrophages *(119,120)*, mediate immune suppression by T-suppressor cells *(121)*, inhibit production of cytotoxic lymphokines *(122)*, and stimulate production of immunosuppressive lymphokines *(123)*. By reducing PG production, standard NSAIDs and selective COX-2 inhibitors could minimize or abolish the immunosuppressive effects of PGs and restore antitumor immunological rejection mechanisms. Stolina et al. *(124)* reported that specific inhibition of COX-2 resulted in growth inhibition of Lewis lung carcinoma, attributing this effect to the alteration in the balance of IL-10 and IL-12 synthesis, which, in turn, led to marked lymphocytic infiltration of the tumor. Our own studies demonstrated that immunosupression reduced the ability of indomethacin to augment the efficacy of tumor radiation *(125)*, implying that some aspects of antitumor activity of NSAIDs and likely selective COX-2 inhibitors as well are immune mediated.

## 6. COX-2 INHIBITORS IN COMBINATION WITH RADIOTHERAPY

There is a large body of evidence that PGs regulate a variety of protective homeostatic functions guarding cells and tissues from different types of injury, including radiation *(126,127)*, and that PG production is associated with tumor resistance to therapy *(128,129)*. For example, exogenous administration of $PGE_2$ prior to the irradiation of mice increased the survival of intestinal epithelial cells *(130)*. PGs or their stable analogs were shown to protect a variety of other normal cells from radiation, including hematopoietic stem cells *(131)*, dermal cells *(132)*, and spermatogonia. In vitro, PGs were shown to protect both normal and cancer cell lines from radiation injury *(126,128,129,133)*. The radioprotective effect of PG requires ligand-receptor binding, because in vitro protection could not be demonstrated in cells lacking PG receptors or when the receptors were blocked *(131)*. Multiple mechanisms are involved in the cellular protection afforded by PGs. One mechanism is repair of DNA damage as suggested by data showing decreased radioprotection under DNA-repair-deficient conditions *(128,133)*. Another possible mechanism of protection is reduced cellular sensitivity to radiation-induced apoptosis *(134)*. Additionally, PGs could protect tissues from radiation damage by stimulating the regeneration of cells surviving radiation exposure *(134)*. All of these mechanisms of radioprotection provide potential targets for modulating tumor response to radiotherapy.

It was first hypothesized by Furuta et al. *(39,135)* that PGs are as radioprotective for tumors as they are for normal tissues *(115)* and that PG inhibition in tumors improves response to radiotherapy. These initial preclinical investigations, which predated the discovery of COX-2 *(5)*, used indomethacin, a standard NSAID, to inhibit PGs *(39,115)*. The results from these early investigations provided proof of principle that decreasing tumor PG levels improved tumor radioresponse quantified by tumor growth delay, cure rate, and time to recurrence. The magnitude of enhanced tumor radioresponse (1.3–2.0) was dependent on tumor type, radiation schedule, radiation dose and fractionation, and treatment end point. Of potential importance to clinical radiotherapy was the finding that larger radiation enhancement factors were obtained when fractionated, rather than single-dose, radiotherapy was combined with indomethacin or ibuprofen treatment *(115,136)*.

Clinically, modulation of tumor treatment response to radiotherapy using high-dose standard NSAIDs, such as indomethacin, ibuprofen, and pyroxicam, were shown to be of limited utility partly because of toxicity to the gastrointestinal tract, such as ulcer formation, wall perforation, and bleeding. Renewed interest in PG-targeted therapy arose following the discovery of COX-2 in the early 1990s and the observations that this enzyme is absent from virtually all normal tissues with exception of certain structures in the brain, kidney, and uterus. Selective inhibition of COX-2 provided a new opportunity to increase tumor response to therapy while potentially avoiding normal tissue toxicity associated with inhibition of COX-1 expression, which was unavoidable when using NSAIDs.

Using murine tumors, Milas et al. were the first to investigate the in vivo radioenhancing potential of a selective COX-2 inhibitor *(116,136,137)*. Treatment efficacy was quantified by both tumor growth delay and tumor cure (Fig. 2). Treatment with SC-236, a selective COX-2 inhibitor, dramatically enhanced NFSa tumor response to radiation, with enhance-

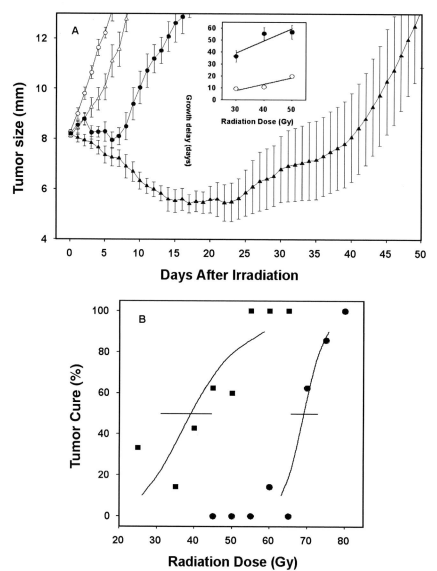

**Fig. 2.** Effect of SC-236 on NFSa tumor growth delay (**A**) and tumor cure (**B**) after irradiation. Leg tumors of 6 mm in diameter were treated with SC-236 (5 mg/kg) in the drinking water for 10 d. (A) Tumors received 30 Gy when 8 mm. O = vehicle, △ = SC-236, ● = 30 Gy, and ▲ = SC-236 plus 30 Gy, Vertical bars represent SE. The inset shows tumor growth delay as a function of radiation dose: O = radiation only, ● = SC-236 plus radiation. (B) Tumor cure as a function of radiation dose. ● = radiation only and ■ = SC-236 plus radiation. Horizontal bars represent 95% confidence intervals at the TCD50 (tumor cure dose 50) dose level. (From ref. *140* with permission.)

ment factors being 3.64 for tumor growth delay and 1.77 for tumor cure *(116)*. Two other tumors studied, murine sarcoma FSa and human glioma U251 xenograft, also showed significant synergistic responses to combined treatment with SC-236 plus radiation *(86–87)*. Radioresponse assayed by tumor growth delay was enhanced by a factor of 1.4 by indomethacin but by factors greater than 2.0 by SC-236 for all three tumors: sarcomas NFSa and FSa, and U251 human glioma. Therefore, SC-236 was a more potent enhancer of tumor radioresponse than the nonspecific inhibitor of COX enzymes indomethacin.

Other selective COX-2 inhibitors, such as NS-398 *(138)* and celecoxib *(139)*, have subsequently also been shown to enhance the effect of radiation both in vitro and in vivo. Pyo et al. *(138)* used NS-398 on rat intestinal epithelial cells stably transfected with COX-2 cDNA in the sense (RIE-S) and antisense (RIE-AS) orientation. The same experiments were repeated with NCI-H460 human lung cancer cells, which express COX-2 constitutively, and HCT-116 human colon cancer cells, which do not express COX-2. NS-398 enhanced the radiosensitivity of RIE-S but not RIE-AS cells. Similarly, NS-398 enhanced the radiosensitivity of H460 cells, but not HCT-116 cells. The radioenhancing ability of NS-398 on xenografts of two human tumors was also tested. The radiation response was enhanced only for the NCI-H460 tumor that expressed COX-2. This effect was attributed to enhancement of radiation-induced apoptosis. In contrast, the radioresponse of HCT-116 tumor xenografts lacking COX-2 was not significantly affected by treatment with NS-398, suggesting that the enhancement of tumor radioresponse by COX-2 inhibition can be achieved only in tumors that express COX-2 enzyme. These data further suggest that it might be possible to predict individual tumor treatment response by assaying the tumor for COX-2 expression or PG profile prior to initiation of radiotherapy. In a study *(141)* of the human head and neck squamous cell carcinoma (HNSCC) cell line HEp3, a radiosensitizing effect of NS-398 was observed using a clonogenic survival assay. Radiation alone upregulated COX-2 protein expression, but the induced upregulation was prevented by NS-398. However, there was no significant corresponding increase in COX-2 mRNA at 48 h after radiation, suggesting that the observed change in COX-2 expression was posttranscriptional. Similar findings have been demonstrated using human prostate carcinoma DU145 *(142)*.

To achieve therapeutic gain by radiation-modulating agents, the tumor response must be greater than that of normal tissues exposed to both treatments. Kishi et al. *(136)* demonstrated preferential enhancement of tumor vs normal tissue radioresponse by specific inhibition of the COX-2 enzyme. Treating the FSa tumor with both SC-236 and radiation enhanced tumor growth delay by a factor of 2.14 and tumor cure by a factor of 1.87, but resulted in no biologically significant increase in normal tissue toxicity of intestinal epithelium and skin. In another study, the combination of a COX-2 inhibitor with local thoracic irradiation showed no increase in the occurrence of radiation-induced pneumonitis *(143)*. Therefore, these results support the general concept of enhanced therapeutic gain when radiotherapy is combined with specific COX-2 inhibition.

## 7. MECHANISMS OF INCREASED TUMOR RADIORESPONSE

The mechanisms by which COX-2 inhibitors enhance tumor radioresponse are multiple and include direct interaction with tumor cells and indirect actions via modulation of the tumor cell microenvironment. In vitro findings obtained using clonogenic cell survival clearly showed that COX-2 inhibitors increase cell radiosensitivity *(138,139,144)*. The effect was attributed to the ability of these agents to inhibit DNA repair from sublethal radiation damage *(137,144)*, to increase cell susceptibility to radiation-induced apoptosis *(138)* and to arrest cells in the radiosensitive phases of the cell division cycle *(144)*. Inhibition of DNA repair was suggested by removal of the "shoulder" region on the radiation survival curve for cells exposed to COX-2 inhibitors *(138,144)* (Fig. 3). This

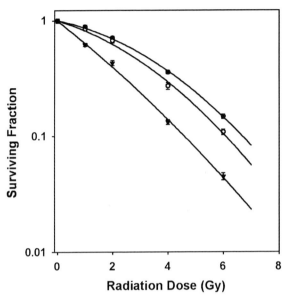

**Fig. 3.** Effect of SC-236 on radiosensitivity of NFSA cells in culture. Cells were treated with SC-236 (10 and 50 μ*M*) for 3 d before irradiation. Then, the cells were trypsinized and plated in specified numbers. Twelve days later, the colonies were counted and the survival curves were constructed with normalized values for the cytotoxicity induced by SC-236 alone. (●) Control; (○) SC-236, 10 μ*M*; (▼) SC-236, 50 μ*M*. Values shown are the means ± SE for three independent experiments. (From ref. *145*. Copyright 2004 with permission of Elsevier.)

mechanism was subsequently confirmed by showing that in the so-called "split-dose experiment," cells treated with a COX-2 inhibitor were less able to recover from radiation damage during the interfraction interval than cells not exposed to the COX-2 inhibitor *(144)*. Induction of apoptosis and cell cycle redistribution were two additional mechanisms considered to play a role in COX-2 inhibitor-induced increased cell radiosensitization, but the results are inconsistent. Although some studies showed an increase in radiation-induced apoptosis *(138)*, others showed no such increase *(137,144)*. Raju et al. *(144)* demonstrated that SC-236 arrested cells in the radiosensitive G2/M phases of the cell cycle, whereas other investigators found no significant cell cycle redistribution by SC-236 *(137)* or other COX-2 inhibitors *(139)*. At the molecular level, the G2/M arrest was associated with downregulation in the expression of cyclin-A, cyclin-B, as well as cyclin-dependent kinase-1 (cdk-1, also known as cdc-2). The reasons for the inconsistencies in the above findings are unknown.

Antiangiogenic actions of COX-2 inhibitors are considered to be an important mechanism underlying increased tumor radioresponse. It has long been known that PGs are angiogenic factors *(110,111)*. Recent investigations suggest a link between COX-2 and VEGF and that PGs can stimulate angiogenesis directly or indirectly through VEGF production. Cells negative for COX-2 demonstrate decreased expression of VEGF *(29)*. COX-2-generated PGs can enhance bFGF-induced angiogenesis through induction of VEGF *(113)*. PGs can induce IL-6, which, in turn, stimulates the production of VEGF *(114)*. Both standard NSAIDs and selective COX-2 inhibitors inhibit angiogenesis *(45,115,116,136)*.

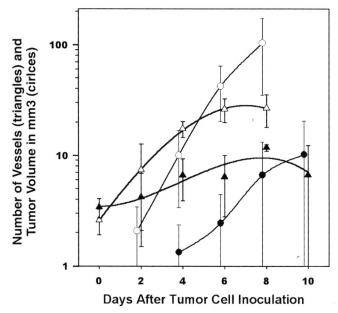

**Fig. 4.** Effect of SC-236 on tumor angiogenesis. The number of newly formed blood vessels was recorded after intradermal injection of $10^6$ NFSa cells in mice treated with vehicle (△) or SC-236 (▲) given at a dose of 6 mg/kg in the drinking water for 9 consecutive days starting 1 d after tumor cell inoculation. Inhibition of tumor angiogenesis was associated with delay in tumor growth, (○), vehicle, or (●), SC-236. Vertical bars are SE of the mean values. (From ref. *116*. By permission of Oxford University Press.)

Figure 4 shows that the COX-2 inhibitor SC-236 reduces newly formed vessels at the site of tumor cell injection and that this reduction is associated with tumor growth retardation. Similarly, Masferrer et al. *(45)* demonstrated that celecoxib was a potent inhibitor of angiogenesis induced by bFGF. In contrast, administration of a selective COX-1 inhibitor or a regioisomer of celecoxib that does not inhibit COX-2 had no inhibitory effect on bFGF-induced neoangiogenesis. Tumor growth was attenuated in *COX-2 –/–* mice compared with wild type or *COX-1 –/–*. Genetic ablation or pharmaceutical inhibition of COX-2 led to decreased production of VEGF, which might explain the reduction of tumor growth in *COX-2 –/–* mice *(112)*. Another selective COX-2 inhibitor, rofecoxib, inhibited in vitro proliferation and capillary tube formation of human umbilical vein (HUVEC) endothelial cells *(139)*. This effect was even more pronounced when rofecoxib was combined with radiation, thus demonstrating an interaction between the two agents.

The combination of antiangiogenic agents, including COX-2 inhibitors, with radiation can enhance tumor response to radiation *(146–148)* by several mechanisms. Antiangiogenic agents inhibit proangiogenic factors produced by tumors, including VEGF, FGF, and, in the case of selective COX-2 inhibitors, PGs. VEGF increases blood vessel permeability that could reduce fluid accumulation and pressure in the extracapillary space and, consequently, impair blood flow and oxygen supply to tumor cells. Therefore, administration of antiangiogenic agents could prevent these effects of VEGF. There is a report that treatment with antiangiogenic agents does enhance tumor oxygenation *(146)*, which could result in tumor cell loss by apoptosis induced by antiangiogenic agents, including

COX-2 inhibitors. This mechanism of improved tumor oxygenation has been well documented to occur after tumor treatment with chemotherapeutic agents (149). Improved tumor oxygenation would improve response to radiotherapy because well-oxygenated cells are generally 2.5–3 times more radiosensitive than hypoxic cells. Another potential mechanism for improvement of tumor radioresponse by antiangiogenic agents is that these agents could cause vascular collapse in tumors and massive necrosis of tumor cells, as is the case for combretastatin (150) and C225 anti-epidermal growth factor receptor antibody (151).

Furthermore, because angiogenic substances, such as VEGF (147) and FGF (152), exhibit radioprotective properties, their inhibition could result in enhanced tumor response to radiation. As already elaborated, PGs are potent radioprotective agents and their inhibition would result in tumor radiosensitization. Treatment with selective COX-2 inhibitors reduced PGs levels in cultured cells (144) and in tumors in vivo (136), and this reduction was associated with enhanced cell and tumor radioresponse. Furthermore, radiation seems to increase the expression of COX-2 protein (139,153) and synthesis of $PGE_2$ in tumor cells (139,144), suggesting that these changes represent a cell survival response to radiation stress. Addition of SC-236 or celecoxib not only abolished the radiation-induced increase in $PGE_2$ but also reduced the level of $PGE_2$ further, to the level in tumor cells treated by the inhibitors only (139,144). Thus, reduction in PG levels deprives cells of the radiation protection afforded by these molecules and leads to increased radiation damage.

Another mechanism for the increase in tumor radioresponse caused by COX-2 inhibitors is immunostimulation. PGs, especially $PGE_2$, suppress the immune system by affecting various facets of immunological reaction, which could then facilitate tumor growth and adversely impact the efficacy of tumor radiotherapy (115). NSAIDs and selective COX-2 inhibitors were shown to restore immunoreactivity (115,123). Also, we previously reported that the indomethacin-induced enhancement of tumor radioresponse was partly mediated by immunological mechanisms (115). Thus, it is likely that selective COX-2 inhibitors involve the immune system as a mechanism for their efficacy when combined with radiotherapy or other cytotoxic treatments.

Finally, COX-2 inhibitors could modulate various microenvironmental factors present within the tumor that are conducive to tumor cell proliferation. For example, COX-2 inhibitors could interfere with EGFR-mediated signaling pathways (154) and hence inhibit tumor cell growth and enhance tumor response to radiation. The blockade of EGFR with C225 anti-EGFR antibody (151) or treatment with tyrosine kinase inhibitors that block EGFR signaling pathways (155) was shown to significantly enhance tumor response to radiotherapy.

## 8. COX-2 INHIBITORS
## IN COMBINATION WITH CHEMOTHERAPY

COX-2 inhibitors have been shown to potentiate cytotoxic actions of a number of chemotherapeutic agents in vitro and to improve their antitumor efficacy in vivo. Hida et al. (62) reported that nimesulide, a COX-2 inhibitor, induced apoptosis and enhanced cytotoxicity of cisplatin and etoposide in lung cancer cells. In another study (156), a concentration-dependent synergistic effect of COX-2 inhibitors combined with anthracyclines (doxorubicin, daunorubicin, and epirubicin) as well as when combined with VP-16 (etoposide) and vincristine was observed. In vivo studies demonstrated that COX-2 inhibitors

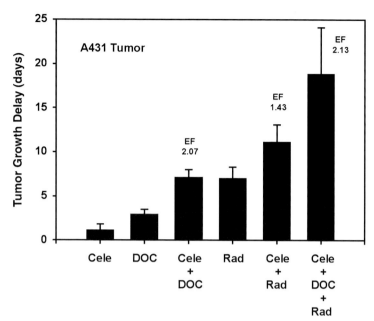

**Fig. 5.** Effect of celecoxib on tumor growth delay of A431 xenographs in nude mice treated with docetaxel and radiation. Celecoxib (Cele) was given as 25 mg/kg by gavage twice a day for 20 d, beginning when tumors were 6 mm. Mice were treated with a single intravenous bolus of 10 mg/kg docetaxel (DOC), 10 Gy local tumor irradiation (Rad), or both when tumors grew to 8 mm. When the two agents were combined, docetaxel was administered 24 h before irradiation. Bars represent the delay in tumor growth induced by the treatments (lines, SE). EFs (enhancement factors) represent the increase in celecoxib enhancement of tumor growth delay when combined with docetaxel, radiation, or docetaxel plus radiation. (From ref. *159*. Copyright 2004 from Elsevier.)

not only augment the antitumor efficacy of various chemotherapeutic drugs *(40)* but also improve their antimetastatic efficiency *(157)*. A study by Trifan et. al. *(158)* showed that celecoxib enhanced antitumor efficacy of irinotecan while reducing diarrhea, a serious side effect of this drug. Thus, as in the case of radiotherapy, combining selective COX-2 inhibitors with chemotherapy has a high potential to increase therapeutic gain. Using human A431 tumor xenografts in mice, we recently reported that celecoxib enhanced the antitumor efficacy of docetaxel or radiation and that the greatest effect was achieved when all three agents were combined (Fig. 5) *(159)*. Mechanistically, the improvement of antitumor efficacy of chemotherapeutic agents by COX-2 inhibitors is commonly attributed to the augmentation of apoptotic cell death. However, other mechanisms, the same or similar to those involved in augmentation of tumor response to radiation, are likely to be involved here as well.

It is generally accepted that P-glycoprotein 170 (MDR1/Pgp170) expression in tumors results in poor response to chemotherapy because of its ability to export chemotherapeutic agents. There is some evidence that inhibition of COX-2 could interfere with multidrug resistance (MDR) factors. Overexpression of COX-2 was reported to increase the production and function of P-glycoprotein or MDR-1 (the product of ABCB1, an efflux pump for chemotherapeutic drugs responsible for multidrug resistance) in cell culture *(160)*, and this effect was minimized by a selective COX-2 inhibitor. Also, COX-2 expression was found to correlate with P-glycoprotein (ABCB1) in human breast cancer *(161)*. Ratnasinghe et al. *(161)* investigated expression of COX-2, MDR1/Pgp170, protein kinase C (PKC), and activator protein 1 (AP1) in a series of increasingly resistant human MCF-7 breast cancer cells compared to wild type using immunohistochemistry, Western blots, Northern blots, reverse transcription–polymerase chain reaction (RT-PCR), and Southern blots. Immunohistochemical analyses of human breast tumor specimens revealed a strong correlation between expression of COX-2 and MDR1/Pgp170. In drug-resistant cell lines that overexpress MDR1/Pgp170, there was also significant upregulation of COX-2 expression. In addition, PKC and AP1 subunits c-Jun and c-Fos were also upregulated. It was thus hypothesized that increased prostaglandin production by COX-2 induces PKC and the expression of transcriptional factor c-Jun, which, in turn, induces the expression of MDR1/Pgp170. The authors suggested that pretreatment with selective COX-2 inhibitors might be useful in the prevention of multidrug resistance in response to cancer chemotherapy and should be further evaluated. Although the clinical significance of these findings awaits further investigation, it is reasonable to anticipate that selective COX-2 inhibitors would enhance the effect of chemotherapeutic drugs by reducing multidrug resistance.

Clearly, ample evidence suggests that COX-2 represents a promising molecular target for cancer therapy and that overcoming the adverse impact of COX-2 on tumor response to cytotoxic therapies should improve both tumor radiotherapy and chemotherapy. Compared to standard NSAIDs, the advantage of the use of selective COX-2 inhibitors is not only in their higher ability to enhance tumor radioresponse or chemoresponse but also in their lower potency to cause gastrointestinal tract complications such as ulcer formation and bleeding *(162)*. However, there are concerns that selective COX-2 inhibitors might be prothrombotic and increase the risk of myocardial infarction as recently shown in a study that demonstrated a significantly higher risk of myocardial infarction in patients receiving rofecoxib vs naproxen *(163)*. However, the results of a similar study of celecoxib vs ibuprofen or diclofenac *(164)*, and data from a meta-analysis of aspirin primary prevention trials suggested that differences in the rates of myocardial infarction between rofecoxib and naproxen might have been the result of an unexpectedly low rate of myocardial infarction in patients receiving naproxen. Thus, the risk of increased myocardial infarction is currently thought to be low in patients with a low risk of cardiac event *(165)*.

## 9. SELECTIVE COX-2 INHIBITORS
## IN CLINICAL TRIALS OF CANCER THERAPY

Based on encouraging findings from preclinical investigations showing that selective COX-2 inhibitors potentiate tumor response to cytotoxic agents, including radiation and chemotherapeutic drugs, a number of clinical trials combining these inhibitors with radiotherapy, chemotherapy, or radiochemotherapy have been initiated. At the University of Texas MD Anderson Cancer Center, a phase I study combining thoracic radiation with celecoxib for patients with unfavorable performance status, inoperable/unresectable, non-small-cell lung carcinoma (NSCLC) was completed *(166)*. The study was designed to determine the maximum tolerated dose (MTD) of celecoxib when used concurrently with standard fractionation thoracic radiotherapy for patients with poor prognosis NSCLC. It included three separate patient groups. Group I was comprised of patients with locally advanced cancer who presented with obstructive pneumonia or minimal metastatic disease. These patients received palliative radiotherapy with 45 Gy total dose delivered in 15 fractions. The patients in group II presented with inoperable early stage tumors, and these patients received definitive radiation therapy consisting of 66 Gy total dose delivered in 33 fractions. Group III included patients who received induction chemotherapy followed by radiotherapy to 63 Gy total dose in 35 fractions. Three-dimensional conformal treatment planning was used for all patients. Celecoxib in the escalation dose schedule of 200 mg, 400 mg, 600 mg, and 800 mg was administered orally in two equally divided doses daily starting 5 d prior to and continuing through the course of radiotherapy. Three to four patients of each group were assigned to each dose level of celecoxib. Forty-seven patients were enrolled in this protocol (19 in group I, 22 in group II, and 6 in group III), with the 800-mg dose level completed only in group I and group II. The main toxicities observed consisted of grades 1 and 2 nausea and esophagitis. Two patients in group II, one on 200 mg and the other on 400 mg celecoxib dose schedule, developed grade 3 pneumonitis 1 mo after radiotherapy plus celecoxib treatment. One patient developed hypertension 2 wk after starting 400 mg celecoxib twice daily that did not normalize following discontinuation of the drug, and the event was considered grade 3 drug toxicity. These results suggest that celecoxib can be safely administered concurrently with thoracic radiotherapy. Importantly, the local progression-free survival rate for all patients on the study was 67% at 20 mo, a result similar to that after concurrent chemoradiotherapy, which is highly encouraging.

The Radiation Therapy Oncology Group (RTOG) initiated a phase I/II study (RTOG 0213) *(167)* combining celecoxib concurrently with 66 Gy total-dose radiotherapy in the treatment of patients with inoperable stage IIB or unresectable stage IIIA or IIIB NSCLC. Celecoxib is administered daily at an escalated dose from 200 mg twice a day to 400 mg twice a day, starting 5 d prior to initiation of radiation therapy, and the treatment with celecoxib is continued for 2 yr or until disease progression. This clinical trial is ongoing.

A phase II trial that combined celecoxib with docetaxel in the treatment of recurrent NSCLC was reported recently *(168)*. Patients included in this study were those who had not responded to one or two previous chemotherapy regimens and were then treated with docetaxel, at a dose of 75 mg/m$^2$ given at a 3-wk interval, and daily celecoxib, at a dose of 400 mg bid starting 5 d prior to initiation of treatment with docetaxel. Preliminary data obtained on the 15 evaluable patients enrolled in the study are encouraging, with partial response in 2 (15%) patients, stable disease in 3 (23%) patients, and 8 patients with disease progression.

Altorki et al. *(169)* reported the final results of a phase II trial using celecoxib in combination with carboplatin and paclitaxel as neoadjuvant therapy in patients with resectable stage IB to IIIA NSCLC. PGE$_2$ analysis on the primary tumor and normal tissue was performed before and after neoadjuvant chemotherapy. Twenty-nine patients were enrolled and 26 (12 IB, 4 IIB, and 10 IIIA) were evaluable. No unexpected chemotherapy related toxicity was reported in this study. This neoadjuvant regimen produced objective response in 17 (65%) patients, including 5 (19%) complete responses. Tumors were downstaged in 13 patients. PGE$_2$ production in the primary tumor was significantly higher before treatment, and it decreased to the normal tissue level after the neoadjuvant therapy with celecoxib. These data suggested that the addition of celecoxib 400 mg bid might enhance tumor response to paclitaxel and carboplatin in patients with NSCLC, and this dose of celecoxib was sufficient to normalize the increase in PGE$_2$ levels in NSCLC after treatment with this chemotherapy regimen *(169)*. The results of this study demonstrated that it is safe and feasible to add celecoxib to chemotherapy, although proof of antitumor efficacy would require a randomized trial.

The preliminary results of a phase II study in which celecoxib was combined with concurrent chemoradiotherapy for patients with stage III NSCLC were reported *(170)*. Chemoradiotherapy consisted of 63 Gy total-dose radiation given in 35 fractions and concurrent administration of paclitaxel and carboplatin. Among nine evaluable patients accrued, there were three grade 3 or 4 esophagitis, two grade 3 pneumonitis, and two grade 5 possible treatment-related pneumonitis cases. The investigators concluded that concurrent administration of celecoxib with chemoradiotherapy is feasible.

In a prospective clinical study reported by Blanke et al. *(171)*, 22 patients with previously untreated unresectable or metastatic colorectal cancer were treated with celecoxib along with a chemotherapy regimen consisting of irinotecan, 5-flurouracil, and leucovorin. Partial tumor response was achieved in 28% of patients, whereas only 17% of patients had obvious tumor progression. Grade 3 and 4 neutropenia occurred significantly less frequently than expected, suggesting that the use of selective COX-2 inhibitors might reduce chemotherapy-related toxicity. Consistent with these findings, Sweeney *(172)*, Trifan *(158)*, and Lin *(173)* found less myelosuppression, equal or less diarrhea, and less hand and food syndrome when celecoxib was part of the chemotherapy regimen containing irinotecan.

In a clinical pilot study *(174)*, the safety and efficacy of oral metronomic low-dose treosulfan chemotherapy in combination with the COX-2 inhibitor rofecoxib as a compound with antiangiogenic potential, a therapeutic regimen optimally targeting endothelial cells instead of tumor cells, were assessed in 12 pretreated advanced melanoma patients. Patients received combined daily treosulfan chemotherapy (500 mg) with rofecoxib (25 mg). Endothelial cells were analyzed for proliferation, apoptosis, and cytotoxicity in response to increasing concentrations of treosulfan, either in the absence or presence of COX-2 inhibitor, to determine whether inhibition of COX-2 enhanced the effect of treosulfan on cell function. Simultaneous inhibition of COX-2 significantly increased the extent to which treosulfan suppressed cell proliferation, without inducing cytotoxicity. Only grade 2 hematologic toxicity was observed. An increase in response rates was observed without prolongation in overall survival. It was suggested that this regimen scheduled to primarily target endothelial cells might potentially provide a palliative alternative that preserves quality of life in the absence of significant treatment-related toxicity in patients with metastatic melanoma. In addition to the above studies, a number of other trials have been proposed or are ongoing (Table 3).

## 10. CONCLUSIONS

Recent advances in molecular biology and pathogenesis of cancer have identified a number of molecular determinants and signaling pathways that function abnormally in tumor cells and thus play a significant role in aggressive biological behavior of cancer and its resistance to therapy. Counteracting these determinants offers great promise for improving tumor therapy. As discussed in this chapter, COX-2 is one of these determinants. This enzyme is responsible for production of PGs in tumors, and through PGs or PG-independent mechanisms, it influences development of tumors, biological behavior of tumors, and tumor response to therapy. Increasing evidence suggests that COX-2 expression in tumors is associated with aggressive tumor growth, increased propensity of tumors to metastasize, tumor resistance to standard treatments, including radiotherapy and chemotherapy, and poor patient prognosis.

Because of these adverse actions, COX-2 represents a potential and appealing target for cancer therapy. Significant preclinical evidence shows that selective inhibitors of

Table 3
Ongoing/Proposed Therapeutic Clinical Trials of COX-2 Inhibitors

| Population | Phase | N | COX-2 Inhibitor |
|---|---|---|---|
| Colorectal cancer | | | |
|   Stage I to II colorectal cancer | III | 1200 | Celecoxib, 3 yr |
|   Stage II or III colorectal cancer | III | 5000 | Rofecoxib, 2 or 5 yr |
|   Advanced colorectal cancer | II | 23 | Celecoxib + irinotecan/ 5-FU/ leucovorin/glutamine |
|   Stage III colorectal cancer | III | 1400 | Celecoxib +5-FU/leucovorin, 3 yr |
|   Stage IV colorectal cancer | III | 700 | Celecoxib + irinotecan/5-FU/ capecitabine/leucovorin, to PD |
| Breast cancer (BC) | | | |
|   Metastatic BC or recurrent BC | II | 132 | Celecoxib, 1 yr (low or high dose) |
|   Postmenopausal w/BC | III | 7000 | Celecoxib, 3 yr |
|   Postmenopausal w/BC ER-negative tumors ER-positive tumors | III | 2700 | Celecoxib, 3 yr |
|   Metastatic breast cancer | III | 195 | Celecoxib + hormone therapy Celecoxib (L/H dose) + standard chemotherapy |
|   Metastatic breast cancer | II | 12–37 | Celecoxib + trastuzumab |
|   Postoperative breast cancer | III | 6800 | Exemestane or anastrazole ± celecoxib |
| Non-small-cell lung cancer | | | |
|   Stage IIB or unresectable IIIA or IIIB | I/II | 128 | Celecoxib + radiation |
|   Locally advanced NSCLC | II | 100 | Celecoxib + radiation |
|   Recurrent NSCLC | II | 64 | Celecoxib + docetaxel |
|   Stage IIIB or IV NSCLC | II | 21–39 | Celecoxib + docetaxel |
|   Early stage NSCLC | II | 23 | Celecoxib + paclitaxel/carboplatin |
|   Locally advanced NSCLC | II | 16 | Celecoxib + carboplatin/paclitaxel ± radiation |
| Other malignancies | | | |
|   Inoperable hepatocellular cancer | I | 8 | Celecoxib + thalidomide |
|   Brainstem glioma | I | 15 | Rofecoxib + radiation |
|   Localized prostate cancer | I | 60–70 | Celecoxib (4+ wk)+ surgery |
|   Locally advanced cervical cancer | I/II | 62 | Celecoxib + radiation/fluorouracil/ cisplatin, 1 yr |
|   Esophageal cancer | II | 17+ | Celecoxib (5 wk) + radiation/ fluorouracil |

COX-2 are effective in preventing carcinogenesis, slowing the growth of established tumors, and inhibiting metastatic spread. These antitumor actions of COX-2 inhibitors are exerted through multiple mechanisms, including inhibition of tumor cell proliferation, induction of apoptosis, inhibition of neoangiogenesis, and stimulation of antitumor immune responses. These effects are associated with reduction in PG production by tumors, implying that inhibition of PGs is a major underlying mechanism.

As a single-modality treatment, selective COX-2 inhibitors generally have modest antitumor efficacy, commonly expressed by slowed tumor growth. However, these agents are more effective in improving tumor response to other cancer treatment modalities, including radiotherapy and chemotherapy. Preclinical studies, using both animal tumors and human tumor xenografts, demonstrated that selective COX-2 inhibitors increase tumor response to radiation, more than that achieved with common NSAIDs. Moreover, selective COX-2 inhibitors do not appreciably enhance normal tissue response to radiation and might even be protective against some chemotherapy-induced normal tissue toxicity. Thus, selective COX-2 inhibitors can provide significant therapeutic gain when combined with radiotherapy and/or chemotherapy.

The preclinical findings on COX-2 and its inhibitors have been rapidly translated to clinical trials testing chemopreventive or therapeutic potential of these agents. A number of clinical studies have been initiated in which COX-2 inhibitors are combined with radiotherapy, chemotherapy, or chemoradiotherapy, and initial results show that these inhibitors can be safely combined with other standard treatments. Although encouraging results in tumor response were observed in some studies, the impact of COX-2 inhibitors on tumor treatment outcome, however, still requires rigorous testing in well-designed clinical trials.

## REFERENCES

1. Herskovic A, Martz K, al-Sarraf M, et al. Combined chemotherapy and radiotherapy compared with radiotherapy alone in patients with cancer of the esophagus. N Engl J Med 1992; 326:1593–1598.
2. Brizel DM, Albers ME, Fisher SR, et al. Hyperfractionated irradiation with or without concurrent chemotherapy for locally advanced head and neck cancer. [comment]. N Engl J Med 1998; 338:1798–1804.
3. Morris M, Eifel PJ, Lu J, et al. Pelvic radiation with concurrent chemotherapy compared with pelvic and para-aortic radiation for high-risk cervical cancer. [comment]. N Engl J Med 1999; 340:1137–1143.
4. Furuse K, Fukuoka M, Kawahara M, et al. Phase III study of concurrent versus sequential thoracic radiotherapy in combination with mitomycin, vindesine, and cisplatin in unresectable stage III non-small-cell lung cancer. J Clin Oncol 1999; 17:2692–2699.
5. Fu JY, Masferrer JL, Seibert K, et al. The induction and suppression of prostaglandin H2 synthase (cyclooxygenase) in human monocytes. J Biol Chem 1990; 265:16,737–16,740.
6. Williams CS, DuBois RN. Prostaglandin endoperoxide synthase: why two isoforms? Am J Physiol 1996; 270:G393–G400.
7. O'Banion MK. Cyclooxygenase-2: molecular biology, pharmacology, and neurobiology. Crit Rev Neurobiol 1999; 13:45–82.
8. Kujubu D, Fletcher B, Varnum B, et al. TIS10, a phorbol ester tumor promoter-inducible mRNA from Swiss 3T3 cells, encodes a novel prostaglandin synthase/cyclooxygenase homologue. J Biol Chem 1991; 266:12,866–12,872.
9. Xie W, Chipman J, Robertson D. Expression of a mitogen-responsive gene encoding prostaglandin synthase is regulated by mRNA splicing. PNAS 1991; 88:2692–2696.
10. Garavito R. The cyclooxygenase-2 structure: new drugs for an old target? Nat Struct Biol 1996; 3:897–901.
11. Otto J, DeWitt D, Smith W. N-Glycosylation of prostaglandin endoperoxide synthases-1 and -2 and their orientations in the endoplasmic reticulum. J Biol Chem 1993; 268:18,234–18,242.
12. Nieder C, Milas L, Ang K. Modification of radiation response. New York: Springer-Verlag, 2003.
13. Marnett J. Cyclooxygenase mechanisms. Curr Opin Chem Biol 2000; 4:545–552.
14. Bakhle Y. COX-2 and cancer: a new approach to an old problem. Br J Pharmacol 2001; 134:1137–1150.
15. Dannhardt G, Kiefer W. Cyclooxygenase inhibitors-current status and future prospects. Eur J Med Chem 2001; 36:109–126.
16. Liao Z, Komaki R, Mason K, et al. Role of cyclooxygenase-2 inhibitors in combination with radiation therapy in lung cancer. Clin Lung Cancer 2003; 4:356–365.
17. Gilman AG. G proteins: transducers of receptor-generated signals. Annu Rev Biochem 1987; 56:615–649.
18. Smith WL. The eicosanoids and their biochemical mechanisms of action. Biochem J 1989; 259:315–324.
19. Lemberger T, Desvergne B, Wahli W. Peroxisome proliferator-activated receptors: a nuclear receptor signaling pathway in lipid physiology. Annu Rev Cell Dev Biol 1996; 12:335–363.
20. Kliewer S, Forman B, Blumberg B, et al. Differential expression and activation of a family of murine peroxisome proliferator-activated receptors. PNAS 1994; 91:7355–7359.

21. Forman B, Tontonoz P, Chen J, et al. 15-Deoxy-delta 12, 14-prostaglandin J2 is a ligand for the adipocyte determination factor PPAR gamma. Cell 1995; 83:803–812.

22. Forman B, Chen J, Evans R. Hypolipidemic drugs, polyunsaturated faty acids, and eicosanoids are ligands for peroxisome proliferator-activated receptors alpha and delta. PNAS 1997; 94:4312–4317.

23. Lim H, Gupta RA, Ma W-G, et al. Cyclo-oxygenase-2-derived prostacyclin mediates embryo implantation in the mouse via PPARdelta. Genes Dev 1999; 13:1561–1574.

24. Giovannucci E, Rimm E, Stampfer M, et al. Aspirin use and the risk for colorectal cancer and adenoma in male health professionals. Ann Intern Med 1994; 121:241–246.

25. Bansal P, Sonnenberg A. Risk factors of colorectal cancer in inflammatory bowel disease. Am J Gastroenterol 1996; 91:44–48.

26. Thun M, Namboodiri M, Calle E, et al. Aspirin use and risk of fatal cancer. Cancer Res 1993; 53:1322–1327.

27. Schreinemachers DM, Everson RB. Aspirin use and lung, colon, and breast cancer incidence in a prospective study. Epidemiology 1994; 5:138–146.

28. Eberhart C, Coffey R, Radhika A, et al. Up-regulation of cyclooxygenase 2 gene expression in human colorectal adenomas and adenocarcinomas. Gastroenterology 1994; 107:1183–1188.

29. Koki A, Leahy KM, Masferrer JL. Potential utility of COX-2 inhibitors in chemoprevention and chemotherapy. Expert Opin Invest Drugs 1999; 8:1623–1638.

30. Oshima M, Dinchuk JE, Kargman SL, et al. Suppression of intestinal polyposis in Apc delta716 knockout mice by inhibition of cyclooxygenase 2 (COX-2). Cell 1996; 87:803–809.

31. Liu CH, Chang S-H, Narko K, et al. Overexpression of cyclooxygenase-2 is sufficient to induce tumorigenesis in transgenic mice. J Biol Chem 2001; 276:18,563–18,569.

32. Jacoby RF, Seibert K, Cole CE, et al. The cyclooxygenase-2 inhibitor celecoxib is a potent preventive and therapeutic agent in the Min mouse model of adenomatous polyposis. Cancer Res 2000; 60:5040–5044.

33. Oshima M, Murai N, Kargman S, et al. Chemoprevention of intestinal polyposis in the Apcdelta716 mouse by rofecoxib, a specific cyclooxygenase-2 inhibitor. Cancer Res 2001; 61:1733–1740.

34. Fischer SM, Lo HH, Gordon GB, et al. Chemopreventive activity of celecoxib, a specific cyclooxygenase-2 inhibitor, and indomethacin against ultraviolet light-induced skin carcinogenesis. Mol Carcinog 1999; 25:231–240.

35. Harris RE, Alshafie GA, Abou-Issa H, et al. Chemoprevention of breast cancer in rats by celecoxib, a cyclooxygenase 2 inhibitor. Cancer Res 2000; 60:2101–2103.

36. Alshafie G, Abou-Issa H, Seibert K, et al. Chemotherapeutic evaluation of celecoxib, a cyclooxygenase-2 inhibitor, in a rat mammary tumor model. Oncol Rep 2000; 7:1377–1378.

37. Dannenberg A, Subbaramaiah K. Targeting cyclooxygenase-2 in human neoplasia: rationale and promise. Cancer Cell 2003; 4:431–436.

38. Steinbach G, Lynch PM, Phillips RK, et al. The effect of celecoxib, a cyclooxygenase-2 inhibitor, in familial adenomatous polyposis. N Engl J Med 2000; 342:1946–1952.

39. Furuta Y, Hall ER, Sanduja S, et al. Prostaglandin production by murine tumors as a predictor for therapeutic response to indomethacin. Cancer Res 1988; 48:3002–3007.

40. Tang D, Honn KV. Eicosanoids and tumor cell metastasis. In: Tang DG, Honn KV, eds. Prostaglandin inhibitors in tumor immunotherapy. Boca Raton, FL: CRC Press, 1994:73–108.

41. Bennett A, Berstock DA, Raja B, et al. Survival time after surgery is inversely related to the amounts of prostaglandins extracted from human breast cancers. [proceedings]. Br J Pharmacol 1979; 66:451.

42. Rigas B, Goldman IS, Levine L. Altered eicosanoid levels in human colon cancer. J Lab Clin Med 1993; 122:518–523.

43. Soslow R, Dannenberg A, Rush D, et al. COX-2 is expressed in human pulmonary, colonic, and mammary tumors. Cancer 2000; 89:2637–2645.

44. Zhang Z, DuBois RN. Par-4, a proapoptotic gene, is regulated by NSAIDs in human colon carcinoma cells. Gastroenterology 2000; 118:1012–1017.

45. Masferrer JL, Leahy KM, Koki AT, et al. Antiangiogenic and antitumor activities of cyclooxygenase-2 inhibitors. Cancer Res 2000; 60:1306–1311.

46. Sheehan KM, Sheahan K, O'Donoghue DP, et al. The relationship between cyclooxygenase-2 expression and colorectal cancer. JAMA 1999; 282:1254–1257.

47. Cianchi F, Cortesini C, Bechi P, et al. Up-regulation of cyclooxygenase 2 gene expression correlates with tumor angiogenesis in human colorectal cancer. Gastroenterology 2001; 121:1339–1347.

48. Uefuji K, Ichikura T, Mochizuki H. Expression of cyclooxygenase-2 in human gastric adenomas and adenocarcinomas. J Surg Oncol 2001; 76:26–30.

49. Saukkonen K, Nieminen O, van Rees B, et al. Expression of cyclooxygenase-2 in dysplasia of the stomach and in intestinal-type gastric adenocarcinoma. Clin Cancer Res 2001; 7:1923–1931.

50. Sung JJY, Leung WK, Go MYY, et al. Cyclooxygenase-2 expression in *Helicobacter pylori*-associated premalignant and malignant gastric lesions. Am J Pathol 2000; 157:729–735.

51. Buskens C, Van Rees B, Sivula A, et al. Prognostic significance of elevated cyclooxygenase 2 expression in patients with adenocarcinoma of the esophagus. Gastroenterology 2002; 122:1800–1807.

52. Zimmerman K, Sarbia M, Weber A, et al. Cyclooxygenase-2 expression in human esophageal carcinoma. Cancer Res 1999; 59:198–204.

53. Wilson K, Fu S, Ramanujam K, et al. Increased expression of inducible nitric oxide synthase and cyclooxygenase-2 in Barrett's esophagus and associated adenocarcinomas. Cancer Res 1998; 58:2929–2934.

54. Tucker ON, Dannenberg AJ, Yang EK, et al. Cyclooxygenase-2 expression is up-regulated in human pancreatic cancer. Cancer Res 1999; 59:987–990.

55. Merati K, said Siadaty M, Andea A, et al. Expression of inflammatory modulator COX-2 in pancreatic ductal adenocarcinoma and its relationship to pathologic and clinical parameters. Am J Clin Oncol 2001; 24:447–452.

56. Niijima M, Yamaguchi T, Ishihara T, et al. Immunohistochemical analysis and in situ hybridization of cyclooxygenase-2 expression in intraductal papillary-mucinous tumors of the pancreas. Cancer 2002; 94:1565–1573.

57. Koshiba T, Hosotani R, Miyamoto Y, et al. Immunohistochemical analysis of cyclooxygenase-2 expression in pancreatic tumors. Int J Pancreatol 1999; 26:69–76.

58. Kokawa A, Kondo H, Gotoda T, et al. Increased expression of cyclooxygenase-2 in human pancreatic neoplasms and potential for chemoprevention by cyclooxygenase inhibitors. Cancer 2001; 91:333–339.

59. Shiota G, Okubo M, Noumi T, et al. Cyclooxygenase-2 expression in hepatocellular carcinoma. Hepatogastroenterology 1999; 46:407–412.

60. Bae SH, Jung ES, Park YM, et al. Expression of cyclooxygenase-2 (COX-2) in hepatocellular carcinoma and growth inhibition of hepatoma cell lines by a COX-2 inhibitor, NS-398. Clin Cancer Res 2001; 7:1410–1418.

61. Wolf H, Saukkonen K, Anttila S, et al. Expression of cyclooxygenase-2 in human lung carcinoma. Cancer Res 1998; 58:4997–5001.

62. Hida T, Yatabe Y, Achiwa H, et al. Increased expression of cyclooxygenase 2 occurs frequently in human lung cancers, specifically in adenocarcinomas. Cancer Res 1998; 58:3761–3764.

63. Achiwa H, Yatabe Y, Hida T, et al. Prognostic significance of elevated cyclooxygenase 2 expression in primary, resected lung adenocarcinomas. Clin Cancer Res 1999; 5:1001–1005.

64. Hasturk S, Kemp B, Kalapurakal S, et al. Expression of cyclooxygenase-1 and cyclooxygenase-2 in bronchial epithelium and nonsmall cell lung carcinoma. Cancer 2002; 94:1023–1031.

65. Lee L, Pan C, Cheng C, et al. Expression of cyclooxygenase-2 in prostate adenocarcinoma and benign prostatic hyperplasia. Anticancer Res 2001; 21:1291–1294.

66. Gupta V, Jaskowiak N, Beckett M, et al. Vascular endothelial growth factor enhances endothelial cell survival and tumor radioresistance. Cancer J Sci Am 2002; 8:47–54.

67. Zha S, Gage WR, Sauvageot J, et al. Cyclooxygenase-2 is up-regulated in proliferative inflammatory atrophy of the prostate, but not in prostate carcinoma. Cancer Res 2001; 61:8617–8623.

68. Boström P, Aaltonen V, Söderström K, et al. Expression of cyclooxygenase-1 and -2 in urinary bladder carcinomas In vivo and In vitro and prostaglandin E2 synthesis in cultured bladder cancer cells. Pathology 2001; 33:469–474.

69. Shirahama T. Cyclooxygenase-2 expression is up-regulated in transitional cell carcinoma and its preneoplastic lesions in the human urinary bladder. Clin Cancer Res 2000; 6:2424–2430.

70. Ristimaki A, Nieminen O, Saukkonen K, et al. Expression of cyclooxygenase-2 in human transitional cell carcinoma of the urinary bladder. Am J Pathol 2001; 158:849–853.

71. Mohammed SI, Bennett PF, Craig BA, et al. Effects of the cyclooxygenase inhibitor, piroxicam, on tumor response, apoptosis, and angiogenesis in a canine model of human invasive urinary bladder cancer. Cancer Res 2002; 62:356–358.

72. Komhoff M, Guan Y, Shappell HW, et al. Enhanced expression of cyclooxygenase-2 in high grade human transitional cell bladder carcinomas. Am J Pathol 2000; 157:29–35.

73. Half E, Tang XM, Gwyn K, et al. Cyclooxygenase-2 expression in human breast cancers and adjacent ductal carcinoma in situ. Cancer Res 2002; 62:1676–1681.

74. Subbaramaiah K, Norton L, Gerald W, et al. Cyclooxygenase-2 is overexpressed in HER-2/neu-positive breast cancer. Evidence for involvement of AP-1 and PEA3. J Biol Chem 2002; 277:18,649–18,657.

75. Kulkarni S, Rader JS, Zhang F, et al. Cyclooxygenase-2 is overexpressed in human cervical cancer. Clin Cancer Res 2001; 7:429–434.

76. Kim Y, Kim G, Cho N, et al. Overexpression of cyclooxygenase-2 is associated with a poor prognosis in patients with squamous cell carcinoma of the uterine cervix treated with radiation and concurrent chemotherapy. Cancer 2002; 95:531–539.

77. Ryu H-S, Chang K-H, Yang H-W, et al. High cyclooxygenase-2 expression in stage IB cervical cancer with lymph node metastasis or parametrial invasion. Gynecol Oncol 2000; 76:320–325.

78. Sales KJ, Katz AA, Davis M, et al. Cyclooxygenase-2 expression and prostaglandin E2 synthesis are up-regulated in carcinomas of the cervix: a possible autocrine/paracrine regulation of neoplastic cell function via EP2/EP4 receptors. J Clin Endocrinol Metab 2001; 86:2243–2249.

79. Gaffney DK, Holden J, Davis M, et al. Elevated cyclooxygenase-2 expression correlates with diminished survival in carcinoma of the cervix treated with radiotherapy. Int J Radiat Oncol Biol Phys 2001; 49: 1213–1217.

80. Ferrandina G, Legge F, Ranelletti F, et al. Cyclooxygenase-2 expression in endometrial carcinoma: correlation with clinicopathologic parameters and clinical outcome. Cancer 2002; 95:801–807.

81. Denkert C, Kobel M, Pest S, et al. Expression of cyclooxygenase 2 is an independent prognostic factor in human ovarian carcinoma. Am J Pathol 2002; 160:893–903.

82. Matsumoto Y, Ishiko O, Deguchi M, et al. Cyclooxygenase-2 expression in normal ovaries and epithelial ovarian neoplasms. Int J Mol Med 2001; 8:31–36.

83. Chan G, Boyle JO, Yang EK, et al. Cyclooxygenase-2 expression is up-regulated in squamous cell carcinoma of the head and neck. Cancer Res 1999; 59:991–994.

84. Denkert C, Kobel M, Berger S, et al. Expression of cyclooxygenase 2 in human malignant melanoma. Cancer Res 2001; 61:303–308.

85. Thompson E, Gupta A, Vielhauer G, et al. The growth of malignant keratinocytes depends on signaling through the PGE(2) receptor EP1. Neoplasia 2001; 3:402–410.

86. Ristimaki A, Sivula A, Lundin J, et al. Prognostic significance of elevated cyclooxygenase-2 expression in breast cancer. Cancer Res 2002; 62:632–635.

87. Subbaramaiah K, Dannenberg A. Cyclooxygenase 2: a molecular target for cancer prevention and treatment. Trends Pharmacol Sci 2003; 24:96–102.

88. Sano H, Kawahito Y, Wilder RL, et al. Expression of cyclooxygenase-1 and -2 in human colorectal cancer. Cancer Res 1995; 55:3785–3789.

89. Hao X, Bishop A, Wallace MB, et al. Early expression of cyclo-oxygenase-2 during sporadic colorectal carcinogenesis. J Pathol 1999; 187:295–301.

90. Khuri FR, Wu H, Lee JJ, et al. Cyclooxygenase-2 overexpression is a marker of poor prognosis in stage I non-small cell lung cancer. Clin Cancer Res 2001; 7:861–867.

91. Yamauchi T, Watanabe M, Hasegawa H, et al. The role of COX-2 expression in colorectal cancer. Proc Am Assoc Cancer Res 2000:41.

92. Murata H, Kawano S, Tsuji S, et al. Cyclooxygenase-2 overexpression enhances lymphatic invasion and metastasis in human gastric carcinoma. Am J Gastroenterol 1999; 94:451–455.

93. Kargman SL, O'Neill GP, Vickers PJ, et al. Expression of prostaglandin G/H synthase-1 and -2 protein in human colon cancer. Cancer Res 1995; 55:2556–2559.

94. Ang KK, Berkey BA, Tu X, et al. Impact of epidermal growth factor receptor expression on survival and pattern of relapse in patients with advanced head and neck carcinoma. Cancer Res 2002; 62:7350–7356.

95. Kozaki K, Koshikawa K, Tatematsu Y, et al. Multi-faceted analyses of a highly metastatic human lung cancer cell line NCI-H460-LNM35 suggest mimicry of inflammatory cells in metastasis. Oncogene 2001; 20:4228–4234.

96. Kakiuchi Y, Tsuji S, Tsujii M, et al. Cyclooxygenase-2 activity altered the cell-surface carbohydrate antigens on colon cancer cells and enhanced liver metastasis. Cancer Res 2002; 62:1567–1572.

97. Niki T, Kohno T, Iba S, et al. Frequent co-localization of Cox-2 and Laminin-5 {gamma}2 chain at the invasive front of early-stage lung adenocarcinomas. Am J Pathol 2002; 160:1129–1141.

98. Tsubouchi Y, Mukai S, Kawahito Y, et al. Meloxicam inhibits the growth of non-small cell lung cancer. Anti-cancer Res 2000; 20:2867–2872.

99. Fulton AM. Interactions of natural effector cells and prostaglandins in the control of metastasis. J Natl Cancer Inst 1987; 78:735–741.

100. Gee J, Lee I, Fischer S, et al. COX-2 selective inhibitor celecoxib induces growth inhibition and apoptosis in bladder carcinoma. Proc Am Assoc Cancer Res 2002; 43:643–644.
101. Zweifel B, Ornberg R, Woerner M, et al. Inhibition of prostaglandins by celecoxib results in suppression of tumor growth and reduces VEGF level in human head and neck xenograft model. Proc Am Assoc Cancer Res 2002; 43:77.
102. Marnett L. Generation of mutagens during arachidonic acid metabolism. Cancer Metastasis Rev 1994; 1994:303–308.
103. Eling TE, Curtis JF. Xenobiotic metabolism by prostaglandin H synthase. Pharmacol Ther 1992; 53: 261–273.
104. Prescott S, White R. Self-promotion? Intimate connections between APC and prostaglandin H synthase-2. Cell 1996; 87:783–786.
105. Wiese FW, Thompson PA, Kadlubar FF. Carcinogen substrate specificity of human COX-1 and COX-2. Carcinogenesis 2001; 22:5–10.
106. Watson AJ. Chemopreventive effects of NSAIDs against colorectal cancer: regulation of apoptosis and mitosis by COX-1 and COX-2. Histol Histopathol 1998; 13:591–597.
107. Smith M-L, Hawcroft G, Hull MA. The effect of non-steroidal anti-inflammatory drugs on human colorectal cancer cells: evidence of different mechanisms of action. Eur J Cancer 2000; 36:664–674.
108. Tsujii M, DuBois RN. Alterations in cellular adhesion and apoptosis in epithelial cells overexpressing prostaglandin endoperoxide synthase 2. Cell 1995; 83:493–501.
109. Dempke W, Rie C, Grothey A, et al. Cyclooxygenase-2: a novel target for cancer chemotherapy? J Cancer Res Clin Oncol 2001; 127:41–47.
110. Form DM, Auerbach R. PGE2 and angiogenesis. Proc Soc Exp Biol Med 1983; 172:214–218.
111. Ziche M, Jones J, Gullino PM. Role of prostaglandin E1 and copper in angiogenesis. J Natl Cancer Inst 1982; 69:475–482.
112. Williams CS, Tsujii M, Reese J, et al. Host cyclooxygenase-2 modulates carcinoma growth. J Clin Invest 2000; 105:1589–1594.
113. Majima M, Hayashi I, Muramatsu M, et al. Cyclo-oxygenase-2 enhances basic fibroblast growth factor-induced angiogenesis through induction of vascular endothelial growth factor in rat sponge implants. Br J Pharmacol 2000; 130:641–649.
114. Rak J, Filmus J, Kerbel RS. Reciprocal paracrine interactions between tumour cells and endothelial cells: the 'angiogenesis progression' hypothesis. Eur J Cancer 1996; 32A:2438–2450.
115. Milas L, Furuta Y, Hunter N, et al. Dependence of indomethacin-induced potentiation of murine tumor radioresponse on tumor host immunocompetence. Cancer Res 1990; 50:4473–4477.
116. Milas L, Kishi K, Hunter N, et al. Enhancement of tumor response to γ-radiation by an inhibitor of cyclo-oxygenase-2 enzyme. J Natl Cancer Inst 1999; 91:1501–1504.
117. Leahy KM, Ornberg RL, Wang Y, et al. Cyclooxygenase-2 inhibition by celecoxib reduces proliferation and induces apoptosis in angiogenic endothelial cells in vivo. Cancer Res 2002; 62:625–631.
118. Dicker A, Williams T, Grant D. Targeting angiogenic processes by combination rofecoxib and ionizing radiation. Am J Clin Oncol 2001; 24:438–442.
119. Leung KH, Mihich E. Prostaglandin modulation of development of cell-mediated immunity in culture. Nature 1980; 288:597–600.
120. Brunda M, Herberman R, Holden H. Inhibition of murine natural killer cell activity by prostaglandins. J Immunol 1980; 124:2682–2687.
121. Fulton AM, Levy JG. The possible role of prostaglandins in mediating immune suppression by nonspecific T suppressor cells. Cell Immunol 1980; 52:29–37.
122. Kambayashi T, Alexander HR, Fong M, et al. Potential involvement of IL-10 in suppressing tumor-associated macrophages. Colon-26-derived prostaglandin E2 inhibits TNF-alpha release via a mechanism involving IL-10. J Immunol 1995; 154:3383–3390.
123. Huang M, Stolina M, Sharma S, et al. Non-small cell lung cancer cyclooxygenase-2-dependent regulation of cytokine balance in lymphocytes and macrophages: up-regulation of interleukin 10 and down-regulation of interleukin 12 production. Cancer Res 1998; 58:1208–1216.
124. Stolina M, Sharma S, Lin Y, et al. Specific inhibition of cyclooxygenase 2 restores antitumor reactivity by altering the balance of IL-10 and IL-12 synthesis. J Immunol 2000; 164:361–370.
125. Milas L, Nishiguchi I, Hunter N, et al. Radiation protection against early and late effects of ionizing irradiation by the prostaglandin inhibitor indomethacin. Adv Space Res 1992; 12:265–271.
126. Hanson WR. Eicosanoid-induced radioprotection and chemoprotection:Laboratory studies and clinical applicatons. In: Bump EA, Malaker K, eds. Radioprotectors: chemical, biological and clinical perspectives. Boca Raton, FL: CRC, 1998:197–221.

127. Milas L, Hunter NR, Mason KA, et al. Role of reoxygenation in induction of enhancement of tumor radioresponse by paclitaxel. Cancer Res 1995; 55:3564–3568.
128. van Buul PP, van Duyn-Goedhart A, Sankaranarayanan K. In vivo and in vitro radioprotective effects of the prostaglandin E1 analogue misoprostol in DNA repair-proficient and -deficient rodent cell systems. Radiat Res 1999; 152:398–403.
129. Zaffaroni N, Villa R, Orlandi L, et al. Differential effect of 9 beta-chloro-16, 16-dimethyl prostaglandin E2 (nocloprost) on the radiation response of human normal fibroblasts and colon adenocarcinoma cells. Radiat Res 1993; 135:88–92.
130. Hanson W, Thomas C. 16,16-Dimethyl prostaglandin E2 increases survival of murine intestinal stem cells when given before photon radiation. Radiat Res 1983; 96:393–398.
131. Hanson W, Geng L, Malkinson F. Prostaglandin-induced protection from radiation or doxorubicin is tissue specific and dependent upon receptor expression. Tenth International Congress of Radiation Research. Wurzburg, Germany, 1995:435.
132. Geng L, Hanson WR, Malkinson FD. Topical or systemic 16, 16 dm prostaglandin E2 or WR-2721 (WR-1065) protects mice from alopecia after fractionated irradiation. Int J Radiat Biol 1992; 61:533–537.
133. van Buul PP, van Duyn-Goedhart A, de Rooij DG, et al. Differential radioprotective effects of misoprostol in DNA repair-proficient and -deficient or radiosensitive cell systems. Int J Radiat Biol 1997; 71:259–264.
134. Houchen CW, Stenson WF, Cohn SM. Disruption of cyclooxygenase-1 gene results in an impaired response to radiation injury. Am J Physiol Gastrointest Liver Physiol 2000; 279:G858–G865.
135. Furuta Y, Hunter N, Barkley T Jr, et al. Increase in radioresponse of murine tumors by treatment with indomethacin. Cancer Res 1988; 48:3008–3013.
136. Kishi K, Petersen S, Petersen C, et al. Preferential enhancement of tumor radioresponse by a cyclooxygenase-2 inhibitor. Cancer Res 2000; 60:1326–1331.
137. Petersen C, Petersen S, Milas L, et al. Human glioma cell radiosensitization by a selective COX-2 inhibitor. Clin Cancer Res 2000; 6:2513–2520.
138. Pyo H, Choy H, Amorino GP, et al. A selective cyclooxygenase-2 inhibitor, NS-398, enhances the effect of radiation in vitro and in vivo preferentially on the cells that express cyclooxygenase-2. Clin Cancer Res 2001; 7:2998–3005.
139. Davis T, Hunter N, Trifan OC, et al. COX-2 Inhibitors as radiosensitizing agents for cancer therapy. Am J Clin Oncol 2002; 26:S58–S61.
140. Milas L. Cyclooxygenase-2 (COX-2) enzyme inhibitors and radiotherapy. Am J Clin Oncol 2003;26: S66–S69.
141. Amirghahari N, Harrison L, Smith M, et al. NS 398 radiosensitizes an HNSCC cell line by possibly inhibiting radiation-induced expression of COX-2. Int J Radiat Oncol Biol Phys 2003; 57:1405–1412.
142. Wen B, Deutsch E, Eschwege P, et al. Cyclooxygenase-2 inhibitor NS398 enhances antitumor effect of irradiation on hormone refractory human prostate carcinoma cells. J Urol 2003; 170:2036–2039.
143. Milas L, Mason K, Liao Z, et al. Role of cyclooxygenase-2 (COX-2) and its inhibition in tumor biology and radiotherapy. In: Nieder C, Milas L, Ang K, eds. Modification of radiation response. New York: Springer-Verlag, 2003:241–258.
144. Raju U, Nakata E, Yang P, et al. In vitro enhancement of tumor cell radiosensitivity by a selective inhibitor of cyclooxygenase-2 enzyme: mechanistic considerations. Int J Radiat Oncol Biol Phys 2002; 54:886–894.
145. Komaki R, Liao Z, Milas L. Improvement strategies for molecular targeting: cyclooxygenase-2 inhibitors as radiosensitizers for non-small cell lung cancer. Semin Oncol 2004; 31(1 Suppl 1):47–53.
146. Teicher BA, Holden SA, Dupuis NP, et al. Potentiation of cytotoxic therapies by TNP-470 and minocycline in mice bearing EMT-6 mammary carcinoma. Breast Cancr Res Treat 1995; 36:227–236.
147. Gorski DH, Beckett MA, Jaskowiak NT, et al. Blockade of the vascular endothelial growth factor stress response increases the antitumor effects of ionizing radiation. Cancer Res 1999; 59:3374–3378.
148. Gorski DH, Mauceri HJ, Salloum RM, et al. Potentiation of the antitumor effect of ionizing radiation by brief concomitant exposures to angiostatin. Cancer Res 1998; 58:5686–5689.
149. Mason KA, Kishi K, Hunter N, et al. Effect of docetaxel on the therapeutic ratio of fractionated radiotherapy in vivo. Clin Cancer Res 1999; 5:4191–4198.
150. Li L, Rojiani A, Siemann DW. Targeting the tumor vasculature with combretastatin A-4 disodium phosphate: effects on radiation therapy. Int J Radiat Oncol Biol Phys 1998; 42:335–363.
151. Milas L, Mason K, Hunter N, et al. In vivo enhancement of tumor radioresponse by C225 antiepidermal growth factor receptor antibody. Clin Cancer Res 2000; 6:701–708.

152. Haimovitz-Friedman A, Vlodavsky I, Chaudhuri A, et al. Autocrine effects of fibroblast growth factor in repair of radiation damage in endothelial cells. Cancer Res 1991; 51:2552–2558.
153. Steinauer KK, Gibbs I, Ning S, et al. Radiation induces upregulation of cyclooxygenase-2 (COX-2) protein in PC-3 cells. Int J Radiat Oncol Biol Phys 2000; 48:325–328.
154. Torrance CJ, Jackson PE, Montgomery E, et al. Combinatorial chemoprevention of intestinal neoplasia. Nat Med 2000; 6:1024–1028.
155. Harari PM, Huang SM. Radiation response modification following molecular inhibition of epidermal growth factor receptor signaling. Semin Radiat Oncol 2001; 11:281–290.
156. Duffy C, Elliott C, O'Connor R, et al. Enhancement of chemotherapeutic drug toxicity to human tumour cells in vitro by a subset of non-steroidal anti-inflammatory drugs (NSAIDs). Eur J Cancer 1998; 34: 1250–1259.
157. Manson MM, Holloway KA, Howells LM, et al. Modulation of signal-transduction pathways by chemopreventive agents. Biochem Soc Trans 2000; 28:7–12.
158. Trifan OC, Durham WF, Salazar VS, et al. Cyclooxygenase-2 inhibition with celecoxib enhances antitumor efficacy and reduces diarrhea side effect of CPT-11. Cancer Res 2002; 62:5778–5784.
159. Nakata E, Mason K, Hunter N, et al. Potentiation of tumor response to radiation or chemoradiation by selective cyclooxygenase-2 enzyme inhibitors. Int J Radiat Oncol Biol Phys 2004; 58:369–375.
160. Patel VA, Dunn MJ, Sorokin A. Regulation of MDR-1 (P-glycoprotein) by cyclooxygenase-2. J Biol Chem 2002; 277:38,915–38,920.
161. Ratnasinghe D, Daschner P, Anver M, et al. Cyclooxygenase-2, P-glycoprotein-170 and drug resistance; is chemoprevention against multidrug resistance possible? Anticancer Res 2001; 21:2141–2147.
162. Silverstein FE, Faich G, Goldstein JL, et al. Gastrointestinal toxicity with celecoxib vs nonsteroidal anti-inflammatory drugs for osteoarthritis and rheumatoid arthritis: The CLASS Study: a randomized controlled trial. JAMA 2000; 284:1247–1255.
163. Cleland LG, James MJ, Stamp LK, et al. COX-2 inhibition and thrombotic tendency: a need for surveillance. Med J Aust 2001; 175:214–217.
164. Mukherjee D, Nissen SE, Topol EJ. Risk of cardiovascular events associated with selective COX-2 inhibitors. JAMA 2001; 286:954–959.
165. Howes LG, Krum H. Selective cyclo-oxygenase-2 inhibitors and myocardial infarction: how strong is the link? Drug Safety 2002; 25:829–835.
166. Liao Z, Chen Y, Komaki R, et al. A phase I study combining thoracic radiation (RT) with celecoxib in patients with non-small cell lung cancer (NSCLC). Proc Am Soc Clin Oncol 2003; 22:216.
167. Radiation Therapy Oncology Group, RTOG 0213. A phase I/II trial of a Cox-2 inhibitor, Celebrex (celecoxib), with limited field radiation for intermediate prognosis patients with locally advanced non-small cell cancer, with analysis of prognostic factors. http://www.rtog.org/members/protocols/0213/0213.pdf. Accessed 11/26/2004.
168. Csiki I, Dang T, Gonzalez A, et al. Cyclooxygenase-2 (COX-2) inhibition + docetaxel (Txt) in recurrent non-small cell lung cancer (NSCLC): preliminary results of a phase II trial (THO-0054). Proc Am Soc Clin Oncol 2002; 21:297a (abstract).
169. Altorki NK, Keresztes RS, Port JL, et al. Celecoxib, a selective cyclo-oxygenase-2 inhibitor, enhances the response to preoperative paclitaxel and carboplatin in early-stage non-small-cell lung cancer. J Clin Oncol 2003; 21:2645–2650.
170. Carbone D, Choy H, Csiki I. Serum/plasma VEGF level changes with cyclooxygenase-2 (COX-2) inhibition in combined modality therapy in stage III non-small cell lung cancer (NSCLC): preliminary results of a phase II trial (THO-0059). Proc Am Soc Clin Oncol 2002; 318a (abstract).
171. Blanke C, Benson A, Dragovich T, et al. A phase II trial of celexoxib (CB), irinotecan (I), 5-fluorouracil (5FU), and leucovorin (LCV) in patients (pts) with unresectable or metastatic colorectal cancr (CRC). Proc Am Soc Clin Oncol 2002; 21:127.
172. Sweeney C, Seitz D, Ansari R, et al. A phase II trial of irinotecan (I), 4-fluorouracil (F), leucovorin (L) (IFL), celecoxib and glutamine as first line therapy for advaned colorectal cancer: a Hoosier Oncology Group study. Proc Am Soc Clin Oncol 2002; 21:105b.
173. Lin E, Morris J, Chau N, et al. Celecoxib attenuated capecitabine induced hand-and-foot syndrome (HFS) and diarrhea and improved time to tumor progression in metastatic colorectal cancer (MCRC). Proc Am Soc Clin Oncol 2002; 21:138b.
174. Spieth K, Kaufmann R, Gille J. Metronomic oral low-dose treosulfan chemotherapy combined with cyclooxygenase-2 inhibitor in pretreated advanced melanoma: a pilot study. Cancer Chemother Pharmacol 2003; 52:377–382.

# 38

## Understanding Prostate-Specific Membrane Antigen and Its Implication in Prostate Cancer

*Arundhati Ghosh, PhD*
*and Warren D. W. Heston, PhD*

### Contents

### Summary

Prostate-specific membrane antigen (PSMA) is a novel marker that represents an excellent ideal cell-surface-bound protein for targeted therapy of prostate cancer and vasculotoxic therapy of nonprostate solid cancers. Clinical trials using humanized version of PSMA-specific antibodies that target the external domain of PSMA with imaging or toxic agents have been encouraging. PSMA is expressed in the prostate and is found to be strongly upregulated in prostate cancer and it is the second highest upregulated gene in Gleason grade 4/5 prostate cancer compared to benign prostate hyperplasia. PSMA is negatively regulated by androgen and the PSMA promoter-enhancer has been analyzed in detail and has been used in gene therapy for selective expression of toxic genes in prostate. It appears that calcium might be involved in the signaling for this increased expression. PSMA has to be glycosylated and in a dimer state to be enzymatically active. PSMA has activity as a carboxypeptidase with the preferred substrates neuro-dipeptide NAAG and poly-γ-glutamated folate releasing glutamate upon hydrolysis of the substrate. The released glutamate might have a role in signaling. PSMA is internalized and exhibits a unique internalization motif, MXXXL. PSMA also interacts with actin-binding protein filamin A. Filamin A is also associated with transducing extracellular stress to internal signaling, and PSMA might modify that signaling process.

**Key Words:** Prostate-specific membrane antigen; carboxypeptidase; folate hydrolase; folyl-poly-γ-glutamate; dileucine motif; PSMA enhancer; endocytosis.

From: *Cancer Drug Discovery and Development: The Oncogenomics Handbook*
Edited by: W. J. LaRochelle and R. A. Shimkets © Humana Press Inc., Totowa, NJ

# 1. PSMA/FOLH1/NAALADase/GCPII

Prostate-specific membrane antigen (PSMA) has an important role in prostate carcinogenesis and progression, glutamatergic neurotransmission, and folate absorption *(1)*. Each of these different areas of research activity leads to different names being given to PSMA. Because of its strong expression in the prostate (where its function is unknown), it is named as PSMA; in the central nervous system, where it metabolizes the brain neurotransmitter, *N*-acetyl-aspartyl-glutamate, it is named NAALADase; in the proximal small intestine, its role is to remove γ-linked glutamates from poly-γ-glutamated folate, folate hydrolase (FOLH1) and as a carboxypeptidase, glutamate carboxypeptidase II (GCPII). Our focus in this chapter will be on its biology and role in the prostate and prostate cancer. PSMA is upregulated many-fold in prostate cancers (PCAs), metastatic disease, and hormone-refractory PCAs. PSMA expression is modulated inversely by androgen levels *(2,3)*. Most interestingly, PSMA expression has been found in the neovasculature of most of the solid tumors (not in vasculature of the normal tissues) *(4)*.

## 1.1. PSMA Discovery and Mapping

Prostate-specific membrane antigen is a type II membrane glycoprotein, $M_r \sim 100,000$ Dalton with an intracellular segment (amino acids 1–18), a transmembrane domain (amino acids 19–43) and an extensive extracellular domain (amino acids 44–750) (Fig. 1A). The human PSMA gene was first cloned in Heston's laboratory from lymph node metastatic lesion of adenocarcinoma of prostate (LNCaP) cells *(2)* and was found to be located in chromosome 11p11–12, which encodes for PSMA transcript expression in the prostate *(6–8)*. Another gene highly homologous to PSMA was found to be located at the loci 11q14.3 and is called PSM-like. The PSM-like gene is expressed in different tissues, such as the kidney and liver, but not in the prostate *(9)*

## 1.2. Variants of PSMA

Prostate-specific membrane antigen is alternatively spliced to produce at least three variants (Fig. 1B), most important of which is PSM', the cDNA of which is identical to PSMA except for a 266-nucleotide region near the 5' end of PSMA cDNA (nucleotides 114–380), which codes for the transmembrane region of the protein. Therefore, PSM' is located in the cytoplasm. Su and co-workers *(10)* used RNAse protection assays to examine the expression of PSMA and PSM' in normal vs benign prostate hyperplasia (BPH) vs prostate cancers. They found increasing expression of PSMA in tumors relative to normal controls and generated a tumor index based on the PSMA : PSM' ratio, which is 9–11 in LNCaP cells, 3–6 in prostatic carcinoma, 0.75–1.6 in BPH, and 0.075–0.45 in normal prostate (Table 1). The enzymatic activity of the alternatively spliced version of PSMA : PSM', has not been undisputedly proven. Evidence in support for the cytoplasmic locations of this form in LNCaP cells has been provided by two groups *(12,13)*. However, Barinka et al. *(14)* could not detect any enzymatic activity in this protein by expressing the recombinant intraellular form of this enzyme. The other two variants of PSMA are PSM-C [with transcription start site same as PSMA, splice donor site same as PSM' (nucleotide 114), different splice acceptor site located within intron 1 of PSMA gene, includes a novel exon 1b, which is identical to PSM'] and PSM-D [same donor site as PSM', but acceptor site includes novel exon 1c, has a new translation start site followed by 42 novel amino acids with a motif ala-ala-tyr-

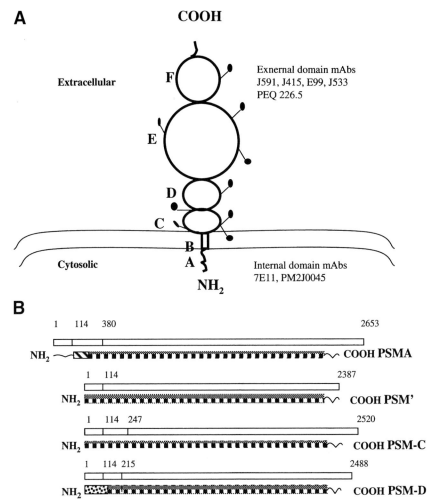

**Fig. 1. (A)** The globular nature of PSMA protein with different domains. Domain A: amino acids 1–19, intracellular, cytoplasmic; domain B: amino acids 20–39, transmembrane; domain C: amino acids 40–144; domain D: amino cells 173–248; domain E: amino acids 275–596; domain F: amino acids 597–756. There are two linker regions between domains C and D (amino acids 145–172) and domains D and E (amino acids 249–274). Domains C, D, E, and F are the extracellular domains. Domain E is the catalytic domain with the zinc-binding and substrate-binding sites. Cellular locations of different epitopes of different PSMA-specific monoclonal antibodies have been shown here. **(B)** Schematic view of the different splice variant of PSMA detected in LNCaP cells. Among the different variants of PSMA, PSM' lacks the intracellular cytoplasmic domain and transmembrane domain, the rest is identical to PSMA. PSM-C, although produced by alternative splicing, has a different splice acceptor site than PSM', encodes a protein identical to PSM'. PSM-D has a unique 42-amino-acid-long domain at the N-terminus and rest is identical to PSM'. The protein sequence is shown by the hatched box. The cDNA sequence of PSMA and its other three variants are shown by the open box. PSMA nucleotide positions are shown according to the Genbank accession number M99487.

ala-cys-thr-gly-cys-leu-ala (found in growth factor cys-knot family of proteins) and rest of the PSMA protein in frame *(1,15)*] (Fig. 1B). The implication of such alternative splice variants in prostate cancer cells is not known at present.

Table 1
Relative Ratio of mRNA and Enzyme Activity of PSMA and PSMA' in Various Tissues

| PSMA/PSMA' | Normal | BPH | PC[a] | LNCaP |
|---|---|---|---|---|
| mRNA ratio | 0.075–0.45 | 0.75–1.6 | 3–6 | 9–11 |
| Enzyme activity/mg of protein | 3.2 | 1.5 | 4.4 | ND[b] |

[a]Prostate cancer.
[b]Not done.
Data from refs. *10* and *11*.

## *1.3. Unique Enzymatic Functions of PSMA*

Prostate-specific membrane antigen is a protein with two unique enzymatic functions, including NAALADase activity (cleaving terminal glutamate from the neuro-dipeptide, *N*-acetyl-aspartyl- glutamate [NAAG] and folate hydrolase activity, which cleaves the terminal glutamates from $\gamma$-linked polyglutamates. NAAG is concentrated in neuronal synapses, whereas folyl-poly-$\gamma$-glutamates are present in dietary components and PSMA protein on the surface of the brush border epithelium of the small intestine enables the generation of folates and subsequent folate uptake. Thus, the question that comes into one's mind is what is a protein like PSMA with such interesting activity profile doing on the surface of prostate cells and why is its expression level enhanced so many-fold in prostate cancer cells? The answer is still unknown, but there are several possible explanations, which we will discuss in this chapter.

The structural similarities between PSMA and other proteins are known. The PSMA gene is highly homologous to the neuropeptidase NAALADase, which releases neuro-transmitter glutamate from neuropeptide NAAG; to human glutamate hydrolase, which is capable of folyl-poly-$\gamma$-glutamate hydrolysis *(16)*; and to I100 (human dipeptidyl peptidase IV), associated with the apical brush border of intestinal epithelial cells *(17,18)*. Human prostate PSMA (FOLH1) and rat NAALADase is classified as GCPII, a member of the M28 peptidase family of metalloproteases *(19)*, with the residues conserved for $Zn^{2+}$ and substrate binding. Human PSMA has about 91% homology to mouse PSMA (folh1) *(20)*. Human, mouse, rat, and porcine folyl-poly-$\gamma$-glutamate carboxypeptidases have 10, 10, 9, and 12 putative glycosylation sites, respectively *(2,21–23)*. PSM' and PSM-like have nine and five potential glycosylation sites, respectively. Mouse, rat, and pig homologs have an additional glycosylation site, which is not present in human forms. Glycosylation of PSMA plays an important role in targeting the protein to the cell membrane, proper protein folding, and enzymatic activity of the protein. Removal of sugar residues partially or completely (enzymatically or by mutagenesis) abolishes the enzyme activity of the protein *(21,24)*. More interestingly, the glycosylation profiles of PSMA obtained from different prostate cancer cell lines were found to be different, leading one to speculate that the different sugar epitopes might play a role in metastasis of prostate cancer. Further work has been carried out in the laboratory to address such a question. Human PSMA has homology to human transferrin receptor. Both are type II glycoproteins and PSMA shares about 54% homology to the transferrin receptor (Tfr) and about 60% with transferrin receptor 2 (Tfr2) *(25)*. The transferrin receptor exists in dimer form because of interstrand sulfhydryl links. PSMA exists in dimeric/monomeric form. A recombinant protein of the extracellular domain of PSMA also exists in readily interconvertible dimer–monomer forms, indicating that the extracellular domain is sufficient for dimerization. PSMA is expressed as a non-

covalent homodimer on the surface of LNCaP cells as well as on the 3T3 cells stably transfected with full-length PSMA (26,27). Like the transferrin receptor, PSMA can undergo
internalization. It is yet to be characterized whether the dimer or monomer can internalize.
It is not understood what induces dimer formation or causes its dissociation to the monomer
form. The difference is important because the dimer (not the monomer) has enzymatic
activity and the dimer (but not monomer) elicited antibodies that efficiently recognized
PSMA-expressing tumor cells.

### 1.3.1. Enzymatic Assays of PSMA

Purification and partial enzymatic characterization of PSMA was established by
Slusher's group (28). The enzyme was detected and partially characterized pharmacologically in multiple prostate cell lines and in prostate tissues of eight mammalian species
(13). First expression and purification of recombinant human GCPII in insect cells using
a baculovirus vector system has been reported by Lodge et al. (29) for production of monoclonal antibodies. There are two assays used for detection of enzymatic activity of this
protein:

1. NAALADase activity, by cleaving Ac-Asp-($^3$H) Glu (30), which is a very sensitive assay,
   enabling one to detect the product at a nanomolar concentration. Recently, another alternative substrate of this enzyme has been identified (14): Ac-Xaa-Met, where Xaa stands
   for Glu, Asp, or Ala, and Met stands for amino acid methionine. Met-containing dipeptides
   are the first examples of substrate without the C-terminal Glu for this enzyme.
2. Folate hydrolase assay, which has been characterized in Heston's laboratory in great detail.
   This assay utilizes methotrexate-di-Glu and methotrexate-tri-Glu as a substrate and subsequent release of glutamate with accumulation of methotrexate at a picomole quantity (31).

## 1.4. Endocytic Function of PSMA

Prostate-specific membrane antigen, like other cell surface receptors, undergoes internalization constitutively, and such spontaneous internalization is enhanced threefold in
a dose-dependent manner by PSMA-specific monoclonal antibody J591 (32). It has been
shown very clearly biochemically (by using biotinylated cell surface PSMA followed by
internalization of the protein), by immunofluorescence analysis or immunoelecton microscopy, that PSMA or the PSMA–antibody complex undergoes internalization through clathrin-coated pits and closely resembles the internalization pathway of transferrin receptor
and finally ends up in the lysosomes. Such constitutive internalization of PSMA might
reflect the recycling of a structural protein or be mediated by binding of a ligand. A detailed
characterization of antibody-mediated PSMA internalization revealed the resemblance
with the epidermal growth factor receptor (EGFR) with its ligand (33). It is well known that
many ligands and their transmembrane receptors are internalized through clathrin-coated
pits (receptor-mediated endocytosis). Formation of antibody–antigen complexes on the
cell surface often results in internalization through a pathway closely resembling the receptor-mediated endocytosis of peptide hormones, growth factors, and natural ligands (34)
(Fig. 2). It can be speculated from these findings that PSMA might have a transport function
for a yet unidentified ligand. A monoclonal antibody such as J591 acts as surrogate ligand-
inducing internalization.

Targeting internalization of receptors through coated pits and their traffic through endo-
cytic compartments are mediated through specific signals or motifs located on the cytoplasmic tail of the receptors. There are two major classes of sorting signal that mediate

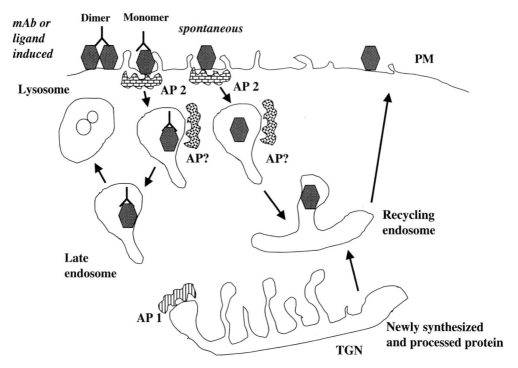

**Fig. 2.** Spontaneous or antibody-induced internalization of PSMA through clathrin-coated pits. The proteins can either recycle through the recycling endosomal compartment (REC) and go to the plasma membrane or they can go to the lysosomes through late endosomes. The cytoplasmic tail of PSMA contains an internalizaton signal, which enables it to internalize into endosomal vesicles. PM, plasma membrane; TGN, trans-Golgi network; AP, adaptor protein.

internalization of membrane proteins from plasma membrane and sort these proteins to endosomes/lysosomes and, finally, to the compartment for peptide loading (*35–37*). These sorting signals are tyrosine-based NPXY and YXXΦ motifs (*37*) and dileucine motif (*36*). Tyrosine motifs are identified in a variety of receptor molecules like the transferrin receptor, low-density lipoprotein receptor, and asialoglycoprotein receptor (*38*). Dileucine (or leucine–isoleucine sequence) motif (Fig. 3A and Color Plate 12 following p. 302) is important for internalization and lysosomal targeting was found in the γ-δ chain of the T-cell receptor, CD4, IFN-γ (*39–41*). Tyrosine-based motifs interact with adaptor complexes AP1, AP2, and AP3 (*42,43*) and dileucine-based motifs bind to the β-subunits of AP1 and AP2; μ-chains of AP1 and AP2 has also been reported to bind to these signals. Apart from this, leucine-based signals of lysosomal protein LIMPII and melanosomal membrane protein tyrosinase have been shown to bind to AP3 (*44*). PSMA has a dileucine motif present at its cytoplasmic tail. Mutation of first leucine (Leu 4) did not change the internalization of monoclonal antibody (mAb) J591; in contrast, conversion of second leucine (Leu 5) resulted in complete loss of internalization indicating that this leucine is important for the internalization (*45*; Ghosh et al., unpublished observation, 2003). This implied that the dileucine motif is responsible for the internalization. However the dileucine motif is generally associated with the basolateral targeting of proteins, and PSMA is found at the apical surface of the cell. In the case of PSMA, the first amino acid methionine located five amino acids upstream of the crucial leucine is involved in the internalization, which makes this signal a unique internalization signal "MXXXL" in PSMA. Amino acid residues adjacent to such motifs have been shown to influence its function. The dileucine signal of CD4 is active when adjacent serine residues are phosphorylated *(46)*. The cytoplasmic tail of PSMA has consensus protein kinase C sequence (Thr 14) and has two other hydroxyl-containing residues (Thr-8, Ser-10), which might serve as phosphorylation acceptor sites. It remains to be seen how mutation of such a residue affects the internalization function of the protein. A detailed mutational analysis has been carried by Rajasekaran's group, which did not have any effect on the internalization function of PSMA. It is known at least in EGFR *(47)* that the dileucine motif and its neighboring residues need to form an amphipathic helix with hydrophilic residues pointing toward one surface and hydrophobic residues pointing toward the other for the interaction with adaptor proteins needed for sorting. The predicted protein structure of the PSMA N-terminal cytoplasmic tail showed that this region (residues $N^3$ to $R^{19}$) has a probability to take up an $\alpha$-helical structure, and the helical wheel projection of this region showed that this helix is an amphipathic $\alpha$-helix with hydrophobic residues projecting toward one surface and hydrophilic residues toward the other (Fig. 3B) *(48)*.

A cytoplasmic leucine-based motif has been shown to be involved in the lysosomal targeting of several membrane proteins *(39,47,49,50)*. PSMA colocalizes with lysosomal marker Lamp1 in LNCaP cells (endogenously express PSMA) or Cos cells expressing transfected PSMA *(45)* or PC3 cells ectopically expressing PSMA (Ghosh et al., unpublished observation), indicating that PSMA is being localized within the lysosome. Furthermore, swapping the MWNLL (the first five amino acids of the PSMA sequence) and MWNLA (fifth leucine has been changed to alanine) to Tac antigen, this group has shown that the wild-type motif could transport the Tac antigen (which is not a lysosome resident) to the lysosome whereas the mutant motif could not, indicating that MXXXL signal in PSMA is, indeed, a lysosomal signal. Knowledge of PSMA's internalization function and regulation can be exploited in cancer therapeutics. A detailed analysis is required to define the putative natural ligand for internalization and what role it plays on the biological function of PSMA. Our lab has shown that substrates and antagonists of the carboxypeptidase function do not alter the rate of internalization, which shows that internalization and enzymatic function are two independent processes. Furthermore, it will be interesting to find out if there is a natural ligand for internalization that could substitute for the mAb in a targeted therapy approach.

## 2. PSMA EXPRESSION IN PROSTATE, BENIGN PROSTATE HYPERPLASIA, AND PROSTATE CANCER

Prostate-specific membrane antigen has been detected in both benign tissue and prostate cancer and is clinically designated as prostate-specific *(2)*. In the past, various methods have been employed to distinguish BPH from among various grades of prostate cancer. By employing *in situ* hybridization, Kawakami et al. *(51)* increased expression of PSMA-specific transcripts in poorly differentiated adenocarcinoma in 15 tumors (from a range of Gleason scores). Similarly, by employing immunohistochemistry analysis with PSMA-specific antibody, Burger et al. *(52)* confirmed that PSMA expression reflects the Gleason score of the tumor with PSMA expression localized in secretary epithelial cells. Bostwick et al. *(53)* has shown intense cytoplasmic immune reactivity for PSMA in every prostate tissue examined. The number of immune-reactive cells increased incrementally from benign epithelium to high-grade prostatic intraepithelial neoplasia (PIN) and prostatic adenocarci-

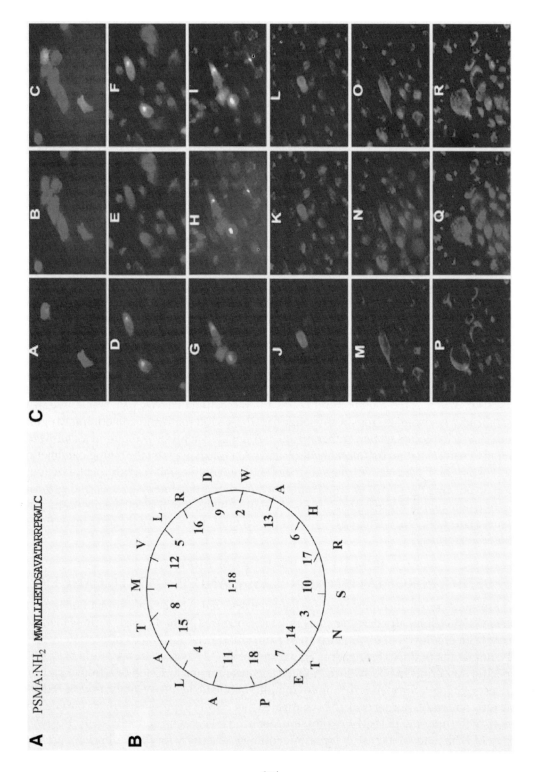

**A** PSMA:NH₂  MWNLLHEIDSAVATARRPRWLC

**B**

**C**

noma. The most extensive and intense staining for PSMA was observed in high-grade carcinoma with immune reactivity in virtually every cell in specimen with Gleason primary pattern 4 or 5 (with greater heterogeneity of staining in primary pattern 3 adenocarcinoma). It has been shown by immunohistochemistry analysis by various other groups that prostate epithelial cells in a large majority of BPH tissues did not express PSMA at a detectable level *(53)*. PSMA enzyme activity (NAALADase) was found to be increased 10-fold in prostate cancer samples as compared to normal prostate and BPH *(11)*. Until now, all reports were on PSMA protein expression in tissue sections. The first report of PSMA as the second most highly expressed gene in prostate cancer (by employing more powerful and advance techniques such as gene-array technology) came from the study of Stamey et al. *(54)*. Molecular profiling of Gleason grade 4/5 cancer (which is the primary cause of failure to cure prostate cancer) was done by taking frozen tissues from nine men with Gleason grade 4/5 cancer and eight men with BPH. Labeled complementary RNA from each of the 17 tissues was applied to HuGene FL probe arrays representing approx 6800 genes. After removing all genes undetectable in BPH and grade 4/5 cancers and transforming the data into a parametric distribution, only those upregulated and downregulated genes were chosen with a $p$ difference in fluorescence between grades 4/5 cancer and BPH of $p < 0.0005$. Further elimination of genes (not expressed in all 8 BPH and 9 grade 4/5

---

**Fig. 3.** *(Opposite page)*    PSMA has a MXXXL motif at its N-terminal cytoplasmic tail, and the first methionine and fifth leucine residues are important for its internalization; the fourth leucine is redundant. PSMA has a dileucine motif at its N-terminal cytoplasmic tail. Dileucine motifs serve as lysosomal targeting signal and usually reside within the cytoplasmic tail of the protein (either N-terminal or C-terminal). **(A)** The peptide sequence N-terminal cytoplasmic sequence is shown here with putative internalization motif (shown in bold). The actual internalization signal of PSMA is the first five amino acids MXXXL. **(B)** The helical wheel projection of the C-terminal tail region (N-terminal 19 amino acid). By using the predict protein program (http://cubic.bioc.columbia.edu/predict-protein), it was found that the N-terminal region contains an α-helical region. Using this sequence, we could make a helical wheel projection by using the site http://www.site.uottawa.ca/~turcotte/resources/Helixwheel and found that one face of the helix contains the hydrophobic residues and the other face of the helix contains the hydrophilic residue, indicating that this region is important for protein–protein interaction. **(C)** Internalization assay of PSMA and its single-leucine and dileucine repeat mutant (L5A and L4AL5A) in PC3 cells. Cover-slip cultures of the PC3 cells expressing PSMA or L5A or L4AL5A have been incubated at 4°C or 37°C with or without J591 for 60 min. The cells were washed and processed for immunofluorescence. The internalized J591 was detected by incubating the cover slips with goat–anti-mouse biotin, followed by streptavidin-FITC; for Lamp1 detection, the cover slips were incubated with polyclonal antibody against Lamp1, followed by detection with goat–anti-rabbit secondary antibody tagged with Texas red. The J591-induced internalization of PSMA and its recycling through endocytic compartment and localization with lysosome has been studied here. Panel A: PC3-PSMA, internalization of J591 at 37°C for 5 min in green; panel B: staining for the lysosomal marker Lamp1 is shown in red; panel C: overlay of A and B showing the colocalization of internalized J591 and Lamp1 in yellow; panel D: J591-induced internalization of PC3-PSMA at 37°C for 60 min shown in green; panel E: staining for Lamp1 shown in red; panel F: overlay of D and E shown in yellow; panel G: PC3-L4A, internalization assay with J591 at 37°C for 60 min shown in green; panel H: staining for the lysosome marker Lamp1 is shown in red; panel I: overlay of G and H; panel J: PC3-L5A, internalization assay with J591 at 37°C for 60 min shown in green; panel K: staining for Lamp1 is shown in red; panel L: the overlay of J and K; panel M: PC3-L4AL5A internalization assay with J591 at 37°C for 60 min shown in green; panel N: staining for Lamp1 is shown in red; panel O: overlay of M and N; panel P: PC3-Ndel19 internalization assay with J591 at 37°C for 60 min shown in green; panel Q: staining for lysosome marker Lamp1 is shown in red; panel R: overlay of P and Q. (*See* Color Plate 12 following p. 302.)

Table 2
Summary of Markers Identified by Array Analysis

| Marker | Genbank Reference no. | Gene Function | Fold Increase in Expression Detected by Arrays* |
|--------|----------------------|---------------|------------------------------------------------|
| δ-Catenin | U96136 | Cell–cell adhesion molecule | 9.5 |
| PSMA | M99487 | Prostate-specific membrane antigen | 4–6 |
| NEK3 | Z29067 | Serine/threonine protein kinase | 5.5 |
| CCK4 | U33635 | Receptor tyrosine kinase | 4.5 |
| TPSP | X87852 | Transmembrane sex protein receptor | 4 |
| PCTK3 | X66362 | Serine/threonine protein kinase | 4 |
| EGR1 | X52541 | Early growth response protein 1-transcription factor | 3.5 |
| PLA2 | M22430 | Phospholipase A2 group IIA-inflammatory response regulator | 3 |

Data from ref. *52*.

tissues) produced a final set of 86 genes, of which 22 were upregulated and 64 were down-regulated. The most upregulated gene found to be Hepsin (a trypsin-like serine protease) and the second most upregulated gene was found to be PSMA *(54)*. Later, Burger et al. *(52)* have shown (by using techniques such as cDNA microarray profiling and real-time reverse transcription–polymerase chain [RT-PCR]) that PSMA is one of the very few markers that could discriminate prostate cancer from BPH, in which cancer cells showed a fourfold to sixfold increase in expression from BPH as detected by arrays (Table 2). There was no overlap between the 17 prostate cancers (of different stages and grades) and 11 BPH samples studied. However in both groups, there were considerable variations among individual samples. Similarly, Zhou et al. *(55)* have shown that δ-catenin (a cell–cell adhesion molecule) was found to be significantly overexpressed in tumors compared to BPH (9.5-fold increase in expression detected by arrays).

## 2.1. Relative Amounts of PSMA/PSM' in Different Tissues

Expression of PSMA and its splice variant PSM' in primary tissues has been analyzed by a number of semiquantitative techniques, including immunohistochemistry, Western blotting, and *in situ* hybridization with specific RNA probes *(10)*. In their studies, Su et al. have shown that PSMA/PSM' expression is highly indicative of disease progression. In primary prostate tumors, PSMA was found to be a dominant transcript, whereas normal and BPH tissues express more PSM' than PSMA. In normal tissues, PSMA/PSM'-specific transcripts were found to be restricted to basal epithelium, with very weak background expression in stromal cells.

## 3. REGULATION OF PSMA EXPRESSION AND ITS IMPLICATION IN PROSTATE CANCER

### 3.1. PSMA–Filamin Interaction

Recently, it has been shown that the cytoplasmic tail of PSMA interacts with the actin-binding protein filamin a (FLNa) *(56)*. PSMA's association with FLNa is necessary for

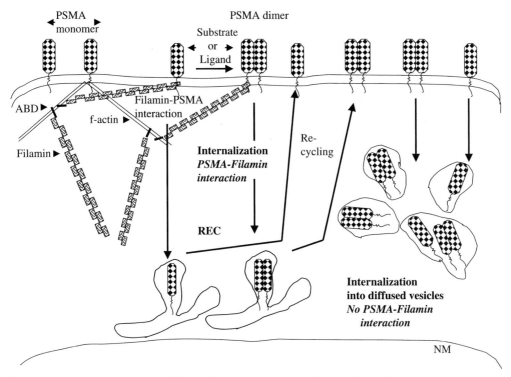

**Fig. 4.** Schematic showing the PSMA–FLNa interaction within the cells and how such an interaction modulates PSMA function. Which form of PSMA undergoes internalization (monomer or dimer form) is not yet known clearly. In the presence of FLNa, PSMA undergoes internalization to the RECs located at the perinuclear region. In the absence of FLNa, PSMA is distributed through the diffused vesicle throughout the cytoplasm. ABD, actin binding domain; REC, recycling endosomal compartment; NM, nuclear membrane.

its localization to the recycling endosomal compartment (REC). In filamin-negative cells, the internalized PSMA accumulates in diffused vesicles throughout the cytoplasm. This distribution can be altered by introducing FLNa in this cell, and the proteins localize into REC. The PSMA–FLNa interaction decreased its rate of internalization by 50%. It could be that linking of PSMA with the actin cytoskeleton by FLNa keeps the proteins attached to the cell membrane and eliminates its ability to bind adaptor proteins, hence the reduction in the internalization rate. A dissociation from FLNa might help in binding of the PSMA cytoplasmic tail with adaptor proteins, which leads to endocytosis. Therefore, FLNa and adaptor proteins could be competing for binding at the same site of PSMA. An internalization motif mutant that could not undergo endocytosis but could bind very strongly to FLNa supported this theory. Figure 4 gives a summary of this event. The importance of phosphorylation of PSMA protein at certain putative phosphorylation sites and its implication on its binding with FLNa remain to be solved.

## 3.2. Regulation of PSMA Expression by PSMA Promoter-Enhancer (Fig. 5)

Prostate-specific membrane antigen has been shown to be increased severalfold in the expression in prostate cancer; its expression is suppressed by androgen. Currently, two regulatory elements controlling PSMA expression have been characterized. The proximal

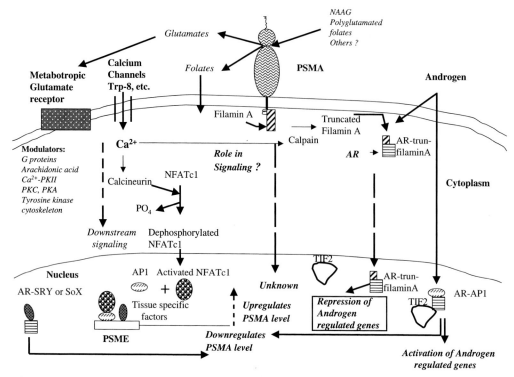

**Fig. 5.** The regulation of PSMA in prostate cancer cells. Negative regulation by androgen receptor and positive regulation by $Ca^{2+}$ is shown. Polyglutamated folates become enzymatically cleaved to deglutamated folates and glutamates. The folates can enter the cells through reduced folate-carrier (RFC) or folate-binding proteins (FBP). The glutamates produced by the PSMA-expressing cells can activate metabotrophic glutamate receptors, which can become activated and alter the resting membrane potential, which causes the efflux of $Cl^-$ ions and influx of $Ca^{2+}$ ions to compensate for the damage of the cells. $Ca^{2+}$ ions can modulate the expression level of PSMA in many ways. Increased $Ca^{2+}$ concentration can activate inactive transcription factor NFATc1 (which is a transcriptional activator of PSMA enhancer [PSME]), or cause activation of calpain, which cleaves FLNa. Truncated FLNa binds to androgen receptor (AR) and localizes to the nucleus and suppresses AR-mediated transactivation. Normally, AR would sequester AP1 or tissue-specific transcription factors (e.g., SRY or SOX), causing inhibition of PSME.

1.2-kb PSMA enhancer (PSME) *(57,58)* (located within the third intron of FOLH1) renders the prostate-specific expression of PSMA. PSME is activated in a prostate-specific manner, negatively regulated by androgen receptor, and its expression is upregulated in prostate cancer. A detailed study showed that proximal 90 bp of PSME contained enhancer element with an AP3 site responsible for elevation of promoter activity of PSME beyond the basal level *(59)*. Furthermore, recent work by this group has shown that $Ca^{2+}$-dependent activation PSME transcription factor NFATc1 isoform binds to AP1. In the presence of the $Ca^{2+}$, NFATc1 protein gets dephosphorylated through $Ca^{2+}$-dependent calcineurin, which drives the translocation of NFAT protein to nucleus and activates the transcription of PSMA (Fig. 4).

Direct repeat regions of PSME harbors nine copies of SRY/SOX sites. SRY, SOX 7, and SOX 18 are reportedly expressed prostate cancer and prostate epithelial cells *(60)*. SRY or SOX might interact with AR-DBD (androgen receptor DNA-binding domain), and as a result, AR sequesters these tissue-specific proteins, causing repression of PSME, which could partially explain the AR-mediated repression of PSME.

$Ca^{2+}$ ions positively regulate PSMA expression. $Ca^{2+}$ influx probably takes place through a CaT-like calcium channel, which is strikingly correlated with the malignancy of prostate cancer as well as PSMA expression *(61)*. How could that start? The possible explanation could involve glutamate receptors. We have observed metabotropic glutamate receptors by gene-array analysis of LNCaP cells (Heston et al., unpublished observation). In prostate cancer cells, such receptors could get activated constitutively by free glutamates (an agonist to such a receptor) released as a byproduct of the folate hydrolase/NAALADase action of PSMA expressed on the cell surface (PSMA level is upregulated many-fold in prostate cancers) and can modulate the function of potassium and calcium channels, which might cause change in resting membrane potential. Such a change in membrane potential could cause oxidative damage to the cells, release of $Cl^-$ ions *(62)*, and continuous influx of $Ca^{2+}$ ions through calcium channels (to compensate for such change in membrane potential).

### 3.3. Gene Therapy Using PSMA Enhancer

Prostate-specific membrane antigen is tissue-specific; that is, PSMA promoter could drive the expression of the luciferase reporter gene specifically in prostate cancer cell lines LNCaP and C4-2, but not other nonprostate cell lines such as breast cancer (MCF-7), lung cancer (H157) and colorectal cancer (HCT8) cell lines in vitro. Expression of suicide gene cytosine deaminase (CD) under the control of the PSMA promoter-enhancer in prostate cancer cells sensitized the cells to 5-fluorocytosine (5-FC) with the inhibitory concentration ($IC_{50}$) <300 µmol/L in vitro. Furthermore, in vivo studies with athymic nude mice carrying transfected to C4-2 cells with the same therapeutic construct (used in in vitro studies) carrying CD gene under regulatory control of the PSMA promoter-enhancer could efficiently sensitize the cells to 5-FC (intraperitoneal injection of 5-FC, 600 mg/kg; twice a day for 3 wk). All C4-2 cell tumors expressing the therapeutic construct were killed by 5-FC, showing in vivo utility of the PSMA promoter/enhancer in a gene therapy situation targeting prostate cancer *(63)*.

## 4. CLINICAL TRIALS OF PROSTATE CANCER USING HuJ591

Prostate Cancer represents an excellent target, especially for monoclonal antibody-based therapy for the following reasons *(64)*:

1. The prostate is a nonessential organ and its destruction will not harm the host, and the identification of tissue-specific antigens for antibody development is easier than elusive tumor-specific antigens.
2. The sites of prostate metastasis being lymph nodes and bone are sites that receive high levels of circulating antibodies.
3. Metastases are typically of small volume, allowing ready access to therapy, and are identified early following primary therapy by elevation in serum prostate-specific antigen (PSA).
4. The PSA serum marker provides a means to monitor therapeutic response.
5. Monoclonal antibodies (mAbs) can mediate antitumor effect by targeting radionuclides, and prostate cancer is relatively radiosensitive.
6. Patients at high risk for subsequent failure from primary therapy can be readily predicted, enabling initiation of therapy while the tumor burden is minimal.

The tissue-specific protein PSMA is an excellent target for imaging and therapy because it is a cell surface protein that presents a large extracellular target and it is expressed at levels that are about a thousand-fold greater than the minimal expression seen in other tissues such as the kidney, liver, proximal small intestine, and salivary gland. Some minimal expression is also observed in the brain, but most agents and especially antibodies do not penetrate the brain because of the blood–brain barrier. To establish PSMA as a potential in vivo target, imaging trials were done with 7E11/CYT 356 *(65,66)* marketed as capromab pentetide (Prostascint; Cytogen Corp, Princeton, NJ). Capromab is the only prostate cancer imaging agent approved by the Food and Drug Administration (FDA), but it has had problems in terms of specificity and sensitivity. The poor quality of the initial antibody was detected because it recognizes an internal epitope of the protein and is binding to areas of tumor necrosis, which is less likely to be found in areas at metastatic sites in the bone *(67)*. Bander's group at Cornell Weil School of Medicine in New York developed monoclonal antibodies against the external domain of PSMA *(32,67)*, namely J591, J415, J533, and E99. Others have developed antibodies as well, such as PEQ226.5 by Hybritech Inc. *(11)*. Among these antibodies, J591 was chosen for clinical development and has been extensively studied in clinical studies *(68–70)*. A major limitation of using a mouse mAb in patients is the development of human anti-mouse antibody (HAMA) response, which prevents repetitive dosing. Therefore, second-generation antibodies such as the humanized version of the J591 was developed by Bander's group based on a technology developed by Biovation Ltd (Aberdeen, UK) *(71)*. Humanized J591 has been used in clinical trials and has demonstrated an ability to image all sites of metastasis, especially bones with nearly 100% specificity and sensitivity *(72)*. Other nonprostate sites of minimal expression are not imaged. Other companies are also developing second-generation antibodies such as the Cytogen/ Progenics joint venture, developing fully human antibodies to the external domain of PSMA. The results of these different groups using these second-generation antibodies are very encouraging and are demonstrating therapeutic activity in delivering radionuclides and cytotoxic agents, resulting in therapeutic responses in both preclinical and early clinical trials *(73)*. The most notable ones are the following.

### 4.1. Phase I Trial of HuJ591

The objectives of this trial were to define the toxicity and maximum tolerated dose of HuJ591, to define the pharmacokinetics of HuJ591, and to determine the incidence of developing a human anti-human antibody (HAHA) response to HuJ591. The mAb was trace labeled with "Indium ($^{111}$In)" using a DOTA chelate. DOTA can be a molecular cage and holds $^{111}$In radiometal.

### 4.2. Phase II Trial of HuJ591 in Combination With Low-Dose Interleukin-2

Interleukin (IL)-2 is a useful agent because it can be an immune stimulant, specifically cancer immunotherapy. IL-2 functions to augment the reticuloendothelial system to recognize antigen–antibody complexes by its effects on natural killer (NK) cells and macrophages. By stimulating NK cells to release interferon-$\gamma$, granulocyte–macrophage colony-stimulating factor, and tumor necrosis factor-$\alpha$, these cytokines will increase the cell surface density of Fc receptors as well as the phagocytic capacities of these cells, thereby enhancing the effector arms of humoral and cellular immune responses. Based on this rationale, a phase II trial of mAb J591 in combination with a daily low dose of subcutaneous IL-2 was initiated. Patients received daily a low-dose subcutaneous rIL-2 ($1.2 \times 10^6$ IU/mL daily) continuously beginning on d 1. Following 3 wk of IL-2, patients received 25 mg/m$^2$ HuJ591 for 3 consecutive weeks. IL-2 was continued for 2 additional weeks for a total of 8 wk (one cycle). Patients who responded to therapy or had stable disease were eligible for additional cycles of therapy. Two studies indicated that weekly-administered HuJ591 was well tolerated, specifically targeted prostate cancer, and appeared to result in PSA stabilization in some patients.

### 4.3. Phase I Trial of Radiolabeled HuJ591

Based on the success of mAbs in targeting radiation therapies directly to tumor cells in the malignancies, two phase I clinical trials were initiated in patients with hormone refractory prostate cancer using β-emitting radiometals $^{90}$Y and $^{177}$Lu linked to HuJ591 via a DOTA chelate.

### 4.4. Clinical Trials of the Solid Tumor Malignancies

This study is based on the fact that PSMA is expressed in the neovasculature of numerous solid tumors. However, PSMA is not expressed by normal vascular endothelium in benign tissues or neoplastic epithelial cells of nonprostate malignancies. It has been demonstrated by immunohistochemistry using CD34 immunostaining, by RT-PCR, and by *in situ* hybridization, showing mRNA transcripts for PSMA in multiple nonprostate solid tumor malignancies. A phase I dose escalation trial of $^{111}$I-labeled mAb HuJ591 was initiated *(73)* and patients entering the study had a variety of solid tumors, including renal, bladder, colon, pancreatic, breast, and lung. Patients with these tumors were similar to those with prostate cancer in that they tolerated mAb HuJ591 well, with no development of HAHA.

## 5. ROLE OF FOLATE HYDROLASE IN PROSTATE CANCER

Folic acid is integral to the various metabolic processes within the body involving one-carbon transfers in DNA synthesis, DNA methylation, and formation of methionine which when decarboxylated is used in polyamine synthesis *(74,75)*. Our initial thinking was that PSM', the alternative spliced form of PSMA, might put the prostate at risk of folate deficiency because as a folate hydrolase, it would allow for deglutamation of the poly-γ-glutamated folates, which are the intracellular storage form of folates. Given that PSM' is less glycosylated being an intracellular protein, we now consider it likely that PSM' does not have folate hydrolase activity. At present, the probable function of the intracellular form PSM' is not known. Outside of the cell, PSMA does bind and hydrolyze poly-γ-glutamated folate. However, serum contains folate in a form that is not poly-γ-glutamated and is ready for transport into tissues. In the normal prostate, PSMA is at the apical surface; it is possible that it is exposed to a glutamated form of folate at this surface in the prostate cells. In cancers, it is not uncommon to have dead and dying cells in the tumor. Because these cells would release their stored folate as poly-γ-glutamated folate, it is possible that PSMA enables cells to capture this folate by removing the γ-linked glutamates, thus freeing folate, which then can be taken into the cell by folate-binding proteins or folate carrier systems. Tumors grow under adverse conditions such as increased interstitial pressure inside tumors because they lack lymphatics, and the cell death that occurs because of hypoxia. This may provide a rationale for why PMSA is expressed on tumor neovasculature in that it may be involved in helping to capture the poly-γ-glutamated folates being released from dead and dying cells. Also, because PSMA does internalize, it might be that it has some transport property for poly-γ-glutamated folates that is as yet not understood.

## REFERENCES

1. O'Keefe DS, Bachich D, Heston WDW. Prostate specific membrane antigen. In: Chung L, Issacs, WB, Simons JW, eds. Prostate cancer, biology, genetics and the new therapeutics. Totowa, NJ: Humana, 2001: 307–326.
2. Israeli RS, Powell CT, Fair WR, Heston WD. Molecular cloning of a complementary DNA encoding a prostate-specific membrane antigen. Cancer Res 1993; 53:227–230.
3. Wright GL Jr, Grob BM, Haley C, et al. Upregulation of prostate-specific membrane antigen after androgen-deprivation therapy. Urology 1996; 48:326–334.
4. Silver DA, Pellicer I, Fair WR, Heston WD, Cordon-Cardo C. Prostate-specific membrane antigen expression in normal and malignant human tissues. Clin Cancer Res 1997; 3:81–85.
5. Gong MC, Chang SS, Sadelain M, Bander NH, Heston WD. Prostate-specific membrane antigen (PSMA)-specific monoclonal antibodies in the treatment of prostate and other cancers. Cancer Metastasis Rev 1999; 18:483–490.
6. Leek J, Lench N, Maraj B, et al. Prostate-specific membrane antigen: evidence for the existence of a second related human gene. Br J Cancer 1995; 72:583–588.
7. O'Keefe DS, Su SL, Bacich DJ, et al. Mapping, genomic organization and promoter analysis of the human prostate-specific membrane antigen gene. Biochim Biophys Acta 1998; 1443:113–127.
8. Rinker-Schaeffer CW, Hawkins AL, Su SL, et al. Localization and physical mapping of the prostate-specific membrane antigen (PSM) gene to human chromosome 11. Genomics 1995; 30:105–108.
9. O'Keefe DS, Bacich DJ, Heston WD. Comparative analysis of prostate-specific membrane antigen (PSMA) versus a prostate-specific membrane antigen-like gene. Prostate 2004; 58:200–210.
10. Su SL, Huang IP, Fair WR, Powell CT, Heston WD. Alternatively spliced variants of prostate-specific membrane antigen RNA: ratio of expression as a potential measurement of progression. Cancer Res 1995; 55:1441–1443.
11. Lapidus RG, Tiffany CW, Isaacs JT, Slusher BS. Prostate-specific membrane antigen (PSMA) enzyme activity is elevated in prostate cancer cells. Prostate 2000; 45:350–354.
12. Grauer LS, Lawler KD, Marignac JL, Kumar A, Goel AS, Wolfert RL. Identification, purification, and subcellular localization of prostate-specific membrane antigen PSM' protein in the LNCaP prostatic carcinoma cell line. Cancer Res 1998; 58:4787–4789.
13. Tiffany CW, Lapidus RG, Merion A, Calvin DC, Slusher BS. Characterization of the enzymatic activity of PSM: comparison with brain NAALADase. Prostate 1999; 39:28–35.
14. Barinka C, Rinnova M, Sacha P, et al. Substrate specificity, inhibition and enzymological analysis of recombinant human glutamate carboxypeptidase II. J Neurochem 2002; 80:477–487.
15. Schmittgen TD, Teske S, Vessella RL, True LD, Zakrajsek BA. Expression of prostate specific membrane antigen and three alternatively spliced variants of PSMA in prostate cancer patients. Int J Cancer 2003; 107:323–329.
16. Yao R, Schneider E, Ryan TJ, Galivan J. Human gamma-glutamyl hydrolase: cloning and characterization of the enzyme expressed in vitro. Proc Natl Acad Sci USA 1996; 93:10,134–10,138.
17. Shneider BL, Thevananther S, Moyer MS, et al. Cloning and characterization of a novel peptidase from rat and human ileum. J Biol Chem 1997; 272:31,006–31,015.
18. Darmoul D, Lacasa M, Baricault L, et al. Dipeptidyl peptidase IV (CD 26) gene expression in enterocyte-like colon cancer cell lines HT-29 and Caco-2. Cloning of the complete human coding sequence and changes of dipeptidyl peptidase IV mRNA levels during cell differentiation. J Biol Chem 1992; 267: 4824–4833.
19. Rawlings ND, Barrett AJ. Structure of membrane glutamate carboxypeptidase. Biochim Biophys Acta 1997; 1339:247–252.
20. Bacich DJ, Pinto JT, Tong WP, Heston WD. Cloning, expression, genomic localization, and enzymatic activities of the mouse homolog of prostate-specific membrane antigen/NAALADase/folate hydrolase. Mamm Genome 2001; 12:117–123.
21. Ghosh A, Heston WD. Role of carbohydrate moieties on folate hydrolase activity of prostate specific membrane antigen. Am Assoc Cancer Res 2003a.

22. Bzdega T, Turi T, Wroblewska B, et al. Molecular cloning of a peptidase against *N*-acetylaspartylgluta-mate from a rat hippocampal cDNA library. J Neurochem 1997; 69:2270–2277.

23. Halsted CH, Ling EH, Luthi-Carter R, Villanueva JA, Gardner JM, Coyle JT. Folylpoly-gamma-glu-tamate carboxypeptidase from pig jejunum. Molecular characterization and relation to glutamate carboxy-peptidase II. J Biol Chem 1998; 273:20,417–20,424.

24. Ghosh A, Heston WD. Role of carbohydrate residues on the folate hydrolase activity of the prostate spe-cific membrane antigen. Prostate 2003; 57(2):140–151.

25. Kawabata H, Yang R, Hirama T, et al. Molecular cloning of transferrin receptor 2. A new member of the transferrin receptor-like family. J Biol Chem 1999; 274:20,826–20,832.

26. Schulke N, Varlamova OA, Donovan GP, et al. The homodimer of prostate-specific membrane antigen is a functional target for cancer therapy. Proc Natl Acad Sci USA 2003; 100:12,590–12,595.

27. Schulke N, Donovan, GP, Morrissey, DM, et al. Human prostate specific membrane antigen (PSMA) is naturally expressed as a non-covalent dimer. In: AACR Preceedings, new discoveries in prostate cancer biology and treatment. 2001:A47.

28. Slusher BS, Robinson MB, Tsai G, Simmons ML, Richards SS, Coyle JT. Rat brain *N*-acetylated alpha-linked acidic dipeptidase activity. Purification and immunologic characterization. J Biol Chem 1990; 265:21,297–21,301.

29. Lodge PA, Childs RA, Monahan SJ, et al. Expression and purification of prostate-specific membrane antigen in the baculovirus expression system and recognition by prostate-specific membrane antigen-specific T cells. J Immunother 1999; 22:346–355.

30. Robinson MB, Blakely RD, Couto R, Coyle JT. Hydrolysis of the brain dipeptide *N*-acetyl-L-aspartyl-L-glutamate. Identification and characterization of a novel *N*-acetylated alpha-linked acidic dipeptidase activity from rat brain. J Biol Chem 1987; 262:14,498–14,506.

31. Pinto JT, Suffoletto BP, Berzin TM, et al. Prostate-specific membrane antigen: a novel folate hydrolase in human prostatic carcinoma cells. Clin Cancer Res 1996; 2:1445–1451.

32. Liu H, Rajasekaran AK, Moy P, et al. Constitutive and antibody-induced internalization of prostate-spe-cific membrane antigen. Cancer Res 1998; 58:4055–4060.

33. Haigler HT. Receptor-mediated endocytosis of epidermal growth factor. Methods Enzymol 1983; 98: 283–290.

34. Pastan IH, Willingham MC. Receptor-mediated endocytosis of hormones in cultured cells. Annu Rev Physiol 1981; 43:239–250.

35. Nordeng TW, Gorvel JP, Bakke O. Intracellular transport of molecules engaged in the presentation of exogenous antigens. Curr Topics Microbiol Immunol 1998; 232:179–215.

36. Sandoval IV, Bakke O. Targeting of membrane proteins to endosomes and lysosomes. Trends Cell Biol 1994; 4:292–297.

37. Marks MS, Ohno H, Kirchhausen T, Bonifacino JS. Protein sorting by tyrosine-based signals: adapting to the Ys and wherefores. Trends Cell Biol 1997; 7:124–128.

38. Trowbridge IS, Collawn JF, Hopkins CR. Signal-dependent membrane protein trafficking in the endo-cytic pathway. Annu Rev Cell Biol 1993; 9:129–161.

39. Letourneur F, Klausner RD. A novel di-leucine motif and a tyrosine-based motif independently mediate lysosomal targeting and endocytosis of CD3 chains. Cell 1992; 69:1143–1157.

40. Shin J, Dunbrack RL Jr, Lee S, Strominger JL. Signals for retention of transmembrane proteins in the endo-plasmic reticulum studied with CD4 truncation mutants. Proc Natl Acad Sci USA 1991; 88:1918–1922.

41. Farrar MA, Schreiber RD. The molecular cell biology of interferon-gamma and its receptor. Annu Rev Immunol 1993; 11:571–611.

42. Hirst J, Robinson MS. Clathrin and adaptors. Biochim Biophys Acta 1998; 1404:173–193.

43. Traub LM, Kornfeld S. The trans-Golgi network: a late secretory sorting station. Curr Opin Cell Biol 1997; 9:527–533.

44. Honing S, Sandoval IV, von Figura K. A di-leucine-based motif in the cytoplasmic tail of LIMP-II and tyrosinase mediates selective binding of AP-3. EMBO J 1998; 17:1304–1314.

45. Rajasekaran S, Anilkumar, G, Oshima E, et al. A novel cytoplasmic tail MXXXL motif mediates the internalization and lysosomal targeting of prostate specific membrane antigen. Mol Biol Cell 2003; 14: 4835–4845.

46. Pitcher C, Honing S, Fingerhut A, Bowers K, Marsh M. Cluster of differentiation antigen 4 (CD4) endo-cytosis and adaptor complex binding require activation of the CD4 endocytosis signal by serine phosphory-lation. Mol Biol Cell 1999; 10:677–691.

47. Kil SJ, Hobert M, Carlin C. A leucine-based determinant in the epidermal growth factor receptor juxta-membrane domain is required for the efficient transport of ligand-receptor complexes to lysosomes. J Biol Chem 1999; 274:3141–3150.

48. Ghosh A, Heston WD. Tumor target prostate specific membrane antigen (PSMA) and its regulation in prostate cancer. J Cell Biochem 2004; 91:528–539.

49. Haft CR, Klausner RD, Taylor SI. Involvement of dileucine motifs in the internalization and degradation of the insulin receptor. J Biol Chem 1994; 269:26,286–26,294.

50. Dittrich E, Haft CR, Muys L, Heinrich PC, Graeve L. A di-leucine motif and an upstream serine in the interleukin-6 (IL-6) signal transducer gp130 mediate ligand-induced endocytosis and down-regulation of the IL-6 receptor. J Biol Chem 1996; 271:5487–5494.

51. Kawakami M, Nakayama J. Enhanced expression of prostate-specific membrane antigen gene in prostate cancer as revealed by in situ hybridization. Cancer Res 1997; 57:2321–2324.

52. Burger MJ, Tebay MA, Keith PA, et al. Expression analysis of delta-catenin and prostate-specific membrane antigen: their potential as diagnostic markers for prostate cancer. Int J Cancer 2002; 100:228–237.

53. Bostwick DG, Pacelli A, Blute M, Roche P, Murphy GP. Prostate specific membrane antigen expression in prostatic intraepithelial neoplasia and adenocarcinoma: a study of 184 cases. Cancer 1998; 82: 2256–2261.

54. Stamey TA, Warrington JA, Caldwell MC, et al. Molecular genetic profiling of Gleason grade 4/5 prostate cancers compared to benign prostatic hyperplasia. J Urol 2001; 166:2171–2177.

55. Zhou J, Liyanage U, Medina M, et al. Presenilin 1 interaction in the brain with a novel member of the Armadillo family. Neuroreport 1997; 8:2085–2090.

56. Anilkumar G, Rajasekaran SA, Wang S, Hankinson O, Bander NH, Rajasekaran AK. Prostate-specific membrane antigen association with filamin A modulates its internalization and NAALADase activity. Cancer Res 2003; 63:2645–2648.

57. O'Keefe DS, Uchida A, Bacich DJ, et al. Prostate-specific suicide gene therapy using the prostate-specific membrane antigen promoter and enhancer. Prostate 2000; 45:149–157.

58. Watt F, Martorana A, Brookes DE, et al. A tissue-specific enhancer of the prostate-specific membrane antigen gene, FOLH1. Genomics 2001; 73:243–254.

59. Lee SJ, Kim HS, Yu R, et al. Novel prostate-specific promoter derived from PSA and PSMA enhancers. Mol Ther 2002; 6:415–421.

60. Takash W, Canizares J, Bonneaud N, et al. SOX7 transcription factor: sequence, chromosomal localisation, expression, transactivation and interference with Wnt signalling. Nucleic Acids Res 2001; 29: 4274–4283.

61. Wissenbach U, Niemeyer BA, Fixemer T, et al. Expression of CaT-like, a novel calcium-selective channel, correlates with the malignancy of prostate cancer. J Biol Chem 2001; 276:19,461–19,468.

62. Shuba YM, Prevarskaya N, Lemonnier L, et al. Volume-regulated chloride conductance in the LNCaP human prostate cancer cell line. Am J Physiol Cell Physiol 2000; 279:C1144–C1154.

63. Uchida A, O'Keefe DS, Bacich DJ, Molloy PL, Heston WD. In vivo suicide gene therapy model using a newly discovered prostate-specific membrane antigen promoter/enhancer: a potential alternative approach to androgen deprivation therapy. Urology 2001; 58:132–139.

64. Bander NH, Nanus DM, Milowsky MI, Kostakoglu L, Vallabahajosula S, Goldsmith SJ. Targeted systemic therapy of prostate cancer with a monoclonal antibody to prostate-specific membrane antigen. Semin Oncol 2003; 30:667–676.

65. Kahn D, Williams RD, Manyak MJ, et al. [111]Indium–capromab pendetide in the evaluation of patients with residual or recurrent prostate cancer after radical prostatectomy. The ProstaScint Study Group. J Urol 1998; 159:2041–2046; discussion 2046–2047.

66. Kahn D, Williams RD, Haseman MK, Reed NL, Miller SJ, Gerstbrein J. Radioimmunoscintigraphy with In-111-labeled capromab pendetide predicts prostate cancer response to salvage radiotherapy after failed radical prostatectomy. J Clin Oncol 1998b; 16:284–289.

67. Liu H, Moy P, Kim S, et al. Monoclonal antibodies to the extracellular domain of prostate-specific membrane antigen also react with tumor vascular endothelium. Cancer Res 1997; 57:3629–3634.

68. McDevitt MR, Barendswaard E, Ma D, et al. An alpha-particle emitting antibody ([213Bi]J591) for radioimmunotherapy of prostate cancer. Cancer Res 2000; 60:6095–6100.

69. Smith-Jones PM, Vallabahajosula S, Goldsmith SJ, et al. In vitro characterization of radiolabeled monoclonal antibodies specific for the extracellular domain of prostate-specific membrane antigen. Cancer Res 2000; 60:5237–5243.

70. Smith-Jones PM, Vallabhajosula S, Navarro V, Bastidas D, Goldsmith SJ, Bander NH. Radiolabeled mono-clonal antibodies specific to the extracellular domain of prostate-specific membrane antigen: pre-clinical studies in nude mice bearing LNCaP human prostate tumor. J Nucl Med 2003; 44:610–617.
71. Hamilton AA, Manuel DM, Grundy JE, et al. A humanized antibody against human cytomegalovirus (CMV) gpUL75 (gH) for prophylaxis or treatment of CMV infections. J Infect Dis 1997; 176:59–68.
72. Bander NH, Trabulsi EJ, Kostakoglu L, et al. Targeting metastatic prostate cancer with radiolabeled mono-clonal antibody J591 to the extracellular domain of prostate specific membrane antigen. J Urol 2003; 170:1717–1721.
73. Nanus DM, Milowsky MI, Kostakoglu L, et al. Clinical use of monoclonal antibody HuJ591 therapy: targeting prostate specific membrane antigen. J Urol 2003; 170:S84–S88; discussion S88–S89.
74. Eto I, Krumdieck CL. Role of vitamin B12 and folate deficiencies in carcinogenesis. Adv Exp Med Biol 1986; 206:313–330.
75. Jennings E. Folic acid as a cancer-preventing agent. Med Hypotheses 1995; 45:297–303.

# 39

# Development of a Radiolabeled Monoclonal Antibody to Prostate-Specific Membrane Antigen

*Stanley J. Goldsmith, MD,*
*Shankar Vallabhajosula, PhD,*
*Matthew I. Milowsky, MD,*
*David M. Nanus, MD, Lale Kostakoglu, MD,*
*and Neil H. Bander, MD*

## CONTENTS

## SUMMARY

Despite advances in the diagnosis and therapy of prostate carcinoma, it remains a serious medical problem accounting for a large number of malignancies in men each year. Although earlier detection is now possible, many patients develop advanced metastatic disease even when there is no evidence of spread at the time of initial diagnosis and treatment. These metastatic sites could initially be controlled by hormonal therapy but ultimately become resistant and the disease enters an aggressive stage for which there is currently no satisfactory therapy. In response to this perceived need, monoclonal antibodies have been considered a direct biological modifier of the disease and a vehicle to deliver radioactive metals and other cytotoxic agents to disseminated tumor sites. J591 is a monoclonal antibody that recognizes the internal portion of PSMA, a prostate-specific membrane antigen that is regularly expressed, almost exclusively, on prostate cancer tissue. The antibody has been "humanized" to reduce immune responses to it and labeled with radioactivity. Gamma-ray-emitting labeled forms of this antibody have

From: *Cancer Drug Discovery and Development: The Oncogenomics Handbook*
Edited by: W. J. LaRochelle and R. A. Shimkets © Humana Press Inc., Totowa, NJ

demonstrated a high degree of binding and β-emitting labeled forms have demonstrated antitumor effects in animal models. Several of the radiolabeled forms are undergoing clinical trials in humans.

**Key Words:** Prostate cancer; monoclonal antibodies; PSMA; Y-90 [yttrium-90]; Lu-177 [lutetium-177].

## 1. INTRODUCTION

In 2004, prostate cancer accounted for approx 33% (230,000) of the new cases of cancer in men in the United States and approx 10% (29,900) of the deaths from cancer in men *(1)*. Of the newly diagnosed cases of prostate cancer, approx 25% have evidence of regional or distant disease at the time of diagnosis *(2)*. During most of the last 60 yr, this disease was managed with hormonal therapy, a treatment to which most prostate cancers initially respond, but this treatment is not curative. Currently, in patients with disease limited to the prostate, initial treatment includes surgery, conformal external beam radiotherapy, and brachytherapy with radioactive seed implantation *(3)*. Of patients who undergo definitive therapy for clinically localized prostate cancer, 30–50% develop systemic disease *(4)*.

The introduction of the serum prostate-specific antigen (PSA) assay has made possible earlier detection and diagnosis of prostate cancer, but treatment still needs to be improved in order to prolong survival. During recent years, tumor-specific antibodies have been developed in an effort to treat patients with disseminated prostate cancer that has become resistant to hormonal therapy. These monoclonal antibodies (mAbs) have direct antitumor effects, including antibody-dependent cellular toxicity and complement fixation that make them potentially useful therapeutic agents. In addition, mAbs can be used to deliver cytotoxins or radionuclides directly to tumor tissue.

## 2. SUITABILITY OF PROSTATE CANCER AS TARGET FOR mAb-BASED THERAPY

Prostate cancer is ideally suited as a target for mAb-based therapy for several reasons *(5)*: (1) Organ- or tissue-specific antigens of this nonessential organ, rather than cancer-specific antigens, can be targeted; (2) bone marrow and lymph nodes, the most frequent sites of prostate cancer metastases, have been demonstrated to be responsive to mAb therapies in other tumor types; (3) prostate cancer is relatively radiosensitive and is, therefore, likely to be a good target for radionuclide-bearing mAbs; (4) the typically small volume of prostate cancer metastases allow ready antibody penetration and access to antigen; (5) relapse and/or metastatic disease is readily detected early by using the serum PSA assay before clinical manifestations become evident and while tumors are still small and can be readily targeted by mAbs; (6) patients at high risk can be predicted by clinically validated measures before PSA failure, and mAb therapy can be initiated in these patients while the tumor burden is still small; and (7) the potential therapeutic efficacy of early clinical trials with mAbs can be rapidly evaluated by a surrogate marker such as PSA.

## 3. PROSTATE-SPECIFIC MEMBRANE ANTIGEN

Just as prostate cancer seems to be an ideal target for mAb therapy in general, prostate-specific membrane antigen (PSMA), the most well-studied, highly restricted prostate cell surface antigen *(6–11)*, seems to be an ideal specific cellular target because it is expressed by all prostate cancers *(8,9,12–14)*. It is an integral type II cell surface transmembrane

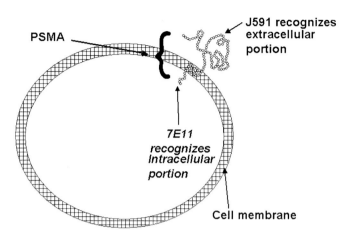

**Fig. 1.** Schematic representation of PSMA demonstrating extracellular, transmembrane, and intracellular portions. J591 recognizes the extracellular portion of the antigen molecule, whereas 7E11 recognizes the intracellular portion. In viable cells, the extracellular epitope is more readily exposed to circulating antibodies. After binding, the J591 and extracellular epitope are internalized.

glycoprotein (Fig. 1) *(15,16)*, and its level of expression is increased with increased tumor dedifferentiation *(9,13,17)*, and in metastatic and hormone-refractory cancers *(8,9,13,14, 17,18)*. In addition to expression by prostate cells, it can be expressed also by nonprostate tissues such as small intestine, proximal renal tubules, and salivary glands *(10)*, albeit at levels 100- to 1000-fold less than in prostate tissue *(11)*. PSMA expression was also found on the vascular endothelium of solid tumors and sarcomas, but not of normal tissues *(8, 10,13,17–22)*. PSMA, therefore, represents a potential target for antiangiogenic therapies.

## 4. DEVELOPMENT OF PSMA-SPECIFIC mAbs

The first PSMA-specific mAb to be developed was 7E11-C5.3 *(6)*, which was later commercialized and used as an imaging agent (ProstaScint®; Cytogen Corporation). The finding that 7E11 bound to an epitope of PSMA located on the inner cytoplasmic surface of the cell *(23,24)* explains the observation that 7E11 binds to fixed cells but not intact cells, as well as the observation that 7E11 does not detect bone marrow metastases. Necrotic cells expose the intracellular components and permit 7E11 binding. Because bone marrow metastases tend to be well vascularized, few if any cells are necrotic and, hence, the intracellular cytosolic domain of PSMA is not exposed.

Subsequently, Liu et al. developed four murine (mu) mAbs that bind to the extracellular domain of PSMA *(19)*: muJ591 (IgG1), muJ415 (IgG1), muJ533 (IgG1), and muE99 (IgG3). These four mAbs bind to approx $1.0–1.3 \times 10^6$ PSMA sites per permeabilized LNCaP cell and $0.6–0.8 \times 10^6$ PSMA sites per viable LNCaP cell. Two epitopes were identified on the extracellular domain of PSMA; muJ591, muJ533, and muE99 bound to one of the epitopes and muJ415 bound to the other. muJ591 and muJ415 bound to viable cultured LNCaP (PSMA-positive) prostate cancer cells with high affinity ($K_d = 1.83 \pm 1.21$ nmol/L and $K_d = 1.76 \pm 0.69$ nmol/L, respectively) *(25)*. After binding, the PSMA–antibody complexes are rapidly internalized *(26)*, increasing the potential utility of PSMA as a target for the delivery of cytotoxins or mAb-conjugated isotopes that would then be sequestered intracellularly.

Most mAbs are prepared from murine hybridoma cells, but repeated dosing of murine mAbs in patients might elicit the formation of human anti-mouse antibodies (HAMA), a response that, even when subclinical, alters the pharmacokinetics of subsequently injected antibody and severely reduces its therapeutic potential. Reactions to HAMA binding of the administered antibody could lead to a severe allergic reaction with its associated sequelae *(3)*. To prevent the formation of HAMA, murine mAbs have been "humanized"; that is, they have been rendered nonimmunogenic by re-engineering the molecule. A large portion of the murine molecular background is replaced by an equivalent human IgG sequence without disturbing the immunorecognition component initially encoded by the murine hybridoma cells.

Accordingly, muJ591 was humanized and the so-called huJ591 was prepared using a process developed by Biovation, Ltd. (Aberdeen, UK) *(27)*. Subsequently, the humanized antibody was covalently linked to a chelating agent, 1,4,7,10-tetraazacyclododecane-*N, N',N'',N'''*-tetra-acetic acid (DOTA). An average of six DOTA molecules can be attached to humanized J591 without apparent loss of immunoreactivity. A variety of radiometals can be linked to the mAb. These include $^{111}$In, a γ-emitter used for dosimetry and as an imaging agent for radioimmunoscintigraphy, $^{90}$Y, a high-energy pure β-emitter that cannot be imaged by a gamma camera but is useful for its therapeutic potential, and $^{177}$Lu, a β-emitter that also emits a γ-ray and thus can be used as an imaging agent to confirm and quantify distribution as well as a therapeutic agent. These various radiometals yield specific activities of 280 MBq $^{111}$In/mg DOTA-J591 and 360 MBq $^{90}$Y/mg DOTA-J591 *(25)*. $^{111}$In-DOTA-J591 demonstrated high cellular retention of radioactivity, with a biphasic release of radioactivity into the medium: 5–10% of the injected dose had an apparent half-life of 1 h and the remaining 90–95% of the radioactivity had an apparent half-life of 520 h *(25)*. The biodistribution of the radiolabeled mAbs injected into patients is affected by the total number of antibody molecules in the injectate. Accordingly, initial trials in humans were performed at varying total protein doses to determine the optimal amount of carrier antibody to administer in order to maximize tumor dose and minimize normal organ, particularly the liver, uptake *(28)*.

The rate of blood clearance of $^{111}$In-DOTA-muJ591 in nude mice bearing LNCaP tumors indicated that the plasma half-life of muJ591 is 2.3 d *(29)*, which is shorter than the retention time of $^{111}$In-DOTA-muJ591 in the tumor in which it becomes trapped. In other studies of nude mice-bearing LNCaP tumors, administration of 5.5–7.4 MBq of $^{90}$Y/mg DOTA-huJ591 and 7.4–11.1 MBq of $^{177}$Lu/DOTA-huJ591 resulted in a significant antitumor response *(30,31)*.

Studies in mouse LNCaP xenograft models showed that (1) antitumor responses were evident with all radionuclides and exhibited a dose–response relationship, (2) the maximum tolerated dose of $^{177}$Lu-huJ591 was higher than that for $^{90}$Y-huJ591, and (3) fractionated dosing permitted the delivery of higher cumulative doses of $^{90}$Y or $^{177}$Lu and resulted in higher response rates (>80% of mice were apparently rendered tumor-free with fractionated dosing of $^{177}$Lu-huJ591) and longer survival (150 d vs 52 d [control] for fractionated dosing of $^{90}$Y-huJ591) *(5)* (Fig. 2).

## 5. CLINICAL STUDIES

In the first phase I clinical trial of huJ591 designed to assess dose-limiting toxicity, maximum tolerated dose, pharmacokinetics, and organ dosimetry *(32)*, 53 patients with

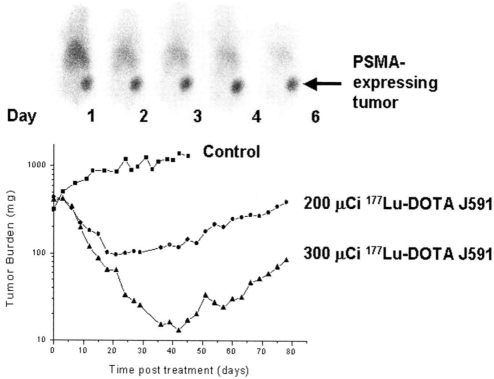

**Fig. 2. Top**: Sequential gamma camera imaging of nude mouse with LNCAP tumor expressing PSMA in left thigh demonstrating good localization of radiometal [[111]In] DOTA-J591; similar images were obtained with [177]Lu-DOTA J591. Activity cephalad to tumor represents nonspecific hepatic uptake and cardiac blood pool, both of which gradually clear over time. **Bottom**: Weight of tumor grafts in nude mice vs time, demonstrating antitumor effect of incremental doses of [177]Lu-DOTA-J591 in nude mice. Similar results were demonstrated with incremental doses of [90]Y-DOTA-J591.

progressing metastatic or recurrent hormone-independent prostate cancer underwent conventional imaging and later received [111]In-DOTA-huJ591 for imaging followed by either [90]Y-DOTA-J591 for therapy ($n = 29$) or [177]Lu-DOTA-huJ591 ($n = 24$). Conventional imaging showed that 46 (87%) of the 53 patients had evidence of metastatic disease. Radiolabeled huJ591 localization identified bone or soft tissue lesions (defined as metastatic disease) in 42 (98%) of 43 evaluable patients. Bone lesions were accurately targeted in 32 (94%) of 34 evaluable patients and soft tissue lesions in 13 (72%) of 18 evaluable patients (Figs. 3 and 4). Conventional imaging showed no evidence of bone metastasis in 18 patients, whereas huJ591 imaging showed no evidence of bone metastasis in 16 patients. The two apparently false-positive huJ591 scans (compared to bone scans) were later shown by magnetic resonance imaging (MRI) to be true positives. huJ591 scans also identified additional sites of apparent nodal disease, but these could not be considered evaluable because of the lack of corroborating evidence from computed tomography (CT) or MRI.

Ten patients in this study *(32)* received multiple doses of radiolabeled huJ591 followed by repeat imaging. J591 consistently and specifically targeted PSMA-expressing tumors and no other tissues. In addition, no systemic adverse or serological immune response to

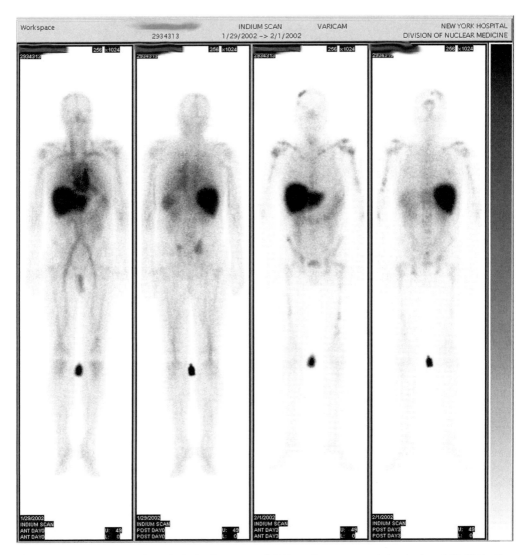

**Fig. 3.** Anterior and posterior whole-body scans at d 0 (day of intravenous injection) and d 3 (72 h after injection) of 5.0 mCi of [111]In-DOTA-J591. Within hours of injection, there is already nonspecific uptake in the liver. Nevertheless, on d 0, note considerable cardiac blood pool and great vessel activity representing circulating radiolabeled antibody. On d 3, the cardiac blood pool and great vessel activity has cleared and there is diffuse uptake in marrow activity at sites of tumor activity (skull, humeri, pelvis, and femurs). The intense activity between the knees is a standard used to convert counts to microcuries to determine the percent injected dose in areas of uptake. [111]In-DOTA-J591 is used for biodistribution studies and imaging as a surrogate for [90]Y-DOTA-J591, which cannot be imaged effectively because it is a pure β-emitter.

huJ591 was observed despite multiple administrations. These results indicate that huJ591 might be useful as an imaging agent and suggest that (1) huJ591 could direct an immune system response toward tumor sites and (2) huJ591 could deliver radionuclides or cytotoxins directly to tumor sites without affecting normal tissues.

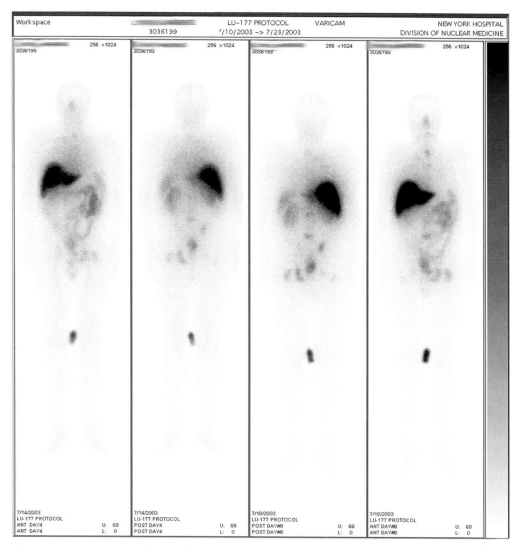

**Fig. 4.** Anterior and posterior whole-body scans on d 4 and d 8 following a 30-mCi/m² dose ¹⁷⁷Lu-DOTA-J591 (dose escalation trial). In addition to nonspecific liver uptake, note foci of specific uptake in tumor sites in multiple vertebral bodies, right iliac crest (posteriorly), left ischium, and femoral neck.

The use of huJ591 as a vehicle for the transport and delivery of cytotoxins to tumors is being explored by conjugating DM1, a derivative of maytansine, a cytotoxic tubulin-inhibiting compound, to huJ591 *(5)*. Conjugated DM1 is not active until it is internalized intracellularly and released from the antibody. The first phase I study to determine the dose-limiting toxicity, maximum tolerated dose, and pharmacokinetics of DM1-J591 is in progress.

Also in progress is a phase I dose escalation trial of ¹¹¹In-DOTA-huJ591 to determine whether huJ591 could target nonprostate solid tumor neovasculature without binding to the vasculature of normal tissue and to characterize the pharmacokinetics and biodistribution of huJ591, as well as to determine whether a human antihuman antibody (HAHA) response to huJ591 was mounted in patients with refractory solid tumor malignancies. [111]In-DOTA-huJ591 was localized to tumor sites, including metastatic sites in viscera, soft tissue, and bone, in 15 of 19 patients, and no patient developed HAHA *(33)*.

The collective data thus far indicate that radiolabeled-DOTA- or cytotoxin-conjugated huJ591 has promise for imaging and for therapeutic targeting of PSMA-expressing tumors and tumor neovasculature. As the results from more clinical studies are generated, these varied roles of J591 will be further elucidated.

# REFERENCES

1. American Cancer Institute. Cancer facts and figures 2004. Atlanta, GA: American Cancer Society, 2004.
2. Stanford JL, Stephenson RA, Coyle LM, Cerhan J, Correa R, Eley JW, et al. Prostate cancer trends 1973–1995, SEER Program. Bethesda, MD: National Cancer Institute, 1999.
3. Goldsmith SJ, Bander NH. Monoclonal antibody therapy. In: Khalkhali I, Maublant J, Goldsmith SJ, eds. Nuclear oncology: diagnosis and therapy. Philadelphia: Lippincott Williams & Wilkins, 2001:433–439.
4. Pound CR. Evaluation and treatment of men with biochemical prostate-specific antigen recurrence following definitive therapy for clinically localized prostate cancer. Rev Urol 2001; 3:72.
5. Bander NH, Nanus DM, Milowsky MI, Kostakoglu L, Vallabahajosula S, Goldsmith SJ. Targeted systemic therapy of prostate cancer with a monoclonal antibody to prostate-specific membrane antigen. Semin Oncol 2003; 30:667–677.
6. Horoszewicz JS, Kawinski E, Murphy GP. Monoclonal antibodies to a new antigenic marker in epithelial prostatic cells and serum of prostatic cancer patients. Anticancer Res 1987; 7:927–935.
7. Israeli RS, Powell CT, Fair WR, Heston WD. Molecular cloning of a complementary DNA encoding a prostate-specific membrane antigen. Cancer Res 1993; 53:227–230.
8. Israeli RS, Powell CT, Corr JG, Fair WR, Heston WD. Expression of the prostate-specific membrane antigen. Cancer Res 1994; 54:1807–1811.
9. Wright GL Jr, Haley C, Beckett ML, Schellhammer PF. Expression of prostate-specific membrane antigen (PSMA) in normal, benign and malignant prostate tissues. Urol Oncol 1995; 1:18–28.
10. Troyer JK, Beckett ML, Wright GL Jr. Detection and characterization of the prostate-specific membrane antigen (PSMA) in tissue extracts and body fluids. Int J Cancer 1995; 62:552–558.
11. Sokoloff RL, Norton KC, Gasior CL, Marker KM, Grauer LS. A dual-monoclonal sandwich assay for prostate-specific membrane antigen: levels in tissues, seminal fluid and urine. Prostate 2000; 43:150–157.
12. Bostwick DB, Pacelli A, Blute M, Roche P, Murphy GP. Prostate specific membrane antigen in prostatic intraepithelial neoplasia and adenocarcinoma: a study of 184 cases. Cancer 1998; 82:2256–2261.
13. Wright L Jr, Grob B, Haley C, Grossman K, Newhall K, Petrylak D, et al. Upregulation of prostate-specific membrane antigen after androgen-deprivation therapy. Urology 1998; 48:326–334.
14. Sweat SD, Pacelli A, Murphy GP, Bostwick DG. Prostate-specific membrane antigen expression is greatest in prostate adenocarcinoma and lymph node metastases. Urology 1998; 52:637–640.
15. Grauer LS, Lawler KD, Marignac JL, Kumar A, Goel AS, Wolfert RL. Identification, purification, and subcellular localization of prostate-specific membrane antigen PSM' protein in the LNCaP prostatic carcinoma cell line Cancer Res 1998; 58:4787–4789.
16. Leek J, Lench N, Maraj B, Bailey A, Carr IM, Andersen S, et al. Prostate-specific membrane antigen: evidence for rhe existence of a second related human gene. Br J Cancer 1995; 72:583–588.
17. Silver DA, Pellicer I, Fair WR, Heston WDW, Cordon-Cardo C. Prostate-specific membrane antigen expression in normal and malignant human tissues. Clin Cancer Res 1997; 3:81–85.
18. Murphy GP, Elgamal AA, Su SL, Bostwick DG, Holmes EH. Current evaluation of the tissue localization and diagnostic utility of prostate specific membrane antigen. Cancer 1998; 83:2259–2269.
19. Liu H, Moy P, Xia Y, Kim S, Rajasekaran AK, Navarro V, et al. Monoclonal antibodies to the extracellular domain of prostate-specific membrane antigen also react with tumor vascular endothelium. Cancer Res 1997; 57:3629–3634.
20. Chang SS, Reuter VE, Heston WD, Bander NH, Grauer LS, Gaudin PB. Five different anti-prostate-specific membrane antigen (PSMA) antibodies confirm PSMA expression in tumor-associated neovasculature. Cancer Res 1999; 59:3192–3198.

21. Dumas F, Gala JL, Berteau F, Brasseur F, Eschwege P, Paradis V, et al. Molecular expression of PSMA mRNA and protein in primary renal tumors. Int J Cancer 1999; 80:799–803.
22. Chang SS, O'Keefe DS, Bacich DJ, Reuter VE, Heston WDW, Gaudin PB. Prostate specific membrane antigen is produced in tumor-associated neovasculature. Clin Cancer Res 1999; 5:2674–2681.
23. Troyer JK, Feng Q, Beckett ML, Wright GL Jr. Biochemical characterization and mapping of the 7E11-C5.3 epitope of the prostate-specific membrane antigen. Urol Oncol 1995; 1:29–37.
24. Troyer JK, Beckett MI, Wright GL Jr. Location of prostate-specific membrane antigen in the LNCaP prostate carcinoma cell line. Prostate 1997; 30:232–242.
25. Smith-Jones PM, Vallabahajosula S, Goldsmith SJ, Navarro V, Hunter CJ, Bastidas D, et al. In vitro characterization of radiolabeled monoclonal antibodies specific for the extracellular domain of prostate-specific membrane antigen. Cancer Res 2000; 60:5237–5243.
26. Liu H, Rajasekaran AK, Moy P, Xia Y, Kim S, Navaro V, et al. Constitutive and antibody-induced internalization of prostate-specific membrane antigen. Cancer Res 1998; 58:4055–4060.
27. Hamilton A, King S, Liu H, Moy P, Bander N, Carr F. A novel humanized antibody against prostate specific membrane antigen (PSMA) for in vivo targeting and therapy. Proc Am Assoc Cancer Res 1998; 39:440.
28. Goldsmith SJ, Kostakoglu L, Vallabhajosula S, Smith-Jones PM, Bremer S, Spangler T, et al. Evaluation of an antibody I-131 J591 in the treatment of prostate cancer. J Nucl Med 2000; 40:80P (abstract).
29. Smith-Jones PM, Vallabhajosula S, Navarro V, Bastidas D, Goldsmith SJ, Bander NH. Radiolabeled mono-clonal antibodies specific to the extracellular domain of prostate-specific membrane antigen: preclinical studies in nude mice bearing LNCaP human prostate tumor. J Nucl Med 2003; 44:610–617.
30. Smith-Jones PM, Vallabhajosula S, Navarro V, Goldsmith SJ, Bander NH. $^{90}$Y-huJ591 MAb specific to PSMA: radioimmunotherapy (RIT) studies in nude mice with prostate cancer LNCaP tumor. Eur J Nucl Med 2000; 8:951 (abstract).
31. Smith-Jones PM, Navarro V, Omer SS, Bander NH, Goldsmith SJ, Vallabhajosula S. comparative antitumor effects of $^{90}$Y-DOTA-J591 and $^{177}$Lu-DOTA-J591 in nude mice bearing LNCaP tumors. J Nucl Med 2001; 42(Suppl):151P–152P (abstract).
32. Bander NH, Trabulsi EJ, Kostakoglu L, Yao D. Vallabhajosula S, Smith-Jones P, et al. Targeting metastatic prostate cancer with radiolabeled monoclonal antibody J591 to the extracellular domain of prostate specific membrane antigen. J Urol 2003; 170:1717–1721.
33. Milowsky MI, Rosmarin AS, Cobham MV, et al. Anti-PSMA mAb HuJ591 specifically targets tumor vascular endothelial cells in patients with advanced solid tumor malignancies. Proc Am Soc Clin Oncol 2002; 21:19 (abstract).

# 40 Monoclonal Antibody Strategies for Targeting HER2

*Joan Albanell, MD, Jeffrey S. Ross, MD,*
*Linda Pronk, MD, and Pere Gascon, MD*

## CONTENTS

## SUMMARY

The HER family is composed of four receptors, HER1 to HER4, is dysregulated, and/or shows abnormal signaling activity in a broad range of human tumors. The essential role of HER2 in the HER signaling network led to the development of anti-HER2 monoclonal antibodies (mAb) for cancer therapy. In particular, the humanized antibody trastuzumab (Herceptin™) has antitumor activity against HER2-overexpressing breast tumors and is widely used for the treatment of women with HER2-overexpressing breast cancers. However, trastuzumab activity relies on the presence of HER2 overexpression and it is not active against tumors that express moderate or normal levels of HER2.

Importantly, there is a large population of breast cancers and many other tumors that have normal (nonoverexpressed) HER2 expression yet show abnormal HER signaling activity. In such tumors, HER2 functions as a preferred coreceptor to form heterodimers with HER1 (EGFR), HER3, or HER4. For this reason, a humanized mAb, called pertuzumab (2C4; Omnitarg™), that targets HER2—the preferred pairing partner—was developed and is now in clinical development. Importantly, pertuzumab is directed at an extracellular region of HER2—the dimerization domain—and blocks HER2 from dimerizing with other receptors and prevents the activation of HER signaling cascades. Pertuzumab represents the first in a new class of targeted therapeutics known as HER dimerization inhibitors (HDIs). Given the good preclinical activity of pertuzumab and its potential

From: *Cancer Drug Discovery and Development: The Oncogenomics Handbook*
Edited by: W. J. LaRochelle and R. A. Shimkets © Humana Press Inc., Totowa, NJ

to target a broad range of human tumors, including those with low HER2 expression, the antibody was recently moved to the clinic. Phase I trials with pertuzumab have shown promising results and phase Ib and II trials are ongoing against a variety of tumor types. Current results and ongoing strategies with these anti-HER2 antibodies are discussed.

**Key Words:** HER2; trastuzumab; pertuzumab; EGFR; monoclonal antibodies; HER dimerization inhibitors; biological therapy.

## 1. INTRODUCTION

The human epidermal growth factor receptor-2 (HER-2)/*neu* (c-*erbB*-2) gene is localized to chromosome 17q and encodes HER2, a transmembrane tyrosine kinase receptor protein that is a member of the epidermal growth factor receptor (EGFR) or HER family *(1)*. The HER family is composed of four receptors, HER1 to HER4, and is involved in normal cell-to-cell and cell-to-stroma communication primarily. However, this receptor family is dysregulated and/or shows abnormal signaling activity in a broad range of human tumors and, in particular, the HER2 receptor plays a critical role in malignancy. HER2 is a ligand-orphan receptor expressed in many human tumors and overexpressed in 15–30% of breast cancers. The primary cause of HER2 overexpression in breast cancer is the amplification of the HER-2/*neu* gene, an event rarely identified in other malignancies. HER2 amplifies the signal provided by other receptors of the HER family by forming heterodimers. The essential role of HER2 in the HER signaling network led to the development of anti-HER2 monoclonal antibodies (mAbs) for cancer therapy *(2–5)*. In particular, the humanized mAb trastuzumab (Herceptin™) *(6)* has antitumor activity against HER2-overexpressing breast tumors and is widely used for the treatment of women with HER2-overexpressing breast cancers *(7,8)*. Trastuzumab is the only anti-HER2 antibody that has been approved for cancer therapy. However, trastuzumab activity relies on the presence of HER2 overexpression and it is not active against tumors that express moderate or normal levels of HER2 *(3)*.

Importantly, there is a large population of breast cancers and many other tumors that have normal (nonoverexpressed) HER2 expression yet show abnormal HER signaling activity. In such tumors, HER2 functions as a preferred coreceptor to form heterodimers with HER1 (EGFR), HER3, or HER4 *(9–12)*. HER dimers initiate intracellular signaling events that ultimately mediate cancer cell growth, proliferation, and survival. For this reason, a humanized mAb, called pertuzumab (2C4; Omnitarg™), that targets HER2—the preferred pairing partner—was developed and is now in clinical development. Importantly, pertuzumab and trastuzumab bind to distinct regions within the extracellular domain of the HER2 protein. Pertuzumab is directed at an extracellular region of HER2—the dimerization domain —and blocks HER2 from dimerizing with other receptors and prevents the activation of HER signaling cascades. Pertuzumab represents the first in a new class of targeted therapeutics known as HER dimerization inhibitors (HDIs). Pertuzumab has antitumor effects in cells with either normal (low) or overexpressed levels of HER2 protein. In vitro and in vivo antitumor activity has been reported in a range of tumor models *(13)*. Phase I trials with pertuzumab have shown promising results and phase Ib and II trials are ongoing against a variety of tumor types *(14)*.

Trastuzumab and pertuzumab are mAbs that act by targeting HER2's role as an oncogene and possibly also by inducing a host immune response. Because of their current clinical relevance and their even greater future clinical potential, they will be discussed

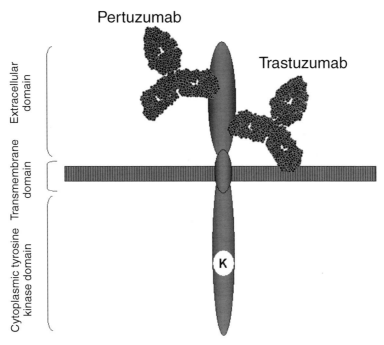

**Fig. 1.** HER2 and binding regions for mAbs. HER2 is composed of an extracellular domain and an intracellular domain that has tyrosine kinase activity (K). The epitopes to which the anti-HER2 monoclonal antibodies pertuzumab and trastuzumab bind are schematically represented. (From ref. 2.)

in detail in this chapter. To increase further the potency of anti-HER2 antibodies, mAbs can be used also as targeted delivery weapons for a wide variety of effector agents *(15)*. Ongoing strategies in this direction will also be discussed.

## 2. HER2 BIOLOGY

To put in perspective how different antibodies (trastuzumab and pertuzumab) targeting a single receptor, HER2, exert distinct antitumor effects, it is appropriate to review the biology of the HER network and the mechanisms of HER2 activation.

The structure of the receptors of the HER family consists of an extracellular ligand-binding domain, a transmembrane lipophylic segment, and an intracellular protein tyrosine kinase domain with a regulatory carboxyl-terminal segment (Fig. 1) *(1)*. HER2, like the other receptors of the family, is inactive when is present in a monomeric state. The activation of all HER proteins requires the formation of dimers or oligomers *(16)*.

HER2 activation can occur in two ways; ligand independent or ligand dependent. For example, ligand-independent HER activation occurs as a result of HER2 overexpression (Fig. 2) *(17,18)*, resulting in the formation of HER2/HER2 homodimers. This homodimerization process would be dependent on the high concentration of receptors at the cell surface and occurs without the need of ligand or a different HER family member as a coreceptor. In support of the role of HER2 overexpression in tumorigenesis, it was shown that the introduction of HER2 into non-neoplastic cells causes their malignant transformation *(19)*. Also, transgenic mice expressing *neu* develop mammary tumors *(20)*. From a clinical

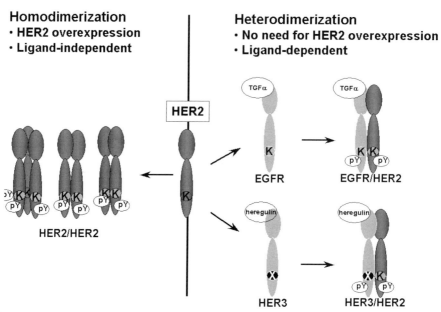

**Fig. 2.** Ligand-independent and ligand-dependent mechanisms of HER2 activation. K, tyrosine kinase; pY, phosphorylation of tyrosine residues that are indicative of receptor activation; X, kinase death domain of HER3. *See* text for further details.

point of view, HER2 overexpression and activation also occurs in a proportion of human tumors *(3,17)*. The most comprehensive studies have been conducted in breast cancer showing that HER2 is overexpressed, most commonly by gene amplification, in 25–30% of human breast cancers *(21)*. In an overview of 80 studies involving 26,309 patients, 72 (90%) of the studies and 24,314 (92%) of the cases revealed that either HER2/*neu* gene amplification or HER2 protein overexpression predicted breast cancer outcome on either univariate or multivariate analysis *(22)*. In 51 (71%) of the 72 studies that featured multivariate analysis of outcome data, the adverse prognostic significance of HER-2/*neu* gene, message, or protein overexpression was independent of all other prognostic variables *(22)*. HER2 overexpression has been also reported in other tumor types such as ovarian, gastric, colon, and non-small-cell lung carcinoma, but the results are less consistent than what has been reported in breast cancer (for review, see ref. *23*).

A second mechanism of HER2 activation is the formation of ligand-dependent HER2-containing heterodimers (Fig. 2). The formation of HER2-containing heterodimers relies initially on the binding of a ligand to the non-HER2 receptor partner, such as HER1 (EGFR), HER3, or HER4 *(1,24–27)*. Once a ligand binds to HER1, HER3, or HER4, the receptor undergoes a conformational change and becomes "open" and available to dimerize with HER2. At least six different ligands, known as EGF-like ligands, bind to the EGFR (HER1). These ligands include epidermal growth factor (EGF), transforming growth factor-α (TGF-α), amphiregulin, heparin binding EGF (HB-EGF), betacellulin, and epiregulin. A second class of ligands, collectively termed heregulins (also known as neu differentiation factors and neuregulins), bind directly to HER3 and/or HER4. Notably, HER2 is the only ligand-orphan receptor of the family but, instead, is the preferred coreceptor for the EGFR, HER3, and HER4. Recent studies of the HER2 structure revealed that HER2 constitutively exists

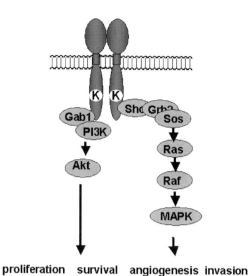

proliferation survival angiogenesis invasion

**Fig. 3.** HER (ErbB) receptor activation triggers a series of intracellular signaling pathways that regulate essential cellular processes. Additional pathways not shown in the schema are also regulated by these receptors.

in the "open" or active conformation. This structure provides a clear explanation of why HER2 is the preferred pairing partner of the other HER receptors (Franklin et al. in press). Additionally, this preference for heterodimerization within the HER receptor family explains how HER2 signals in the absence of a cognate ligand *(12)*. The heterodimers between HER2 and the other HER receptors have relatively high ligand affinity and potent signaling activity and are synergistic for cell transformation *(11,28,29)*. The best example of the ability of HER2 to transactivate signaling initiated by ligands that bind to other HER receptors is that the HER2/HER3 heterodimers exhibit an extremely potent mitogenic activity, whereas HER3 homodimers are inactive *(9,30,31)*. This mechanism of ligand-dependent HER2 activation (heterodimerization) could be more general in tumors compared to the one related to HER2 overexpression. Many studies have confirmed the expression of HER2 and other HER receptors and their ligands in many tumor types (see ref. *23* for review). For instance, HER2 and the EGFR are frequently coexpressed in breast cancer and their overexpression is associated with a more aggressive clinical behavior. HER3 is overexpressed in about 20% of breast cancers and the frequent coexpression of HER2 and HER3 suggests a role for the heterodimer in carcinogenesis in vivo *(30)*.

Following receptor dimerization, activation of the intrinsic protein tyrosine kinase activity and tyrosine autophosphorylation occur *(16)*. The formation of specific dimeric complexes of HER (ErbB) receptors and the consequent activation of different intracellular signaling pathways is viewed as the result of the cellular expression of each receptor and the availability of ligands in each individual cell *(11,32)*. There are many signaling pathways activated by HER dimers, such as Ras-Raf-mitogen-activated protein kinase (MAPK), PI3K-Akt, PLC-$\gamma$1, Src, STATs, and others (Fig. 3). The best characterized to date are the Ras-Raf-MAPK pathway *(32–34)* and the phosphatidylinositol-3 kinase

(PI3K)/Akt. These pathways ultimately regulate essential cellular functions such as proliferation, survival, angiogenesis, and invasion (Fig. 3).

## 3. ANTI-HER2 MONOCLONAL ANTIBODIES TARGETING HER2-OVEREXPRESSING CANCER CELLS: FOCUS ON TRASTUZUMAB

### 3.1. Mechanisms of Action of Trastuzumab

Trastuzumab is a recombinant humanized anti-HER2 mAb directed at the HER2 ectodomain, in the juxtamembrane region, that is selectively active against tumor cells that overexpress HER2 (6,35) (Fig. 1). 4D5, the parental murine version of trastuzumab, exhibited a clear relationship between the level of HER2 receptor expression and sensitivity to the growth inhibitory effects of the mAb 4D5 (2,36). In cells with moderate or low expression of HER2, both trastuzumab and 4D5 display little or no antitumor activity (36,37). In contrast, these antibodies display a potent antiproliferative effect against tumor cells with high expression of HER2 (37). Interestingly, the sensitivity to the growth inhibitory effects of trastuzumab is highly dependent not only on the presence of HER2 protein overexpression but also on HER2 gene amplification (38).

A key effect for the selective antitumor activity of trastuzumab (and other nonclinical anti-HER2 antibodies) against HER2-overexpressing cells seems to be their ability to downmodulate the levels of HER2 at the cell surface (39–43). It is presumed that the removal of HER2 from the plasma membrane reduces the availability of the receptor for dimerization, which, in turn, diminishes the HER2-initiated growth signals (Fig. 4). Along this line, trastuzumab results in the blockade of the two major signaling transduction pathways of HER2, as shown by the inhibition of MAPK and Akt phosphorylation (38). Akt appears to play a major role in trastuzumab activity because when cells were genetically manipulated to have an activated form of Akt, trastuzumab was without effect (38). Interestingly, it takes several hours of exposure to trastuzumab to see these effects. This observation thus supports the notion that it is likely necessary to induce receptor downregulation before the signaling pathways are affected by trastuzumab and that trastuzumab does not directly block receptor activation and signaling transduction. An additional property of trastuzumab is the prevention of HER2 cleavage (42,44,45). It is attractive to hypothesize that inhibition of HER2 cleavage by trastuzumab might have therapeutic value by preventing the formation of the potentially deleterious truncated HER2 intracellular and activated fragments. The potential clinical relevance of this finding is that a HER2 truncated, intracellular fragment is phosphorylated in human breast cancer tumors and is linked to poor prognosis (46)

Altogether, the effects of trastuzumab on receptor downmodulation and the resulting consequences on signaling pathways and cell cycle regulatory molecules are primarily associated with cytostatic effects in cultures of tumor cells that overexpress HER2. Cell cycle analysis of cells treated with trastuzumab reveal a partial block in G1 and a reduction of cells undergoing the S-phase (41). The induction of apoptosis varies among cell lines (38,47).

In contrast to the mainly cytostatic effect of trastuzumab in cultured cells, studies using human breast cancer xenografts revealed a cytotoxic effect, with common tumor eradication. The greater in vivo effect might be the result of the antiangiogenic (48) and immunostimulatory properties (6) of trastuzumab, which only have an effect in in vivo animal models (41). Considering that trastuzumab is bivalent and the concentration of HER2 protein at the cell surface of HER2-overexpressing cells is very high, an avidity component

## Trastuzumab

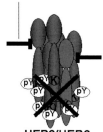

**HER2/HER2**

Targets HER2 overexpression
• Receptor downmodulation
• Blocks HER2 cleavage
• Angiogenesis inhibition
• ADCC important
• Proof-of-concept established
in patients with HER2 3+
breast cancer

## Pertuzumab

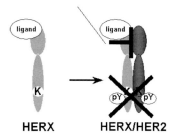

**HERX        HERX/HER2**

Targets ligand-activated HERX-HER2
dimerization
• Prevents heterodimer formation
• Inhibits MAPK and Akt signaling
• Activity is independent of HER2
expression level
• May have wider application and may
inhibit the growth of a number of
tumor types

**Fig. 4.** Summary of the mechanism of action of anti-HER2 antibodies trastuzumab and pertuzumab. HERX, EGFR, HER3, or HER4. ADCC, antibody-dependent cellular cytotoxicity; MAPK, mitogen-activated protein kinase; pY, phosphorylation of tyrosine residues indicative of receptor activation; X, kinase death domain of HER3.

also likely contributes to the near-irreversible binding of trastuzumab to cells that overexpress HER2. Based on this observation, it has been proposed that the trigger of antibody-dependent cellular cytotoxicity (ADCC) might be an additional explanation for the selective antitumor action of trastuzumab toward HER2-overexpressing cells compared to cells with low or moderate HER2 expression *(41)*. Recent evidence has provided support for a substantial role of ADCC in the in vivo antitumor activity of trastuzumab *(49)*.

In addition to its antitumor activity as single agents, anti-HER2 antibodies can markedly enhance or promote sensitivity to the antitumor effects of chemotherapeutic agents such as doxorubicin, paclitaxel, docetaxel, etoposide, and cisplatin, to cite a few examples *(37, 50,51)*. In in vivo models, the combination of various chemotherapeutic agents with trastuzumab has resulted in an enhancement of the tumoricidal effects of chemotherapy and in a striking rate of tumor eradication. The simplest explanation for the enhanced activity of chemotherapy and trastuzumab is that it is the result of the summation of effects of two anticancer drugs that act on different targets. Trastuzumab acts on the HER2 receptor signaling pathway and chemotherapy acts on other targets (DNA, tubulin, topoisomerases, etc.). However, the magnitude of the enhanced antitumor activity with certain combinations might be well beyond a simple summation of effects and further mechanistic explanations have been elucidated *(52,53)*.

### 3.2. Pivotal Clinical Studies

HER2-overexpression in human cancers occurs in 15–30% of breast cancers but is very uncommon in other tumor types. Therefore, and given that trastuzumab activity is limited to HER2-overexpressing cells, the clinical development of this antibody focused on HER2-overexpressing breast cancer. The critical trials that led to trastuzumab approval are reviewed in the following subsections.

### 3.2.1. TRASTUZUMAB AS A SINGLE AGENT

In a pivotal phase II trial, trastuzumab was administered using the standard schedule (4 mg/kg intravenous [iv] loading dose followed by weekly doses of 2 mg/kg) as a single agent to 222 patients with previously treated, HER2-positive, metastatic breast cancer (7). In that study, the response rates were 15%, determined by the response evaluation committee and 20%, determined by investigators, with a median response duration of 9 mo and median survival of 13 mo. In a subsequent study in women with HER2-overexpressing breast cancer who had not previously received chemotherapy for their metastatic disease (i.e., first line), trastuzumab was also active (54). The response rate was 26% and the clinical benefit rate was 38% in all assessable patients and 48% in the subset whose tumors expressed the highest HER2 protein levels (immunohistochemistry [IHC] score of 3+). The median survival of the patients was 24 mo, suggesting that trastuzumab alone as first-line therapy for metastatic disease does not adversely affect long-term outcome. The investigators assessed the standard dose of trastuzumab as well as a higher dose of trastuzumab. However, no apparent benefit of a higher trastuzumab dose was observed, as assessed by the efficacy end points used in the trial (54).

One major advantage of trastuzumab compared to the majority of chemotherapeutic agents is the safety profile (55). As expected for a targeted agent, toxicities typically associated with chemotherapy, such as myelotoxicity, mucositis, and alopecia, rarely occur in patients treated with trastuzumab as a single agent (7,54,56). The most common treatment-related adverse events occur after the first infusion and consist of chills, fever, and nausea. These events are much less frequent after the second and subsequent infusions. Because of the increased risk of cardiotoxicity of anthracycline–trastuzumab combinations (see Section 3.2.2), trastuzumab-associated cardiac events have been thoroughly investigated. In data pooled from patients included in trastuzumab trials, the incidence of heart failure was 2.7% in patients treated with antibody alone. Notably, patients at risk can often be identified prior to therapy, as the majority had a history of cardiac disease, cardiac risk factors (NYHA class 2), left ventricular ejection fraction (LVEF) <50%, or prior anthracycline therapy (high cumulative dose). These symptoms typically improved with standard treatment, with or without discontinuation of trastuzumab (57,58).

### 3.2.2. TRASTUZUMAB IN COMBINATION WITH CHEMOTHERAPY

The pivotal combination therapy trial was a randomized study evaluating the benefit of trastuzumab in combination with chemotherapy for women with HER2-overexpressing metastatic breast cancer (8). Four hundred sixty-nine patients who had not received anthracyclines as adjuvant therapy were randomly assigned to receive an anthracycline (doxorubicin or epirubicin) plus cyclophosphamide (AC) alone or in combination with trastuzumab. Patients who had received anthracyclines as adjuvant therapy were randomly assigned to receive paclitaxel alone or with trastuzumab. The response rate was 42% for AC alone in anthracycline-naive patients and 17% for paclitaxel in anthracycline-exposed patients; the response rate was higher when trastuzumab was added to AC (56%, $p = 0.02$) or paclitaxel (41%, $p = 0.001$). The median duration of survival was 25.1 mo for trastuzumab and chemotherapy, 26.8 mo for trastuzumab and AC, and 22.1 mo for trastuzumab and paclitaxel. The survival gain was observed despite of the fact that 66% of patients originally

Table 1
Randomized Results of Taxanes Alone or Plus Trastuzumab

|  | Slamon, 2001 | | Extra, 2004 | |
| --- | --- | --- | --- | --- |
|  | T + P (n = 68) | P (n = 77) | T + D (n = 92) | D (n = 94) |
| ORR (%) | 49 | 17 | 61 | 34 |
| TTP (mo) | 7.1 | 3.0 | 10.6 | 6.1 |
| OS (mo) | 24.8 | 17.9 | 27.7 | 18.3 |

*Abbreviations:* T, trastuzumab; P, paclitaxel; D, docetaxel; ORR, overall
response rate; TTP, time to progression; OS, overall survival.

assigned to chemotherapy alone crossed over to receive trastuzumab in an extension trial. This trial also demonstrated that the administration of trastuzumab was associated with relatively few serious adverse events. However, an increased incidence of cardiac dysfunction, particularly in patients receiving concomitant anthracycline and trastuzumab therapy, was observed. Class III or IV cardiac dysfunction occurred in 27% of the anthracycline and cyclophosphamide plus trastuzumab-treated group compared to 8% of the group given an anthracycline and cyclophosphamide alone. Searching for mechanisms, studies have demonstrated that HER2 and HER4 with its ligand heregulin are necessary for normal development of the heart, and knockout mice that lack the HER2/*neu* gene expression in their cardiac myocytes develop progressive dilated cardiomyopathy *(59,60)*. This led to focusing on the development of nonanthracycline-containing regimens.

Because of the synergy between docetaxel and trastuzumab in preclinical studies *(50, 61)*, the data of the pivotal study *(8)* and the promising activity and safety profile of this combination in phase II trials *(62–65)*, another randomized study was conducted in 118 women with HER2+ metastatic breast cancer to compare docetaxel alone or with trastuzumab *(66)*. The response rate was 34% for docetaxel alone and 61% for docetaxel plus trastuzumab ($p = 0.0002$). Importantly, survival was improved with the combined treatment; the median duration of survival was 27.7 mo for trastuzumab and docetaxel and 18.3 mo for docetaxel alone ($p = 0.0002$) (Table 1) *(66)*.

### 3.3. Trastuzumab Use in Standard Practice

Trastuzumab has a very favorable risk : benefit ratio as a monotherapy and in combination with taxanes; as a result, trastuzumab was approved in many countries for patients with advanced breast cancer whose tumors overexpress HER2 *(3,7,8,67,68)*. The two approved indications of trastuzumab are as a single agent in pretreated patients or in first-line therapy in combination with paclitaxel. Considering the recent study showing that trastuzumab also dramatically increases survival when added to docetaxel, in October 2003 trastuzumab plus docetaxel was filed with the European Agency for the Evaluation of Medicinal Products (EMEA) *(66)*.

The best method to identify patients who might respond to trastuzumab therapy has been a source of controversy *(3,22)*. Commonly, overexpression of HER2 is considered as IHC 3+ or IHC2+ and gene amplification as assayed by fluorescence *in situ* hybridization (FISH+). Most laboratories are either screening all cases with IHC and triaging selected cases for FISH testing or using FISH as the only method for HER-2/neu testing. Compared with IHC, FISH is more expensive, time-consuming, and labor-intensive. On the other hand, FISH has an objective and quantitative scoring system. More importantly, data from trastuzumab pivotal trials suggest that FISH is a superior method for selecting patients likely to benefit from trastuzumab therapy (69–71). Consequently, FISH has been advocated to confirm some or all positive IHC results or even as the only modality of testing based on cost-effective analysis, considering also the cost of using trastuzumab in IHC false-positive patients (72). A newer technique, such as the chromogenic in situ hybridization method (CISH technique), features the advantages of both IHC (routine microscope, lower cost, familiarity) and FISH (built-in internal control, subjective scoring, the more robust DNA target), but is not, to date, Food and Drug Administration (FDA)-approved for the selection of patients for trastuzumab treatment (3,22).

### 3.4. Areas of Trastuzumab Research

Despite trastuzumab becoming a new standard in HER2-overexpressing metastatic breast cancer, there are many active areas of research:

1. Scheduling: The standard schedule is a weekly administration, but there is emerging evidence suggesting that a three-weekly regimen may be as effective and more convenient (73–75).
2. Optimal chemotherapeutic combinations: Trastuzumab has shown encouraging activity and tolerability when combined with multiple agents, including (but not limited to) paclitaxel, docetaxel, anthracyclines (at the cost of a cardiotoxicity risk), vinorelbine, capecitabine, platinum salts, gemcitabine, or liposomal anthracyclines (76–85). Predominantly based on preclinical data that suggested a powerful synergistic interaction between trastuzumab and both platinum and docetaxel, randomized, multicenter, phase III trials in the metastatic and adjuvant setting are currently underway to test the hypothesis that synergistic combinations of docetaxel, platinums, and trastuzumab will result in superior safety as well as efficacy (83). Improved combinations might emerge (65).
3. Use in the neoadjuvant (86) and adjuvant settings (87).
4. Combination with hormonal treatments (88,89).
5. Combination with novel biological agents such as HER receptor tyrosine kinase inhibitors, antiangiogenic agents, cyclooxygenase-2 (COX-2) inhibitors, proteasome inhibitors, or immunomodulators, to name a few (90–94).
6. Optimal duration of treatment: Clinical trials are addressing a new paradigm in oncologic therapy, that is, whether continuing treatment beyond progression would be of value (95).
7. Clinical trials in tumors other than breast cancer (96,97).
8. Understanding and overcoming trastuzumab resistance (98).
9. Predictive medicine (3,22).

## 4. ANTI-HER2 MONOCLONAL ANTIBODIES TARGETING LIGAND-ACTIVATED HER2: FOCUS ON PERTUZUMAB

### 4.1. Mechanisms of Action of Pertuzumab

Trastuzumab is effective in the treatment of breast cancers with HER2 protein overexpression or with HER2 gene amplification. However, more that 70–85% of breast cancers and the majority of many other malignancies have normal levels (moderate or low) of HER2 expression. Many tumors also coexpress other receptors of the HER family such

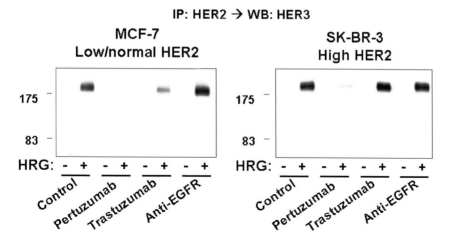

Adapted from Agus et al. (2002) Cancer Cell 2:127 (Ref. 12)

**Fig. 5.** Pertuzumab, but not trastuzumab, blocks ligand-dependent HER2/HER3 association. Adapted from ref. *13*. HRG, heregulin; EGFR, epidermal growth factor receptor.

as the EGFR or HER3, or their ligands *(23,99)*. Ligands are commonly produced by stromal cells leading to paracrine mechanisms of receptor activation. In such tumors, HER2 might be activated as the result of the formation of ligand-dependent heterodimers.

Although trastuzumab has a poor ability to disrupt the formation of ligand-dependent HER2 heterodimers, pertuzumab efficiently blocks the crosstalk between HER2 and its family members. Pertuzumab targets an extracellular domain of HER2—the dimerization domain—that, unlike trastuzumab, results in sterical hindrance of HER2 for recruitment into HER–ligand complexes *(2,13,43,100,101)* (Fig. 1), hence allowing an effective disruption of HER2 ligand-dependent activation (Figs. 4 and 5).

A series of elegant experiments showed that pertuzumab was much more effective in disrupting the formation of ligand-dependent HER2-heterodimeric complexes as compared to trastuzumab *(13)*. The use of HER2/HER3 heterodimers as a model is particularly interesting, because the HER3 receptor contains an inactive tyrosine kinase domain and HER2 is a ligandless receptor; therefore, the formation of dimers of HER2/HER3 following addition of the HER3 ligand heregulin is a prerequisite for signaling activity *(9)*. When the ability of the two antibodies was assayed in terms of signaling, pertuzumab was very effective in blocking heregulin-mediated HER3/HER2 signaling, whereas trastuzumab was poorly effective. This was concluded from assays that assessed the phosphorylation of HER2 , MAPK, Akt, and GSK3 (a downstream marker of Akt kinase activity) following a short exposure to ligand and antibodies *(13)*. Pertuzumab also blocked TGF-α-mediated MAPK activation, indicating that the antibody also interferes with EGFR–HER2 dimers. The short exposure time to the antibodies in such experiments did not allow for trastuzumab-mediated downmodulation and, as a consequence, the results reflect the ability of the antibodies tested to act on ligand-driven signaling. Similar results have been reported in a panel of ovarian cancer cell lines *(102)*. In another study, pertuzumab also inhibited ligand-dependent activation of signal transduction pathways in colorectal cancer cells, except for TGF-α-mediated MAPK activation *(103)*. Additional downstream events inhibited by pertuzumab are the heregulin-induced phosphorylation of JAK1 and STATs *(104)*.

Initial studies have investigated the antitumor activity of pertuzumab against breast and prostate tumor xenografts that do not have HER2 overexpression and, therefore, would not be adequate targets for treatment with trastuzumab *(13,101)*. In these studies, it has been shown that the in vitro and in vivo growth of several breast and prostate tumor animal models is inhibited by pertuzumab treatment. The antitumor activity in vivo was seen both in tumor xenografts with normal or overexpressed levels of HER2. In tumor xenografts overexpressing HER2, the antitumor effects of pertuzumab or murine 4D5 (the precursor of trastuzumab) were similar. This observation led the authors to propose that pertuzumab shares the inhibitory activity of trastuzumab in tumor systems whose growth is driven by ligand-independent HER2 activation (i.e., related to HER2 overexpression) *(13)*. In prostate cancer models, pertuzumab was effective in both androgen-dependent and androgen-independent tumors *(13,101)*, supporting a role for this antibody in the treatment of these malignancies. An additional finding was that, in contrast with the important role for ADCC for trastuzumab in vivo activity in animal models, monovalent versions of pertuzumab that do not have an intact Fc region retain the antitumor potential of the antibody *(13)*. In another study, pertuzumab was also active against lung tumor xenografts *(105)*. Additional studies have also shown that the in vivo activity of pertuzumab in tumor xenografts is independent of tumor type and degree of HER2 overexpression *(106)*.

Pertuzumab, in addition to its activity as a single agent, might augment the activity of other antitumor treatments. Of note, the distinct mechanism of action of pertuzumab and trastuzumab raised the interest of combination studies (Fig. 4). In experiments using cotreatment with pertuzumab and trastuzumab, there was an enhanced antitumor activity against breast cancer xenografts in animals treated with both antibodies *(105)*. Pertuzumab has been also tested in combination with small-molecule HER receptor tyrosine kinase inhibitors. For example, the EGFR tyrosine kinase inhibitor erlotinib (Tarceva) augmented the antitumor activity of pertuzumab against human breast tumor cells that have an autocrine HER loop *(107)*. Further in vivo animal studies with lung or breast tumor xenografts have shown that the antitumor and biological effects of pertuzumab and erlotinib are additive or synergistic when compared to each agent alone *(108)*. Studies combining pertuzumab with standard chemotherapeutic agents or with other biological agents are also promising *(109)*.

Given the good preclinical activity of pertuzumab and its potential to target a broad range of human tumors, including those with low HER2 expression, the antibody was humanized for clinical use.

## 4.2. Clinical Studies

In a recent phase I dose escalation study, 21 patients with advanced tumors received pertuzumab using a three-weekly schedule at doses ranging from 0.5 mg/kg to 15 mg/kg *(14)*. Partial responses were observed in 14% of patients (3/21), and an additional 24% of patients (5/21) achieved stable disease lasting for more than 3 mo in this study. Partial responders included one patient with ovarian cancer, who received 5 mg/kg of pertuzumab; one with prostate cancer, who received 15 mg/kg of pertuzumab; and one patient with a pancreatic neuroendocrine cancer who received 15 mg/kg of pertuzumab *(14)*. Two of these patients (ovarian and pancreatic cancer) remained in remission and received pertuzumab for over a year since the start of therapy. Pertuzumab was well tolerated at doses up to 15 mg/kg, as a majority of adverse events were of grade 1 and 2, with the most frequently reported adverse events being vomiting, nausea, fatigue, rash, anemia, abdominal pain, and diarrhea. Skin rash and diarrhea occurred in about one-third of the patients. No significant declines of left ventricular ejection fraction below 50% were noted in the first two cycles. At later time-points, one patient experienced a drop in left ventricular activity to < 50% following a myocardial infarction. There was one dose-limiting toxicity, a gastrointestinal bleeding in a patient with a pre-existing esophageal varix. Pharmacokinetic studies showed that the antibody terminal half-life was approx 3 wk (similar to trastuzumab) and that biologically relevant serum concentrations were achieved without need of reaching the maximal tolerated dose *(14,110)*.

Based on these promising results, phase II studies have been initiated in ovarian cancer, prostate cancer, non-small-cell lung cancer and breast cancer (non-HER2-overexpressing). Furthermore, phase Ib trials are ongoing on the combination of pertuzumab and capecitabine and of pertuzumab and docetaxel. Another critical focus of research is the identification of markers that could predict a response to this novel antibody. Along this line, a recent preclinical study indicates that the presence of HER2/HER3 heterodimers predicts the antitumor effects of pertuzumab in different human xenograft models *(111)*.

## 5. OTHER MONOCLONAL ANTIBODY STRATEGIES FOR TARGETING HER2

Chemically coupling antibodies to toxins or radionuclides is the most widely investigated means for increasing the antitumor activity of mAbs and there are several examples of the clinical utility of this strategy involving antibodies against several targets *(15)*. In the HER2 field, this area is still in preclinical development *(112)*. One example of this approach is Herceptin–DM-1 ("armed" trastuzumab), an immunoconjugate that consists of a combination of trastuzumab with a highly potent microtubule toxin, maytansinoid *(113)*. In laboratory experiments, Herceptin–DM-1 exhibited a higher antitumor potency than trastuzumab, and the cytotoxicity of the DM-1 was restricted to HER2-expressing cells.

An additional strategy in development is the use of bispecific antibodies. Bispecific antibodies that bind to two different antigens might selectively deliver cytotoxic effectors, such as immune effector cells, radionuclides, drugs, and toxins, to tumour cells in vivo. Antibody 520C9xH22 (MDX-H210) is a partially humanized bispecific antibody containing Fab fragments of a mAb (520C9) targeting HER2-expressing tumor cells and a mAb (H22) targeting Fc gamma RI (CD64) *(114–121)*. The Fc gamma receptor mediates phagocytosis and cytolysis of HER2-overexpressing breast cancer cells by macrophages. MDX-H210 has been in clinical trials for metastatic cancers, such as breast and ovarian cancers that overexpress HER2. Granulocyte colony-stimulating factor (G-CSF) and interferon were found to enhance the immune-based cytotoxic potential of MDX-H210 and, therefore, were coadministered with MDX-H210 in several phase I trials. Available data from phase I studies revealed that MDX-H210 is biologically active and can stabilize patients with HER2-overexpressing tumors.

Another strategy to improve delivery and selectivity is the development of chemotherapy-loaded anti-HER2 liposomes *(122,123)*. This strategy combines the tumor-targeting properties of anti-HER2 antibodies such as trastuzumab with the drug delivery properties of sterically stabilized liposomes. In in vivo models, it has been shown that anti-HER2 immunoliposomes are bound and internalized in HER2-overexpressing cells and result in intracellular drug delivery. There are strong preclinical bases to suggest that anti-HER2 liposomes might enhance the therapeutic index of selected chemotherapeutic agents against HER2-overexpressing cancers.

# REFERENCES

1. Yarden Y, Sliwkowski MX. Untangling the ErbB signalling network. Nat Rev Mol Cell Biol 2001; 2(2): 127–137.
2. Fendly BM, Winget M, Hudziak RM, Lipari MT, Napier MA, Ullrich A. Characterization of murine monoclonal antibodies reactive to either the human epidermal growth factor receptor or HER2/neu gene product. Cancer Res 1990; 50:1550–1558.
3. Ross J, Fletcher J, Linette G, et al. The Her-2/neu gene and protein in breast cancer 2003: biomarker and target of therapy. Oncologist 2003; 8(4):307–325.
4. Shepard HM, Lewis GD, Sarup JC, et al. Monoclonal antibody therapy of human cancer: taking the HER2 protooncogene to the clinic. J Clin Immunol 1991; 11(3):117–127.
5. Albanell J, Baselga J. The ErbB receptors as targets for breast cancer therapy. J Mamm Gland Biol Neoplasia 1999; 4(4):337–351.
6. Carter P, Presta L, Gorman CM, et al. Humanization of an anti-p185HER2 antibody for human cancer therapy. Proc Natl Acad Sci USA 1992; 89:4285–4289.
7. Cobleigh MA, Vogel CL, Tripathy D, et al. Multinational study of the eficacy and safety of human-ized anti-HER2 monoclonal antibody in women who have HER2-overexpressing metastatic breast cancer that has progressed after chemotherapy for metastatic disease. J Clin Oncol 2000; 17(9):2639–2648.
8. Slamon DJ, Leyland-Jones B, Shak S, et al. Use of chemotherapy plus a monoclonal antibody against HER2 for metastatic breast cancer that overexpresses HER2. N Engl J Med 2001; 344(11):783–792.
9. Sliwkowski MX, Schaefer G, Akita RW, et al. Coexpression of erbB2 and erbB3 proteins reconstitutes a high affinity receptor for heregulin. J Biol Chem 1994; 269(20):14,661–14,665.
10. Lewis GD, Lofgren JA, McMurtrey AE, et al. Growth regulation of human breast and ovarian tumor cells by heregulin: evidence for the requirement of ErbB2 as a critical component in mediating heregulin responsiveness. Cancer Res 1996; 56(6):1457–1465.
11. Pinkas-Kramarski R, Soussan L, Waterman H, et al. Diversification of Neu differentiation factor and epidermal growth factor signaling by combinatorial receptor interactions. EMBO J 1996; 15(10):2452–2467.
12. Graus-Porta D, Beerli RR, Daly JM, Hynes NE. ErbB-2, the preferred heterodimerization partner of all ErbB receptors, is a mediator of lateral signaling. EMBO J 1997; 16(7):1647–1655.
13. Agus D, Akita R, Fox W, et al. Targeting ligand-activated ErbB2 signaling inhibits breast and prostate tumor growth. Cancer Cell 2002; 2(2):127.
14. Agus D, Gordon M, Taylor C, et al. Clinical activity in a phase I trial of HER-2-targeted rhuMAb 2C4 (pertuzumab) in patients with advanced solid malignancies (AST). Proc ASCO 2003; 22 (abstract 771).
15. Carter P. Improving the efficacy of antibody-based cancer therapies. Nat Rev Cancer 2001; 1(2):118–129.
16. Lemmon MA, Schlessinger J. Regulation of signal transduction and signal diversity by receptor oligo-merization. Trends Biochem Sci 1994; 19:459–463.
17. Thor AD, Liu S, Edgerton S, et al. Activation (tyrosine phosphorylation) of ErbB-2 (HER-2/neu): a study of incidence and correlation with outcome in breast cancer. J Clin Oncol 2000; 18(18):3230–3239.
18. Samanta A, LeVea CM, Dougall WC, Qian X, Greene MI. Ligand and p185c-neu density govern receptor interactions and tyrosine kinase activation. Proc Natl Acad Sci USA 1994; 91(5):1711–1715.
19. Hudziak RM, Schlessinger J, Ullrich A. Increased expression of the putative growth factor receptor p185HER2 causes transformation and tumorigenesis of NIH3T3 cell. Proc Natl Acad Sci USA 1987; 84:7159–7163.
20. Katsumata M, Okudaira T, Samanta A, et al. Prevention of breast tumour development in vivo by down-regulation of the p185neu receptor. Nat Med 1995; 1(7):644–648.
21. Slamon DJ, Clark GM, Wong SG, Levin WJ, Ullrich A, McGuire WL. Human breast cancer: correla-tion of relapse and survival with amplification of the HER-2/neu oncogene. Science 1987; 235:177–182.
22. Ross J, Linette G, Stec J, et al. Breast cancer biomarkers and molecular medicine. Expert Rev Mol Diagn 2003; 3(5):573–585.
23. Salomon D, Brandt R, Ciardiello F, Normanno N. Epidermal growth factor-related peptides and their receptors in human malignancies. Crit Rev Oncol Hematol 1995; 19(3):183–232.
24. Karunagaran D, Tzahar E, Beerli RR, et al. ErbB-2 is a common auxiliary subunit of NDF and EGF receptors: implications for breast cancer. EMBO J 1996; 15(2):254–264.

25. Tzahar E, Pinkas-Kramarski R, Moyer JD, et al. Bivalence of EGF-like ligands drives the ErbB signaling network. EMBO J 1997; 16(16):4938–4950.

26. Klapper LN, Glathe S, Vaisman N, et al. The ErbB-2/HER2 oncoprotein of human carcinomas may function solely as a shared coreceptor for multiple stroma-derived growth factors. Proc Natl Acad Sci USA 1999; 96:4995–5000.

27. Klapper LN, Kirschbaum MH, Sela M, Yarden Y. Biochemical and clinical implications of ErbB/HR signaling network of growth factor receptors. Adv Cancer Res 1999:25–79.

28. Pinkas-Kramarski R, Alroy I, Yarden Y. ErbB receptors and EGF-like ligands: cell lineage determination through combinatorial signaling. J Mamm Gland Biol Neoplasia 1997; 2(2):97–108.

29. Lenferink AE, Pinkas-Kramarski R, van de Poll ML, et al. Differential endocytic routing of homo- and hetero-dimeric ErbB tyrosine kinases confers signaling superiority to receptor heterodimers. EMBO J 1998; 17(12):3385–3397.

30. Alimandi M, Romano A, Curia MC, et al. Cooperative signaling of ErbB3 and ErbB2 in neoplastic transformation and human mammary carcinomas. Oncogene 1995; 10(9):1813–1821.

31. Citri A, Skaria KB, Yarden Y. The deaf and the dumb: the biology of ErbB-2 and ErbB-3. Exp Cell Res 2003; 284(1):54–65.

32. Yarden Y. Biology of HER2 and its importance in breast cancer. Oncology 2001; 61(Suppl 2):1–13.

33. Gee JM, Robertson JF, Ellis IO, Nicholson RI. Phosphorylation of ERK1/2 mitogen-activated protein kinase is associated with poor response to anti-hormonal therapy and decreased patient survival in clinical breast cancer. Int J Cancer 2001; 95(4):247–254.

34. Albanell J, Codony-Servat J, Rojo F, et al. Activated extracellular signal-regulated kinases: association with epidermal growth factor receptor/transforming growth factor alpha expression in head and neck squamous carcinoma and inhibition by anti-epidermal growth factor receptor treatments. Cancer Res 2001; 61(17):6500–6510.

35. Cho HS, Mason K, Ramyar KX, et al. Structure of the extracellular region of HER2 alone and in complex with the Herceptin Fab. Nature 2003; 421(6924):756–760.

36. Lewis GD, Figari I, Fendly B, et al. Differential responses of human tumor cell lines to anti-p185HER2 monoclonal antibodies. Cancer Immunol Immunother 1993; 37(4):255–263.

37. Baselga J, Norton L, Albanell J, Kim YM, Mendelsohn J. Recombinant humanized anti-HER2 antibody (Herceptin) enhances the antitumor activity of paclitaxel and doxorubicin against HER2/neu overexpressing human breast cancer xenografts. Cancer Res 1998; 58(13):2825–2831.

38. Yakes FM, Chinratanalab W, Ritter CA, King W, Seelig S, Arteaga CL. Herceptin-induced inhibition of phosphatidylinositol-3 kinase and Akt Is required for antibody-mediated effects on p27, cyclin D1, and antitumor action. Cancer Res 2002; 62(14):4132–4141.

39. Drebin JA, Link VC, Stern DF, Weinberg RA, Greene MI. Down-modulation of an oncogene protein product and reversion of the transformed phenotype by monoclonal antibodies. Cell 1985; 41:695–706.

40. Klapper LN, Vaisman N, Hurwitz E, Pinkas-Kramarski R, Yarden Y, Sela M. A subclass of tumor-inhibitory monoclonal antibodies to ErbB-2/HER2 blocks crosstalk with growth factor receptors. Oncogene 1997; 14(17):2099–2109.

41. Sliwkowski MX, Lofgren JA, Lewis GD, Hotaling TE, Fendly BM, Fox J. Nonclinical studies addressing the mechanism of action of trastuzumab (Herceptin®). Semin Oncol 1999; 26(Suppl 12):60–70.

42. Molina MA, Codony-Servat J, Albanell J, Rojo F, Arribas J, Baselga J. Trastuzumab (herceptin), a humanized anti-Her2 receptor monoclonal antibody, inhibits basal and activated Her2 ectodomain cleavage in breast cancer cells. Cancer Res 2001; 61(12):4744–4749.

43. Albanell J, Codony J, Rovira A, Mellado B, Gascon P. Mechanism of action of anti-HER2 monoclonal antibodies: scientific update on trastuzumab and 2C4. Adv Exp Med Biol 2003; 532:253–268.

44. Codony-Servat J, Albanell J, Lopez-Talavera JC, Arribas J, Baselga J. Cleavage of the HER2 ectodomain is a pervanadate activable process that is inhibited by the tissue inhibitor of metalloproteases TIMP-1 in breast cancer cells. Cancer Res 1999; 59:1196–1201.

45. Christianson TA, Doherty JK, Lin YJ, et al. NH2-terminally truncated HER-2/neu protein: relationship with shedding of the extracellular domain and with prognostic factors in breast cancer. Cancer Res 1998; 15(58(22)):5123–5129.

46. Molina MA, Saez R, Ramsey EE, et al. NH(2)-terminal truncated HER-2 protein but not full-length receptor is associated with nodal metastasis in human breast cancer. Clin Cancer Res 2002; 8(2):347–353.

47. Anido J, Albanell J, Rojo F, Codony-Servat J, Arribas J, Baselga J. Inhibition by ZD1839 (Iressa) of epidermal growth factor (EGF) and heregulin Induced signaling pathways in human breast cancer cells. Proc Am Soc Clin Oncol 2001; 20:1712A.

48. Izumi Y, Xu L, di Tomaso E, Fukumura D, Jain RK. Tumour biology: herceptin acts as an anti-angio-genic cocktail. Nature 2002; 416(6878):279–280.

49. Clynes RA, Towers TL, Presta LG, Ravetch JV. Inhibitory Fc receptors modulate in vivo cytoxicity against tumor targets. Nat Med 2000; 6(4):443–446.

50. Pegram MD, Lopez A, Konecny G, Slamon DJ. Trastuzumab and chemotherapeutics: drug interactions and synergies. Semin Oncol 2000; 27(6 Suppl 11):21–25; discussion 92–100.

51. Pegram M, Hsu S, Lewis G, et al. Inhibitory effects of combinations of HER-2/neu antibody and chemo-therapeutic agents used for the treatment of human breast cancers. Oncogene 1999; 18(13):2241–2251.

52. Yu D, Jing T, Liu B, et al. Overexpression of ErbB2 blocks taxol-induced apoptosis by upregulation of $p21^{cip1}$, which inhibits $p34^{cdc2}$ kinase. Mol Cell 1998; 2:581–591.

53. Lee S, Yang W, Lan KH, et al. Enhanced Sensitization to taxol-induced apoptosis by Herceptin pre-treatment in ErbB2-overexpressing breast cancer cells. Cancer Res 2002; 62(20):5703–5710.

54. Vogel CL, Cobleigh MA, Tripathy D, et al. Efficacy and safety of trastuzumab as a single agent in first-line treatment of HER2-overexpressing metastatic breast cancer. J Clin Oncol 2002; 20(3):719–726.

55. Vogel CL, Franco SX. Clinical experience with trastuzumab (herceptin). Breast J 2003; 9(6):452–462.

56. Baselga J, Tripathy D, Mendelsohn J, et al. Phase II study of weekly intravenous recombinant human-ized anti-$p185^{HER2}$ monoclonal antibody in patients with HER2/neu-overexpressing metastatic breast cancer. J Clin Oncol 1996; 14:737–744.

57. Perez EA, Rodeheffer R. Clinical cardiac tolerability of trastuzumab. J Clin Oncol 2004; 22(2):322–329.

58. Seidman A, Hudis C, Pierri MK, et al. Cardiac dysfunction in the trastuzumab clinical trials experience. J Clin Oncol 2002; 20(5):1215–1221.

59. Ozcelik C, Erdmann B, Pilz B, et al. Conditional mutation of the ErbB2 (HER2) receptor in cardio-myocytes leads to dilated cardiomyopathy. Proc Natl Acad Sci USA 2002; 99(13):8880–8885.

60. Negro A, Brar BK, Lee KF. Essential roles of Her2/erbB2 in cardiac development and function. Recent Prog Horm Res 2004; 59:1–12.

61. Pegram MD. Docetaxel and Herceptin: foundation for future strategies. Oncologist 2001; 6(Suppl 3): 22–25.

62. Montemurro F, Choa G, Faggiuolo R, et al. A phase II study of three-weekly docetaxel and weekly trastuzumab in HER2-overexpressing advanced breast cancer. Oncology 2004; 66(1):38–45.

63. Raff JP, Rajdev L, Malik U, et al. Phase II study of weekly docetaxel alone or in combination with trastuzumab in patients with metastatic breast cancer. Clin Breast Cancer 2004; 4(6):420–427.

64. Tedesco KL, Thor AD, Johnson DH, et al. Docetaxel combined with trastuzumab is an active regimen in HER-2 3+ overexpressing and fluorescent in situ hybridization-positive metastatic breast cancer: a multi-institutional phase II trial. J Clin Oncol 2004; 22(6):1071–1077.

65. Montemurro F, Valabrega G, Aglietta M. Trastuzumab-based combination therapy for breast cancer. Expert Opin Pharmacother 2004; 5(1):81–96.

66. Extra J, Cognetti F, Maraninchi D, et al. Trastuzumab (Herceptin) plus docetaxel versus docetaxel alone as first-line treatment of HER2-positive metastatic breast cancer (MBC): results of a randomised multi-center trial. Eur J Cancer 2004; 2(Suppl):125 (abstract).

67. Nahta R, Esteva FJ. HER-2-targeted therapy: lessons learned and future directions. Clin Cancer Res 2003; 9(14):5078–5084.

68. Albanell J, Baselga J. Trastuzumab, a humanized anti-HER2 monoclonal antibody, for the treatment of breast cancer. Drugs Today (Barc) 1999; 35(12):931–946.

69. Mass R, Sanders C, Charlene K, Johnson L, Everett T, Anderson S. The concordance between the clinial trials assay and fluorescence in situ hybridization in the Herceptin pivotal trials. Proc Am Soc Clin Oncol 2000; 19:291 (abstract).

70. Mass R, Press M, Anderson S, Murphy M, Slamon D. Improved survival benefit from herceptin (trastuzu-mab) in patients selected by fluorescence in situ hybridization (FISH). Proc Am Soc Clin Oncol 2001: 85 (abstract).

71. Vogel C, Cobleigh M, Tripathy D, Mass R, Murphy M, Stewart SJ. Superior outcomes with Herceptin (trastuzumab) (H) in fluorescence in situ hybridization (FISH)-selected patients. Proc Am Soc Clin Oncol 2001: 86 (abstract).

72. Elkin EB, Weinstein MC, Winer EP, Kuntz KM, Schnitt SJ, Weeks JC. HER-2 testing and trastuzumab therapy for metastatic breast cancer: a cost-effectiveness analysis. J Clin Oncol 2004; 22(5):854–863.

73. Carbonell X, Castaneda-Soto N, Clemens M, et al. Efficacy and safety of 3-weekly herceptin (H) mono-therapy in women with HER2-positive metastatic breast cancer (MBC): preliminary data from a phase II study. Proc Am Soc Clin Oncol 2002 (abstract).

74. Cobleigh M, Frame D. Is trastuzumab every three weeks ready for prime time? J Clin Oncol 2003; 21 (21):3900–3901.

75. Leyland-Jones B, Gelmon K, Ayoub JP, et al. Pharmacokinetics, safety, and efficacy of trastuzumab administered every three weeks in combination with paclitaxel. J Clin Oncol 2003; 21(21):3965–3971.

76. Bell R. Ongoing trials with trastuzumab in metastatic breast cancer. Ann Oncol 2001; 12(Suppl 1): S69–S73.

77. Burris HA, 3rd. Docetaxel (Taxotere) plus trastuzumab (Herceptin) in breast cancer. Semin Oncol 2001; 28(1 Suppl 3):38–44.

78. Burstein HJ, Kuter I, Campos SM, et al. Clinical activity of trastuzumab and vinorelbine in women with HER2-overexpressing metastatic breast cancer. J Clin Oncol 2001; 19(10):2722–2730.

79. Fountzilas G, Tsavdaridis D, Kalogera-Fountzila A, et al. Weekly paclitaxel as first-line chemotherapy and trastuzumab in patients with advanced breast cancer. A Hellenic Cooperative Oncology Group phase II study. Ann Oncol 2001; 12(11):1545–1551.

80. Fujimoto-Ouchi K, Sekiguchi F, Tanaka Y. Antitumor activity of combinations of anti-HER-2 antibody trastuzumab and oral fluoropyrimidines capecitabine/5'-dFUrd in human breast cancer models. Cancer Chemother Pharmacol 2002; 49(3):211–216.

81. Hortobagyi GN. Overview of treatment results with trastuzumab (Herceptin) in metastatic breast cancer. Semin Oncol 2001; 28(6 Suppl 18):43–47.

82. Jahanzeb M, Mortimer JE, Yunus F, et al. Phase II trial of weekly vinorelbine and trastuzumab as first-line therapy in patients with HER2(+) metastatic breast cancer. Oncologist 2002; 7(5):410–417.

83. Crown J, Pegram M. Platinum–taxane combinations in metastatic breast cancer: an evolving role in the era of molecularly targeted therapy. Breast Cancer Res Treat 2003; 79(Suppl 1):S11–S18.

84. Miller KD, Sisk J, Ansari R, et al. Gemcitabine, paclitaxel, and trastuzumab in metastatic breast cancer. Oncology (Huntingt) 2001; 15(2 Suppl 3):38–40.

85. Bianchi G, Albanell J, Eiermann W, et al. Pilot trial of trastuzumab starting with or after the doxorubicin component of a doxorubicin plus paclitaxel regimen for women with HER2-positive advanced breast cancer. Clin Cancer Res 2003; 9(16 Pt 1):5944–5951.

86. Spigel DR, Burstein HJ. Trastuzumab regimens for HER2-overexpressing metastatic breast cancer. Clin Breast Cancer 2003; 4(5):329–337; discussion 38–39.

87. Tan AR, Swain SM. Ongoing adjuvant trials with trastuzumab in breast cancer. Semin Oncol 2003; 30 (5 Suppl 16):54–64.

88. Jones A. Combining trastuzumab (Herceptin) with hormonal therapy in breast cancer: what can be expected and why? Ann Oncol 2003; 14(12):1697–1704.

89. Argiris A, Wang CX, Whalen SG, DiGiovanna MP. Synergistic interactions between tamoxifen and trastuzumab (Herceptin). Clin Cancer Res 2004; 10(4):1409–1420.

90. Mann M, Sheng H, Shao J, et al. Targeting cyclooxygenase 2 and HER-2/neu pathways inhibits colorectal carcinoma growth. Gastroenterology 2001; 120(7):1713–1719.

91. Willett CG, Boucher Y, di Tomaso E, et al. Direct evidence that the VEGF-specific antibody bevacizumab has antivascular effects in human rectal cancer. Nat Med 2004; 10(2):145–147.

92. Moulder SL, Arteaga CL. A phase I/II trial of trastuzumab and gefitinib in patients with metastatic breast cancer that overexpresses HER2/neu (ErbB-2). Clin Breast Cancer 2003; 4(2):142–145.

93. Repka T, Chiorean EG, Gay J, et al. Trastuzumab and interleukin-2 in HER2-positive metastatic breast cancer: a pilot study. Clin Cancer Res 2003; 9(7):2440–2446.

94. Adams J, Palombella VJ, Sausville EA, et al. Proteasome inhibitors: a novel class of potent and effective antitumor agents. Cancer Res 1999; 59(11):2615–2622.

95. Tripathy D, Slamon DJ, Cobleigh M, et al. Safety of treatment of metastatic breast cancer with trastuzumab beyond disease progression. J Clin Oncol 2004; 22(6):1063–1070.

96. Langer CJ, Stephenson P, Thor A, Vangel M, Johnson DH. Trastuzumab in the treatment of advanced non-small-cell lung cancer: is there a role? Focus on Eastern Cooperative Oncology Group Study 2598. J Clin Oncol 2004; 22:1180–1187.

97. Rosell R. Toward customized trastuzumab in HER-2/neu-overexpressing non-small-cell lung cancers. J Clin Oncol 2004; 22:1171–1173.

98. Albanell J, Baselga J. Unraveling resistance to trastuzumab (Herceptin): insulin-like growth factor-I receptor, a new suspect. J Natl Cancer Inst 2001; 93(24):1830–1832.

99. Witton CJ, Reeves JR, Going JJ, Cooke TG, Bartlett JM, Pathol J. Expression of the HER1–4 family of receptor tyrosine kinases in breast cancer. J Pathol 2003; 200(3):290–297.

100. Lee H, Akita RW, Sliwkowski MX, Maihle NJ. A naturally occurring secreted human ErbB3 receptor isoform inhibits heregulin-stimulated activation of ErbB2, ErbB3, and ErbB4. Cancer Res 2001; 61(11): 4467–4473.

101. Mendoza N, Phillips GL, Silva J, Schwall R, Wickramasinghe D. Inhibition of ligand-mediated HER2 activation in androgen-independent prostate cancer. Cancer Res 2002; 62(19):5485–5488.

102. Toptal K, Balter I, Akita R, Bargiacchi F, Lewis G, Sliwkowski M. Targeting ErbB2/HER2's role as a coreceptor with rhuMAb2C4 inhibits ErbB/HER ligand-dependent signaling and proliferation of ovarian tumor cell lines. Proc Am Assoc Cancer Res 2003; 44 (abstract).

103. Jackson J, St Clair P, Sliwkowski M, Brattain M. Blockade of ErbB2 activation with the anti-ErbB2 monoclonal antibody 2C4 has divergent downstream signaling and growth effects following stimulation by epidermal growth factor or heregulin. Proc Am Assoc Cancer Res 2002; 43:4123a.

104. Liu J, Kern JA. Neuregulin-1 activates the JAK-STAT pathway and regulates lung epithelial cell proliferation. Am J Respir Cell Mol Biol 2002; 27(3):306–313.

105. Lewis-Phillips G, Totpal K, Kang K, Crocker L, Schwall R, Sliwkowski M. In vitro and in vivo efficacy of a novel HER2 antibody, rhuMAb 2C4, on human breast and lung tumor cells. Proc Am Assoc Cancer Res 2002; 43:3556a.

106. Friess T, Bauer S, Burger A, Fiebig H, Allison D, Müller H-J. In vivo activity of recombinant humanized monoclonal antibody 2C4 in xenografts is independent of tumor type and degree of HER2 overexpression. In: AACR-NCI-EORTC Meeting, 2002.

107. Totpal K, Lewis G, Balter I, Sliwkowski M. Augmentation of rhuMAb2C4 induced growth inhibition by TARCEVA™ the EGFR tyrosine kinase inhibitor on human breast cancer cell line. Proc Am Assoc Cancer Res 2002; 43:3889a.

108. Friess T, Scheuer W, Hasmann M. Combination treatment with erlotinib (Tarceva) and pertuzumab (Omnitarg) against different human xenografts is superior to monotherapy as measured by tumor growth and tumor serum markers. In: AACR–NCI–EORTC meeting, 2003: (abstract).

109. Friess T, Juchem R, Scheuer W, Hasmann M. Additive antitumor activity by combined treatment with recombinant humanized monoclonal antibody 2C4 and standard chemotherapeutic agents in NSCLC xenografts is independent of HER2 overexpression. Proc Am Soc Clin Oncol 2003; 22:238 (abstract).

110. Allison D, Malik M, Qureshi F, et al. Pharmacokinetics of HER2-targeted rhuMAb 2C4 (pertuzumab) in patients with advanced solid malignancies: phase Ia results. Proc Am Soc Clin Oncol 2003; 22:197 (abstract).

111. Bossenmaier B, Hasmann M, Koll H, Fiebig H, Akita R, Sliwkowski M. Presence of HER2/HER3 heterodimers predicts antitumor effects of pertuzumab (Omnitarg) in different human xenograft models. Proc Am Assoc Cancer Res 2004; 45:1232–1233 (abstract).

112. Palm S, Enmon RM Jr, Matei C, et al. Pharmacokinetics and biodistribution of (86)Y-trastuzumab for (90)Y dosimetry in an ovarian carcinoma model: correlative MicroPET and MRI. J Nucl Med 2003; 44(7):1148–1155.

113. Schwall R, Dugger D, Erickson. SL, et al. Potent preclinical efficacy of Herceptin–DM1 against HER-2-overexpressing breast tumors in vivo. Clin Cancer Res 2001; 7:3784s (abstract).

114. Pullarkat V, Deo Y, Link J, et al. A phase I study of a HER2/neu bispecific antibody with granulocyte-colony-stimulating factor in patients with metastatic breast cancer that overexpresses HER2/neu. Cancer Immunol Immunother 1999; 48(1):9–21.

115. Keler T, Graziano RF, Mandal A, et al. Bispecific antibody-dependent cellular cytotoxicity of HER2/neu-overexpressing tumor cells by Fc gamma receptor type I-expressing effector cells. Cancer Res 1997; 57 (18):4008–4014.

116. Posey JA, Raspet R, Verma U, et al. A pilot trial of GM-CSF and MDX-H210 in patients with erbB-2-positive advanced malignancies. J Immunother 1999; 22(4):371–339.

117. Schwaab T, Lewis LD, Cole BF, et al. Phase I pilot trial of the bispecific antibody MDXH210 (anti-Fc gamma RI X anti-HER-2/neu) in patients whose prostate cancer overexpresses HER-2/neu. J Immunother 2001; 24(1):79–87.

118. Wallace PK, Kaufman PA, Lewis LD, et al. Bispecific antibody-targeted phagocytosis of HER-2/neu expressing tumor cells by myeloid cells activated in vivo. J Immunol Methods 2001; 248(1–2):167–182.

119. James ND, Atherton PJ, Jones J, Howie AJ, Tchekmedyian S, Curnow RT. A phase II study of the bispecific antibody MDX-H210 (anti-HER2 × CD64) with GM-CSF in HER2+ advanced prostate cancer. Br J Cancer 2001; 85(2):152–156.

120. Lewis LD, Beelen AP, Cole BF, et al. The pharmacokinetics of the bispecific antibody MDX-H210 when combined with interferon gamma-1b in a multiple-dose phase I study in patients with advanced cancer. Cancer Chemother Pharmacol 2002; 49(5):375–384.
121. Repp R, van Ojik HH, Valerius T, et al. Phase I clinical trial of the bispecific antibody MDX-H210 (anti-FcgammaRI x anti-HER-2/neu) in combination with Filgrastim (G-CSF) for treatment of advanced breast cancer. Br J Cancer 2003; 89(12):2234–2243.
122. Park JW, Hong K, Kirpotin DB, et al. Anti-HER2 immunoliposomes: enhanced efficacy attributable to targeted delivery. Clin Cancer Res 2002; 8(4):1172–1181.
123. Park JW, Kirpotin DB, Hong K, et al. Tumor targeting using anti-HER2 immunoliposomes. J Control Release 2001; 74(1-3):95–113.

# 41 From XenoMouse® Technology to Panitumumab (ABX-EGF)

*Xiaodong Yang, MD, PhD, Lorin Roskos, PhD, C. Geoffrey Davis, PhD, and Gisela Schwab, MD*

## CONTENTS

SUMMARY

Recent success of antibody therapeutics in oncology has revived a keen interest in the development of monoclonal antibodies (mAbs) for the treatment of cancer. To date, eight mAbs have been approved in the United States for the treatment of hematological malignancies or solid tumors. The increased success has been largely attributed to advances in antibody technology such as chimerization and humanization of mAbs and the development of fully human antibodies allowing for reduction in immunogenicity and creation of antibodies of desired affinity and isotype. XenoMouse® technology is a technology that allows for the generation of fully human mAbs in transgenic mice. Using this technology, the anti-epidermal growth factor receptor (EGFR) antibody, panitumumab, has been created.

Panitumumab (ABX-EGF) is a fully human IgG2 anti-EGFR mAb. Panitumumab binds EGFR with high affinity, inhibits ligand-dependent receptor activation, and effectively inhibits the growth of multiple human tumor xenografts in mouse models. To date, in phase 1 and phase 2 clinical studies, panitumumab has been generally well tolerated, exhibited no immunogenicity, and demonstrated low interpatient and intrapatient pharmacokinetic variability. Objective responses have been observed in patients with metastatic colorectal cancer and advanced renal cell carcinoma.

**Key Words:** Panitumumab; ABX-EGF; EGFR; mAb; cancer; XenoMouse; targeted therapy; IgG2.

From: *Cancer Drug Discovery and Development: The Oncogenomics Handbook*
Edited by: W. J. LaRochelle and R. A. Shimkets © Humana Press Inc., Totowa, NJ

# 1. INTRODUCTION

More than a quarter century after the discovery of monoclonal antibodies (mAbs) by Kohler and Milstein, the therapeutic utility of mAbs is now being realized *(1)*. MAbs have been approved as effective therapies for the treatment of human diseases, including cancer. The therapeutic potential of mAbs mainly stems from their specific and high-affinity binding to targets coupled with their diversity of effector function. The first generation of mAb products was of murine origin. These antibodies have had limited therapeutic utility primarily because of their inherent immunogenicity in humans. Patients who received murine mAbs rapidly developed an immune response to the mouse protein, known as human anti-mouse antibody (HAMA) response *(2,3)*. HAMA responses can lead to reduced potency and efficacy of the mAb by enhancing its clearance rate and might cause a safety risk, including allergies and anaphylaxis, with repeated administrations.

Considerable efforts have been expended to advance and improve antibody technology. One major effort has focused on reducing the immunogenicity by making murine antibodies more humanlike. With relatively simple antibody engineering techniques, murine antibodies can be chimerized by linking the murine antibody variable region to human constant regions. This results in a "chimeric" antibody *(4)*. Two of the eight mAbs now approved for oncology indications, rituximab (Rituxan, anti-CD20 mAb) and cetuximab (Erbitux, anti-EGFR mAb), are chimeric antibodies *(5–7)*. Chimeric mAbs retain approx 34% of murine protein sequences. With more sophisticated recombinant DNA techniques, the actual antigen-binding pocket of the murine antibody can be "implanted" into the framework of the human antibody constant region by inserting the murine antibody complementarity determining regions (CDRs) sequences into the human variable gene framework. Such "humanized" mAbs retain as little as 5% of murine protein sequences *(8)*. Trastuzumab (Herceptin, the anti-ErbB2 mAb) and bevacizumab (Avastin, anti-vascular endothelial cell growth factor [VEGF] mAb) are humanized mAbs *(9,10)*. Chimeric and humanized mAbs have improved therapeutic utility and markedly reduced immunogenicity compared with murine mAbs, but they might still be immunogenic and allergenic in a portion of patients *(11–14)*. With further advances in antibody technology, the generation of fully human mAbs has now become a reality. Two major approaches are now readily available to make fully human mAbs. One approach is to apply display technologies using phage, ribosomes, or yeast that display human antibody variable regions on the surface as a tool to screen and generate human mAbs *(15)*. Alternatively, transgenic mice that have been genetically engineered to produce human antibody have been developed. The XenoMouse® technology represents a success of the transgenic mouse approach.

XenoMouse mice are genetically engineered mice in which the genes encoding the murine endogenous antibody have been functionally replaced by the genes encoding human antibody counterparts (Fig. 1). XenoMouse mice carry the majority of the human antibody variable region repertoire and can undergo class switching from IgM to IgG isotypes as well as somatic hypermutation and affinity maturation. This supports the formation of broad and diverse primary and secondary antibody responses upon immunization with human antigens. Thus, XenoMouse mice offer a powerful platform technology for the rapid generation of therapeutic mAbs *(16)*. Using this technology, fully human mAbs against cancer targets have been developed and shown to have antitumor activity. This has been exemplified by the development of panitumumab, a fully human mAb against EGFR.

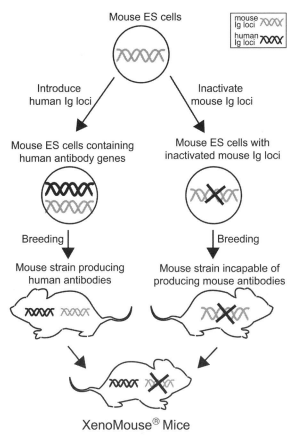

**Fig. 1.** Creation of XenoMouse mice. The endogenous mouse immunoglobulin (Ig) heavy-chain and kappa light-chain loci were inactivated in mouse embryonic stem (ES) cells using gene-targeting technology to remove the JH genes and the JK region genes. In parallel, the majority of the human heavy, kappa and lambda light-chain loci were cloned into yeast artificial chromosomes, which were then used to generate transgenic mice. Thus, in XenoMouse mice, the mouse antibody genes are functionally replaced by human antibody genes.

Epidermal growth factor receptor is a 170-kDa, type I transmembrane glycoprotein and a receptor tyrosine kinase. EGFR is a member of the ErbB receptor family comprised of ErbB1 or EGFR, ErbB2 (HER2/neu), ErbB3 (HER3), and ErbB4 (HER4). EGFR can be activated through a series of events initiated by binding to its ligands, epidermal growth factor (EGF) and transforming growth factor-α (TGF-α). Ligand binding induces receptor dimerization, which, in turn, activates receptor tyrosine kinase activity and induces EGFR tyrosine autophosphorylation. Activation of EGFR triggers a cascade of downstream signaling pathways that mediate a variety of cellular responses, including cell proliferation, differentiation, survival, motility, adhesion, and repair *(17)*. Two major pathways are involved in EGFR-mediated signaling. Activation of Ras following EGFR tyrosine phosphorylation initiates a multistep phosphorylation event, leading to the activation of mitogen-activating protein kinases (MAPKs), ERK1 and ERK2. ERK1 and ERK2 control and regulate transcription of molecules that are involved in cell transformation, proliferation,

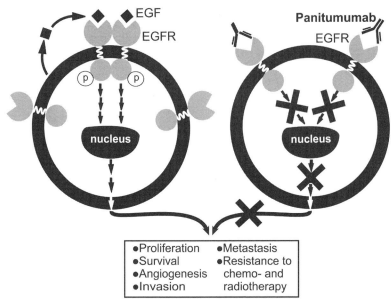

**Fig. 2.** Targeting EGFR as an anticancer therapy with panitumumab. Panitumumab binds to the EGFR with high affinity and blocks ligand binding. The blockade of ligand binding by panitumumab inhibits EGFR tyrosine phosphorylation, tumor growth, and metastasis. p, phosphorylation.

and survival *(18)*. Another important signaling route is phosphatidylinositol-3-kinase (PI3K) and the downstream protein–serine/threonine kinase Akt. Akt transduces intracellular signals that are linked to cell survival, proliferation, and motility *(19,20)*. In tumor cells, EGFR activation and its signaling pathway are often deregulated, which leads to malignant transformation, growth, angiogenesis, invasion and metastasis, and resistance to chemotherapy and radiotherapy (Fig. 2) *(17)*.

The rationale for targeting EGFR as an anticancer therapy is threefold. First, EGFR is frequently overexpressed in many human epithelial carcinomas, including colorectal cancer, ovarian carcinoma, prostate cancer, and cancers of the breast, lung, head and neck, bladder, and kidney *(21–23)*. Second, studies have shown that increased EGFR expression in tumors correlates with poor clinical prognosis and outcome *(24)*. Third, overexpression of the receptor is often associated with increased production of ligands—in particular TGF-α—by the same tumor cells *(25)*. This establishes an autocrine regulatory loop that stimulates EGFR and amplifies its signaling pathway.

Several potential strategies for targeting EGFR as a cancer therapy have been devised and implemented. These include mAbs that block ligand binding and receptor signaling *(6,26)*, mAbs conjugated with radionuclides, toxin, or prodrugs as tumor-targeting agents *(27)*, and small-molecule tyrosine kinase inhibitors (TKis) that inhibit receptor tyrosine kinase activity *(28,29)*.

Both mAbs and small molecule TKis are at the most advanced development stages. The recent approvals of gefinitib (Iressa, EGFR TKi), for the treatment of patients with locally advanced or metastatic non-small-cell lung cancer after failure of both platinum-based and docetaxel chemotherapies, and of cetuximab (Erbitux, mAb against EGFR), as monotherapy or in combination with irinotecan for the treatment of EGFR-expressing, metastatic colorectal carcinoma in patients who are refractory to irinotecan-based chemotherapy, have further validated targeting the EGFR in human cancer therapy *(30,31)*.

Panitumumab is a fully human IgG2κ mAb that binds EGFR with high affinity ($K_d$ = 50 p*M*) *(26)*. It blocks EGFR binding to its ligands EGF and TGF-α, and it inhibits EGF-induced EGFR tyrosine phosphorylation and tumor cell proliferation in vitro (Fig. 2). In vivo studies demonstrated that panitumumab not only inhibited tumor growth but also eradicated large established tumors in xenograft models *(26,32)*. Panitumumab is currently being studied in multiple phase II clinical trials for the treatment of metastatic colorectal carcinoma, advanced renal cell carcinoma, and non-small-cell lung cancer. Pivotal trials for evaluation of efficacy of panitumumab in patients with advanced metastatic colorectal cancer have been initiated.

In this chapter, we describe the origin and properties of XenoMouse technology and the development of panitumumab using this technology. A discussion of the panitumumab preclinical and clinical data follows.

## 2. DEVELOPMENT OF XENOMOUSE TECHNOLOGY

The first step toward the creation of the XenoMouse animals that produce human antibodies was to inactivate the endogenous mouse antibody genes. This was achieved through the use of gene-targeting technology to knock out specific segments of the mouse immunoglobulin (Ig) heavy-chain and light-chain loci; the J regions of the mouse heavy-chain and of the mouse κ light-chain loci were deleted. Consequently, the double-deleted mouse strains exhibited arrested B-cell development and lack of mouse antibody responses and provided a genetic background for introduction of the human Ig transgenes *(33,34)*.

The more challenging steps were to clone the germline human Ig heavy-chain and kappa light chain loci onto yeast artificial chromosomes (YACs) and introduce the human Ig genes carried on YACs into the mouse genome. Retaining as much of the complexity of the human antibody loci as possible was critically important for ensuring that XenoMouse mice could produce a broad and diverse repertoire of antibodies that recognize a wide spectrum of human antigens. This was accomplished by cloning large segments of the human Ig loci in their germline configuration into YACs. Next, the human Ig loci on YACs were successfully introduced and integrated into the mouse genome by fusing the yeast spheroplasts with mouse embryonic stem (ES) cells *(35,36)*. XenoMouse animals were thereafter created by successive breeding of human-Ig YAC-bearing transgenic mice against the double-deleted genetic background (Fig. 1). Consequently, the XenoMouse animals possess, on the heavy-chain locus, 34 functional V genes, all of the D genes, all of the J genes, and the downstream Cμ, Cδ, and appropriate Cγ constant region genes. On the kappa light-chain locus, the XenoMouse animals possess 18 functional V genes, all of the J genes, as well as the Cκ constant region gene *(36)*. The human heavy-chain locus undergoes normal class switch in XenoMouse mice. Multiple strains of XenoMouse mice that are constrained to class switching from IgM to either IgG1, IgG2, or IgG4 were developed. The available selection of IgG subclasses depends on the strain of mouse. This facilitates the selection and generation of mAbs with a preferred isotype. Interestingly, the human antibody genes introduced in the mouse germline appear to be fully compatible with the mouse recombination machinery that controls and regulates both class switching and somatic hypermutation. Thus, the XenoMouse animals show a diverse, human adultlike antibody repertoire with CDR3 regions of a length more like human than mouse *(37)*. Recently, the XenoMouse strains have been further improved by introduction of the entire human Ig lambda light-chain locus on a YAC transgene to increase their antibody repertoire. As a result of these manipulations, it is possible to consistently derive human mAbs from XenoMouse mice that contain kappa and lambda light chains that are of low nanomolar or subnanomolar affinity *(38)*.

## 3. THERAPEUTIC POTENTIAL OF PANITUMUMAB

### 3.1. Discovery of Panitumumab

To develop a fully human anti-EGFR mAb, XenoMouse–IgG2 mice were immunized with human epidermoid cervical carcinoma A431 cells that express over one million copies of EGFR per cell on the cell surface. An IgG2 isotype was chosen to avoid potential toxicity resulting from recruitment of antibody effector functions such as antibody-dependent cell-mediated cytotoxicity (ADCC) and complement-dependent cytotoxicity (CDC) to normal tissues that express EGFR. The mice were immunized intraperitoneally or subcutaneously with A431 cells in complete Freund's adjuvant and boosted with three to five additional injections of the same cells in incomplete Freund's adjuvant. Using standard hybridoma technology, the spleen or lymph node cells from immunized mice were fused with myeloma cells. The resulting hybridomas producing specific antibodies were selected through screening by enzyme-linked immunosorbent assay (ELISA).

Out of 22 XenoMouse mice immunized, a panel of 70 EGFR-specific antibodies was identified. Thirty-eight antibodies were evaluated for their neutralization activity and 15 out of the 38 mAbs blocked binding of EGF to the receptor *(39)*. DNA sequence analysis of the transcripts encoding the eight neutralizing antibodies revealed striking similarities in their heavy-chain V gene usage (either VH4-31 or VH4-61), kappa light-chain gene usage (utilization of the Vκ 018 gene by 7/8 mAbs), and an aspartate residue mutation in CDR1 of the heavy chain suggesting a highly stringent structural requirement for these antibodies to bind EGFR with high affinity and effectively block ligand binding. The antibody clone E7.6.3 was chosen as panitumumab primarily based on its high potency as well as its superior productivity in serum-free medium *(26,39,41)*.

### 3.2. Preclinical Development of Panitumumab

Panitumumab has been evaluated in an extensive series of in vitro assays and in vivo human tumor xenograft models. Panitumumab causes cell cycle arrest at the G0/G1 interphase in vitro and inhibits tumor colony formation *(40)*. Upon binding to the receptor, panitumumab is rapidly internalized, resulting in a,marked downregulation of cell surface EGFR in A431 cells *(40,41)*. When the effect on EGFR signaling was evaluated, panitumumab was found to inhibit EGF-induced EGFR tyrosine phosphorylation. Panitumumab also inhibited proliferation of A431 cells and of the breast cancer cell line MDA-468 in vitro *(26)*. The fact that no exogenous EGF was added to the culture suggests that panitumumab blocks autocrine growth stimulation and thus inhibits EGF/TGF-α-mediated tumor activation and proliferation. Interestingly, treatment of the prostate cancer cell line DU145 with panitumumab in vitro resulted in inhibition of VEGF and interleukin-8 production, suggesting that the antitumor activity of panitumumab could also result from indirect inhibition of tumor angiogenesis *(42,43)*.

Panitumumab was able to prevent the formation of A431 tumor xenografts in vivo and was similarly effective in established A431 tumor xenografts, producing complete eradication of tumors as large as 1.2 cm$^3$. These effects were long lasting (no recurring tumors detected with more than 8 mo of follow-up) and dose dependent (26). Complete tumor eradication in these animals could result from the fact that panitumumab is able to penetrate the tumor mass and saturate EGFR expressed in the tumor tissue in a time- and dose-dependent fashion (44). Moreover, panitumumab therapy in combination with chemotherapeutic agents such as doxorubicin demonstrated additive antitumor activity in the A431 tumor model (45). In addition to inhibiting tumor cell proliferation, panitumumab showed inhibitory activity on tumor development and was able to prevent metastasis of human breast cancer MDA-231 cells in a severe combined immunodeficient (SCID) mouse model (46).

Using xenograft models, the antitumor effect of panitumumab was also observed in multiple human tumors derived from different tissues expressing various levels of EGFR. These include tumors from breast (MDA-468), kidney (SK-RC-29), pancreas (BxPC-3, and HS766T), prostate (PC3), ovary (IGROVI), and colon (HT-29). These data suggest that panitumumab could inhibit the growth of not only the tumors that express extremely high EGFR levels, such as A431 ($1.2 \times 10^6$ receptors per cell) and MDA-MB-468 ($1.6 \times 10^6$ receptors per cell), but also other human carcinomas that express lower EGFR levels such as HS766T ($17 \times 10^3$ receptors per cell) and HT-29 ($9 \times 10^3$ receptors per cell) (47).

As a result of its effects on the EGFR and the downstream cellular functions, panitumumab might exert its antitumor activity by a number of different mechanisms. This could involve the downregulation of EGFR expression by induction of receptor internalization, inhibition of proliferation by blocking EGFR signaling pathways and induction of cell cycle arrest, and inhibition of angiogenesis (32). Finally, the antibody effector functions, namely ADCC and CDC, are unlikely to account for its antitumor effects because panitumumab is human IgG2, an isotype that essentially lacks effector functions.

### 3.3. Clinical Development of Panitumumab

Currently available clinical data from phase I and II studies evaluating single-agent therapy with panitumumab are described. In aggregate, available data suggest that panitumumab is generally well tolerated, does not require routine premedication, and is associated with a low incidence of infusion-related reactions (< 1%). Pharmacokinetic variability is low and no HAHA development has been observed in the patients tested to date. Antitumor activity has been observed in patients with solid tumors, specifically in patients with advanced renal cell carcinoma and colorectal cancer.

A multicenter phase I clinical trial was conducted in patients with EGFR-positive cancers to evaluate the safety, pharmacokinetics, and clinical effect of panitumumab. This was a monotherapy, open-label, and dose-escalating clinical trial in patients with late-stage renal cell, prostate, non-small-cell lung, pancreatic, colorectal, or gastroesophageal cancers, who had relapsed or progressed on standard antitumor therapy for their malignancy. All patients were prescreened for EGFR expression in their tumor tissues using immunohistochemistry. The EGFR detection in tumor tissues had to display the following staining characteristics: 2+ or 3+ in ≥10% of evaluated tumor cells. A central laboratory using a validated EGFR immunohistochemistry kit developed by DAKO Cytomation Corporation determined the levels of EGFR expression in patient tumor samples.

At an interim analysis, 43 patients were enrolled in this phase I trial with cancer types including renal ($n = 10$), prostate ($n = 13$), non-small-cell lung ($n = 7$), pancreatic ($n = 3$), gastroesophageal ($n = 3$), and colorectal ($n = 7$) cancer. Cohorts of patients received four intravenous panitumumab infusions with doses ascending per cohort ranging from 0.01 to 2.5 mg/kg once weekly *(32)*. Clinical responses were evaluated 4 wk after the fourth dose of panitumumab and patients were followed for safety evaluation for an additional 5 wk after the fourth panitumumab dose. Panitumumab was well tolerated with low pharmacokinetic variability. No HAHA formation was detected. Transient acneiform skin rash was the main toxicity thought to be related to panitumumab. All patients who received at least one dose of 2.0 or 2.5 mg/kg developed NCI CTC version 2.0, grade $\geq 1$ skin rashes. Biological activity of panitumumab was seen in several patients with responsive or stable disease observed at wk 8 following initiation of treatment. One patient with gastroesophageal cancer (0.1-mg/kg dose level) had stable disease for 7 mo; one patient with prostate cancer (0.75-mg/kg dose level) had a minor response lasting for 6 mo, with three or four lesions regressing 38% to 76% and prostate-specific antigen (PSA) levels decreasing by 60%; one patient with colorectal cancer (1.5-mg/kg dose level) had stable disease for 4 mo; and another colorectal cancer patient (2.5-mg/kg dose level) had a partial response *(48)*.

Several phase II trials have been initiated on the basis of these phase I data in multiple tumor types that are known to express EGFR and results from two phase II studies evaluating panitumumab monotherapy in patients with advanced renal cell cancer and colorectal cancer are summarized next.

Panitumumab is being evaluated in a two-part phase II trial in patients with metastatic renal cell carcinomas who had failed or were unable to tolerate previous therapy with IL-2 or interferon. Data from part 1 of this phase II monotherapy trial have been reported *(49, 50)*. Eighty-eight patients received at least one dose of panitumumab at 1.0 mg/kg (22 patients), 1.5 mg/kg (22 patients), 2.0 mg/kg (23 patients), or 2.5 mg/kg (21 patients). EGFR expression was documented by immunohistochemistry in 91% of available tumor samples. The majority of patients had received one or more prior regimens of systemic tumor therapy, with 56% having received one or two and 33% of patients having received three or more prior regimens. Only 11% of patients had received no prior biotherapy or chemotherapy. Tumor response was assessed at the end of the first 8-wk treatment period and responses were confirmed 4 wk later. Three partial responses (one each from the 1.0-, 1.5-, and 2.5-mg/kg dose levels) and two minor responses (one each from the 1.0- and 2.5-mg/kg dose levels) were observed. One of the patients showing a partial response in his lung metastases had a stable primary tumor. Fifty percent of patients had stable disease at the end of the first 8-wk treatment period. Similar to the phase I study, a transient acneiform skin rash was the primary drug-related toxicity, observed in 70%, 91%, 95%, or 100% of patients treated with at least three doses of panitumumab at the 1.0-, 1.5-, 2.0-, or 2.5-mg/kg dose levels, respectively. Asthenia, abdominal pain, back pain, constipation, cough, and dyspnea occurred in a dose-independent fashion *(49,50)*. No HAHA responses have been detected in patients treated with panitumumab to date, consistent with low intrapatient variability of panitumumab exposure. Pharmacokinetic analysis showed that EGFR-mediated clearance of panitumumab was saturated at doses greater than 2 mg/kg. Serum trough panitumumab concentrations at the dose of 2.5 mg/kg exceeded serum panitumumab concentrations that resulted in regression of A431 tumors in xenograft models *(51)*. Interestingly, similar to the phase I study, a 100% skin rash incidence was also observed at the 2.5-mg/kg/wk dose level, supporting saturation of EGFR at this dose level.

A multi-institutional phase II study of panitumumab monotherapy in patients with advanced metastatic colorectal cancer has been conducted, and interim results were reported by Meropol et al. *(52)*. This study included patients with EGFR-expressing colorectal cancer who had failed prior therapy with fluorouracil (with or without leucovorin) and either irinotecan or oxaliplatin, or both. Panitumumab was administered at a dose of 2.5 mg/kg given by intravenous infusion weekly in 8-wk treatment cycles. Assessment of tumor response was performed at the end of the first 8-wk treatment cycle. Patients with responding or stable disease were eligible for continued panitumumab treatment for up to five additional cycles or until disease progression, whichever occurred first. The interim analysis of the study evaluating the response rate at wk 8 of cycle 1 of the first 44 patient enrolled in the study indicated that approx 9% of patients (intent-to-treat analysis) or 10% of efficacy evaluable patients (defined as having received at least 5 of the first 8 planned doses of panitumumab) exhibited partial responses to panitumumab. Stable disease was observed in approx 55% of patients enrolled in the study *(52)*. Additionally, panitumumab was generally well tolerated in this study, with a similar adverse event profile as described earlier. The most frequently reported adverse event was a reversible acneiform or maculopapular skin rash observed in all patients. Adverse events reported in ≥25% of patients included fatigue, nausea, abdominal pain, diarrhea, vomiting, and constipation.

Other phase II studies are in progress to further evaluate the safety and efficacy of panitumumab.

## 4. CONCLUSION

MAb treatment has become an important therapeutic modality for cancer. The increased success of mAbs in human therapy has largely resulted from advances in antibody technology. The availability of fully human mAbs to human antigens could further advance the use of therapeutic mAbs in the clinic. Fully human antibodies allow repeated administrations with little risk of immunogenic or allergic responses and thus increase their safety for use in chronic disease as well as many malignant diseases.

The XenoMouse-derived fully human anti-EGFR mAb panitumumab has demonstrated attractive preclinical characteristics with high binding affinity and effective inactivation of EGFR in vitro, along with promising preclinical efficacy data in vivo. Panitumumab has exhibited favorable safety and pharmacokinetic profiles. Preliminary data from phase I and phase II studies in patients with metastatic colorectal cancer and advanced renal cell carcinoma show encouraging antitumor activity. These data provided the basis for initiation of pivotal studies evaluating the efficacy and safety of panitumumab in patients with advanced metastatic colorectal cancer who have developed progressive disease or relapsed while on or after prior fluoropyrimidine, irinotecan, and oxaliplatin chemotherapy.

## ACKNOWLEDGMENTS

Development of panitumumab is jointly sponsored by Amgen, Inc. and Abgenix, Inc.

## REFERENCES

1. Kohler G, Milstein C. Continuous cultures of fused cells secreting antibody of predefined specificity. Nature 1975; 256:495–497.
2. Dillman RO. Human antimouse and antiglobulin responses to monoclonal antibodies. Antibody Immunocon Radiopharm 1990; 3:1–15.
3. Isaacs JD. The antiglobulin response to therapeutic antibodies. Semin Immunol 1990; 2:449–456.

4. Morrison S, Oi VT. Chimeric immunoglobulin genes. In: Hongo T, Alt FW, Rabbitts TH (eds.). Immuno-globulin genes. London: Academic, 1989:260–274.

5. Grillo-Lopez AJ, White CA, Varns C, Shen D, Wei A, McClure A, et al. Overview of the clinical development of rituximab: first monoclonal antibody approved for the treatment of lymphoma. Semin Oncol 1999; 26(5 Suppl 14):66–73.

6. Baselga J. The EGFR as a target for anticancer therapy-focus on cetuximab. Eur J Cancer 2001; 37(Suppl 4):S16–S22.

7. Herbst RS, Shin DM. Monoclonal antibodies to target epidermal growth factor receptor-positive tumors: a new paradigm for cancer therapy. Cancer 2002; 94:1593–1611.

8. Riechmann L, Clark M, Waldmann H, Winter G. Reshaping human antibodies for therapy. Nature 1988; 332:323–327.

9. Baselga J. Clinical trials of Herceptin (trastuzumab). Eur J Cancer 2001; 37(Suppl 1):S18–S24.

10. Miller KD, Rugo HS, Cobleigh MA, Marcom PK, Chap LI, et al. Phase III trial of capecitabine (Xeloda®) plus bevacizumab (Avastin®) versus capecitabine alone in women with metastatic breast cancer (MBC) previously treated with an anthracycline and a taxane. In: 26th Annual San Antonio Breast Cancer Symposium 2002; 12:11.

11. Robert F, Ezekiel MP, Spencer SA, et al. Phase I study of anti-epidermal growth factor receptor antibody cetuximab in combination with radiation therapy in patients with advanced head and neck cancer. J Clin Oncol 2001; 19:3234–3243.

12. Scott AM, Wiseman G, Welt S, Adjei A, Lee FT, et al. A phase I dose-escalation study of sibrotuzumab in patients with advanced or metastatic fibroblast activation protein-positive cancer. Clin Cancer Res 2003; 9:1639–1647.

13. Weinblatt ME, Maddison PJ, Bulpitt KJ, Hazleman BL, Urowitz MB, Sturrock RD, et al. Campath-1H, a humanized monoclonal antibody, in refractory rheumatoid arthritis. An intravenous dose-escalation study. Arthritis Rheum 1995; 38:1589–1594.

14. Welt S, Ritter G, Williams C Jr, Cohen LS, John M, Jungbluth A, et al. Phase I study of anticolon cancer humanized antibody A33. Clin Cancer Res 2003; 9:1338–1346.

15. Kretzschmar T, von Ruden T. Antibody discovery: phage display. Curr Opin Biotechnol 2002; 3:598–602.

16. Green L. Antibody engineering via genetic engineering of the mouse: XenoMouse strains are vehicles for the facile generation of therapeutic human monoclonal antibodies. J Immunol Methods 1999; 231:11–23.

17. Yarden Y, Sliwkowski M. Untangling the ErbB signaling network. Nat Rev Mol Cell Biol 2001; 2: 127–137.

18. Lewis TS, Shapiro PS, Ahn NG. Signal transduction through MAP kinase cascades. Adv Cancer Res 1998; 74:49–139.

19. Chan TO, Rittenhouse SE, Tisichlis PN. AKT/PKB and D3 phosphinositide-regulated kinases: kinase activation by phosphoinositide-dependent phosphorylation. Annu Rev Biochem 1999; 68:965–1014.

20. Vivanco I, Sawyers CL. The phosphatidylinositol 3-kinase-Akt pathway in human cancer. Nat Rev Cancer 2002; 2:489–501.

21. Modjtahedi H, Dean C. The receptor for EGF and its ligands: expression, prognostic value and target for therapy in cancer. Intl J Oncol 1994; 4:277–296.

22. Gullick WJ. Prevalence of aberrant expression of the epidermal growth factor receptor in human cancers. Br Med Bull 1991; 47:87–98.

23. Salomon DS, Brandt R, Ciardiello F, Normanno N. Epidermal growth factor-related peptides and their receptors in human malignancies. Crit Rev Oncol Hematol 1995; 19:183–232.

24. Neal DE, Marsh C, Bennett MK, et al. Epidermal-growth-factor receptors in human bladder cancer: comparison of invasive and superficial tumours. Lancet 1985; 1:366–368.

25. Di Marco E, Pierce JH, Fleming TP, et al. Autocrine interaction between TGF alpha and the EGF-receptor: quantitative requirements for induction of the malignant phenotype. Oncogene 1989; 4:831–838.

26. Yang XD, Jia XC, Corvalan JR, Wang P, Davis C, Jakobovits A. Eradication of established tumors by a fully human monoclonal antibody to the epidermal growth factor receptor without concomitant chemotherapy. Cancer Res 1999; 59:1236–1243.

27. Azemar M, Scmidt M, Arlt F, et al. Recombinant antibody toxins specific for ErbB2 and EGF receptor inhibit the in vivo growth of human head and neck cancer cells and cause rapid regression in vivo. Int J Cancer 2000; 86:269–275.

28. Ciardiello F, Caputo R, Bianco R, et al. Inhibition of growth factor production and angiogenesis in human cancer cells by ZD1839 ('Iressa'), a selective epidermal growth factor receptor tyrosine kinase inhibitor. Clin Cancer Res 2001; 7:1459–1465.

29. Hightower M. Erlotinib (OSI-774, Tarceva), a selective epidermal growth factor receptor tyrosine kinase inhibitor, in combination with chemotherapy for advanced non-small-cell lung cancer. Clin Lung Cancer 2003; 4(6):336–338.

30. AstraZeneca UK Ltd. Iressa™ (gefitinib tablets) product package insert. AstraZeneca, Wilmington, DE, 2003.

31. Imclone Systems and Bristol-Myers Squibb. Erbitux™ (Cetuximab) product package insert. Imclone Systems Inc., Branchburg, NJ, and Bristol-Myers Squibb Company, Princeton, NJ, 2004.

32. Foon KA, Yang XD, Weiner LM, et al. Preclinical and clinical evaluations of ABX-EGF, a fully human anti-epidermal growth factor receptor antibody. Int J Radiat Oncol Biol Phys 2004; 58:984–990.

33. Jakobovits A, Vergara GJ, Kennedy JL, et al. Analysis of homozygous mutant chimeric mice: deletion of the immunoglobulin heavy-chain joining region blocks B-cell development and antibody production. Proc Natl Acad Sci USA 1993; 90:2551–2555.

34. Green LL, Jakobovits A. Regulation of B cell development by variable gene complexity in mice reconstituted with human immunoglobulin yeast artificial chromosomes. J Exp Med 1998; 188:483–495.

35. Jakobovits A, Moore AL, Green LL, et al. Germ-line transmission and expression of a human-derived yeast artificial chromosome. Nature 1993; 362:255–258.

36. Mendez MJ, Green LL, Corvalan JR, et al. Functional transplant of megabase human immunoglobulin loci recapitulates human antibody response in mice. Nat Genet 1997; 15:146–156.

37. Gallo ML, Ivanov VE, Jakobovits A, Davis CG. The human immunoglobulin loci introduced into mice: V(D)and J gene segment usage similar to that of adult humans. Eur J Immunol 2000; 30:534–540.

38. Kellermann SA, Green L. Antibody discovery: the use of transgenic mice to generate human monoclonal antibodies for therapeutics. Curr Opin Biotechnol 2002; 13:593–597.

39. Davis CG, Gallo ML, Corvalan JRF. Transgenic mice as a source of fully human antibodies for the treatment of cancer. Cancer Metastasis Rev 1999; 18:421–425.

40. Yang XD, Wang P, Fredlin P, Jia XC, Oppenheim JJ, Davis CG. Preclinical evaluation of ABX-EGF as a potent anti-tumor agent. Proc Annu Meet Am Assoc Cancer Res 2002; 43:1004 (abstract).

41. Yang XD, Jia XC, Corvalan JR, Wang P, Davis CG. Therapeutic potential of ABX-EGF, a fully human anti-EGF receptor monoclonal antibody, for cancer treatment. Proc Am Soc Clin Oncol 2000; 19:41a.

42. Yang XD, Wang P, Fredlin P, Davis CG. ABX-EGF, a fully human anti-EGF receptor monoclonal antibody: inhibition of prostate cancer in vitro and in vivo. Proc Annu Meet Am Assoc Cancer Res 2002; 21: 116b (abstract).

43. Wang P, Fredlin P, Davis CG. Yang XD. Human anti-EGF receptor monoclonal antibody ABX-EGF: a potential therapeutic for the treatment of prostate cancer. Proc Annu Meet Am Assoc Cancer Res 2002; 43:913 (abstract).

44. McDorman K, Freemen DJ, Bush T, Cerretti D, Fanslow W, Starnes C, et al. ABX-EGF tumor penetration and EGFR saturation correlate with pharmacokinetic, pharmacodynamic, and antitumor activity in an A431 xenograft model system. Proc Annu Meet Am Assoc Cancer Res. 2004; 45(Suppl):109 (abstract).

45. Lynch DH, Yang XD. Therapeutic potential of ABX-EGF: a fully human anti-epidermal growth factor receptor monoclonal antibody for cancer treatment. Semin Oncol 2002; 29(1 Suppl 4):47–50.

46. Salcedo R, Martins-Green M, Gertz B, Oppenheim JJ, Murphy WJ. Combined administration of antibodies to human interleukin 8 and epidermal growth factor receptor results in increased antimetastatic effects on human breast carcinoma xenografts. Clin Cancer Res 2002; 8:2655–2665.

47. Yang XD, Jia XC, Corvalan JR, Wang P, Davis CG. Development of ABX-EGF, a fully human anti-EGF receptor monoclonal antibody, for cancer therapy. Crit Rev Oncol Hematol 2001; 38:17–23.

48. Figlin RA, Belldegrun AS, Crawford J, et al. ABX-EGF, a fully human anti-epidermal growth factor receptor (EGFR) monoclonal antibody (mAb) in patients with advanced cancer: phase 1 clinical results. Proc Am Soc Clin Oncol 2002; 21:10a.

49. Rowinsky E, Schwartz G, Dutcher J, et al. ABX-EGF, a fully human anti-epidermal growth factor receptor (EGFr) monoclonal antibody: phase 2 clinical trial in renal cell cancer (RCC). In: 14th EORTC-NCI-AACR Symposium on Molecular Targets and Cancer Therapeutics, Frankfurt, 2002:1.

50. Rowinsky F, Schwartz G, Gollob J, Thompson J, Vogelzang N, Figlin R, et al. Safety, pharmacokinetics, and activity of ABX-EGF, a fully human anti-epidermal growth factor receptor monoclonal antibody in patients with metastatic renal cell cancer. J Clin Oncol 2004; 22:3003–3015.

51. Roskos L, Lohner M, Osbern K, Pasumarti R, Lu H, Funelas C, et al. Optimal dosing of ABX-EGF in cancer patients. Int J Cancer 2002; 13(Suppl):444.

52. Meropol NJ, Berlin J, Hecht JR, et al. Multicenter study of ABX-EGF monotherapy in patients with metastatic colorectal cancer. Proc Am Soc Clin Oncol 2003; 22:256.

# 42 Development and Evaluation of Cancer Therapeutic Agents Targeting TRAIL Receptor 1 and 2

*Robin C. Humphreys, PhD*

## Contents

## Summary

Novel biological agents are being developed as cancer therapeutics to target the signaling pathway that mediates programmed cell death. The ability to directly signal apoptosis and the relatively restricted tumor cell expression of the tumor necrosis factor-related apoptosis-inducing ligand (TRAIL) cell surface receptors reflect their potential as specific, therapeutic cancer targets. Therapeutic agents being developed to activate this pathway include agonist human and chimeric TRAIL receptor monoclonal antibodies and the ligand TRAIL. This chapter will summarize the current knowledge of the targets in the TRAIL cell death pathway and the status of the agents being developed to activate this pathway.

**Key Words:** Monoclonal antibody; TRAIL; TRAIL-R1; TRAIL-R2; apoptosis; TNF.

## 1. INTRODUCTION

The use of systemic or nontargeted therapies to treat cancer has been the mainstay of cancer therapy for more than 50 yr. Current cancer chemotherapeutic agents disrupt normal physiological processes, including proliferation, DNA synthesis, and mitosis. The abrogation or obstruction of these processes can induce cell death or growth arrest of the tumor cell. The efficacy of these drugs against tumor growth and metastasis has been well characterized *(1,2)*. New chemotherapeutic agents, improved drug design, and dose scheduling have generated significant enhancement in survival for cancer patients. Unfortunately, the majority of these agents are neither specific for tumor cells nor any of the immortalizing or transforming molecular signals, leading to the disruption of growth and differentiation

From: *Cancer Drug Discovery and Development: The Oncogenomics Handbook*
Edited by: W. J. LaRochelle and R. A. Shimkets © Humana Press Inc., Totowa, NJ

pathways in normal cells and precipitating broad nonspecific toxicity. Importantly, one of the undesirable consequences of chemotherapeutic treatment is the induction of chemoresistance within surviving tumor cells. These resistance mechanisms include the inactivation of DNA mismatch repair, induction of multidrug-resistant phenotypes that eliminate toxic agents from the cell, and mutations in the TP53 gene that prevent induction of DNA damage- and cell cycle checkpoint-induced apoptosis (3).

With the objective of enhancing anticancer therapy and avoidance of additional toxicity, targeted therapies have been designed to modulate the activity of specific cell surface receptors, intracellular signaling moieties, and transcription factors. Recently, several targeted agents have been approved for the treatment of cancer that specifically target cell surface receptors and attenuate proliferation signals or induce programmed cell death. Antibodies, like anti-ErbB2, herceptin and anti-CD20 rituximab, have demonstrated the ability to inhibit tumor cell growth or induce cell death without a significant increase in systemic toxicity. A variety of new agents are being developed to specifically exploit the ability to induce cell death or attenuate the cell death inhibitory mechanisms within a tumor cell, including agonistic apoptosis-inducing antibodies or small molecules that inactivate antiapoptotic proteins (4,5).

The ability to activate programmed cell death, or apoptosis, is an inherent property of every eukaryotic cell and can be induced by specific extrinsic and intrinsic signals. A variety of external and internal stimuli, in response to DNA damage, viral transformation, cytotoxic stress, or lack of survival signals from growth factors and the extracellular milieu, can initiate the apoptotic cascade leading to cell death. The direct extrinsic signaling of cell death is mediated through a group of related ligands and their cognate type I cell surface receptors that are members of the tumor necrosis factor (TNF) superfamily (TNFSF) cell surface receptors. The members of this apoptosis-inducing family include TNFR1, FAS, tumor necrosis factor-related apoptosis-inducing ligand (TRAIL)-R1 (DR4, TRAIL receptor 1, TNFSFR10a) and TRAIL-R2 (DR5, TRAIL receptor 2, TNFSFR10b). In response to the ligands TNF-α, FASL, and TRAIL, the receptors TNFR1, FAS, and TRAIL-R1 and TRAIL-R2, respectively, have demonstrated the ability to potently induce apoptosis in virally and oncogenically transformed cells, cytokine-activated T- and B-lymphocytes, natural killer (NK) cell, and monocytes (6,7). Activation of these receptor-mediated signaling pathways has been the objective of a number of novel targeted therapies, including recombinant ligands and agonist antibodies directed against the receptors. Unfortunately, systemic treatment with TNF-α or agonist–FAS antibodies elicits fatal inflammatory reaction or hepatotoxic injury, respectively, that precludes them from use as systemic therapeutics (8–11). Recent preclinical safety evaluations of the TRAIL ligand have not demonstrated a similar systemic toxicity in rodents or primates (12).

The trimeric TRAIL receptors, TRAIL-R1 and TRAIL-R2, in response to binding of the trimerized TRAIL ligand, initiate a signaling cascade leading to cell death that is independent of p53 and the intrinsic cell death pathway utilized by some chemotherapeutic agents. Consequently, activation of the TRAIL receptor-dependent pathway could bypass acquired chemotherapy resistance, mediated through the intrinsic pathway, in tumor cells. A broad array of human tumor cell lines are sensitive to TRAIL in vitro and in vivo and possess high-level expression of these death receptors (12). Many normal cell types have been tested for in vitro responsiveness to TRAIL ligand, in its native nontagged form. TRAIL failed to induce significant apoptosis in lung fibroblasts, colon smooth muscle cells, renal proximal tubule epithelium, umbilical vein endothelium, microvascular endothelium, and astrocytes *(12–14)*. With TRAIL-R1 and TRAIL-R2 cell surface expression chiefly restricted to tumor cells and studies demonstrating that short-term treatment of primates with the ligand TRAIL is systemically safe, preclinical studies and clinical evaluation of the suitability of these receptors as targets for cancer therapy have been initiated. The ability to specifically enforce the elimination of tumor cells, without additional systemic toxicity, and the ability to potentially bypass chemotherapeutic resistance mechanisms make these death receptors attractive targets for cancer therapy.

## 2. LIGANDS AND RECEPTORS OF THE TNF SUPERFAMILY

The founding member of the TNF superfamily was identified as a soluble serum factor isolated from lipopolysaccharide (LPS)-treated mice that could induce necrosis of murine and engrafted human tumors *(15,16)*. Isolation of purified TNF-$\alpha$ and cloning of the cDNA *(17)* permitted unequivocal demonstration of the ability of TNF-$\alpha$ to inhibit the growth of transformed tumor cell lines in vitro and in vivo *(18–20)*. Successive TNF superfamily ligands have demonstrated the ability to induce apoptosis in virally or oncogenically transformed cells, human tumor cell lines and activated lymphocytes, NK cells, and monocytes (TRAIL, TNF-$\alpha$, TNF-$\beta$, FASL, DR6). The other 14 nonapoptosis-inducing TNF ligands possess a broad array of immunomodulatory and growth stimulatory capabilities, including stimulation and proliferation of B-cells (BLYS,) and T-cells (CD40L, LIGHT, OX40L, 4-1-BBL) and regulation of bone metabolism (RANKL) (reviewed in refs. *7* and *21*).

Identification of the TNF-$\alpha$ receptor was initiated by the discovery that TNF-$\alpha$ and TNF-$\beta$, the second of the TNF ligands to be identified (renamed LT-$\beta$), could bind to a single class of interferon-inducible receptors on human tumor cells *(22)*. TNF-$\alpha$ and LT-$\beta$ were able to bind to and activate TNFR1 and TNFR2. Identification and cloning of these two receptors revealed a theme that persists throughout the TNFSF: that some TNF ligands can interact with multiple receptors, implying a functional overlap or redundancy among the ligands (Table 1). Cloning of the TNF-$\alpha$ receptors lead to the subsequent addition of 27 structurally related receptors to the TNFRSF. The TNFSF ligands and receptors are now classified according to a standardized nomenclature that indicates to which receptor each ligand can bind (see Table 1).

TRAIL was identified through searches of expressed sequence tag (EST) databases for sequences containing homology to FasL and TNF-$\alpha$ *(23,24)*. TRAIL is a type II membrane protein that is cleaved by an extracellular cysteine protease releasing the soluble ligand in a homotrimeric subunit structure *(25–27)*. Despite the readily detectable presence of TRAIL mRNA in many normal human tissues and cells, including prostate, lung, lymphocytes, and spleen, expression of membrane-bound TRAIL is restricted to a narrow population of immune cells. Cell surface expression of TRAIL has been detected in interleukin (IL)-15- or IL-2-activated NK cells, virally infected T-cells, interferon-activated monocytes and dendritic cells, as well as CD3+ T-cells and can confer tumoricidal activity to monocytes and NK cells *(28–36)*. The soluble and membrane-bound form of TRAIL induced apoptosis in a wide variety of human tumor cells both in vitro and in vivo without affecting the viability of normal cells *(12,13,30)*.

There are five distinct but closely related receptors that are capable of interacting with the ligand TRAIL, only two of which, TRAIL-R1 (DR4, TNFSF10a) and TRAIL-R2 (DR5, TNFSF10b), have the capability to transmit intracellular death signals through their cytoplasmic death domains. All of the TRAIL receptors were identified shortly after the cloning

Table 1
Receptors and Ligands of the TNF Super Family

| Receptor TNFSF No. | Receptor Name (Other Names) | Ligand (TNFRSF No.) | Known Roles/Signaling Events |
|---|---|---|---|
| 1A | TNFR I[DD] | TNF-α (2) LT-α (1) | Apoptosis |
| 1B | TNFR II | TNF-α (2) LT-α (1) | Apoptosis |
| 3 | LTβR | LT-β (3) LIGHT (14) | Immune modulation |
| 4 | OX-40 | OX-40L (4) | Inflammation |
| 5 | CD40 | CD40L (5) | Lymphocyte activation |
| 6 | FAS (CD95)[DD] | FasL (6) | Apoptosis |
| 6B | DcR3 (TR6) | TL1A FasL (6) LIGHT (14) | Immune modulation |
| 7 | CD27 | CD27L (7) | Lymphocyte proliferation |
| 8 | CD30 | CD30L (8) | Lymphocyte proliferation |
| 9 | 4-1BB | 4-1BBL (9) | T-cell, monocyte activation |
| 10A | TRAILR1 (DR4)[DD] | TRAIL (10) | Apoptosis |
| 10B | TRAILR2 (DR5)[DD] | TRAIL (10) | Apoptosis |
| 10C | TRAILR3 (DcR1) | TRAIL (10) | Apoptosis decoy |
| 10D | TRAILR4 (DcR2) | TRAIL (10) | Apoptosis decoy |
| 11A | RANK | TRANCE (11) | Bone metabolism |
| 11B | OPG | TRAIL (10) TRANCE (11) | Bone metabolism |
| 12 | FN14 | TWEAK (12) | Apoptosis endothelial proliferation |
| 13B | TACI | BLYS (13B) APRIL (13) | B-cell homeostasis |
| 13C | BR3 (BAFFR) | BLYS (13B) | B-cell homeostasis |
| 14 | HVEM | LIGHT (14) LT-α (1) | T-cell activation |
| 16 | NGFR (p75NTR)[DD] | NGF | Proliferation apoptosis |
| 17 | BCMA | BLYS (13B) APRIL (13) | B-cell homeostasis |
| 18 | GITR (AITR) | GITRL (18) | Inflammation |
| 19 | TROY | Unknown | Olfactory development? |
| 19L | RELT | Unknown | Lymphocyte activation |
| 21 | DR6[DD] | Unknown | Unknown |
| 25 | DR3[DD] | TL1A | Endothelial proliferation inflammation |
| Not defined | EDAR[DD] | EDA1 | Ectodermal development |
| Not defined | XEDAR | EDA2 | Skeletal muscle development? |

*Note:* The superscript DD indicates that the receptor contains a complete cytoplasmic death domain.

of the ligand TRAIL *(14,23,24,37–40)*. The decoy receptors DcR3 and DcR4 contain either a truncated or absent death domain, respectively *(14,37,41–43)*. Osteoptegrin (OPG), a soluble receptor for the ligand RANKL, can also bind TRAIL, although some evidence suggests that this binding is weak at physiological temperatures *(44,45)*. The two TRAIL decoy (DcR1,TNFRSF10C) (DcR2,TNFRSF10D) receptors are believed to be involved in protecting normal cells from the proapoptotic effects of TRAIL, but their expression is not widespread nor predictive of a lack of sensitivity to TRAIL in all cases (46).

Cell surface expression analysis by flow cytometry of primary human cells, using various antibody reagents, have indicated weak but detectable TRAIL-R1 and TRAIL-R2 receptor expression on the surface of a limited number of normal cells, including, hepatocytes, keratinocytes, astrocytes, and osteoblasts (46–50). Relatively high-level expression of TRAIL-R1 and TRAIL-R2 has been primarily restricted to the surface of tumor cells. Primary human tumor cell populations isolated from the brain (51,52), melanoma (53), ovary (54), leukemia (55), sarcoma (56), and lung (57) have detectable cell surface expression of TRAIL-R1 and TRAIL-R2. Tumor cell lines derived from the colon (58), breast (12), melanoma (53), brain (52), ovary (59,60), thyroid (61), lung (62), pancreas (63), liver (64), and sarcoma (56) have detectable TRAIL-R1 and TRAIL-R2 and are sensitive to the effects of TRAIL and TRAIL agonist mAbs in vitro and in vivo (65).

Expression analysis revealed mRNA for TRAIL-R1 and TRAIL-R2 is present in a majority of normal human cells, both epithelial and mesenchymal. Transcripts for the death and decoy receptors have been identified in tumor cells from diverse tissue origins. Importantly, the presence of mRNA for either TRAIL-R1 or TRAIL-R2 does not appear to correlate with expression of detectable TRAIL receptors on the surface of the cell (46).

The TRAIL receptors are type I receptors that possess an extracellular domain rich in cysteine residues that are critical for maintaining the structure of the ligand interaction domain and the trimeric structure of the receptor, a common feature of the TNFRSF (66). Both TRAIL-R1 and TRAIL-R2 contain a conserved cytoplasmic protein interaction domain called the "death domain." This domain can be found in all TNFSFRs that mediate apoptosis. The "death domain" couples the receptor–ligand complex to cytoplasmic adaptor proteins, most notably FADD (Fas-associated death domain) (37,67–69). FADD recruits one of the cytoplasmic cysteine proteases, caspase-8 or caspase-10, to the receptor–ligand complex also known as the DISC or "death-inducing signaling complex" (70). Although the precise mechanism of ligand-initiated signaling through the DISC is unknown, ligand binding to the TRAIL receptor results in the cleavage of the pro-form of caspase-8. This active protease dissociates form the DISC and targets secondary signaling molecules, including the pro-form of the executioner caspase-3, caspase-6, and caspase-7. Caspase-3 is one of three executioner caspases that directly mediates cleavage and inactivation of signaling and structural proteins leading to cell death. The activation of the intrinsic cell death pathway, in response to loss of growth survival signals, hypoxia, radiation, cell cycle defects, and DNA damage, is dependent on the loss of mitochondrial membrane integrity. TRAIL binding to the TRAIL receptor can lead to activation of the intrinsic cell death pathway, as well. This is accomplished through caspase-8 cleavage of the proapoptotic protein BID (71). BID interacts with other proapoptotic proteins, BAX and BAK, promoting their association with the mitochondrial membrane. BAX and BAK induce mitochondrial release of cytochrome-c, SMAC/DAIBLO, and formation of the caspase-9-activating complex, known as the apoptosome, leading to activation of caspase-9 and caspase-3 (72,73). The activation of the intrinsic pathway by TRAIL receptor engagement is independent of the tumor suppressor p53. Consequently, in tumor cells that, in response to chemotherapeutic or radiation treatment, have an inactive p53, TRAIL or agonist TRAIL receptor antibodies can bypass the intrinsic cell death pathway and induce apoptosis (74).

Signaling pathways other than those leading to the induction of the caspase cascade and apoptosis have been discovered for TRAIL and the TRAIL receptors. The ligation of TRAIL with TRAIL-R1 and TRAIL-R2 can initiate signaling through the nuclear factor (NF)-κB and JNK pathways (75–78). The cytoplasmic adaptor proteins TRADD (TNFR-associated death domain) mediate these interactions between the TRAIL receptors and the transcription factor NF-κB or receptor-associated protein kinases like RIP (76,79). Interestingly, the ability to activate NF-κB signaling is the same for both receptors, but TRAIL-R1 and TRAIL-R2 differentially activate the JNK/p38 pathway. Some studies have suggested that activation of the NF-κB pathway is a mechanism of synergy between TRAIL and chemotherapeutic agents (80,81); other reports have suggested that RIP does not play a role in TRAIL-mediated apoptosis (76). Evidence from these studies suggests that TRAIL can influence cellular processes other than apoptosis. TRAIL has been implicated in endothelial cell proliferation (82) and in the maturation of monocytes (77,83). In transformed and primary keratinocytes, activation of TRAIL-R1 induced inflammation and IL-8 secretion as well as caspase activation (84). It is unclear what impact the activation of these non-apoptotic pathways have on the survival of the cell (85). These results suggest the TRAIL receptors activate a potentially complex signaling network that might mediate both proapoptotic, antiapoptotic, and growth signals (reviewed in refs. 86 and 87).

## 3. NOVEL THERAPEUTICS
## TARGETING THE TRAIL CELL DEATH PATHWAY

Several novel therapeutic agents are being developed to target the TRAIL pathway. Currently, the most advanced of these agents are agonist monoclonal antibodies, either human or chimeric or humanized mouse, directed against either TRAIL-R1 or TRAIL-R2, and recombinant forms of the ligand TRAIL. All of these agents are either in early clinical development (human TRAIL receptor agonist monoclonal antibodies) or in late-stage preclinical development (TRAIL, mouse TRAIL receptor agonist monoclonal antibodies).

The potency of the ligand TRAIL on human tumor cells has been demonstrated primarily in human cell lines in vitro and in xenograft models and primary tissues transplanted into immunocomprimised mice. TRAIL, either alone or in combination with chemotherapeutic agents, has demonstrated in vitro efficacy against cell lines derived from a broad array of human tumors, including those derived from the colon, brain, uterus, ovary, liver, breast, prostate, kidney, lung, thyroid, leukemic, lymphoma, and myeloma lineages (6,12,23,56,80,83,86,88–99). This broad and potent spectrum of activity against many different types of human cancer cell lines suggests that this agent might be effective across a wide range of human cancers. Of significance, TRAIL treatment of chemoresistant or radioresistant tumor cell lines enhances the cytotoxic effect of chemotherapy, including adriamycin-resistant myeloma, radioresistant lymphoma, and taxane- and platinum-insensitive breast and osteosarcoma cell lines (59,62,95,97,99–107). In cell lines that possess resistance to TRAIL-mediated apoptosis, chemotherapy agents can improve the cytotoxic effects of TRAIL (91,104,108). The resistance to TRAIL-mediated apoptosis in these tumor cell lines is controlled by intracellular inhibitors of the extrinsic and intrinsic pathways, including FLICE-like inhibitory protein (FLIP) (53,65,109,110), X-linked inhibitor of apoptosis (XIAP) (111,112), and BAX (113,114). Novel biologic reagents are being developed to overcome these TRAIL-resistant phenotypes. Proteosome inhibitors like PS-341 in combination with TRAIL have shown an effect on TRAIL-resistant multiple myeloma *(115,116)*. Decreasing FLIP levels with small interfering RNA (siRNA) *(117)* or modulation of Bcl-2 expression with histone deacetylase inhibitors *(118,119)* have also demonstrated enhancement of TRAIL activity in human tumor cells. These studies demonstrate that chemotherapy and TRAIL-receptor-activating therapeutic agents could be combined to enhance antitumor activity in chemoresistant and TRAIL-resistant resistant tumor types, increasing the potential usefulness of the TRAIL receptors as a cancer therapeutic target.

Importantly, clinical patient samples have been evaluated with TRAIL in xenograft models and in ex vivo cultures *(55,85,93,120–124)*. TRAIL has demonstrated potent apoptosis activity on patient samples either alone or in combination with chemotherapeutic agents in AML, ALL, CML, NHL, and multiple myeloma. In published reports of TRAIL's effects on CLL samples, very little response was observed with TRAIL alone, but cytotoxicity could be enhanced in combination with actinomycin D *(110,125)*. Responses within a tumor type were noticeably variable with cytotoxic effects ranging between 10% and 80% in 10–70% of the evaluated samples. The results from the available data suggest that patient tumors, although not affected with the same efficiency as immortalized tumor cell lines, are still susceptible to TRAIL alone or in combination with chemotherapy. In these studies, both primary patient samples and human cell lines display a consistent lack of correlation between sensitivity to the ligand TRAIL and the cell surface expression of TRAIL-R1 or TRAIL-R2.

The absence of detectable apoptosis activity in normal cells after treatment with soluble TRAIL has been shown for primary cells from the lung, bone, liver, endothelium breast, brain, and kidney *(12,47)*. Importantly, short-term treatment of mouse, monkey, and chimpanzee with soluble, recombinant, $Zn^{2+}$-stabilized TRAIL has demonstrated the tolerability of the ligand. No detectable toxicities were observed in these nonclinical safety studies. Earlier forms of TRAIL were generated with epitope tags *(126)*. These epitope tagged forms also enhanced the toxicity of TRAIL on normal cells. HIS-tagged, leucine-zipper or antibody crosslinked forms of TRAIL have demonstrated the ability to induce apoptosis in normal hepatocytes in vitro *(49,127)*. TRAIL can induce apoptosis in bacterially activated hepatocytes, in stellate cells from the liver and pancreas, or in mouse models of hepatitis or pancreatitis *(50,128)*. Membrane-bound TRAIL has been shown to induce liver damage in adenoviral-transfected hepatocytes in vivo *(127)*. To date, only interferon-activated normal cells or cells with an activated inflammation pathway appear to be responsive to soluble recombinant TRAIL treatment, arguing that it could be a safe and effective therapeutic agent.

Human Genome Sciences is developing two fully human agonist, monoclonal antibodies, specifically targeted to either the TRAIL-R1 (HGS-ETR1) or TRAIL-R2 (HGS-ETR2) *(129)*. Each antibody is specific for its cognate human receptor and does not crossreact with any other TRAIL receptor, including the decoy receptors DcR1 and DcR2. These antibodies were isolated from phage display libraries, in collaboration with Cambridge Antibody Technology, as single-chain (scFv) antibody molecules that displayed the ability to inhibit TRAIL binding to either TRAIL-R1 or TRAIL-R2 and loss of cell viability in human tumor cells. These single chains were converted into complete $IgG_1$ molecules, HGS-ETR1 and HGS-ETR2. Both antibodies have demonstrated their ability to activate apoptosis in human tumor cell lines in vitro and in vivo *(130–132)*.

The effectiveness of the HGS-ETR1 and HGS-ETR2 antibodies in impacting tumor cell viability has been demonstrated in a broad range of human tumor cell lines, including

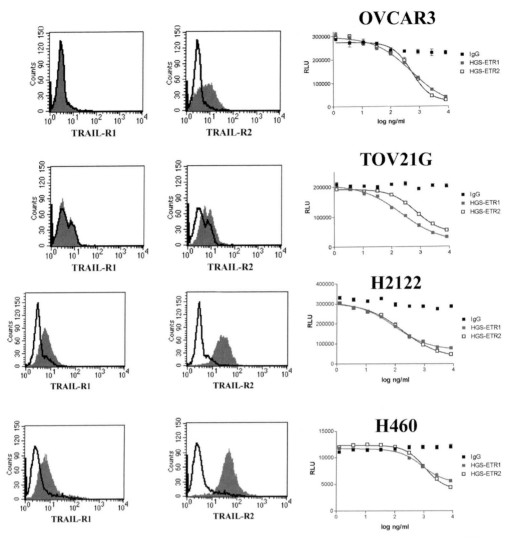

**Fig. 1.** HGS-ETR1 and HGS-ETR2 reduce the viability of human ovarian and lung tumor cell lines. FACS analysis: (left panels) The level of cell surface expression of TRAIL-R1 or TRAIL-R2 (DR4 or DR5) (solid gray peak) vs an isotype control antibody (open peak). Cell-Glo cytotoxicity assay: (right panels) Cell viability curves for human tumor cell lines; ovarian (OVCAR3, TOV21G), and lung (H460, H2122) treated with HGS-ETR1 (light grey square) or HGS-ETR2 (open square) or an isotype control antibody (black square). Data points are the mean ± SEM of three determinations.

lung, colon, breast, glioma, non-Hodgkin's lymphoma, and ovary. Examples of this activity are shown in Fig. 1A for non-small-cell lung cancer (NSCLC) and ovarian cell lines. In the ovarian cell lines shown, no cell surface expression of TRAIL-R1 could be detected by flow cytometry. Despite this low level of receptor expression, HGS-ETR1 is still able to induce apoptosis. This supports the observation made in other tumor lines that receptor expression does not necessarily correlate with sensitivity to apoptosis induction. The appearance of Annexin V-positive cells, a hallmark of the early stage of apoptosis, under these same conditions confirms that the HGS-ETR1 and HGS-ETR2 antibodies alter cell

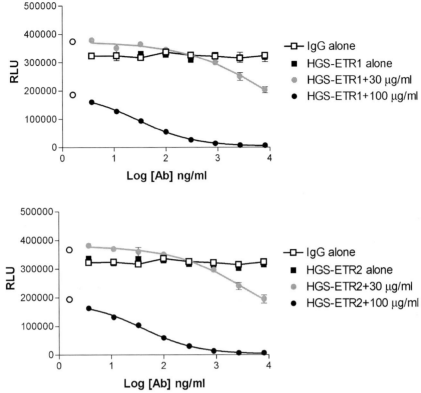

**Fig. 2.** HGS-ETR1 or HGS-ETR2 in combination with carboplatin synergistically reduces the viability of ovarian ES-2 tumor cells. ES-2 cells were treated with control antibody (open squares), HGS-ETR1, or HGS-ETR2 in increasing doses either alone (black square) or in combination with fixed concentrations of carboplatin (30 and 100 µg/mL, gray and black, respectively). Following 2 d of treatment, cell viability was determined with a Cell-Glo cytoxicity assay. Open circles: chemotherapeutic drug alone. Data points are the mean ± SEM of three determinations.

viability through the induction of apoptosis *(132)*. In combination with several chemotherapeutic agents, including folate, platinum, and taxane agents, enhanced in vitro cytotoxicity was observed in breast, lung, and ovarian tumor cell lines (an example is shown in Fig. 2). As expected, both antibodies activated the caspase cascade and cleavage of down-stream substrates *(132,133)*.

In vivo experiments have demonstrated significant single-agent activity for both antibodies against a variety of solid tumors. The antibodies are able to potently inhibit tumor growth in multiple settings, in various subcutaneous and orthotopic xenograft models, including the colon, lung, and breast *(130–133)*. An example of the effect of HGS-ETR1 and HGS-ETR2 treatment on the growth of subcutaneous NSCLC and colon tumor cell line xenografts is shown in Figs. 3A and 3B. Immunohistochemical analysis of HGS-ETR2-treated tumors for apoptotic cells revealed the presence of apoptotic bodies throughout the tumor mass, suggesting that the antibody induces changes in tumor volume through apoptosis and that the antibody can readily penetrate this large solid tumor (Fig. 4). HGS-ETR1 and HGS-ETR2 have demonstrated activity against leukemia and lymphoma cell

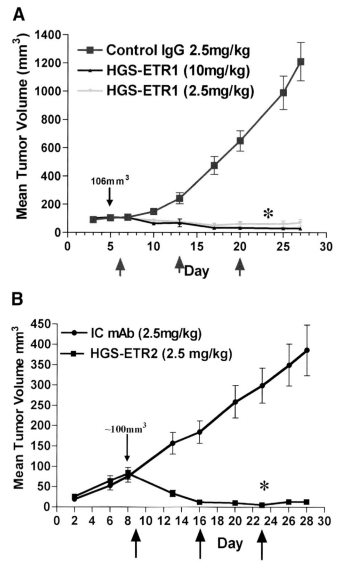

**Fig. 3.** (**A**) HGS-ETR1 induces regression of subcutaneous NSCLC tumors (H2122) in nude mice. $n = 10$ for all treatment groups. Arrows indicate days of treatment. $*p < 0.0001$. Effect of HGS-ETR1 at 2.5 mg/kg and 10 mg/kg on tumor growth compared to IC mAb. IC mAb is an isotype control antibody. (**B**) HGS-ETR2 induces rapid regression of 100-mm³ colon (COLO205) tumors in nude mice. $n = 10$ for all treatment groups. $*p < 0.0001$. Effect of HGS-ETR2 at 2.5 mg/kg on tumor growth compared to IC mAb. Arrows indicate days of treatment.

lines and patient samples *(134)*. These two TRAIL-receptor-targeted monoclonal antibodies have a broad spectrum of antitumor capability coupled with the ability to enhance the activity of chemotherapeutic reagents. Both antibodies are currently in clinical safety trials.

An agonist mouse monoclonal antibody to human TRAIL-R2 (TRA-8) was generated by immunization of mice with the extracellular domain of human TRAIL-R2 fused to the

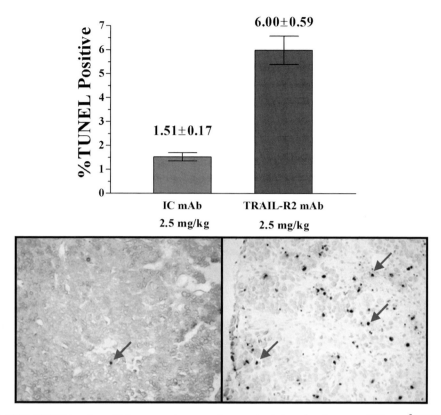

**Fig. 4.** HGS-ETR2 treatment triggers an increase in apoptosis in subcutaneous 400-mm³ COLO205 tumors. TUNEL analysis reveals apoptotic cells indicated by black, pyknotic nuclei (arrows) in control (left panel) and HGS-ETR2-treated tumors (right panel) 5 d after first dose of antibody. Magnification is ×400. Bar graph: quantitation of apoptosis levels in HGS-ETR2 treated 400-mm³ COLO205 tumors vs control treated tumors. ($n = 3$ for both groups. $*p < 0.001$; HGS-ETR2 compared to IC mAb.)

Fc portion of human IgG1. With a reported $K_d$ of 3 n$M$, the antibody bound specifically to TRAIL-R2, induced apoptosis in Jurkat cells, and showed an associated increase in activated caspase-8, caspase-3, and caspase-9. TRA-8 induced apoptosis in several different T-cell leukemia, B-cell lymphoma, and glioma lines. The TRA-8 antibody demonstrated enhanced antitumor activity in combination with chemotherapeutic agents against human tumor cell lines (80,135). In TRA-8-resistant glioma lines sensitivity was restored after overexpression of Bax mediated by adenoviral transfer (136). TRA-8 inhibited tumor growth in leukemic and astrocytoma xenograft models. Although mRNA expression of TRAIL-R1, TRAIL-R2, and DcR2 was detectable in all normal primary T- and B-cells and astrocytes, FACS-detectable cell surface expression of TRAIL-R2 was not observed. Not surprisingly, neither TRA-8 nor TRAIL was able to induce apoptosis in these cells. Immunohistochemical analysis of TRAIL-R2 expression using TRA-8 revealed scattered positive expression in the spleen but an absence of detectable expression in the liver, lung, and breast tissue. Deficient cell surface expression in normal cells was supported by the absence of detectable TRAIL-R2 protein in liver, lung, kidney, spleen, testes, ovary, heart, and pancreas tissue lysates. Thus, this mouse monoclonal antibody can induce apoptosis in human tumor cells without apparent effects on normal primary cells, including hepatocytes *(127)*.

The TRAIL receptor pathway plays a significant role in the induction of programmed cell death in transformed cells. Novel agents—agonist TRAIL receptor monoclonal antibodies and the recombinant ligand TRAIL—have been developed to exploit the capability of this pathway to induce programmed cell death in human tumor cells. These therapeutic proteins have been evaluated extensively for efficacy in vitro and in preclinical xenograft models, either alone or in combination with chemotherapeutic agents. Biochemical studies have revealed interactions among the TRAIL receptors, adaptor proteins, and downstream effectors molecules. Understanding the mechanism of programmed cell death signaling within the extrinsic pathway is not completely understood and requires continued study. The TRAIL receptor pathway appears to impinge upon other signaling networks and plays a role in regulating cellular events other than apoptosis. Safety studies in primates and rodents have demonstrated the tolerability of the recombinant ligand, and evaluation of the safety of the agonist antibodies is ongoing. The clinical evaluation of the safety and efficacy of the agonist monoclonal antibodies is expected to produce potent targeted, therapeutics for the treatment of cancer and fulfill the potential of genomics-based drug design and development. Hopefully, the objectives of these novel agents to kill tumor cells, complement current chemotherapy regimens, and bypass chemoresistance without significant nonspecific systemic toxicity will be realized and translated into improved cancer therapy for patients.

## REFERENCES

1. Decatris MP, Sundar S, O'Byrne KJ. Platinum-based chemotherapy in metastatic breast cancer: current status. Cancer Treat Rev 2004; 30(1):53–81.
2. Spira AI, Ettinger DS. The use of chemotherapy in soft-tissue sarcomas. Oncologist 2002; 7(4):348–359.
3. Perona R, Sanchez-Perez I. Control of oncogenesis and cancer therapy resistance. Br J Cancer 2004; 90(3):573–577.
4. Ludwig DL, Pereira DS, Zhu Z, Hicklin DJ, Bohlen P. Monoclonal antibody therapeutics and apoptosis. Oncogene 2003; 22(56):9097–9106.
5. Hu W, Kavanagh JJ. Anticancer therapy targeting the apoptotic pathway. Lancet Oncol 2003; 4(12): 721–729.
6. Srivastava RK. TRAIL/Apo-2L: mechanisms and clinical applications in cancer. Neoplasia 2001; 3(6): 535–546.
7. Ashkenazi A. Targeting death and decoy receptors of the tumour-necrosis factor superfamily. Nat Rev Cancer 2002; 2(6):420–430.
8. Nagaki M, Sugiyama A, Osawa Y, et al. Lethal hepatic apoptosis mediated by tumor necrosis factor receptor, unlike Fas-mediated apoptosis, requires hepatocyte sensitization in mice. J Hepatol 1999; 31(6): 997–1005.
9. Nagata S. A death factor—the other side of the coin. Behring Inst Mitt 1996; 97:1–11.
10. Mueller H. Tumor necrosis factor as an antineoplastic agent: pitfalls and promises. Cell Mol Life Sci 1998; 54(12):1291–1298.
11. Bradham CA, Plumpe J, Manns MP, Brenner DA, Trautwein C. Mechanisms of hepatic toxicity. I. TNF-induced liver injury. Am J Physiol 1998; 275(3 Pt 1):G387–G392.
12. Ashkenazi A, Pai RC, Fong S, et al. Safety and antitumor activity of recombinant soluble Apo2 ligand. J Clin Invest 1999; 104(2):155–162.
13. Walczak H, Miller RE, Ariail K, et al. Tumoricidal activity of tumor necrosis factor-related apoptosis-inducing ligand in vivo. Nat Med 1999; 5(2):157–163.
14. Sheridan JP, Marsters SA, Pitti RM, et al. Control of TRAIL-induced apoptosis by a family of signaling and decoy receptors. Science 1997; 277(5327):818–821.

15. O'Malley WE, Achinstein B, Shear MJ. Journal of the National Cancer Institute, Vol. 29, 1962: action of bacterial polysaccharide on tumors. II. Damage of sarcoma 37 by serum of mice treated with Serratia marcescens polysaccharide, and induced tolerance. Nutr Rev 1988; 46(11):389–391.

16. Carswell EA, Old LJ, Kassel RL, Green S, Fiore N, Williamson B. An endotoxin-induced serum factor that causes necrosis of tumors. Proc Natl Acad Sci USA 1975; 72(9):3666–3670.

17. Pennica D, Hayflick JS, Bringman TS, Palladino MA, Goeddel DV. Cloning and expression in *Escherichia coli* of the cDNA for murine tumor necrosis factor. Proc Natl Acad Sci USA 1985; 82(18):6060–6064.

18. Rutka JT, Giblin JR, Berens ME, et al. The effects of human recombinant tumor necrosis factor on glioma-derived cell lines: cellular proliferation, cytotoxicity, morphological and radioreceptor studies. Int J Cancer 1988; 41(4):573–582.

19. Kramer SM, Aggarwal BB, Eessalu TE, et al. Characterization of the in vitro and in vivo species preference of human and murine tumor necrosis factor-alpha. Cancer Res 1988; 48(4):920–925.

20. Sugarman BJ, Aggarwal BB, Hass PE, et al. Recombinant human tumor necrosis factor-alpha: effects on proliferation of normal and transformed cells in vitro. Science 1985; 230(4728):943–945.

21. Gardnerova M, Blanque R, Gardner CR. The use of TNF family ligands and receptors and agents which modify their interaction as therapeutic agents. Curr Drug Targets 2000; 1(4):327–364.

22. Aggarwal BB, Eessalu TE, Hass PE. Characterization of receptors for human tumour necrosis factor and their regulation by gamma-interferon. Nature 1985; 318(6047):665–667.

23. Pitti RM, Marsters SA, Ruppert S, Donahue CJ, Moore A, Ashkenazi A. Induction of apoptosis by Apo-2 ligand, a new member of the tumor necrosis factor cytokine family. J Biol Chem 1996; 271(22): 12,687–12,690.

24. Wiley SR, Schooley K, Smolak PJ, et al. Identification and characterization of a new member of the TNF family that induces apoptosis. Immunity 1995; 3(6):673–682.

25. Mariani SM, Krammer PH. Differential regulation of TRAIL and CD95 ligand in transformed cells of the T and B lymphocyte lineage. Eur J Immunol 1998; 28(3):973–982.

26. Hymowitz SG, Christinger HW, Fuh G, et al. Triggering cell death: the crystal structure of Apo2L/TRAIL in a complex with death receptor 5. Mol Cell 1999; 4(4):563–571.

27. Hymowitz SG, O'Connell MP, Ultsch MH, et al. A unique zinc-binding site revealed by a high-resolution X-ray structure of homotrimeric Apo2L/TRAIL. Biochemistry 2000; 39(4):633–640.

28. Johnsen AC, Haux J, Steinkjer B, et al. Regulation of APO-2 ligand/trail expression in NK cells-involvement in NK cell-mediated cytotoxicity. Cytokine 1999; 11(9):664–672.

29. Kayagaki N, Yamaguchi N, Nakayama M, et al. Involvement of TNF-related apoptosis-inducing ligand in human CD4+ T cell-mediated cytotoxicity. J Immunol 1999; 162(5):2639–2647.

30. Griffith TS, Wiley SR, Kubin MZ, Sedger LM, Maliszewski CR, Fanger NA. Monocyte-mediated tumoricidal activity via the tumor necrosis factor-related cytokine, TRAIL. J Exp Med 1999; 189(8): 1343–1354.

31. Mariani SM, Krammer PH. Surface expression of TRAIL/Apo-2 ligand in activated mouse T and B cells. Eur J Immunol 1998; 28(5):1492–1498.

32. Martinez-Lorenzo MJ, Alava MA, Gamen S, et al. Involvement of APO2 ligand/TRAIL in activation-induced death of Jurkat and human peripheral blood T cells. Eur J Immunol 1998; 28(9):2714–2725.

33. Zamai L, Ahmad M, Bennett IM, Azzoni L, Alnemri ES, Perussia B. Natural killer (NK) cell-mediated cytotoxicity: differential use of TRAIL and Fas ligand by immature and mature primary human NK cells. J Exp Med 1998; 188(12):2375–2380.

34. Fanger NA, Maliszewski CR, Schooley K, Griffith TS. Human dendritic cells mediate cellular apoptosis via tumor necrosis factor-related apoptosis-inducing ligand (TRAIL). J Exp Med 1999; 190(8): 1155–1164.

35. Lum JJ, Pilon AA, Sanchez-Dardon J, et al. Induction of cell death in human immunodeficiency virus-infected macrophages and resting memory CD4 T cells by TRAIL/Apo2l. J Virol 2001; 75(22):11,128–11,136.

36. Katsikis PD, Garcia-Ojeda ME, Torres-Roca JF, Tijoe IM, Smith CA, Herzenberg LA. Interleukin-1 beta converting enzyme-like protease involvement in Fas-induced and activation-induced peripheral blood T cell apoptosis in HIV infection. TNF-related apoptosis-inducing ligand can mediate activation-induced T cell death in HIV infection. J Exp Med 1997; 186(8):1365–1372.

37. Pan G, Ni J, Wei YF, Yu G, Gentz R, Dixit VM. An antagonist decoy receptor and a death domain-containing receptor for TRAIL. Science 1997; 277(5327):815–818.

38. Chaudhary PM, Eby M, Jasmin A, Bookwalter A, Murray J, Hood L. Death receptor 5, a new member of the TNFR family, and DR4 induce FADD-dependent apoptosis and activate the NF-kappaB pathway. Immunity 1997; 7(6):821–830.

39. Walczak H, Degli-Esposti MA, Johnson RS, et al. TRAIL-R2: a novel apoptosis-mediating receptor for TRAIL. EMBO J 1997; 16(17):5386–5397.

40. Wu GS, Burns TF, Zhan Y, Alnemri ES, El-Deiry WS. Molecular cloning and functional analysis of the mouse homologue of the KILLER/DR5 tumor necrosis factor-related apoptosis-inducing ligand (TRAIL) death receptor. Cancer Res 1999; 59(12):2770–2775.

41. Mongkolsapaya J, Cowper AE, Xu XN, et al. Lymphocyte inhibitor of TRAIL (TNF-related apoptosis-inducing ligand): a new receptor protecting lymphocytes from the death ligand TRAIL. J Immunol 1998; 160(1):3–6.

42. Degli-Esposti MA, Smolak PJ, Walczak H, et al. Cloning and characterization of TRAIL-R3, a novel member of the emerging TRAIL receptor family. J Exp Med 1997; 186(7):1165–1170.

43. Marsters SA, Sheridan JP, Pitti RM, et al. A novel receptor for Apo2L/TRAIL contains a truncated death domain. Curr Biol 1997; 7(12):1003–1006.

44. Truneh A, Sharma S, Silverman C, et al. Temperature-sensitive differential affinity of TRAIL for its receptors. DR5 is the highest affinity receptor. J Biol Chem 2000; 275(30):23,319–23,325.

45. Emery JG, McDonnell P, Burke MB, et al. Osteoprotegerin is a receptor for the cytotoxic ligand TRAIL. J Biol Chem 1998; 273(23):14,363–14,367.

46. Leverkus M, Neumann M, Mengling T, et al. Regulation of tumor necrosis factor-related apoptosis-inducing ligand sensitivity in primary and transformed human keratinocytes. Cancer Res 2000; 60(3):553–559.

47. Atkins GJ, Bouralexis S, Evdokiou A, et al. Human osteoblasts are resistant to Apo2L/TRAIL-mediated apoptosis. Bone 2002; 31(4):448–456.

48. Dorr J, Bechmann I, Waiczies S, et al. Lack of tumor necrosis factor-related apoptosis-inducing ligand but presence of its receptors in the human brain. J Neurosci 2002; 22(4):RC209.

49. Jo M, Kim TH, Seol DW, et al. Apoptosis induced in normal human hepatocytes by tumor necrosis factor-related apoptosis-inducing ligand. Nat Med 2000; 6(5):564–567.

50. Mundt B, Kuhnel F, Zender L, et al. Involvement of TRAIL and its receptors in viral hepatitis. FASEB J 2003; 17(1):94–96.

51. Frank S, Kohler U, Schackert G, Schackert HK. Expression of TRAIL and its receptors in human brain tumors. Biochem Biophys Res Commun 1999; 257(2):454–459.

52. Song JH, Song DK, Pyrzynska B, Petruk KC, Van Meir EG, Hao C. TRAIL triggers apoptosis in human malignant glioma cells through extrinsic and intrinsic pathways. Brain Pathol 2003; 13(4):539–553.

53. Song JH, Song DK, Herlyn M, Petruk KC, Hao C. Cisplatin down-regulation of cellular Fas-associated death domain-like interleukin-1beta-converting enzyme-like inhibitory proteins to restore tumor necrosis factor-related apoptosis-inducing ligand-induced apoptosis in human melanoma cells. Clin Cancer Res 2003; 9(11):4255–4266.

54. Arts HJ, de Jong S, Hollema H, ten Hoor K, van der Zee AG, de Vries EG. Chemotherapy induces death receptor 5 in epithelial ovarian carcinoma. Gynecol Oncol 2004; 92(3):794–800.

55. Clodi K, Wimmer D, Li Y, et al. Expression of tumour necrosis factor (TNF)-related apoptosis-inducing ligand (TRAIL) receptors and sensitivity to TRAIL-induced apoptosis in primary B-cell acute lymphoblastic leukaemia cells. Br J Haematol 2000; 111(2):580–586.

56. Bouralexis S, Clayer M, Atkins GJ, et al. Sensitivity of fresh isolates of soft tissue sarcoma, osteosarcoma and giant cell tumour cells to Apo2L/TRAIL and doxorubicin. Int J Oncol 2004; 24(5):1263–1270.

57. Odoux C, Albers A, Amoscato AA, Lotze MT, Wong MK. TRAIL, FasL and a blocking anti-DR5 antibody augment paclitaxel-induced apoptosis in human non-small-cell lung cancer. Int J Cancer 2002; 97(4):458–465.

58. van Geelen CM, de Vries EG, Le TK, van Weeghel RP, de Jong S. Differential modulation of the TRAIL receptors and the CD95 receptor in colon carcinoma cell lines. Br J Cancer 2003; 89(2):363–373.

59. Cuello M, Ettenberg SA, Nau MM, Lipkowitz S. Synergistic induction of apoptosis by the combination of trail and chemotherapy in chemoresistant ovarian cancer cells. Gynecol Oncol 2001; 81(3):380–390.

60. Vignati S, Codegoni A, Polato F, Broggini M. Trail activity in human ovarian cancer cells: potentiation of the action of cytotoxic drugs. Eur J Cancer 2002; 38(1):177–183.

61. Mitsiades N, Poulaki V, Tseleni-Balafouta S, Koutras DA, Stamenkovic I. Thyroid carcinoma cells are resistant to FAS-mediated apoptosis but sensitive tumor necrosis factor-related apoptosis-inducing ligand. Cancer Res 2000; 60(15):4122–4129.

62. Frese S, Brunner T, Gugger M, Uduehi A, Schmid RA. Enhancement of Apo2L/TRAIL (tumor necrosis factor-related apoptosis-inducing ligand)-induced apoptosis in non-small cell lung cancer cell lines by chemotherapeutic agents without correlation to the expression level of cellular protease caspase-8 inhibitory protein. J Thorac Cardiovasc Surg 2002; 123(1):168–174.

63. Ibrahim SM, Ringel J, Schmidt C, et al. Pancreatic adenocarcinoma cell lines show variable susceptibility to TRAIL-mediated cell death. Pancreas 2001; 23(1):72–79.

64. Shin EC, Ahn JM, Kim CH, et al. IFN-gamma induces cell death in human hepatoma cells through a TRAIL/death receptor-mediated apoptotic pathway. Int J Cancer 2001; 93(2):262–268.

65. Griffith TS, Chin WA, Jackson GC, Lynch DH, Kubin MZ. Intracellular regulation of TRAIL-induced apoptosis in human melanoma cells. J Immunol 1998; 161(6):2833–2840.

66. Marsters SA, Frutkin AD, Simpson NJ, Fendly BM, Ashkenazi A. Identification of cysteine-rich domains of the type 1 tumor necrosis factor receptor involved in ligand binding. J Biol Chem 1992; 267(9):5747–5750.

67. Kuang AA, Diehl GE, Zhang J, Winoto A. FADD is required for DR4- and DR5-mediated apoptosis: lack of trail-induced apoptosis in FADD-deficient mouse embryonic fibroblasts. J Biol Chem 2000; 275(33):25,065–25,068.

68. Kischkel FC, Lawrence DA, Chuntharapai A, Schow P, Kim KJ, Ashkenazi A. Apo2L/TRAIL-dependent recruitment of endogenous FADD and caspase-8 to death receptors 4 and 5. Immunity 2000; 12(6): 611–620.

69. Schneider P, Thome M, Burns K, et al. TRAIL receptors 1 (DR4) and 2 (DR5) signal FADD-dependent apoptosis and activate NF-kappaB. Immunity 1997; 7(6):831–836.

70. Kischkel FC, Lawrence DA, Tinel A, et al. Death receptor recruitment of endogenous caspase-10 and apoptosis initiation in the absence of caspase-8. J Biol Chem 2001; 276(49):46,639–46,646.

71. Luo X, Budihardjo I, Zou H, Slaughter C, Wang X. Bid, a Bcl2 interacting protein, mediates cytochrome c release from mitochondria in response to activation of cell surface death receptors. Cell 1998; 94(4):481–490.

72. Tang D, Lahti JM, Kidd VJ. Caspase-8 activation and bid cleavage contribute to MCF7 cellular execution in a caspase-3-dependent manner during staurosporine-mediated apoptosis. J Biol Chem 2000; 275(13):9303–9307.

73. McDonnell MA, Wang D, Khan SM, Vander Heiden MG, Kelekar A. Caspase-9 is activated in a cytochrome c-independent manner early during TNFalpha-induced apoptosis in murine cells. Cell Death Differ 2003; 10(9):1005–1015.

74. Wang S, El-Deiry WS. TRAIL and apoptosis induction by TNF-family death receptors. Oncogene 2003; 22(53):8628–8633.

75. Muhlenbeck F, Haas E, Schwenzer R, et al. TRAIL/Apo2L activates c-Jun NH2-terminal kinase (JNK) via caspase-dependent and caspase-independent pathways. J Biol Chem 1998; 273(49):33,091–33,098.

76. Lin Y, Devin A, Cook A, et al. The death domain kinase RIP is essential for TRAIL (Apo2L)-induced activation of IkappaB kinase and c-Jun N-terminal kinase. Mol Cell Biol 2000; 20(18):6638–6645.

77. Secchiero P, Milani D, Gonelli A, et al. Tumor necrosis factor (TNF)-related apoptosis-inducing ligand (TRAIL) and TNF-alpha promote the NF-kappaB-dependent maturation of normal and leukemic myeloid cells. J Leukocyte Biol 2003; 74(2):223–232.

78. Secchiero P, Melloni E, Heikinheimo M, et al. TRAIL regulates normal erythroid maturation through an ERK-dependent pathway. Blood 2004; 103(2):517–522.

79. Muhlenbeck F, Schneider P, Bodmer JL, et al. The tumor necrosis factor-related apoptosis-inducing ligand receptors TRAIL-R1 and TRAIL-R2 have distinct cross-linking requirements for initiation of apoptosis and are non-redundant in JNK activation. J Biol Chem 2000; 275(41):32,208–32,213.

80. Ohtsuka T, Buchsbaum D, Oliver P, Makhija S, Kimberly R, Zhou T. Synergistic induction of tumor cell apoptosis by death receptor antibody and chemotherapy agent through JNK/p38 and mitochondrial death pathway. Oncogene 2003; 22(13):2034–2044.

81. Vivo C, Liu W, Broaddus VC. c-Jun N-terminal kinase contributes to apoptotic synergy induced by tumor necrosis factor-related apoptosis-inducing ligand plus DNA damage in chemoresistant, p53 inactive mesothelioma cells. J Biol Chem 2003; 278(28):25,461–25,467.

82. Secchiero P, Gonelli A, Carnevale E, et al. TRAIL promotes the survival and proliferation of primary human vascular endothelial cells by activating the Akt and ERK pathways. Circulation 2003; 107(17): 2250–2256.

83. Secchiero P, Gonelli A, Mirandola P, et al. Tumor necrosis factor-related apoptosis-inducing ligand induces monocytic maturation of leukemic and normal myeloid precursors through a caspase-dependent pathway. Blood 2002; 100(7):2421–2429.

84. Leverkus M, Sprick MR, Wachter T, et al. TRAIL-induced apoptosis and gene induction in HaCaT keratinocytes: differential contribution of TRAIL receptors 1 and 2. J Invest Dermatol 2003; 121(1): 149–155.

85. Ehrhardt H, Fulda S, Schmid I, Hiscott J, Debatin KM, Jeremias I. TRAIL induced survival and proliferation in cancer cells resistant towards TRAIL-induced apoptosis mediated by NF-kappaB. Oncogene 2003; 22(25):3842–3852.

86. LeBlanc HN, Ashkenazi A. Apo2L/TRAIL and its death and decoy receptors. Cell Death Differ 2003; 10(1):66–75.

87. Thorburn A. Death receptor-induced cell killing. Cell Signal 2004; 16(2):139–144.

88. Muhlethaler-Mottet A, Bourloud KB, Auderset K, Joseph JM, Gross N. Drug-mediated sensitization to TRAIL-induced apoptosis in caspase-8-complemented neuroblastoma cells proceeds via activation of intrinsic and extrinsic pathways and caspase-dependent cleavage of XIAP, Bcl-x(L) and RIP. Oncogene 2004; 23(32):5415–5425.

89. Wang LL, Zhang MH, Xu CG. [Synergistic effect of Apo2L and chemotherapeutic agents on leukemia cells]. Zhonghua Xue Ye Xue Za Zhi 2003; 24(11):593–595.

90. Singh TR, Shankar S, Chen X, Asim M, Srivastava RK. Synergistic interactions of chemotherapeutic drugs and tumor necrosis factor-related apoptosis-inducing ligand/Apo-2 ligand on apoptosis and on regression of breast carcinoma in vivo. Cancer Res 2003; 63(17):5390–5400.

91. Bouralexis S, Findlay DM, Atkins GJ, Labrinidis A, Hay S, Evdokiou A. Progressive resistance of BTK-143 osteosarcoma cells to Apo2L/TRAIL-induced apoptosis is mediated by acquisition of DcR2/ TRAIL-R4 expression: resensitisation with chemotherapy. Br J Cancer 2003; 89(1):206–214.

92. Asakuma J, Sumitomo M, Asano T, Hayakawa M. Selective Akt inactivation and tumor necrosis actor-related apoptosis-inducing ligand sensitization of renal cancer cells by low concentrations of paclitaxel. Cancer Res 2003; 63(6):1365–1370.

93. Naka T, Sugamura K, Hylander BL, Widmer MB, Rustum YM, Repasky EA. Effects of tumor necrosis factor-related apoptosis-inducing ligand alone and in combination with chemotherapeutic agents on patients' colon tumors grown in SCID mice. Cancer Res 2002; 62(20):5800–5806.

94. Kelly MM, Hoel BD, Voelkel-Johnson C. Doxorubicin pretreatment sensitizes prostate cancer cell lines to TRAIL induced apoptosis which correlates with the loss of c-FLIP expression. Cancer Biol Ther 2002; 1(5):520–527.

95. Nagane M, Huang HJ, Cavenee WK. The potential of TRAIL for cancer chemotherapy. Apoptosis 2001; 6(3):191–197.

96. Chen XP, He SQ, Wang HP, Zhao YZ, Zhang WG. Expression of TNF-related apoptosis-inducing Ligand receptors and antitumor tumor effects of TNF-related apoptosis-inducing Ligand in human hepatocellular carcinoma. World J Gastroenterol 2003; 9(11):2433–2440.

97. Jazirehi AR, Ng CP, Gan XH, Schiller G, Bonavida B. Adriamycin sensitizes the adriamycin-resistant 8226/Dox40 human multiple myeloma cells to Apo2L/tumor necrosis factor-related apoptosis-inducing ligand-mediated (TRAIL) apoptosis. Clin Cancer Res 2001; 7(12):3874–3883.

98. Mitsiades CS, Treon SP, Mitsiades N, et al. TRAIL/Apo2L ligand selectively induces apoptosis and overcomes drug resistance in multiple myeloma: therapeutic applications. Blood 2001; 98(3):795–804.

99. Keane MM, Ettenberg SA, Nau MM, Russell EK, Lipkowitz S. Chemotherapy augments TRAIL-induced apoptosis in breast cell lines. Cancer Res 1999; 59(3):734–741.

100. Nagane M, Pan G, Weddle JJ, Dixit VM, Cavenee WK, Huang HJ. Increased death receptor 5 expression by chemotherapeutic agents in human gliomas causes synergistic cytotoxicity with tumor necrosis factor-related apoptosis-inducing ligand in vitro and in vivo. Cancer Res 2000; 60(4):847–853.

101. Clayer M, Bouralexis S, Evdokiou A, Hay S, Atkins GJ, Findlay DM. Enhanced apoptosis of soft tissue sarcoma cells with chemotherapy: a potential new approach using TRAIL. J Orthop Surg (Hong Kong) 2001; 9(2):19–22.

102. Liu W, Bodle E, Chen JY, Gao M, Rosen GD, Broaddus VC. Tumor necrosis factor-related apoptosis-inducing ligand and chemotherapy cooperate to induce apoptosis in mesothelioma cell lines. Am J Respir Cell Mol Biol 2001; 25(1):111–118.

103. Mitsiades N, Mitsiades CS, Poulaki V, Anderson KC, Treon SP. Concepts in the use of TRAIL/Apo2L: an emerging biotherapy for myeloma and other neoplasias. Expert Opin Invest Drugs 2001; 10(8): 1521–1530.

104. Evdokiou A, Bouralexis S, Atkins GJ, et al. Chemotherapeutic agents sensitize osteogenic sarcoma cells, but not normal human bone cells, to Apo2L/TRAIL-induced apoptosis. Int J Cancer 2002; 99(4): 491–504.

105. Voelkel-Johnson C. An antibody against DR4 (TRAIL-R1) in combination with doxorubicin selectively kills malignant but not normal prostate cells. Cancer Biol Ther 2003; 2(3):283–290.

106. Belka C, Schmid B, Marini P, et al. Sensitization of resistant lymphoma cells to irradiation-induced apoptosis by the death ligand TRAIL. Oncogene 2001; 20(17):2190–2196.

107. Johnston JB, Kabore AF, Strutinsky J, et al. Role of the TRAIL/APO2-L death receptors in chlorambucil- and fludarabine-induced apoptosis in chronic lymphocytic leukemia. Oncogene 2003; 22(51): 8356–8369.

108. Arizono Y, Yoshikawa H, Naganuma H, Hamada Y, Nakajima Y, Tasaka K. A mechanism of resistance to TRAIL/Apo2L-induced apoptosis of newly established glioma cell line and sensitisation to TRAIL by genotoxic agents. Br J Cancer 2003; 88(2):298–306.

109. Harper N, Farrow SN, Kaptein A, Cohen GM, MacFarlane M. Modulation of tumor necrosis factor apoptosis-inducing ligand-induced NF-kappa B activation by inhibition of apical caspases. J Biol Chem 2001; 276(37):34,743–34,752.

110. MacFarlane M, Harper N, Snowden RT, et al. Mechanisms of resistance to TRAIL-induced apoptosis in primary B cell chronic lymphocytic leukaemia. Oncogene 2002; 21(44):6809–6818.

111. Kang J, Kisenge RR, Toyoda H, et al. Chemical sensitization and regulation of TRAIL-induced apoptosis in a panel of B-lymphocytic leukaemia cell lines. Br J Haematol 2003; 123(5):921–932.

112. Ng CP, Bonavida B. X-linked inhibitor of apoptosis (XIAP) blocks Apo2 ligand/tumor necrosis factor-related apoptosis-inducing ligand-mediated apoptosis of prostate cancer cells in the presence of mitochondrial activation: sensitization by overexpression of second mitochondria-derived activator of caspase/direct IAP-binding protein with low pI (Smac/DIABLO). Mol Cancer Ther 2002; 1(12):1051–1058.

113. He Q, Huang Y, Sheikh MS. Proteasome inhibitor MG132 upregulates death receptor 5 and cooperates with Apo2L/TRAIL to induce apoptosis in Bax-proficient and -deficient cells. Oncogene 2004; 23(14): 2554–2558.

114. LeBlanc H, Lawrence D, Varfolomeev E, et al. Tumor-cell resistance to death receptor—induced apoptosis through mutational inactivation of the proapoptotic Bcl-2 homolog Bax. Nat Med 2002; 8(3): 274–281.

115. Mitsiades N, Mitsiades CS, Poulaki V, et al. Biologic sequelae of nuclear factor–kappaB blockade in multiple myeloma: therapeutic applications. Blood 2002; 99(11):4079–4086.

116. Johnson TR, Stone K, Nikrad M, et al. The proteasome inhibitor PS-341 overcomes TRAIL resistance in Bax and caspase 9-negative or Bcl-xL overexpressing cells. Oncogene 2003; 22(32):4953–4963.

117. Siegmund D, Hadwiger P, Pfizenmaier K, Vornlocher HP, Wajant H. Selective inhibition of FLICE-like inhibitory protein expression with small interfering RNA oligonucleotides is sufficient to sensitize tumor cells for TRAIL-induced apoptosis. Mol Med 2002; 8(11):725–732.

118. Zhang XD, Gillespie SK, Borrow JM, Hersey P. The histone deacetylase inhibitor suberic bishydroxamate: a potential sensitizer of melanoma to TNF-related apoptosis-inducing ligand (TRAIL) induced apoptosis. Biochem Pharmacol 2003; 66(8):1537–1545.

119. Rosato RR, Almenara JA, Dai Y, Grant S. Simultaneous activation of the intrinsic and extrinsic pathways by histone deacetylase (HDAC) inhibitors and tumor necrosis factor-related apoptosis-inducing ligand (TRAIL) synergistically induces mitochondrial damage and apoptosis in human leukemia cells. Mol Cancer Ther 2003; 2(12):1273–1284.

120. Jones DT, Ganeshaguru K, Mitchell WA, et al. Cytotoxic drugs enhance the ex vivo sensitivity of malignant cells from a subset of acute myeloid leukaemia patients to apoptosis induction by tumour necrosis factor receptor-related apoptosis-inducing ligand. Br J Haematol 2003; 121(5):713–720.

121. Plasilova M, Zivny J, Jelinek J, et al. TRAIL (Apo2L) suppresses growth of primary human leukemia and myelodysplasia progenitors. Leukemia 2002; 16(1):67–73.

122. Wuchter C, Krappmann D, Cai Z, et al. In vitro susceptibility to TRAIL-induced apoptosis of acute leukemia cells in the context of TRAIL receptor gene expression and constitutive NF-kappa B activity. Leukemia 2001; 15(6):921–928.

123. Hussain A, Doucet JP, Gutierrez M, et al. Tumor necrosis factor-related apoptosis-inducing ligand (TRAIL) and Fas apoptosis in Burkitt's lymphomas with loss of multiple pro-apoptotic proteins. Haematologica 2003; 88(2):167–175.

124. Zhao S, Asgary Z, Wang Y, Goodwin R, Andreeff M, Younes A. Functional expression of TRAIL by lymphoid and myeloid tumour cells. Br J Haematol 1999; 106(3):827–832.

125. Olsson A, Diaz T, Aguilar-Santelises M, et al. Sensitization to TRAIL-induced apoptosis and modulation of FLICE-inhibitory protein in B chronic lymphocytic leukemia by actinomycin D. Leukemia 2001; 15(12):1868–1877.

126. Lawrence D, Shahrokh Z, Marsters S, et al. Differential hepatocyte toxicity of recombinant Apo2L/TRAIL versions. Nat Med 2001; 7(4):383–385.

127. Ichikawa K, Liu W, Zhao L, et al. Tumoricidal activity of a novel anti-human DR5 monoclonal antibody without hepatocyte cytotoxicity. Nat Med 2001; 7(8):954–960.

128. Hasel C, Durr S, Rau B, et al. In chronic pancreatitis, widespread emergence of TRAIL receptors in epithelia coincides with neoexpression of TRAIL by pancreatic stellate cells of early fibrotic areas. Lab Invest 2003; 83(6):825–836.

129. Dobson C, Edwards B, Main S, Minter R, Williams L. Generation of human therapeutic anti-TRAIL-R1 agonistic antibodies by phage display. In: AACR Annual Proceedings, 2002.

130. Humphreys RC, Alderson RF, Bayever E, et al. HGS-ETR2 TRAIL R2-mAb, a human agonistic monoclonal antibody to tumor necrosis factor-related apoptosis inducing ligand receptor 2, affects tumor growth and induces apoptosis in human tumor xenograft models in vivo. In: 94th AACR Annual Meeting 2003; 44:123.

131. Johnson RL, Gillotte D, Poortman C, et al. Human agonistic anti-TRAIL receptor antibodies, HGS-ETR1 and HGS-ETR2, induce apoptosis in ovarian tumor lines and their activity is enhanced by taxol and carboplatin. In: Proceedings of the AACR 2004:45.

132. Johnson RL, Huang X, Fiscella M, et al. Human agonistic anti-TRAIL receptor antibodies, HGS-ETR1 and HGS-ETR2, induce apoptosis in diverse hematological tumor lines. Blood 2003; 102(11):891a.

133. Alderson RF, Birse CE, Connolly K, et al. HGS-ETR2 TRAIL-R2 mAb, a human agonistic monoclonal antibody to tumor necrosis factor-related apoptosis inducing ligand receptor 2, induces apoptosis in human tumor cells. In: Proceedings of 94th AACR Annual Meeting 2003; 44:192.

134. Georgakis GV, Li Y, Humphreys R, et al. Activity of selective agonistic monoclonal antibodies to TRAIL death receptors R1 and R2 in primary and cultured tumor cells of hematological origin. Blood 2003; 102(11):228a.

135. Ohtsuka T, Zhou T. Bisindolylmaleimide VIII enhances DR5-mediated apoptosis through the MKK4/JNK/p38 kinase and the mitochondrial pathways. J Biol Chem 2002; 277(32):29,294–29,303.

136. Kaliberov S, Stackhouse MA, Kaliberova L, Zhou T, Buchsbaum DJ. Enhanced apoptosis following treatment with TRA-8 anti-human DR5 monoclonal antibody and overexpression of exogenous Bax in human glioma cells. Gene Ther 2004; 11(8):658–667.

# 43

# Clinical Studies of Immunotherapy With Rituximab (Rituxan®) and Radioimmunotherapy With Ibritumomab Tiuxetan (Zevalin®) in B-Cell Lymphoid Malignancies

*Arturo Molina,* MD

## Contents

## Summary

The introduction of the monoclonal antibody rituximab has expanded the treatment options for patients with B-cell non-Hodgkin's lymphoma (NHL). In patients with indolent B-cell lymphomas, rituximab is highly effective both as a single agent and in combination with chemotherapy regimens. Ongoing studies evaluating maintenance rituximab therapy and new combinations suggest clinical outcomes defined primarily by improvements in progression-free survival. In chronic leukemia, the use of rituximab in combination with chemotherapy has led to improved response rates and durable remissions. Studies in aggressive NHL indicate that the addition of rituximab to first-line chemotherapy is associated with improved clinical benefit, and ongoing studies are better defining the optimal use of rituximab in this setting.

Radioimmunotherapy with Y-90 ibritumomab tiuxetan has been shown to be safe and effective for the treatment of patients with relapsed or refractory low-grade, follicular, or transformed B-cell NHL. Of importance, radioimmunotherapy does not preclude the use of other NHL therapies in these patients. This chapter will provide an extensive review of clinical trials with rituximab and Y-90 ibritumomab tiuxetan for the treatment of patients with B-cell NHL.

**Key Words:** Immunotherapy; radioimmunotherapy; rituximab; ibritumomab tiuxetan; B-cell lymphoid malignancies; Non-Hodgkin's lymphoma.

From: *Cancer Drug Discovery and Development: The Oncogenomics Handbook*
Edited by: W. J. LaRochelle and R. A. Shimkets © Humana Press Inc., Totowa, NJ

# 1. RITUXIMAB

The monoclonal antibody rituximab (Rituxan®) has been extensively evaluated in clinical trials, both as a single agent and in combination with chemotherapy, for the treatment of indolent and aggressive B-cell lymphomas, chronic lymphocytic leukemia (CLL), and other lymphoproliferative disorders. In addition, rituximab is an essential component of the ibritumomab tiuxetan (Zevalin®) radioimmunotherapy regimen.

Rituximab is approved in the United States for the treatment of patients with relapsed or refractory low-grade or follicular CD20-positive B-cell non-Hodgkin's lymphoma (NHL). A recent expansion of the labeled indication includes treatment of patients with relapsed or refractory low-grade or follicular NHL with bulky disease (defined as a lesion > 10 cm), retreatment of patients with a prior response to rituximab, and an extended treatment schedule consisting of rituximab 375 mg/m$^2$ weekly for 8 wk. Rituximab is approved in the European Union and other countries under the trade name MabThera®, where it is indicated for the treatment of patients with stage III/IV follicular, chemoresistant, or relapsed NHL and in combination with chemotherapy for the treatment of diffuse aggressive NHL.

## 1.1. Mechanism of Action

Rituximab is a chimeric $IgG_1$ kappa monoclonal antibody, engineered to combine murine light- and heavy-chain variable region sequences with human light- and heavy-chain constant region sequences. Rituximab is specifically directed against the CD20 antigen, a transmembrane protein involved in cell cycle progression and differentiation and is present on greater than 90% of B-cell NHLs [1,2]. CD20 is also normally expressed during B-cell development, from pre-B-cells through activated B-cells, but it is not present on stem cells or fully differentiated plasma cells [2–3].

Exposure to rituximab results in rapid and sustained depletion of CD20-positive B-cell populations. Multiple mechanisms of action appear to be involved, including antibody-dependent cellular cytotoxicity (ADCC), complement-dependent cytolysis (CDC), and initiation of apoptosis [4–11]. Recent studies have suggested that the therapeutic activity of rituximab can, in part, be directly related to interactions between the antibody and cellular Fc receptors involved in ADCC [12–14].

Antibody-dependent cellular cytotoxicity is mediated through immune effector cells, such as monocytes, macrophages, and natural killer (NK) cells, via binding of cellular Fcγ receptors to the Fc portion of IgG [15]. Engagement of FcγRIII, a subclass of Fcγ receptors, activates and promotes ADCC activity. A genetic dimorphism results in either a phenylalanine (F) or a valine (V) residue at position 158 on the receptor, which is in a region that directly interacts with $IgG_1$ [16]. FcγRIII receptors that are homozygous for valine (V/V) have an increased affinity for $IgG_1$ compared to either heterozygous (F/V) or homozygous phenylalanine (F/F) receptors [17]. Studies have indicated that rituximab response rates are higher and event-free survival is longer in B-cell follicular NHL patients with homozygous FcγRIII V/V receptors compared to patients with heterozygous or homozygous F/F receptors. As such, these data also suggest that ADCC is a critical mechanism related to therapeutic outcomes in these patients.

Rituximab also binds with human C1q, leading to complement-dependent cytolysis of B-lymphocytes [4]. Resistance to rituximab therapy in CLL cells might, in part, be mediated through the presence of cell surface complement inhibitors CD55 and CD5 [11]. Binding of rituximab to the CD20 antigen on the surface of B-cells can result in direct cellular effects, including phosphorylation of tyrosine kinases, leading to inhibition of cell proliferation and induction of apoptosis (5–10).

The mechanisms by which rituximab affects B-cell depletion continue to be defined and it has yet to be determined which specific mechanisms might most influence clinical outcomes. Indeed, it remains possible that different mechanisms could be predominant for specific hematologic malignancies, within particular sites of the body or among individual patients.

Rituximab can synergistically enhance the cytotoxicity of traditional chemotherapeutic agents, including doxorubicin, cisplatin, fludarabine, and vinblastine, an effect apparently mediated through downregulation of bcl-2 (18–20). The combination of rituximab with glucocorticoids can synergistically enhance antiproliferative and apoptotic effects through increased CDC activity (21). In addition, the use of cytokines such as interleukin-2 (IL-2) and IL-12 in combination with rituximab might be effective in enhancing immune responsiveness, thereby increasing responsiveness to rituximab (6,22,23).

## 1.2. Rituximab for the Treatment of NHL

### 1.2.1. RITUXIMAB IN INDOLENT NHL

**1.2.1.1. Single-Agent Therapy.** The first clinical trials of rituximab administered the antibody as a single agent in patients with relapsed or refractory B-cell NHL (Table 1). These studies showed that rituximab administered at a dose of 375 mg/m$^2$ weekly for 4 wk had substantial efficacy and was well tolerated in these patients (24,25). An early, pivotal study was a single-arm multicenter trial of a standard dose of rituximab, 375 mg/m$^2$ weekly for 4 wk, in 166 patients with relapsed or refractory low-grade or follicular B-cell NHL (26,27). These patients were heavily pretreated, having received a median of three prior therapies. The overall response rate was 48% (6% complete response and 42% partial responses), with a median response duration of 11.2 mo and a median time to progression in responding patients of 13.1 mo. Although standard response criteria were not available at the time that this study was conducted, a subsequent analysis applying the newly adopted International Workshop Response Criteria (IWRC) (37) assessed the overall response rate in the trial at 57% (38). Subsequent clinical trials have confirmed the efficacy of a standard 4-wk course of rituximab, reporting overall response rates ranging from 46% to 59% in patients with relapsed or refractory B-cell NHL and an overall response rate of 39% in patients with relapsed B-cell NHL and bulky disease (28–31).

The use of extended dosing schedules of rituximab has also proven to be effective in patients with relapsed or refractory indolent NHL. Rituximab 375 mg/m$^2$ administered weekly for 6 or 8 wk was well tolerated and resulted in overall response rates of 57–76% (32,33). Retreatment with a standard course of rituximab is also feasible in patients who have previously responded to rituximab. In one study evaluating 57 such patients, retreatment produced an overall response rate of 40%, with a median response duration of over 15 mo, which was longer than the 9.8-mo response duration observed with these patients in the initial rituximab course (34,35).

Scheduled maintenance therapy is emerging as a therapeutic option. Patients with recurrent follicular NHL or small lymphocytic lymphoma (SLL) with either a clinical response or stable disease following a standard course of rituximab were randomized to receive either maintenance rituximab (rituximab 375 mg/m$^2$ weekly for 4 wk, repeated every 6 mo for four courses) or retreatment with a standard course of rituximab at the time of disease pro-

Table 1

Single-Agent Rituximab in Relapsed or Refractory Low-grade or Follicular NHL

| Study | Population | Dose and Schedule | Patients (N)[a] | Response |
|---|---|---|---|---|
| Maloney 1997 (24) | Relapsed low-grade B-cell NHL | Rituximab 125 mg/m$^2$, 250 mg/m$^2$, 375 mg/m$^2$ or 500 mg/m$^2$ weekly × 4 | 14[b,c] | ORR = 40% (40% PR) Median DR not available |
| Maloney 1997 (25) | Relapsed low-grade B-cell NHL | Rituximab 375 mg/m$^2$ weekly × 4 | 37 | ORR = 46% (8% CR, 38% PR) Median DR = 8.6 mo |
| McLaughlin 1998 (26,27) | Relapsed or refractory low-grade or follicular B-cell NHL | Rituximab 375 mg/m$^2$ weekly × 4 | 166 | ORR = 48% (6% CR, 42% PR) Median DR = 11.2 mo |
| Foran 2000 (28) | Relapsed or refractory follicular NHL | Rituximab 375 mg/m$^2$ weekly × 4 | 70 | ORR = 46% (3% CR, 43% PR) Median DR = 11 mo |
| Feuring-Buske 2000 (29) | Relapsed advanced-stage follicular lymphoma | Rituximab 375 mg/m$^2$ weekly × 4 | 30[b,c] | ORR = 47% (17% CR, 30% PR) Median DR = 5.8 mo |
| Walewski 2001 (30) | Recurrent indolent lymphoma | Rituximab 375 mg/m$^2$ weekly × 4 | 34[b] | ORR = 59% (24% CR, 35% PR) Median TTP = 16 mo |
| Davis 1999 (31) | Relapsed or refractory, bulky disease, low-grade NHL | Rituximab 375 mg/m$^2$ weekly × 4 | 31 | ORR = 39% (3% CR, 35% PR) Median DR = 5.9 mo |
| Piro 1999 (32) | Relapsed or refractory follicular, low-grade NHL | Rituximab 375 mg/m$^2$ weekly × 8 | 37 | ORR = 57% (14% CR, 43% PR) Median DR = 13.4+ mo |

| Study | Patient population | Treatment | N | Results |
|---|---|---|---|---|
| Avilés 2001 (33) | Relapsed or refractory follicular NHL | Rituximab 375 mg/m² weekly × 6 | 17 | ORR = 76% (47% CR, 29% PR) Median DR not available |
| Davis 2000 (34,35) | Rituximab-relapsed low-grade or follicular NHL | Rituximab 375 mg/m² weekly × 4 | 57[b] | ORR = 40% (11% CR, 30% PR) Median DR = 15.7+ mo |
| Hainsworth 2004 (36) | Recurrent follicular NHL or SLL | Rituximab 375 mg/m² weekly × 4; responding and stable disease patients randomized to: 1. Maintenance rituximab 375 mg/m² weekly × 4 every 6 mo × 4 or 2. Retreatment with rituximab 375 mg/m² weekly × 4 at time of progression | 114 | With first course: ORR/SD = 47% Maintenance or retreatment (n = 90): Maintenance ORR = 52% (27% CR, 25% PR) Median PFS = 31 mo Retreatment ORR = 35% (4% CR, 31% PR) Median PFS = 8 mo |

ORR, overall response rate; PR, partial response; DR, duration of response; CR, complete response; SLL, small lymphocytic lymphoma; SD, stable disease; PFS, progression-free survival.

[a]Intent-to-treat population, unless noted otherwise.

[b]Evaluable patients.

[c]Subset of patients with follicular or low-grade NHL.

gression *(36)*. Preliminary results from 114 patients had 47% achieving a clinical response or stable disease following an initial course of rituximab. A total of 90 patients received either maintenance therapy or retreatment, with an overall response rate of 52% and median progression-free survival time of 31 mo in the maintenance group, compared to an overall response rate of 35%, with a median progression-free survival time of 8 mo in the retreatment group. Further follow-up time will determine the full comparative benefit of maintenance vs retreatment strategies in these relapsed or refractory NHL patients *(36)*.

First-line treatment with single-agent rituximab in patients with follicular or low-grade B-cell NHL has produced overall response rates ranging from 47% to 73% (Table 2) *(39–44)*. Therapy with rituximab can also produce durable molecular responses. The t(14;18) (q32;q21) translocation is the most common bcl-2 gene rearrangement in lymphoid malignancies. In one study of patients with low tumor burden, a single course of standard rituximab therapy rendered 17 of 30 patients with an initially detectable bcl-2 gene rearrangement negative by polymerase chain reaction (PCR) in the peripheral blood at study day 50, with 9 of these patients also having PCR-negative bone marrows. A significant relationship was noted between molecular and clinical response ($p < 0.0001$), and an early molecular remission was associated with a more favorable progression-free survival time ($p < 0.005$) within the first year compared to those patients with a persistent bcl-2 rearrangement *(39)*.

Maintenance therapy with rituximab in patients who achieve a response or have stable disease after first-line treatment with rituximab produces prolonged remissions in a substantial proportion of patients. With maintenance therapy consisting of a standard 4-wk course of rituximab repeated every 6 mo for 4 courses, Hainsworth et al. reported an improvement in overall response rate in 62 patients, from 47% to 73%, with the complete response rate increasing from 7% to 37% *(41)*. Median progression-free survival is currently 37 mo, with a 5-yr progression-free survival rate of 34% *(42,43)*.

Ghielmini et al. randomized patients achieving a clinical response or stable disease following a single course of standard rituximab as either first-line therapy or for relapsed or refractory follicular B-cell NHL to either rituximab, delivered as a single infusion of rituximab 375 mg/m$^2$ delivered every 8 wk (mo 3, 5, 7, and 9) or observation *(44)*. Overall response rates to initial therapy were 67% in 57 first-line patients and 46% in 128 relapsed or refractory patients. In the 151 patients randomized to either maintenance or observation, median event-free survival was 23 mo in the maintenance group and 12 mo in the observation group ($p = 0.02$). In first-line patients, median event-free survival was 36 mo with maintenance rituximab compared to 19 mo for observation ($p = 0.009$). Overall, for patients responding to the rituximab-induction phase, event-free survival with maintenance therapy was 36 mo, more than double the 16-mo event-free survival time seen in patients randomized to observation ($p = 0.004$) *(44)*.

Rituximab has also demonstrated significant activity in other indolent lymphoma subsets, including Waldenstrom's macroglobulinemia (lymphoplasmacytic lymphoma) and extranodal marginal zone/mucosa-associated lymphoid tissue (MALT) lymphomas (Table 3) *(45–50)*. In a retrospective analysis of 30 patients with Waldenstrom's macroglobulinemia treated with a standard 4-wk course of rituximab, 8 patients (27%) had achieved a partial response and 10 patients (33%) achieved a minor response, with a median time to treatment failure of 8 mo *(45)*. Three studies have since prospectively evaluated rituximab for the treatment of Waldenstrom's macroglobulinemia. In two trials, first-line or relapsed or refractory patients received an initial standard course of rituximab, followed by a second course 6 mo later in patients without disease progression. Overall response rates ranged

Table 2

Single-Agent Rituximab in as First-line Therapy in Low-Grade or Follicular NHL

| Study | Population | Dose and Schedule | Patients (N)[a] | Response |
|---|---|---|---|---|
| Colombat 2001 (39) | Follicular NHL with low tumor burden | Rituximab 375 mg/m² weekly × 4 | 49[b] | ORR = 73% (26% CR, 47% PR) Median DR not available |
| Gutheil 2000 (40) | Low-grade or follicular NHL | Rituximab 375 mg/m² weekly × 4 | 20 | ORR = 50% Median DR not available |
| Hainsworth 2002 (41–43) | Low-grade follicular NHL and CLL | Rituximab 375 mg/m² weekly × 4; After evaluation at 6 wk, rituximab was repeated in responding and stable disease patients every 6 mo for maximum 4 courses | 62 | With first course: ORR = 47% (7% CR, 40% PR) ≥ 1 course (n = 55): ORR = 73% (37% CR, 37% PR) Median PFS = 37 mo 5-yr PFS = 34% |
| Ghielmini 2004 (44) | Follicular NHL, first-line or relapsed or refractory | Rituximab 375 mg/m² weekly × 4; responding and stable disease patients randomized to 1. Observation or 2. Repeated single infusion every 8 wk (mo 3, 5, 7, and 9) | 185[b] | With first course: ORR = 67% in 57 first-line patients; 46% in 128 relapsed or refractory patients. Median event-free survival: 23 mo in maintenance arm, 12 mo in observation arm |

PFS, progression-free survival.
[a]Intent-to-treat population, unless noted otherwise.
[b]Evaluable patients.

683

Table 3
Single-Agent Rituximab in Other Indolent Lymphoma Subtypes

| Study | Population | Dose and Schedule | Patients (N)[a] | Response |
|---|---|---|---|---|
| Treon 2001 (45) | First-line, relapsed, or refractory Waldenstrom's macroglobulinemia | Retrospective analysis of multiple trials; Rituximab 375 mg/m$^2$ weekly × 4, median 4 infusions (range 1–11) | 30[b] | ORR = 27% (27% PR, 33% minor response) Median time to treatment failure in responders = 8 mo |
| Dimopoulos 2002 (46) | First-line, relapsed, or refractory Waldenstrom's macroglobulinemia | Rituximab 375 mg/m$^2$ weekly × 4; if no disease progression at 6 mo, repeat course | 27 | ORR = 44% (44% PR) Median TTP = 16 mo |
| Treon 2002 (47) | First-line, relapsed, or refractory Waldenstrom's macroglobulinemia | Rituximab 375 mg/m$^2$ weekly × 4; if no disease progression at 6 mo, repeat course | 22[b] | ORR = 73% (50% PR, 23% minor response) Median time to treatment failure in responding patients not reached |
| Gertz 2004 (48) | First-line, relapsed, or refractory Waldenstrom's macroglobulinemia | Rituximab 375 mg/m$^2$ weekly × 4 | 69 | First-line (n = 34): ORR = 35% (35% PR) Median DR = 27 mo Relapsed/refractory (n = 35): ORR = 20% (20% PR) Median DR not available |
| Conconi 2001 (49) | First-line, relapsed, or refractory MALT | Rituximab 375 mg/m$^2$ weekly × 4 | 34[b] | ORR = 73% (44% CR, 29% PR) ORR = 87% in 23 first-line patients; 45% in 11 relapsed or refractory patients Median DR = 10.5 mo |
| Martinelli 2004 (50) | First-line, relapsed, or refractory gastric MALT | Rituximab 375 mg/m$^2$ weekly × 4 | 26[b] | ORR = 73% (42% CR, 31% PR) Median DR not available |

TTP, time to progression.
[a]Intent-to-treat population, unless noted otherwise.
[b]Evaluable patients.

from 44% to 73% *(45,46)*. The third study, an Eastern Cooperative Oncology Group (ECOG) pilot trial, administered a single course of standard rituximab therapy, with preliminary results indicating overall response rates of 35% and 20% as first-line therapy and in relapsed or refractory patients, respectively *(48)*.

Preliminary reports on predictive factors associated with response to rituximab in patients with Waldenstrom's macroglobulinemia suggest that patients with baseline IgM levels <6000 mg/dL and patients with FcγRIII (V/V) or (V/F) phenotypes are more likely to respond *(51,52)*.

In patients with untreated or relapsed extranodal marginal zone B-cell and MALT lymphomas, single-agent rituximab appears to have substantial activity (Table 3). Overall response rates of 87% and 45% were reported for patients receiving first-line therapy or treatment for relapsed or refractory MALT lymphoma, respectively, with a median duration of response of 10.5 mo *(49)*. In gastric MALT lymphoma, 73% of patients responded to a standard course of rituximab *(50)*.

**1.2.1.2. Rituximab in Combination With Chemotherapy.** A number of clinical trials have evaluated rituximab either in sequence or in combination with chemotherapy, including CHOP (cyclophosphamide, doxorubicin, vincristine, prednisone) and other alkylator-based chemotherapy regimens *(53–63)* as well as fludarabine-based chemotherapy regimens *(65–77)* in patients with indolent NHL (Tables 4 and 5). Compared to single agent rituximab, these regimens have generally demonstrated higher response rates and longer responses in indolent NHL.

In a sequential treatment scheme, Maloney et al. administered six cycles of CHOP chemotherapy to patients as first-line therapy for follicular lymphoma *(53)*. Patients responding to CHOP received further therapy with a standard course of rituximab 375 mg/m$^2$ weekly for 4 wk. The overall response rate in 84 evaluable patients was 72%, with improvements in response in 16 patients (19%) following rituximab.

Rambaldi et al. evaluated the benefit of adding sequential rituximab to CHOP for achieving and maintaining molecular remissions in first-line follicular lymphoma patients *(54)*. The study enrolled 128 patients with bcl-2 rearrangements in either peripheral blood or bone marrow at baseline. After six cycles of CHOP, the overall response rate was 94%. Patients responding to CHOP but with persistent bcl-2 rearrangements went on to receive a standard course of rituximab. Of these 77 patients, 74% were bcl-2 negative at 28 wk. With extended follow-up, patients maintaining a durable bcl-2-negative status had a 5-yr failure-free survival rate of 54% compared to 29% in patients who either never achieved or lost molecular negativity *(55)*. In the 41 patients who achieved a bcl-2-negative status following CHOP alone, the 5-yr failure-free survival rate was 45%.

Because rituximab has demonstrated synergistic activity with a number of chemotherapy agents, several studies have evaluated administering rituximab in combination with chemotherapy for indolent lymphoma (Table 4). In an early study, Czuczman et al. combined rituximab with CHOP as follows: rituximab 375 mg/m$^2$ was administered weekly for two doses prior to the first cycle of CHOP, a single dose of rituximab 375 mg/m$^2$ was administered 2 d before cycles three and five of CHOP, and two doses of rituximab 375 mg/m$^2$ were administered weekly following the sixth and final cycle of CHOP. In the intent-to-treat population of 40 patients, the overall response rate was 95%, with 55% complete responses and 45% partial responses *(56)*. Two patients did not receive therapy; thus, the overall response rate in the 38 evaluable patients was 100%. After nearly 9 yr of follow-up, the median time to progression in evaluable patients was reached at 82 mo *(57)*. Seven of

Table 4

Rituximab in Combination with Chemotherapy in Indolent Lymphoma

| Study | Population | Dose and Schedule | Patients (N)[a] | Response |
|---|---|---|---|---|
| Maloney 2001 (53) | First-line follicular NHL | CHOP × 6<br>If CR or PR, then rituximab 375 mg/m² weekly × 4 | 84[b] | ORR = 72%<br>(54% CR/CRu, 18% PR)<br>2-yr PFS = 76%<br>2-yr OS = 95% |
| Czuczman 2001 (56,57) | First-line, relapsed or refractory low-grade B-cell NHL | Rituximab 375 mg/m² + CHOP[c] × 6 | 38[b] | ORR = 100%<br>(58% CR, 42% PR)<br>Median TTP = 82 mo |
| Hainsworth 2002 (58) | First-line follicular NHL | Rituximab 375 mg/m² weekly × 4, followed by R+CHOP × 3 or R+CVP[c] × 3 | 82[b] | ORR = 97%<br>(57% CR, 40% PR)<br>15-mo PFS = 87% |
| Hiddemann 2004 (59) | First-line follicular NHL | Randomized to<br>1. Rituximab 375 mg/m² + CHOP × 6<br>or<br>2. CHOP × 6<br>Responding patients then received interferon-α or ABMT | 394[b] | R+CHOP<br>ORR = 97%<br>(21% CR, 76% PR)<br>Median TTF = 3+ yr<br>CHOP alone<br>ORR = 93%<br>(18% CR, 75% PR)<br>Median TTF = 2.6 yr |
| Marcus 2004 (60) | First-line follicular NHL | Randomized to<br>1. Rituximab 375 mg/m² + CVP × 8<br>or<br>2. CVP × 8 | 321 | R+CVP (n = 162)<br>ORR = 81%<br>(41% CR/CRu, 40% PR)<br>Median TTF = 27 mo<br>CVP alone (n = 159)<br>ORR = 57%<br>(10% CR/CRu, 47% PR)<br>Median TTF = 7 mo |

| Study | Patient population | Treatment | N | Results |
|---|---|---|---|---|
| Patel 2001 (*61*) | Relapsed or refractory low-grade NHL | Rituximab 375 mg/m$^2$ + CD$^c$; median 6 cycles | 10 | ORR = 100% (40% CR, 60% PR) Median DR not reached at 10+ mo |
| Herold 2001 (*62*) | Advanced follicular, lymphoplasmacytic, or mantle cell lymphoma | Randomized to 1. Rituximab 375 mg/m$^2$ + MCP$^c$ × 8 or 2. MCP × 8 | 106$^b$ | ORR = 81% in all patients (40% CR, 41% PR) Median DR not available |
| Martinelli 2002 (*63*) | First-line or relapsed low-grade NHL | Chl$^c$ daily × 6 wk with rituximab 375 mg/m$^2$ weekly × 4; If CR or PR, then Chl daily for 2 wk × 4 with rituximab × 4 | 29 | ORR = 93% (50% CR, 43% PR) |

CR, complete response; CRu, complete response unconfirmed; PFS, progression-free survival; OS, overall survival; ABMT, autologous bone marrow transplant.
[a]Intent-to-treat population, unless noted otherwise.
[b]Evaluable patients.
[c]CHOP, cyclophophamide/doxorubicin/vincristine/prednisone; CVP, cyclophosphamide/vincristine/prednisone; CD, cyclophosphamide/dexamethasone; MCP, mitoxantrone/chlorambucil/prednisolone; Chl, chlorambucil.

eight patients initially positive for bcl-2 rearrangements tested negative following therapy; three of these patients have remained bcl-2 negative and in continuous complete remission, two patients have reverted to bcl-2 positivity but also remain in continuous complete remission, and two patients with partial responses who reverted to bcl-2 positivity have had disease progression *(57,64)*.

The combination of a standard 4-wk course of rituximab followed by rituximab combined with a short course of chemotherapy, either CHOP or CVP (cyclophosphamide, vincristine, prednisone) for three cycles as first-line treatment for follicular NHL, has also been shown to be effective. An overall response rate of 97% in 82 evaluable patients was reported, with 87% of patients having no evidence of disease progression at 15 mo *(58)*.

Early reports of two large randomized studies have confirmed a clinical benefit of combining rituximab with either CHOP or CVP as first-line therapy for follicular NHL. In a study conducted by the German Low Grade Lymphoma Study Group, the combination of rituximab with six courses of CHOP resulted in a modest increase in overall response rate, 97% vs 93% for CHOP alone *(59)*. However, patients who received CHOP plus rituximab had a significantly improved time to treatment failure, with a median not yet reached after a 3-yr follow-up time compared to 2.6 yr for CHOP alone ($p < 0.0007$). Significant improvements in both overall response rate and time to progression were seen with the addition of rituximab to eight cycles of CVP compared to CVP alone. As reported by Marcus et al., the combination of eight cycles of CVP with rituximab resulted in an overall response rate of 81% compared to 57% for CVP alone ($p < 0.0001$) and an improved median time to treatment failure of 27 mo compared to 7 mo, respectively ($p < 0.0001$) *(60)*. Toxicity profiles of rituximab in combination with CHOP or CVP regimens have been similar to those observed with chemotherapy alone.

Rituximab in combination with other chemotherapy regimens, including cyclophosphamide and dexamethasone, mitoxantrone, chlorambucil, and prednisolone, and single agent chlorambucil has been evaluated in phase II studies in patients with indolent NHL, with overall response rates ranging from 81% to 100% *(51–63)*.

Rituximab has been studied both in combination and in sequence with fludarabine-based regimens in patients with indolent NHL (Table 5) *(65–77)*. The combination of fludarabine and rituximab produced an overall response rate of 90%, with a median duration of response exceeding 15 mo *(65)*. Sequential therapy with FMD (fludarabine, mitoxantrone, dexamethasone) followed by a standard course of rituximab as either first-line therapy or for relapsed or refractory indolent NHL produced an overall response rate of 94%, and in 64 evaluable patients greater than age 60, the overall response rate was 89%, with improvements in the proportion of patients achieving a complete response following rituximab *(66,67)*.

Early results are available for a randomized trial evaluating combination vs sequential FND with rituximab, both followed by maintenance interferon, as first-line therapy for stage IV indolent NHL. Although not statistically different, overall response rates and 3-yr failure-free survival rate favor the combination arm, 100% vs 95% and 77% vs 64%, respectively *(68)*.

For first-line follicular NHL therapy, a randomized trial is comparing a standard course of rituximab following clinical response to either CHOP or FM (fludarabine, mitoxantrone). In a preliminary report, the overall response rates following CHOP and FM were 94% and 93%, respectively, with improvements in molecular responses in both arms following rituximab *(70)*. In patients with relapsed or refractory follicular or mantle cell lymphoma, the combination of FCM (fludarabine, mitoxantrone, cyclophosphamide) with rituximab produced a significantly higher response rate, 82% vs 61%, and a superior progression-free and overall survival time compared with FCM alone *(71)*.

Additional phase II trials of fludarabine-based chemotherapy in combination or in sequence with rituximab as either first-line therapy or in relapsed or refractory indolent NHL have consistently reported overall response rates in the 80–100% range *(69,72–77)*.

There has been concern with the potential for increased infectious complications when using rituximab with fludarabine because of the depletion of both B-cells and T-cells. In a review of the safety of FMD in combination with rituximab, there was a modest increase in the incidence of neutropenia but no apparent increase in infectious complications compared that expected with FMD alone *(78)*.

These studies indicate the combination of rituximab and CVP and CHOP or related chemotherapy regimens as well as fludarabine-based chemotherapy regimens are highly active as first-line therapy and in relapsed or refractory indolent lymphomas. Long-term follow-up results of randomized trials will further define the benefits of combination vs sequential therapies.

### 1.2.2. RITUXIMAB IN B-CELL CHRONIC LYMPHOCYTIC LEUKEMIA

**1.2.2.1. Single-Agent Therapy.** In early clinical trials, the response rates of patients with CLL or small lymphocytic lymphoma (SLL) to a standard 4-wk course of rituximab ranged from 13% to 25% *(26,79,80)*, much lower than that seen typically seen with other indolent NHL subtypes. The density of the CD20 antigen on the surface of B-cell CLL cells is substantially lower than that observed in follicular and other B-cell lymphoma subtypes, and could, in part, explain lower clinical sensitivities of CLL to standard rituximab therapy *(81–83)*. In addition, low levels of soluble CD20 can be detected in the plasma of CLL patients, which could interfere with cellular binding of rituximab *(84)*. In pharmacokinetic studies, rituximab serum concentrations in patients with CLL were lower compared to those observed in other indolent lymphoma patients, and lower rituximab serum concentrations were associated with lower response rates *(85)*. Also of interest, a recent Fcγ receptor study in CLL cells suggests that ADCC might not be a predominant mechanism of action of rituximab in this disease *(86)*. Given the above observations, it was theorized that higher plasma concentrations of rituximab might improve efficacy in CLL, and studies using intensified or escalated rituximab doses were conducted (Table 6).

Because patients with high circulating numbers of lymphoma cells are at increased risk for infusion-related averse effects, Byrd et al. devised a stepped approach for rituximab administration in CLL patients *(87)*. Following an initial rituximab dose of 100 mg/m$^2$, patients were stepped up to doses of either 250 mg/m$^2$ or 375 mg/m$^2$ delivered on d 3 and thrice-weekly thereafter for 4 wk. Clinical activity improved, with an overall response rate of 45% and a median response duration of 10 mo. The intensified therapy was reasonably well tolerated, although an increased incidence of infusion-related adverse reactions were noted, consistent with previous reports of rituximab in CLL. O'Brien et al. administered weekly rituximab in escalating doses, with an initial dose of 375 mg/m$^2$ followed by weekly doses ranging from 500 mg/m$^2$ to 2250 mg/m$^2$ for 3 wk. They achieved an overall response rate of 36% with six of eight patients (75%) responding at the highest dose level *(88)*. Mild to moderate grade 1 to 2 toxicity, including fever, chills, nausea, and vomiting, occurred more frequently at the highest rituximab dose.

Extended infusion schedules and maintenance therapy with rituximab has also produced improved clinical results in first-line CLL patients, with an 8-wk course of rituximab 375

Table 5
Rituximab in Combination with Chemotherapy in Indolent Lymphoma; Fludarabine-Based Regimens

| Study | Population | Dose and Schedule | Patients (N)[a] | Response |
|---|---|---|---|---|
| Czuczman 2001 (65) | First-line, relapsed, or refractory low-grade lymphoma | Rituximab 375 mg/m$^2$ × 1, followed by rituximab 375 mg/m$^2$ + F[c] × 6 | 40 | ORR = 90% (82.5% CR/CRu, 7.5% PR) Median DR = 15+ mo |
| Vitolo 2001 (66) | First-line or relapsed follicular or indolent NHL | FMD[c] × 4, followed by rituximab 375 mg/m$^2$ weekly × 4 | 16[b] | After FMD ORR = 94% (37.5% CR, 19% CRu, 37.5% PR) After R ORR = 94% (75% CR, 6% CRu, 12% PR) Median DR not available |
| Vitolo 2004 (67) | First-line advanced follicular NHL, patients > 60 yr | FMD × 4, followed by rituximab 375 mg/m$^2$ weekly × 4 | 64[b] | ORR = 89% (72% CR, 12% CRu, 5% PR) |
| McLaughlin 2004 (68) | First-line stage IV indolent lymphoma | Randomized to 1. Rituximab 375 mg/m$^2$ + FMD × 6 then FMD × 2 or 2. FMD × 8, followed by rituximab 375 mg/m$^2$ weekly × 6 Interferon maintenance for 1 yr in both arms 3-yr FFS = 64% 3-yr OS = 95% | 149[b] | 2-yr PFS = 62% R+FMD (n = 76) ORR = 100% (92% CR/CRu, 8% PR) 3-yr FFS = 77% 3-yr OS = 95% FMD then R (n = 73) ORR = 95% (85% CR/CRu, 10% PR) |
| Hagemeister 2002 (69) | Chemotherapy-resistant indolent NHL | Rituximab 375 mg/m$^2$ + FMD, median 3 cycles | 21[b] | ORR = 90% (57% CR, 33% PR) Median DR not available |

690

| Study | Patient population | Treatment regimen | n | Results |
|---|---|---|---|---|
| Zinzani 2002 (70) | First-line follicular NHL | Randomized to 1. FM[c] × 6 or 2. CHOP × 6 If CR or PR, then rituximab 375 mg/m² weekly × 4 | 93[b] | After FM (n = 47) ORR = 94% (68% CR, 26% PR) After CHOP (n = 46) ORR = 93% (37% CR, 56% PR) Molecular responses following R: 59% with FM, 40% with CHOP |
| Dreyling 2004 (71) | Relapsed or refractory follicular or mantle cell NHL | Randomized to 1. Rituximab 375 mg/m² + FCM × 4 or 2. FCM × 4 | 126[b] | R+FCM (n = 64) ORR = 82% (37% CR, 46% PR) FCM (n = 62) ORR = 61% (14% CR, 47% PR) |
| Gregory 2004 (72) | First-line advanced low-grade NHL | FM × 4 to 6, followed by rituximab 375 mg/m² weekly × 4 | 36[b] | ORR = 80% (44% CR, 36% PR) Median DR of CR = 18 mo |
| Cohen 2002 (73) | First-line advanced follicular NHL | FC[c] × 4 to 6, followed by rituximab 375 mg/m² weekly × 4 | 33 | ORR = 88% (85% CR, 3% PR) 2-yr PFS = 63% 2-yr OS = 89% |
| Sacchi 2004 (74) | Relapsed follicular NHL | Rituximab 375 mg/m² + FC × 4 | 39[b] | ORR = 97% (75% CR, 19% PR) Median DR = 26 mo |
| Leo 2002 (75) | Relapsed follicular NHL | Rituximab 375 mg/m² + FC × 2, then FC × 4 | 11[b] | ORR = 100% (55% CR, 45% PR) Median DR not available |
| Ebeling 2002 (76) | First-line or relapsed low-grade NHL | Rituximab 375 mg/m² + FCD[c], maximum 5 cycles | 14 | ORR = 93% (79% CR, 14% PR) Median DR not available |

[a]Intent-to-treat population, unless noted otherwise.
[b]Evaluable patients.
[c]F, fludarabine; FMD, fludarabine/mitoxantrone/dexamethasone; FCM, fludarabine/cyclpohosphamide/mitoxantrone; FM, fludarabine/mitoxantrone; FC, fludarabine/cyclophosphamide; FCD, fludarabine/cyclophosphamide/dexamethasone; CHOP, cyclophopshamide/doxorubicin/vincristine/prednisone.

691

**Table 6**
**Single-Agent Rituximab in B-Cell CLL**

| Study | Population | Dose and Schedule | Patients (N)[a] | Response |
|---|---|---|---|---|
| McLaughlin 1998 (26) | Relapsed or refractory SLL | Rituximab 375 mg/m² weekly × 4 | 30[c] | ORR = 13% |
| Foran 2000 (79) | Relapsed or refractory SLL | Rituximab 375 mg/m² weekly × 4 | 28[b,c] | ORR = 14% (14% PR) |
| Huhn 2001 (80) | Relapsed or refractory CLL | Rituximab 375 mg/m² weekly × 4 | 28[b] | ORR = 25% (25% PR) |
| Byrd 2001 (87) | First-line or relapsed CLL/SLL | Randomized to Rituximab 100 mg/m², followed by 250 mg/m² thrice-weekly × 4 wk or Rituximab 100 mg/m², followed by 375 mg/m² thrice-weekly × 4 wk | 33 | Median DR = 20 wk ORR = 45% (3% CR, 42% PR) Median DR = 10 mo |
| O'Brien 2001 (88) | First-line, relapsed, or refractory CLL or other mature B-cell lymphoid leukemias | Rituximab 375 mg/m² wk 1, followed by weekly doses of 500 to 2250 mg/m² × 3 | 45[b] | All patients ORR = 40% Median TTP in responders = 8 mo In CLL (n = 39[b]) ORR = 36% (36% PR) |
| Thomas 2001 (89) | First-line, early stage CLL | Rituximab 375 mg/m² weekly × 8 | 21[b] | ORR = 90% (19% CR, 19% nodular PR, 48% PR) |
| Hainsworth 2004 (90) | First-line CLL/SLL | Rituximab 375 mg/m² weekly × 4; After evaluation at 6 wk, rituximab repeated in responding and stable disease patients every 6 mo for maximum 4 courses | 43[b] | Median DR not available ORR = 58% (9% CR, 47% PR) Median PFS = 19 mo |

[a]Intent-to-treat population, unless noted otherwise.
[b]Evaluable patients.
[c]Subset of patients with CLL/SLL

692

mg/m$^2$ producing a 90% overall response rate in earlier-stage patients (89), and maintenance therapy with repeated standard courses of rituximab producing an overall response rate of 58% with a median progression-free survival time of 19 mo (90). Still, in all of these studies, complete response rates remained relatively low, and the focus of investigation has turned toward rituximab–chemotherapy combinations.

**1.2.2.2. Rituximab in Combination With Chemotherapy.** Combinations of rituximab with cyclophosphamide and dexamethasone have produced promising results (91,92). Preliminary results of one trial reported an overall response rate of 77%, with 36% complete responses in 22 heavily pretreated CLL patients (Table 7) (91).

Far more common have been investigations of rituximab and fludarabine-based therapies for patients with CLL (Table 7). A randomized phase III trial conducted by the Cancer and Leukemia Group B (CALGB) compared concurrent vs sequential therapy with fludarabine and rituximab as first-line therapy in CLL. The overall response rate with concurrent therapy was 90%, with 47% complete responses, compared to response rates of 77% and 28%, respectively, with sequential therapy (93). Median progression-free and overall survival times had not yet been reached at the time of the initial report and have remained similar after an updated median follow-up time of 43 mo (94). A retrospective review of previous CALGB trials revealed that the addition of rituximab to fludarabine significantly increased overall and complete response rates, as well as progression-free and overall survival times compared to fludarabine alone (94). These investigators also found that the addition of rituximab to fludarabine did not increase the risk of infection in CLL patients (95).

In phase II studies, the use of four cycles of fludarabine followed by a standard course of rituximab reported an overall response rate of 87% (96), whereas an escalated dose schedule of rituximab with FC (fludarabine, cyclophosphamide) reported overall response rates of 73% in patients with relapsed or refractory CLL and 100% for first-line therapy of CLL (97,98). Additional first-line CLL trials are evaluating a sequential fludarabine, high-dose cyclophosphamide, and rituximab regimen, as well as chlorambucil followed by rituximab in older CLL patients, with promising early response rates (99,100).

The use of chemotherapy, particularly fludarabine-based therapies, in combination with rituximab for the treatment of CLL has substantially improved overall response rates and complete response rates over either rituximab or fludarabine alone. Further study will better define the clinical benefits of combination vs sequential regimens.

### 1.2.3. RITUXIMAB IN AGGRESSIVE NHL

**1.2.3.1. Single-Agent Therapy.** As a single agent, rituximab is active in the treatment of refractory aggressive NHL, producing overall response rates of 33–37% in diffuse large-cell lymphoma (DLCL) and mantle cell lymphoma (MCL) (Table 8) (101–103). With single-agent activity established, studies evaluating rituximab in combination with chemotherapy for aggressive NHL soon followed.

**1.2.3.2. Rituximab in Combination With Chemotherapy.** CHOP chemotherapy remains a standard of care for patients with aggressive NHL. The addition of rituximab to CHOP chemotherapy can further improve clinical outcomes (Table 9) (104–108). The benefit of the addition of rituximab to CHOP in elderly patients DLCL was demonstrated in a randomized trial reported by Coiffier et al. comparing eight cycles of CHOP with rituximab 375 mg/m$^2$ to CHOP alone (104,105). Overall response rates favored CHOP plus rituximab compared to CHOP alone, 82% compared to 69%, with a significantly higher

**Table 7**
**Rituximab in Combination With Chemotherapy in B-Cell CLL**

| Study | Population | Dose and Schedule | Patients (N)[a] | Response |
|---|---|---|---|---|
| Gupta 2002 (91) | Relapsed or refractory advanced CLL | Rituximab 375 mg/m² + CD[c]; median 4 cycles | 22 | ORR = 77% (36% CR, 41% PR) After 27+ mo median OS not yet reached |
| Byrd 2003 (93) | First-line CLL | Randomized to<br>1. Rituximab 375 mg/m² + F[c] × 6, followed by rituximab 375 mg/m² weekly × 4<br>or<br>2. F × 6, followed by rituximab 375 mg/m² weekly × 4 | 104[b] | R+F (n = 51) ORR = 90% (47% CR, 43% PR) F followed by R (n = 53) ORR = 77% (28% CR, 49% PR) |
| Schulz 2002 (96) | First-line, relapsed, or refractory CLL; no prior anthracycline or fludarabine therapy | Rituximab 375 mg/m² + F × 4 | 31[b] | ORR = 87% (23% CR, 10% CRu, 55% PR) |
| Weirda 2003 (97) | Relapsed or refractory CLL | Rituximab 375 mg/m² + FC[c] × 1, followed by rituximab 500 mg/m² + FC[c] × 5 | 179[b] | Median DR = 75 wk ORR = 73% (25% CR, 16% nodular PR, 32% PR) |
| Keating 2003 (98) | First-line CLL | Rituximab 375 mg/m² + FC[c] × 1, followed by rituximab 500 mg/m² + FC[c] × 5 | 202[b] | Median DR not available ORR = 100% 68% CR, (18% nodular PR, 14% PR) |
| Lamanna 2003 (99) | First-line CLL | F, followed by HDC[c], × 3, followed by rituximab 375 mg/m² weekly × 4 | 21[b] | Median DR not available ORR = 86% (57% CR, 10% nodular PR, 19% PR) |
| Mauro 2003 (100) | First-line CLL | Chl + P[c] × 6, If CR or PR, then rituximab 375 mg/m² weekly × 4 | 19[b] | Median DR = not available ORR = 86% (68% CR, 32% PR) Median PFS = 16 mo |

[a]Intent-to-treat population, unless noted otherwise.
[b]Evaluable patients.
[c]CD, cyclophosphamide/dexamethasone; F, fludarabine; FC, fludarabine/cyclophosphamide; HDC, high-dose cyclophosphamide; Chl, chlorambucil, P, prednisone.

694

**Table 8**
**Single-Agent Rituximab in Aggressive NHL**

| Study | Population | Dose and Schedule | Patients (N)[a] | Response |
|-------|-----------|-------------------|------------------|----------|
| Coiffier 1998 (101) | Relapsed or refractory diffuse large-cell lymphoma (DLCL), mantle cell lymphoma (MCL), or other aggressive B-cell lymphoma | Randomized to<br>1. Rituximab 375 mg/m$^2$ weekly × 8<br>or<br>2. Rituximab 375 mg/m$^2$ × 1, followed by rituximab 500 mg/m$^2$, weekly × 7 | 52[b] | ORR = 33%<br>(10% CR, 23% PR)<br>In DLCL (n = 30),<br>ORR = 37%<br>In MCL (n = 12),<br>ORR = 33%<br>Median DR not available |
| Foran 2000 (102) | First-line or relapsed MCL | Rituximab 375 mg/m$^2$ weekly × 4 | 81[b] | ORR = 37%<br>(14% CR, 23% PR)<br>Median DR = 1 yr |
| Igarashi 2002 (103) | Relapsed or refractory aggressive NHL | Rituximab 375 mg/m$^2$ weekly × 8 | 57[b] | ORR = 37%<br>(12% CR, 25%PR)<br>Median DR not available |

[a]Intent-to-treat population, unless noted otherwise.
[b]Evaluable patients.

695

Table 9
Rituximab in Combination With Chemotherapy in Aggressive NHL

| Study | Population | Dose and Schedule | Patients (N)[a] | Response |
|---|---|---|---|---|
| Coiffier 2002 (104,105) | First-line diffuse large-cell lymphoma (DLCL); patients > 60 yr | Randomized to<br>1. Rituximab 375 mg/m$^2$ + CHOP[c] × 8<br>or<br>2. CHOP × 8 | 202 (R+CHOP) 197 (CHOP) | R+CHOP<br>ORR = 82%<br>(75% CR, 7% PR)<br>3-yr EFS = 53%<br>CHOP alone<br>ORR = 69%<br>(63% CR, 6% PR)<br>3-yr EFS = 35% |
| Vose 2001 (107,108) | First-line advanced aggressive NHL | Rituximab 375 mg/m$^2$ + CHOP × 8 | 33 | ORR = 94%<br>(61% CR, 33% PR)<br>PFS at 60+ mo = 87% |
| Habermann 2003 (109) | First-line diffuse large-cell lymphoma (DLCL); patients > 60 yr | Randomized to<br>1. Rituximab 375 mg/m$^2$ × 5 + CHOP × 8<br>or<br>2. CHOP × 8; second randomization to maintenance R or observation | 540[b] | R+CHOP<br>ORR = 77%<br>CHOP alone<br>ORR = 76% |
| Wilson 2002 (110) | First-line, relapsed, or refractory aggressive NHL | Rituximab 375 mg/m$^2$ + EPOCH[d]; minimum 6 cycles | 34[b] | First line (n = 20)<br>ORR = 85% (85% CR)<br>12-mo PFS = 85%<br>Relapsed or refractory (n = 14)<br>ORR = 85%<br>(64% CR, 21% PR) |
| Howard 2002 (111) | First-line mantle cell lymphoma (MCL) | Rituximab 375 mg/m$^2$ + CHOP × 6 | 40 | ORR = 96%<br>(48% CR, 48% PR)<br>Median PFS = 17 mo |
| Venugopal 2003 (112) | First-line aggressive NHL | Rituximab 375 mg/m$^2$ + CHOP + GM-CSF × 6 | 27[b] | ORR = 74%<br>(48% CR, 26% PR)<br>Median DR of CR = 16 mo |

| Study | Patient population | Regimen | N | Results |
|---|---|---|---|---|
| Kewalramani 2004 (113) | Relapsed or refractory aggressive NHL | Rituximab 375 mg/m² + ICE$^c$ × 3 | 34$^b$ | ORR = 78% (53% CR, 25% PR) Median DR not available |
| Venugopal 2003 (114) | Relapsed or refractory aggressive NHL | Rituximab 375 mg/m² + ESHAP$^c$ + GM-CSF × 6 | 6$^b$ | ORR = 84% (67% CR, 17% PR) Median DR not available |
| Hiddemann 2001 (115) | Relapsed or refractory follicular, immunocytoma or MCL | Randomized to 1. Rituximab 375 mg/m² + FCM$^c$ × 4 or 2. FCM × 4 | 94$^b$ | R+FCM ORR = 83% FCM alone ORR = 58% |
| Levine 2002 (116) | First-line or relapsed MCL | FM$^c$ × 3, then rituximab 375 mg/m² + FM$^c$ × 3, then rituximab 375mg/m² weekly × 3 | 12$^b$ | ORR = 92% (92% CR) Median DR = 15+ mo |
| Romagura 2001 (117) | First-line MCL | Rituximab 375 mg/m² + HCVAD$^d$ × 6 | 75$^b$ | ORR = 92% (89% CR, 3% PR) 2-yr OS = 90% |
| Thomas 2001 (118) | Front-line Burkitt's, Burkitt's-like leukemia or lymphoma | Rituximab 375 mg/m² with HCVAD and high-dose methotrexate with and cytarabine | 19$^b$ | ORR = 89% |

[a]Intent-to-treat population, unless noted otherwise.
[b]Evaluable patients.
[c]CHOP, cyclophosphamide/doxorubicin/vincristine/prednisone; EPOCH, etoposide/vincrinstine/doxorubicin/cyclophosphamide/prednisone; ICE, ifosamide/etopside/carboplatin; ESHAP, etoposide/methylprednisolone/cytarabine/cisplatin; FCM, fludarabine/cyclophosphamide/mitoxantrone; FM, fludarabine/mitoxantrone; HCVAD, fractionated cyclophosphamide/vincristine/doxorubicin/dexamethasone.

complete response rate for the combination 76% vs 63%, ($p = 0.005$). Significant improvements in both 3-yr event-free survival (53% vs 35%, $p = 0.00008$) and 3-yr overall survival (62% vs 51%, $p = 0.008$) were also seen with the combination vs CHOP alone *(105)*. The incidence of grade 3 and grade 4 toxicities with CHOP and rituximab were consistent with those expected with CHOP alone.

In a subset of patients with bcl-2 overexpression ($n = 193$), CHOP with rituximab also proved superior, producing an overall response rate of 78% vs 60% for CHOP alone ($p = 0.01$) *(105)*. Multivariate analyses confirmed a clinical benefit for CHOP plus rituximab over CHOP alone in both event-free and overall survival in this patient subset, suggesting that the combination decreases the rate of chemotherapy failure in patients with bcl-2 overexpression.

As first-line therapy, administration of rituximab with CHOP produced an overall response rate of 94% with 61% complete responses in a phase II trial in patients with advanced aggressive NHL, with a progression-free survival rate of 87% at a median follow-up time of over 5 yr *(107,108)*. As first-line therapy in MCL, CHOP plus rituximab produced an overall response rate of 96% *(111)*.

Rituximab in combination with CHOP in older patients with DLCL has also been evaluated by the Eastern Cooperative Oncology Group (ECOG). Patients were first randomized to receive either CHOP with rituximab or CHOP alone, followed by a second randomization to maintenance rituximab therapy or observation. Unlike the trial reported by Coiffier et al., in which rituximab accompanied each cycle of CHOP, the ECOG trial administered two doses of rituximab before chemotherapy and one dose with CHOP cycles 3, 5, and 7 *(109)*. Preliminary results revealed no difference in response rate or time to treatment failure between patients randomized to initial therapy with rituximab plus CHOP vs CHOP alone. However, maintenance therapy with rituximab was associated with a statistically significant improvement in time to treatment failure in patients receiving CHOP alone. In an analysis of CHOP vs CHOP with rituximab in patients not receiving maintenance therapy, the addition of rituximab significantly improved time to treatment failure. Taken together, these results provide further evidence that the addition of rituximab improves clinical outcomes in the first-line treatment of diffuse aggressive NHL.

In addition to the CHOP regimen, rituximab was evaluated with several other regimens as first-line therapy and in relapsed or refractory aggressive NHL. Combinations of rituximab with EPOCH (etoposide, vincristine, doxorubicin, cyclophosphamide, prednisone), ICE (ifosfamide, etoposide, carboplatin), ESHAP (etoposide, methylprednisolone, cytarabine, cisplatin), FCM (fludarabine, cyclophosphamide, mitoxantrone, FM (fludarabine, mitoxantrone), and HCVAD (fractionated cyclophosphamide, vincristine, doxorubicin, dexamethasone) have produced response rates ranging from 81% to 92% (Table 9) *(110,113–118)*.

## 1.3. Safety

Treatment with rituximab results in rapid and sustained depletion of CD20-positive B-cells *(26)*. B-cell recovery occurs 9–12 mo following therapy, although as mature plasma cells are unaffected by rituximab, immunoglobulin production is not substantially decreased. The most common adverse events associated with rituximab are mild to moderate infusion-related reactions. These typically occur with the first dose and might include fever, chills, nausea, headache, fatigue, angioedema, and pruritis. Hypotension and bronchospasm are less common. Infrequently, deaths within 24 h of rituximab administration have occurred in association with an infusion reaction complex. Approximately 80% of these reactions

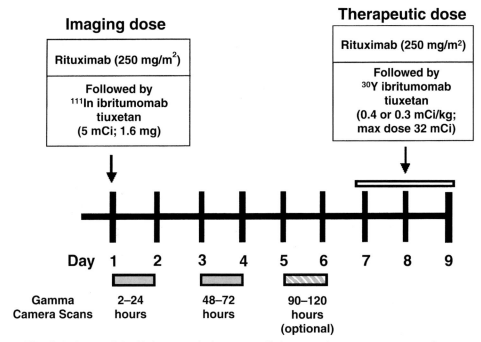

**Fig. 1.** Schema of the ibritumomab tiuxetan radioimmunotherapy treatment regimen.

were with the first dose of rituximab. Rarely, severe mucocutaneous reactions have been associated with rituximab, which in some patients has been fatal (<0.01% incidence) *(119)*. Tumor lysis syndrome has occurred at a rate of 0.1–0.15%, and patients with high circulating malignant cells counts are at greater risk. Transient grade 3 or 4 neutropenia and thrombocytopenia has occurred in 6% and 2% of patients, respectively.

## 2. IBRITUMOMAB TIUXETAN

Radioimmunotherapy with $^{90}$Y–ibritumomab tiuxetan (Zevalin) is approved for the treatment of relapsed or refractory low-grade, follicular or CD20+ transformed B-cell NHL, including rituximab-refractory follicular NHL. This immunoconjugate combines the murine IgG1 kappa monoclonal antibody ibritumomab, directed against the CD20 antigen, with the high-affinity chelator tiuxetan. Covalently bound to ibritumomab, the tiuxetan chelator provides stable linkage between the antibody and the radioisotopes indium-111 ($^{111}$In) and yttrium-90 ($^{90}$Y).

The ibritumomab tiuxetan regimen (Fig. 1) incorporates rituximab, $^{111}$In–ibritumomab tiuxetan, and $^{90}$Y–ibritumomab tiuxetan. Rituximab is administered prior to radiolabeled ibritumomab tiuxetan to optimize biodistribution *(120,121)*. Imaging studies to assess biodistribution are performed with $^{111}$In–ibritumomab tiuxetan, with $^{90}$Y–ibritumomab tiuxetan administered as the radioimmunotherapeutic. The regimen is delivered over 7–9 d as outpatient therapy. $^{90}$Y–ibritumomab tiuxetan is administered at a dose of 0.4 mCi/kg (14.8 MBq/kg) for patients with platelet counts greater than or equal to 150,000/mm$^3$ and 0.3 mCi/kg (11.1 MBq/kg) for patients with platelet counts of 100,000–149,000/mm$^3$. The maximum administered dose of $^{90}$Y–ibritumomab tiuxetan is 32.0 mCi (1184 MBq). Patients with platelet counts less than 100,000/mm$^3$ should not receive $^{90}$Y–ibritumomab tiuxetan.

## 2.1. Mechanism of Action

Yitrium-90 is a pure β-emitter, having a physical half-life of 64 h and an effective path length of approx 5 mm (122). The immunoconjugate targets CD20-positive B-cells and also emits crossfire radiation to nearby cells. Crossfire activity might be of particular benefit in treating bulky or poorly vascularized tumors.

## 2.2. Ibritumomab Tiuxetan in the Treatment of NHL

Radioimmunotherapy with the ibritumomab tiuxetan therapeutic regimen has produced response rates of 74–83% in patients with relapsed or refractory low-grade, follicular, or CD20+ transformed B-cell NHL (Table 10) (123–127).

Long-term follow-up of the phase I/II dose finding showed an overall response rate of 73%, with a total 51% of patients achieving a complete response (CR)/CR unconfirmed (CRu) using the International Workshop Response Criteria (IWRC). Durable remissions were observed in follicular and diffuse aggressive NHL, with some responses lasting longer than 6 yr (128).

In a randomized multicenter phase III trial comparing ibritumomab tiuxetan radioimmunotherapy with rituximab in patients with relapsed or refractory low-grade, follicular, or CD20+ transformed B-cell NHL, radioimmunotherapy produced higher a overall response rate, 80% vs 56% ($p = 0.002$) and a higher CR/CRu rate, 34% vs 20% ($p = 0.04$) compared to rituximab (123). The enrolled patients had received a median of two prior therapies (range: one to six), and 45% of patients had tumors of 5 cm or larger, with 8% of patients having bulky tumors of 10 cm or larger. Duration of response favored the ibritumomab tiuxetan regimen, at 13.9 mo vs 11.8 mo for rituximab, but this trial was not powered to show a statistically significant difference (124). Median time to next therapy for the ibritumomab tiuxetan arm was 17.6 mo compared to 12.4 mo for rituximab.

In patients with relapsed or refractory low-grade, follicular, or CD20+ transformed B-cell NHL and baseline mild thrombocytopenia, defined as a platelet count of 100,000–149,000/mm$^3$, radioimmunotherapy with a reduced dose of ibritumomab tiuxetan ($^{90}$Y–ibritumomab tiuxetan 0.3 mCi/kg) produced an overall response rate of 83%, with a 47% CR/CRu rate (125,126). The median duration of response was 12.9 mo and the median time to next therapy was 14.6 mo (125,126). Ibritumomab tiuxetan radioimmunotherapy is also effective in patients with rituximab-refractory NHL, producing an overall response rate of 74%, with 15% complete responses and a median response duration of 6.4 mo (127).

Analysis of 211 patients enrolled in clinical studies, including those above, revealed that 37% of patients achieved a long-term durable response, defined as a response duration of 12 mo or greater (128). In patients achieving a CR/CRu, the median duration of response approaches 2 yr, with some patients in continuous complete response for over 6 yr (129). Data also indicate that higher response rates and longer response durations are achieved when ibritumomab tiuxetan radioimmunotherapy is used as the first therapy for relapsed disease (130). Age does not appear to impact response, as an analysis of patients age 65 yr or older compared to those less than 65 yr enrolled revealed no differences in overall response rates or safety profiles between age groups (131).

In a review of 152 follicular NHL patients treated with ibritumomab tiuxetan, the overall response rate was 83%, with response rates of 84%, 82%, and 77% for follicular center grades 1, 2, and 3, respectively (132). Data indicate that radioimmunotherapy with ibritu-

Table 10
Radioimmunotherapy With Ibritumomab Tiuxetan in NHL

| Study | Population | Dose and Schedule | Patients (N)[a] | Response |
|---|---|---|---|---|
| Witzig 2002 (121,123) | Relapsed or refractory low-grade, follicular or CD20+ transformed B-cell NHL | Randomized to 1. $^{90}$Y–ibritumomab tiuxetan 0.4 mCi/kg or 2. Rituximab 375 mg/m$^2$ weekly × 4 | 143 | $^{90}$Y–ibritumomab tiuxetan (n =73) ORR = 80% (30% CR, 4% CRu, 45% PR) Median DR = 13.9 mo Rituximab (n = 70) ORR = 56% (16% CR, 4% CRu, 36% PR) Median DR = 11.8 mo |
| Wiseman 2002 (125) | Relapsed or refractory low-grade, follicular or CD20+ transformed B-cell NHL | $^{90}$Y–ibritumomab tiuxetan 0.3 mCi/kg | 30 | ORR = 83% (37% CR, 6% CRu, 40% PR) Median DR = 12.9 mo |
| Witzig 2002 (126,128) | Rituximab-refractory follicular NHL | $^{90}$Y–ibritumomab tiuxetan 0.4 mCi/kg | 57 | ORR = 74% (15% CR, 59% PR) Median DR = 11.5 mo |

[a]Intent-to-treat population.

momab tiuxetan is also effective in patients with transformed histologies, mantle cell lymphoma, MALT, and aggressive NHL *(133–136)*.

Studies have also begun to evaluate sequential doses of ibritumomab tiuxetan radioimmunotherapy and its use in transplant regimens *(137–139)*. Preliminary results indicate that retreatment with ibritumomab tiuxetan radioimmunotherapy is feasible and its use in combination with conditioning chemotherapy regimens with autologous stem cell transplant is promising. Studies are also evaluating low-dose ibritumomab tiuxetan in combination with radiation therapy as a means of enhancing targeting and specificity *(140)*.

## *2.3. Safety*

Treatment with ibritumomab tiuxetan radioimmunotherapy is predominantly associated with transient hematologic toxicity. An integrated safety analysis of 349 patients found that grade 4 neutropenia, thrombocytopenia, and anemia to occur in 30%, 10%, and 4% of patients, respectively. Nadir counts generally occurred 7–9 wk following treatment *(141)*. Neutropenia was generally uncomplicated, with only 7% of patients requiring hospitalization for infection or febrile neutropenia.

Nonhematologic adverse events tend to be infusion-related, including asthenia, chills, nausea, and fever. They are typically mild to moderate and are consistent with that expected with rituximab. Serum IgG and IgA levels remain within normal ranges following therapy, although serum IgM levels might transiently decline. In 211 patients evaluated, human anti-mouse antibodies (HAMA) and human anti-chimeric antibodies (HACA) were noted in 1% and 0.5% of patients, respectively. Treatment with ibritumomab tiuxetan radioimmunotherapy does not appear to be associated with an increased incidence of secondary myelodysplastic syndrome (MDS) or acute myelogenous leukemia (AML) *(142)*.

Prior treatment with ibritumomab tiuxetan radioimmunotherapy does not preclude the use of subsequent NHL therapies, including chemotherapy, rituximab immunotherapy, and high-dose therapy, and ibritumomab tiuxetan radioimmunotherapy can also be used in patients following transplant, albeit at a reduced dose *(143–148)*.

## REFERENCES

1. Anderson KC, Bates MP, Slaughenhoupt BL, et al. Expression of human B cell-associated antigens on leukemias and lymphomas: a model of human B cell differentiation. Blood 1984; 63:1424–1433.
2. Nadler LM, Ritz, J, Hardy R, et al. A unique cell surface antigen identifying lymphoid malignancies of B cell origin. J Clin Invest 1981; 67:134–140.
3. Stashenko P, Nadler LM, Hardy R, Schlossman SF. Characterization of a human B lymphocyte-specific antigen. J Immunol 1980; 125:1678–1685.
4. Reff ME, Carner K, Chambers KS, et al. Depletion of B cells in vivo by a chimeric mouse human monoclonal antibody to CD20. Blood 1994; 83:435–445.
5. Flieger D, Renoth S, Beier I, et al. Mechanism of cytotoxicity induced by chimeric mouse human monoclonal antibody IDEC-C2B8 in CD20-expresing lymphoma cell lines. Cell Immunol 2000; 204:55–63.
6. Maloney DG, Smith B, Appelbaum FR. The anti-tumor effect of monoclonal anti-CD20 antibody (MAB) therapy includes direct anti-proliferative activity and induction of apoptosis in CD20 positive non-Hodgkin's lymphoma (NHL) cell lines. Blood 1996; 88:637a.
7. Maloney DG, Smith B, Rose A. Rituximab: mechanism of action and resistance. Semin Oncol 2002; 29(1 Suppl 2):2–9.
8. Shan D, Ledbetter JA, Press OW. Signaling events involved in anti-CD20-induced apoptosis of malignant human B cells. Cancer Immunol Immunother 2000; 48:673–683.
9. Shan D, Ledbetter JA, Press OW. Apoptosis of malignant human B cells by ligation of CD20 with monoclonal antibodies. Blood 1998; 91:1644–1652.

10. Mathas S, Rickers A, Bommert K, et al. Anti-CD20- and B-cell receptor-mediated apoptosis: evidence for shared intracellular signaling pathways. Cancer Res 2000; 60:7170–7176.

11. Bannerji R, Pearson M, Flinn IW, et al. Cell surface complement inhibitors CD55 and CD59 may mediate chronic lymphocytic leukemia (CLL) resistance to rituximab therapy. Blood 2000; 96:164a.

12. Cartron G, Dacheux L, Salles G, et al. Therapeutic activity of humanized anti-CD20 monoclonal antibody and polymorphism in IgG Fc receptor FcγRIIIa gene. Blood 2002; 99(3):754–758.

13. Weng WK, Levy R. analysis of IgG Fc receptor FcγRIIIa polymorphism in relapsed follicular non-Hodgkin's lymphoma treated with rituximab. Blood 2002; 99(11):353a.

14. Ghielmini M, Schmitz SFH, Leger-Falandry C, et al. The genotype of the IgG Fc receptor is predictive of event-free survival after treatment with rituximab in patients with follicular lymphoma participating in study SAKK 35/98. Blood 2003; 102:409a.

15. Clynes RA, Towers TL, Presta LG, Ravetch JV. Inhibitory Fc receptors modulate in vivo cytotoxicity against tumor targets. Nat Med 2000; 6:443–446.

16. Sondermann P, Huber R, Oosthuizen V, Jacob U. The 3.2-A crystal structure of the human IgG1 Fc fragment-FcγRIII complex. Nature 2000; 406:267–273.

17. Koene HR, Kleijer M, Algra J, et al. FcγRIIIa-158V/F polymorphism influences the binding of IgG by natural killer cell FcγRIIIa, independently of the FcγRIIIa-48L/R/H phenotype. Blood 1997; 90: 1109–1114.

18. Demidem A, Lam T, Alas S, et al. Chimeric anti-CD20 (IDEC-C2B8) monoclonal antibody sensitizes a B cell lymphoma cell line to cell killing by cytotoxic drugs. Cancer Biother Radiopharm 1997; 12: 177–185.

19. Alas S, Bonavida B, Emmanouilides C. Potentiation of fludarabine cytotoxicity on non-Hodgkin's lymphoma by pentoxifylline and rituximab. Anticancer Res 2000; 20:2961–2966.

20. Alas S, Emmanouilides C, Bonavida B. Inhibition of interleukin 10 by rituximab results in down-regulation of Bcl-2 and sensitization of B-cell non-Hodgkin's lymphoma to apoptosis. Clin Cancer Res 2001; 7:709–723.

21. Rose AL, Smith BE, Maloney DG. Glucocorticoids and rituximab in vitro: direct antiproliferative and apoptotic effects. Blood 2002; 100:1765–1773.

22. Friedberg JW, Neuberg D, Gribben JG, et al. Combination immunotherapy with rituximab and interleukin 2 in patients with relapsed or refractory follicular non-Hodgkin's lymphoma. Br J Haematol 2002; 117:828–834.

23. Ansell SM, Witzig TE, Kurtin PJ, et al. Phase I study of interleukin-12 in combination with rituximab in patients with B-cell non-Hodgkin's lymphoma. Blood 2002; 99:67–74.

24. Maloney DG, Grillo-López AJ, Bodkin DJ, et al. IDEC-C2B8: results of a phase I multiple-dose trial in patients with relapsed non-Hodgkin's lymphoma. J Clin Oncol 1997; 15:3266–3274.

25. Maloney DG, Grillo-López AJ, White CA, et al. IDEC-C2B8 (rituximab) anti-CD20 monoclonal antibody therapy in patients with relapsed low-grade non-Hodgkin's lymphoma. Blood 1997; 90:2188–2195.

26. McLaughlin P, Grillo-López A J, Link BK, et al. Rituximab chimeric anti-CD20 monoclonal antibody therapy for relapsed indolent lymphoma: half of patients respond to a four-dose treatment program. J Clin Oncol 1998; 16:2825–2833.

27. Grillo-López AJ, Shen D, Lee D, et al. Rituximab: sustained remissions in patients (pts) with relapsed or refractory low grade or follicular non-Hodgkin's lymphoma (LG/NHL). Blood 2000; 96:238b.

28. Foran JM, Gupta RK, Cunningham D, et al. A UK multicentre phase II study of rituximab (chimaeric anti-CD20 monoclonal antibody) in patients with follicular lymphoma, with PCR monitoring of molecular response. Br J Haematol 2000; 109:81–88.

29. Feuring-Buske M, Kneba M, Unterhalt M, et al. IDEC-C2B8 (rituximab) anti-CD20 antibody treatment in relapsed advanced-stage follicular lymphomas: results of a phase-II study of the German Low-Grade Lymphoma Study Group. Ann Hematol 2000; 79:493–500.

30. Walewski J, Kraszewska E, Mioduszewska O, et al. Rituximab (Mabthera, Rituxan) in patients with recurrent indolent lymphoma: evaluation of safety and efficacy in a multicenter study. Med Oncol 2001; 18:141–148.

31. Davis TA, White CA, Grillo-López AJ, et al. Single-agent monoclonal antibody efficacy in bulky non-Hodgkin's lymphoma: results of a phase II trial of rituximab. J Clin Oncol 1999; 17:1851–1857.

32. Piro LD, White CA, Grillo-López AJ, et al. Extended rituximab (anti-CD20 monoclonal antibody) therapy for relapsed or refractory low-grade or follicular non-Hodgkin's lymphoma. Ann Oncol 1999; 10:655–661.

33. Avilés A, Talavera A, Diaz-Maqueo JC, et al. Evaluation on a six-dose treatment of anti CD 20 mono-clonal antibody in patients with refractory follicular lymphoma. Cancer Biother Radiopharm 2001; 16: 159–162.

34. Davis TA, Grillo-López AJ, White CA, et al. Rituximab anti-CD20 monoclonal antibody therapy in non-Hodgkin's lymphoma: safety and efficacy of re-treatment. J Clin Oncol 2000; 18:3135–3143.

35. Davis TA, Grillo-López AJ, McLaughlin P, et al. Repeated treatments (ReRx) with rituximab in patients (pts) with relapsed or refractory low-grade or follicular non-Hodgkin's lymphoma (LG/F NHL) pro-vide longer response duration (DR) compared to prior chemotherapy. Blood 2000; 96:235b.

36. Hainsworth JD Litchy S, Greco AF. Schedules rituximab maintenance therapy versus retreatment at progression in patients with indolent non-hodgkin's lymphoma (NHL) responding to single-agent rituxi-mab: a randomized trial of the Minnie Pearl Cancer Research Network. Blood 2003; 102:69a.

37. Cheson BD, Horning SJ, Coiffier B, et al. Report of an international workshop to standardize response criteria for non-Hodgkin's lymphomas. J Clin Oncol 1999; 17:1244–1253.

38. Grillo-López AJ, McLaughlin P, Cheson BD, et al. First report on the application of new response cri-teria (RC) proposed for NHL: the rituximab pivotal trial. Proc Am Soc Clin Oncol 1999; 18:13a.

39. Colombat P, Salles G, Brousse N, et al. Rituximab (anti-CD20 monoclonal antibody) as single first-line therapy for patients with follicular lymphoma with a low tumor burden: clinical and molecular eval-uation. Blood 2001; 97:101–106.

40. Gutheil JC, Finucane D, Rodriquez F, et al. Phase II study of rituximab (Rituxan) in patients with pre-viously untreated low-grade or follicular non-Hodgkin's lymphoma. Proc Am Soc Clin Oncol 2000; 19:22a.

41. Hainsworth JD, Burris HA, Morrissey LH, et al. Rituximab monoclonal antibody as initial systemic therapy for patients with low-grade non-Hodgkin lymphoma. Blood 2000; 95:3052–3056.

42. Hainsworth JD, Litchy S, Burris HA, et al. Rituximab as first-line and maintenance therapy for patients with indolent non-Hodgkin's lymphoma. J Clin Oncol 2002; 20:4261–4267.

43. Hainsworth JD, Litchy S, Morrissey L, et al. Rituximab as first-line and maintenance therapy for indolent non-Hodgkin's lymphoma: long term follow-up of a Minnie Pearl Cancer Research Network phase II trial. Blood 2003; 102:411a.

44. Ghielmini M, Schmitz SFU, Cogliatti S, et al. Prolonged treatment with rituximab in patients with follic-ular lymphoma significantly increases event-free survival and response duration compared with the stan-dard weekly × 4 schedule. Blood 2004; 103:4416–4423.

45. Treon SP, Agus DB, Link B, et al. CD20-directed antibody-mediated immunotherapy induces responses and facilitates hematologic recovery in patients with Waldenstrom's macroglobulinemia. J Imunother 2001; 24:272–279.

46. Dimopoulos MA, Zervas A, Zomas A, et al. Treatment of Waldenstrom's macroglobulinemia with rituxi-mab. J Clin Oncol 2002; 20:2327–2333.

47. Treon SP, Emmanouilides CE, Kimby E, et al. Extended rituximab therapy is highly active and facili-tates hematological recovery in patient with lymphoplasmacytic lymphoma (Waldenstrom's macroglo-bulinemia, WM). Proc Am Soc Clin Oncol 2002; 21:268a.

48. Gertz MA, Rue M, Blood E, et al. Rituximab for Waldenstrom's macroglobulinemia (WM) (E3A98): an ECOG phase II pilot study for untreated or previously patients. Blood 2003; 102:148a.

49. Conconi A, Martinelli G, Thiéblemont C, et al. Clinical activity of rituximab in extranodal marginal zone B-cell lymphoma pf MALT type. Blood 2003; 102:2741–2747.

50. Martinelli G, Laszlo D, Conconi A, et al. Anti-CD20 monoclonal antibody (rituximab) in gastric extra-nodal marginal zone (MALT) non-Hodgkin's lymphoma (NHL) patients: clinical and biological results (phase II study). Blood 2003; 102:410a.

51. Treon SP, Fox EA, Hansen M, et al. Polymorphisms in Fc gamma RIIIa (CD16) receptor expression are associated with clinical response to rituximab in Waldenstrom's macroglobulinemia. Blood 2002; 100:573a.

52. Treon SP, Emmanouilides C, Kimby E, et al. Pre-therapy serum IgM levels predict clinical response to extended rituximab in Waldenstrom's macroglobulinemia. Blood 2002; 100:813a.

53. Maloney DG, Press OW, Braziel RM, et al. A phase II trial of CHOP followed by rituximab chimeric monoclonal anti-CD20 antibody for treatment of newly diagnosed follicular non-Hodgkin's lymphoma: SWOG 9800. Blood 2001; 98:843a.

54. Rambaldi A, Lazzari M. Manzoni C, et al. Monitoring of minimal residual disease after CHOP and rituxi-mab in previously untreated patients with follicular lymphoma. Blood 2002; 99:856–862.

55. Rambaldi A, Carlotti E, Baccarani M, et al. Long term improvement of clinical outcome of follicular lymphoma patients achieving a molecular response after sequential CHOP and rituximab treatment: predictive value of real time quantitative PCR to identify responding patients. Blood 2003; 102:409a.

56. Czuczman MS, Grillo-López AJ, White CA, et al. Treatment of patients with low-grade B-cell lymphoma with the combination of chimeric anti-CD20 monoclonal antibody and CHOP chemotherapy. J Clin Oncol 1999; 17:268–276.

57. Czuczman M, Grillo-López AJ, LoBuglio AI, et al. Patients with low-grade NHL treated with rituximab + CHOP experience prolonged clinical and molecular remission. Blood 2004; 102:411a.

58. Hainsworth JD, Burris HA III, Yardley DA, et al. Rituximab plus short duration chemotherapy as first-line treatment for follicular non-Hodgkin's lymphoma (NHL): a Minnie Pearl Cancer Research Network phase II trial. Proc Am Soc Clin Oncol 2002; 21:268a.

59. Hiddemann W, Dreyling MH, Forstpointner R, et al. Combined immuno-chemotherapy (R-CHOP) significantly improves time to treatment failure in first-line therapy of follicular lymphoma—results of a prospective randomized trial of the German Low Grade Study Group (GLSG) Blood 2003; 102:104a.

60. Marcus R, Imrie K, Belch A, et al. an international randomized, open-label, phase III trial comparing rituximab assed to CVP chemotherapy to CVP chemotherapy alone in untreated stage III/IV follicular non-Hodgkin's lymphoma. Blood 2003; 102:28a.

61. Patel D, Gupta NK, Mehrotra B, et al. Rituximab, cyclophosphamide and Decadron (RCD) combination is an effective salvage regimen for previously treated low grade lymphoma. Proc Am Soc Clin Oncol 2001; 20:228b.

62. Herold M, Fiedler R, Pasold R, et al. Efficacy and toxicity of rituximab plus mitoxantrone, chlorambucil, prednisolone (MCP) versus MCP alone in advance indolent NHL—interim results of a clinical phase III study of the East German Study Group Hematology/Oncology (OSHO). Blood 2001; 98:601a.

63. Martinelli G, Laszlo D, Mancuso P, et al. Rituximab plus chlorambucil in low-grade non Hodgkin's lymphomas (NHL): clinical results of a phase II study. Blood 2002; 100:777a.

64. Czuczman MS, Grillo-López AJ, McLaughlin P, et al. Clearing of cells bearing the bcl-2 [t(14;18)] translocation from blood and marrow of patients treated with rituximab alone or in combination with CHOP chemotherapy. Ann Oncol 2001; 12:109–114.

65. Czuczman MS, Fallon A, Mohr A, et al. Phase II study of rituximab plus fludarabine in (pts) with low-grade lymphoma (LGL): final report. Blood 2001; 98:601a.

66. Vitolo U, Boccomini C, Astolfi M, et al. Chemoimmunotherapy with fludarabine + mitoxantrone + dexamethasone (FND) and rituximab in indolent non-Hodgkin's lymphoma (NHL): a pilot study to evaluate feasibility, safety, clinical and molecular response. Blood 2001; 98:251b.

67. Vitolo U, Boccomini C, Ladetto M, et al. A brief course of chemo-immunotherapy FND + rituximab is effective to induce a high clinical and molecular response in elderly patients with advanced stage follicular lymphoma (FL) at diagnosis. Blood 2003; 102:400a.

68. McLaughlin P, Rodriguez MA, Hagemeister FB, et al. Stage IV indolent lymphoma: a randomized study of concurrent vs. sequential use of FND chemotherapy (fludarabine, mitoxantrone, dexamethasone) and rituximab (R) monoclonal antibody therapy, with interferon maintenance. Proc Am Soc Clin Oncol 2003; 22:564.

69. Hagemeister FB, McLaughlin P, Clemons M, et al. FND (fludarabine, mitoxantrone, dexamethasone)-R (rituximab) for patients (pts) with relapsed (rel) or chemotherapy resistant (CTR) indolent lymphomas (IL): a preliminary report. Blood 2002; 100:305b.

70. Zinzani PL. A multicenter randomized trial of fludarabine and mitoxantrone (FM) plus rituximab versus CHOP plus rituximab as first-line treatment in patients with follicular lymphoma (FL). Blood 2002; 100:93a.

71. Dreyling MH, Forstpointner R, Repp R, et al. Combined immuno-chemotherapy (R-FCM) results in superior remission and survival rates in recurrent follicular and mantle cell lymphoma—final results of a prospective randomized trial of the German Low Grade Study Group (GLSG). Blood 2003; 102: 103a.

72. Gregory SA, Venugopal P, Adler SS, et al. Phase II study of fludarabine phosphate and mitoxantrone followed by anti-CD20 monoclonal antibody in the treatment of patients with newly diagnosed low-grade non-Hodgkin's lymphoma (LGNHL): interim results. Blood 2003; 102:412a.

73. Cohen A, Polliack A, Ben-Bassat I, et al. Results of a phase II study employing a combination of fludarabine, cyclophosphamide and rituximab (FCR) as primary therapy for patients with advanced follicular lymphoma (FL): the Israel Cooperative Lymphoma Group. Blood 2002; 100:360a.

74. Sacchi S, Tucci A, Merli F, et al. Efficacy controla and long-term follow-up of patients (pts) treated with FC plus rituximab for relapsed follicular lymphoma patients. Blood 2003; 102:295b.

75. Leo E, Scheuer L, Kraemer A, Kerowgan M, Leo, et al. Unexpected hematotoxicity associated with a combination of rituximab, fludarabine and cyclophosphamide in the treatment of relapsed follicular lymphoma. Blood 2002; 100:301b.

76. Ebelin P, Schuett P, Seeber S, Nowrousian MR. Combined therapy with rituximab, fludarabine, cyclophosphamide, and dexamethasone (R-FCD) in patients with low-grade-lymphoma. Blood 2002; 100: 298b.

77. Treon SP, Wasi P, Emmanouilides C, et al. Combination therapy with rituximab and fludarabine is highly active in Waldenstrom's macroglobulinemia. Blood 2002; 100:211a.

78. McLaughlin P, Hagemeister F B, Rodriguez MA, et al. Safety of fludarabine, mitoxantrone, and dexamethasone combined with rituximab in the treatment of stage IV indolent lymphoma. Semin Oncol 2000; 27(6 Suppl 12):37–41.

79. Foran JM, Rohatiner AZ, Cunningham D, et al. European phase II study of rituximab (chimeric anti-CD20 monoclonal antibody) for patients with newly diagnosed mantle-cell lymphoma and previously treated mantle-cell lymphoma, immunocytoma, and small B-cell lymphocytic lymphoma. J Clin Oncol 2000; 18:317–324.

80. Huhn D, von Schilling C, Wilhelm M, et al. Rituximab therapy of patients with B-cell chronic lymphocytic leukemia. Blood 2001; 98:1326–1331.

81. Almasri NM, Duque RE, Iturraspe J, et al. Reduced expression of CD20 antigen as a characteristic marker for chronic lymphocytic leukemia. Am J Hematol 1992; 40:259–263.

82. Ginaldi L, De Martinis M, Matutes E, et al. Levels of expression of CD19 and CD20 in chronic B cell leukaemias. J Clin Pathol 1998; 51:364–369.

83. Huh YO, Keating MJ, Saffer HL, et al. Higher levels of surface CD20 expression on circulating lymphocytes compared with bone marrow and lymph nodes in B-cell chronic lymphocytic leukemia. Am J Clin Pathol 2001; 116:437–443.

84. Manshouri T, Do KA, Wang X, et al. Circulating CD20 is detectable in the plasma of patients with chronic lymphocytic leukemia and is of prognostic significance. Blood 2003; 101:2507–2513.

85. Berinstein NL, Grillo-López AJ, White CA, et al. Association of serum rituximab (IDEC-C2B8) concentration and anti-tumor response in the treatment of recurrent low-grade or follicular non-Hodgkin's lymphoma. Ann Oncol 1998; 9:995–1001.

86. Farag SS, Flinn IW, Modali R, et al. Fcgamma RIIIa and Fc gamma RIIa polymorphisms do not predict response to rituximab in B-cell chronic lymphocytic leukemia. Blood 2004; 103:1472–1474.

87. Byrd JC, Murphy T, Howard RS, et al. Rituximab using a thrice weekly dosing schedule in B-cell chronic lymphocytic leukemia and small lymphocytic lymphoma demonstrates clinical activity and acceptable toxicity. J Clin Oncol 2001; 19:2153–2164.

88. O'Brien S, Kantarjian H, Thomas DA, et al. Rituximab dose-escalation trial in chronic lymphocytic leukemia. J Clin Oncol 2001; 19:2165–2170.

89. Thomas DA, O'Brien S, Giles FJ, et al. Single agent Rituxan in early stage chronic lymphocytic leukemia (CLL). Blood 2001; 98:364a.

90. Hainsworth JD, Litchy S, Barton, et al. Rituximab as first-line and maintenance therapy for patients with chronic lymphocytic leukemia (CLL) or small lymphocytic lymphoma (SLL): a Minnie Pearl Cancer Research Network phase II trial. Proc Am Soc Clin Oncol 2003; 22:580.

91. Gupta NK, Kavuru S, Patel DV, et al. Long-term results from a monthly regimen of rituximab (R), cyclophosphamide (C) and dexamethasone (D) in advanced chronic lymphocytic leukemia (CLL). Proc Am Soc Clin Oncol 2002; 21:275a.

92. Poretta TA, Devereux L, Grana G, et al. Rituximab, cyclophosphamide, and dexamethasone provide hematologic and immunologic response in patients with relapsed refractory chronic lymphocytic leukemia and associated autoimmune activity. Proc Am Soc Clin Oncol 2001; 20:225b.

93. Byrd JC, Peterson BL, Morrison VA, et al. Randomized phase 2 study of fludarabine with concurrent versus sequential treatment with rituximab in symptomatic, untreated patients with B-cell chronic lymphocytic leukemia: results from Cancer and Leukemia Group B 9712 (CALGB 9712). Blood 2003; 101: 6–14.

94. Byrd JC, Rai KR, Peterson BL, et al. The addition of rituximab to fludarabine significantly improves progression-free survival and overall survival in previously untreated chronic lymphocytic leukemia (CLL) patients. Blood 2003; 102:73a.

95. Morrison VA, Byrd JC, Peterson BL, et al. Adding rituximab to fludarabine therapy for patients with untreated chronic lymphocytic leukemia (CLL) does not increase the risk of infections: Cancer and Leukemia Group B (CALGB) 9712. Blood 2003; 102:440a.

96. Schultz H, Klein SK, Rehwald U, et al. Phase 2 study of a combined immunochemotherapy using rituximab and fludarabine in patients with chronic lymphocytic leukemia. Blood 2002; 100:3115–3120.

97. Wierda W, Garcia-Manero G, O'Brien S, et al. Molecular remissions in patients with relapsed or refractory CLL treated with combined fludarabine, cyclophosphamide, and rituximab. Proc Am Soc Clin Oncol 2003; 22:581.

98. Keating MJ. Manshouri T, O'Brien S, et al. A high proportion of true complete remission can be obtained with a fludarabine, cyclophosphamide, rituximab (FCR) combination in chronic lymphocytic leukemia. Proc Am Soc Clin Oncol 2003; 22:569.

99. Lamana N, Weiss MA, Maslak PG, et al. Sequential therapy with fludarabine, high dose cyclophosphamide, and rituximab induces a high incidence of complete response in patients with chronic lymphocytic leukemia (CLL). Blood 2003; 102:440a.

100. Mauro FR, Gentile M, DePropris MS, et al. Postremissional rituximab administration for the treatment of older chronic lymphocytic leukemia (CLL) patients responsive to first line therapy with chlorambucil and prednisone. Blood 2003; 102:647a.

101. Coiffier B, Haioun C, Ketterer N, et al. Rituximab (anti-CD20 monoclonal antibody) for the treatment of patients with relapsing or refractory aggressive lymphoma: a multicenter phase II study. Blood 1998; 92:1927–1932.

102. Foran JM, Cunningham D, Coiffier B, et al. Treatment of mantle-cell lymphoma with rituximab (chimeric monoclonal anti-CD20 antibody): analysis of factors associated with response. Ann Oncol 2000; 11(Suppl 1):S117–S121.

103. Igarashi T, Itoh K, Kobayashi Y, et al. Phase II and pharmacokinetic study of rituximab with eight weekly infusions in relapsed aggressive B-cell non-Hodgkin's lymphoma (B-NHL). Proc Am Soc Clin Oncol 2002; 21:286a.

104. Coiffier B, LePage E, Briere J, et al. CHOP chemotherapy plus rituximab compared with CHOP alone in elderly patients with diffuse large-B-cell lymphoma. N Engl J Med 2002; 346:235–242.

105. Coiffier B, Herbrecht R, Tilly H, et al. GELA study comparing CHOP and R-CHOP in elderly patients with DLCL: 3-year median follow-up with an analysis according to comorbidity factors. Proc Am Soc Clin Oncol 2003; 22:596.

106. Mounier N, Briere J, Gisselbrecht C, et al. Rituximab plus CHOP (R-CHOP) overcomes bcl-2-associated resistance to chemotherapy in elderly patients with diffuse large B-cell lymphoma (DLBCL). Blood 2003; 101:4279–4284.

107. Vose JM, Link BK, Grossbard ML, et al. Phase II study of rituximab in combination with CHOP chemotherapy in patients with previously untreated, aggressive non-Hodgkin's lymphoma. J Clin Oncol 2001; 19:389–397.

108. Vose JM, Link BK, Grossbard M, et al. Long term follow-up of a phase II study of rituximab in combination with CHOP chemotherapy in patients with previously untreated non-Hodgkin's lymphoma. Blood 2002; 100:361a.

109. Habermann TM, Weller EA, Morrison VA, et al. Phase III trial of rituximab CHOP (R-CHOP) versus CHOP with a second randomization to maintenance rituximab (MR) or observation in patients 60 years of age or older with diffuse large B-cell lymphoma (DLBCL) Blood 2003; 102:6a.

110. Wilson WH, Gutierrez M, O'Connor P, et al. The role of rituximab and chemotherapy in aggressive B-cell lymphoma: a preliminary report of dose-adjusted EPOCH-R. Semin Oncol 2002; 29(1 Suppl 2):41–47.

111. Howard OM, Gribben JG, Neuberg DS, et al. Rituximab and CHOP induction therapy for newly diagnosed mantle-cell lymphoma: molecular complete responses are not predictive of progression-free survival. J Clin Oncol 2002; 20:1288–1294.

112. Venugopal P, Gregory SA, Wooldridge JE, et al. Phase II study of rituximab in combination with CHOP chemotherapy and GMCSF in patients with previously untreated aggressive non-Hodgkin's lymphoma. Blood 2002; 100:314b.

113. Kewalramani T, Zelenetz A, Bertino J, et al. Rituximab significantly increases the complete response rate in patients with relapsed or primary refractory DLBCL receiving ICE as second-line therapy (SLT). Blood 2002; 98:346a.

114. Vengugopal P, Gregory SA, Showel J, et al. ESHAP combined with rituximab and GMCSF is highly active in relapsed/refractory aggressive lymphoma. Blood 2002; 100:314b.

115. Hiddemann W, Unterhald M, Dreyling M, et al. The addition of rituximab (R) to combination chemotherapy (CT) significantly improves the treatment of mantle cell lymphomas (MCL): results of two prospective randomized studies by the German low Grade Lymphoma Study Group (GLSG). Blood 2002; 100:92a.

116. Levine AM, Espina BM, Mohrbacher A, et al. Fludarabine, mitoxantrone and Rituxan: an effective regimen for the treatment of mantle cell lymphoma. Blood 2002; 100:361a.

117. Romaguera J, Cabanillas F, Dang NH, et al. Mantle cell lymphoma (MCL)—high rates of complete response (CR) and prolonged failure-free survival (FFS) with Rituxan–hyperCVAD (R-HCVAD) without stem cell transplant (SCT). Blood 2001; 98:726a.

118. Thomas DA, Cortes J, Giles FJ, et al. Rituximab and hyper-CVAD for adult Burkitt's (BL) or Burkitt's-like (BLL) lymphoma. Blood 2002; 100:763a.

119. Grillo-López AJ, Hedrick E, Rashford M, Benyunes M. Rituximab: ongoing and future clinical development. Semin Oncol 2002; 29(1 Suppl 2):105–112.

120. Knox SJ, Goris ML, Trisler K, et al. Yttrium-90-labeled anti-CD20 monoclonal antibody therapy of recurrent B-cell lymphoma. Clin Cancer Res 1996; 2:457–470.

121. Witzig TE, White CA, Wiseman G A, et al. Phase I/II trial of IDEC-Y2B8 radioimmunotherapy for treatment of relapsed or refractory CD20+ B-cell non-Hodgkin's lymphoma. J Clin Oncol 1999; 17: 3793–3803.

122. Wagner HN, Wiseman GA, Marcus CS, et al. Administration guidelines for radioimmunotherapy of non-Hodgkin's lymphoma with $^{90}$Y-labeled anti-CD20 monoclonal antibody. J Nucl Med 2002; 43: 267–272.

123. Witzig TE, Gordon LI, Cabanillas F, et al. Randomized controlled trial of yttrium-90-labeled ibritumomab tiuxetan radioimmunotherapy versus rituximab immunotherapy for patients with relapsed or refractory low-grade, follicular, or transformed B-cell non-Hodgkin's lymphoma. J Clin Oncol 2002; 20: 2453–2463.

124. Gordon LI, Witzig TE, Murray JL, et al. Yttrium-90 ibritumomab tiuxetan radioimmunotherapy produces high response rates and durable remissions in patients with relapsed or refractory low grade, follicular or transformed B-cell NHL: final results of a randomized controlled trial. Proc Am Soc Clin Oncol 2003; 22:576.

125. Wiseman GA, Gordon L, Multani PS, et al. Ibritumomab tiuxetan radioimmunotherapy for patients with relapsed or refractory non-Hodgkin's lymphoma and mild thrombocytopenia: a phase II multicenter trial. Blood 2002; 99:4336–4342.

125a. Schilder RJ, Molina A, Bartlett N, et al. Follow-up results of a phase II study of ibritumomab tiuxetan radioimmunotherapy in patients with relapsed or refractory low-grade, follicular, or transformed B-cell non-Hodgkin's lymphoma and mild thrombocytopenia. Cancer Biother Radiopharm 2004; 19:478–481.

126. Witzig TE, Flinn IW, Gordon LI, et al. Treatment with ibritumomab tiuxetan radioimmunotherapy in patients with rituximab refractory follicular non-Hodgkin's lymphoma. J Clin Oncol 2002; 20:3262–3269.

127. Gordon LI, Molina A, Witzig et al. Durable responses after ibritumomab tiuxetan radioimmunotherapy for CD20+ B-cell lymphoma: long term follow-up of a phase I/II study. Blood 2004; 103:4429–4431.

128. Witzig TE, Molina A, Gordon LI, et al. Yttrium-90 ibritumomab tiuxetan radioimmunotherapy (RIT) induces durable remissions in patients with relapsed or refractory B-cell non-Hodgkin's lymphoma. Drugs Today (Barc) 2004; 40:111–119.

129. Witzig TE, Emmanouilides C, Molina A, et al. Yttrium-90 ibritumomab tiuxetan radioimmunotherapy (RIT) induces durable complete responses (CR/CRu) in patients with relapsed or refractory B-cell non-Hodgkin's lymphoma. Proc Am Soc Clin Oncol 2003; 22:597.

130. Emmanouilides C, Murray JL, Vo K, et al. Earlier treatment with yttrium 90 ibritumomab tiuxetan (Zevalin) radioimmunotherapy is associated with higher response rates and longer durations of response in patients with previously treated B-cell non-Hodgkin's lymphoma. Blood 2003; 102:306b.

131. Emmanouilides C, Witzig T, Gordon L, et al. Zevalin radioimmunotherapy (RIT) is safe and effective in geriatric patients with low grade, follicular or CD20+ transformed (L/G/F/T) non-Hodgkin's lymphoma (NHL). Proc Am Soc Clin Oncol 2002; 21:286a.

132. Witzig TE, Gordon LI, Gaston I, et al. $^{90}$Y ibritumomab tiuxetan (Zevalin) radioimmunotherapy of follicular NHL: results by follicular subtype. Proc Am Soc Clin Oncol 2002; 21:266a.

133. Bartlett NL, Witzig TE, Gordon LI, et al. $^{90}$Y ibritumomab tiuxetan (Zevalin) radioimmunotherapy for transformed B-cell non-Hodgkin's lymphoma (NHL) patients. Proc Am Soc Clin Oncol 2002; 21:14a.

134. Younes A, Pro B, Delpassand E, et al. A phase II study of 90 yttrium-ibritumomab tiuxetan for the treatment of patients with relapsed and refractory mantle cell lymphoma (MCL). Blood 2003; 102:406a.
135. Witzig TE, Gordon LI, Emmanouilides C, et al. Safety and efficacy of Zevalin in four patients with mucosal associated lymphoid tissue (MALT) lymphoma. Blood 2001; 98:254b.
136. Gordon LI, Witzig TE, Emmanouilides CE, et al. $^{90}$Y ibritumomab tiuxetan (Zevalin) in aggressive non-Hodgkin's lymphoma; analysis of response and toxicity. Proc Am Soc Clin Oncol 2002; 21:15b.
137. Witzig TE, Wiseman GA, Geyer SM, et al. Phase I trial of two-sequential doses of Zevalin radioimmunotherapy for relapsed low-grade B-cell non-Hodgkin's lymphoma. Blood 2003; 102:406a.
138. Nademanee A, Molina A, Forman SJ, et al. A phase I/II trial of high-dose radioimmunotherapy (RIT) with Zevalin in combination with high-dose etoposide (VP-16) and cyclophosphamide (CY) followed by autologous stem cell transplant (ASCT) in patients with poor-risk or relapsed B-cell non-Hodgkin's lymphoma. Blood 2002; 100:182a.
139. Winter JN, Inwards D, Erwin W, et al. Zevalin dose-escalation followed by high-dose BEAM and autologous peripheral blood progenitor cell (PBPC) transplant in non-Hodgkin's lymphoma: early outcomes results. Blood 2002; 100:411a.
140. Macklis RM, White CA. Rationale and feasibility of combined radiotherapy and anti-CD20 immunotherapy in CD20+ B cell NHL. In: American Society for Therapeutic Radiology and Oncology, 2002.
141. Witzig TE, White CA, Gordon LI, et al. Safety of yttrium-90 ibritumomab tiuxetan radioimmunotherapy for relapsed low-grade, follicular, or transformed non-Hodgkin's lymphoma. J Clin Oncol 2003; 21(7):1263–1270.
142. Czuczman M, Witzig TE, Gaston I, et al. Zevalin radioimmunotherapy is not associated with an increased incidence of secondary myelodysplastic syndrome (MDS) or acute myelogenous leukemia (AML). Blood 2002; 100(11):357a.
143. Ansell SM, Ristow KM, Habermann TM, et al. Subsequent chemotherapy regimens are well tolerated after radioimmunotherapy with yttrium-90 ibritumomab tiuxetan for non-Hodgkin's lymphoma. J Clin Oncol 2002; 20:3885–3890.
144. Schilder RJ, Witzig T, Gordon L, et al. $^{90}$Y ibritumomab tiuxetan (Zevalin) radioimmunotherapy does not preclude effective delivery of subsequent therapy for lymphoma. Proc Am Soc Clin Oncol 2002; 21:267a.
145. Saleh F, Saleh M, Witzig T, et al. Rituximab administration subsequent to ibritumomab tiuxetan (Zevalin) radioimmunotherapy. Proc Am Soc Clin Oncol 2002; 21:8a.
146. Gordon L, Witzig T, Schilder R, et al. High-dose therapy can be safety and successfully administered after Zevalin treatment. Proc Am Soc Clin Oncol 2002; 21:216b.
147. Vose JM, Bierman PJ, Lynch JC, et al. Phase I clinical trial of Zevalin (90-Y-ibritumomab) in patients with B-cell non-Hodgkin's lymphoma (NHL) with relapsed disease following high-dose chemotherapy and autologous stem cell transplantation. Blood 2003; 102:30a.

# VII   Informatics Strategies and Initiatives

# 44

## Informatics Strategies and Initiatives Used in Cancer Research

*Martin D. Leach, PhD*

### SUMMARY

The use of genomics technologies for cancer research has resulted in a vast amount of data that need to be handled and organized using informatics approaches. Through the use of controlled vocabularies and ontologies, biological data can be annotated in a consistent manner so that scientists can more easily integrate datasets and collaborate. Datasets are being coded using Extensible Markup Language (XML) to aid in the communication and transfer of data. Numerous software applications have been built to facilitate the analysis and visualization of research data and some of these have incorporated features that facilitate data uniformity and sharing. To aid with postgenomics analysis, grid-computing initiatives are providing the computational horsepower so that complex patterns and analyses can be performed on the large datasets. In this chapter, we give a brief overview of the methodologies used and resources available for bioinformaticists wishing to explore cancer biology datasets.

**Key Words:** Oncology; bioinformatics; ontology; XML; grid computing; software.

## 1. INTRODUCTION

**Question**: How much "knowledge" is actually generated using genomics technologies?
**Answer**: *Not much.*

From: *Cancer Drug Discovery and Development: The Oncogenomics Handbook*
Edited by: W. J. LaRochelle and R. A. Shimkets © Humana Press Inc., Totowa, NJ

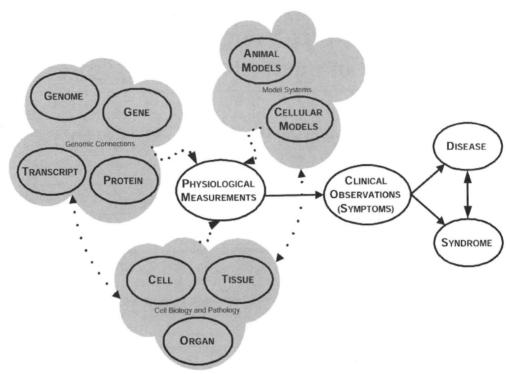

**Fig. 1.** Schematic showing the relationship among genomics-based data, cell biology and pathology, model systems used for studying biology, and the physiological measurements made from each of these disciplines and their connection to disease indication.

Through the use of these technologies a vast amount of data is generated. Data are the first step in the knowledge creation process where data are created and processed to form information, information is layered with other data and verified to form facts, and facts form the underlying basis of knowledge. Genomics technologies create sequencing, gene expression, and proteomics datasets and it is through the process of integrating these forms of information and associating them with peer-reviewed scientific publications, the knowledgebase of individual scientists, and background knowledge from their discipline that these data will be transformed eventually into knowledge.

The goal of cancer research is to identify the underlying mechanisms and intervention points to stop the disease. Figure 1 is a schematic of the relationship of genomics to disease and clearly illustrates that there are a number of steps and gaps to traverse before scientists can link genomics data to clinical observations and disease diagnoses such as cancer. Informatics scientists are bridging the gap between genomic data and the clinic through a number of annotation, organization, classification, and data integration approaches. As a field, this is being described as "systems biology" and the result is the creation, layering, and integration of information onto the physiological networks among genes, proteins, cells, tissues, organs, and the nervous system of an organism.

The role of informatics in genomics has evolved alongside the evolution and extinction of genomic technologies. In the early stages of genomics, bioinformatics was specifically focused on the analysis of sequence from expressed sequence tag (EST) sequencing projects. The National Cancer Institute (NCI) initiated the Cancer Genome Anatomy Project (CGAP) in 1997, generating a large EST dataset from cancerous tissues, normal tissues, and related cell lines *(1)*. This dataset has subsequently been combined with many other EST sequence datasets collated by the National Center for Biotechnology Information in the dbEST database *(2)*. Use of EST sequencing technology created one of the first informatics challenges where bioinformaticists were asked to reduce the data analysis space by clustering related sequences and removing redundancy. The product of this task was the generation of the UniGene clusters *(3)*. With the consolidation of these data, bioinformaticists could begin the work of layering tissue source data to get basic gene expression profiles from the EST sequence data. Following the clustering, bioinformatics scientists set out to assemble the clusters into contigs so that splice variants could be distinguished, then came the search for disease- and tissue-specific splice variants. With the consolidation of the sequence data into contigs, subtle differences could be seen between the "consensus" sequence and some of the underlying sequences, this resulted in additional exploration of single-nucleotide polymorphisms (SNPs), haplotype identification, and subsequent association with diseases.

Information gleaned from sequencing projects required validation from alternate expression profiling technologies. Expression profiling technologies, including the serial analysis of gene expression (SAGE) *(4)* and microarray hybridization, were used to generate quantitative expression data vs the qualitative expression data from prior sequencing projects *(5)*. Following the lead of technology development, informatics techniques and analyses provided insight into understanding cancer gene expression *(5,6)*.

Data are now being generated in staggering amounts and biologists are now presented with a glut of bewildering "data" that they wish to convert into information for their knowledge base. These burgeoning genomics data are just a fraction of the global expansion of data generated in cancer research. Scientists are now realizing that more data reduction tools are needed, as well as better ways of clustering, accessing, and integrating data beyond algorithmic approaches. To address these issues, bioinformaticists need common methods and standards for organizing, annotating, analyzing, communicating, and managing of data, information, and knowledge.

There a number of major informatics initiatives that are tackling the problem of bringing data together, organizing data through central ontologies and classification systems, and providing numerous interfaces to the information through a multitude of software applications that allow specific questions to be asked on specific data types. Two major initiatives include those at the UK National Cancer Research Institute (NCRI) and the US National Cancer Institute (NCI). A coordination unit has been setup at the NCRI that is working with the NCI and the European Bioinformatics Institute so that global standards are developed and applied globally to research datasets. Both initiatives have a matrix approach for the organized informatics attack on cancer.

The NCRI has identified many informatics approaches and organizes them into nine sources of information ranging from DNA to Epidemiology & Population Studies and eight challenges and approaches for organizing and analyzing these information sources of data *(7)*. Table 1 shows the subset of informatics strategies and approaches that are being applied to genomics and proteomics data by the NCRI. The NCI has developed a similar matrix of informatics applications and projects spanning the research continuum for oncology research like the UK-based NCRI. On July 11, 2003, the NCI announced the start of a cancer-based biomedical informatics network, called the Cancer Biomedical Informatics

**Table 1**
**Subset of the "Genomics" Portion of the NCRI Matrix of Informatics Projects**

| | Data Elements | Controlled Vocabularies and Ontologies | Data-Exchange Formats | Protocol Standardization | Implementation | Data Mining | Privacy-enhancing Technologies/ Security | Knowledge Management |
|---|---|---|---|---|---|---|---|---|
| DNA | GO<br>GONG<br>caBIG–caDSR<br>caBIG–EVS | GO<br>caBIG–caBIO<br>GONG | caBIG–caBIO<br>DAG_edit<br>DAML+OIL<br>OWL<br>Relevant XML | caBIG–caLIMS<br>NIST<br>LGC | caBIG–caBIO<br>GeneCensus<br>KEGG<br>NDB<br>LSID<br>Ensembl<br>Transfac<br>dbSNP | dbSNP<br>GeneCensus<br>KEGG<br>BIOGopher<br>BIOMoby | caBIG–caBIO | caBIG–cMAP |
| Functional genomics | MIAME<br>GMOD<br>caBIG–caDSR<br>caBIG–EVS | GO<br>GONG<br>SOFG<br>MGED | GO<br>DAG_edit<br>DAML+OIL<br>OWL<br>Relevant XML<br>GONG | caBIG–caLIMS<br>National Physical Laboratory<br>LGC | BIOgopher<br>MyGrid<br>MAGE-OM<br>Transfac<br>GMOD<br>HapMap<br>DECIPHER<br>GXD<br>GEDP | Discovery Net<br>Bio-Logical<br>SCIpath | caBIG–caBIO | MyGrid<br>caBIG–CMAP<br>Bio-Logical<br>Tambis |
| Proteomics | E-Protein<br>Intact<br>MSD<br>HUPO<br>PSI<br>UNIPROT | E-Protein | E-Protein<br>DAG_Edit<br>DAML+OIL<br>OWL<br>Relevant XML<br>HUPO<br>PSI<br>AGML | HUPO<br>LGC<br>NIST | Pedro<br>Swiss Model<br>DMM<br>Dali<br>SCOP<br>CATH<br>Intact<br>PDB<br>MSD<br>LSID<br>ISPIDER | HUPO<br>Dali<br>MSD<br>MyGrid<br>ISPIDER | – | MSD<br>ISPIDER |

Additional information and a brief description of each of these projects are shown in Table 2.

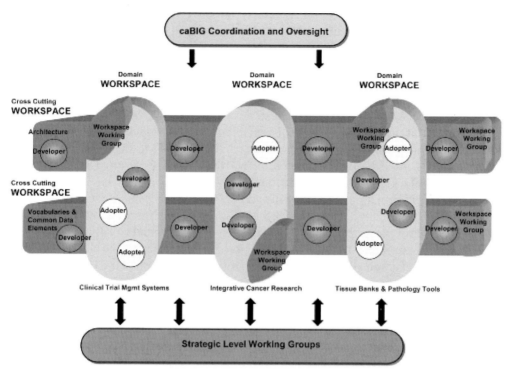

**Fig. 2.** The 'pilot' workspaces that have been setup as part of the US Cancer Biomedical Informatics Grid (caBIG). Three domain workspaces covering clinical trial management systems, integrative cancer research, and tissue banks and pathology are being addressed in the caBIG pilot project. Across each of these domains, informatics scientists are utilizing, adapting, and creating solutions for necessary informatics architecture and standards for vocabularies and common data elements. A number of working groups have been set up in each of these areas and developers and adopters have been identified to work on projects. (Reproduced with kind permission from the NCI caBIG Project Team, ref. *39*.)

Grid (caBIG). The goal of caBIG is to unify informatics projects across the cancer research space integrating as much work from the National Cancer Institute Center for Bioinformatics (NCICB), National Center for Biotechnology Information (NCBI), and other governmental, academic, and NCI-sponsored clinical centers. In the current "pilot" state, the areas covered include Clinical Trial Management Systems, Integrative Cancer Research, and Tissue Banks & Pathology Tools (Fig. 2). Spanning each of these areas are informatics projects for Vocabularies & Common Data Elements and Architecture. Work initiated with other NCICB and NCI initiatives will be rolled into caBIG.

The NCRI and NCI share the adoption and exploration of a number of informatics approaches, some of which will be discussed in the subsequent sections of this chapter.

## 2. DATA ELEMENTS, CONTROLLED VOCABULARIES, ONTOLOGIES, AND DATA EXCHANGE FORMATS

We are all familiar with the sharing of information on the internet via the World Wide Web (WWW), but we take for granted the underlying uniform and ubiquitous way the information is organized, delivered, and then interpreted by web browsers. What you see on your screen is an "interpretation" of Hypertext Markup Language (HTML) that is delivered by a web server upon request. HTML is a specialized way of demarking text such as used by the publishing industry and was the basis of early word-processing computers and applications. For example, my text demarks the term "my text" to be made bold upon parsing of the HTML and delivery onto the screen by the web browser. Uniformity is also required in cancer research for the organization and exchange of information among researchers, and informatics scientists are addressing this challenge through the use of Extensible Markup Language (XML). XML is an emerging standard for the representation of any form of data elements or metadata *(8)*. Unlike HTML, XML is not "one language," but, it is, instead, a more "generic" method that is used to construct a specific XML representation of a given set of information. XML in its original form has allowed scientists to organize information into uniformly acceptable ways so that the data can be parsed and interpreted by virtually anyone. In fact, the latest versions of Microsoft Internet Explorer support the reading, parsing, and basic visualization of the structure and organization of an XML dataset. An example of XML delimited biological information can be seen in Fig. 3. As shown in the example, the XML structure allows organization of the information that is easily interpreted by a human and, subsequently, by software written to parse it. However, XML has several limitations: (1) It allows only hierarchical organization of information; (2) it is extremely verbose and adds overhead to the size of data files transferred when requested; and (3) although easily readable and interpretable, XML still requires software to parse the XML and display it in a form that is "acceptable" to the researcher. Many forms of XML, tools for XML generation, editing, and visualization have been developed that are applicable to cancer research *(10)*.

A number of markup languages have also been created for delimiting a scientific database, but most of these are instances of XML. The Bioinformatics Sequence Markup Language (BSML) organization has developed an XML-based standard for the representation and integration of many forms of bioinformatics data *(11)*. Many groups are using this standard for the sharing of information, however, not many groups are generating scientific data in this standard. On the other hand, the Generalized Analytical Markup Language (GAML) has been to be adopted by a number of key instrument vendors that provide tools for the exportation of experimental data in this format *(12)*.

Extensible Markup Language is a method of organizing information into a simple-to-understand structure, but work is required to control the right content that is put into XML structures. The construction and adoption of controlled vocabularies allows the uniformity of content. Controlled vocabularies are typically constructed as hierarchical classification trees with terms that are recognizable to the scientists. A simple hierarchical classification, however, is limited to a simple parent–child relationship of the data element being classified. Ontologies are being used in biological research, as these allow a more complex set of relationships to be constructed between entries in a classification tree. Ontologies also use a framework-based method of classifying data but are typically Directed Acyclic Graphs (DAGs). DAGs have the advantage of allowing objects to be arranged so that multiple parent–child relationships can be constructed.

---

**Fig. 3.** *(Opposite page)*    The complement component C2 complex entry from the Gene Ontology™ database showing (**A**) the underlying XML representation used and (**B**) one interpretation of the XML data into a series of hyperlinks leading to additional information as specified in the XML.

**A**

```xml
<?xml version="1.0" encoding="UTF-8"?>
<!DOCTYPE go:go PUBLIC "-//Gene Ontology//Custom XML/RDF Version 2.0//EN" "http://www.godatabase.org/dtd/go.dtd">

<go:go xmlns:go="http://www.geneontology.org/dtds/go.dtd#" xmlns:rdf="http://www.w3.org/1999/02/22-rdf-syntax-ns#">
<rdf:RDF>
    <go:term rdf:about="http://www.geneontology.org/go#GO:0005603">
        <go:accession>GO:0005603</go:accession>
        <go:name>complement component C2 complex</go:name>
        <go:association rdf:parseType="Resource">
            <go:evidence evidence_code="TAS">
                <go:dbxref rdf:parseType="Resource">
                    <go:database_symbol>PMID</go:database_symbol>
                    <go:reference>6199794</go:reference>
                </go:dbxref>
            </go:evidence>
            <go:gene_product rdf:parseType="Resource">
                <go:name>CO2_HUMAN</go:name>
                <go:dbxref rdf:parseType="Resource">
                    <go:database_symbol>uniprot</go:database_symbol>
                    <go:reference>P06681</go:reference>
                </go:dbxref>
            </go:gene_product>
        </go:association>
        <go:association rdf:parseType="Resource">
            <go:evidence evidence_code="TAS">
                <go:dbxref rdf:parseType="Resource">
                    <go:database_symbol>PMID</go:database_symbol>
                    <go:reference>6199794</go:reference>
                </go:dbxref>
            </go:evidence>
            <go:gene_product rdf:parseType="Resource">
                <go:name>CO2_HUMAN</go:name>
                <go:dbxref rdf:parseType="Resource">
                    <go:database_symbol>uniprot</go:database_symbol>
                    <go:reference>P06681</go:reference>
                </go:dbxref>
            </go:gene_product>
        </go:association>
    </go:term>
</rdf:RDF>
</go:go>
```

**B**

| GO:0005603 | complement component C2 complex | | |
|---|---|---|---|
| | CO2_HUMAN | UniProt | TAS |
| | CO2_HUMAN | UniProt | TAS |

719

A number of ontology editors and browsers have been developed to aid with the construction, editing, maintenance, propagation, and integration of ontologies for scientific research. A comprehensive list of these can be found at http://www.geneontology.org/GO.tools.html or in the recent review article by Bard et al. *(13)*. Two of the most popular ontology editors are DAG_edit and Protégé 2000. DAG_edit is a Java-based application that was originally built as a tool for editing ontologies created for the Drosophila Genome project and is freely accessible from the Sourceforge website *(14)*. Protégé 2000 supports the construction and editing of complex hierarchies and DAGs. However, Protégé 2000 has many additional functions because it is an extensible platform for knowledge-based systems development *(15,16)*.

The Gene Ontology™ (GO) is a project that is the product of the GO Consortium and is attempting to build a controlled vocabulary that can be applied to all organisms *(9,17)*. The GO currently provides three classification networks that provide annotations for structured classification of Molecular Function, Biological Processes, and Cellular Components. As a general ontology, the GO ontology is one of the most popular used throughout all areas of research. Upon examination, the GO ontology "Oncogenesis" was a biological process used in the classification scheme but has subsequently been made obsolete without any replacement. The GO ontology is best used for the classification of individual genes and mapping of its relationship to additional biological functions, processes, and cellular components. An example of the GO classification of Mas proto-oncogene receptor activity is shown in Fig. 4.

The Gene Ontology Next Generation (GONG) has set out to enrich the content of the GO project and extend the function of GO from being a frame-based graph of relationships to a network that incorporates logic between the relationships *(18,19)*. The methodology initially used the DAML + OIL language, based on the DARPA Agent Markup Language (DAML) with a combined Ontology Inference Layer (OIL). An ontology from the Microarray Gene Expression Data (MGED) society currently uses DAML. The MGED ontology is used for describing samples used in microarray experiments *(20,21)*. The MGED ontology is actively being used for cancer research as part of the NCI caBIG initiative as a means of creating a reference "bridge" between the microarray datasets and oncology terms used by the NCI.

The MGED Society has also been developing a data content standard for describing the Minimum Information About a Microarray Experiment (MIAME) that is needed for easy and reproducible interpretation of microarray experiments *(22)*. To encode the data, the Microarray Gene Expression Markup Language (MAGE-ML) has been developed using XML *(23)*. The MIAME standard has been widely adopted, and data submissions are required from a number of leading cancer and general scientific journals such as *Science, Nature, EMBO, Cell, The Lancet, The American Physiological Society, Journal of the National Cancer Institute, Physiological Genomics, Cancer Genomics & Proteomics,*

**Fig. 4.** *(Opposite page)* Visualization of the Mas proto-oncogene receptor activity that is organized as a biological function in the GO ontology. The diagram shows how the Mas proto-oncogene receptor activity is organized within the biological function network. The support of multiparent classification can be seen, where class A orphan receptor activity is classified as being a grouping under both rhodopsin-like receptor activity and G protein-coupled receptor activity (unknown ligand). GO entry unique identifiers are shown in the top right-hand corner of each box. The visualization was generated from the QuickGO server located at http://www.ebi.ac.uk/ego/.

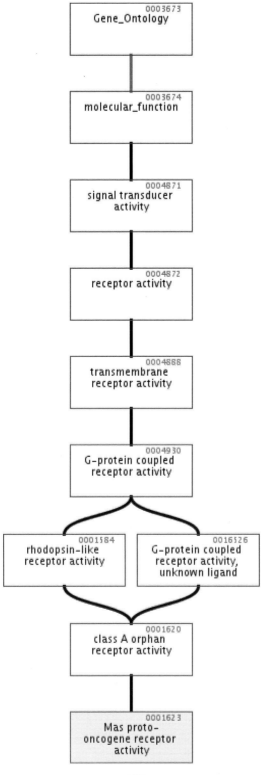

and *Cancer Research*. In addition to scientific journals, two major gene expression sites have adopted or are supportive of the MIAME standard; the NCI Gene Expression Data Portal (GEDP) developed for the microarray community of cancer researchers and the NCBI Gene Expression Omnibus website that is a central repository integrating many forms of expression data *(24,25)*.

DAML + OIL-based ontologies have recently been superceded by the Ontology Web Language (OWL). OWL, like DAML + OIL, has been developed to facilitate the publishing and sharing of ontologies on the WWW *(26)*. OWL is derived from DAML + OIL and is being used as the "next generation" method of representing and organizing ontologies. A number of biological ontologies that have been converted or created using this new format include the following:

- The National Cancer Institute Thesaurus. This is a very large file of many cancer or research-related terms used by the NCI (http://www.mindswap.org/2003/CancerOntology/).
- BioPax, a data exchange format for biological pathways (http://www.biopax.org).
- The TAMBIS biological and chemical ontology. http://www.cs.man.ac.uk/~horrocks/OWL/Ontologies/tambis-full.owl. (Note: This is rather limited, as only one biological process "transcription" is included in this ontology. The classification of chemical terms is quite in depth.)

Additional OWL ontology examples for nonbiological uses can be found at http://protege.stanford.edu/plugins/owl/ontologies.html.

OWL ontologies can be readily manipulated and edited with software applications such as Protégé 2000 that has been fitted with an OWL plug-in *(15)*. Figure 5 shows an example of the NCI OWL-based ontology. Where logical expressions are created between objects in this ontology they can be seen displayed in the "Asserted" and "Inferred" tabs, as shown in the center panel of Fig. 5.

## 3. PROTOCOL STANDARDIZATION IN INFORMATICS FOR CANCER RESEARCH

Standardization in bioinformatics and genomics comes in two flavors: (1) standardization of the file formats created, used, and shared between scientists for the exchange of scientific database, as described in Section 2, and (2) standardization of the process for the generation, capture, and analysis of scientific data. Much effort has gone into the standardization of protocols for clinical research for cancer but has not advanced far for oncogenomic research. This is predominantly because standardization for discovery projects tends to be free-flowing. Constraining research scientists tends to result in push back and failure to use the informatics systems offered to them. Smaller organizations tend to be more successful in getting scientists to adopt the use of informatics systems. However, if informatics scientists cannot rapidly respond to change or rapidly customize the systems as needed, researchers fall back to using their own methods for tracking and organizing

**Fig. 5.** *(Opposite page)* Screenshot of Protégé ontology editor (v2.1b) using a plug-in for displaying and manipulating semantic OWL ontologies. The National Cancer Institute OWL ontology is shown in the left-hand panel. The oncogene ERB_A is shown highlighted in the left-hand panel and a number of asserted conditions are shown in the central Asserted Panel indicating properties of the ERB_A oncogene.

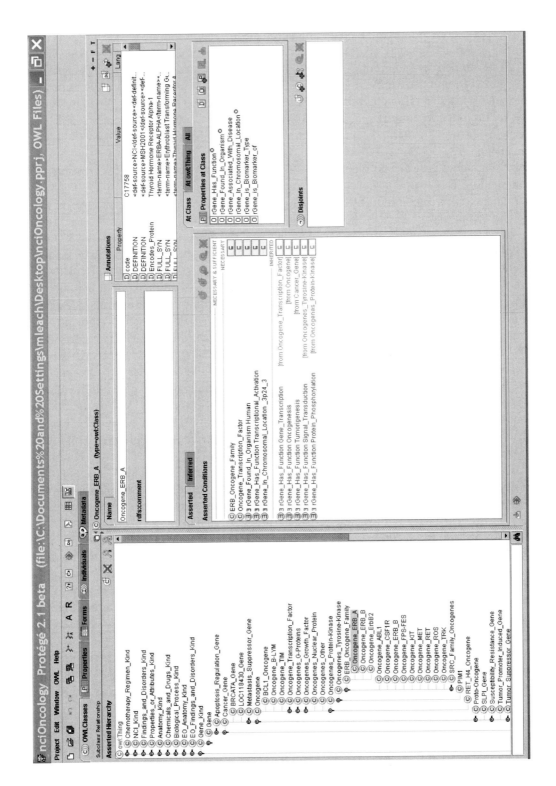

their experiments, usually with Microsoft Excel spreadsheets for tracking and Microsoft Powerpoint or Word for the display and summary of results.

For genomics data analysis and process organization, several commercial products have been developed for generating and automating the data analysis pipeline. The Visual Integrated Bioinformatics Environment (VIBE) allows creation of analytical pipelines by building a graphical flowchart of the analytical process (INCOGEN, Inc., Williamsburg, VA). Through a recent phase II award from the National Cancer Institute, INCOGEN is using its software for the analysis of protein chip data. The Pipeline Pilot™ pipeline (Scitegic, San Diego, CA) and TurboWorx Builder™ (TurboWorx, Inc., Shelton, CT) are similar systems, with both generic and specialized modules for bioinformatics process creation and automation. These systems have not generated any general standards that are applicable to the cancer research community, but they do allow for standardization of processes within an organization.

In an effort to standardize the way data are generated in cancer research, the Science Applications International Corporation (SAIC) in cooperation with the National Cancer Institute has developed the Cancer Laboratory Information Management System (caLIMS). caLIMS is a web-based system that supports user and laboratory administration, equipment operation, inventory management, project creation, electronic data capture, and presentation of results. caLIMS is an open-source project and is freely downloadable from the NCI website at http://lpglims.nci.nih.gov/. The caLIMS architecture is built using Java software and allows communication with a central database, delivering data for software processing or visualization via a web browser. This multipurpose suite for setting up experimental projects, performing data entry, and generating crude visualization of data is quite extensive, rivaling some commercial LIMS development environments. However, caLIMS lacks features for automated data analysis. Future releases of caLIMS are planned to extend the system from an organized project creation and electronic data capture system into a system that will automate data analysis and quality control.

Use of such an electronic data capture (EDC) system where data entry is the main form of data collection would be the perfect solution in an ideal world. In reality, data are generated on many different instruments, in a multitude of formats, many of which are proprietary. Extraction of data or metadata from data files generated becomes a difficult and time-consuming task as the complexity of the organization and number of technologies used increase. Many systems support "delimited" text dumps that can then be readily imported into applications such as Microsoft Excel or Word. Where image data might be available, images typically are exported as TIFFs, GIFs, or JPEGs and are associated with the data file. What follows is a nightmare—managing hundreds of thousands of files instead of managing the data in a database. Some of the more successful systems such as the GeneScape® platform (CuraGen Corporation, New Haven, CT) support the "Microsoft" world of files, integrating them with other electronically captured data derived from experiments.

As an alternative, some organizations rely on managing their scientific data in the ubiquitous Portable Document Format (PDF) established by Adobe Systems (San Jose, CA). The documents created in the PDF format still have to be managed as a file system or, in some cases, within a document management system such as Documentum (Documentum Inc., Pleasanton, CA). PDF documents are created by sending data from any application to a custom PDF print driver. The PDF print driver processes the data instead of spooling the data to a printer, and the data are converted into a PDF formatted document. PDF files are viewable using the Acrobat PDF viewer. Although uniformity is created in data files generated using this method, the extraction of information from a PDF requires manual editing or the purchase of expensive PDF processing software. PDFs are better suited for archiving information and are the mode of choice for scientists collating, locking down, and archiving clinical trial data.

To address both uniformity of data files generated and their reuse and manipulation, Nugenesis Technologies (Westborough, MA) has developed their Scientific Data Management System (SDMS). As with PDFs, the SDMS system captures data from a print stream and converts it to an extended Windows metafile. The typical Windows metafile is file that can be created on Microsoft platforms that can be viewed and used by multiple applications. Nugenesis's value addition is providing tools for extracting desired images, text, tables, and data from the extended Windows metafile. This allows data to be integrated from multiple experiments generated in multiple formats into customized reports. As with PDFs the Nugenesis system requires file or database management and this is provided with their suite of products.

## 4. BIOINFORMATICS IMPLEMENTATIONS AND DATA MINING IN CANCER RESEARCH

Many informatics applications have been built for the visualization, mining, and extraction of biological data. The list is so vast that it is beyond the scope of this chapter to describe each of these in detail. In addition, many genomic resources for cancer biologists have already been described previously in this volume by Ling et al. (27). Tables 1 and 2 summarize additional bioinformatics applications and methodologies that have been identified for use by the UK National Cancer Research Institute. As part of caBIG and initiated prior to the start of this new initiative, the National Cancer Institute Center for Bioinformatics (NCICB) has been generating an excellent set of tools, guidelines, applications, and systems accessible from their website and servers.

To facilitate interaction and integration of data from multiple sources, the NCICB has developed a core suite of standards, schema, objects, and software called the caCORE. The caCORE is the NCICB informatics infrastructure backbone. caCORE is an open-source platform that the NCI has used to build its research information management systems. It is built from the three major components: caDSR, caEVS, and caBIO. An Application Programming Interface (API) has been developed and is supported in a number of programming languages. Data communication protocols predominantly handle XML-based data. A number of applications have been built upon the caCORE platform, including BIOgopher and BioBrowser (see Table 2). A comprehensive technical description of caCORE can be found at ftp://ftp1.nci.nih.gov/pub/cacore/caCORE2.0_Tech_Guide.pdf.

As part of the overall cancer Biomedical Informatics Grid (caBIG), the National Cancer Institute (NCI), together with members of the cancer research community, have developed common data elements (CDEs) that will be used to describe metadata in NCI-sponsored research. A CDE is based on the ISO/IEC 11179 specification developed by the National Institute of Standards and Technology (NIST). The Cancer Data Standards Repository (caDSR) is a database and toolset used to create, edit, and deploy the CDEs (28). The caDSR brings together the CDEs in one place so that they can be shared and reused among research groups at a number of NCI-sponsored research facilities (29).

The NCI Enterprise Vocabulary Services (EVS) is a collaborative project of the NCICB and the NCI Office of communications (30). The result of this collaboration is the development of the NCI Thesaurus and NCI Metathesaurus (31,32). The NCI Thesaurus is a bio-

Table 2
Description of Informatics Tools Identified by the NCRI Currently Used in Cancer Research or Under Investigation for Cancer Research

| Description | URL | Comment |
|---|---|---|
| BIOgopher | http://biogopher.nci.nih.gov/BIOgopher/index.jsp | The National Cancer Institute (NCI)—Integration/ Annotation tool |
| Bio-Logical | http://www.nesc.ac.uk/action/projects/project_action. cfm?title=167 | Database technology for knowledge discovery in functional genomics |
| BIOMoby | http://www.biomoby.org | An open-source web-based protocol for integration of biological information |
| caBIG-caBIO | http://ncicb.nci.nih.gov/core/caBIO | The Cancer Biomedical Information Grid (caBIG)– Cancer Bioinformatics Infrastructure Objects |
| caBIG–caDSR | http://ncicb.nci.nih.gov/core/caDSR | Cancer Data Standards Repository |
| caBIG–caLIMS | http://lpglims.nci.nih.gov/ | NCI–Laboratory Information Management System |
| caBIG–cMAP | http://cmap.nci.nih.gov/ | NCI–Cancer Molecular Analysis Project |
| caBIG–EVS | http://ncicb.nci.nih.gov/core/EVS | NCI–Enterprise Vocabulary Services |
| CATH | http://www.biochem.ucl.ac.uk/bsm/cath/ | Classic, Architecture, Topology and Homologous Superfamily protein domain classified database |
| DAG_edit | http://geneontology.sourceforge.net/ | DAG Software from The Gene Ontology Project |
| DALI | http://www.ebi.ac.uk/dali/index.html | Server for comparing protein structures in three dimensions |
| DAML + OIL | http://www.w3.org/TR/2004/REC-owl-ref-20040210/ | Darpa Agency Markup Language and Ontology Inference Layer |
| dbSNP | http://www.ncbi.nlm.nih.gov/SNP/ | Database of Single-Nucleotide Polymorphisms |
| DECIPHER | http://www.sanger.ac.uk/PostGenomics/decipher/ | Database of Chromosomal Imbalance and Phenotype in Humans using Ensembl Resources |
| Discovery Net | http://www.discovery-on-the.net/new/index.php | e-Science Platform of the Imperial College London |
| DMM | http://molmovdb.mbb.yale.edu/molmovdb | Database of Macromolecular Movements |
| E-Protein | http://www.e-protein.org | Grid-based annotation pipeline for proteomes |
| Ensembl | http://www.ensembl.org | Ensembl Genome Browser |
| GEDP | http://gedp.nci.nih.gov/dc/index.jsp | NCI–Gene Expression Data Portal |
| GeneCensus | http://bioinfo.mbb.yale.edu/genome/ | Comparative Genome Analysis tool |
| GMOD | http://www.gmod.org | Generic Model Organism Project |
| GO | http://www.geneontology.org | Gene Ontology |
| GONG | http://gong.man.ac.uk/ | Gene Ontology Next Generation |
| GXD | http://www.informatics.jax.org/mgihome/GXD/about GXD.shtml | Gene Expression Database |

| | | |
|---|---|---|
| HapMap | http://www.hapmap.org/index.html.en | Human genome haplotype mapping project |
| HUPO | http://www.hupo.org/ (http://211.32.65.137/) | Initiative to consolidate national and regional proteome organizations |
| IntAct | http://www.ebi.ac.uk/intact/ | Protein–protein interaction database and standards for representation and annotation |
| KEGG | http://www.genome.ad.jp/kegg/kegg2.html | Kyoto Encyclopedia of Genes and Genomes |
| LSID | http://www-124.ibm.com/developerworks/opensource/lsid/?Open&ca=daw-ws-dr | Life Sciences Identifier Project |
| MAGE-OM | http://www.mged.org/Workgroups/MAGE/mage.html | MGED—Microarray and Gene Expression Object Model |
| MGED | http://www.mged.org | The Microarray Gene Expression Data Society (MGED) |
| MIAME | http://www.mged.org/Workgroups/MIAME/miame.html | MGED—Minimum Information About a Microarray Experiment |
| MSD | http://www.ebi.ac.uk/msd/index.html | Macro Molecular Structure Database |
| MyGrid | http://www.mygrid.org.uk | UK-based in silico biology grid-computing project |
| NDB | http://ndbserver.rutgers.edu/about_ndb/index.html | Nuclei Acid Database |
| NIST | http://www.cstl.nist.gov/div831/biotech/workshops.html | National Institute of Standards and Technology—Biotechnology Division |
| NPL | http://www.npl.co.uk | UK National Physical Laboratory for national standards |
| OWL | http://www.w3.org/TR/2004/REC-owl-ref-20040210/ | Ontology Web Language |
| PDB | http://www.pdb.org | Protein Data Bank—repository of three-dimensional biological macromolecular structure data |
| Pedro | http://pedrodownload.man.ac.uk/index.shtml | Tool for generating data entry forms from an XML schema |
| PSI | http://psidev.sourceforge.net/ | Proteomics Standards Initiative |
| SCIpath | http://www.ucl.ac.uk/oncology/MicroCore/microcore.htm | Systems Complexity Interface for Pathways—suite of programs developed by University College London Department of Oncology |
| SCOP | http://scop.mrc-lmb.cam.ac.uk/scop/ | Structural Classification of Proteins Database |
| SOFG | http://www.sofg.org | Standards and Ontologies for Functional Genomics |
| SwissModel | http://www.expasy.org/swissmod/SWISS-MODEL.html | Protein Structure homology-modeling server |
| TAMBIS | http://imgproj.cs.man.ac.uk/tambis/ | Transparent Access to Multiple Bioinformatics Information Sources—project to provide a single web-based interface for biological information sources |
| Transfac® | http://www.gene-regulation.com/pub/databases.html | Eukaryotic Transcription Factor database |
| UniProt | http://www.pir.uniprot.org/ | Central repository/catalog of information on proteins |

727

medical thesaurus providing access to the clinical, translational, basic research, and administrative terminology used by the NCI *(33)*. The NCI Metathesaurus is more diverse and contains over 50 biomedical source vocabularies from the National Library of Medicine's Unified Medical Language System (UMLS) Metathesaurus, a number of NCI cancer-specific vocabularies, and proprietary vocabularies *(34,35)*.

The Cancer Bioinformatics Infrastructure Objects (caBIO) provides a set of predefined data structures, programming interfaces, and customized data sources for the development of software applications for cancer researchers *(36)*. Over 25 major data sources that are used by molecular biologists and clinical researchers are available through the programmatic interfaces of caBIO *(37)*. The caBIO objects have been implemented as Java beans and include Java classes that represent biological and bioinformatics concepts or entities. Several applications have been written using caBIO, including BIOgopher and BIO Browser. The BIO Browser requires a brief mention, as it utilizes caBIO, caDSR, and caMOD (cancer model) data sources and communicates to a central CABIO server using XML-based communication protocols.

## 5. OTHER INFORMATICS CONCERNS FOR CANCER RESEARCH

As with any vast amount of information generated through genomics processes, computational analyses of such data can be rather time-consuming or computationally expensive. A number of initiatives have utilized or are using grid computing approaches for biological and cancer research. In July 9, 2001, the NCI and Cray Inc. announced a collaboration for utilizing a grid of computers for sequence analysis and mapping of data to the human genome. This grid computing approach showed to researchers how a distributed computing environment would be beneficial to cancer research. More recently, a number of additional grid initiatives have begun for *in silico* biological computing. Some of these projects include the following:

- The Asia Pacific BioGrid Initiative (http://www.apgrid.org/)
- The North Carolina BioGrid (http://www.ncbiogrid.org/)
- The Canadian BioGrid (http://www.cbr.nrc.ca)
- The Japanese BioGrid (http://www.biogrid.jp/)
- The EUROGRID Bio-GRID (http://www.eurogrid.org/wp1.html)
- The UK-based MyGrid Project (http://www.mygrid.org.uk), and
- The Biomedical Informatics Research Network (http://www.nbirn.net/)—currently being applied for imaging in neuroscience

A number of tools that are being used to enable grid computing, such as the publicly available Globus Toolkit from The Globus Alliance (http://www.globus.org) or the commercially available Sun ONE Grid Engine from Sun Microsystems (Santa Clara, CA), ensure that data security is managed as part of these distributed computing environments.

## 6. SUMMARY

Ater reading this chapter you are probably just as bewildered by the number of informatics initiatives as you are by the volume of genomic datasets. Some standards are clearly emerging for cancer and other areas of science: XML is becoming the "method" of choice for delimiting data and communicating the data among software; MIAME and MAGE-ML for microarray data are required for data submissions and publication in many high-profile journals; OWL is emerging in the latest wave of ontologies and controlled vocabularies. There are many ways to test a scientific hypothesis and there will always be many tools and methodologies used to generate and dissect data needed for research.

As mentioned at the outset of this chapter, the creation of pathways and the layering of information onto network or pathway diagrams hold the key to understanding the underlying mechanism and intervention points for cancer. As common languages and classifications are developed and applied in cancer research, we get closer to being able to traverse the data integration gaps. Although not fully utilizing the ontologies and technologies mentioned in this chapter, several groups have attempted to organize genomic data around a networked pathway model of oncology through integrating data. Gene Network Sciences (Ithaca, NY) has built a model of oncology that combines data from over 10,000 articles, animal knockout/knockdown measurements, mRNA expression measurements, protein expression levels, phenotypic measurements, and includes many key cancer networks. Similarly, Ingenuity Systems (Mountain View, CA) has developed an integrated pathways-based way of integrating genomic data and literature information and is working with the CaP Cure Prostate Cancer Foundation *(38)*.

In closing, bioinformatics plays an important role in organizing and cataloging genomic data that has been generated for cancer research. Genomics data alone will not generate enough information to build a clear picture of oncogenesis. With the postgenomics romp into "systems biology" and layering of genomics and postgenomics data, such as in vivo data, clinical data, and information from published articles will informatics scientists be able build truly representative descriptions of the underlying mechanisms of cancer?

## REFERENCES

1. Krizman DB, Wagner L, Lash A, Strausberg RL, Emmert-Buck MR. The Cancer Genome Anatomy Project: EST sequencing and the genetics of cancer progression. Neoplasia 1999; 1(2):101–106.
2. Boguski MS, Lowe TM, Tolstoshev CM. dbEST—database for "expressed sequence tags." Nat Genet 1993; 4(4):332–333.
3. Schuler GD. Pieces of the puzzle: expressed sequence tags and the catalog of human genes. J Mol Med 1997; 75(10):694–698.
4. Velculescu VE, Zhang L, Vogelstein B, Kinzler KW. Serial analysis of gene expression. Science 1995; 270(5235):484–487.
5. Scherf U, Ross DT, Waltham M, et al. A gene expression database for the molecular pharmacology of cancer. Nat Genet 2000; 24(3):236–244.
6. Ross DT, Scherf U, Eisen MB, et al. Systematic variation in gene expression patterns in human cancer cell lines. Nat Genet 2000; 24(3):227–235.
7. National Cancer Research Institute website: http://www.cancerinformatics.org.uk/planning_matrix. htm. Accessed 1/7/05.
8. XML Organization website: http://www.xml.org. Accessed 1/7/05.
9. Gene Ontology Consortium website: http://www.geneontology.org. Accessed 1/7/05.
10. NCRI Cancer Informatics website: http://www.cancerinformatics.org.uk/xml.htm. Accessed 1/7/05.
11. Bioinformatics Sequence Markup Language website: http://www.bsml.org. Accessed 1/7/05.
12. Generalized Analytical Markup Language website: http://www.gaml.org. Accessed 1/7/05.
13. Bard JB, Rhee SY. Ontologies in biology: design, applications and future challenges. Nat Rev Genet 2004; 5(3):213–222.
14. Gene Ontology Project website: http://geneontology.sourceforge.net/. Accessed 1/7/05.
15. Noy NF, Sintek M, Decker S, Crubezy M, Fergerson RW, Musen MA. Creating semantic web contents with Protege-2000. IEEE Intell Syst 2001; 16(2):60–71.
16. Musen MA, Eriksson H, Gennari JH, Tu SW, Puerta AR. PROTEGE-II: a suite of tools for development of intelligent systems from reusable components. In: Proceedings of the Annual Symposium on Computer Applications in Medical Care 1994:1065.

17. Harris MA, Clark J, Ireland A, et al. The Gene Ontology (GO) database and informatics resource. Nucleic Acids Res 2004; 32: Database Issue D258–D261.
18. Gene Ontology Next Generation website: http://gong.man.ac.uk. Accessed 1/7/05.
19. Wroe CJ, Stevens R, Goble CA, Ashburner M. A methodology to migrate the gene ontology to a description logic environment using DAML + OIL. Pac Symp Biocomput 2003:624–635.
20. MGED Sample Ontology website: http://mged.sourceforge.net/. Accessed 1/7/05.
21. Stoeckert CJ Jr, Causton HC, Ball CA. Microarray databases: standards and ontologies. Nat Genet 2002; 32(Suppl):469–473.
22. Brazma A, Hingamp P, Quackenbush J, et al. Minimum information about a microarray experiment (MIAME)—toward standards for microarray data. Nat Genet 2001; 29(4):365–371.
23. Spellman PT, Miller M, Stewart J, et al. Design and implementation of microarray gene expression markup language (MAGE-ML). Genome Biol 2002; 3(9):RESEARCH0046-1-0046.9.
24. NCI Gene Expression Data Portal website: http://gedp.nci.nih.gov.
25. NCBI Gene Expression Omnibus website: http://www.ncbi.nlm.nih.gov/geo/. Accessed 1/7/05.
26. W3C Ontology Web Language website: http://www.w3.org/TR/2004/REC-owl-ref-20040210/. Accessed 1/7/05.
27. Ling XB, Cutler G, Hoey T. Genomic resources for cancer biologists. In: LaRochelle WJ, Shimkets RA, eds. The Oncogenomics Handbook. Totowa, NJ: Humana, 2004:3–18.
28. NCI Data Standards Repository website: http://ncicb.nci.nih.gov/core/caDSR. Accessed 1/7/05.
29. Warzel DB, Andonaydis C, McCurry B, Chilukuri R, Ishmukhamedov S, Covitz P. Common Data Element (CDE) Management and Deployment in Clinical Trials. In: Proceedings of the AMIA Symposium 2003:1048.
30. NCI Enterprise Vocabulary Services website: http://ncicb.nci.nih.gov/core/EVS. Accessed 1/7/05.
31. Golbeck J, Fragoso G, Hartel F, Hendler J, Oberthaler J, Parsia B. The National Cancer Institute's Thesaurus and Ontology. J Web Seman 2003; 1:75–80.
32. Covitz PA, Hartel F, Schaefer C, et al. caCORE: a common infrastructure for cancer informatics. Bioinformatics 2003; 19(18):2404–2412.
33. NCI Thesaurus website: http://nciterms.nci.nih.gov/NCIBrowser/Startup.do. Accessed 1/7/05.
34. National Library of Medicine UMLS Metathesaurus source web page: http://www.nlm.nih.gov/research/umls/umlsdoc.html. Accessed 1/7/05.
35. NCI Metathesaurus website: http://ncimeta.nci.nih.gov/indexMetaphrase.html. Accessed 1/7/05.
36. NCI Cancer Bioinformatics Infrastructure Objects website: http://ncicb.nci.nih.gov/core/caBIO. Accessed 1/7/05.
37. NCI caBIO Data Sources web page: http://ncicb.nci.nih.gov/core/caBIO/technical_resources/system_architecture/caBIO/data_sources. Accessed 1/7/05.
38. CaP Cure Prostate Cancer Foundation website: http://www.capcure.org. Accessed 1/7/05.
39. NCI caBIG website: http://cabig.nci.nih.gov/workspaces. Accessed 1/7/05.

# Index